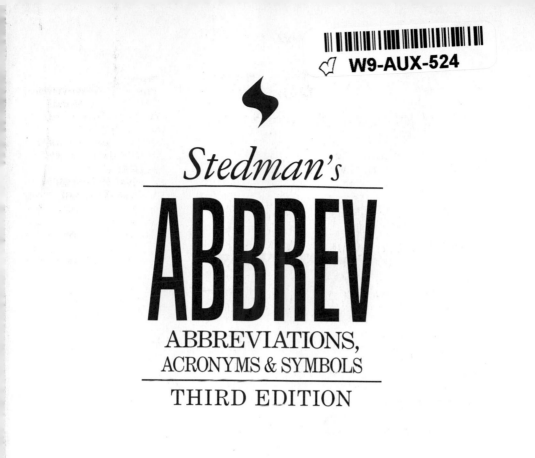

Stedman's

ABBREV

ABBREVIATIONS,
ACRONYMS & SYMBOLS

THIRD EDITION

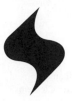

Stedman's

ABBREV

ABBREVIATIONS,
ACRONYMS & SYMBOLS

THIRD EDITION

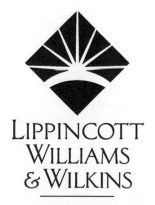

LIPPINCOTT
WILLIAMS
& WILKINS

Publisher: Julie K. Stegman
Series Managing Editor: Trista A. DiPaula
Art Program Project Manager: Jennifer Clements
Assistant Production Manager: Kevin Iarossi
Typesetter: Peirce Graphic Services, Inc.
Printer & Binder: Quebecor World

Copyright © 2003 Lippincott Williams & Wilkins
351 West Camden Street
Baltimore, Maryland 21201-2436

Printed in the United States of America

Third Edition, 2003

Library of Congress Cataloging-in-Publication Data

Stedman's abbreviations, acronyms & symbols.—3rd ed.
    p. ; cm.
    ISBN 0-7817-4403-2 (alk. paper)
    1. Medicine—Abbreviations—Dictionaries.   2. Medicine—Acronyms—
Dictionaries.
    [DNLM: 1. Medicine—Abbreviations. W 13 S8119 2003]   I. Title: Stedman's
abbreviations, acronyms, and symbols.   II. Title: Abbreviations, acronyms, &
symbols. III. Lippincott Williams & Wilkins.
    R123.S69 2003
    610'.148—dc21
              2002156021

08 07 06
4 5 6 7 8 9 10

Contents

Acknowledgments

An important part of our editorial process is the involvement of medical transcriptionists—as advisors, reviewers, and/or editors.

We extend special thanks to Ellen Atwood, as well as Susan Bartolucci and Andrea Linderman for editing the manuscript and helping resolve many difficult questions.

We also extend thanks to Ellen Atwood and Jeanne Bock, CRS, MT for working on the appendix. Additional thanks to Helen Littrell for performing the final prepublication review. Another important contributor to this edition is Lisa Kairis.

And, as always, Barb Ferretti played an integral role in the process by reviewing the content files for format, updating the database, and providing a final quality check. Special thanks also goes to Lisa Fahnestock for her assistance with the database work.

As with all our *Stedman's* word references, this resource incorporates the suggestions and expertise of our many contacts in the medical transcriptionist community. Thanks to all of our advisory board participants, reviewers, and editors; AAMT meeting attendees; and others who have written us with requests and comments—keep talking, and we'll keep listening.

Editor's Preface

Epi! Bag 'em! D5, BP, crit, lytes STAT! MS in the field. PERRL. GCS is 12. Using such language, a team of medical professionals communicates rapidly, as dramatized by emergency room and "doctor shows." So what about the folks watching the TV? They can zip to the 7–11 for a 6-pack or to the fridge for some chips. Would the preceding plain English, non-medical sentence be comprehensible to a person speaking only Russian or Japanese? What about healthcare when things are not so urgent? Think about the routines - vitals, T-max, labs, UA, RSV, TAHBSO. These are all examples of how we tend to speak or write among ourselves or our peers. We shorten words. We use abbreviations. We make up new words that our crowd understands.

Using medical language, trained health care professionals, can communicate regardless of country or language of origin. The specialized language-within-a-language of medical abbreviations has evolved, not just in the ER, but in all aspects of healthcare—from research to administration—as a simpler, faster, easier way to say things. Not found in ordinary dictionaries, with many of them not even being found in medical dictionaries, the above medical abbreviations and some 75,000 others will be found in this comprehensive compilation of medical abbreviations and their expansions.

Proper interpretation, expansion, and application of abbreviations are all critical to patient well-being; to health professionals and educators, as well as to medical transcriptionists, medical records, and other medical assisting staff. Misused or wrongly expanded abbreviations make literally life or death differences - was that H20 or H2O2? Is this dosage 40 mEq or 40 mg? In addition, erroneous expansion of an inaccurate abbreviation can make an individual's medical record a minefield of potential and exponential error. Does this μg really mean a microgram, or did Dr. Smith's pen leak again?

The cradle-to-grave healthcare professional, who could easily evaluate and correct errors in medical documentation, is as extinct as the dinosaurs; one patient and her records are evaluated by tens of specialists and ancillary personnel for even common ailments. Documentation of patient care has become an industry in itself. Orders are written, nursing notes faithfully record details of patient's care and activities; charts are compiled, H&Ps are dictated and transcribed. Insurance companies, lawyers, oversight committees, and quality assurance divisions all rely on patient records. Acronyms and abbreviations proliferate in records as they pass through their life cycle.

New terms and abbreviations from staggering quantities of new drugs, treatments, concepts, products, basic bits of life's chemistry and genetics, new species and discoveries flood into medical language daily. Some of these new abbreviations conflict with or duplicate the old ones; some are used one time, in an obscure journal. The expansions and meanings of these abbreviations vary according to specialty. What a cardiothoracic surgeon means by triple-A differs from the interpretation of a biochemist, and their stockbrokers mean something else entirely.

Why a book of abbreviations, acronyms, symbols? Medical language is built on a dead language (Latin) with bits and pieces of many other languages, and then all those made-up words are squished into short forms! A tourist usually carries along a phrase book when visiting a new country. So too, this book is a guide into the strange and complicated foreign language of medicine and science, and its subset, abbreviations, acronyms, and symbols.

As usual, we have relied on many contributors from various specialties around the world, who glean new terms and give us great ideas. For this Third Edition, rather than simply adding more and more, we decided to analyze new terms carefully, retaining the reliable and verifiable. We have removed the redundant and antiquated, improved the ordering sequence, and highlighted slang terms. Please be sure to look at the Explanatory Notes for details of usage, capitalization and mixed case, and other improvements designed to facilitate ease of use and understanding.

Books like this are a reflection and compilation of the ideas, thoughts, efforts, and input of many people. Along with those named in the Publisher's Preface, all the others who contributed—customers sending in

comments and queries, the technical and publishing people, and the staff
at Lippincott Williams & Wilkins—to them, my heartfelt thanks and ap-
preciation. It is refreshing to work with people who take pride in getting
it right and getting it done.

Ellen Atwood
January, 2003

Publisher's Preface

Stedman's Abbreviations, Acronyms & Symbols, Third Edition, offers an authoritative assurance of quality and exactness to the healthcare community including practitioners, educators, students, and the wordsmiths of the healthcare professions — medical transcriptionists, medical editors and copyeditors, health information management personnel, and court reporters. In addition, this reference offers valuable abbreviations, acronyms, symbols and their meanings to many other areas such as insurance companies, law firms, and others who work or are exposed to medical terminology and medical documentation.

We have received many requests to update *Stedman's Abbreviations, Acronyms, & Symbols.* We realized that the healthcare community needed an updated, current reference for the abbreviations, acronyms, and symbols relevant to the broad spectrum of healthcare settings. *Stedman's Abbreviations, Acronyms & Symbols, Third Edition* is a compilation of more than 75,000 clinically relevant abbreviations, acronyms, and symbols. As the product of expanded, ongoing reviews of medical and allied health literature since the publication of the second edition in 1999, this Third Edition incorporates terms gleaned from dictionaries, style manuals, approved lists from teaching hospitals, nomenclatures, glossaries, and other compendia.

A major focus of this effort, from design specifications to construction of individual entries, involved presenting sought-after information in a format that would facilitate efficient loading, easy reading, and quick comprehension. Novices as well as seasoned professionals are encouraged to read the following descriptions of this reference's organization, format, and style to make the most of its features.

The creation of new abbreviations and usage changes outpace compilation of them. Thousands of new abbreviations appear monthly, many of them simply reworking of existing material to the individual specifications of untold numbers of medical specialty journals. We have carefully culled these specialty abbreviations, focusing on quality and usability. We at Lippincott Williams & Wilkins strive to provide you with the most up-to-date and accurate word references available. Your use of this reference will prompt new editions, which we will publish as often as updates and revisions justify. We welcome your suggestions for improvements, changes, corrections, and additions—whatever will make this *Stedman's* product more useful to you. Please complete the postpaid card in this book, and send your recommendations care of "Stedman's" at Lippincott Williams & Wilkins.

Explanatory Notes

In keeping with our goals of accuracy and quality, several major changes were incorporated into this new third edition. These include creating specialty sections, simplifying the ordering scheme, eliminating antiquated Latin phrases, identifying slang, and culling dubious terms and gratuitous abbreviations of common terms.

As in the second edition, the appendices contain the graphic representations of symbols used in medicine and science, as noted in the table of contents. In order to keep the A-Z portion manageable while incorporating categories of terms previously excluded and expanding the scope to non-USA English-speaking countries, we created four new appendices:

- Professional Titles and Degrees
- Professional Associations and Organizations
- Chemotherapy and Other Drug Regimens
- Clinical Trials

These appendices follow the same ordering scheme explained elsewhere, and the terms within are readily recognizable as belonging to a specific category.

Organization and Order

This book lists all types of abbreviations in the same order, making no distinction among or identification of the various types of abbreviations, initialisms, acronyms, or symbols, other than those symbols in the appendices. For simplicity, all the examples and explanations herein are referred to as "abbreviation." Slang terms are distinguished within the text by red ink, but otherwise follow the same ordering scheme.

Entries in the A–Z portion of the book are alphabetized letter by letter as written. Standard punctuation such as diacritics, hyphens, commas, parentheses, ampersands, colons, slashes, and spaces are treated as if they are not there unless they are the only distinction between similar groups of letters. Normal typeface precedes italics.

A

A

Å

AS

A/S

a

a

(a)

Within the letter-by-letter alphabetization, accompanying numbers are numerically sequenced, arabic first, then roman, in this order:

- Leading numbers, regardless of position (superscript, normal, subscript)
- Numbers within an abbreviation
- Trailing numbers, regardless of position (superscript, normal, subscript)
- A range of numbers is ordered by the first number of the range.

A1

A$_1$

AI-III

2A

A$_2$

^{3}A

A250

CN

CNI-XII

DW

D5W

DWA

For mixed case with or without standard (ignored) punctuation, the first alphabetic character provides the ordering:

A-A

A-a

a-A

a/A

aa

mm

mmHg

SPECIAL CHARACTERS (other than Greek): These are largely found in the appendices. Within the A–Z portion, special characters contained in an uppercase alphabetic or alphanumeric abbreviation are sequenced after the regular uppercase letter-by-letter ordering (including numerals), and before the lower case of the same letter-by-letter sequence. Lower case plus special characters will be found following the lower case sequence. These special characters follow the standard computerized ordering protocols. Not all alphabetic sections will contain alphanumeric combined with special character combinations and no example is given here. For special-character-only and non-alphanumeric symbols, consult the specialized appendices. Please note that the special characters in the appendices do not follow an alphanumeric sequence; they are listed in a logical fashion. Please see below for the Greek alphabet and how Greeks are used.

Format and Style

Each entry consists of a boldface short form (abbreviation) and its "expansions" or meaning(s) following, listed alphabetically, indented, and in lightface. When there is more than one expansion, each resides on its own line, letter-by-letter in alphabetical order.

ABG
  air-bone gap
  aortoiliac bypass graft
  arterial blood gas
  axiobuccogingival

If the expansion requires more space, it wraps to the next line with extra indentation.

POEMS
  polyneuropathy, organomegaly, endocrinopathy,
    M protein, and skin changes (syndrome)
  polyneuropathy, organomegaly, endocrinopathy,
    monoclonal gammopathy, and skin changes

CROSS-REFERENCES: There are two types of cross-references.

Variants arise when different short forms are used for one expansion or meaning. Rather than having separate entries for each variation, the closely similar abbreviations are combined on one line, separated by a comma, alphabetized only by the first or preferred form, with expansion(s) listed as usual.

BX, Bx
  biopsy

Not all obvious variant forms will be presented in the above format, especially those abbreviations with multiple expansions. If every single term does not use all of the variant abbreviations, no combination will be made.

(*See also*) highlights forms of an abbreviation that have the same or similar meaning. For example:

DPT
>diphtheria, pertussis, and tetanus (vaccine) (*See also* DTP, DTaP, DTPa)

D-stix
>Dextrostix (*See also* DSX)

Periods are ignored in alphabetization.

Periods are used in lower case English or Latin abbreviations if the shortened version is also a regular word:

add.	**addict.**	**anal.**

Periods are no longer used in upper case English degrees or titles:

MD	**RN**	**BS**

Mixed case terms usually have periods in the United States, but not in other English-speaking countries. This style can be highly variable, so please follow your institution's guidelines.

Mr.	**Dr.**	**Jr.**

Periods are used in most lower case Latin abbreviations, but never upper case.

b.i.d.	**BID**
q.d.	**QD**
p.o.	**PO**

BRACKETS: Brackets [ ] contain information about a term's origin (etymology), and immediately follow the expanded form. Enclosed within the brackets are the language of origin and the foreign word of origin in italics:

Languages are signified: L., Latin; G., Greek; Ger., German; Fr., French; Sp., Spanish; It., Italian

HD
hard corn [L. *heloma durum*]

PARENTHESES: Parentheses used within the abbreviation are simply a part of that abbreviation and are ignored in ordering.

PAA
P(A-aDO$_2$)
p(A-a)O2
pAAT

Used with the expansion, parentheses have several functions:

Enclose explanatory material to provide further information:

A
absolute (temperature)
(start of) anesthesia

Clarify usage that otherwise might be ambiguous:

BEPTI
bionomics, environment, *Plasmodium,* treatment, and immunity (malaria epidemiology)

Provide a mini-definition:

Gy
gray (unit of absorbed dose of ionizing radiation)

Identify the generic name of a drug:

CAM
cyclophosphamide, Adriamycin (doxorubicin), and methotrexate

Brackets and parentheses and the material they contain are ignored in alphabetization.

PREFERENCES AND STYLE: *Stedman's Abbreviations, Acronyms & Symbols Third Edition* acknowledges the wide variety of preferences among institutions, associations, and users. Stedman's collects current examples from the literature and this book, as do others in the series, reflects preferences and usage across a wide spectrum of users and organizations in English-speaking countries.

CAPITAL LETTERS AND MIXED CASE: For reasons of clarity and space, we have not included every possible combination of the abbreviations that have several versions, such as all capitals, all lower case, initial capital letter. In many instances, lower-case abbreviations with an initial capital letter have been traced back to an index or table that automatically capitalizes the first letter and thus are not reflective of usage. However, if your workplace or supervisor prefers initial capitals on particular terms, it is not "wrong" to follow that style. Simply find the lower case abbreviation and make the first letter capital.

abd hyst   **Abd hyst**

Some terms are normally mixed case:

pH

mmHg

EtOH

Some caretaker and nursing notations prefer all drugs, generic and brand, be capitalized and that all abbreviations begin with a capital letter. Again, follow your local guidelines for variations in format.

PLURALS: We have retained plural expansions only when more than one, or plurality, is described by the expansion. Plural forms of singular abbreviations have been discarded. To make a plural, simply add a lower case "s" to the abbreviation:

ABG (singular)   **ABGs** (plural)

COLONS AND SLASHES (VIRGULE): The preferred scientific notation to express ratio is the colon:

A:V

In nontechnical settings and in some disciplines, the slash (virgule) is frequently used:

S/N

We have both types in this edition and have taken care to include the identification "ratio" in the expansion. If you find a ratio abbreviation using a colon but your workplace prefers a slash, just substitute as appropriate.

SLANG: Slang terms are commonly short forms or actual abbreviations. Slang terms, sometimes dictated or written in rough drafts, are not appropriate in formal documents, and should always be expanded or replaced with the corresponding expansion or translation.

We have identified slang by printing the expansion in red ink. This method preserves the cross-references so useful in Stedman's word books, and makes it easy to identify the slang usage when a short form has a number of expansions.

So no matter if the short form itself is the slang term:

crit   **bili**

    hematocrit   bilirubin

Or if the slang term is one of many expansions:

ABG

    air-bone gap

    aortoiliac bypass graft

    arterial blood gas

    axiobuccogingival

Or a non-slang expansion that has a slang counterpart:

AP

    auscultation and palpation

    apical pulse

apothecary
appendectomy (*See also* appy)
apex
appendiceal perforation

You will be able to easily identify and determine proper usage.

SCIENTIFIC NOTATION: Certain units of measure, scientific notation, amino acids, and elements have universally recognized or preferred abbreviations.

To the degree possible, we have reserved (or limited) the expansions of these abbreviations to the universally accepted meanings.

UNITS OF MEASURE
Initial Capital and Upper Case Abbreviations

ampere	A	gray	Gy
becquerel	Bq	henry	H
celsius	C	hertz	Hz
coulomb	C	newton	N
curie	Ci	pascal	Pa
Fahrenheit	F	Siemens	S
farad	F	Tesla	T
joule	J	Volt	V
liter	L	Watt	W

AMINO ACID ABBREVIATIONS
Each amino acid has two recognized abbreviations, a trivial name, and a letter symbol:

Amino Acid	Name	Symbol	Amino Acid	Name	Symbol
alanine	Ala	**A**	arginine	Arg	**R**
asparagine	Asn	**N**	aspartic acid	Asp	**D**
cysteine	Cys	**C**	glutamine	Gln	**Q**
glutamic acid	Glu	**E**	glycine	Gly	**G**
histidine	His	**H**	isoleucine	Ile	**I**

Amino Acid	Name	Symbol	Amino Acid	Name	Symbol
leucine	Leu	**L**	lysine	Lys	**K**
methionine	Met	**M**	phenylalanine	Phe	**F**
proline	Pro	**P**	serine	Ser	**S**
threonine	Thr	**T**	tryptophan	Trp	**W**
tyrosine	Tyr	**Y**	valine	Val	**V**

GREEK CHARACTERS: Greek characters that are part of an abbreviation are alphabetized as written in English, except for those used as symbols.

ALPase   **del**
α, alpha   **Δ, delta**
ALPI   **DEM**

BET   **galv**
bet.   **γ, gamma**
β, beta   **GAMG**
betaLP

GREEKS USED AS SYMBOLS: Certain Greek characters are used as a universally recognized symbol. These will be found in two places:

alphabetically per English language when used as a character
OME
Ω, omega {Greek character}
OMF

alphabetically as the English translation of the symbolic word
OHL
Ω Ohm {Greek character used as symbol}
OHN

GREEK MU (μ): The Greek character μ is written mu, and will be found following MT and before MV. This character also symbolizes "micro" when used with a unit of measure and as such will be found alphabetically in the sequence m-i-c-r-o. Both the Greek symbol and fully spelled out English version are provided.

microbiol
μg, microgram
μf, microfarad
μm, micron
MICU

Greek Alphabet

Upper case	Lower case	Greek name	English equivalent
A	α	alpha	a
B	β	beta	b
Γ	γ	gamma	g
Δ	δ	delta	d
E	ε	epsilon	e
Z	ζ	zeta	z
H	η	eta	h
Θ	θ	theta	th
I	ι	iota	i
K	κ	kappa	k
Λ	λ	lambda	l
M	μ	mu	m
N	ν	nu	n
Ξ	ξ	xi	x
O	o	omicron	o
Π	π	pi	p
P	ρ	rho	r
Σ	σ	sigma	s
T	τ	tau	t
Υ	υ	upsilon	u
Φ	φ	phi	ph
X	χ	chi	ch
Ψ	ψ	psi	ps
Ω	ω	omega	o

Please note that some Greek characters have more than one configuration. We have chosen the most common.

Elements and Their Symbols

Element	Symbol	Element	Symbol
Actinium	Ac	Erbium	Er
Silver	Ag	Einsteinium	Es
Aluminum	Al	Europium	Eu
Americium	Am	Fluorine	F
Argon	Ar	Iron	Fe
Arsenic	As	Fermium	Fm
Astatine	At	Francium	Fr
Gold	Au	Gallium	Ga
Boron	B	Gadolinium	Gd
Barium	Ba	Germanium	Ge
Beryllium	Be	Hydrogen	H
Bohrium	Bh	Helium	He
Bismuth	Bi	Hafnium	Hf
Berkelium	Bk	Mercury	Hg
Bromine	Br	Holmium	Ho
Carbon	C	Hassium	Hs
Calcium	Ca	Iodine	I
Cadmium	Cd	Indium	In
Cerium	Ce	Iridium	Ir
Californium	Cf	Potassium	K
Chlorine	Cl	Krypton	Kr
Curium	Cm	Lanthanum	La
Cobalt	Co	Lithium	Li
Chromium	Cr	Lawrencium	Lr
Cesium	Cs	Lutetium	Lu
Copper	Cu	Mendelevium	Md
Dubnium	Db	Magnesium	Mg
Dysprosium	Dy	Manganese	Mn

Element	Symbol	Element	Symbol
Molybdenum	Mo	Sulfur	S
Meitnerium	Mt	Antimony	Sb
Nitrogen	N	Scandium	Sc
Sodium	Na	Selenium	Se
Niobium	Nb	Seaborgium	Sg
Neodymium	Nd	Silicon	Si
Neon	Ne	Samarium	Sm
Nickel	Ni	Tin	Sn
Nobelium	No	Strontium	Sr
Neptunium	Np	Tantalum	Ta
Oxygen	O	Terbium	Tb
Osmium	Os	Technetium	Tc
Phosphorus	P	Tellurium	Te
Protactinium	Pa	Thorium	Th
Lead	Pb	Titanium	Ti
Palladium	Pd	Thallium	Tl
Promethium	Pm	Thulium	Tm
Polonium	Po	Uranium	U
Praseodymium	Pr	Ununbium	Uub
Platinum	Pt	Ununnilium	Uun
Plutonium	Pu	Unununium	Uuu
Radium	Ra	Vanadium	V
Rubidium	Rb	Tungsten	W
Rhenium	Re	Xenon	Xe
Rutherfordium	Rf	Yttrium	Y
Rhodium	Rh	Ytterbium	Yb
Radon	Rn	Zinc	Zn
Ruthenium	Ru	Zirconium	Zr

References

In addition to the manufacturers' literature we gather at various medical meetings, scientific reports from hospitals, and the lists of our MT Editorial Advisory Board members (from their daily transcription work), we used the following sources for new terms in *Stedman's Abbreviations, Acronyms & Symbols, Third Edition.*

Books

The AAMT Book of Style, 2nd Edition. Modesto, CA: AAMT, 2002.

Drake E. Sloane's Medical Word Book, 4th Edition. Philadelphia: Saunders, 2001.

Jablonski S. Cardiology Acronyms and Abbreviations. Baltimore: Lippincott Williams & Wilkins, 2001.

Lance LL. Quick Look Drug Book. Baltimore: Lippincott Williams & Wilkins, 2002.

Marcucci L. Marcucci's Handbook of Medical Eponyms. Baltimore: Lippincott Williams & Wilkins, 2001.

Mitchell-Hatton SL. Davis Book of Medical Abbreviations. Philadelphia: F.A. Davis Company, 1991.

Sloane SB. Medical Abbreviations & Eponyms. Philadelphia: Saunders, 1997.

Stedman's Abbreviations, Acronyms & Symbols, 2nd Edition. Baltimore: Lippincott Williams & Wilkins, 1999.

Stedman's Alternative Medicine Words. Baltimore: Lippincott Williams & Wilkins, 2000.

Stedman's Anatomy & Physiology Words, 2nd Edition. Baltimore: Lippincott Williams & Wilkins, 2002.

Stedman's Cardiovascular & Pulmonary Words, 3rd Edition. Baltimore: Lippincott Williams & Wilkins, 2001.

Stedman's Concise Medical Dictionary for the Health Professions, Illustrated 4th Edition. Baltimore: Lippincott Williams & Wilkins, 2001.

Stedman's Dermatology & Immunology Words, 2nd Edition. Baltimore: Lippincott Williams & Wilkins, 2002.

Stedman's Endocrinology Words. Baltimore: Lippincott Williams & Wilkins, 2001.

Stedman's Equipment Words, 3rd Edition. Baltimore: Lippincott Williams & Wilkins, 2001.

Stedman's GI & GU Words, 3rd Edition. Baltimore: Lippincott Williams & Wilkins, 2002.

Stedman's Internal Medicine & Geriatric Words. Baltimore: Lippincott Williams & Wilkins, 2002.

Stedman's Medical Dictionary, 27th Edition. Baltimore: Lippincott Williams & Wilkins, 2000.

Stedman's OB-GYN & Genetics Words, 3rd Edition. Baltimore: Lippincott Williams & Wilkins, 2001.

Stedman's Oncology Words, 3rd Edition. Baltimore: Lippincott Williams & Wilkins, 2000.

Stedman's Ophthalmology Words, 2nd Edition. Baltimore: Lippincott Williams & Wilkins, 2000.

Stedman's Organisms & Infectious Disease Words. Baltimore: Lippincott Williams & Wilkins, 2001.

Stedman's Orthopaedic & Rehab Words, 3rd Edition. Baltimore: Lippincott Williams & Wilkins, 1999.

Stedman's Pathology & Lab Medicine Words, 3rd Edition. Baltimore: Lippincott Williams & Wilkins, 2002.

Stedman's Pediatric Words. Baltimore: Lippincott Williams & Wilkins, 2001.

Stedman's Plastic Surgery/ENT/Dentistry Words, 2nd Edition. Baltimore: Lippincott Williams & Wilkins, 1999.

Stedman's Psychiatry/Neurology/Neurosurgery Words, 2nd Edition. Baltimore: Lippincott Williams & Wilkins, 1999.

Stedman's Radiology Words, 3rd Edition. Baltimore: Lippincott Williams & Wilkins, 2000.

Stedman's Surgery Words, 2nd Edition. Baltimore: Lippincott Williams & Wilkins, 2002.

Vera Pyle's Current Medical Terminology, 8th Edition. Modesto, CA: Health Professions Institute, 2000.

Journals

Latest Word. Philadelphia: Saunders, 1999–2002.

Perspectives on the Medical Transcription Profession. Modesto, CA: Health Professions Institute, 1999–2002.

A

abnormal (*See also* AB, ABN, abn, abnor, abnorm)
abortus
absolute temperature (*See also* T)
absorbance (*See also* abs)
acceptor
accommodation (*See also* a, ACC, acc, accom)
acetone
acetum (vinegar)
acid (*See also* a, AC)
acidophil
acidophile
acidophilic
Acinetobacter
acromion
actin
activity (radiation)
adenine (*See also* Ade)
adenoma
adenosine
adrenaline (*See also* Adr)
adult
aesthetic
age
akinetic
alanine (*See also* Ala)
albumin (5%, followed by amount in mL) (*See also* AL, ALB, abl)
alive
allergologist
allergy (*See also* Al, alg, ALL)
alpha (cell) alternate
alpha (first letter of Greek alphabet), uppercase
alveolar
alveolar gas (subscript)
ambulatory (*See also* AM, AMB, amb, ambul)
amp
ampere (*See also* a)
amphetamine
ampicillin (*See also* AM, AMP)
amyloid
anaphylaxis
androsterone
anesthesia (*See also* AN, ANA, anes, anesth)
angioplasty
angle (*See also* ang)
anisotropic (band in striated muscle)
annum (year)
anode (*See also* a, AN, An)

ante (before)
anterior (*See also* a, AN, ANT, ant.)
antrectomy
anxiety
apex, pl. apices
apical
aqueous
area (*See also* a, S)
argon
arterial
artery [L. *arteria*] (*See also* a, ART, art.)
Asian
assessment
asymmetric (*See also* a, AS)
atomic weight
atrium (*See also* At)
atropine (*See also* ATRO)
auricle
auris
auscultation
axial (*See also* a, ax.)
axilla (*See also* ax.)
axillary (temperature) (*See also* (a))
blood group in the ABO system
ear [L. *auris*]
Helmholtz energy
mass number
(start of) anesthesia
(start of) anesthetic
subspinale (point A in cephalometrics)
total acid
total acidity (*See also* a)
water [L. *aqua*] (*See also* a, aq.)
year [L. *annum*]

A1

alpha-1

A₁

aortic first sound
first auditory area

AI–III

angiotensin I, II, III

A₂

aortic second sound
second auditory area

A₄

androstenedione

A250

5% albumin, 250 mL

A1000

5% albumin, 1000 mL

A

Ångström (*See also* A)

A *(continued)*
> angstrom
> cumulated activity

A+
> blood type A positive

A-
> blood type A negative

(a)
> axillary temperature *(See also* A)

a
> absorptivity *(See also a)*
> acceleration *(See also* α, acc, accel)
> accommodation *(See also* A, ACC, acc, accom)
> acid *(See also* A, AC)
> acidity *(See also* AC)
> agar
> alpha (first letter of Greek alphabet)
> ampere *(See also* A)
> angular acceleration
> annum
> anode *(See also* A, AN, An)
> anterior *(See also* A, AN, ANT, ant.)
> area *(See also* A, S)
> arterial
> arterial blood (subscript)
> asymmetric *(See also* A, AS)
> atto-
> auris *(See also* aur)
> axial *(See also* A, ax.)
> thermodynamic activity
> total acidity *(See also* A)

ā
> before [L. *ante*] *(See also* a., bef, ante)

a.
> artery [L. *arteria*] *(See also* A, ART, art.)
> before [L. *ante*] *(See also* ā, bef, ante)
> water [L. *aqua*] *(See also* A, aq.)

a
> absorptivity *(See also* a)

AA
> abampere *(See also* aA)
> Academic Alertness
> acetabular anteversion
> acetic acid
> achievement age
> active alcoholic
> active-assisted (range of motion) *(See also* AAROM)
> active-assistive
> active avoidance
> acupuncture analgesia

acute appendicitis
acute asthma
adenine arabinoside *(See also* ara-A)
adenylic acid
adjuvant arthritis
adrenal androgen
adrenocortical autoantibody
African American
aggregated albumin
agranulocytic angina
alcohol abuse
allergic alveolitis
alopecia areata
aminoacetone
amino acid
aminoacyl
amplitude of accommodation
amyloid A
amyloid-associated
anaplastic astrocytoma
anesthesia *(See also* A, AN, ANA, anes, anesth)
anterior apical
antiarrhythmic agent
anticipatory avoidance
antigen aerosol
aortic amplitude
aortic aneurysm
aortic arch
aplastic anemia
arachidonic acid
arm-ankle (pulse ratio)
Ascaris antigen
ascending aorta *(See also* Asc-A, AO, ASCAo)
atlantoaxial *(See also* A-A)
atomic absorption
audiologic assessment
Australia antigen *(See also* AU, Au Ag)
autoanalyzer
axonal arborization

A-A
> atlantoaxial *(See also* AA)

A&A
> aid and attendance
> arthroscopy and arthrotomy
> awake and aware

A/A
> automobile accident

A-a
> alveolar-arterial (gradient)
> aortic artery

aA
> abampere *(See also* AA)
> arterial to alveolar (gradient)
> azure A

aa.
  arteria
  arteries [L. *arteriae*]
AAA
  abdominal aortic aneurysm
  abdominal aortic aneurysmectomy
  achalasia-addisonism-alacrimia
  acquired aplastic anemia
  acute anxiety attack
  addiction, autoimmune diseases, and
    aging
  amalgam (*See also* aaa)
  androgenic anabolic agent
  aneurysm of ascending aorta
  antigen-extracted allogenic
  aromatic amino acid
  diagnostic arthroscopy, operative
    arthroscopy, and possible
    operative arthrotomy
aaa
  amalgam (*See also* AAA)
AAAAA
  aphasia, agnosia, apraxia, agraphia,
    and alexia
AAAD
  aromatic amino acid decarboxylase
AAAE
  amino acid activating enzyme
AAAF
  albumin autoagglutinating factor
AA-AMP
  amino acid adenylate
    (adenomonophosphate)
AAB
  action against burns
  aminoazobenzene
AABCC
  alertness (consciousness), airway,
    breathing, circulation, and cervical
    spine
AABR
  automated auditory brainstem
    response
AAC
  acute acalculous cholecystitis
  antibiotic-associated colitis
  antimicrobial agent-induced colitis
  antimicrobial agents and
    chemotherapy
  augmentative and alternative
    communication

a-1-ac
  alpha-1 antichymotrypsin
AACA
  acylaminocephalosporanic acid
AACD
  abdominal aortic counterpulsation
    device
  age-associated cognitive decline
AACE
  antigen-antibody crossed
    electrophoresis
AACG
  acute angle-closure glaucoma
AACI
  arachidonic acid cascade inhibitor
AACLR
  arthroscopic anterior cruciate
    ligament reconstruction
AACSH
  adrenal androgen corticotropic
    stimulating hormone
AAD
  acid-ash diet
  acroangiodermatitis
  acute agitated delirium
  alloxazine adenine dinucleotide
  antiarrhythmic drug
  antibiotic-associated diarrhea
  aromatic acid decarboxylase
  atlantoaxial dislocation
AADC
  amino acid decarboxylase
  aromatic l-amino acid decarboxylase
AAdC
  anterior adductor of the coxa
AADI
  anterior atlantodental interval
(A-a)D$_{N2}$
  difference in nitrogen tension
    between mixed alveolar gas and
    mixed arterial blood
(A-a)D$_{O2}$
  difference in partial pressures of
    oxygen in mixed alveolar gas
    and mixed arterial blood
AADP
  amyloid A-degrading protease
AADPPO
  alveolar-arterial difference in partial
    pressure of oxygen
AAE
  acquired angioedema

NOTES

AAE *(continued)*
  active assistive exercise *(See also A/AEX)*
  acute allergic encephalitis
  annuloaortic ectasia
AAECS
  amino acid-enriched cardioplegic solution
A/AEX
  active assistive exercise *(See also AAE)*
AAF
  acetamidofluorene
  acetic acid-alcohol-formalin (fixative)
  altered auditory feedback
  ascorbic acid factor
2-AAF
  2-acetamidofluorene
AAG
  allergic angiitis and granulomatosis
  $alpha_1$-acid glycoprotein *(See also AGP)*
  antral atrophic gastritis
  autoantigen
AAGS
  adult adrenogenital syndrome
AAH
  acute alcoholic hepatitis
  atypical adenomatous hyperplasia
AAI
  activating adjusting instrument
  acute adrenal insufficiency
  acute alveolar injury
  Adolescent Alienation Index
  arm-ankle indices
  atrial demand-inhibited (pacemaker)
  atrial inhibited (pacemaker)
  axial acetabular index
AAIB
  $alpha_1$-aminoisobutyrate
AAIN
  acute allergic interstitial nephritis
AAK
  allo activated killer (cell)
AAL
  anterior axillary line
AAM
  acute aseptic meningitis
  aggressive angiomyxoma
  amino acid mixture
AAMD
  atrophic age-related macular degeneration
AAME
  acetylarginine methyl ester
AAMI
  age-associated memory impairment

AAML
  atypical angiomyolipoma of the kidney
AAMRS
  automated ambulatory medical record system
AAMS
  acute aseptic meningitis syndrome
AAN
  AIDS-associated nephropathy
  alpha-amino nitrogen
  amino acid nitrogen
  analgesic-associated nephropathy
  attending's admission notes
AA-NAT
  arylalkylamine *N*-acetyltransferase
AAO
  amino acid oxidase
  awake, alert, oriented
$(A-a)O_2$
  alveolar-arterial oxygen gradient
AAOC
  antacid of choice
AAOx3
  alert, awake, and oriented to time, place, and person
AAP
  achromatic automated perimetry
  air at atmospheric pressure
  $alpha_1$-antiprotease
  assessment adjustment pass
  attenuated adenomatous polyposis
$A-aP_{CO2}$
  alveolar-arterial carbon dioxide difference
a-2AP
  a-2 antiplasmin
AAPBDS
  anomalous arrangement of pancreaticobiliary ductal system
AAPC
  antibiotic-associated pseudomembranous colitis
AAPF
  anti-arteriosclerosis polysaccharide factor
AAPMC
  antibiotic-associated pseudomembranous colitis
$AaPO_2$
  alveolar-arterial PO_2 difference
  arterial to alveolar oxygen tension ratio
AAPSA
  age-adjusted prostate-specific antigen
AAR
  active avoidance reaction
  acute articular rheumatism

antigen-antibody reaction
antigen-antiglobulin reaction
Australia antigen radioimmunoassay

AARF

atlantoaxial rotatory fixation

AAROM

active ankle joint complex range
of motion
active-assisted range of motion
(*See also* AA)

AAS

acid aspiration syndrome
acute abdominal series
alcoholic abstinence syndrome
amino-alkylsilane
androgenic-anabolic steroid
aneurysm of atrial septum
anthrax antiserum
aortic arch syndrome
atlantoaxial subluxation
atomic absorption spectrophotometer
atomic absorption spectrophotometry
atypical absence seizure

aa seq

amino acid sequence

AASH

adrenal androgen-stimulating
hormone

AASP

acute atrophic spinal paralysis
ascending aorta synchronized
pulsation

AAT

Aachen aphasia test
academic aptitude test
activity as tolerated
acute abdominal tympany
alanine aminotransferase
alkylating agent therapy
alpha1-antitrypsin (*See also* A1AT)
aminoazotoluene
androgen ablation therapy
animal-assisted therapy
atrial triggered (pacemaker)
atypical antibody titer
auditory apperception test
automatic atrial tachycardia

A1AT, A₁AT

alpha1-antitrypsin (*See also* AAT)

a-2AT

alpha2-antitrypsin

AATD

alpha1-antitrypsin disease

AAU

acute anterior uveitis

AAV

ANCA-associated vasculitis

AAV 1–5

adenoassociated virus 1–5

AAV-CF

adenoassociated virus for cystic
fibrosis

AAVNRT

atypical atrioventricular nodal
reentrant tachycardia

AAVT

acral arteriovenous tumor

AAVV

accumulated alveolar ventilatory
volume

AAW

anterior aortic wall

AB

abdominal
abnormal (*See also* A, ABN, abn,
abnor, abnorm)
abortion
abortus
Ace bandage
active bilaterally
aid to the blind
air bleed
Alcian blue
anterior basal
antibiotic (*See also* ATB, anti bx,
ABx)
antibody (*See also* ab)
antigen binding
apex beat
apnea and bradycardia (*See also*
A&B)
asbestos body
asthmatic bronchitis
axiobuccal (*See also* ab)
blood group in ABO system

3AB

3-aminobenzamide

A>B

air greater than bone (conduction)

A/B

acid-base ratio

NOTES

A&B
    apnea and bradycardia (*See also* AB)
aB
    azure B
a-b
    air-bone
ab
    about
    antibody (*See also* AB)
    axiobuccal (*See also* AB)
ABA
    abscissic acid
    allergic bronchopulmonary aspergillosis
    antibacterial activity
    applied behavioral analysis
    applied behavior analysis
    Apraxia Battery for Adults
ABAb
    anti-beta-1-adrenoreceptor antibody
ABAER
    automated brainstem auditory evoked response
A band
    the dark-staining zone of a striated muscle
AbAP
    antibody-against-panel
ABB
    acute bronchitis/bronchiolitis
ABBI
    advanced breast biopsy instrumentation
ABBQ
    Acquired Immunodeficiency Syndrome Beliefs and Behavior Questionnaire
abbr, abbrev
    abbreviated
    abbreviation
ABC
    abacavir
    abbreviated blood count
    absolute band count
    absolute basophil count
    absolute bone conduction
    acalculous biliary colic
    acid balance control
    aconite-belladonna-chloroform
    Activities-Specific Balance Confidence Scale
    airway, breathing, circulation
    all but code (resuscitation order)
    alternative birth center
    aneurysmal bone cyst
    antigen-binding capacity
    apnea, bradycardia, and cyanosis

    applesauce, bananas, and cereal (diet)
    argon beam coagulator
    artificial beta cells
    aspiration biopsy cytology
    assessment of basic competency
    avidin-biotin complex
    avidin-biotin horseradish peroxidase complex
    avidin-biotin-peroxidase method
    axiobuccocervical
A&BC
    air and bone conduction
ABC and C&C
    airway, breathing, circulation, cervical spine, and consciousness level
ABCD
    airway, breathing, circulation, differential
    amphotericin B colloid dispersion
    Arizona Battery for Communication Disorders of Dementia
    asymmetry, border, color, and diameter (of melanoma)
    avidin-biotin complex assay
ABCDE
    airway, breathing, circulation, disability, exposure
    pentavalent botulism toxin
ABCIC
    airway, breathing, circulation, intravenous crystalloid
ABCIL
    antibody-mediated cell-dependent immunolympholysis
ABCT
    ATP-binding cassette transporter
ABD
    abdomen (*See also* abd, abdom)
    adynamic bone disease
    after bronchodilator
    aged, blind, and disabled
    aggressive behavioral disturbance
    autologous blood donation
    automated border detection
    average body dose
abd
    abdomen (*See also* ABD, abdom)
    abdominal (*See also* abdom)
    abduction (*See also* abduc)
    abductor (muscle)
ABDCT
    atrial bolus dynamic computed tomography
abd hyst
    abdominal hysterectomy (*See also* AH)

A

abdom
    abdomen (*See also* abd, ABD)
    abdominal (*See also* abd)
abd poll
    abductor pollicis (muscle)
abduc
    abduction (*See also* abd)
ABE
    acute bacterial endocarditis
    adult basic education
    botulism equine trivalent antitoxin
ABECB
    acute bacterial exacerbation of
      chronic bronchitis
ABEP
    auditory brainstem-evoked potential
ABER
    abducted and externally rotated
aber
    aberrant
ABES
    Adaptive Behavior Evaluation Scale
ABF
    aortobifemoral (bypass)
ABG
    air-bone gap
    aortoiliac bypass graft
    arterial blood gas
    axiobuccogingival
abg
    addictive behavior group
ABG PCT
    arterial blood gas point-of-care test
ABH
    angina bullosa haemorrhagica
    Ativan, Benadryl, Haldol
ABI
    ankle-brachial index
    atherothrombotic brain infarction
    auditory brainstem implant
ABIC
    Adaptive Behavior Inventory for
      Children
ABID
    antibody identification
ABIG
    absence of immunoglobulin G
ABK
    aphakic bullous keratopathy
ABL, abl
    abetalipoproteinemia
    acute basophilic leukemia

    African Burkitt lymphoma
    allograft-bound lymphocyte
    angioblastic lymphadenopathy
    antigen-binding lymphocyte
    axiobuccolingual
ABLB
    alternate binaural loudness balance
ABLC
    amphotericin B lipid complex
ABLE
    Adult Basic Learning Examination
ABM
    adjusted body mass
    adult bone marrow
    alveolar basement membrane
    autologous bone marrow
ABMA
    antibasement membrane antibody
ABMD
    anterior basement membrane
      dystrophy
ABMR
    autologous bone marrow rescue
ABMS
    autologous bone marrow support
A/B MS
    apnea/bradycardia mild stimulation
ABMT
    allogeneic bone marrow transplant
    allogeneic bone marrow
      transplantation
    autologous blood and marrow
      transplantation
    autologous bone marrow transplant
    autologous bone marrow
      transplantation
ABMV
    Abu Mina virus
ABN, abn
    abnormal (*See also* A, AB, abnor,
     abnorm)
    abnormality
    advance beneficiary notice
AbN
    antibody nitrogen
ABNC
    abnormal curve
ABN F%
    abnormal forms percent (sperm
     count)
ABNG
    AB negative (blood type)

NOTES

ABNMP
  alpha-benzyl-*N*-methyl
    phenethylamine
abnor, abnorm
  abnormal (*See also* A, AB, ABN,
    abn)
ABO
  absent bed occupancy
  blood group system of groups A,
    AB, B, and O
ABO-HD
  ABO hemolytic disease
ABP
  ambulatory blood pressure
  androgen binding protein
  antigen binding protein
  arterial blood pressure
  automated boundary protection
  avidin-biotin peroxidase
ABPA
  acute bronchopulmonary asthma
  allergic bronchopulmonary
    aspergillosis
AB/PAS
  Alcian blue and periodic acid-
    Schiff
ABPC
  antibody-producing cell
ABPE
  acute bovine pulmonary edema
ABPI
  ankle-brachial pressure index
ABPM
  allergic bronchopulmonary mycosis
  ambulatory blood pressure monitor
  ambulatory blood pressure
    monitoring
ABR
  abortus-Bang-ring (test)
  absolute bedrest
  anterior band remover
  auditory brainstem response
ABr
  agglutination test for brucellosis
abr, abras
  abrasion
ABRS
  acute bacterial rhinosinusitis
ABRV
  Abras virus
ABS
  abdominal surgery
  abnormal brainstem
  absent (*See also* abs)
  absorbed
  absorption (*See also* absorb.)
  acrylonitrile-butadiene-styrene
  acute brain syndrome

  Adaptive Behavior Scale
  admitting blood sugar
  adult bovine serum
  aging brain syndrome
  alkylbenzene sulfonate
  aloin, belladonna, strychnine
    (laxative)
  amniotic band sequence
  antibody screen
  anti-B serum
  arterial blood sample
  arterial blood supply
  at bedside
abs
  absent (*See also* ABS)
  absolute
  absorbance (*See also* A)
absc
  abscess
  abscissa
AbSD
  abductor spasmodic dysphonia
ABSe
  ascending bladder septum
absorb.
  absorption (*See also* ABS)
ABSR
  auditory brainstem response
A/B SS
  apnea/bradycardia self-stimulation
abst, abstr
  abstract
ABT
  alcohol breath tester
  aminopyrine breath test
ABT-538
  ritonavir
abt
  about
ABTX
  alpha-bungarotoxin
ABU
  aminobutyrate
  asymptomatic bacteriuria
ABV
  Aransas Bay virus
  arthropod-borne virus
ABW
  actual body weight
ABx, abx
  antibiotic (*See also* ATB, AB, anti
    bx)
ABY
  acid bismuth yeast (medium)
ABZ
  albendazole
AC
  abdominal circumference

abdominal compression
absorption coefficient
absorptive cell
abuse case
accommodative convergence
acetate
acetylcholine (*See also* AcCh, ACH, ACh)
acetylcysteine
acid (*See also* A, a)
acidified complement
acidity (*See also* a)
Acinetobacter calcoaceticus
aconitine
acromioclavicular
activated charcoal
acupuncture clinic
acute (*See also* ac)
acute cholecystitis
adenocarcinoma (*See also* ACA)
adenylate cyclase
adenylyl cyclase
adherent cell
adrenal cortex
adrenocorticoid
air chamber
air changes
air conduction
alcoholic cirrhosis
all culture (broth)
alternating current
ambulatory care
ambulatory controls
anchored catheter
anesthesia circuit
angiocellular
anodal closure
antecubital
anterior chamber (of eye) (*See also* A/C)
anterior circulation
anterior column
anterior commissure
anterior cruciate
antibiotic concentrate
anticoagulant
anticomplement
anticomplementary
antiinflammatory corticoid
antiphlogistic corticoid
aortic closure
aortocoronary

arm circumference
arterial capillary
ascending colon
assist control
atriocarotid
auriculocarotid
autoclave
axiocervical
before meals [L. *ante cibum*] (*See also* a.c.)

A2C

apical two-chamber

AC-17

carbazochrome sodium sulfonate

A-C

adult-versus-child
aortocoronary (bypass)

A/C

anterior chamber (of eye) (*See also* AC)
assist/control
assisted-control ventilation

Ac

accelerator (globulin)
acetyl
actinium

aC

abcoulomb
azure C

a.c.

before meals [L. *ante cibum*] (*See also* AC)

ac

acute (*See also* AC)
antecubital
anterior chamber
assisted control
axiocervical

ACA

abnormal coronary artery
accessory conduction ablation
acrodermatitis chronica atrophicans
acute cerebellar ataxia
adenine-cytosine-adenine
adenocarcinoma (*See also* AC)
adenylate cyclase activity
aminocaproic acid
ammonia, copper, arsenic
amyotrophic choreoacanthocytosis
anomalous coronary artery
anterior cerebral artery
anterior choroidal artery

NOTES

ACA *(continued)*
    anterior communicating aneurysm
    anterior communicating artery *(See also* ACoA, AComA)
    anticanalicular antibody
    anticardiolipin antibody *(See also* ACLA)
    anticentromere antibody
    anticentromere autoantibody
    anticollagen autoantibody
    anticomplement activity
    anticytoplasmic antibody
    asthma care algorithm
    automatic clinical analyzer

7-ACA
    aminocephalosporanic acid

AC/A
    accommodative
    convergence/accommodation ratio

AcAcOH
    acetoacetic acid

ACAD
    allograft coronary artery disease
    asymptomatic coronary artery disease
    atherosclerotic carotid artery disease
    atherosclerotic coronary artery disease

A-CAH
    autoimmune chronic active hepatitis

ACAID
    anterior chamber-associated immune deviation

ACAN, ACANTH
    acanthocyte
    acanthrocyte (obsolete)

ACAO
    acylcoenzyme A oxidase

ACAPI
    anterior cerebral artery pulsatility index

ACAS
    asymptomatic carotid artery stenosis

Ac-5-ASA
    N-acetyl-5-ASA

ACASH
    Automated Child/Adolescent Social History

ACAT
    acyl-coenzyme A:cholesterol acyltransferase
    aged care assessment team
    automated computerized axial tomography

ACAV
    Acara virus

ACB
    albumin cobalt binding

    alveolar-capillary block
    antibody-coated bacteria
    aortocoronary bypass
    arterialized capillary blood
    asymptomatic carotid bruit

AC&BC
    air conduction and bone conduction

ACBE
    air contrast barium enema

ACBG
    aortocoronary bypass graft

ACC
    acalculous cholecystitis
    accident *(See also* acc, accid)
    accommodation *(See also* A, a, acc, accom)
    acetylcoenzyme A carboxylase
    acinar cell carcinoma
    acute care center
    adenoid cystic carcinoma
    administrative control center
    adrenocortical carcinoma
    alveolar cell carcinoma
    ambulatory care center
    amylase/creatinine clearance
    anodal closure contraction *(See also* AnCC)
    anterior central curve
    antitoxin-containing cell
    aplasia cutis congenita
    articular chondrocalcinosis
    automated cell count

acc
    acceleration *(See also* a, α, accel)
    accelerator
    accident *(See also* ACC, accid)
    accommodation *(See also* A, a, ACC, accom)
    according

accel
    acceleration *(See also* a, α, acc)

AcCh
    acetylcholine *(See also* AC, ACH, ACh)

ACCHN
    adenoid cystic carcinoma of head and neck

AcChR
    acetylcholine receptor

AcCHS
    acetylcholinesterase *(See also* AChE)

ACCI
    Adult Career Concerns Inventory

accid
    accident *(See also* ACC, acc)

ACCL, accl
    anodal closure contraction

ACCLA
anticardiolipin lupus anticoagulant

AcCoA
acetylcoenzyme A (*See also* acetyl-CoA)

accom
accommodation (*See also* A, a, ACC, acc)

ACCR
amylase/creatinine clearance ratio

ACCS
acute change clinical score

ACCSCI
acute central cervical spinal cord injury

accum
accumulated
accumulation

accur.
accurately [L. *accuratissime*]

ACD
absolute cardiac dullness
acid-citrate-dextrose
active compression-decompression
adult celiac disease
advanced care directive
allergic contact dermatitis
alopecia, contracture, dwarfism
alpha-chain disease
anemia of chronic disease
angiokeratoma corporis diffusum
annihilation coincidence detection
anterior cervical diskectomy
anterior chamber diameter
anterior chest diameter
anticonvulsant drug (*See also* AED)
arrhythmia control device
Assessment of Career Development
(citric) acid-citrate (trisodium) -
dextrose (solution)

AcD
alive with disease

AC-DC, ac/dc
alternating current or direct current
bisexual

ACDF
adult child of dysfunctional family
anterior cervical diskectomy and fusion

ACDK
acquired cystic disease of the kidney

ACDM
Assessment of Career Decision Making

ACDV
Acado virus

ACE
acetonitrile
actinium emanation
acute care for the elderly
acute cerebral encephalopathy
acute coronary event
adrenocortical extract
advanced combined encoder
aerobic chair exercises
aerosol cloud enhancer
alcohol, chloroform, and ether (mixture)
angiotensin-converting enzyme
antegrade colonic enema
antegrade continence enema
autologous-cultured epithelium

ace
accessory cholera enterotoxin

ace.
acentric

ACE-II
angiotensin-converting enzyme II

ACED
anhydrotic congenital ectodermal dysplasia

ACE-DD
angiotensin converting enzyme DD

ACEDS
angiotensin-converting enzyme dysfunction syndrome

ACEH
acid cholesterol ester hydrolase

ACEI
angiotensin-converting enzyme inhibitor

AcEst
acetyl esterase

acetyl-CoA
acetylcoenzyme A (*See also* AcCoA)

ACF
aberrant crypt focus
accessory clinical findings
acute care facility
advanced communications function
anterior cervical fusion

NOTES

ACF (*continued*)
  area correction factor
  asymmetric crying facies
ACFM
  automated cardiac flow
    measurement
ACFn
  additional cost of false negatives
ACFp
  additional cost of false positives
ACFS
  anterior cervical plate fixation
    system
ACG
  angiocardiogram
  angiocardiography
  angle-closure glaucoma
  aortocoronary graft
  apexcardiogram
  apexcardiography
  Assessment of Core Goals
AcG
  accelerator globulin (factor V)
ACH
  acetylcholine (*See also* AC, AcCh,
    ACh)
  achalasia
  active chronic hepatitis
  adrenocortical hormone
  air changes per hour
  amyotrophic cerebellar hypoplasia
  arm girth, chest depth, and hip
    width (nutritional index)
ACh
  acetylcholine (*See also* AC, AcCh,
    ACH)
Ach
  acetaldehyde
  acetylcholine
AChA
  anterior choroidal artery
AChE
  acetylcholinesterase (*See also*
    AcCHS)
AChEI
  acetylcholinesterase inhibitor
ACHOO
  autosomal dominant compelling
    helioophthalmic outburst
    (syndrome)
AChR
  acetylcholine receptor
AChRAb
  acetylcholine receptor antibody
AC&HS
  before meals and at bedtime [L.
    antecibum + hora somni]

ACI
  acoustic comfort index
  acute coronary insufficiency
  adenylate cyclase inhibitor
  adrenocortical insufficiency
  aftercare instructions
  asymptomatic cardiac ischemia
  autologous chondrocyte implantation
  average cost of illness
ACID
  Arithmetic, Coding, Information,
    and Digit Span
ACIDS
  acquired cellular immunodeficiency
    syndrome
ACIF
  anticomplement immunofluorescence
AC IOL, ACIOL
  anterior chamber intraocular lens
ACIP
  acute canine idiopathic
    polyneuropathy
ACIS
  automated cellular imaging system
ACJ
  acromioclavicular joint
ACKD
  acquired cystic kidney disease
ACL
  accessory collateral ligament
  Achievement Checklist
  acromegaloid features, cutis verticis
    gyrata, corneal leukoma
  Adjective Check List
  anal canal length
  anterior cruciate ligament
ACl
  aspiryl chloride
aCL
  anticardiolipin
ACLA, ACLAb
  anticardiolipin antibody (*See also*
    ACA)
ACLC
  Assessment of Children's Language
    Comprehension
ACLE
  acute cutaneous lupus
    erythematosus
ACLF
  adult congregate living facility
ACLR
  anterior capsulolabral reconstruction
  anterior cruciate ligament repair
ACLS
  advanced cardiac life support
ACM
  acute cerebrospinal meningitis

acute confusional migraine
albumin-calcium-magnesium
alveolar capillary membrane
anticardiac myosin
Arnold-Chiari malformation
automated cardiac flow
measurement

ACME
aphakic cystoid macular edema

ACMF
arachnoid cyst of the middle fossa

ACML
atypical chronic myeloid leukemia

ACMP
alveolar-capillary membrane
permeability

ACMT
artificial circus-movement
tachycardia

ACMV
assist-controlled mechanical
ventilation

ACN
acute conditioned neurosis

ACO
acute coronary occlusion
alert, cooperative, and oriented
Assessment of Conceptual
Organization

ACOA
adult child of alcoholic

ACoA, A-comm
anterior communicating artery (*See
also* ACA, AComA)

ACOM
automated cardiac output
measurement

AComA
anterior communicating artery (*See
also* ACoA, ACA)

ACOP
Adriamycin, Cytoxan, Oncovin,
prednisone

acor
apex cornea

acous
acoustic
acoustics

ACP
absorbable collagen paste
accessory conduction pathway

acid phosphatase (*See also* AcP,
AC-PH, ac phos, AP)
acyl carrier protein
anodal closure picture
anterior cervical plate
aspirin-caffeine-phenacetin

AcP
acid phosphatase (*See also* ACP,
AC-PH, ac phos, AP)

ACPA
anticytoplasmic antibody

AC-PC
anterior commissure-posterior
commissure

ACPE
acute cardiogenic pulmonary edema

AC-PH, ac phos
acid phosphatase (*See also* ACP,
AcP, AP)

ACPL
antibody-conjugated paramagnetic
liposome

ACPP
adrenocortical polypeptide

ACPS
acrocephalopolysyndactyly

acq
acquired
acquisition

ACR
abnormally contracting regions
absolute catabolic rate
adenomatosis of colon and rectum
anterior chamber reformation
anticonstipation regimen
axillary count rate

Acr
acriflavine
acrylic

ACRF
ambulatory care research facility

ACS
abdominal compartment syndrome
acetyl strophanthidin
acrocallosal syndrome
acrocephalosyndactyly, type I–V
acute chest syndrome
acute confusional state
acute coronary syndrome
acute mountain sickness
Advanced Cardiovascular Systems
Advanced Catheter System

NOTES

ACS *(continued)*
Alcon Closure System
ambulatory care services
anodal closure sound
anterior compartment syndrome
anterior cricoid split
antireticular cytotoxic serum
aperture current setting
arterial cannulation support
automated corneal shaper

AcS
acetylstrophanthidin

ACSL
automatic computerized solvent
litholysis

ACST
asymptomatic carotid surgery trial

ACSV
aortocoronary-saphenous vein (graft)

ACSVBG
aortocoronary-saphenous vein bypass
graft

ACT
achievement through counseling and
treatment
acid clearance test
actinomycin
activated clotting time
activated coagulation time
adaptive control of thought
adenylate cyclase toxin
advanced coronary treatment
allergen challenge test
alternate cover test
antichymotrypsin
anticoagulant therapy
antrocolic transposition
anxiety control training
asthma care training
atropine coma therapy
axial computed tomography

act.
active
activity (*See also* activ, α)

ACTA
automatic computed transverse axial
(scanning)

ACTe
anodal closure tetanus

ACTeRS
ADD-H: Comprehensive Teacher's
Rating Scale, Second Edition

Act Ex
active exercise

ACTH
adrenocorticotropic hormone
(corticotropin)

ACTH-RF
adrenocorticotropic hormone-releasing
factor

activ
activity (*See also* act., α)

ACTN
adrenocorticotropin

ACTP
adrenocorticotropic polypeptide

ActR
activin receptor

ActRI
activin receptor I

ActRII
activin receptor II

ActRIB
activin receptor IB

ActRIIB
activin receptor IIB

ACTRS
Abbreviated Conners Teacher
Rating Scale

ACTS
acute cervical traumatic sprain or
syndrome
Auditory Comprehension Test for
Sentences

ACU
acquired cold urticaria
acute care unit
ambulatory care unit

ACUTENS
acupuncture and transcutaneous
electrical nerve stimulation

ACV
acute cardiovascular (disease)
acyclovir
assist/control ventilation
atrial/carotid/ventricular

ACVB
aortocoronary venous bypass

ACVD
acute cardiovascular disease
atherosclerotic cardiovascular disease
autoimmune collagen vascular
disease

ACVRD
arteriosclerotic cardiovascular renal
disease

AC/W
acetone in water

acyl-CoA
acylcoenzyme A

AD
abdominal diameter
above diaphragm
absorbed dose
accident dispensary

acetate dialysis
achievement drive
active disease
acute dermatomyositis
addict
addiction (*See also* addict.)
adenoid degeneration (agent)
adherent
adjuvant disease
admitting diagnosis
adult disease
advanced directive
aerodynamic mass diameter
aerosol bolus dispersion
aerosol deposition
affective disorder
after discharge
alcohol dehydrogenase
Aleutian disease (of mink) (*See also* AMD)
alveolar duct
Alzheimer dementia
Alzheimer disease
analgesic dose
androstenedione
anodal duration
anterior displacement
anterior division
antidepressant
antigenic determinant
aortic diameter
aortic dissection
appropriate disability
arthritic dose
Asperger disorder
atopic dermatitis
attentional disturbance
auris dexter
autogenic drainage
autonomic dysreflexia
autosomal dominant
average day
average deviation
axiodistal
axis deviation

A/D
analog-to-digital (converter)

A&D
admission and discharge
alcohol and drugs
ascending and descending
vitamins A and D

A.D.
right ear [L. *auris dextra*] (*See also* a.d.)

a.d.
alternating days (every other day) [L. *alternis dies*]
as desired
right ear [L. *auris dextra*] (*See also* A.D.)

ad
adduction (*See also* ADD)
adductor
adenovirus
adipocyte
adrenal
anisotropic disk
axiodistal

ad.
let there be added [L. *addetur*] (*See also* add.)

ADA
adenosine deaminase
Americans with Disabilities Act
anterior descending artery
antideoxyribonucleic acid antibody
approved dietary allowance

ADA #
American Diabetes Association diet number

ADAD
Adolescent Drug and Alcohol Diagnostic Assessment

ADAM
aerosol-derived airway morphometry
amniotic deformity, adhesion, mutilation (syndrome)
a disintegrin and matrilysin

ADAP
AIDS Drug Assistance Program

ADAS
Alzheimer Disease Assessment Scale

ADAS-Cog, ADAS-cog
Alzheimer Disease Assessment Scale, cognitive subscale

ADase
adenosine deaminase

ADASI
Atopic Dermatitis Area and Severity Index

ADAU
adolescent drug abuse unit

NOTES

15

ADB
anti-DNase B

ADC
affective disorders clinic
Aid to Dependent Children
AIDS dementia complex
albumin, dextrose, and catalase
(medium)
ambulance design criteria
analog-to-digital converter
anodal duration contraction
antral diverticulum of the colon
anxiety disorder clinic
apparent diffusion coefficient
average daily census
axiodistocervical

AdC
adenylate cyclase
adrenal cortex

ADCC
acute disorder of cerebral
circulation
antibody-dependent cell cytotoxicity
antibody-dependent cell-mediated
cytotoxicity
antibody-dependent cellular
cytotoxicity

ADCHF
acutely decompensated congestive
heart failure

ADD
adduction (*See also* ad)
adenosine deaminase
alcohol and drug dependency (unit)
angled delivery device
attention deficit disorder
average daily dose

ADD1
adipocyte determination and
differentiation factor-1

add.
addition
let there be added [L. *addetur*]
(*See also* ad.)

ADDBRS
Attention Deficit Disorder Behavior
Rating Scale

addend.
to be added [L. *addendus*]

ADDES
Attention Deficit Disorders
Evaluation Scale

ADD-HA
attention deficit disorder with
hyperactivity (*See also* ADHD)

addict.
addiction (*See also* AD)
addictive

AdDNV
Acheta domestica densovirus

ADDU
alcohol and drug dependence unit

ADE
acute disseminated encephalomyelitis
(*See also* ADEM)
antibody-dependent enhancement
apparent digestible energy

Ade
adenine (*See also* A)

ADEAR
Alzheimer's Disease Education and
Referral

AdeCbl
adenosyl cobalamin

ADEE
age-dependent epileptic
encephalopathy

ADEM
acute disseminated encephalomyelitis
(*See also* ADE)

ADEPT
antibody-directed enzyme prodrug
therapy

adeq
adequate

ADF
aortoduodenal fistula

AD/FHD
acetabular depth to femoral head
diameter

ADFN
albinism-deafness (syndrome)

ADFU
agar diffusion for fungus

ADG
adjustable-depth (gauge needle)
atrial diastolic gallop
axiodistogingival

ADH
adhesion (*See also* adh)
alcohol dehydrogenase
antidiuretic hormone
atypical ductal hyperplasia

adh
adhesion (*See also* ADH)
adhesive

AdHCC
advanced hepatocellular carcinoma

ADHD, ADD-H
attention deficit hyperactivity
disorder (*See also* ADD-HA)

ADHD-PI
attention deficit hyperactivity
disorder-predominantly inattentive

ad hoc
informal

temporary
for this (purpose) [L. *ad hoc*]

ADI

absolute dose intensity
acceptable daily intake
Adolescent Diagnostic Interview
Adolescent Drinking Index
allowable daily intake
antral diverticulum of the ileum
artificial diverticulum of the ileum
atlantodens interval
autism diagnostic interview
autosomal-dominant ichthyosis
axiodistoincisal

ADICOL

advanced insulin infusion with a
control loop

ADI-R

Autism Diagnostic Interview-Revised

ADJ

adjustable dynamic joint

adj

adjacent
adjoining
adjunct
adjuvant

ADK

adenosine kinase
automated disposable keratome

ADKC

atopic dermatitis with
keratoconjunctivitis

ADL

activities of daily living (*See also*
ADLs)
adrenoleukodystrophy
Amsterdam Depression List

ADLC

antibody-dependent lymphocyte-
mediated cytotoxicity

ad lib.

as desired [L. *ad libitum*]

ADLR

advanced design LINAC
radiosurgery

ADLs

activities of daily living (*See also*
ADL)

ADM

abductor digiti minimi (muscle)
administration (*See also* admin)

administrative medicine
administrator
admission
admit
apparent distribution mass
atypical diabetes mellitus

AdM

adrenal medulla

ADMA

asymmetric dimethylarginine

ADMCKD

autosomal dominant medullary
cystic kidney disease

Adm Dr

admitting doctor

ADME

absorption, distribution, metabolism,
and excretion

admin

administer
administration (*See also* ADM)

ADMLX

adhesion molecule like from the X-
chromosome

Adm Ph

admitting physician

ADMR

average daily metabolic rate

ADMX

adrenal medullectomy

ADN

antideoxyribonuclease (*See also*
ADNase)
aortic depressor nerve

adn

adenoid
adenoidectomy

ADNase

antideoxyribonuclease (*See also*
ADN)

ADNase-B

antideoxyribonuclease B (*See also*
ADN-B, anti-DNase B)

ad naus.

to the point of producing nausea
[L. *ad nauseam*]

ADN-B

antideoxyribonuclease B (*See also*
anti-DNase B, ADNase-B)

ADNR

anterior displacement no reduction

NOTES

ADO
adolescent medicine
axiodistoocclusal
Ado
adenosine
ADOD
arthrodentoosteodysplasia
AdoDABA
adenosyl-diaminobutyric acid
ADODM
adult-onset diabetes mellitus
AdoHcy
S-adenosylhomocysteine (*See also* SAH)
AdoHcyase
S-adenosylhomocysteine hydrolase
adol
adolescent
AdoMet
S-adenosyl-methionine
ADOS
Autism Diagnostic Observation Schedule
autosomal dominant Opitz syndrome
Adox
oxidized adenosine
ADP
adenopathy
adenosine diphosphate
adenosine 5′-diphosphate
administrative psychiatry
ammonium dihydrogen phosphate
approved drug product
area diastolic pressure
arterial demand pacing
automatic data processing
ADPA
aggressive digital papillary adenoma
ADPase
adenosine diphosphatase
adenosine 5′-diphosphatase
ADP/ATP
adenosine 5′-diphosphate/adenosine triphosphate
ADPKD
autosomal dominant polycystic kidney disease
ADPL
average daily patient load
ADPR
adenosine diphosphate ribose
ADPV
anomaly of drainage of pulmonary vein
ADQ
abductor digiti quinti (muscle)
adequate

ADR
acceptable dental remedies
acute dystonic reaction
adverse drug reaction
airway dilation reflex
allergic drug reaction
ataxia-deafness-retardation (syndrome)
Adr
adrenaline (*See also* A)
adr
adrenal
adrenalectomy (*See also* ADX)
ADRBR
adrenergic beta-receptor
ADROM
ankle dorsiflexion range of motion
adRP
autosomal-dominant retinitis pigmentosa
ADRS
Alzheimer Disease Rating Scale
ADRV
adult diarrhea rotavirus
ADS
acute death syndrome
acute diarrheal syndrome
Alcohol Dependence Scale
alternative delivery system
anatomical dead space
anonymous donor sperm
anterior drawer sign
antibody deficiency syndrome
antidiuretic substance
AdSD
adductor spasmodic dysphonia
ADSI
Atopic Dermatitis Severity Index
ADSQC
adenosquamous cell carcinoma
ADSV
Arboledas virus
ADT
accepted dental therapeutics
adenosine triphosphate
admission, discharge, transfer
agar-gel diffusion test
alternate day therapy
androgen deprivation therapy
anethol dithiolethione
anterior drawer test
anticipate discharge tomorrow
any desired thing
Auditory Discrimination Test
automated dithionite test
ADTe
anodal duration tetanus

ADTP
    adolescent day treatment program
    alcohol dependence treatment
      program

ADU
    acute duodenal ulcer
    addictive disease unit

A-DV
    arterial/deep venous difference

ADV, Adv
    adefovir dipivoxil
    adenovirus
    adventitia

A/DV
    arterial/deep venous

adv
    advanced
    advice
    advise

ADVIRC
    autosomal-dominant
      vitreoretinochoroidopathy

ADW
    assault with deadly weapon

A5D5W
    5% alcohol and 5% dextrose in
      water

ADWOR
    anterior disk displacement without
      reduction

ADWR
    anterior displacement with reduction

ADX
    adrenalectomized
    adrenalectomy (*See also* adr)

AE
    above elbow (amputation) (*See also*
      AEA)
    accident and emergency
      (department) (*See also* A&E)
    accurate empathy
    acrodermatitis enteropathica
    activation energy
    acute exacerbation
    adrenal epinephrine
    adult erythrocyte
    aftereffect
    agarose electrophoresis
    air embolism
    air entry
    alcoholic embryopathy
    androstanediol

    anoxic encephalopathy
    antiembolitic
    antiepileptic
    antitoxin unit [Ger. *Antitoxineinhei*]
    apoenzyme
    aryepiglottic (fold)
    atherosclerotic encephalopathy

AE1
    antikeratin

A&E
    accident and emergency
      (department) (*See also* AE)

AEA
    above-elbow amputation (*See also*
      AE)
    adrenal epithelioid angiosarcoma
    alcohol, ether, and acetone
      (solution)
    allergic extrinsic alveolitis
    antiendomysium antibody

AEB
    as evidenced by
    atrial ectopic beat
    avian erythroblastosis

AEC
    absolute blood eosinophil count
    3-amino-9-ethylcarbazole
    ankyloblepharon, ectodermal defect,
      and cleft lip and/or palate
    aortic ejection click
    at earliest convenience
    automatic exposure control

AECA
    antiendothelial cell antibody
    antiendothelial cell autoantibody

AECB
    acute exacerbation of chronic
      bronchitis

AECD
    allergic eczematous contact
      dermatitis
    automatic external cardioverter-
      defibrillator

AECG
    ambulatory electrocardiogram
    ambulatory electrocardiography

AECP
    antiepiligrin cicatricial pemphigoid

AECS
    acute exertional compartment
      syndrome

NOTES

AECUS
atypical endocervical cells of undetermined significance

AED
aerodynamic equivalent diameter
antiepileptic (anticonvulsant) drug
antihidrotic ectodermal dysplasia
automated external defibrillator
automatic external defibrillator

AEDP
automated external defibrillator pacemaker

aEEG
amplitude-integrated electroencephalogram

AEEU
admission, entrance, and evaluation unit

AEF
allogenic effect factor
amyloid-enhancing factor
aryepiglottic fold
auditory-evoked magnetic field

AEFI
acute esophageal food impaction

AEG
acute erosive gastritis
air encephalogram
air encephalography
atrial electrogram

Ae-H
anterograde conduction

AEI
atrial emptying index

AEIOU TIPS
alcohol, epilepsy, insulin, overdose, uremia, trauma, infection, psychiatric, stroke

AEL
acute erythroleukemia

AELT
ascites euglobulin lysis time

AEM
ambulatory electrocardiographic monitoring
ambulatory electrogram monitor
analytical electron microscope
analytical electron microscopy
antiepileptic medication
avian encephalomyelitis

AEN
aseptic epiphyseal necrosis

AENNS
Albert Einstein Neonatal Developmental Scale

AEO
apraxia of eyelid opening

AEP
acute edematous pancreatitis
appropriateness evaluation protocol
artificial endocrine pancreas
auditory evoked potential
average evoked potential

AEq
age equivalent

AER
abduction-external rotation
acoustic evoked response
acute exertional rhabdomyolysis
agranular endoplasmic reticulum
aided equalization response
albumin excretion rate
aldosterone excretion rate
apical ectodermal ridge
auditory evoked response
automatic endoscopic reprocessor
average electroencephalic response
average evoked response

aer
aerosol

AERA
average evoked response audiometry

AERD
atheroembolic renal disease

AerM
aerosol mask

AERP
atrial effective refractory period

AerT
aerosol tent

AES
acetone-extracted serum
anal endosonography
anterior esophageal sensor
antiembolic stockings
antral ethmoidal sphenoidectomy
aortic ejection sound
Auger electron spectroscope

AESOP
automated endoscopic system for optimal positioning

AESP
applied extrasensory projection

AEST
aeromedical evacuation support team

A-esu
statampere (*See also* statA)

AET
absorption-equivalent thickness
atrial ectopic tachycardia

AETT
acetyl ethyl tetramethyl tetralin

AEU

allercoat enzyme allergosorbent unit

AEVS

automated eligibility verification system

AEX

aerobic exercise

AF

abnormal frequency

acid fast

adult female

afebrile (*See also* AFEB)

aflatoxin (*See also* AFT)

albumose-free (tuberculin)

aldehyde fuchsin

alleged father

amaurosis fugax

ameloblastic fibroma

aminophylline

amniotic fluid

anchoring fibril

angiogenesis factor

anteflexed

anteflexion

anterior fontanelle

anterior frontal

anterofrontal

antibody forming

antifibrinogen

antifungal

aortic flow

aortofemoral

apical foramen

arcuate fasciculus

artificially fed

ascitic fluid (*See also* ascit fl)

atrial fibrillation (*See also* AFib, At Fib, ATR FIB, atr fib.)

atrial flutter (*See also* AFL)

atrial fusion

attenuation factor

attributable fraction

audiofrequency (*See also* af)

auricular fibrillation (*See also* AUR FIB, aur fib.)

AF-1

antifertility factor-1

A-F

air-fluid (level)

ankle-foot (orthosis)

antifibrinogen

aF

abfarad

af

audio frequency (*See also* AF)

AFA

acromegaloid facial appearance

advanced first aid

alcohol-formaldehyde-acetic acid (fixative or solution)

AFAFP

amniotic fluid alpha fetoprotein

A-FAIR

arrhythmia-insensitive flow-sensitive alternating inversion recovery

AFB

acid-fast bacillus

aflatoxin B

air-fluidized bed

aortofemoral bypass

aspirated foreign body

AFBG

aortofemoral bypass graft

AFBN

acute focal bacterial nephritis

AFC

acid-fast culture

adult foster care

air-filled cushion

allergic fungal sinusitis

antibody-forming cell

AFCI

acute focal cerebral ischemia

AFCL

atrial fibrillation cycle length

AFD

accelerated freeze-drying

AFDC

Aid to Families with Dependent Children

AFE

amniotic fluid embolism

amniotic fluid embolization

AFEB

afebrile (*See also* AF)

AFF

atrial fibrillation-flutter

atrial filling fraction

AF/F

atrial fibrillation and/or flutter

aff

afferent

NOTES

AFFN
acrofrontofacionasal

AFG
aflatoxin G
alpha-fetoglobulin
amniotic fluid glucose
auditory figure-ground

aFGF, a-FGF
acidic fibroblast growth factor (*See also* FGFa)

AFH
angiofollicular hyperplasia
angiomatoid fibrous histiocytoma
anterior facial height

AFI
acute febrile illness
amaurotic familial idiocy
amniotic fluid index

AFib
atrial fibrillation (*See also* AF, At Fib, ATR FIB, atr fib.)

AFIS
amniotic fluid infection syndrome

AFL
antifatty liver (factor)
antifibrinolysin
artificial limb
atrial flutter (*See also* AF)

AFLH, AFLNH
angiofollicular lymphoid hyperplasia

AFLP
acute fatty liver of pregnancy
amplicon fragment length polymorphism

AFM
aflatoxin M
atomic force microscopy

AFN
afunctional neutrophil

AFND
acute febrile neutrophilic dermatosis

AFO
ankle-foot orthosis

AFORMED
alternating failure of response mechanical to electrical depolarization

AFP
acute flaccid paralysis
adiabatic fast passage
alpha-fetoprotein (*See also* aFP)
anterior faucial pillar
ascending frontal parietal
atrial filling pressure
atypical facial pain

aFP
alpha-fetoprotein (*See also* AFP)

AFP-EIA
alpha-fetoprotein enzyme immunoassay

AFPP
acute fibropurulent pneumonia

AFQ
aflatoxin Q

AFQT
Armed Forces Qualification Test

AFR
aqueous flare response
ascorbic free radical
atrial flutter response

AFRAX
autism-fragile X (syndrome)

AFRD
acute febrile respiratory disease

AFRI
acute febrile respiratory illness

AFS
acid-fast smear
acromegaloid facial syndrome
aldehyde-fuchsin stain
allergic fungal sinusitis
antifibroblast serum

AFT
aflatoxin (*See also* AF)
agglutination-flocculation test
autologous fat transfer

AFT$_3$
absolute free triiodothyronine

AFT$_4$
absolute free thyroxine

AFTC
apparent free testosterone concentration

AFTN
autonomously functioning thyroid nodule

AFTP
ascitic fluid total protein

AFUD
American Foundation for Urologic Diseases

AFV
amniotic fluid volume

AFVSS
afebrile, vital signs stable

AFX
air/fluid exchange
atypical fibroxanthoma

AG
abdominal girth
agarose
albumin-globulin (ratio)
aminoglutethimide (*See also* AGL)
aminoglycoside
analytical grade

angular gyrus
anion gap
antigen (*See also* ag, AGN)
antiglobulin
antigravity
atrial gallop (*See also* ag)
attached gingiva
axiogingival
azurophilic granule

AG-1343
nelfinavir

A:G, A/G
albumin-globulin (ratio) (*See also*
ALB/GLOB, AB)

Ag
silver [L. *argentum*]

ag
antigen (*See also* AG, AGN)
atrial gallop (*See also* AG)

AGA
accelerated growth area
acetylglutamate
acute gonococcal arthritis
allergic granulomatosis and angiitis
androgenetic alopecia
antigliadin antibody
antiglomerular antibody
anti-IgA autoantibody
appropriate for gestational age
aspartylglucosamide

Ag-Ab
antigen-antibody (complex)

AGAG
acidic glycosaminoglycans

AGAS
accelerated graft atherosclerosis
acetylglutamate synthetase

AGC
absolute granulocyte count
anatomic graduated component
automatic gain control

AGCT
adult granulosa cell tumor
Army General Classification Test

AGCUS
atypical glandular cells of
undetermined significance (*See also*
AGUS)

AGD
agar/agarose-gel diffusion (method)
antigonadotropic decapeptide

AGDD
agar-agarose-gel double diffusion
(method)

AGE
acrylamide gel electrophoresis
acute gastroenteritis
advanced glycation end-product
advanced glycosylation end-product
(*See also* AGEP)
angle of greatest extension
arterial gas embolism

AGED
automated general experimental
device

AGEP
acute generalized exanthematous
pustulosis
advanced glycosylation end product
(*See also* AGE)

AGF
adrenal growth factor
angle of greatest flexion
autologous growth factor

AGG
agammaglobulinemia

agg
aggregation

agg, aggl, agglut
agglutinate
agglutination (*See also* AGL)

AGGS
anti-gas gangrene serum

AGH
amenorrhea, galactorrhea,
hypothyroidism

AGHE
Association for Gerontology in
Higher Education

agit.
shake [L. *agita*]

AGL
acute granulocytic leukemia
agglutination (*See also* agg)
aminoglutethimide (*See also* AG)
anterior glenoid labrum

A-GLACTO-LK
alpha-galactoside leukocyte

AGLMe
N-alpha-acetylglycyl-L-lysine

AGM
absorbent gelling material

NOTES

AGMK, AGMk
African green monkey kidney (cell)
AGML
acute gastric mucosal lesion
AGN
acute glomerulonephritis
agnosia (*See also* agn)
antigen (*See also* AG, ag)
agn
agnosia (*See also* AGN)
AgNO₃

silver nitrate
AgNOR
argyrophil organizer region protein
silver-staining nucleolar organizer
region
AGP
acute gallstone pancreatitis
agar-gel precipitation (test) (*See
also* AGPT)
alpha₁-acid glycoprotein (*See also*
AAG)
AGPNHL
aggressive good prognosis non-
Hodgkin lymphoma
AGPT
agar-gel precipitation test (*See also*
AGP)
AGR
aniridia, ambiguous genitalia,
mental retardation
anticipatory goal response
AGS
adrenogenital syndrome
antiglucagon
audiogenic seizures
AGT
abnormal glucose tolerance
activity group therapy
acute generalized tuberculosis
adrenoglomerulotropin (*See also*
AGTr)
aminoglutethimide
angiotensinogen test
antiglobulin test
AGTH
adrenoglomerulotropin hormone
AGTr
adrenoglomerulotropin (*See also*
AGT)
AGTT
abnormal glucose tolerance test
AGU
aspartylglucosaminuria
aspartylglycosaminuria

AGUS
atypical glandular cells of
undetermined significance (*See also*
AGCUS)
AGUV
Aguacate virus
AGVHD
acute graft-versus-host disease
AH
abdominal hysterectomy (*See also*
abd hyst)
absorptive hypercalciuria
accidental hypothermia
acetohexamide
acid hydrolysis
acute hepatitis
adenomatous hyperplasia
adrenal hypoplasia
after-hyperpolarization (*See also*
AHP)
agnathia holoprosencephaly
alcoholic hepatitis
amenorrhea and hirsutism
amenorrhea and hyperprolactinemia
aminohippurate
anterior hypothalamus
antihyaluronidase
Arachis hypogaea
arcuate hypothalamus
arterial hypertension
artificial heart
ascites hepatoma
assisted hatching
astigmatic hypermetropia
ataxic hemiparesis
atrium-His bundle
atypical hyperplasia
autonomic hyperreflexia
axillary hair
A&H
accident and health (policy)
A-h
ampere-hour
aH
abhenry
ah
hyperopic astigmatism
AHA
acetohydroxamic acid
acquired hemolytic anemia
acute hemolytic anemia
alpha hydroxy acid
anterior hypothalamic area
antiheart antibody
antihistone antibody
area health authority
arthritis-hives-angioedema (syndrome)
aspartylhydroxamic acid

Australian hepatitis antigen
autoimmune hemolytic anemia
AHA.SOC
American Heart Association Stroke
Outcome Classification
AHB
alpha-hydroxybutyric dehydrogenase
AHBC
hepatitis B core antibody
AHC
academic health care
acute hemorrhagic conjunctivitis
acute hemorrhagic cystitis
adrenal hypoplasia congenita
alternating hemiplegia of childhood
antihemophilic factor C
AHCy
S-adenosylhomocysteine
AHD
acquired hepatocerebral degeneration
acute heart disease
antihypertensive drug
arteriohepatic dysplasia
arteriosclerotic heart disease
atherosclerotic heart disease
autoimmune hemolytic disease
AHDMS
automated hospital data
management system
AHDP
azacycloheptane diphosphonate
AHDS
Allen-Herndon-Dudley syndrome
AHE
acute hemorrhagic edema
acute hemorrhagic encephalomyelitis
AHEC
area health education center
AHEI
acute hemorrhagic edema of
infancy
AHES
artificial heart energy system
AHF
accelerated hyperfractionation
acute heart failure
antihemophilic factor (factor VIII)
Argentinian hemorrhagic fever
AHFS
American Hospital Formulary
Service

AHG
aggregated human globulin
antihemophilic globulin
antihuman globulin
AHG-CDC
antiglobulin-enhanced complement-
dependent cytotoxicity
AHGG
aggregated human gamma globulin
AHGS
acute herpetic gingival stomatitis
AHGXM
antihuman globulin crossmatch
AHH
alpha-hydrazine analog of histidine
analog of histidine
anosmia and hypogonadotropic
hypogonadism (syndrome)
arylhydrocarbon hydroxylase
AHHD
arteriosclerotic hypertensive heart
disease
AHI
acetabular head index
acromiohumeral interval
active hostility index
acute HIV-1 infection
anterior horn index
apnea-hypopnea index
Arthritis Helplessness Index
AHIP
assisted health insurance plan
AHIS
automated hospital information
system
AHJ
artificial hip joint
AHL
aggressive histology lymphoma
apparent half-life
AHLE
acute hemorrhagic leukoencephalitis
AHLG
antihuman lymphocyte globulin
AHLS
antihuman lymphocyte serum
AHLT
auxiliary heterotopic liver
transplantation
AHM
ambulatory Holter monitor

NOTES

AHM *(continued)*
　　ambulatory Holter monitoring
　　anterior hyaloid membrane
AHMA
　　antiheart muscle autoantibody
AHMO
　　anterior horizontal mandibular
　　　osteotomy
AHN
　　adenomatous hyperplastic nodule
AHO
　　acute hematogenous osteomyelitis
AHP
　　acute hemorrhagic pancreatitis
　　after-hyperpolarization (*See also*
　　　AH)
　　afterspike hyperpolarization
　　air at high pressure
　　American Hand Prosthetics
AHPCT
　　autologous hematopoietic progenitor
　　　cell transplantation
AHPO
　　anterior hypothalamic preoptic
　　　(area)
AHR
　　acute humoral rejection
　　airway hyperreactivity
　　airway hyperresponsiveness
　　autonomic hyperreflexia
AhR
　　aryl hydrocarbon receptor
AHRF
　　acute hypoxemic respiratory failure
AHS
　　adaptive hand skills
　　African horse sickness
　　allopurinol hypersensitivity
　　　syndrome
　　alveolar hypoventilation syndrome
　　antiepileptic drug hypersensitivity
AHSDF
　　area health service development
　　　fund
AHSV 1–9
　　African horse sickness virus 1–9
AHT
　　aggregation half-time
　　alternating hypertropia
　　amiodarone-iodine-induced
　　　thyrotoxicosis
　　antihyaluronidase titer
　　augmented histamine test
　　autoantibodies to human
　　　thyroglobulin
AHTG
　　antihuman thymocyte globulin

AHTP
　　antihuman thymocyte plasma
AHTS
　　antihuman thymus serum
AHU
　　acute hemolytic uremic (syndrome)
　　arginine, hypoxanthine, and uracil
AHuG
　　aggregated human immunoglobulin
　　　G
AHV
　　Abu Hammad virus
　　avian herpesvirus
aHyl
　　allohydroxylysine
AHYS
　　acquired hyperostosis syndrome
AI
　　accidental injury
　　accidentally incurred
　　acetabular index
　　acute inflammation
　　adiposity index
　　aggregation index
　　allergy and immunology (*See also*
　　　A&I)
　　allergy index
　　anal index
　　angiogenesis inhibitor
　　angiotensin inhibitor
　　anxiety index
　　aortic incompetence
　　aortic insufficiency
　　apical impulse
　　apnea index
　　apoptotic index
　　articulation index
　　artificial insemination
　　artificial intelligence
　　atherogenic index
　　atrial insufficiency
　　autoimmune
　　autoimmunity
　　axioincisal
A-I
　　aortoiliac
A&I
　　allergy and immunology (*See also*
　　　AI)
AIA
　　adjuvant-induced arthritis
　　allergen-induced asthma
　　allylisopropylacetamide
　　amylase inhibitor activity
　　antigen-induced arthritis
　　antiimmunoglobulin antibody
　　antiinsulin antibody (*See also* AI-
　　　Ab)

aspirin-induced asthma
aspirin-intolerant asthma
automated image analysis

AI-Ab
antiinsulin antibody (*See also* AIA)

AIB
aminoisobutyric acid (*See also* AIBA)
avian infectious bronchitis

AIBA
aminoisobutyric acid (*See also* AIB)

AIBF
anterior interbody fusion

AIBH
ACTH-independent bilateral macronodular hyperplasia

AIC
aminoimidazole carboxamide

AICA
anterior internal cerebellar artery

AI-CAH
autoimmune-type chronic active hepatitis

AICAR
aminoimidazole carboxamide ribonucleotide
aminoimidazole carboxamide ribotide

AICC
antiinhibitor coagulant complex

AICD
activation-induced cell death
automatic implantable cardioverter-defibrillator
automatic internal cardioverter-defibrillator

AICF
autoimmune complement fixation

AICS
acute ischemic coronary syndrome
artery of inferior cavernous sinus

AID
acute infectious disease
acute ionization detector
antiinflammatory drug
argon ionization detector
artificial insemination donor
artificial insemination by donor
autoimmune deficiency
autoimmune disease
automatic implantable defibrillator
average interocular difference

AIDH
artificial insemination donor, husband

AIDP
acute inflammatory demyelinating polyneuropathy
acute inflammatory demyelinating polyradiculoneuropathy
acute inflammatory demyelinating polyradiculopathy

AIDS
acquired immune deficiency syndrome
acquired immunodeficiency syndrome
acute infectious disease series
Assessment of Intelligibility of Dysarthric Speech

AIDS-HAQ
acquired immunodeficiency syndrome health assessment questionnaire

AIDS-KS
acquired immunodeficiency syndrome with Kaposi sarcoma

AIDSLINE
online information on acquired immunodeficiency syndrome

AIE
autoimmune enteropathy

AIED
autoimmune inner ear disease

AIEP
amount of insulin extractable from pancreas

AIF
anemia-inducing factor
antiinflammatory
antiinvasion factor
aortic-iliac-femoral

AIF-1
anemia-inducing factor-1

AIFD
acute intrapartum fetal distress

AIG
antiimmunoglobulin

AIgA
absence of immunoglobulin A

AIGF
androgen-induced growth factor

AIgM
absence of immunoglobulin M

NOTES

A-IGP
activity-interview group psychotherapy

AIH
anterior interhemispheric approach
aortic intramural hematoma
artificial insemination, homologous
artificial insemination, husband
autoimmune hepatitis

AIHA
autoimmune hemolytic anemia

AIHD
acquired immune hemolytic disease

AII
acute intestinal infection

AIIS
anterior inferior iliac spine

AIL
acute infectious lymphocytosis
angiocentric immunoproliferative lesion
angioimmunoblastic lymphadenopathy
angioimmunoblastic lymphoma

AILD
alveolar-interstitial lung disease
angioimmunoblastic lymphadenopathy with dysproteinemia

AILE, aIle
alloisoleucine

AILT
amiloride-inhibitable lithium transport

AIM
Ace intramedullary (nail)
aerosol inhalation monitor
area of interest magnification
artificial intelligence in medicine

AIMD
abnormal involuntary movement disorder

AIMO
anterior inferior mandibular osteotomy

AIMS
Abnormal Involuntary Movements Scale
Alberta Infant Motor Scale
arthritis impact measurement scale

AIN
acute interstitial nephritis
anal intraepithelial neoplasia
anterior interosseous nerve
autoimmune neutropenia

AINS
antiinflammatory nonsteroidal (agent)

A Insuf
aortic insufficiency

AIO
all-in-one
amyloid of immunoglobulin origin

AIOD
aortoiliac occlusive disease

AION
anterior ischemic optic neuropathy

AIP
acute idiopathic pericarditis
acute infectious polyneuritis
acute inflammatory polyneuropathy
acute intermittent porphyria
acute interstitial pneumonia
acute interstitial pneumonitis
aldosterone-induced protein
automated immunoprecipitation
average intravascular pressure

A/I-PACG
acute intermittent primary angle-closure glaucoma

AIPC
androgen-independent prostate cancer

AIPE
acute idiopathic peripheral facial nerve palsy

AIR
accelerated idioventricular rhythm (See also AIVR)
acute insulin response
aminoimidazole ribonucleotide
5-aminoimidazole ribose 5′-phosphate
5-aminoimidazole ribotide
average impairment rating

AIRA
antiinsulin receptor antibody

AIRE
autoimmune regulator
autoimmune regulatory

AIRF
alteration in respiratory function

AIROM
active integral range of motion

AIRS
Amphetamine Interview Rating Scale

AIS
Abbreviated Injury Scale
Abbreviated Injury Score
acute ischemic stroke
adenocarcinoma in situ
adolescent idiopathic scoliosis
Advanced Interventional Systems
amniotic infection syndrome
amputation index score

androgen insensitivity syndrome
anterior interosseous nerve
  syndrome
antiinsulin serum
AISA
acquired idiopathic sideroblastic
  anemia
AIS/ISS
Abbreviated Injury Score/Injury
  Severity Score
AIS/MR
Alternative Intermediate Services
  for the Mentally Retarded
AIT
acute intensive treatment
administrator-in-training
adoptive immunotherapy
auditory integration training
AITD
autoimmune thyroid disease
AITN
acute interstitial tubular nephritis
AITP
autoimmune thrombocytopenia
autoimmune thrombocytopenic
  purpura
AITT
arginine/insulin tolerance test
AIU
absolute iodine uptake
antigen-inducing unit
AIVR
accelerated idioventricular rhythm
  (*See also* AIR)
AIVV
anterior internal vertebral vein
AJ, A/J
ankle jerk
AJC
ankle joint complex
AJPBD
anomalous junction of the
  pancreatobiliary duct
AJR
abnormal jugular reflex
AJS
acute joint syndrome
AK
above knee (amputation) (*See also*
  AKA)
acne keloidalis
actinic keratosis

adenosine kinase
adenylate kinase
amebic keratitis
applied kinesiology
artificial kidney
astigmatic keratotomy
AKA
above-knee amputation (*See also*
  AK)
alcoholic ketoacidosis
all known allergies
alpha-allokainic acid
also known as
antikeratin antibody
AKAV
Akabane virus
AKD
atypical Kawasaki disease
AKE
acrokeratoelastoidosis
active knee extension
A/kg
amperes per kilogram
AKP
alkaline phosphatase (*See also*
  ALK-P, alk phos, alk p'tase, ALP,
  AlPase, AP, KA, P'ase)
AKR
aldo-keto reductase
AKS
alcoholic Korsakoff syndrome
arthroscopic knee surgery
auditory and kinesthetic sensation
AKU
alkaptonuria
AL
absolute latency
acinar lumina
acute leukemia
adaptation level
albumin (5%, followed by amount
  in mL) (*See also* A, ALB, abl)
alcoholism (*See also* alc)
alignment mark
amyloidosis
annoyance level
anterolateral
antihuman lymphocytic (globulin)
argininosuccinate lysate
argon laser
arterial line (*See also* A-line, art.
  line, ART)

NOTES

AL (*continued*)
   avian leukosis
   axial length
   axiolingual
   left ear [L. *auris laeva*] (*See also* a.l., AS, a.s.)
   lethal antigen

Al
   allantoic
   allergic
   allergy (*See also* A, alg, ALL)
   aluminum

a.l.
   left ear [L. *auris laeva*] (*See also* AL, AS, a.s.)

ALA
   Activity Loss Assessment
   alpha lactalbumin
   alpha linolenic acid (*See also* LNA)
   alpha lipoic acid
   aminolevulinic acid
   anterior lip of the acetabulum
   antilymphocyte antibody
   axiolabial (*See also* ALa)
   delta-aminolevulinic acid

5-ALA
   5-aminolevulinic acid

ALa
   axiolabial (*See also* ALA)

Ala
   alanine (*See also* A)

AL-Ab
   antilymphocyte antibody

ALAC
   antibiotic-loaded acrylic cement

ALAD
   abnormal left axis deviation
   aminolevulinic acid dehydrase (*See also* ALA-D)

ALA-D
   aminolevulinic acid dehydrase (*See also* ALAD)

ALAG, ALaG
   axiolabiogingival

ALAL, ALaL
   axiolabiolingual

ALA-PDT
   5-aminolevulinic acid photodynamic therapy

ALARA
   as low as reasonably achievable (radiation exposure)

ALARM
   adjustable leg and ankle repositioning mechanism

ALAS
   aminolevulinic acid synthetase

ALAT
   alanine aminotransferase

ALAX
   apical long axis

ALB
   albumin (*See also* A, AL, abl)
   avian lymphoblastosis

alb.
   white [L. *albus*]

ALB/GLOB
   albumin-globulin (ratio) (*See also* A:G, AG)

ALBPSQ
   Acute Low Back Pain Screening Questionnaire

ALC
   absolute lymphocyte count
   acetyl-L-carnitine
   acute lethal catatonia
   alcohol (*See also* alc)
   alcoholic liver cirrhosis
   allogeneic lymphocyte cytotoxicity
   alternate level of care
   Alternative Lifestyle Checklist
   approximate lethal concentration
   avian leukosis complex
   axiolinguocervical

alc
   alcohol (*See also* ALC)
   alcoholic
   alcoholism (*See also* AL)

ALCA
   anomalous left coronary artery

ALCAPA
   anomalous left coronary artery from pulmonary artery
   anomalous origin of left coronary artery from pulmonary artery

ALCEQ
   Adolescent Life Change Event Questionnaire

ALCL
   anaplastic large cell lymphoma

ALCR, AlcR
   alcohol rub

AlCr
   aluminum crown

AL/CR ratio
   axial length/corneal radius ratio

ALD
   adrenoleukodystrophy
   alcoholic liver disease
   aldolase (*See also* Ald)
   aldosterone (*See also* ALDOST)
   anterior latissimus dorsi
   appraisal of language disturbances
   assistive listening device

Ald
    aldolase *(See also* ALD)
ALD-AMN
    adrenoleukodystrophy-
      adrenomyeloneuropathy
ALDH
    aldehyde dehydrogenase
ALDOST
    aldosterone *(See also* ALD)
ALE
    active life expectancy
    allowable limits of error
ALEC
    artificial lung-expanding compound
ALEP
    atypical lymphoepithelioid cell
      proliferation
ALEV
    Alenquer virus
ALF
    acute liver failure
    anterior long fiber
ALFT
    abnormal liver function test
ALG
    Annapolis lymphoblast globulin
    antilymphocyte globulin
    axiolinguogingival
alg
    allergy *(See also* A, Al, ALL)
ALGOL
    algorithm-oriented language
ALH
    angiolymphoid hyperplasia
    anterior lobe hormone
    anterior lobe of hypophysis
    atypical lobular hyperplasia
ALHE
    angiolymphoid hyperplasia with
      eosinophilia
ALI
    acute lung injury
    argon laser iridotomy
A-line
    arterial line *(See also* AL, art. line,
      ART)
ALIP
    abnormal location of immature
      myeloid precursor
ALK, alk
    alkaline
    alkylating (agent)

    automated lamellar keratoplasty
    automated laser keratomileusis
ALK-E
    automated lamellar keratoplasty-
      excimer
ALK-P, alk phos, alk p'tase
    alkaline phosphatase *(See also* AKP,
      ALP, AlPase, AP, KA, P'ase)
ALL
    acute lymphoblastic leukemia
    acute lymphocytic leukemia
    allergic *(See also* Al)
    allergy *(See also* A, Al, alg)
    anterior longitudinal ligament
    antihypertensive and lipid lowering
ALLA
    acute lymphocytic leukemia antigen
ALLD
    arthroscopic lumbar laser
      diskectomy
ALLO
    atypical Legionella-like organism
allo-BMT
    allogeneic bone marrow
      transplantation
allo-HSCT
    allogenic hematopoietic stem cell
      transplantation
ALM
    acral lentiginous melanoma
    alveolar living material
ALMCA
    anomalous left main coronary
      artery
ALME
    acetyl-lysine methyl ester
ALMI
    anterior lateral myocardial infarct
    anterior lateral myocardial infarction
ALMN
    adrenoleukomyeloneuropathy
ALMV
    Almpiwar virus
    anterior leaflet of the mitral valve
ALN
    alendronate
    anterior lymph node
    axillary lymph node
ALND
    axillary lymph node dissection
ALNM
    axillary lymph node metastasis

NOTES

ALO
 Aerococcus-like organism
 average lymphocyte output
 axiolinguoocclusal

Al₂O₃
 aluminum oxide

ALOS
 average length of stay

ALP
 acute leukemia protocol
 acute lupus pericarditis
 acute lupus pneumonitis
 alkaline phosphatase (*See also* AKP,
  ALK-P, alk phos, alk p'tase,
  AlPase, AP, KA, P'ase)
 ankle ligament protector
 anterior lobe of pituitary
 antileukoproteinase
 argon laser photocoagulation

AlPase
 alkaline phosphatase (*See also* AKP,
  ALK-P, alk phos, alk p'tase, ALP,
  AP, KA, P'ase)

α, alpha
 acceleration (*See also* a, acc, accel)
 activity (*See also* activ, act.)
 alpha (first letter of Greek
  alphabet), lowercase
 alpha particle
 Bunsen solubility coefficient
 constituent of alpha protein plasma
  fraction
 first in alpha series or group
 heavy chain of immunoglobulin A
 optical rotation
 probability of type I error
  (statistics)
 specific absorption coefficient

[α]
 specific optical rotation

alpha₂-AP
 alpha₂antiplasmin

alpha-APA
 alpha-anilinophenyl-acetamide

alpha₁-AT
 alpha₁-antitrypsin
 alpha₁-proteinase inhibitor

alpha₂β₁
 alpha-2-beta-1 integrin cell-surface
  collagen

alpha-BSM
 alpha bone substitute material

alpha-cat
 alpha-catenin

alpha-GLUC
 alpha-glucosidase

alpha-GST
 alpha-glutathione S-transferase

alpha-HCD
 alpha-heavy-chain disease

alpha-hCG
 alpha-human chorionic gonadotropin

3-alpha-HSD
 3-alpha-hydroxysteroid
  dehydrogenase

alpha-IFN
 alpha-interferon

alpha-KG
 alpha-ketoglutarate

alpha-KIC
 alpha-ketoisocaproic acid

alpha-LP
 alpha-lipoprotein

alpha₂M
 alpha₂-macroglobulin

alpha-MHC
 alpha-myosin heavy chain

alpha-MSH
 alpha-melanocyte-stimulating
  hormone

alpha-NREM
 alpha-nonrapid eye movement

1-alpha-OHase
 25-hydroxy-vitamin D 1α-
  hydroxylase

alpha₁PI
 alpha₁-protease inhibitor
 human α₁-proteinase inhibitor

5-alpha-R
 5-alpha-reductase

alpha-T
 alpha-tocopherol

ALPI
 alkaline phosphatase isoenzymes
 argon laser peripheral iridoplasty

ALPP
 abdominal leak-point pressure

AL protein
 immunoglobulin light chain-origin
  amyloid deposit

ALPS
 alcoholism, leukopenia,
  pneumococcal sepsis
 anterior locking plate system
 Aphasia Language Performance
  Scale
 autoimmune lymphoproliferative
  syndrome
 autologous leukapheresis, processing,
  and storage (container)

ALPSA
 anterior labroligamentous periosteal
  sleeve avulsion
 anterior labrum periosteal sleeve
  avulsion

ALPZ
  alprazolam
ALRI
  acute lower respiratory infection
  anterolateral rotational instability
ALRTI
  acute lower respiratory tract
    infection
ALS
  acid-labile subunit
  advanced life support
  afferent loop syndrome
  amyotrophic lateral sclerosis
  androgen insensitivity syndrome
  angiotensin-like substance
  anterolateral sclerosis
  anticipated lifespan
  antilymphocyte serum
  antiviral lymphocyte serum
  atypical lichenoid stomatitis
ALSD
  Alzheimer-like senile dementia
ALS-PD
  amyotrophic lateral sclerosis-
    parkinsonism dementia (complex)
ALT
  alanine aminotransferase
  alanine transaminase
  anterolateral tract
  argon laser trabeculoplasty (*See also*
    ALTP)
  avian laryngotracheitis
alt
  alternate
  altitude
ALT/AST
  ratio of serum alanine
    aminotransferase to serum
    aspartate aminotransferase
ALTB
  acute laryngotracheobronchitis
ALTE
  apparent life-threatening event
ALTEE
  acetyl-L-tyrosine ethyl ester
ALTP
  argon laser trabeculoplasty (*See also*
    ALT)
ALT-RCC
  autolymphocyte-based treatment for
    renal cell carcinoma

ALTS
  acute lumbar trauma syndrome
ALTV
  Altamira virus
ALU
  arithmetic and logic unit
ALV
  Abelson leukemia virus
  adeno-like virus
  ascending lumbar vein
  avian leukosis virus
alv
  alveolar
  alveolus
ALVAD
  abdominal left ventricular assist
    device
ALVM
  alveolar mucosa
ALVT
  aortic and left ventricular tunnel
alv vent
  alveolar ventilation (*See also* $\mathring{V}_A$)
alvx
  alveolectomy
ALW
  arch-loop-whorl (system)
ALX40-4C
  N-alpha-acetyl-nona-D-argine amide
A-LYM
  atypical lymphocyte
AM
  acrylamide
  actomyosin
  acute myelofibrosis
  adrenomedullin
  adult male
  adult monocyte
  aerospace medicine
  alternative medicine
  alveolar macrophage
  alveolar mucosa
  amacrine cell
  amalgam (*See also* AMAL)
  ambulatory (*See also* A, AMB,
    amb, ambul)
  amethopterin
  ametropia (*See also* am.)
  ammeter
  amperemeter
  ampicillin (*See also* A, AMP)

NOTES

AM (*continued*)
 amplitude modulation (*See also* A-mode)
 anovular menstruation
 anterior midpapillary
 anteromeatal
 arithmetic mean
 arousal mechanism
 arterial malformation
 arterial mean
 articulation manipulation
 atrial myxoma
 Austin Moore (prosthesis)
 aviation medicine (*See also* AV, AVM)
 axiomesial
 before noon [L. *ante meridiem*] (*See also* a.m.)
 meter angle
 mixed astigmatism
 myopic astigmatism (*See also* ASM, AsM, am.)

A/m
 amperes per meter

Am
 americium
 amnion
 amyl

^{241}Am
 americium-241

A-m^2
 ampere-square meter

a-2M
 a-2 macroglobulin

a.m.
 before noon [L. *ante meridiem*] (*See also* AM)

am
 ammeter

am.
 ametropia (*See also* AM)
 amplitude
 meter angle
 myopic astigmatism (*See also* ASM, AsM, AM)

AMA
 actual mechanical advantage
 against medical advice
 antimitochondrial antibody
 antimyosin antibody
 antithyroid microsomal antibody
 augmentation of mandibular angle
 autoregressive moving average

AMAC
 adults molested as children

AMAD
 Assessment Measure for Atopic Dermatitis
 morning admission

AMA-Fab
 antimyosin monoclonal antibody with Fab fragment

AMAG
 adrenal medullary autograft
 autoimmune metaplastic atrophic gastritis

AMAL
 amalgam (*See also* AM)

AMAN
 acute motor-axonal neuropathy

AMAP
 as much as possible

AMAT
 antimalignant antibody test

A-MAT
 amorphous material

AMAV
 Amapari virus

AMB
 ambulate (*See also* amb, ambul)
 ambulatory (*See also* A, AM, amb, ambul)
 amphotericin B (*See also* AmB)
 anomalous muscle bundle
 avian myeloblastosis

AmB
 amphotericin B (*See also* AMB)

amb
 ambient
 ambiguous (*See also* ambig)
 ambulance
 ambulate (*See also* AMB, ambul)
 ambulatory (*See also* A, AM, AMB, ambul)

AmBd
 amphotericin B deoxycholate

AMBER
 advanced multiple-beam equalization radiography

AMBI
 acute multiple brain infarcts

ambig
 ambiguous (*See also* amb)

AmB-induced reduction GFR
 amphotericin B-induced reduction glomerular filtration rate

AMBL
 acute myeloblastic leukemia (*See also* AML)

AMBRI
 atraumatic, multidirectional, bilateral rehabilitation inferior

ambul
> ambulate (*See also* AMB, amb)
> ambulation
> ambulatory (*See also* A, AM, AMB, amb)

AMBV
> Anhembi virus

AMC
> antibody-mediated cytotoxicity
> antimalaria campaign
> arm muscle circumference
> arthrogryposis multiplex congenita
> ataxia-microcephaly-cataract
> automated mixture control
> automatic mode conversion
> axiomesiocervical

AMCHA
> aminomethylcyclohexane-carboxylic acid

AMCN
> anteromedial caudate nucleus

AM/CR
> amylase to creatinine ratio

AMD
> acid maltase deficiency
> acromandibular dysplasia
> adrenomyelodystrophy
> age-related macular degeneration
> Aleutian mink disease (*See also* AD)
> alpha-methyldopa
> arthroscopic microdiskectomy
> articular motion device
> axiomesiodistal

AME
> apparent mineralocorticoid excess (syndrome)
> aseptic meningoencephalitis
> Austin Medical Equipment

AMEAE
> acute monophasic experimental autoimmune encephalomyelitis

AMEGL, AMegL
> acute megakaryoblastic leukemia

AMERIND
> American Indian Sign Language

AMES
> age, (distant) metastases, extent and size

Ameslan
> American Sign Language (*See also* ASL)

AMet
> adenosyl-l-methionine

AMF
> antimuscle factor
> autocrine motility factor

AMFH
> angiomatoid malignant fibrous histiocytoma

AM/FM
> alopecia mucinosa/follicular mucinosis

AMFR
> autocrine motility factor receptor

AMG
> acoustic myography
> aminoglycoside
> amyloglucosidase
> antimacrophage globulin
> autometallography
> axiomesiogingival

A₂MG
> alpha₂-macroglobulin

AMH
> antimüllerian hormone
> automated medical history

Amh
> mixed astigmatism with myopia predominating

AMHT
> automated multiphasic health testing

AMI
> acquired monosaccharide intolerance
> acute myocardial infarction
> amitriptyline
> anterior myocardial infarct
> anterior myocardial infarction
> antibody-mediated immunity
> Athletic Motivation Inventory
> axiomesioincisal

AMIS
> antibody-mediated immune suppression

AMK
> anatomic modular knee

AMKL
> acute megakaryoblastic leukemia

AML
> acute monoblastic leukemia
> acute monocytic leukemia (*See also* AMOL, mLa)
> acute mucosal lesion

NOTES

AML *(continued)*
    acute myeloblastic leukemia (*See also* AMBL)
    acute myelocytic leukemia
    acute myelogenous leukemia
    acute myeloid leukemia
    anatomic medullary locking
    angiomyolipoma
    anterior mitral leaflet
    automated multitest laboratory

AMLA
    antimyolemmal antibody

AMLB
    alternate monaural loudness balance (test)

AMLC
    adherent macrophage-like cell
    autologous mixed lymphocyte culture

AMLR
    auditory middle-latency response
    autologous mixed lymphocyte reaction

AMLS
    antimouse lymphocyte serum

AMLV-RT
    avian myeloblastosis leukemia virus reverse transcriptase

AMM
    agnogenic myeloid metaplasia
    ammonia (*See also* amm, ammon.)
    antibody to murine cardiac myosin

amm
    ammonia (*See also* AMM, ammon.)

AMML, AMMOL, AMMoL
    acute myelomonoblastic leukemia
    acute myelomonocytic leukemia

ammon.
    ammonia (*See also* AMM, amm)

AMN
    acquired melanocytic nevus
    adrenomyeloneuropathy
    alloxazine mononucleotide
    anterior median nucleus
    atypical melanocytic nevus

amnio
    amniocentesis

AMN SC
    amniotic fluid scan

AMO
    Allergan Medical Optics
    axiomesioocclusal

A-mode
    amplitude mode
    amplitude modulation (*See also* AM)

AMOL
    acute monoblastic leukemia

    acute monocytic leukemia (*See also* AML, mLa)

AMOR, amor, AMORP, amorp
    amorphous (sediment)

AMP
    accelerated mental processes
    acid mucopolysaccharide
    adenosine 5′-monophosphate
    adenosine monophosphate (adenylic acid)
    amphetamine
    ampicillin (*See also* A, AM)
    amprenavir
    ampule (*See also* ampul.)
    amputation
    assisted medical procreation
    average mean pressure

amp
    amplification
    amputee

AMPA
    α-amino-3-hydroxy-5-methylisoxazole-4-propionic acid

AMP-c
    cyclic adenosine monophosphate (*See also* cAMP)

AMPD1
    adenosine monophosphate deaminase 1

AMPH
    amphetamine

amph
    amphoric (respiratory sound)

amp-hr
    ampere-hour

AMP-HSA
    ampicillin-human serum albumin

AMPK
    AMP-activated protein kinase

AMPPE
    acute multifocal placoid pigment epitheliopathy

AMPPPE
    acute multifocal posterior placoid pigment epitheliopathy

A-M pr
    Austin Moore prosthesis

AMPS
    acid mucopolysaccharide

AMP-S
    adenylosuccinic acid

AMPT
    alpha-methyl-para-tyrosine
    alpha-methyl-*p*-tyrosine

ampul.
    ampule [L. *ampulla*] (*See also* AMP)

AMR
abnormal muscle response
acoustic muscle reflex
activity metabolic rate
alopecia mental retardation
(syndrome)
alternating motion rate

AMRI
anteromedial rotatory instability

AMRO
Amsterdam Rotterdam

AMRS
automated medical record system

AMRV
Almeirim virus

AMS
ablepharon macrostomia syndrome
accelerator mass spectrometry
Access Management Survey
acute mountain sickness
aggravated in military service
altered mental status
amylase
antimacrophage serum
antimigration system
aseptic meningitis syndrome
atypical measles syndrome
auditory memory span
automated multiphasic screening
automatic mode switching

AMSA
amsacrine
anterior middle superior alveolar

AMSAN
acute motor-sensory axonal
neuropathy

AMSIT
appearance, mood, sensorium,
intelligence, and thought process
(portion of mental status
examination)

AMT
active motion testing
acute miliary tuberculosis
air medical transportation
amethopterin
alpha-methyltyrosine
3'-amino-3'-deoxythymidine
amitriptyline
amphetamine
Anxiety Management Training

amt
amount

AMTDT
amplified *Mycobacterium tuberculosis* direct test

AMTP
alpha-methyltryptophan

AMTR
anteromedial temporal lobe
resection

AMTV
Arumowot virus

amu
atomic mass unit

AMuLV
Abelson murine leukemia virus
amphotropic murine leukemia virus

AMV
alveolar minute ventilation
assisted mechanical ventilation
avian myeloblastosis virus

AMV2
avian myelocytomatosis virus

AMVI
acute mesenteric vascular
insufficiency

aMVL
anterior mitral valve leaflet

AMX
amoxicillin

AMX/CL
amoxicillin/clavulanate

AMY
amylase

AMY-SP
amylase urine spot (test)

AN
acanthosis nigricans
acne neonatorum
acoustic neuroma
adult, normal
aminonucleoside
amyl nitrate
anesthesia (*See also* A, AA, ANA,
anes, anesth)
aneurysm
anisometropia (*See also* An)
anodal (*See also* An)
anode (*See also* A, a, An)
anorexia nervosa
antenatal
anterior (*See also* A, a, ANT, ant.)

NOTES

AN *(continued)*
> antineuraminidase
> aseptic necrosis
> atrionodal
> autonomic neuropathy
> avascular necrosis

A/N
> artery and/or nerve
> as needed

A$_n$
> normal atmosphere

An
> actinon
> anatomic
> anatomy response
> aniridia
> anisometropia (*See also* AN)
> anodal (*See also* AN)
> anode (*See also* A, a, AN)

ANA
> acetylneuraminic acid
> anesthesia (*See also* A, AA, AN, anes, anesth)
> anesthetic (*See also* anes, anesth)
> antinuclear antibody (*See also* ANuA)
> articular/nonarticular
> aspartyl naphthylamide

ANAD
> anorexia nervosa and associated disorders

ANA-FL
> antinuclear antibody fluid

ANAG
> acute narrow angle glaucoma

anal.
> analgesia
> analgesic
> analysis
> analyst
> analytic

ANAP
> agglutination negative, absorption positive (reaction)
> anionic neutrophil-activating peptide

ANAS, anast
> anastomosis

anat
> anatomical
> anatomist
> anatomy

ANB
> avascular necrosis of bone

ANC
> absolute neutrophil count
> acid neutralization capacity
> acid-neutralizing capacity

ANCA
> antineutrophil cytoplasmic antibody
> antineutrophil cytoplasmic autoantibody
> antineutrophilic cytoplasmic antibody

ANCA-SVV
> antineutrophilic cytoplasmic autoantibody-small vessel vasculitis

AnCC
> anodal closure contraction (*See also* ACC)

anch
> anchored

ANCOVA
> analysis of covariance

AND
> administratively necessary days
> algoneurodystrophy
> anterior nasal discharge

and.
> androgen

ANDA
> Abbreviated New Drug Application

andro, andros
> androsterone

ANDTE, AnDTe
> anodal duration tetanus

ANDV
> Andasibe virus

anes, anesth
> anesthesia (*See also* A, AA, AN, ANA)
> anesthesiology
> anesthetic (*See also* ANA)

ANESR
> apparent norepinephrine secretion rate

AnEx, an ex
> anodal excitation

ANF
> alpha-naphthoflavone
> antineuritic factor
> antinuclear factor
> atrial natriuretic factor

ANG
> angiogenin
> angiogram (*See also* ang)
> angiography (*See also* ang)
> angiotensin

Ang-2
> angiopoietin-2

ang
> angiogram (*See also* ANG)
> angiography (*See also* ANG)
> angle (*See also* A)
> angular

ANGEL
angiolipoma, (posttraumatic) neuroma, glomus (tumor), eccrine (spiradenoma), and leiomyoma (cutis)

Ang GR
angiotensin generation rate

ang pect
angina pectoris

ANH
acute normovolemic hemodilution
artificial nutrition and hydration
atrial natriuretic hormone

anh
anhydrous

ANHV
Anhanga virus

ANI
acute nerve irritation
autoimmune neutropenia of infancy

ANIS, ANISO
anisocytosis
Anorexia Nervosa Inventory for Self-Rating

ANIT
alpha-naphthyl-isothiocyanate

ank
ankle

ANKENT
ankylosis and ankylosing enthesopathy

ANLL
acute nonlymphoblastic leukemia
acute nonlymphocytic leukemia
acute nonlymphoid leukemia

ANM
auxiliary nurse midwife

ANN
alloimmune neonatal neutropenia
artificial neural network
axillary node negative

ann.
annual

ANNA
antineuronal nuclear antibody

ann fib
annulus fibrosus

annot.
annotation

ANoA
antinucleolar antibody

AnOC
anodal opening contraction (*See also* AOC)

ANOTHER
alopecia, nail (dystrophy), ophthalmic (complication), thyroid (dysfunction), hypohidrosis, ephelides, enteropathy, respiratory (tract infection)

ANOVA
analysis of variance

ANP
acute necrotizing pancreatitis
A-norprogesterone
atrial natriuretic peptide
atrial natriuretic polypeptide
autonomic nerve preservation
axillary node positive

A-NPP
absorbed normal pooled plasma

ANQ
Adult Neuropsychological Questionnaire

ANRBC
absolute nucleated red blood cell

ANRL
antihypertensive neural renomedullary lipids

ANS
acanthion
antenatal corticosteroid treatment
anterior nasal spine
antineutrophilic serum
autonomic nervous system

ANSD
autonomic nervous system dysfunction

ANT
acoustic noise test
adenosine nucleotide translocator
aminoglycoside2′-0-nucleotidyltransferase
aminonitrothiazole
anterior (*See also* A, a, AN, ant.)
antimycin (*See also* ant.)

ant.
anterior (*See also* A, a, AN, ANT)
antimycin (*See also* ANT)

antag
antagonist

ant ax line
anterior axillary line

NOTES

ante
>before [L. *ante*] (*See also* bef, a., ā)

anti.
>antidote

ANTI A:AGT
>anti-blood group A antiglobulin test

anti-BrDU, anti-BrDu
>anti-bromodeoxyuridine

anti-BSA
>antibovine serum albumin

anti bx
>antibiotic (*See also* ATB, AB, ABx)

anti-c100
>antibody to c100

anti-CEA
>anticarcinoembryonic antigen

anti-CMV
>anticytomegalovirus

anticoag
>anticoagulant

anti-CP9
>antibody to core peptide 9

anti-CP10
>antibody to core peptide 10

anti-DNA
>anti-deoxyribonucleic acid

anti-DNase B
>antideoxyribonuclease B (*See also* ADN-B, ADNase-B)

anti-dsDNA
>anti-double-stranded deoxyribonucleic acid

anti-E2
>envelope 2 antigen

anti-EBV
>anti-Epstein-Barr virus

anti-EMA
>antiendomysial antibody

anti-ENA
>antiextractable nuclear antibody

anti-GAD
>antiglutamic acid decarboxylase

anti-GBM, anti-GMB
>antiglomerular basement membrane

anti-GOR
>antibody to GOR

anti-HA
>antihepatitis antigen

anti-HAA
>antibody to hepatitis-associated antigen

anti-HAV
>antibody to hepatitis A virus

anti-HB$_c$, anti-HB$_s$, anti-HBc, anti-HBs
>antibody to hepatitis B core antigen
>hepatitis B surface antibody

anti-HCV
>antibody to hepatitis C virus

anti-HDV
>antibody to hepatitis D virus

anti-HEV
>antibody to hepatitis E virus

anti-HTLV-I
>antibody to human T-lymphoctropic virus type I

anti-IgE
>antiimmunoglobulin E

anti-IL-2R Ab
>antiinterleukin-2 antibody

anti-log
>antilogarithm

anti-MPO
>antimyeloperoxidase

anti-MPO Ab
>antimyeloperoxidase antibody

anti-NADase
>antinicotinamide adenine dinucleotidase

anti-PCAM
>antiplatelet endothelial cell adhesion molecule

anti-PCNA
>antiproliferating cell nuclear antigen

anti-PNM Ab
>anti-peripheral nerve myelin antibody

anti-RNP
>antiribonucleoprotein

anti-RSV
>antirespiratory syncytial virus

anti-S
>anti-sulfanilic acid

anti-Scl-70
>antiscleroderma-70 antibody
>antitopoisomerase-1

anti-Sm
>anti-Smith (antibody)

anti-SMA
>antismooth muscle actin

anti-SM/RNP
>antibody-smooth muscle/ribonucleoprotein

anti-Tac
>humanized anti-human IL-2 receptor antibody

anti-Tg
>antithyroglobulin

anti-TPO
>antithyroperoxidase

anti-TSH
antithyroid-stimulating hormone
anti-vWF
anti-von Willebrand factor
ANTR
apparent net transfer rate
ant. sag D
anterior sagittal diameter
ant. sup. spine
anterior-superior spine
ANTU
α-naphthylthiourea
ANTV
Antequera virus
ANuA
antinuclear antibody (See also ANA)
ANUG
acute necrotizing ulcerative gingivitis
ANUV
Ananindeua virus
ANX, anx
anxiety
anxious
anx neur
anxiety neurosis
anx react
anxiety reaction
A-O
acoustic-optic
atlantooccipital (joint)
AO
abdominal aorta
academic orientation
achievement orientation
acid output
acridine orange (dye or test)
airway obstruction
American Optical
ankle orthosis
anodal opening
anterior oblique
aorta (See also Ao)
aortic opening
arthroophthalmopathy
ascending aorta (See also Asc-A, AA, ASCAo)
atlantooccipital
atomic orbital
atrioventricular valve opening
auriculoventricular valve opening

average optical density
avoidance of others
axioocclusal
A&O
alert and oriented
A/O
analog to digital
Ao
aorta (See also AO)
AOA
abnormal oxygen affinity
average orifice area
AOAA
aminooxyacetic acid
AO:AC
aortic valve opening to aortic valve closing ratio
AOA-MCA
alternative occipital artery middle cerebral artery
AOAP
as often as possible
AOB
accessory olfactory bulb
alcohol on breath
AoBP
aortic blood pressure
AOBS
acute organic brain syndrome
AOC
abridged ocular chart
advanced ovarian cancer
amyloxycarbonyl
anodal opening contraction (See also AnOC)
antacid of choice
aortic opening click
area of concern
AOCD
anemia of chronic disease
AOCl
anodal opening clonus
AOCLD
acute on chronic liver disease
AOD
adult-onset diabetes mellitus (See also AODM)
alcohol and other drugs
alleged onset date
arterial occlusive disease
arterial oxygen desaturation
auriculoosteodysplasia

NOTES

AODA
alcohol and other drug abuse

AODM
adult-onset diabetes mellitus (*See also* AOD)

AODP
alcohol and other drug problems

AODT
Animal and Opposite Drawing Technique

AoG
androsterone glucuronide

ao-il
aorta-iliac

AOIVM
angiographically occult intracranial vascular malformation

AOL
acroosteolysis
anterior oblique ligament

AOM
acute otitis media
alternatives of management
ambulatory oximetry monitoring
azoxymethane

AoMP
aortic mean pressure

AOP
aminooxypentane
anodal opening picture
aortic pressure
apnea of prematurity

AoP
left ventricle to aorta pressure gradient

AOPP
advanced oxidation protein product

AOP-RANTES
aminooxypentane regulated-on-activation normal T-expressed and secreted

AoPW
aortic posterior wall

AOR
auditory oculogyric reflex

aor regurg
aortic regurgitation (*See also* AR)

aort sten
aortic stenosis (*See also* AS, A sten)

AOS
acridine orange staining
anodal opening sound
anterior oesophageal sensor
aortic ostial stenosis

AOSC
acute obstructive suppurative cholangitis

AOSD
adult-onset Still disease

AOT
accessory optic tract
adenomatoid odontogenic tumor
antiovotransferrin

AOTe
anodal opening tetanus

AOU
amount of use
apparent oxygen utilization

AOV
aortic valve

AOVM
angiographically occult vascular malformation

A&Ox3
alert and oriented to person, place, and time

A&Ox4
alert and oriented to person, place, time, and date

AOZ
anterior optical zone

A-P
abdominoperineal (resection) (*See also* AP)
analytic-psychologic
anterior-posterior

AP
abdominoperineal (resection) (*See also* A-P)
accelerated phase
accessory pathway
acid phosphatase (*See also* ACP, AcP, AC-PH, ac phos)
acinar parenchyma
action potential
activator protein
active pepsin
acute pancreatitis
acute phase
acute pneumonia
acute proliferative
adductor pollicis
adenomatous polyp
adenomatous polyposis
adolescent psychiatry
aerosol pentamidine
after parturition
alkaline phosphatase (*See also* AKP, ALK-P, alk phos, alk p'tase, ALP, KA, P'ase)
alum-precipitated (vaccine)
alveolar permeability
aminopeptidase
aminopyrine
anatomic profile

A

angina pectoris
antepartum [L. *ante partum*]
anterior pituitary
anterior and posterior
anteroposterior
antidromic potential
antiparkinsonian (*See also* APK)
antiplasmin
antipyrine
antral peristalsis
aortic pressure
aortic pulmonary
apical pulse
apothecary (*See also* ap, apoth)
appendectomy (*See also* appy)
appendiceal perforation
appendicitis
appendix
area postrema
arithmetic progression
arterial pressure
artificial pneumothorax
aspiration pneumonitis
assessment and plan (*See also* A&P)
assessment and planning
association period
atherosclerotic plaque
atrial pacing
atrioventricular pathway
atrium pace
attending physician
axiopulpal
pokeweed antiviral protein

AP1
activator protein 1

A₂P₂

A_2P_2
aortic second sound, pulmonary second sound

$A_2 < P_2$
second aortic sound less than second pulmonic sound

$A_2 = P_2$
second aortic sound equals second pulmonic sound

$A_2 > P_2$
second aortic sound greater than second pulmonic sound

3-AP
3-acetylpyridine (nicotinic antagonist)

4-AP
4-aminopyridine

8AP
eighth nerve action potential

A/P
ascites-plasma (ratio)

A&P
abdominal and perineal
active and present
anatomy and physiology
anterior and posterior
assessment and plan (*See also* AP)
auscultation and palpation
auscultation and percussion

Ap
apex

ap
apothecary (*See also* apoth, AP)

a.p.
prior to [L. *a priori*]

APA
air pollution adaptation
aldosterone-producing adenoma
aminopenicillanic acid
antiparietal antibody
antipernicious anemia (factor)
antiphospholipid antibody
atypical polypoid adenomyoma

6-APA
6-aminopenicillanic acid

APAA
anterior parietal artery aneurysm

APAAP
alkaline phosphatase antialkaline phosphatase

APAB
antiphospholipid antibody

APACG
acute primary angle-closure glaucoma

APACHE
Acute Physiology and Chronic Health Evaluation (score, system)

APACHE II
Acute Physiology and Chronic Health Evaluation II

APAD
anterior-posterior abdominal diameter

APAF
antipernicious anemia factor

NOTES

43

APA-LMP
> atypical polypoid adenomyofibroma of low malignant potential

APAP
> auto-titrating continuous positive airway pressure

APAS
> annular phased array system

APAT
> Accounting Program Admission Test

APB
> abductor pollicis brevis (muscle)
> atrial premature beat
> auricular premature beat

A.P.B.
> All-Purpose Boot

APBD
> anomalous pancreaticobiliary duct

APBDJ
> anomalous pancreaticobiliary duct junction

APBDU
> anomalous pancreaticobiliary ductal union

APBF
> accessory pulmonary blood flow

APBSCT
> autologous peripheral blood stem cell transplantation

APBU
> anomalous pancreaticobiliary union

APC
> absolute phagocyte count
> absolute plasma concentration
> acetylsalicylic acid, phenacetin, and caffeine
> activated protein C
> acute pharyngoconjunctival (fever)
> adenoidal-pharyngeal-conjunctival (agent or virus)
> adenomatous polyposis coli
> all-purpose capsule
> alternative patterns of complement
> ambulatory payment classification group
> anterior-posterior compression
> antigen-presenting cell
> antiphlogistic corticoid
> aperture current
> apneustic center (of brain)
> argon plasma coagulation
> argon plasma coagulator
> aspirin-phenacetin-caffeine
> atrial premature complex
> atrial premature contraction

APCA
> antiparietal cell antibody

APCC, APC-C
> aspirin-phenacetin-caffeine-codeine

APCD
> acquired prothrombin complex deficiency (syndrome)
> adult polycystic kidney disease (See also APKD)

APCF
> acute pharyngoconjunctival fever

APCKD
> adult-type polycystic kidney disease

APCR
> activated protein C resistance

APD
> acquired perforating dermatosis
> action potential duration
> acute polycystic disease
> adult polycystic disease
> afferent pupillary defect
> airway pressure disconnect
> anteroposterior diameter (See also A-PD)
> antipsychotic drug
> atrial premature depolarization
> auditory processing disorder
> autoimmune progesterone dermatitis
> automated percutaneous diskectomy
> automated peritoneal dialysis

A-PD (See also APD)
> anteroposterior diameter (See also APD)

APDC
> anxiety and panic disorder clinic

APDCC
> antropyloroduodenal common chamber

APDER
> anterior-posterior dual energy radiography

APDI
> Adult Personal Data Inventory

APDT
> acellular pertussis vaccine with diphtheria and tetanus toxoid

APE
> acetone powder extract
> acute polioencephalitis
> acute psychotic episode
> acute pulmonary edema
> Advanced Placement Examination
> airway pressure excursion
> aminophylline, phenobarbital, and ephedrine
> anterior pituitary extract
> asthma of physical effort
> avian pneumoencephalitis

APEC
asymmetric periflexural exanthem of childhood

APECED
autoimmune polyendocrinopathy, candidiasis, ectodermal dysplasia
autoimmune polyendocrinopathy, candidiasis, ectodermal dystrophy

APELL
Assessment Program of Early Learning Levels

ApEn
approximate entropy

APERP
accessory pathway effective refractory period

APEUV
Apeu virus

APF
acidulated phosphofluoride
anabolism-promoting factor
animal protein factor
antiperinuclear factor

APG
acid-precipitated globulin
ambulatory patient group
animal pituitary gonadotropin
Apgar (score)

APGAR
adaptability, partnership, growth, affection, and resolve (family screening, not Apgar score of newborn physical status)
American Pediatric Gross Assessment Record

APGL
alkaline phosphatase activity of granular leukocytes

APGN
acute postinfectious glomerulonephritis

APH
adult psychiatric hospital
alcohol-positive history
antepartum hemorrhage
anterior pituitary hormone

aph
aphasia

AP/HC
accreditation program/hospice care

AP/HHC
accreditation program/home health care

APHLT
auxiliary partial heterotopic liver transplantation

APHP
anti-*Pseudomonas* human plasma

APHSCS
autologous peripheral hematopoietic stem cell support

API
Activity Pattern Indicator
Adult Personality Inventory
alkaline protease inhibitor
analytical profile index
ankle-arm pressure index
arterial pressure index
Autonomy Preference Index

A1PI
alpha-1 proteinase inhibitor

APIB
Assessment of Preterm Infants Behavior

APIE
assessment plan, implementation, and evaluation

APIP
additional personal injury protection

APIVR
artificial pacemaker-induced ventricular rhythm

APK
antiparkinsonian (*See also* AP)

APKD
adult polycystic kidney disease (*See also* APCD)

APKG
acute primary keratotic gingivostomatitis

APL
abductor pollicis longus (muscle)
accelerated painless labor
acquired progressive lymphangioma
acute promyelocytic leukemia (*See also* FAB M3, APro L)
animal placenta lactogen
anterior pituitary-like (hormone)
antiphospholipid

AP&L, AP&Lat
anteroposterior and lateral (radiologic view)

NOTES

45

aPL, APLA
antiphospholipid antibody
APLD
adult polycystic liver disease
automated percutaneous lumbar
diskectomy
APLS
Adult Performance Level Survey
advanced pediatric life support
aPLS
antiphospholipid antibody syndrome
AP/LTC
accreditation program/long-term care
APM
acid-precipitable material
alternating pressure mattress
anterior papillary muscle
anterior and posterior medialization
anteroposterior movement
aspartame
APMET
aggressive papillary middle ear
tumor
APMPPE
acute posterior multifocal placoid
pigment epitheliopathy
APN
acute pyelonephritis
average peak noise
APO
adductor pollicis obliquus (muscle)
adverse patient occurrences
airway peroxidase
aphoxide (See also TEPA)
apomorphine
apoprotein
apo
apoenzyme
apolipoprotein
apo AI
apolipoprotein AI
apo B
apolipoprotein B
apobec-1
apo B mRNA-editing catalytic
polypeptide-1
apo C
apolipoprotein C
ApoDCIS
apocrine ductal carcinoma in situ
Apo E
apolipoprotein E
Apo E4
apolipoprotein E epsilon 4
ApoHyp
apocrine hyperplasia
APOIV
Apoi virus

APOLT
auxiliary partial orthotopic liver
transplant
auxiliary partial orthotopic liver
transplantation
APOPPS
adjustable postoperative protective
prosthetic socket
APORF
acute postoperative renal failure
apoth
apothecary (See also ap, AP)
APP
acute-phase protein
addiction-prone personality
Advanced Placement Program
alum-precipitated pyridine
aminopyrazolopyrimidine
amyloid precursor protein
antiplatelet plasma
appendix (See also app, appx)
aqueous procaine penicillin
automated physiologic profile
average pixel projection
avian pancreatic polypeptide
app
appendix (See also APP, appx)
applied
approximate (See also appr, approx)
AP/PA
anteroposterior/posteroanterior
appar
apparatus
apparent
AP-PCR
arbitrary-primed polymerase chain
reaction
APPG
aorticopulmonary paraganglioma
aqueous procaine penicillin G
appl
appliance
applicable
application
applied
applan.
flattened [L. applanatus]
APPM
antegrade perfusion pressure
measurement
appoint.
appointment (See also appt)
appr, approx
approximate (See also app)
approximately
approximation
APPT
Adolescent and Pediatric Pain Tool

appt
appointment (*See also* appoint.)
appx
appendix (*See also* APP, app)
appy
appendectomy (*See also* AP)
APQ
average perturbation quotient
APR
abdominoperineal resection
absolute proximal reabsorption
accelerator-produced
  radiopharmaceuticals
acute phase reactant
acute phase reaction
acute phase response
amebic prevalence rate
anatomic porous replacement
anterior pituitary resection
auropalpebral reflex
aprax
apraxia
APRE
acute phase response element
APRIL
A proliferation-inducing ligand
APRO
aprobarbital
AProL
acute progranulocytic leukemia
acute promyelocytic leukemia (*See
  also* APL, FAB M3)
APRP
acidic proline-rich protein
acute-phase reactant protein
APRT
abdominopelvic radiotherapy
adenine phosphoribosyltransferase
APRV
airway pressure release ventilation
APS
acute physiology score
adenosine phosphosulfate
adenosine 5'-phosphosulfate
Adult Protective Services
Adult Psychiatric Service
air plasma spray
air pollution syndrome
anterior pararenal space
anterior plate system
antiphospholipid antibody syndrome
antiphospholipid syndrome

arterioportal vein shunting
attending physician's statement
autoimmune polyglandular syndrome
automated patient system
APS-1
autoimmune polyglandular syndrome
  type 1
6-APS
6-aminopenicillanic acid
APSAC
anisoylated plasminogen
  streptokinase activator complex
APSD
Alzheimer presenile dementia
aorticopulmonary septal defect
aortopulmonary septal defect
APSGN
acute poststreptococcal
  glomerulonephritis
APSQ
Abbreviated Parent Symptom
  Questionnaire
APSR
acute paranoid schizophrenic
  reaction
APT
Age Projection Test
alum-precipitated toxoid
antiplatelet trial
atopy patch test
automatic peak tracking
AP-T
apical transverse
APTA
aneurysm of persistent trigeminal
  artery
APTC
anteroposterior talocalcaneal angle
APTD
Aid to Permanently and Totally
  Disabled
APTT, aPTT
activated partial thromboplastin time
APTX
acute parathyroidectomy
APUD
amine precursor uptake and
  decarboxylation (cell)
APV
amprenavir
ANCA-positive vasculitis
average peak velocity

NOTES

APVC
anomalous pulmonary venous connection

APVD
anomalous pulmonary venous drainage

APVR
anomalous pulmonary venous return

APW
aortopulmonary window

AQ
accomplishment quotient
achievement quotient
acoustic quantification
any quantity
aphasia quotient

aq.
aqueous (*See also* aqu)
water [L. *aqua*] (*See also* A, a)

AQLQ
Asthma Quality of Life Questionnaire

AQP
aquaporin

AQP2
aquaporin-2

AQS
additional qualifying symptoms

aqu
aqueous (*See also* aq.)

A-R
apical-radial (pulse) (*See also* AR, A/R)

AR
abnormal record
achievement ratio
Achilles reflex
acoustic reflex
acoustic rhinometry
actinic reticuloid (syndrome)
active resistance
acute rejection
adherence ratio
admitting room
adrenergic receptor
airway resistance (*See also* R_A, RAW, R_{AW}, R (AW))
alarm reaction
alcohol related
aldose reductase
allergic rhinitis
alloy restoration
amphiregulin
amplitude ratio
analytical reagent
androgen receptor
ankle reflex
anterior root
aortic regurgitation (*See also* aor regurg)
apical-radial (pulse) (*See also* A-R, A/R)
Argyll Robertson (pupil)
arsphenamine (*See also* Ars, ARS)
articulare (craniometric point) (*See also* Ar)
artificially ruptured
artificial respiration
assisted respiration
atrial rate
atrial regurgitation
at risk
atrophic rhinitis
attack rate
aural rehabilitation
autoradiography
autorefraction
autorefractor
autosomal recessive

A/R
accounts receivable
apical/radial (pulse) (*See also* AR, A-R)

A&R
adenoidectomy with radium
advised and released

Ar
argon
articulare (craniometric point) (*See also* AR)

ARA
acetylene reduction activity
adenosine regulating agent
antireticulin antibody
aortic root angiogram
Axenfeld-Reiger anomaly

ara-A, ara-a
adenine arabinoside (*See also* AA)

ARAD
abnormal right axis deviation

ARAS
ascending reticular-activating system

ARB
adrenergic receptor binder
angiotensin II receptor blocker
angiotensin receptor blocker
any reliable brand

arb
arbitrary (unit)

ARBD
alcohol-related birth defect

ARBOR
arthropod-borne (virus)

ARBOW
artificial rupture of bag of waters

ARBV
　　Arbia virus
ARC
　　abnormal retinal correspondence
　　accelerating rate calorimetry
　　active renin concentration
　　AIDS-related complex
　　alcohol rehabilitation center
　　anomalous retinal correspondence
　　antigen-reactive cell
　　antirotation cable
　　anxiety rating for children
　　arcuate nucleus of the
　　　hypothalamus
　　arcuate nucleus (of brain)
　　average response computer
ARCA
　　acquired red-cell aplasia
ARCD
　　acquired renal cystic disease
arch.
　　archives
ARCO
　　antigen-reactive cell opsonization
ARCP
　　alcohol-related chronic pancreatitis
ARCS
　　azoospermia, renal anomaly,
　　　cervicothoracic spine dysplasia
ARD
　　absolute reaction of degeneration
　　acid-related disorder
　　acute radiation disease
　　acute respiratory disease
　　acute respiratory distress
　　allergic respiratory disease
　　anisotropically rotational diffusion
　　anorectal dressing
　　antibiotic removal device
　　antimicrobial removal device
　　aphakic retinal detachment
　　arthritis and rheumatic diseases
　　atopic respiratory disease
ARDS
　　acute respiratory distress syndrome
　　adult respiratory distress syndrome
ARE
　　active-resistive exercises
　　AIDS-related encephalitis

AREDYLD
　　acrorenal field defect, ectodermal
　　　dysplasia, and lipoatrophic
　　　diabetes
ARF
　　acute renal failure
　　acute respiratory failure
　　acute rheumatic fever
　　Adjective Rating Form
　　area resource file
ArF
　　argon fluoride
ARFC
　　active rosette-forming T cell
ARF/CRF
　　acute renal failure and chronic
　　　renal failure
ARG
　　alkaline reflux gastritis
Arg
　　arginine (*See also* R)
arg-gly-asp
　　arginine-glycine-aspartic acid
ARGNO
　　antibiotic-resistant gram-negative
　　　organism
ARGO
　　Adjustable Advanced Reciprocating
　　　Gait Orthosis
ARHL
　　age-related hearing loss
ARHNC
　　advanced resected head and neck
　　　cancer
ARHS
　　acute right heart syndrome
ARI
　　acute renal insufficiency
　　acute respiratory infection
　　airway reactivity index
　　aldose reductase inhibitor
　　anxiety reaction, intense
ARIA
　　acetylcholine receptor-inducing
　　　activity
　　automated radioimmunoassay
ARIC
　　acrosome reaction with ionophore
　　　challenge
ARIF
　　assisted reduction and internal
　　　fixation

NOTES

ARK
adrenergic receptor kinase
ARK-1
adrenergic receptor kinase 1
ARKD
autosomal recessive kidney disease
ArKr
argon-krypton [laser]
ARKV
Arkonam virus
ARL
AIDS-related lymphoma
average remaining lifetime
ARLD
alcohol-related liver disease
ARLL
AIDS-related lymphoma of the
lung
ARM
adrenergic receptor material
aerosol rebreathing method
age-related maculopathy
allergy relief medicine
alternating range of motion
anorectal manometry
anxiety reaction, mild
atomic resolution microscopy
ARMD
age-related macular degeneration
ARMS
acoustic respiratory motion sensor
Adverse Reaction Monitoring
System
alveolar rhabdomyosarcoma
amplification refractory mutation
system
ARMS-PCR
amplification refractory mutation
system-polymerase chain reaction
ARN
acute renal necrosis
acute retinal necrosis (syndrome)
arcuate nucleus
ARND
alcohol-related neurodevelopmental
disorder
ARNT
aryl hydrocarbon receptor nuclear
translocator
AROA
autosomal recessive ocular albinism
AROAV
Aroa virus
AROM
active range of motion
artificial rupture of membranes
ARP
abbreviated rapid processing

absolute refractory period
acute recurrent pancreatitis
alcohol rehabilitation program
Aptitude Research Project
assay reference plasma
assimilation regulatory protein
at-risk period
automaticity recovery phase
ARPES
angular resolved photoelectron
spectroscopy
ARPF
anterior release posterior fusion
ARPKD, AR-PKD
autosomal recessive polycystic
kidney disease
ARPTH
autosomal recessive renal proximal
tubulopathy and hypercalciuria
ARR
absolute risk reduction
aortic root replacement
arr
arrest
arrested
arrive
ARREST
AngioRad radiation for restenosis
ARROM
active resistive range of motion
arry
arrhythmia
ARS
Academic Readiness Scale
acquiescent response scale
acute repetitive seizure
acute retroviral syndrome
adult recovery services
AIDS-related syndrome
alizarin red S (dye)
amylase-resistant starch
angiographic reference system
antirabies serum
arsphenamine (*See also* AR, Ars)
arylsulfatase
Ars
arsphenamine (*See also* AR, ARS)
ARS-A, ARS A, Ars-A
arylsulfatase A (*See also* ASA,
AsA)
ARSA
aberrant right subclavian artery
ARSACS
autosomal recessive spastic ataxia
of Charlevoix-Saguenay
ARS-B, ARS B, Ars-B
arylsulfatase B (*See also* AsB)

ARS-C, Ars-C
  arylsulfatase C (*See also* AsC)
ARSM
  acute respiratory system
    malfunction
ART
  absolute retention time
  Achilles (tendon) reflex text
  acoustic reflex test
  acoustic reflex threshold
  acoustic response technology
  active-release technique
  algebraic reconstruction technique
  androgen replacement therapy
  antiretroviral treatment
  arrest-and-reversal treatment
  arrhythmia research technology
  arterial (line) (*See also* AL, A-line,
    art. line)
  artery (*See also* A, a, art.)
  articulation treatment
  assisted reproductive technique
  assisted reproductive technology
  asymmetry, range of motion
    abnormality, tissue texture
    abnormality
  autologous reactive T cell
  automated reagin test
  automaticity recovery time
art.
  arterial
  artery (*See also* A, a, ART)
  articulation
  artificial (*See also* artif)
arth.
  arthritis
  arthrotomy
arthro
  arthroscopy
ARTI
  acute respiratory tract illness
artif
  artificial (*See also* art.)
art. line
  arterial line (*See also* AL, A-line,
    ART)
ARTMA
  advanced real-time motion analysis
ARTS
  arterial revascularization therapy
    study

Art T
  art therapy
ARUV
  Aruac virus
ARV
  acquired immunodeficiency
    syndrome-related virus
  Adelaide River virus
  AIDS-associated retrovirus
  AIDS-related virus
  anterior right ventricular (wall)
  antiretroviral
ARV-A, B, C, D, E, F
  Aquareovirus A–F
ARVC
  arrhythmogenic right ventricular
    cardiomyopathy
ARVD
  arrhythmogenic right ventricular
    dysplasia
ARVDD-1
  type 1 autosomal recessive vitamin
    D dependency
ARW
  accredited rehabilitation worker
ARWY
  airway
AS
  above scale
  acetylstrophanthidin
  acidified serum
  acoustic stimulation
  active sarcoidosis
  active sleep
  acute salpingitis
  Adams-Stokes (disease or
    syndrome)
  additive solution
  adolescent suicide
  aerosol sensitization
  aerosol steroid
  affective style
  alimentary sleep
  Alport syndrome
  alveolar sac
  alveolar space
  amphetamine sulfate
  amyloid substance
  anabolic steroid
  anal sphincter
  androgen suppression
  androsterone sulfate

NOTES

AS *(continued)*
   Angelman syndrome
   angiosarcoma
   ankylosing spondylitis *(See also* ASP)
   annulospiral
   anovulatory syndrome
   anterior synechia
   anterosuperior
   antiserum
   antisocial
   antistreptolysin
   antral spasm
   anxiety sensitivity
   anxiety state
   aortic sac
   aortic sound
   aortic stenosis *(See also* A sten, aort sten)
   aqueous solution
   aqueous suspension
   arteriosclerosis *(See also* asc, ASCL, ATS)
   artificial sweetener
   aseptic meningitis
   Asperger syndrome
   asthma astrocyte
   astigmatism *(See also* As, AST, Ast)
   asymmetric *(See also* A, a)
   atherosclerosis *(See also* Athsc, ATS)
   atrial sense
   atrial septum
   atrial stenosis
   atropine sulfate
   audiogenic seizure
   autologous stem
   left ear [L. *auris sinistra*] *(See also* AL, a.l., a.s.)
   sickle cell trait (heterozygous genotype for hemoglobin) *(See also* A/S)

A-S
   ascendance-submission

A/S
   sickle cell trait (heterozygous genotype for hemoglobin) *(See also* AS)

A(s)
   asplenia syndrome

As
   arsenic
   astigmatism *(See also* AS, AST, Ast)
   asymptomatic
   atmosphere, standard

A·s
   ampere-second

aS
   absiemens

a.s.
   left ear [L. *auris sinistra*] *(See also* AL, a.l., AS)

ASA
   acetylsalicylic acid (aspirin)
   active systemic anaphylaxis
   Adams-Stokes attack
   Adaptive Speech Alignment
   anterior spinal artery
   anticoagulation regimen of aspirin
   argininosuccinate
   argininosuccinic acid
   arylsulfatase A *(See also* ARS-A, AsA)
   aspirin-sensitive asthma
   atrial septal aneurysm

4-ASA
   4-aminosalicylic acid

5-ASA
   5-aminosalicylic acid

AsA
   arylsulfatase A *(See also* ARS-A, ASA)

Asa
   arsenate

ASA I
   healthy patient with localized pathologic process

ASA I–V
   American Society of Anesthesiologists' patient classifications I to V, followed by "E" for emergency operations

ASA II
   patient with mild to moderate systemic disease

ASA III
   patient with severe systemic disease limiting activity but not incapacitating

ASA IV
   patient with incapacitating systemic disease

ASA V
   moribund patient not expected to live

ASAA
   acquired severe aplastic anemia

ASAC
   acidified serum, acidified complement

ASA-G
   guaiacolic acid ester of acetylsalicylic acid

ASAH
>aneurysmal subarachnoid hemorrhage
>antibiotic-sterilized aortic valve homograft

ASAI
>aortic stenosis and aortic insufficiency (murmurs)

ASAL
>argininosuccinic acid lyase

ASAP
>as soon as possible
>atypical small acinar proliferation of prostate
>(Vanderbilt University) Asthma, Sinus and Allergy Program

ASAS
>argininosuccinate synthetase

ASB
>anencephaly-spinal bifida (syndrome)
>anesthesia standby
>Anxiety Scale for the Blind
>Aptitude Tests for School Beginners
>asymptomatic bacteriuria

AsB
>arylsulfatase B (*See also* ARS-B, Ars-B)

A-SBFM
>Andresen Six-Basic-Factors-Model (Questionnaire)

ASBS
>arteriosclerotic brain syndrome

ASC
>acetylsulfanilyl chloride
>acute suppurative cholangitis
>adenosine-coupled spleen cell
>altered state of consciousness
>ambulatory surgery center
>anterior subcapsular cataract
>antibody-secreting cell
>antigen-sensitive cell
>antimony-sulfur colloid
>ascorbic acid
>asthma symptom checklist

AsC
>arylsulfatase C (*See also* ARS-C, Ars-C)

asc
>anterior subcapsular
>arteriosclerosis (*See also* AS, ASCL, ATS)
>arteriosclerotic
>ascending

ASCA
>anti-*Saccharomyces cerevisiae* antibody
>Anxiety Scales for Children and Adults

Asc-A
>ascending aorta (*See also* AA, AO, ASCAo)

ASCAD
>arteriosclerotic coronary artery disease
>atherosclerotic coronary artery disease

ASCAo
>ascending aorta (*See also* Asc-A, AO, AA)

ASCCC
>advanced squamous cell cervical carcinoma

ASCI
>acute spinal cord injury

ASCII
>American Standard Code for Information Interchange

ascit fl
>ascitic fluid (*See also* AF)

ASCL
>arteriosclerosis (*See also* AS, asc, ATS)

ASCR
>autologous stem cell rescue

ASCS
>acute sickle chest syndrome
>autologous stem cell support

ASCT
>autologous stem cell transplantation

ASCURD
>arteriosclerotic cardiovascular renal disease

ASCUS
>atypical squamous cells of uncertain significance
>atypical squamous cells of undetermined significance

ASCVD
>arteriosclerotic cardiovascular disease
>atherosclerotic cardiovascular disease

ASD
>acute stress disorder

NOTES

ASD (*continued*)
    adult/adolescent spectrum of (HIV) disease
    aldosterone secretion defect
    Alzheimer senile dementia
    anterior sagittal diameter
    antisiphon device
    arthritis syphilitica deformans
    atrial septal defect
    autism spectrum disorder

ASD2
    secundum atrial septal defect

ASDH
    acute subdural hematoma

ASDO
    anterior segmental dentoalveolar osteotomy

ASDOS
    atrial septal defect occlusion system

ASE
    acute stress erosion
    axilla, shoulder, elbow (bandage)

ASES
    Adult Self-Expression Scale
    American shoulder and elbow system

ASEx
    anterosuperior external ilium movement

ASF
    African swine fever
    aniline-sulfur-formaldehyde (resin)
    anterior spinal fusion
    asialofetuin

ASFP
    ascending frontoparietal

ASFR
    age-specific fertility rate

ASFV
    African swine fever virus

ASG
    advanced stage group

ASGB
    adjustable silicone gastric banding

AS/GP
    antiserum, guinea pig

ASGPR
    antiasialoglycoprotein receptor

ASG system
    Adhesion Scoring Group

ASH
    aldosterone-stimulating hormone
    ankylosing spinal hyperostosis
    antistreptococcal hyaluronidase
    asymmetric septal hypertrophy

A & Sh
    arm and shoulder

ASHCVD
    atherosclerotic hypertensive cardiovascular disease

ASHD
    arteriosclerotic heart disease
    atherosclerotic heart disease
    atrial septal heart disease

ASHN
    acute sclerosing hyaline necrosis

AS/Ho
    antiserum, horse

ASI
    acromial spur index
    active specific immunotherapy
    addiction severity index
    Anxiety Sensitivity Index
    Anxiety Status Inventory
    arthroscopic screw installation

asialo-galacto-Tg
    asialo-galacto-thyroglobulin

asialo-hCG
    asialo-human chorionic gonadotropin

ASIC
    application-specific integrated circuit

A-SICD
    Adapted Sequenced Inventory of Communication Development

a-SiC:H
    amorphous hydrogenated silicon carbide

ASICT
    amplitude-summation interferential current therapy

ASIL
    anal squamous intraepithelial lesion

ASIn
    anterosuperior internal ilium movement

ASIQ
    Adult Suicidal Ideation Questionnaire

ASIS
    anterior superior iliac spine

ASK
    antistreptokinase

ASKA
    antiskeletal antibody

ASL
    American Sign Language (*See also* Ameslan)
    ankylosing spondylitis, lung
    anterolateral sclerosis
    antistreptolysin

ASLC
    acute self-limited colitis

ASLD
    adenylosuccinate lyase deficiency

ASLO, ASL-O
   antistreptolysin-O (*See also* ASO, ASTO)
ASLT
   antistreptolysin test
ASLV
   avian sarcoma and leukosis virus (Rous virus)
ASM
   airway smooth muscle
   anterior scalenus muscle
   appendicular skeletal muscle
   myopic astigmatism (*See also* AsM, AM, am.)
AsM
   myopic astigmatism (*See also* ASM, AM, am.)
ASMA
   alpha smooth muscle actin
   antismooth muscle antibody
ASMC
   arterial smooth muscle cell
ASMD
   atonic sclerotic muscle dystrophy
ASMI
   anteroseptal myocardial infarct
   anteroseptal myocardial infarction
As/Mk
   antiserum, monkey
ASMR
   age-standardized mortality ratio
ASMT
   American Society for Medical Technology
asmt
   assessment
ASN
   alkali-soluble nitrogen
   arteriosclerotic nephritis
   automatic single-needle monitor
Asn
   asparagine (*See also* N)
ASO
   adenocarcinoma of the uterus with sarcomatous overgrowth
   AIDS service organization
   aldicarb sulfoxide
   allele-specific oligonucleotide
   ankle stabilizing orthosis
   antistreptolysin-O (*See also* ASLO, ASL-O, ASTO)
   arteriosclerosis obliterans

   atherosclerosis obliterans
   automatic stop order
As₂O₃
   arsenic trioxide
ASOR
   asialoorosomucoid
ASO-RAD
   arteriosclerotic renal artery disease
ASOT
   antistreptolysin-O titer
ASP
   abnormal spinal posture
   acute suppurative parotitis
   acute symmetric polyarthritis
   African swine pox
   aged substrate plasma
   alkali-stable pepsin
   amnesic shellfish poisoning
   ankylosing spondylitis (*See also* AS)
   antisocial personality
   aortic systolic pressure
   area systolic pressure
   aspartic acid (*See also* asp)
   aspiration (*See also* asp)
   automatic signal processing
asp
   asparate
   aspartic acid (*See also* ASP)
   aspiration (*See also* ASP)
asp.
   aspirate
ASPAT
   antistreptococcal polysaccharide A test
AS-PCR
   allele-specific polymerase chain reaction
ASPD
   anterior superior pancreaticoduodenal
   antisocial personality disorder
ASPECT
   Ackerman-Schoendorf Scales for Parent Evaluation of Custody
ASPED
   angel-shaped phalangoepiphyseal dysplasia
asper
   aspergillosis
ASPG
   antispleen globulin

NOTES

Asp/Glu-Tyr
aspartic acid/glutamic acid-tyrosine
ASPI
Adolescent Problem Severity Index
ASPS
alveolar soft part sarcoma
ASPVD
arteriosclerotic peripheral vascular disease
atherosclerotic pulmonary vascular disease
ASQ
abbreviated symptom questionnaire
Ages and Stages Questionnaire
anxiety scale questionnaire
Attitude to School Questionnaire
Attributional Style Questionnaire
ASR
adrenal-to-spleen ratio
aldosterone secretion rate
aldosterone secretory rate
analyte-specific reagent
atrial septal resection
AS/Rab
antiserum, rabbit
ASRD
aspirin-sensitive respiratory disease
ASS
Aarskog-Scott syndrome
acute serum sickness
acute spinal stenosis
anterior-superior spine
argininosuccinate synthetase
Asthma Severity Score
ASSAS
aminopterin syndrome sine aminopterin
ASSC
acute splenic sequestration crisis
AS-SCORE
assessing severity: age of patient, systems involved, stage of disease, complications, response to therapy
ASSI
Accurate Surgical and Scientific Instruments (Corporation)
Assn, assn
association (*See also* Assoc, assoc)
Assoc, assoc
associate
association (*See also* Assn, assn)
assocd
associated (with)
ASSQ
autism spectrum screening questionnaire

ASSR
adult situational stress reaction
adult situation stress reaction
asst
assistant
AST
above selected threshold
acoustic stimulation test
alcohol sniff test
angiotensin sensitivity test
anterior spinothalamic tract
antistreptolysin titer
Aphasia Screening Test
aspartate aminotransferase
aspartate transaminase
astemizole
astigmatism (*See also* AS, As, Ast)
atrial overdrive stimulation rate
audiometry sweep test
AST2
antistreptozyme
Ast
astigmatism (*See also* AS, As, AST)
ASTA
anti-alpha-staphylolysin
A sten
aortic stenosis (*See also* AS, aort sten)
Asth
asthenopia
ASTI
acute soft tissue injury
antispasticity index
ASTM
augmented soft tissue mobilization
ASTO
antistreptolysin-O (*See also* ASLO, ASL-O, ASO)
AS TOL, as tol
as tolerated
ASTZ
antistreptozyme (test)
ASU
acute stroke unit
ambulatory surgical unit
ASV, AS-V, A/SV
adaptive support ventilation
anodic stripping voltammetry
antisiphon valve
antisnake venom
arteriosuperficial venous (difference)
avian sarcoma virus
ASVAB
Armed Services Vocational Aptitude Battery
ASVD
arteriosclerotic vascular disease

ASVIP
  atrial-synchronous ventricular-
    inhibited pacemaker
ASVS
  arterial stimulation and venous
    sampling
ASW
  artificial seawater
asw
  artificially sweetened
Asx
  amino acid that gives aspartic acid
    after hydrolysis
  asymptomatic
ASYM, asym
  asymmetric
  asymmetry
AT
  abdominal tympany
  Achard-Thiers (syndrome)
  achievement test
  Achilles tendon
  activity therapy
  activity training
  acute thrombosis
  adaptive thermogenesis
  adenosine triphosphate
  adipose tissue
  adjunctive therapy
  adjuvant therapy
  air temperature
  air trapping
  allergy treatment
  amegakaryocytic thrombocytopenia
  aminotransferase
  aminotriazole
  amitriptyline
  anaerobic threshold
  anaphylatoxin
  anionic trypsinogen
  anterior tibia
  antithrombin
  antitrypsin
  antral transplantation
  apoptotic index
  applanation tension
  applanation tonometry (*See also* T
    APPL, TAP)
  assistive technology
  ataxia-telangiectasia (*See also* A-T)
  atraumatic
  atresia, tricuspid

  atrial tachycardia
  atropine
  attenuate
  attenuation
  autoimmune thrombocytopenia
  autologous transplant
  axonal terminal
  old tuberculin [Ger. *alt Tuberkulin*]
AT I
  angiotensin I
AT 3
  antithrombin 3
AT$_7$
  hexachlorophene
AT$_{10}$
  dihydrotachysterol
At
  astatine
  atrial (*See also* ATR)
  atrium (*See also* A)
^{211}At
  Astatine-211
a.t.
  air tight
  ampere turn
at.
  atom
  atomic
A-T
  ataxia-telangiectasia (*See also* AT)
ATA
  acquired tufted angioma
  alimentary toxic aleukia
  aminotriazole
  anterior temporal artery
  antithymic activity
  antithyroglobulin antibody
  antithyroid antibody
  anti-*Toxoplasma* antibody
  atmosphere absolute (*See also* ata)
  aurin tricarboxylic acid
ata
  atmosphere absolute (*See also* ATA)
ATAI
  acute traumatic aortic injury
ATB
  antibiotic (*See also* AB, anti bx,
    ABx)
  atrial tachycardia with block
  atypical tuberculosis
ATBC
  alpha tocopherol beta carotene

NOTES

ATC
    activated thymus cell
    aerosol treatment chamber
    aggressive thyroid carcinoma
    alcoholism therapy classes
    anaplastic thyroid carcinoma
    antituberculous chemoprophylaxis
    around the clock

ATCC
    American Type Culture Collection

ATCL
    angioimmunoblastic T-cell
      lymphoma

ATCS
    active trabecular calcification
      surface
    anterior tibial compartment
      syndrome

ATD
    Alzheimer-type dementia
    Amplatz thrombectomy device
    androstatrienedione
    anthropomorphic test dummy
    antithyroid drug
    aqueous tear deficiency
    asphyxiating thoracic dystrophy
    assistive technology device
    autoimmune thyroid disease

A-TDA
    aminothiadiazole

ATDLG
    antithoracic duct lymphocytic
      globulin

ATDP
    Attitudes Toward Disabled Persons

ATDR
    atrial tachycardia detection rate

ATE
    acute toxic encephalopathy
    adipose tissue extract
    autologous tumor extract

ATEE, ATEe
    N-acetyl-l-tyrosine ethyl ester

ATEM
    analytic transmission electron
      microscope

ATEN
    atenolol

A tetra P
    adenosine tetraphosphate

ATF
    activating transcription factor
    anterior talofibular ligament
    ascites tumor fluid
    ascitic tumor fluid

ATFC
    alternative temporal forced choice

At Fib, at. fib.
    atrial fibrillation (*See also* AF,
      AFib, ATR FIB, atr fib.)

ATFL
    anterior talofibular ligament

AT III FUN
    antithrombin III functional

ATG
    adenine-thymine-guanine
    antihuman thymocyte globulin
    antithymocyte globulin (*See also*
      ATGAM)
    antithyroglobulin

ATGAM, Atgam
    antithymocyte globulin (*See also*
      ATG)

AT/GC
    adenine-thymine/guanine-cytosine
      (ratio)

ATH
    acetyltyrosine hydrazide
    anthropometric total hip

ATHC
    allotetrahydrocortisol

ATHR
    angina threshold heart rate

Athsc
    atherosclerosis (*See also* AS, ATS)

ATI
    abdominal trauma index

AT-I, -II, -III
    angiotensin I–III

ATIS
    HIV/AIDS Treatment Information
      Service

ATL
    Achilles tendon lengthening
    acute tumor lysis
    adult T-cell leukemia (*See also*
      ATLL)
    adult T-cell lymphoma (*See also*
      ATLL)
    anterior temporal lobectomy
    anterior tricuspid leaflet
    antitension line
    atypical lymphocytes

ATLA
    adult T-cell leukemia antigen

ATLL
    adult T-cell leukemia/lymphoma
      (*See also* ATL)

ATLS
    acute tumor lysis syndrome
    advanced trauma life support

ATLV
    adult T-cell leukemia virus

ATM
    abnormal tubular myelin

acute transverse myelitis
acute transverse myelopathy
asynchronous transfer mode
ataxia telangiectasia mutated
Awareness Through Movement

atm
atmosphere
(standard) atmosphere

ATMA
antithyroid plasma membrane
antibody

At mA
atrial milliampere

atmos
atmospheric

ATMS
Attitudes Toward Mainstreaming
Scale

ATN
acute tubular necrosis
augmented transition network
tyrosinase-negative oculocutaneous
albinism

ATNC, AT/NC
atraumatic normocephalic

aTNM
(at) autopsy tumor, nodes, and
metastases (staging of cancer)

at. no.
atomic number

ATNR
asymmetric tonic neck reflex

ATOD
alcohol, tobacco, and other drugs

ATODC
atraumatic osteolysis of distal
clavicle

ATON
adductor tenotomy and obturator
neurectomy

AT-P
antitrypsin-Pittsburgh

A-TP
absorbed test plasma

ATP
addiction treatment program
adenosine triphosphate
adenosine 5′-triphosphate
ambient temperature and pressure
antitachycardia pacemaker
antitachycardia pacing

autoimmune thrombocytopenic
purpura

AtP
attending physician

AT-PAS
aldehyde-thionine-periodic acid-Schiff
(test)

ATPase
adenosine triphosphatase

ATPD
ambient temperature and pressure,
dry

ATP-2Na
adenosine triphosphate disodium

ATPS
ambient temperature and pressure,
saturated (with water vapor)

ATP-SPECT
adenosine triphosphate single-photon
emission computed tomography

ATPTX
acute thyroparathyroidectomy

ATR
Achilles tendon reflex
Achilles tendon rupture
alpha thalassemia mental retardation
atrial (*See also* At)
atrial tachy response
attenuated total reflection

atr
atrophy

ATRA
all-trans-retinoic acid

ATRA1
autoimmune thyroid-related antigen-
1

ATR FIB, atr fib.
atrial fibrillation (*See also* AF,
AFib, At Fib)

ATRO
atropine (*See also* A)

AT/RT
atypical teratoid/rhabdoid tumor
(*See also* ATT/RhT)

ATRT-CNS
atypical teratoid/rhabdoid tumor of
the central nervous system

ATRX
X-linked alpha-thalassemia mental
retardation

ATS
acid test solution

NOTES

ATS *(continued)*
  adjustable thigh antiembolism stockings
  anti-rat thymocyte serum
  antitetanus serum
  antithymocyte serum
  anxiety tension state
  arteriosclerosis (*See also* AS, asc, ASCL)
  atherosclerosis (*See also* AS, Athsc)
  autotransfusion

ATSB
  Aptitude Tests for School Beginners

ATT
  anterior talar translation
  arginine tolerance test
  aspirin tolerance time
  atypical teratoid tumor

att
  attending

ATTC
  automated test target calibration

ATTF
  anterior tibiotalar fascicle

ATTR
  attached report

ATT/RhT
  atypical teratoid/rhabdoid tumor (*See also* AT/RT)

ATU
  alcohol treatment unit
  allylthiourea

ATV
  all-terrain vehicle
  anterior terminal vein
  atrioventricular
  avian tumor virus

AtV
  assisted ventilation (*See also* AV)

at. vol
  atomic volume

at. wt
  atomic weight (*See also* AW)

atyp
  atypical

ATZ
  anal transitional zone
  atypical transformation zone

AU
  according to custom [L. *ad usum*]
  advanced ultrasonography
  allergy unit
  antitoxin unit
  arbitrary unit
  atomic unit
  Australia antigen (*See also* AA, Au Ag)
  both ears together [L. *aures unitas*] (*See also* a.u.)
  each ear [L. *auris uterque*] (*See also* a.u.)

AU4
  area under pH4

Au
  gold [L. *aurum*]

¹⁹⁸Au
  colloidal gold (*See also* CG)
  gold-198
  radioactive gold

a.u.
  both ears together [L. *aures unitas*] (*See also* AU)
  each ear [L. *auris uterque*] (*See also* AU)

Au Ag
  Australia antigen (*See also* AA, AU)

AUB
  abnormal uterine bleeding

AuBMT
  autologous bone marrow transplantation

AUC
  area under the curve

AUD, aud
  arthritis of unknown diagnosis
  auditory

AUDIT
  Alcohol Use Disorders Identification Test

aud-vis
  audiovisual (*See also* AV)

AUFS
  absorbance units, full scale

AUG
  acute ulcerative gingivitis
  adenine, uracil, guanine
  adenine, uridine, guanosine

AUGH
  acute upper gastrointestinal hemorrhage

AUGIB
  acute upper gastrointestinal bleeding

AUHAA
  Australia hepatitis-associated antigen

AUI
  alcohol use inventory

AUL
  acute undifferentiated leukemia

AUM
  asymmetric unit membrane

AUO
  amyloid of unknown origin

AuP
  Australia antigen protein

AUQ
Alcohol Usage Questionnaire
AUR
acute urinary retention
aur
auricle
auricular
auris (*See also* a)
AURAV
Aura virus
AUR FIB, aur fib.
auricular fibrillation (*See also* AF)
AUS
acute urethral syndrome
artificial urinary sphincter
auscultation (*See also* aus, ausc, auscul)
aus, ausc, auscul
auscultation (*See also* AUS)
AuSH
Australia serum hepatitis (antigen)
AU/SR
acute undifferentiated schizophrenic reaction
AUTI
asymptomatic urinary tract infection
autoAB
autoantibody
Auto-PBSC BMT
autologous peripheral blood stem cell bone marrow transplantation
auto-PEEP
auto-positive end-expiratory pressure
aux
auxiliary
AV
allergic vasculitis
alveolar duct
anteroventral
anteversion (*See also* Av, av)
anteverted (*See also* Av, av)
anticipatory vomiting
aortic valve
arteriovenous (*See also* A-V)
artificial ventilation
assisted ventilation (*See also* AtV)
atrioventricular (*See also* A-V)
audiovisual (*See also* aud-vis)
auditory-visual
augmented vector
auriculoventricular (*See also* A-V)

aviation medicine (*See also* AM, AVM)
avoirdupois (*See also* Av, av, AVDP, avdp)
A-V
arteriovenous (*See also* AV)
atrioventricular (*See also* AV)
auriculoventricular (*See also* AV)
A/V
alanine/valine
ampere/volt
arterial/venous
artery-to-vein ratio
atrial/ventricular
auricular/ventricular
A:V
arterial-venous (ratio in fundi)
Av, av
anteversion (*See also* AV)
anteverted (*See also* AV)
average (*See also* avg, aver)
avoirdupois (*See also* AV, AVDP, avdp)
aV
abvolt
AVA
antiviral antibody
aortic valve area
aortic valve atresia
Arracacha A virus
arteriovenous anastomosis
availability
AVAD
acute ventricular assist device
AV/AF
anteverted and anteflexed
AVAV
Avalon virus
AVB
Arracacha B virus
atrioventricular block
AVBR
automated ventricular brain ratio
AVC
aberrant ventricular conduction
acrylic veneer crown
allantoin vaginal cream
associative visual cortex
atrioventricular canal
atrioventricular conduction
automatic volume control

NOTES

AVCD
atrioventricular canal defect

$AvCDO_2$
arteriovenous oxygen content difference (*See also* $AVDO_2$)

AVCS
atrioventricular conduction system

AVD
aortic valvular disease
apparent volume of distribution
arteriosclerotic vascular disease
arteriovenous difference
atrioventricular delay

$AVDO_2$, AVD O_2
arteriovenous oxygen content difference (*See also* $AvCDO_2$)

AVDP, avdp
average diastolic pressure
avoirdupois (*See also* AV, Av, av)

AVE
aortic valve echocardiogram
atrioventricular extrasystole

AVEEG
audiovisual electroencephalogram

aver
average (*See also* AV, avg)

AVF
antiviral factor
arteriovenous fistula

aVF
augmented voltage unipolar left foot lead (electrocardiography)

AVFM
arteriovenous fistulous malformation

AVG
ambulatory visit groups (patient classification)
aortic valve gradient

avg
average (*See also* Av, av, aver)

AVGC
autogenous vein graft conduit

AVGCS
autologous vein graft-coated stent

AVGS
autologous vein graft stent

AVH
acute viral hepatitis

AVHB
atrioventricular heart block

AVHD
acquired valvular heart disease

AVI
air velocity index

AV-ICD
atrial and ventricular implantable cardioverter-defibrillator

A-V IMA
arteriovenous internal mammary (fistula)

AVJ
atrioventricular junction

AVJR
atrioventricular junctional rhythm

AVJRe
atrioventricular junctional reentrant

AVJT
atrioventricular functional tachycardia

AVL
anterior vein of the leg

aVL
augmented voltage unipolar left arm lead (electrocardiography)

AVLINE
audiovisuals on-line

AVM
arteriovenous malformation
aviation medicine (*See also* AM, AV)

AVN
acute vasomotor nephropathy
arbitrary valve unit
arteriovenous nicking
atrioventricular nodal (conduction)
atrioventricular node
avascular necrosis

AVNA
atrioventricular node artery

AVND
atrioventricular node dysfunction

AVNFH
avascular necrosis of the femoral head

AVNFRP
atrioventricular node functional refractory period

AVNR
atrioventricular nodal reentry

AVNRT
atrioventricular nodal reentrant tachycardia
atrioventricular nodal reentry tachycardia

AVNT
atrioventricular nodal tachycardia

AVO
atrioventricular opening

$A-VO_2$
arteriovenous oxygen difference

AVP
ambulatory venous pressure
antiviral protein
aqueous vasopressin
arginine vasopressin

arteriovenous passage (time)
ARTMA virtual patient

AVPR2

antidiuretic arginine vasopressin V2 receptor

AVPU

alert, verbal stimulus response, painful stimulus response, unresponsive

AVR

accelerated ventricular rhythm
aortic valve replacement

AVr

antiviral regulator

aVR

augmented voltage unipolar right arm lead (electrocardiography)

AVRB

added viscous resistance to breathing

AVRI

acute viral respiratory infection

AVRP

atrioventricular refractory period

AVRT

atrioventricular reciprocating tachycardia
atrioventricular reentrant tachycardia

AVS

adrenal venous sampling
aneurysm of membranous ventricular septum
aortic valve stenosis
arteriovenous shunt
auditory vocal sequencing

AVSC

aortic valve cusp separation

AVSD

acquired ventricular septal defect
atrioventricular septal defect

A-V shunt

arteriovenous shunt

AVSS

afebrile, vital signs stable

AVSV

aortic valve stroke volume

AVT

Allen vision test
area ventralis of Tsai
arginine oxytocin
arginine vasotocin

atrioventricular tachycardia
atypical ventricular tachycardia

AVTB

absolute volume of trabecular bone

AV3V, Av3V

anteroventral 3rd ventricle

AVVM

angiographically visualized vascular malformation

AvWD

acquired von Willebrand disease

AVXR

acute vascular xenograft rejection

AVZ

avascular zone

AW

abdominal wall
abnormal wave
above waist
abrupt withdrawal
actual weight
alcohol withdrawal
aluminum wafer
alveolar wall
alveolar wash
Anderson-Wilkins
anterior wall
atomic warfare
atomic weight (*See also* at. wt)

A3W

crystalline amino-acid solution

A/W

able to work

A&W

alive and well

aw

airway

AWA

as well as
away without authorization

AWBM

alveolar wall basement membrane

AWD

alive with disease

AWE

advancing wave-like epitheliopathy

AWF

adrenal weight factor

AWG

American wire gauge

NOTES

AWHONN
   Association of Women's Health, Obstetrics, and Neonatal Nursing
AWI
   anterior wall infarction
   authorized walk-in (patient)
AWMI
   anterior wall myocardial infarction
AWO
   airway obstruction
AWOD, AWD
   alive without disease
AWOL
   absent without leave
AWP
   airway pressure
AWRU
   active wrist rotation unit
AWS
   AIDS wasting syndrome
   Alagille-Watson syndrome
   alcohol withdrawal syndrome
AWTA
   aniridia-Wilms tumor association
awu
   atomic weight unit
AX
   alloxan
ax
   axis (*See also* ax.)
ax.
   axial (*See also* A, a)
   axilla (*See also* A)
   axillary
   axis (*See also* ax)
   axon
AXB
   axillary block
AXBF
   axillobifemoral
AXC
   aortic crossclamp
AXF
   advanced x-ray facility
AXG
   adult-type xanthogranuloma
ax. grad
   axial gradient
AX-HSA
   amoxicilloyl-human serum albumin
axial QCT
   computer tomographic methods of axial skeleton
AXL
   axillary lymphoscintigraphy
AXM
   acetoxycycloheximide

AXP
   total adenine ribonucleotide
AXR
   abdominal x-ray
Axs
   ampere per second
AXT
   alternating exotropia
AXUF
   axillounifemoral
AYA
   acute yellow atrophy
AYF
   antiyeast factor
AYP
   autolyzed yeast protein
AZ
   acetazolamide
   acquisition zoom
   Aschheim-Zondek (test) (*See also* A-Z)
   azathioprine (*See also* AZA)
A-Z
   Aschheim-Zondek (test) (*See also* AZ)
Az
   nitrogen [Fr. *azote*]
AZA
   azathioprine (*See also* AZ)
   azelaic acid
AzddUrd
   3′-azido-2′,3′-dideoxyurine
AZF
   azoospermia factor
AZH
   assisted zonal hatching
AZO, azo
   indicates presence of the group -N:N-
AZOOR
   acute zonal occult outer retinopathy
AZR
   alizarin
AZS
   automatic zero set
AZT
   Aschheim-Zondek test
   3′-azido-3′deoxythymidine zidovudine (azidothymidine)
   azidothymidine (zidovudine)
AZTMP
   azidothymidine monophosphate
AZTTP
   azidothymidine triphosphate

B

bacillus
bands
barometric (*See also* BAR, bar)
base (chemistry, of a prism) (*See also* b)
baseline
bath [L. *balneum*]
Baumé scale
behavior
bel
Benoist scale
benzoate
beta (uppercase second letter of Greek alphabet)
bicuspid
bloody
blue (*See also* bl)
body
boils at (*See also* b)
Bolton point (*See also* bb, BO, Bo, BP)
bone
bone marrow-derived (cell or lymphocyte)
born (*See also* b, n.)
boron
both
bound (*See also* BD)
bovine
bregma
bronchial
bronchus
brother (*See also* br, BRO)
bruit
buccal
Bucky (film in cassette in Potter-Bucky diaphragm)
bursa cells
corticosterone (compound B)
gauss (unit of magnetic induction)
magnetic flux density
magnetic induction
supramentale (craniometric point)
tomogram with oscillating Bucky
twice [L. *bis*] (*See also* b., bis.)
whole blood (*See also* QB, WB, W Bld)

b

barn (unit of area for atomic nuclei)
base (*See also* B)
bis
blood (*See also* BL, bl, bld)
boils at (*See also* B)

born (*See also* B, n.)
brain (*See also* BRA)

b.

twice [L. *bis*] (*See also* B, bis.)

B_0

constant magnetic field in nuclear magnetic resonance

B_1

radiofrequency magnetic field in nuclear magnetic resonance
thiamin (vitamin B_1)

B_2

riboflavin (vitamin B_2)

B_6

pyridoxine (vitamin B_6)

B_7

biotin (vitamin B_7)

B_8

adenosine phosphate

B_{12}

cyanocobalamin (vitamin B_{12})

B69

chemically modified protein

BA

bacillary angiomatosis
backache
bacterial agglutination
basilar artery
basion (*See also* Ba, ba)
benzyladenine
best amplitude
betamethasone acetate
bilateral asymmetric
bile acid
biliary atresia
bioactive
biologic activity
blocking antibody
blood agar
blood alcohol
bone age
boric acid
Bourns assist
bovine albumin
brachial artery (pressure)
breathing apparatus
bronchial asthma
bronchoalveolar
buccoaxial
buffered acetone
butyric acid

B<A

bone conduction less than air conduction

B>A
bone conduction greater than air conduction

B&A
before and after
brisk and active

Ba
barium
basion (*See also* BA, ba)

ba
basion (*See also* BA, Ba)
basophil (*See also* bas, baso)

BAA
benzoylarginine amide

BAB
blood agar base

Bab
Babinski (reflex, sign)

BabK
baboon kidney

BABV
Babahoya virus

BAC
bacterial adherent colony
bacterial antigen complex
bacterial artificial chromosome
benzalkonium chloride
blood alcohol concentration
blood alcohol content
bronchoalveolar cells
buccoaxiocervical

Bac, bac.
bacillary [L. *Bacillus*]
bacillus

BACA
bronchioalveolar carcinoma

BaClr
barium chloride

bact
bacteria
bacterial
bacteriologist
bacteriology
bacterium

BAD
biologic aerosol detection

BADGE
Békésy Ascending-Descending Gap Evaluation

BAE
bone-anchored prosthesis
bovine aortic endothelium
bronchial artery embolization

BaE, BaEn
barium enema (*See also* BE)

BAEE
benzoylarginine ethyl ester

BAEP
brainstem auditory evoked potential

BAER, BSAER
brainstem auditory evoked response

BAG
buccoaxiogingival

BAGG
buffered azide glucose glycerol

BAGV
Bagaza virus

BAHA
bone-anchored hearing aid

BAHV
Bahig virus

BAI
basilar artery insufficiency
breath-actuated inhaler

BAIB
beta-aminoisobutyric (acid)

BAIF
bile acid independent flow

BAIT
bacterial automated identification technique

BAKUV
Baku virus

BAKV
Bakau virus

BAL
balance (*See also* bal)
bioartificial liver
blood alcohol level
British anti-Lewisite (therapy)
bronchoalveolar lavage

bal
balance (*See also* BAL)
balsam (*See also* bals)

BALB
binaural alternate loudness balance

BALF
bronchoalveolar lavage fluid

B ALL, B-ALL
B-cell acute lymphoblastic leukemia

BALP
bone-specific alkaline phosphatase

bals
balsam (*See also* bal)

BALT
bronchus-associated lymphoid tissue

BAM, BAm
brachial artery mean (pressure)

BaM
barium meal

Bam
benzamide

BAME
benzoylarginine methyl ester

BAMO
behavioral, anxiety, mood, and other types of disorders

BAN
British approved name

Ba-N
basion-nasion

band, stab
neutrophil

BANS
back, arm, neck, and scalp
budesonide aqueous nasal spray

BANV
Banzi virus

BAO
basal acid output
basilar artery occlusion
brachial artery output

BAO/MAO
ratio of basal acid output to maximal acid output

BAP
bacterial alkaline phosphatase
basic adaptive process
Behavior Activity Profile
Behavioral Assessment of Pain
blood agar plate
bone alkaline phosphatase
bovine albumin in phosphate buffer
brachial artery pressure
brightness area product

BaP
benzoapyrene

BAPN
beta-aminopropionitrile fumarate

BAPP
bacteremia-associated pneumococcal pneumonia

BAPS
Biomechanical Ankle Platform System
bovine albumin phosphate saline

bAPV
baseline average peak velocity

BAQ
brain-age quotient

BAR, bar
bariatrics
barometer
barometric (*See also* B)
beta adrenergic receptor

barb.
barbiturate

BARN
bilateral acute retinal necrosis

BARNY
Body Awareness Resource Network

BARSIT
Barranquilla Rapid Survey Intelligence Test

BARV
Barur virus

BAS
Ballard Assessment Score
balloon atrial septostomy
Barnes Akathisia Scale
behavioral activation system
benzyl antiserotonin
boric acid solution
British Ability Scale

BaS
barium swallow (*See also* BS, b.s.)

bas
basilar
basophil (*See also* ba, baso)
basophilic

BASA
Boston Assessment of Severe Aphasia

BASC
Behavioral Assessment Scale for Children

BASE
b27-arthritis-sacroiliitis-extraarticular features (syndrome)
Brief Aphasia Screening Examination

BASH
body acceleration synchronous with heart rate

BaSO4
barium sulfate

baso
basophil (*See also* ba, bas)

BASO STIP
basophilic stippling

BAT
Basic Aid Training
basic assurance test
best available technology
bilateral advancement transposition
brain adjacent tumor

NOTES

BAT *(continued)*
Brightness Acuity Test
brown adipose tissue

batt
battery

BATV
Batai virus

BAU
biological allergic unit

BAUP
Bovie-assisted uvulopalatoplasty

BAUV
Bauline virus

BAV
balloon aortic valvotomy (*See also* BAVP)
Banna virus
BeAr 328208 virus
bicuspid aortic valve

BAVCP
bilateral abductor vocal cord paralysis

BAVFO
bradycardia after arteriovenous fistula occlusion

BAVP
balloon aortic valvuloplasty

BAW
bronchoalveolar washing

BAYV
Bayou virus

BB
baby boy
backboard
bad breath
bed bath
bed board
beta blockade
beta blocker
BioBreeding (rat)
blanket bath
blood bank (*See also* BLBK, Bld Bk)
blood buffer (base)
blow bottle
blue bloater (emphysema)
body belt
both bones (fractures)
bowel and bladder (function) (*See also* B&B)
breakthrough bleeding (*See also* BTB)
breast biopsy (*See also* B Bx, br bx)
brush border
buffer base
bundle branch

isoenzyme of creatine kinase containing two B subunits (*See also* CK-BB)

B&B
bowel and bladder (*See also* BB)

B/B
backward bending

Bb
Borrelia burgdorferi

bb
Bolton point (*See also* B, BO, Bo, BP)
both bones

BBA
born before arrival

BBB
blood-brain barrier
blood buffer base
bundle branch block

BBBB
bilateral bundle-branch block

BBC
biceps, brachialis, coracobrachialis
bromobenzylcyanide
Brown-Buerger cytoscope

BBD
baby born dead
benign breast disease

BBDS
benign bile duct stricture

BBE
Bacteroides bile esculin (agar)

BBF
bronchial blood flow

BBFD
blood and body fluid precaution

BBI
Bowman-Birk inhibitor

4-1BBL
4-1BB ligand

BBM
banked breast milk
brush border membrane

BB to MM
belly button to medial malleolus

BBN
broadband noise

BBOT, bbot
2,5-bis(5-t-butylbenzoxazol-2-yl)thiophene

BBOV
Bimbo virus

BBOW
bulging bag of waters

BBP
butylbenzyl phthalate

BBPRL
big big prolactin

B

BBR
  bibasilar rale
  bundle-branch reentry
BBRS
  Burks Behavior Rating Scale
BBS
  bashful bladder syndrome
  benign breast syndrome
  BES buffered saline
  bilateral breath sounds
  bombesin
  brown bowel syndrome
BBT
  basal body temperature
  Bingham Button Test
BBTB
  blood-brain-tumor barrier
BBTOP
  Bankson-Bernthal Test of
    Phonology
BBV
  black beetle virus
BB/W
  BioBreeding/Worcester (rat)
B Bx
  breast biopsy (*See also* BB, br bx)
BC
  back care (*See also* bc)
  backcross
  background counts
  bactericidal concentration
  basal cell
  basket cell
  battle casualty
  bed and chair (*See also* B&C)
  behavior control
  beta carotene
  Bilhaut-Cloquet
  biliary colic
  biotin carboxylase
  bipolar cell
  birth control
  bladder cancer
  blast crisis
  blastic crisis
  blood cardioplegia
  blood center
  blood count
  blood culture (*See also* BlC)
  board certified
  bone conduction
  Bowman capsule

  brachiocephalic
  bronchial carcinoma
  buccal cartilage
  buccocervical
  buffy coat
  bulbus chordae
B/C
  because
  blood urea nitrogen/creatinine
    (ratio)
B&C
  bed and chair (*See also* BC)
  biopsy and curettage
  board and care
  breathed and cried
bc
  back care (*See also* BC)
b/c
  benefit/cost (ratio)
BCA
  balloon catheter angioplasty
  Barrett adenocarcinoma
  basal cell atypia
  bell-clapper anomaly
  bicinchoninic acid
  blood color analyzer
  brachiocephalic artery
  branchial cleft anomaly
  breast cancer antigen
BCAA
  branched-chain amino acid
BCAT
  brachiocephalic arterial trunk
BCAVD
  bilateral congenital absence of vas
    deferens
BCB
  blood-cerebrospinal fluid barrier
  brilliant cresyl blue (stain)
BCBL
  body cavity-based lymphoma
BCBR
  bilateral carotid body resection
BCC
  basal cell carcinoma (*See also*
    BCCa)
  benign cellular changes
  biliary cholesterol concentration
  birth control clinic
bcc
  body-centered-cubic

NOTES

BCCa
 basal cell carcinoma (*See also* BCC)

BCCI
 Barclay Classroom Climate Inventory

BCCP
 biotin carboxyl carrier protein

BCCV
 Black Creek Canal virus

BCD
 bad conduct discharge
 basal cell dysplasia
 binary-coded decimal
 blepharocheilodontic
 borderline of cardiac dullness

BCDDP
 Breast Cancer Detection Demonstration Project

BCDF
 B-cell differentiation factor

BCDL
 Brachmann-Cornelia de Lange

BCE
 basal cell epithelioma
 B-cell enriched
 benign childhood epilepsy
 bubble chamber equipment

B-cell CLL/SLL
 B-cell chronic lymphocytic leukemia/small lymphocytic lymphoma

BCF
 basophil chemotactic factor
 bioconcentration factor
 breast cyst fluid

BCFA
 branched-chain fatty acid

BCFP
 breast cyst fluid protein

BCG
 Bacille bilié de Calmette-Guérin
 Bacille Calmette-Guérin (vaccine)
 ballistocardiogram
 ballistocardiograph
 ballistocardiography
 bicolor guaiac (test)
 bilateral cystogram
 bromcresol green

bCgA
 bovine chromogranin A

BCGF
 B-cell growth factor

BCH
 basal cell hyperplasia
 benign cephalic histiocytosis
 benign coital headache

BCHA
 bone conduction hearing aid

BchE
 butylcholinesterase

bChl, Bchl
 bacterial chlorophyll

BCI
 blunt cardiac injury
 blunt carotid injury

BCKA
 branched-chain keto acid

BCKD
 branched chain alpha ketoacid dehydrogenase

BCL
 basic cycle length
 B-cell lymphoma
 Békésy comfortable loudness

BCLL, B-CLL
 B-cell chronic lymphocytic leukemia

BCLP
 bilateral cleft lip and palate

BCLPD
 B-cell chronic lymphoproliferative disorder

BCLS
 basic cardiac life support (system)

BCM
 birth control medication
 blood-clotting mechanism (effects)
 body cell mass

BCME
 bischloromethyl ether

BCN
 basal cell nevus
 bilateral cortical necrosis

BCNS
 basal cell nevus syndrome

BCO
 balloon coronary occlusion
 biliary cholesterol output

BCOC
 bowel care of choice

BCP
 basic calcium phosphate
 biochemical profile
 birth control pill
 blood cell profile
 bromcresol purple

BCP-LBL
 B-cell precursor lymphoblastic leukemia

BCPS
 battery-charging power supply

BCR
 B-cell antigen receptor
 B-cell reactivity

behavior control room
birth control regimen
breakpoint cluster region (*See also* bcr)
bromocriptine (*See also* Brc, BRO)
bulbocavernosus reflex

bcr
breakpoint cluster region (*See also* BCR)

BCR-ABL
breakpoint cluster region-Abelson murine leukemia (virus)

BCR-negative
breakpoint cluster region negative

BCR-positive
breakpoint cluster region positive

BCRS
Brief Cognitive Rating Scale

BCRT
Beast Cancer Risk tool

BCRx
birth control drug

BCS
battered child syndrome
blood cell separator
Budd-Chiari syndrome

BCSI
breast cancer screening indicator

BCSR
bone-contacting surface ratio

BCSS
Basic Clinical Scoring System
breast cancer-specific survival

BCT
benign cystic teratoma
brachiocephalic trunk
breast conservation therapy
breast-conserving therapy

BCU
burn care unit

BCV
Bunyip Creek virus

BCVA
best-corrected visual acuity

BCW
biologic and chemical warfare

BCYE
buffered charcoal yeast extract

BD
band neutrophil
barbital dependent
barbiturate dependence

base deficit
base-down prism
base (of prism) down
basophilic degeneration
beclomethasone dipropionate
Becton Dickinson (catheter, guidewire, spinal needle)
behavioral disorder
belladonna
below diaphragm
benzidine
benzodiazepine
bicarbonate dialysis
bile duct
binocular deprivation
birth date
birth defect
black death
block design (test)
blood donor
blue diaper (syndrome)
board (*See also* Bd)
borderline dull
bound (*See also* B)
brain death
brain dysfunction
bronchial drainage
bronchodilator
buccodistal

B&D
bondage and discipline

Bd
board (*See also* BD)

bd
band
bundle

BDA
balloon dilation angioplasty
bile duct adenoma

BDAE
Boston Diagnostic Aphasia Examination

BDAV
Bandia virus

BDB
bis-diazotized-benzidine

BD/BS
bile duct-to-portal space ratio

BDC
burn dressing change

BDCL
basic drive cycle length

NOTES

BDCS
Behavioral Dyscontrol Scale
BDD
blistering distal dactylitis
body dysmorphic disorder
BDE
bile duct epithelia
BDG
bidirectional Glenn procedure
bilirubin diglucuronide
buccal developmental groove
buffered desoxycholate glucose
BDGF
bone-derived growth factor
BDH
biologically designed hip
BDI
Baseline Dyspnea Index
Battelle Developmental Inventory
Beck Depression Inventory
burn depth indicator
BDIBS
Boston Diagnostic Inventory of
Basic Skills
BDID
bystander dominates initial
dominant
BDIS
Behavior Disorders Identification
Scale
BDI SF
Beck Depression Index Short Form
BDL
below detectable levels
below detectable limits
bile duct ligation
BDLS
Brachmann-Cornelia de Lange
syndrome (*See also* CLS, CDL)
BDM
benzphetamine demethylase
border detection method
BDMP
Birth Defects Monitoring Program
bDNA, b-DNA
branched chain deoxyribonucleic
acid
branched deoxyribonucleic acid
BDNF
brain-derived neurotrophic factor
brain-derived neurotropic factor
BDP
beclomethasone dipropionate
benzodiazepine
bilateral diaphragm paralysis
BDR
background diabetic retinopathy

BDRS
Blessed Dementia Rating Scale
BDS
biologic detection system
Blessed Dementia Scale
BDT
bronchodilator
BDTVMI
Beery Developmental Test of
Visual-Motor Integration
BDV
balloon dilation valvuloplasty
border disease virus
Borna disease virus
BDW
buffered distilled water
BE
bacillary emulsion (tuberculin)
bacterial endocarditis (*See also*
BEC)
barium enema (*See also* BaE)
Barrett esophagus
base excess
below-elbow (*See also* BELB, B/E)
bile esculin (test)
board eligible
bovine enteritis
brain edema
bread equivalent
breast examination
bronchoesophagology
B↓E
both lower extremities
B/E, B-E
below-elbow (*See also* BELB, BE)
below-elbow (amputation) (*See also*
BEA)
B&E
brisk and equal
B↑E
both upper extremities
Be
Baumé (scale)
beryllium
BEA
below-elbow amputation (*See also*
B/E)
bromoethylamine
BEAM
brain electrical activity map
brain electrical activity mapping
BeAnV-157575
BeAn 157575 virus
BEAP
bronchiectasis, eosinophilia, asthma,
pneumonia

BEB
    benign essential blepharospasm
    blind esophageal brushing
BEBV
    Bebaru virus
BEC
    bacterial endocarditis (*See also* BE)
    biliary epithelial cell
    blood ethanol content
    bromoergocryptine
BECF
    blood extracellular fluid
BeCoMo
    Bernse Coping Modes
BED
    bioeffect dose
    biologically equivalent dose
    biologic effective dose
BEE
    basal energy expenditure
BEEP
    both end-expiratory pressures
BEF
    bronchoesophageal fistula
    Byrne and Euler formula
bef
    before (*See also* a., ā, ante)
BEFV
    bovine ephemeral fever
beg.
    begin
    beginning
BEH
    benign essential hypertension
beh
    behavior
    behavioral
Beh Sp
    behavior specialist
BEI
    back-scattered electron imaging
    Biological Exposure Indexes
    butanol-extractable iodine
BEIR
    biologic effects of ionizing
      radiation
BEK
    bovine embryonic kidney (cell)
BEL
    blood ethanol level
    bovine embryonic lung

BELB
    below-elbow (*See also* BE, B/E)
BELS
    bioartificial extracorporeal liver
      support system
BELTV
    Belterra virus
BELV
    Belmont virus
BEMA
    bioerodible mucoadhesive
BENAR
    blood eosinophilic nonallergic
      rhinitis
BENESTENT
    Belgium Netherlands stent
BENV
    Benevides virus
    Benfica virus
benz.
    benzidine
    benzoate
BEP
    brain evoked potential
    brainstem evoked potential
BEPI
    beta-endorphin immunoreactivity
BEPTI
    bionomics, environment,
      Plasmodium, treatment, and
      immunity (malaria epidemiology)
BER
    basic electrical rhythm
    benign early repolarization
BERA
    brainstem electric response
      audiometry
BERG
    balloon-assisted, endoscopic,
      retroperitoneal, gasless
BERS
    Behavioral and Emotional Rating
      Scale
BES
    balanced electrolyte solution
    British Engineering System
BES-2
    Behavior Evaluation Scale-2
BESM
    bovine embryo skeletal muscle
BESP
    bovine embryonic spleen (cells)

B

NOTES

BET
  benign epithelial tumor
  bleeding esophageal varix
  Brunauer-Emmet-Teller (method)
bet.
  between (*See also* bi)
β, beta
  anomer of carbohydrate
  buffer capacity
  carbon separated from carboxyl by
    one other carbon in aliphatic
    compounds
  constituent of plasma protein
    fraction
  probability of type II error
  β (second letter of Greek
    alphabet), lowercase
  second in series or group
  substituent group of steroid that
    projects above plane of ring
βAR
  beta-adrenergic receptor
βARK
  beta-adrenergic receptor kinase
beta-END
  beta-endorphin
beta$_2$-GPI
  beta$_2$-glycoprotein I
beta-hCG, beta hCG
  beta-human chorionic gonadotropin
beta-HCH
  beta-hexachlorocyclohexane
3betaHSD, 3beta-HSD, 3-beta-HSD
  3-beta-hydroxysteroid dehydrogenase
11-beta-HSD
  11-beta-hydroxysteroid
    dehydrogenase
11-beta-HSD1
  11-beta-hydroxysteroid
    dehydrogenase type 1
11-beta-HSD2
  11-beta-hydroxysteroid
    dehydrogenase type 2
17-beta-HSD
  17-beta-hydroxysteroid
    dehydrogenase
17-beta-HSD1
  17-beta-hydroxysteroid
    dehydrogenase type 1
17-beta-HSD2
  17-beta-hydroxysteroid
    dehydrogenase type 2
17-beta-HSD3
  17-beta-hydroxysteroid
    dehydrogenase type 3
17-beta-HSD4
  17-beta-hydroxysteroid
    dehydrogenase type 4

17-beta-HSD5
  17-beta-hydroxysteroid
    dehydrogenase type 5
beta LP, beta-LPH
  beta lipoprotein
beta$_2$m, beta$_2$M
  beta$_2$-microglobulin
beta-T
  beta-tocopherol
beta-TG
  beta-thromboglobulin
beta-TSH
  beta-thyroid-stimulating hormone
BETS
  benign epileptiform transients of
    sleep
BEV
  beam's eye view
  Berne virus
  bleeding esophageal varices
BeV
  billion electron volts
Bex
  base excess
BF
  bentonite flocculation (test)
  bile flow
  black female
  blastogenic factor
  blister fluid
  blocking factor
  blood flow (*See also* Q_B)
  body fat
  Bolivian hemorrhagic fever
  bone fragment
  bouillon filtrate (tuberculin) (*See
    also* bf)
  boyfriend
  breast fed
  breathing frequency
  buccofacial
  buffered
  burning feet (syndrome)
  butter fat
B/F
  bound/free (antigen ratio)
bf
  bouillon filtrate (tuberculin) (*See
    also* BF)
BFA
  baby for adoption
  bifemoral arteriogram
BFB
  biologic feedback
  bronchial foreign body
BFC
  benign febrile convulsion

B

BFD
    bias flow down
BFDI
    bronchodilation following deep
     inspiration
BFDT
    Békésy Functionality Detection Test
BFEC
    benign focal epilepsy of childhood
bFGF
    basic fibroblast growth factor
BFH
    benign familial hematuria
BFL
    bird fancier's lung
    Börjeson-Forssman-Lehmann
    breast firm and lactating
BFM
    bendroflumethiazide
    benign familial macrocephaly
    Brunnstrom-Fugl-Meyer
BFNC
    benign familial neonatal convulsions
BFO
    balanced forearm orthosis
    ball-bearing forearm orthosis
    blood-forming organ
    buccofacial obturator
BFP
    biologic false-positive
BFQ
    Big Five Questionnaire
BFR
    biologic false-positive reactor
    blood filtration rate
    blood flow rate
    bone formation rate
    buffered Ringer (solution)
BFS
    blood fasting sugar
BFST
    behavioral family systems therapy
BF-STS
    biological false-positive serologic
     test for syphilis
BFT
    bentonite flocculation test
    biofeedback training
    bladder flap tube
BFU
    burst-forming unit

BFU-E
    burst-forming unit-erythroid
BFV
    Barmah Forest virus
    blood flow velocity
BFVW
    blood flow velocity waveform
BG
    baby girl
    background (*See also* BKg)
    basal ganglia (plural)
    basal ganglion (singular)
    basic gastrin
    Bender Gestalt
    beta-galactosidase
    beta-glucuronidase
    bicolor guaiac (test)
    big gastrin
    blood glucose (*See also* BGlu)
    blood group (system)
    bone graft
    Bordet-Gengou (agar, bacillus,
     phenomenon) (*See also* B-G)
    brilliant green
    buccal groove
    buccogingival
B-G
    Bordet-Gengou (agar, bacillus,
     phenomenon) (*See also* BG)
BGA
    blood group antigen
    blue-green algae
BGAg
    blood group antigen
B-GALACTO
    beta-galactosidase
BGC
    basal ganglion calcification
    blood group class
BGCA
    bronchogenic carcinoma
BGCF
    buccal groove of central fossa
BG-corr
    background corrected
BGCT
    benign glandular cell tumor
BGD
    blood group degrading (enzyme)
BGDC
    Bartholin gland duct cyst

NOTES

BGDR
background diabetic retinopathy
BGE
butyl glycidyl ether
BGG
bovine gamma globulin
BGH, bGH
bovine growth hormone
BGIV
Bangui virus
Bg^J
beige (mouse)
BGL
blood glucose level
BGLB
brilliant green lactose broth
BGlu
blood glucose (*See also* BG)
BGM
blood glucose monitoring
BGMR
basal ganglion disorder-mental retardation
BGMV
bean golden mosaic virus
BGNV
Bangoran virus
BGO
bismuth germanate
BGP
beta-glycerophosphatase
biliary glycoprotein
bone Gla protein
brain-type glycogen phosphorylase
BGRS
blood glucose reagent strip
BGS
balance, gait, and station
Baller-Gerold syndrome
blood group substance
BGSA
blood granulocyte-specific activity
BGT
basophil granulation test
Bender-Gestalt test
bungarotoxin
BGTT
borderline glucose tolerance test
BGV
bleeding gastric varix
BH
base hospital
benzalkonium and heparin
bill of health
birth history
Bishop-Harman (instrument)
board of health
Bolton-Hunter (reagent)

borderline hypertensive
both hands
bowel habits
brain hormone
Braxton-Hicks (contraction)
breath holding
bronchial hyperreactivity
Bryan high titer
bundle of His (*See also* BOH)
BH$_4$
tetrahydrobiopterin (cofactor)
BHA
bilateral hilar adenopathy
bound hepatitis antibody
butylated hydroxyanisole
BHAP
bisheteroarylpiperazine
BHB
beta-hydroxybutyrate
bHb
bovine hemoglobin
BHBA
beta-hydroxybutyrate
beta-hydroxybutyric acid
BHC
benzene hexachloride
bHCG, bhCG
beta human chorionic gonadotropin
BHD
bilateral hemisphere damage
Birt-Hogg-Dubé syndrome
B-HEXOS-A-K
beta-hexosaminidase A leukocytes
BHF
Bolivian hemorrhagic fever
BHI
Battery of Health Improvement
beef heart infusion (broth)
biosynthetic human insulin
brain heart infusion (broth)
breath-holding index
BHIA
brain heart infusion agar
BHK
baby hamster kidney (cells)
BHL
bilateral hilar lymphadenopathy
biologic half-life
bHLH
basic helix-loop-helix
BHN
bephenium hydroxynaphthoate
Brinell hardness number
BHP
basic health profile
BHR
basal heart rate

bronchial hyperreactivity
bronchial hyperresponsiveness

BHS

Beck Hopelessness Scale
Behavioral Health Systems
beta-hemolytic streptococcus
breath-holding spell

BHT

beta-hydroxytheophylline
borderline hypertension
breath hydrogen test
butylated hydroxytoluene

BHU

basic health unit

BH/VH

body hematocrit-venous hematocrit
(ratio)

BI

background interval
bacterial index
bactericidal index
bacteriological index
bacteriologic index
Barthel index
base (of prism) in
basilar impression
bifocal (*See also* BIF, bif)
biologic indicator
bodily injury
bone injury
bowel impaction
brain infarct
brain injured
brain injury
burn index

Bi

bismuth

bi

between (*See also* bet.)
bilateral (*See also* BIL, bilat)

BIA

bioelectrical impedance analysis
bioimpedance

BIAV

Bobia virus

BIB, bib

biliointestinal bypass
brought in by

bib.

drink [L. *bibe*]

biblio

bibliography

BIBPD

brought in by police department

BIC

blood isotope clearance
brain injury center

Bic

biceps

BICAO

bilateral internal carotid artery
occlusion

BICAP

bipolar circumactive probe

bicarb

bicarbonate (*See also* HCO$_3$)

BICROS, BiCROS

bilateral contralateral routing of
signals

BID

bibliographic information and
documentation
brought in dead
twice a day [L. *bis in die*] (*See
also* b.i.d.)

b.i.d.

twice a day [L. *bis in die*] (*See
also* BID)

BIDA

butyl iminodiacetic acid

BIDS

bedtime insulin, daytime
sulfonylurea (therapy)
brittle hair, intellectual impairment,
decreased fertility, short stature
(syndrome)

BIE

bayesian image estimation

BIEF

bilateral inferior epigastric artery
flap

BIF, bif

bifocal (*See also* BI)

BIFC

benign infantile familial convulsions

BIGGY

bismuth glycine glucose yeast
(agar)

BIH

basal interhemispheric approach
benign intracranial hypertension
bilateral inguinal hernia

BII

BPH impact index

NOTES

bi isch
between ischial tuberosities

BIL, bil
basal insulin level
biceps interval lesion
bilateral (*See also* bilat, bi)
bilirubin (*See also* bili, bilirub, BR, Bu)
brother-in-law

BILAG
British Isles Lupus Assessment Group index

BIL/ALB
bilirubin to albumin (ratio)

bilat
bilateral (*See also* BIL, bil, bi)

BILAT SLC
bilateral short leg cane

BILAT SXO, bilat sxo
bilateral salpingo-oophorectomy

bili
bilirubin (*See also* BIL, bil, bilirub, BR, Bu)

bili-c
conjugated bilirubin

bilirub
bilirubin (*See also* BIL, bil, bili, BR, Bu)

BIMA
bilateral internal mammary arteries

BiMAB
bispecific monoclonal antibody

BiMAb
I-labeled B-cell-specific anti-CD20 monoclonal antibody

BIMV
Bimiti virus

BIND
bilirubin-induced neurologic dysfunction

BINO
binocular internuclear ophthalmoplegia

BINS
Bayley Infant Neurodevelopmental Screener

biochem
biochemical
biochemistry

BIOD
bony interorbital distance

BIOETHICSLINE
Bioethical Information On-Line

biof
biofeedback

Bi(OH)$_3$
bismuth hydroxide

biol
biologic
biology

bioLH
bioassay of luteinizing hormone

biophys
biophysical
biophysics

BIOSIS
BioScience Information Service

BIP
Background Interference Procedure
bacterial intravenous protein
biparietal (diameter)
bismuth iodoform paraffin
brief infertile period
bronchiolitis with interstitial pneumonitis

BiPAP
bilevel positive airway pressure

BiPD
biparietal diameter (fetal skull)

BIPLED
bilateral independent periodic lateralizing epileptiform discharge

BIPP
bismuth-iodoform-paraffin paste

BIR
backward internal rotation
basic incidence rate

BIRADS
Breast Imaging Reporting and Data System

BIRV
Birao virus

BIS, bis
behavioral inhibition system
bioenergy imbalance syndrome
bone cement implantation syndrome
Brain Information Service
budesonide inhalation suspension
building illness syndrome
sodium bicarbonate in invert sugar

bis.
twice [L.] (*See also* B, b.)

BISF-W
Brief Index of Sexual Functioning for Women

bis-Gd-MP
bis-gadolinium-mesoporphyrine

bis-GMA
bisphenol A-glycidyl methacrylate

Bisp, bisp
bispinous or interspinous (diameter)

bis(POC)
bis(isopropyloxycarboxymethyl)
bis(isopropyloxymethyl)

bis-POM, bis(POM)
bis(piareloyloxymethyl)
bis(POM)PMEA
bispivaloyloxymethyl-
phosohonylmethoxyethyladenine
BITU
benzylthiourea
BIU
barrier isolation unit
BIVAD
bilateral ventricular assist device
BIW, biw, bi wk
biweekly
twice weekly
BIZ-PLT
bizarre platelets
BJ

Bence Jones
biceps jerk
bones and joints (*See also* B&J)
B&J
bones and joints (*See also* BJ)
BJE
bone and joint examination
BJI
bone and joint infection
BJM
bones, joints, and muscles
BJP

Bence Jones protein
Bence Jones proteinuria
BK

bekanamycin
below knee
bovine kidney (cells)
bradykinin
bullous keratopathy
Bk
berkelium
bk
back
BK-A
basophil kallikrein of anaphylaxis
BKA, BK amp
below-knee amputation
BKC
blepharokeratoconjunctivitis
bkf, bkfst, bkft
breakfast (*See also* brkf)
BKG, BKg
background (*See also* BG)

bkly
back lying
BKO
below-knee orthosis
BKS
beekeeper serum
BKTT
below-knee-to-toe (cast)
BKU
base up
BKWC
below-knee walking cast
BKWP
below-knee walking plaster
BL

bacterial levan
basal lamina
baseline
baseline (fetal heart rate)
Bessey-Lowry (unit) (*See also* BLU, B.L. unit)
bifurcation lesion
black light
bland (*See also* bl)
blast cells
bleed
bleeding (*See also* bl)
blind loop
blood (*See also* b, bl, bld)
blood lactate
blood level
blood loss
bone marrow lymphocyte
borderline lepromatous
bronchial lavage
buccolingual
Burkitt lymphoma
butyrolactone
B-L
bursa-equivalent lymphocyte
Bl
black (*See also* blk, bl)
bl
black (*See also* Bl, blk)
bland (*See also* BL)
bleeding (*See also* BL, bldg)
blood (*See also* b, BL, bld)
blue (*See also* B)
BL=BS
bilateral equal breath sounds
BLa
buccolabial

B

NOTES

BLAD
borderline left axis deviation
blad
bladder
BLADES
Bristol Language Development Scale
BLAT
Blind Learning Aptitude Test
BLB
Bessey-Lowry-Brock (method or unit)
black light bulb
Boothby, Lovelace, Bulbulian bulb (syringe)
BLBK
blood bank (*See also* BB, Bld Bk)
BLC
beef liver catalase
BlC, BL CULT, bl cult
blood culture (*See also* BC)
BLCL
Burkitt lymphoma cell line
BLD
basal-cell liquefactive degeneration
basal laminar deposit
benign lymphoepithelial disease
beryllium lung disease
bld
blood (*See also* b, BL, bl)
Bld Bk
blood bank (*See also* BB, BLBK)
bld chem
blood chemistry
bldg
bleeding (*See also* BL, bl)
bld tm
bleeding time (*See also* BT, BLEED, BLT)
BLDY
grossly bloody
BLE
both lower extremities
BLEED
bleeding time (*See also* bld tm, BT, BLT)
BLEL
benign lymphoepithelial lesion
bleph
blepharoplasty
BLES
bovine lavage extract surfactant
BLESS
bath, laxative, enema, shampoo, and shower
BLFD
buccolinguofacial dyskinesia

BLFG
bilateral firm (hand) grips
BL-FST
blood fasting (glucose tolerance test)
BLG
beta-lactoglobulin
blH
biologically active luteinizing hormone
BLHI
Brief Life History Inventory
BLIC
beta lactamase inhibitor combination
BLIP
beta lactamase inhibiting protein
blk
black (*See also* Bl, bl)
BLL
below lower limit
benign lymphoepithelial lesion
bilateral lower lobe
blood lead level
brows, lids, and lashes
Burkitt-like lymphoma
BLLS
bilateral leg strength
BLM
basolateral membrane
bilayer lipid membrane
bimolecular liquid membrane
black lipid membrane
borderline malignancy
buccal-lingual-masticatory
BLMV
Belem virus
BLN
bronchial lymph node
BLNAI
Barclay Learning Needs Assessment Inventory
BlObs
bladder obstruction
BLOT
Bimodality Lung Oncology Team
BLP
beta-lipoprotein
BLPB
beta-lactamase-producing bacteria
BLPD
B-cell lymphoproliferative disorder
BLPO
beta-lactamase-producing organism
BL PR, bl pr
blood pressure (*See also* BP)
BLQ
both lower quadrants

B

BLRA
    beta-lactamase-resistant antimicrobial
BLS
    bare lymphocyte syndrome
    basic life support
    blind loop syndrome
    blood and lymphatic system
BlS
    blood sugar (*See also* BS)
BLSD
    bovine lumpy skin disease
BLST
    Bankson Language Screening Test
BLT, BlT
    balanced ligamentous tension
      treatment
    bilateral lung transplant
    bladder tumor
    bleeding time (*See also* bld tm, BT,
      BLEED)
    blood-clot lysis time
    blood test
    blood type
    blood typing
BLT-2
    Bankson Language Test-2
BLU, B.L. unit
    Bessey-Lowry unit (*See also* BL)
BLUV 1–24
    bluetongue virus 1–24
BLV
    blood volume (*See also* BlV, BV)
    bovine leukemia virus
BlV
    blood viscosity
    blood volume (*See also* BLV, BV)
BLVR
    biliverdin reductase
BM
    bacterial meningitis
    basal medium
    basal membrane
    basal metabolism
    basement membrane
    basilar membrane
    Bergersen medium
    betamethasone
    biomedical
    black male
    blind matching
    blood monocyte
    body mass

    Bohr magneton
    bone marrow
    bowel movement
    breast milk
    buccal mass
    buccomesial
B2M
    beta$_2$-microglobin
BMA
    bismuth subsalicylate, metronidazole,
      and amoxicillin
    bone marrow arrest
    bone marrow aspirate
BmA
    Brugia malayi adult antigen
BMAL1
    brain/muscle ARNT-like protein 1
BMAP
    bone marrow acid phosphatase
BMAV
    Batama virus
BMB
    biomedical belt
    bone marrow biopsy
BMBL
    benign monoclonal B-cell
      lymphocytosis
BMC
    balloon mitral commissurotomy
    blood mononuclear cell (*See also*
      BMNC)
    bone marrow cell
    bone marrow culture
    bone mineral content
BMCL
    blastoid variant of mantel cell
      lymphoma
    blastoma mantel cell lymphoma
BMCMC
    bone marrow-derived cultured mast
      cell
BMD
    Becker muscular dystrophy
    bone marrow depression
    bone mineral densitometry
    bone mineral density
    bovine mucosal disease
BMDC
    Biomedical Documentation Center
BME
    basal medium, Eagle

NOTES

BME *(continued)*
>biundulant meningoencephalitis
brief maximal effort

BMET
>basic metabolic panel

BMF
>bone marrow failure

BMG
>benign monoclonal gammopathy

BMI
>bicuculline methiodide
body mass index

BMIPP
>betamethyliodophenyl pentadecanoic
acid

BMJ
>bones, muscles, joints

BMK, bmk
>birthmark

BML
>bone marrow lymphocytosis

BMLM
>basement membrane-like material

BMLS
>billowing mitral leaflet syndrome

BMM
>bone mineral mass

BMMM
>bone marrow micrometastasis

BMMP
>benign mucous membrane
pemphigoid
bone marrow myeloid precursor

BMN
>bone marrow necrosis

BMNC
>blood mononuclear cell (*See also*
BMC)

BMNR
>bone marrow neutrophil reserve

BMOC
>Brinster medium for ovum culture

Bmod, B-mod
>behavior modification

B-mode
>brightness modulation

BMP
>basic metabolic profile
behavior management plan
bone marrow pressure
bone morphogenetic protein

BMP-2
>bone morphogenetic protein type 2

BMPI
>bronchial mucous proteinase
inhibitor

BMR
>basal metabolic rate

>best motor response
biologic response modifier

BMS
>betamethasone
biomedical monitoring system
biometal surface
burning mouth syndrome

BMST
>Bruce maximal stress test

BMT
>basement membrane thickness
behavioral marital therapy
benign mesenchymal tumor
bilateral myringotomy and tubes
bilateral myringotomy tubes
bismuth, metronidazole, tetracycline
bone marrow transplant
bone marrow transplantation
Buschke Memory Test

BMTN
>bone marrow transplant neutropenia

BMTU
>bone marrow transplant unit

BMU
>basic multicellular unit

BMV
>balloon mitral valvotomy
balloon mitral valvuloplasty

BMZ
>basement membrane zone

BN
>bladder neck
brachial neuritis
bronchial nodes
brown Norway (rat)
bucconasal
bulimia nervosa

BNA
>bronchoscopic needle aspiration

BNAS, BNBAS
>Brazelton Neonatal Assessment
Scale
Brazelton Neonatal Behavioral
Assessment Scale

BNB
>blood-nerve barrier

BNC
>binasal cannula
bladder neck contracture

BNCT
>boron neutron capture therapy

BND
>barely noticeable difference

BNEG
>B negative (blood type)

BNG, BNGase
>bromonaphthyl-beta-galactosidase

B

BNGD
    biopsy-negative graft dysfunction
BNGF
    beta-nerve growth factor
B-NHL
    B-cell non-Hodgkin lymphoma
BNL
    breast needle location
BNMSE
    Brief Neuropsychological Mental
    Status Examination
BNO
    bladder neck obstruction
    bowels not open
    bowels not opened
BNOE
    benign necrotizing otitis externa
BNP
    brain natriuretic peptide
    B-type natriuretic peptide
BNPA
    binasal pharyngeal airway
BNR
    bladder neck resection
BNS
    benign nephrosclerosis
    bladder neck suspension
BNT
    Boston Naming Test
    brain neurotransmitter
BO
    bacterial overgrowth
    base (of prism) out
    base out
    behavior objective
    body odor
    Bolton (craniometric point) (*See
        also* B, bb, Bo, BP)
    bowel (*See also* bo)
    bowel obstruction
    bowels open
    bronchiolitis obliterans
    buccoocclusal
B&O
    belladonna and opium
B/O
    because of
Bo
    Bolton point (*See also* B, bb, BO,
        BP)
bo
    bowel (*See also* BO)

BOA
    behavioral observation audiometry
    born on arrival
    born out of asepsis
BOB
    ball on back
BOBA
    beta-oxybutyric acid
BOBV
    Bobaya virus
BOC
    beats of clonus
    blood oxygen capacity
    butyloxycarbonyl
BOD
    bilateral orbital decompression
    biochemical oxygen demand
    biological oxygen demand
    borderline (*See also* BORD)
    brachymorphism, onychodysplasia,
        dysphalangism
    braided occlusion device
    burden of disease
Bod units
    Bodansky units
BOE
    bilateral otitis externa
BOEA
    ethyl biscoumacetate
BOF
    branchiooculofacial
BOFA
    beta-oncofetal antigen
BOFS
    branchiooculofacial syndrome
BOH
    bundle of His (*See also* BH)
bol
    bolus
BOLD
    blood oxygenation level-dependent
BOLT
    Basic Occupational Literacy Test
BolVX
    Boletus virus X
BOM
    benign ovarian mass
    bilateral otitis media
BOMA
    bilateral otitis media, acute
BOME
    bilateral otitis media with effusion

NOTES

BONG
> body oscillation neuromuscular gain

BOO
> bladder outlet obstruction
> buccinator-orbicularis oris

BOOP
> bronchiolitis obliterans-organizing
>   pneumonia

BOP
> bilateral occipitoparietal
> bromooxyprogesterone
> Buffalo orphan prototype (virus)

BOPP
> boronated porphyrin

BOR
> basal optic root
> before time of operation
> bowels open regularly
> branchiootorenal (syndrome)

BORD
> borderline (*See also* BOD)

BORR
> blood oxygen release rate

BORV
> Boraceia virus

BOS
> base of skull
> Boix-Ochoa score
> bronchiolitis obliterans syndrome

bos 1–10
> *Bos* adenovirus 1–10

BOSS
> Becker orthopaedic spinal system

BOT
> base of tongue
> botulinum toxin

bot
> botany
> bottle

BOTV
> Botambi virus

BOU
> burning on urination

BOUV
> Bouboui virus

BOW
> bag of waters

bowel prep
> bowel preparation

BOWI
> bag of waters intact

BOWR
> bag of waters ruptured

BOZR
> back optic zone radius

BP
> bacillary peliosis
> back pressure

> barometric pressure
> basic protein
> bathroom privileges (*See also* BRP)
> bed pan
> before present
> behavior pattern
> Bell palsy
> benzoyl peroxide
> benzpyrene
> bioequivalence problem
> biotic potential
> biparietal
> biphenyl
> bipolar
> birthplace
> bladder pressure
> blood pressure (*See also* BL PR, bl
>   pr)
> body part
> body plethysmography
> boiling point (*See also* bp)
> Bolton point (*See also* B, bb, BO,
>   Bo)
> borderline personality
> British Pharmacopoeia (*See also*
>   PB)
> bronchopleural
> bronchopulmonary
> buccopulpal
> bullous pemphigus
> bypass

BPI
> bipolar affective disorder, type 1

bp
> base pair
> boiling point (*See also* BP)

BPA
> *Bauhinia purpura* agglutinin
> blood pressure assembly
> boronophenylalanine
> bovine plasma albumin
> bronchopulmonary aspergillosis
> bullous pemphigoid antigen
> burst-promoting activity

BPB
> biliopancreatic bypass
> black-pigmented bacteria
> bone-patellar ligament-bone (*See
>   also* BPLB)
> bone-patellar tendon-bone (*See also*
>   BPTB)
> brachial plexus block
> bromphenol blue

BPC
> Behavior Problem Checklist
> benign pheochromocytoma
> bile phospholipid concentration

B

British Pharmaceutical Codex
bronchial provocation challenge
BPCC
  bilateral percutaneous cervical
    cordotomy
BPCF
  bronchopleurocutaneous fistula
BPCHI
  benign pheochromocytoma with
    histological invasion
BPD
  biparietal diameter
  bipolar disorder (type 1, 2)
  blood pressure decreased
  borderline personality disorder
  bronchopulmonary dysplasia (*See
    also* BPd)
BPd
  bronchopulmonary dysplasia (*See
    also* BPD)
  diastolic blood pressure
BPE
  bacterial phosphatidylethanolamine
  basal promoter element
  benign prostatic enlargement
BPEC
  benign partial epilepsy with
    centrotemporal spike
  bipolar electrocoagulation
BPEIS, BPES
  blepharophimosis, ptosis, epicanthus
    inversus syndrome
BPF
  bradykinin potentiating factor
  Brazilian purpuric fever
  bronchopleural fistula
  burst-promoting factor
BPG
  benign paraganglioma
  benzathine penicillin G
  blood pressure gauge
  bypass graft
BPH
  benign prostatic hyperplasia
  benign prostatic hypertrophy
BPh
  buccopharyngeal
Bph
  bacteriopheophytin
BPI
  bactericidal/permeability-increasing
    protein

Basic Personality Inventory
beef-pork insulin
bipolar illness
Bipolar Psychological Inventory
blood pressure increased
brachial plexus injury
Brief Pain Inventory
BPL
  benign proliferative lesion
  benzylpenicilloyl polylysine (*See
    also* BPO)
  beta-propiolactone
  bone phosphate of lime
BP lar
  blood pressure, left arm
BPLB
  bone-patellar ligament-bone (*See
    also* BPB)
B-PLL
  B-cell prolymphocytic leukemia
BPLN
  bilateral pelvic lymph node
BPLND
  bilateral pelvic lymph node
    dissection
BPM, bpm
  beats per minute
  bipiperidyl mustard
  births per minute
  blood perfusion monitor
  blood pressure monitor
  breaths per minute
  brompheniramine maleate
BPMS
  blood plasma measuring system
BPN
  bacitracin, polymyxin B, and
    neomycin sulfate
  brachial plexus neuropathy
BPO
  basal pepsin output
  benign prostatic obstruction
  benzylpenicilloyl polylysine (*See
    also* BPL)
  bilateral partial oophorectomy
  bile phospholipid output
BPOP
  bizarre parosteal osteochondromatous
    proliferation
BPP
  binding protein protease
  biophysical profile

NOTES

BPP *(continued)*
Bloembergen, Purcell, and Pound (theory)
bovine pancreatic polypeptide
bradykinin potentiating peptide
breast parenchymal pattern

BP&P
blood pressure and pulse

BPPN
benign paroxysmal positioning nystagmus

BPPP
bilateral pedal pulses present

BP,P,R,T
blood pressure, pulse, respiration, and temperature

BPPV
benign paroxysmal positional vertigo

BPQ
Berne pain questionnaire

BPR
blood per rectum
blood pressure recorder
blood production rate

BP rar
blood pressure, right arm

BPRS
Brief Psychiatric Rating Scale

BPRS-C
Brief Psychiatric Rating Scale for Children

BPS
beats per second
bilateral partial salpingectomy
biophysical profile score
biophysical profile scoring
brain protein solvent
breaths per second
bronchopulmonary sequestration

BPs
blood pressure, systolic

BPSA
bronchopulmonary segmental artery

BPSD
bronchopulmonary segmental drainage

BPSV
bovine papular stomatitis

BPT
benign paroxysmal torticollis

BPTB
bone-patellar tendon-bone (*See also* BPB)

bPTH
bovine parathyroid hormone

BPTI
bovine pancreatic trypsin inhibitor
brachial plexus traction injury

BPV
balloon pulmonary valvuloplasty
benign paroxysmal vertigo
benign positional vertigo
bioprosthetic valve
bovine papillomavirus

BP(VET)
British Pharmacopoeia (Veterinary)

Bq
becquerel (SI unit of radionuclide activity)

BQC sol
2,6-dibromoquinone-4-chlorimide solution

BQSV
Barranqueras virus

BR
barrier-reared (experimental animals)
baseline recovery
bathroom
bedrest
bedside rounds
benzodiazepine receptor
bilirubin (*See also* BIL, bil, bili, bilirub, Bu)
biologic response
blink reflex
bowel rest
brachialis
branchial
breathing rate
breathing reserve
bronchial
bronchial responsiveness
bronchitis (*See also* Br)
bronchus
brown (*See also* br, Br)
buccal root

Br
breech
bregma
bridge
bromine
bronchitis (*See also* BR)
brown (*See also* BR, br)
brucellosis

br
boiling range
brachial (*See also* brach)
branch
breath (*See also* brth)
broiled
brother (*See also* B, BRO)
brown (*See also* BR, Br)

BRA
    beta-resorcylic acid
    bilateral renal agenesis
    bone-resorbing activity
    brain (*See also* b)
    brain-reactive antibody

bra
    brassiere

BRAC
    basic rest-activity cycle

brach
    brachial (*See also* br)

brady
    bradycardia

brady-tachy
    bradycardia-tachycardia (syndrome)
    (*See also* BTS)

BRAFE
    brachial, radial, femoral

BRAO
    branch retinal artery occlusion

BRAP
    burst of rapid atrial pacing

BrAP
    brachial artery pressure

BRAT
    bananas, rice, applesauce, toast
    (diet)
    bananas, rice cereal, applesauce,
    toast (diet)

BRATT
    bananas, rice, applesauce, tea, toast
    (diet)

BRB
    blood-retinal barrier
    bright red blood

BRBC
    bovine red blood cell

BRBPR, BRBR
    bright red blood per rectum

br bx
    breast biopsy (*See also* BB, B Bx)

Brc
    bromocriptine (*See also* BCR, BRO)

BRCA
    breast cancer antigen

BRCA1
    breast cancer gene 1

BRCA2
    breast cancer gene 2

BRCM
    below right costal margin

BRD
    baroreflex dysfunction
    bladder retraining drill

BRDS
    Blessed-Roth Dementia Scale

BrDu, BrdU, BrdUrd
    bromodeoxyuridine
    5-bromodeoxyuridine

BRE
    benign rolandic epilepsy

BRET
    bretylium tosylate

BRFSS
    Behavioral Risk Factor Surveillance
    System

BRH
    benign recurrent hematuria

BRI
    Basic Reading Inventory
    Bio-Research Index

BRIC
    benign recurrent intrahepatic
    cholestasis

Brit
    British

BRJ
    brachial radialis jerk

brkf
    breakfast (*See also* bkf, bkfst, bkft)

BRM
    biologic response modifier

BrM
    breast milk

BRMP
    Biological Response Modification
    Program

BRMV
    Berrimah virus

BRN
    Board of Registered Nursing

BRO
    bromocriptine (*See also* BCR, Brc)
    bronchoscopy (*See also* bronch)
    brother (*See also* B, br)

BRO LAC
    bromothymol blue lactose

BROM
    back range of motion

brom
    bromide

B

NOTES

bron
    bronchi
    bronchial
bronch
    bronchoscope
    bronchoscopy (*See also* BRO)
BRP
    bathroom privileges (*See also* BP)
    bilirubin production
BRP-2
    Behavior Rating Profile, Second
        Edition
Brph
    bronchophony
BRR
    baroreceptor reflex response
BRRS
    Bannayan-Riley-Ruvalcaba syndrome
BR RVO
    branch retinal vein occlusion (*See
        also* BRVO)
BR S
    breath sounds (*See also* BS, bs)
BRS
    baroreceptor reflex sensitivity
    baroreflex sensitivity
    Behavior Rating Scale
BRSA
    borderline-resistant *Staphylococcus
        aureus*
brth
    breath (*See also* br)
B-RTO
    balloon-occluded retrograde
        transvenous obliteration
BrU
    bromouracil
BRVO
    branch retinal vein occlusion (*See
        also* BR RVO)
BRW
    Brown-Roberts-Wells (stereotactic
        system)
BRW-PB
    Brown-Roberts-Wells phantom base
BS
    Bacillus subtilis
    barium swallow (*See also* BaS,
        b.s.)
    Bartter syndrome
    bedside
    before sleep
    Behçet syndrome
    Bennett seal
    bilateral symmetric
    bile salt
    Binet-Simon (test)
    bismuth subgallate

    bismuth subsalicylate
    blood sugar (*See also* BlS)
    Bloom syndrome
    borderline schizophrenia
    bowel sounds (*See also* bs)
    breaking strength
    breath sounds (*See also* BR S, bs)
    British Standard
    buffered saline
B&S
    Bartholin and Skene (glands)
    Brown and Sharp (suture)
bs
    bedside
    bowel sounds (*See also* BS)
    breath sounds (*See also* BR S, BS)
b.s.
    barium swallow (*See also* BaS, BS)
BSA
    beef serum albumin
    benzenesulfonic acid
    bismuth-sulfite agar
    bis-trimethylsilylacetamide
    body surface area
    bovine serum albumin
    bowel sounds active
    broad-spectrum antibiotic
BSAB
    Balthazar Scales of Adaptive
        Behavior
BSAG
    Bristol Social Adjustment Guides
BSAP
    bone-specific alkaline phosphatase
    brief, small, abundant (motor-unit
        action) potential
BSAPP
    brief, small, abundant, polyphasic
        potential
BSB
    bedside bag
    body surface burned
BSBC
    buffer-soluble binding component
BS=BL
    breath sounds equal bilaterally
BSBV
    Bushbush virus
BSC
    basosquamous carcinoma
    bedside care
    bedside commode
    bench scale calorimeter
    bile salt concentrate
    bile salt concentration
    Biological Stain Commission
    biosafety cabinet
    burn scar contracture

B

BSCC
basaloid squamous cell carcinoma
BSCP
bovine spinal cord protein
BSCT
breast stimulation contraction test
BSD
baby soft diet
bedside drainage
BSDT
Bryant-Schwan Design Test
BSE
bacillus species enzyme
behavior summarized evaluation
bilateral, symmetrical, equal
bovine spongiform encephalopathy
breast self-examination
BSEP
bile salt export pump
brainstem evoked potential
BSER, BSERA
brainstem evoked response
(audiometry)
BSF
backscatter factor
basal skull fracture
B-lymphocyte stimulatory factor
busulfan
BSFR
basal secretory flow rate
BSG
brachioskeletogenital (syndrome)
BSGA
beta-hemolytic streptococcus group
A
BSH
boron sulfhydryl
broad-spectrum heater
BSI
Behavior Status Inventory
bloodstream infection
body substance isolation
borderline syndrome index
bound serum iron
brainstem injury
Brief Symptom Inventory
BSID
Bayley Scales of Infant
Development
BSID-II
Bayley Scales of Infant
Development-II

BSK
Barbour-Stoenner-Kelly (medium)
BSL
benign symmetric lipomatosis
biosafety level
blood sugar level
BSLE
bullous systemic lupus
erythematosus
BSLM
body surface laplacian mapping
BSM
bile salt metabolism
Bilingual Syntax Measure (Test)
BSM II
Bilingual Syntax Measure II (Test)
BSN
bowel sounds normal
BSNA
bowel sounds normal and active
BSNT
breasts soft and nontender
BSO
bilateral sagittal osteotomy
bilateral salpingo-oophorectomy
bilateral serous otitis
bile salt output
buthionine sulfoximine
BSOM
bilateral serous otitis media
BSP
body segment parameter
bone sialoprotein
bromsulfophthalein (liver function)
BSp
bronchospasm
BSPA
bowel sounds present and active
BSPM
body surface potential mapping
BSPS
Brief Social Phobia Scale
BSQ
Behavior Style Questionnaire
BSQV
Bussuquara virus
BSR
basal skin resistance
blood sedimentation rate
bowel sounds regular
brain stimulation reinforcement

NOTES

89

BSRI
> Bem Sex Role Inventory

BSS
> balanced saline solution
> balanced salt solution
> bedside scale
> Bernard-Soulier syndrome
> bismuth subsalicylate
> black silk suture
> buffered saline solution
> buffered single substrate

BSSE
> bile salt-stimulated esterase

BSSI
> Basic School Skills Inventory

BSSL
> bile salt-stimulated lipase

BSSO
> bilateral sagittal split osteotomy

BSSRO
> bilateral sagittal split ramus
> osteotomies

BST
> bedside testing
> biceps semitendinosus
> blood serologic test
> breast stimulation test
> brief stimulus therapy

BSTFA
> bis-trimethylsilyltrifluoroacetamide

BSU
> Bartholin, Skene, and urethral
> (glands) (See also BUS)
> basic structural unit
> British Standard Unit

BSV
> binocular single vision

BSW
> Bachelor of Social Work

BSYN
> biphasic synovial sarcoma

BT
> *Bacillus thuringiensis*
> base of tongue
> bedtime
> bitemporal
> bitemporal (diameter of fetal head)
> bitrochanteric
> bituberous
> bladder tumor
> bleeding time (See also bld tm,
> BLEED, BLT)
> blood transfusion
> blood type
> blood typing
> blue tetrazolium
> blue tongue
> body temperature

> borderline tuberculoid
> bovine turbinate (cells)
> brain tumor
> breast tumor
> bulbotruncal

BTA
> biological terrain assessment
> bladder tumor antigen
> botulinum toxin A
> brief tone audiometry
> N-benzoyl-1-tyrosine amide

BTB
> breakthrough bleeding (See also
> BB)
> bromothymol blue

BTBC
> Boehm Test of Basic Concepts

BTBV
> beat-to-beat variability

BTC
> basal temperature chart
> betacellulin
> bilateral tubal coagulation
> bladder tumor check
> blood temperature chart
> by the clock

BTD
> bolus thermodilution

BTDS
> benzoylthiamine disulfide

BTE
> Baltimore Therapeutic Equipment
> (work simulator)
> behind the ear
> behind-the-ear (hearing aid)
> bovine thymus extract

BTEA
> Boston Test for Examining
> Aphasia

BTF
> blenderized tube feeding

BTG
> beta-thromboglobulin

BTg
> bovine trypsinogen

BTHI
> Brief Test of Head Injury

BThU
> British thermal unit (See also BTU)

BTI
> biliary tract infection
> bitubal interruption

BTi
> biomagnetometer

BTK
> Bruton tyrosine kinase

BTKV
> Boteke virus

BTL
  bilateral tubal ligation
BTLS
  basic trauma life support
BTM
  benign tertian malaria
  bilateral tympanic membranes
BTMSA
  bis-trimethylsilacetylene
BTO
  balloon test occlusion
  bilateral tubal occlusion
BTP
  biliary tract pain
BT-PABA
  benzoyl-tyrosyl-paraaminobenzoic
    acid
BTPD
  body temperature, pressure, dry
BTPS
  body temperature, ambient pressure,
    and saturated with water vapor
    (gas)
BTR
  Bezold-type reflex
  biceps tendon reflex
  bladder tumor recheck
  bovine trypsin
  buccal triangular ridge
BTS
  bioptic telescopic spectacle
  bithional sulfoxide
  Blalock-Taussig shunt
  blood transfusion service
  blue toe syndrome
  bradycardia-tachycardia syndrome
    (*See also* brady-tachy)
BTSH, bTSH
  bovine thyroid-stimulating hormone
BTU
  British thermal unit (*See also*
    BThU)
BTV 1–24
  bluetongue virus 1–24
BTX
  bactrachotoxin
  benzene, toluene, and xylene
  botulinum toxin
  brevotoxin
  bungarotoxin
BTZ
  benzothiazepine

BU
  base (of prism) up
  base-up prism
  below the umbilicus
  Bethesda unit
  biologic unit
  blood urea
  Bodansky unit
  bromouracil
  burn unit
  busulfan
Bu
  bilirubin (*See also* BIL, bil, bili,
    bilirub, BR)
  butyl
BUA
  blood uric acid
  bone ultrasound attenuation
buc, bucc
  buccal
BUD
  budesonide
BUDS
  bilateral upper dorsal
    sympathectomy
BUE
  both upper extremities
  built-up edge
BUEC
  balloon uterine elevator cannula
BUEV
  Buenaventura virus
BUF
  Buffalo (rat)
BUFA
  baby up for adoption
BUG
  buccal ganglion
BUI
  brain uptake index
BULIT
  bulimia test
BULL
  buccal of upper and lingual of
    lower
bull.
  bulletin
  let it boil [L. *bulliat*]
BUN
  blood urea nitrogen
  bunion

NOTES

B

bun br
  bundle branch
BUN/C, BUN/CR, BUN/Cr
  blood urea nitrogen/creatinine
    (ratio)
BUNV
  Bunyamwera virus
BUO
  bilateral ureteral obstruction
  bilirubin of undetermined origin
  bleeding of undetermined origin
  bruising of undetermined origin
BUQ
  both upper quadrants
BUR
  backup rate (ventilator)
bur
  bureau
Burd
  Burdick (suction)
BUS
  Bartholin, urethral, and Skene
    (glands) (See also BSU)
  busulfan
BUSEG
  Bartholin, urethral, and Skene
    (glands), and external genitalia
BUSTOP
  Burke Stroke Time-Oriented profile
But
  butyrate
  butyric (acid)
but.
  butter [L. butyrum]
BUTV
  Buttonwillow virus
BUV
  backup ventilation
BV
  bacitracin V
  bacterial vaginitis
  bacterial vaginosis
  balloon valvuloplasty
  billion volts
  biologic value
  blood vessel
  blood volume (See also BLV, BlV)
  bronchovesicular
  buccoversion
  bulboventricular
BVA
  best-corrected visual acuity
  bioimpedance venous analysis
BVAD
  biventricular assist device
BVAS
  Birmingham Vasculitis Activity
    Score

BVAT
  Binocular Visual Acuity Test
BVC
  British Veterinary Codex
BVD
  bovine viral diarrhea
BVD-MD
  bovine viral diarrhea mucosal
    disease
BVDs
  underwear
BVDT
  Brief Vestibular Disorientation Test
BVDV1,2
  bovine viral diarrhea virus 1 & 2
BVE
  binocular visual efficiency
  biventricular enlargement
  blood vessel endothelium
  blood volume expander
  blood volume expansion
BVFI
  bilateral vocal fold (cord)
    immobility
BVFP
  bilateral vocal fold (cord) paralysis
BVH
  biventricular hypertrophy
BVI
  blood vessel invasion
BVL
  bilateral vas ligation
BVM
  bag-valve-mask (See also B-V-M)
  bronchovascular markings
B-V-M
  bag-valve-mask (See also BVM)
BVMOT
  Bender Visual-Motor Gestalt Test
BVO
  branch vein occlusion
  brominated vegetable oil
BVP
  back vertex power
  blood vessel prosthesis
  blood volume pulse
  burst of ventricular pacing
BVR
  baboon virus replication
  balloon valvuloplasty registry
  basal vein of Rosenthal
BVRO
  bilateral vertical ramus osteotomy
BVRT
  Benton Visual Retention Test
BVRT-R
  Benton Visual Retention Test,
    Revised

BVS
>biventricular support
>blanked ventricular sense

BVT
>bilateral ventilation tubes

BVU
>bromoisovalerylurea

BW
>bacteriologic warfare
>bandwidth
>bed wetting
>below waist
>biological warfare
>biologic weapon
>birth weight (*See also* BWt)
>bite-wing (radiograph)
>bladder washout
>blood Wassermann
>body water
>body weight (*See also* bw)

B&W
>black and white (milk of magnesia and cascara extract)

bw
>body weight (*See also* BW)

BWA
>bedwetter admission

BWAS
>Barron-Welsh Art Scale

BWAV
>Bwamba virus

BWD
>bacillary white diarrhea

BWFI
>bacteriostatic water for injection

BWGA
>birth weight for gestational age

BWM
>Bad Wildungen Metz (system)

BWS
>battered-woman syndrome

BWST
>black widow spider toxin

BWSV
>black widow spider venom

BWt
>birth weight (*See also* BW)

bwyv
>beet western yellows virus

BX, Bx
>biopsy

BXO
>balanitis xerotica obliterans

BZ, bz
>benzodiazepine (*See also* BZD, BZDZ)
>benzoyl (*See also* Bzl)

BZA
>benzylamine

BZD, BZDZ
>benzodiazepine (*See also* BZ, bz)

BZK
>benzalkonium chloride

Bzl
>benzoyl (*See also* BZ)

BZLZ
>bian zheng lun zhi (pattern diagnosis)

BZQ
>benzquinamide

BZS
>Bannayan-Zonna syndrome

Bz-Ty-PABA
>benzoyltyrosyl-*p*-aminobenzoic acid (test)

NOTES

B

C

ascorbic acid (vitamin C)
bruised [L. *contusus*] (*See also* cont.)
calcitonin-forming (cell)
calculus
calorie (large) (*See also* Cal)
canine (tooth) (*See also* c)
capacitance
carbon
carrier
cast
cathodal
cathode (*See also* CA, cath)
Catholic
Caucasian (*See also* cauc)
cell
Celsius (temperature scale)
centesimal dilution
centigrade
central (*See also* CENT, cent.)
central (electrode placement in electroencephalography)
cerebrospinal (fluid)
certified (*See also* CRT)
cervical (spine)
cesarean (section)
chest (precordial lead in electrocardiography)
cholesterol (*See also* CH, Ch, CHOL, chol, chol.)
chromosome (banding)
class
clear (*See also* cler)
clearance rate (renal)
clonus
Clostridium
closure
clubbing
coarse (bacterial colonies)
cocaine
coefficient
colored (guinea pig)
color sense
complement
complete (*See also* cpl)
complex
compliance
component
compound [L. *compositus*] (*See also* CO, comp, compd, CP, cpd)
concentration (*See also* c, conc, concentr)
conditioned
conditioning
condyle
constant
consultation
contact (*See also* c)
content
contraction (*See also* contr, contrx, CTX, CTXN, Cx)
control
conventionally reared (experimental animal)
convergence
cornea
cornu
correct
cortex (*See also* cort)
costa (rib)
coulomb (*See also* Q, coul)
creatinine (*See also* CR, cr, cre)
cup (*See also* c)
cuspid (secondary dentition)
cuticular
cyanosis
cylinder (*See also* cyl)
cylindrical lens (*See also* cyl)
cytidine
cytochrome
cytosine
heat capacity
hundred [L. *centum*] (*See also* h)
large calorie (*See also* Cal)
molar heat capacity
rib [L. *costa*]
velocity of light
velocity of sound of blood

3C

craniocerebellocardiac

C₃

Collins solution

C-6

hexamethonium

C-10

decamethonium

¹¹C, C-11

carbon-11

¹²C, C-12

carbon-12

¹³C, C-13

carbon-13

¹⁴C, C-14

carbon-14 (isotope)

°C

degree Celsius

c

about [L. *circa*] (*See also* ca)
calorie (small) (*See also* cal)

c *(continued)*
candle (*See also* ca)
canine (tooth) (*See also* C)
capacity (*See also* cap.)
capillary blood (subscript)
carat
centi- (prefix)
circumference
concentration (*See also* C, conc, concentr)
contact (*See also* C)
cubic (*See also* cu)
culture [medium]
cup (*See also* C)
cuspid (primary dentition)
cycle
cyclic
meal [L. *cibus*]
molar concentration
small calorie (*See also* cal)
specific heat capacity

c̄
with [L. *cum*] (*See also* W, w/)

CI, CII, CIII, CIV, CV
DEA controlled substances schedules I through V

CA
anterior commissure [L. *commissura anterior*]
calcium antagonist
California (rabbit)
cancer (*See also* Can)
cancer antigen
caproic acid
capsid
carbohydrate antigen
carbonic anhydrase
carcin
carcinoma
cardiac-apnea (monitor)
cardiac arrest
cardiac arrhythmia
carotid artery
cast
catecholamine (*See also* CAT)
catecholaminergic
cathode (*See also* C, cath)
Caucasian adult
celiac artery
celiac axis
cellulose acetate
central apnea
cerebral aqueduct
cerebral atrophy
chemotactic activity (*See also* CTA)
child abuse
chloroamphetamine
cholic acid

chorioamnionitis
chronic anovulation
chronologic age
citric acid
clotting assay
coagglutination (test)
coefficient of absorption
cold agglutinin
collagen antigen
collagenolytic activity
colloid antigen
commissural associated
common antigen
community acquired
compressed air
conceptional age
conditioned abstinence
conditioned air
condyloma acuminatum
coronary angioplasty
coronary arrest
coronary artery
corpus albicans
corpus amylaceum
cortisone acetate
cricoid arch
croup-associated (virus)
cytotoxic antibody

C&A
conscious and alert

Ca
calcium
can

C3a
C3 anaphylatoxin

ca
about [L. *circa*] (*See also* c)
candle (*See also* c)

CA II
carbonic anhydrase II

CA19-9, CA 19-9
cancer antigen 19-9

^{45}Ca, Ca-45
calcium-45 (radioisotope)

CA125, CA-125
cancer antigen 125
cancer antigen-125 (test)

^{47}Ca, Ca-47
calcium-47

CAA
cardiac allograft atherosclerosis
carotid audiofrequency analysis
cerebral amyloid angiopathy
chloracetaldehyde
circulating anodic antigen
coloanal anastomosis
complementary and alternative approach

computer-assisted assessment
constitutional aplastic anemia
coronary artery aneurysm
crystalline amino acid

CAAS
Children's Attention and
Adjustment Survey

CAAT
computer-assisted axial tomography

CAB
captive air bubble
catheter-associated bacteriuria
cellulose acetate butyrate
combined androgen blockade
Comprehensive Ability Battery
coronary artery bypass

CABA
child and adolescent burden
assessment

CABBS
computer-assisted blood background
subtraction

CaBF
carotid blood flow

CABG
coronary artery bypass graft
coronary artery bypass grafting

CABGS
coronary artery bypass graft
surgery

CaBI
calcium bone index

CaBP
calcium-binding protein

CABS
chronic alcoholic brain syndrome
coronary artery bypass surgery

CAC
cancer (malignant) cell
cardiac-accelerator center
cardiac arrest code
carotid artery canal
chronic active cirrhosis
circulating anticoagulant
cold air challenge
comprehensive ambulatory care
coronary artery calcification
cryptogenic autoimmune cirrhosis

CA/C
convergence accommodation (ratio)

CaCC
cathodal-closure contraction (*See
also* CCC)

CACh
cold air challenge

CACI
computer-assisted continuous
infusion

CaCO₃
calcium carbonate

CACS
cancer, anorexia, cachexia syndrome

CaCx
cancer of cervix

CAD
cadaver
cadaver donor
cadaveric
chronic actinic dermatitis
chronic airway disease
cold agglutinin disease
compressed-air disease
computer-aided diagnosis
computer-assisted diagnosis
congenital abduction deficiency
coronary artery disease

CADASIL
cerebral autosomal dominant
arteriopathy with subcortical
infarcts and leukoencephalopathy

CAD/CAM
computer-aided design/computer-
aided manufacturing
contoured adducted
trochanteric/controlled-alignment
method

CADD
central-axis-depth-dose

CADI
computer-assisted diabetic instruction
(system)

CADL
Communicative Abilities in Daily
Living

CADT
Communication Abilities Diagnostic
Test

CaDTe
cathodal-duration tetanus

CAE
caprine arthritis-encephalitis
cefuroxime axetil (suspension)

NOTES

CAE *(continued)*
  cellulose acetate electrophoresis
  chloroacetate esterase
  contingent aftereffects
  coronary artery embolization
CaE
  calcium excretion
CAEC
  cardiac arrhythmia evaluation center
CAECS
  chronic anterior exertional
    compartment syndrome
CaEDTA, CaEdTA
  calcium disodium edetate
  calcium disodium
    ethylenediaminetetraacetate
  edathamil calcium disodium
CAEP
  chronotropic exercise assessment
    protocol
  cortical auditory evoked potential
CAER
  caerulein
  cortical auditory evoked response
CAEV
  caprine arthritis encephalitis virus
CAF
  cell adhesion factor
  chronic atrial fibrillation
  citric acid fermenters
  contract administration fees
  coronary artery fistula
CaF
  correction of area factor
caf
  caffeine
CAFAS
  Child and Adolescent Functional
    Assessment Scale
CAFET
  computer-aided fluency
    establishment trainer
CAFF
  controlled atrial fibrillation/flutter
CAFT
  Clinitron air-fluidized therapy
CAG
  cholangiogram
  cholangiography
  chronic atrophic gastritis
  continuous ambulatory gamma
    globulin (infusion)
  coronary angiogram
  coronary angiography
  coronary arteriography
CaG
  calcium gluconate

CagA, cagA
  cytotoxin-associated gene (product)
    A
CAGE
  cut down (on drinking), annoyance,
    guilt (about drinking), (need for)
    eyeopener (Ewing & Rooss four-
    question alcohol screening)
CAGEIN
  catheter-guided endoscopic
    intubation
CAH
  Camber axis hinge
  central alveolar hypoventilation (*See
    also* CAHV)
  chronic active hepatitis
  chronic aggressive hepatitis
  combined atrial hypertrophy
  congenital adrenal hyperplasia
  congenital adrenogenital hyperplasia
  cryptogenic autoimmune hepatitis
  cyanacetic acid hydrazide
CaHA
  calcium hydroxyapatite
CAHB
  chronic active hepatitis B
CAHC
  chronic active hepatitis with
    cirrhosis
CAHD
  coronary arteriosclerotic heart
    disease
  coronary atherosclerotic heart
    disease
CAHM
  complex atypical
    hyperplasia/metaplasia
CAHMR
  cataract, hypertrichosis, mental
    retardation
CAHS
  central alveolar hypoventilation
    syndrome
CAHV
  central alveolar hypoventilation (*See
    also* CAH)
CAI
  carbonic anhydrase inhibitor
  Career Assessment Inventory
  catheter-associated infection
  complete androgen insensitivity
  computer-assisted instruction
  cortical arousal index
  Cultural Attitude Inventory
Ca ION
  calcium, ionized

CAIS
complete androgen insensitivity syndrome

CAIV
Caimito virus
cold-attenuated intranasal influenza vaccine

CAIV-T
cold-adapted influenza virus vaccine, trivalent

CAL
café au lait
calcium (test)
calculated average life
callus
calories
chronic airflow limitation
computer-assisted learning
coracoacromial ligament
coronary artery lesion

Cal
calorie (large) (*See also* C)

cal
caliber
calorie
calorie (small) (*See also* c)

Calb, C$_{alb}$, C/alb/
albumin clearance

calc
calculate
calculated

calcif
calcification

cal ct
calorie count

CALD
chronic active liver disease

CALGB
cancer and leukemia group B

CALH
chronic active lupoid hepatitis

calib
calibrated

cal/kg day
calories per kilogram per day

CALLA, cALLA
common acute lymphoblastic leukemia antigen
common acute lymphocytic leukemia antigen

CALM
café-au-lait macule

cal/oz
calories per ounce

CALP
calponin

CALS
Checklist of Adaptive Living Skills

CAM
calf aortic microsome
carminomycin
cell adhesion molecule
cellular adhesion molecule
child-adult mist
chorioallantoic membrane
circulating adhesion molecule
complementary and alternative medicine
computer-assisted (or aided) myelography
Confusion Assessment Method
contralateral axillary metastasis
controlled ankle motion
cystic adenomatous malformation

C$_{am}$
amylase clearance

CaM
calmodulin

CAMAC
computer-automated measurement and control

CAMAK
cataract, microcephaly, arthrogryposis, kyphosis

CAMDEX
Cambridge Mental Disorders in Elderly Examination

CAMFAK
cataract, microcephaly, failure to thrive, kyphoscoliosis

CaMKII
calcium-calmodulin kinase II

CaM-kinase
calmodulin-dependent protein kinase

CAML
calcium-signal modulating cyclophilin B ligand
Coarticulation Assessment in Meaningful Language

CA monitor
cardiac-apnea monitor

CAMP
Childhood Asthma Management Program

NOTES

CAMP *(continued)*
    Christie-Atkins-Munch-Petersen (test)
    computer-assisted menu planning
    concentration of adenosine
        monophosphate
cAMP
    cyclic adenosine monophosphate
        (*See also* AMP-c)
    cyclic 3′,5′-adenosine
        monophosphate
    cyclic adenosine 3′,5′-
        monophosphate
CAMS
    computer-assisted monitoring system
CAMU
    cardiac ambulatory monitoring unit
    coronary arrhythmia monitoring unit
CAMV
    congenital anomaly of mitral valve
CaMV
    cauliflower mosaic virus
CAN
    chronic allograft nephropathy
    continuous albuterol nebulization
    cord (umbilical) around neck
CA/N
    child abuse and neglect
Can
    cancer (*See also* CA)
can.
    cannabis
CANA
    circulation antineuronal antibody
CANC, canc
    cancelled
C-ANCA, cANCA, c-ANCA
    cytoplasmic antineutrophil
        cytoplasmic antibody
CANCERLIT
    Cancer Literature
CANE
    computer-assisted neuroendoscopy
CANP
    calcium-activated neutral protease
C-ANP
    C-type atrial natriuretic peptide
CANS
    central auditory nervous system
    computer-assisted neurosurgical
        navigational system
CANV
    Caninde virus
CAO
    chronic airflow obstruction
    chronic airway obstruction
    coronary artery obstruction
Ca$_{O2}$
    arterial oxygen concentration

CaOC
    cathodal opening contraction (*See
        also* COC)
CaOCl
    cathodal opening clonus (*See also*
        COC, COCL)
CAOD
    coronary artery occlusive disease
CAOM
    chronic adhesive otitis media
CAOS
    computer-assisted orthopedic surgery
Ca ox
    calcium oxalate (crystal)
CAP
    camptodactyly-arthropathy-pericarditis
        (syndrome)
    cancer of prostate
    capillary blood
    capsule (*See also* cap., caps.)
    captopril
    carcinoma of prostate
    carotid Amytal procedure
    catabolite (gene) activator protein
    cell attachment protein
    cellular acetate propionate
    cellulose acetate phthalate
    central apical portion
    Children's Art Project
    chloroacetophenone
    cholesteric analysis profile
    chronic alcoholic pancreatitis
    community-acquired pneumonia
    complement-activated plasma
    compound action potential
    computerized automated psycho-
        physiologic (device)
    continent anal cap
    contraction-associated protein
    coronary artery fistula
    coupled atrial pacing
    cyclic AMP-binding protein
    cystine aminopeptidase
CA4P
    combretastatin A4 prodrug
Ca/P
    calcium to phosphorus ratio
cap.
    capacity (*See also* c)
    capillary
    capsule (*See also* CAP, caps.)
CAPA
    caffeine, alcohol, pepper, and
        aspirin (diet free of)
    cancer-associated polypeptide
        antigen
    Child and Adolescent Psychiatric
        Assessment

CAPB
central auditory processing battery

CAPB gene
cancer of the prostate and brain gene

CAPC
calcium phosphate

CAPD
central auditory processing disorder
chronic ambulatory peritoneal dialysis
continuous abdominoperitoneal dialysis
continuous ambulatory peritoneal dialysis

CAPE
caffeic acid phenethyl ester
Clifton Assessment Procedures for the Elderly
continuous anatomical passive exerciser

CAPERS
Computer-Assisted Psychiatric Evaluation and Review System

CAPP
clinical appraisal of psychosocial problems

CAPPS
Current and Past Psychopathology Scales

CAPR
calcium pyrophosphate

CAPRCA
chronic, acquired, pure red cell aplasia

CAPS
caffeine, alcohol, pepper, and spicy foods (diet free of)
carbamoyl phosphate synthetase
Children of Aging Parents

caps.
capsule (*See also* CAP, cap.)

CAPSO
cautery-assisted palatal stiffening operation

CAP test
cholesteric analysis profile test

CAPV
Capim virus

CAPYA
child and adolescent psychoanalysis

CAQ
Change Agent Questionnaire
Childhood Asthma Questionnaire
Classroom Atmosphere Questionnaire
Clinical Analysis Questionnaire

CAR
cancer-associated retinopathy
cardiac ambulation routine
center of mandibular autorotation
chronic articular rheumatism
computer-assisted research
conditioned avoidance response

CaR
calcium-sensing receptor

car.
carotid

CARA
chronic aspecific respiratory ailment

CARB, carb, carbo
carbohydrate (*See also* carb, carbo, CHO)
carbonate
coronary artery bypass (graft)

CARBAM
carbamazepine (*See also* CBZ)

CARD
cardiac automatic resuscitative device
cardiology (*See also* card., cardiol)
catalyzed reporter deposition

card., cardiol
cardiac
cardiology (*See also* CARD)

CARE Act
Comprehensive AIDS Resources Emergency Act

CARIFS
Canadian Acute Respiratory Illness and Flu Scale

CAROT
carotene

CARS
Childhood Autism Rating Scale
Children's Affective Rating Scale
compensatory antiinflammatory response syndrome

CART
Classification and Regression Tree analysis

NOTES

101

CART (*continued*)
    cocaine and amphetamine regulated
        transcript
    combined antiretroviral therapy
cart
    cartilage
CARTOS
    computer-assisted reconstruction by
        tracing of serial sections
CARTT
    computer-assisted real-time
        transcription
CARV
    Caraparu virus
CAS
    calcarine sulcus
    calcific aortic stenosis
    Cancer Attitude Survey
    carbohydrate-active steroid
    cardiac adjustment scale
    cardiac surgery
    carotid angioplasty and stenting
    carotid artery stenosis
    carotid artery system
    casein
    central anticholinergic syndrome
    cerebral arteriosclerosis
    cerebral atherosclerosis
    Chemical Abstracts Service
    chronic alcohol syndrome
    chronic anovulation syndrome
    cold agglutinin syndrome
    computer-aided surgery
    Concept-Specific Anxiety Scale
    congenital alcoholic syndrome
    congenital anterior staphyloma
    congenital asplenia syndrome
    contralateral acoustic stimulation
    control adjustment strap
    coronary artery scan
    coronary artery spasm
    Creativity Attitude Survey
    Cultural Attitude Scale
Cas
    casualty
cas
    castrated
    castration
CASA
    cancer-associated serum antigen
    Child and Adolescent Services
        Assessment
    computer-assisted self-assessment
    computer-assisted semen analysis
CASE
    computer-assisted sensory
        examination

CA-series dialyzer
    cellulose acetate dialysis device
CASH
    cancer and steroid hormone
    classic abdominal Semm
        hysterectomy
    comprehensive assessment of
        symptoms and history
    cortical androgen-stimulating
        hormone
    cruciform anterior spinal
        hyperextension
CASHD
    coronary arteriosclerotic heart
        disease
    coronary atherosclerotic heart
        disease
CASL-PI MRI
    continuous arterial spin-labeled
        perfusion magnetic resonance
        imaging
CASMD
    congenital atonic sclerotic muscular
        dystrophy
CASP
    contoured anterior spinal plate
Ca-SP
    calcium urine spot (test)
CAS-REGN
    Chemical Abstracts Service Registry
        Number
CASRT
    corrected adjusted sinus (node)
        recovery time
CASS
    California soft spinal system
    computer-aided sleep system
    computer-assisted stereotactic
        surgery
    continuous aspiration of subglottic
        secretions
C-AST
    cytoplasmic aspartate
        aminotransferase
CAST
    Canterbury Alcoholism Screening
        Test
    childhood accidental spiral tibial
        (fracture)
    Children of Alcoholics Screening
        Test
    Children's Apperceptive Story-
        Telling Test
    color allergy screening test
CASTLE
    carcinoma showing thymus-like
        differentiation

CASTNO
number of casts (urinalysis)
CAT
California Achievement Test
capillary agglutination test
catalase (*See also* CAT'ase)
cataract (*See also* cat.)
catecholamine (*See also* CA)
cellular atypia
Children's Apperception Test
Children's Articulation Test
chlormerodrin accumulation test
choline acetyltransferase
chronic abdominal tympany
classified anaphylatoxin
Clinical Adaptive Test
Coblation-assisted tonsillectomy
Cognitive Abilities Test
College Ability Test
computed abdominal tomography
computed axial tomography
computer of average transients
computerized axial tomography
conventional asthma therapy
CAT/5
California Achievement Test, Fifth
Edition
cat.
catalyst
cataract (*See also* CAT)
CAT'ase
catalase (*See also* CAT)
CAT-CAM
contoured adduction trochanteric-
controlled alignment method
CATCH
cardiac abnormality, T-cell deficit,
clefting, hypocalcemia
CATCH-22
cardiac abnormality, abnormal
facies, thymic hypoplasia, cleft
palate, hypocalcemia
cat c̄ IL, cat c̄ IOL
cataract with intraocular lens
CAT/CLAMS
Clinical Adaptive Test/Clinical
Linguistic and Auditory Milestone
Scale
CAT-H
Children's Apperception Test-Human
cath
cathartic

catheter
catheterization
catheterize
cathode (*See also* C, CA)
CATS
cartilaginous autologopus thin septal
(graft)
CAT-S
Children's Apperception Test,
Supplemental
CAT scan
computerized axial tomography scan
CATT
calcium tolerance test
card agglutination trypanosomiasis
test
CATUV
Catu virus
CAU
chronic anterior uveitis
cauc
Caucasian (*See also* C)
caud
caudal (*See also* cd, CD)
caut
cauterization
CAV
cardiac allograft vasculopathy
computer-assisted ventilation
congenital absence of vagina
congenital adrenal virilism
constant angular velocity
cav
cavity
CAVB
complete atrioventricular block
CAVC
common atrioventricular canal
CAVD
cardiac allograft vascular disease
complete atrioventricular dissociation
completion, arithmetic problems,
vocabulary, following directions
(battery)
congenital absence of vas deferens
C(a-VDO$_2$), C(aVDO$_2$)
arteriovenous oxygen difference
CAVH
chronic active viral hepatitis
continuous arteriovenous
hemofiltration

NOTES

C

103

CAVH-B
chronic active viral hepatitis, type B

CAVHD
continuous arteriovenous hemodialysis

CAVHDF
continuous arteriovenous hemodiafiltration

CAVH-NAB
chronic active viral hepatitis, non-A, non-B

CA virus
croup-associated virus

CAVLT
Children's Auditory Verbal Learning Test

CAVLT-2
Children's Auditory Verbal Learning Test-2

CAVM
cerebral arteriovenous malformation

CAVO
common atrioventricular orifice

C(a-v)O$_2$
arteriovenous oxygen content difference

CAVU
continuous arteriovenous ultrafiltration

CAW
carbonaceous activated water
catalyst altered water
central airways

C$_{AW}$, C$_{aw}$
airway conductance (*See also* Gaw)

CAWO
closing abductory wedge osteotomy

CB
calcium blocker
carbenicillin
carbonated beverage
carcinoma of the breast
carotid body
catheterized bladder
ceased breathing
centroblastic
cesarean birth
chair and bed (*See also* C&B)
chest-back (*See also* C-B, C/B)
chocolate blood (agar)
chondroblast
chronic blepharitis
chronic bronchitis
circumflex branch
code blue
color blind
compensated base
conjugated bilirubin
contrast bath
coracobrachial
cord blood
cytochalasin B

C-B, C/B
chest-back (*See also* CB)

C&B
chair and bed (*See also* CB)
crown and bridge (*See also* Cr&Br)

Cb
columbium

cb
cardboard (or plastic film holder without intensifying screens)

CBA
carcinoma-bearing animal
chronic bronchitis with asthma
competitive-binding assay
congenital bronchial atresia
cost-benefit analysis
cutting balloon angioplasty
cytochemical bioassay

CBAB
complement-binding antibody

CBAT
Coulter battery

CBAVD
congenital bilateral absence of the vas deferens

CBB
communications in behavioral biology
Coomassie brilliant blue R-250 (stain)

CBBB
complete bundle branch block

CBC
Camelot Behavioral Checklist
carbenicillin (*See also* CBCN)
cerebrobuccal connective
child behavior characteristics
complete blood (cell) count (*See also* cbc)

cbc
complete blood (cell) count (*See also* CBC)

CBCL
Child Behavior Checklist
cutaneous B-cell lymphoma

CBCL/2-3
Child Behavior Checklist for ages 2-3

CBCME
computer-based continuing medical education

CBCN
carbenicillin (*See also* CBC)

CBD
    cannabidiol
    carotid body denervation
    chronic beryllium disease
    closed bladder drainage
    common bile duct
    community-based distribution

CBDC
    chronic bullous disease of
      childhood

CBDE
    common bile duct exploration

CBDL
    chronic bile duct ligation

CBDM
    common bile duct microlithiasis

CBDS
    Carcinogenesis Bioassay Data
      System
    common bile duct stone

CBE
    clinical breast examination

CBF
    capillary blood flow
    cerebral blood flow
    ciliary beat frequency
    cochlear blood flow
    coronary blood flow
    cortical blood flow

CBFS
    cerebral blood flow studies

CBFV
    cerebral blood flow velocity
    coronary blood flow velocity

CBG
    capillary blood gas
    capillary blood glucose
    cord blood gas
    coronary bypass graft
    corticosteroid-binding globulin
    cortisol-binding globulin

CBG-BC, CB-GBC
    corticosteroid-binding globulin-
      binding capacity

CBG$_v$
    corticosteroid-binding globulin
      variant

CBH
    chronic benign hepatitis
    collimated beam handpiece
    cutaneous basophilic hypersensitivity

CBI
    Career Beliefs Inventory
    continuous bladder irrigation
    convergent beam irradiation

CBIL
    conjugated bilirubin

CBIP
    Cancer Background Interference
      Procedure

CBIPBG
    Cancer Background Interference
      Procedure for Bender Gestalt

CBL
    circulating blood lymphocytes
    (umbilical) cord blood leukocytes

Cbl
    cobalamin

cbl
    chronic blood loss

CBM
    capillary basement membrane
    cryopreserved bone marrow

CBMC
    cord blood mononuclear cell

CBMMP
    chronic benign mucous membrane
      pemphigus

CBMT
    capillary basement membrane
      thickness

CBMW
    capillary basement membrane width

CBN
    cannabinol
    cellular blue nevus
    central benign neoplasm
    chronic benign neutropenia

CBOC
    completion bed occupancy care

CBP
    calcium-binding protein
    carbohydrate-binding protein
    cardiac bypass
    casual blood pressure
    chiropractic biophysics
    chlorobiphenyl
    chronic bacterial prostatitis
    chronic benign pain
    cobalamin-binding protein
    copper-binding protein
    CREB-binding protein

C

NOTES

CBPA
competitive protein-binding assay
CBPP
contagious bovine pleuropneumonia
CBPS
coronary bypass surgery
CBR
carotid bodies resected
chemical, bacteriologic, and radiologic (warfare)
chemically bound residue
complete bedrest
cord blood registry
crude birth rate
C$_{BR}$
bilirubin clearance
CBRAM
controlled partial rebreathing - anesthesia method
CBRF
child behavior rating form
CBRG
cancer biotherapy study group
CBRN
chemical, biological, radiological or nuclear (weapons)
CBS
capillary blood sugar
cervicobrachial syndrome
Charles Bonnet syndrome
child behavioral study
chronic brain syndrome
citrate-buffered saline
colloidal bismuth subcitrate
conjugated bile salts
Cruveilhier-Baumgarten syndrome
culture-bound syndrome
cystathionine beta-synthase
CBT
carotid body tumor
cognitive behavior therapy
computed body tomography
cord blood transplantation
corticobulbar tract
CBTIS
computerized bedside transfusion identification system
CBTP
Cognitive Behavior Therapy Package
CBV
capillary blood (flow) velocity
catheter balloon valvuloplasty
central blood volume
cerebral blood volume
circulating blood volume
corrected blood volume
cortical blood volume

CBV/CBF
cerebral blood volume/cerebral blood flow (ratio)
CBVD
cerebrovascular disease
CBV-DP
carbovir monophosphate
CBW
chemical and biological warfare
critical bandwidth (range of frequencies)
CBWO
closed base wedge osteotomy
CBX
computer-based examination
Cbx
core biopsy
CBZ
carbamazepine (*See also* CARBAM)
Cbz
benzyloxycarbonyl
carbobenzoxy (*See also* Z)
C-C
convexoconcave
CC
calcaneocuboid
calcium cyclamate
canal catheterization
cardiac catheterization
cardiac cycle
cardiovascular clinic
carotid-cavernous
case coordinator
caval catheterization
cell culture
cellular compartment
central compartment
cerebral commissure
cerebral concussion
cervical collar
chest circumference (*See also* cc)
chief complaint (*See also* C/C)
cholangiocarcin
cholecalciferol
chondrocalcinosis
choriocarcinoma (*See also* CCA)
chronic complainer
ciliated cell
circulatory collapse
classical conditioning
clean catch (of urine)
clinical course
clomiphene citrate
closing capacity
coefficient of correlation
colony count
colorectal cancer
columnar cells

commission-certified (stain)
complications and comorbidities
compound cathartic
computer calculated
concave (*See also* Cc, cc)
congenital cardiopathy
consumptive coagulopathy
continuing care
contractile component
contrast cystogram
coracoclavicular
cord compression
coronary collateral
corpus callosum
costochondral
Coulter counter
craniocaudal
craniocervical
creatinine clearance (*See also* C~cr~,
  CrCl, CRC)
critical care
critical condition
crus cerebri
crus communis
cubic centimeter (*See also* cc, c.c.,
  cm^3, cu cm)
cup cell
current complaint
current contents
cytochrome C
with correction (with glasses) (*See
  also* cc)

C1–C7
  cervical vertebrae 1–7
C1–C8
  cervical nerves 1–8
  complement 1–8
C1–C9
  serum complement C1–C9
C&C
  cold and clammy
  confirmed and compatible
C/C
  chief complaint (*See also* CC)
  cholecystectomy and (operative)
    cholangiogram
  complete upper and lower dentures
Cc
  concave (*See also* CC, cc)
cc
  carbon copy
  chest circumference (*See also* CC)

concave (*See also* CC, Cc)
condylocephalic
corrected
cubic centimeter (*See also* CC,
  cm^3, cu cm, c.c.)
with correction (with glasses) (*See
  also* CC)

c̄c̄
  with meals

c.c.
  cubic centimeter (*See also* cc, CC,
    cm^3, cu cm)

C-CA
CCA
  calcium channel antagonist
  central choroidal apposition
  cephalin cholesterol antigen
  chick-cell agglutination (unit)
  chimpanzee coryza agent
  choriocarcinoma (*See also* CC)
  chromated copper arsenak
  circulating cathodic antigen
  circumflex coronary artery
  colitis colon antigen
  common carotid artery
  concentrated care area
  congenital contractural
    arachnodactyly
  constitutional chromosome
    abnormality
CCA-1
  cancer cell-derived blood
    coagulating activity 1
CCAE
  Checklist for Child Abuse
    Evaluation
CCAI
  Clinical Colitis Activity Index
  Cross-Cultural Adaptability
    Inventory
CCA-IMT
  common carotid artery intima-media
    thickness
CCAM
  congenital cystic adenomatoid
    malformation
C-CAM
  cell-cell adhesion molecule
CCAP
  capsule cartilage articular
    preservation

NOTES

CCAS
Comprehensive Career Assessment Scale

CCAT
Canadian Cognitive Abilities Test
conglutinating complement absorption test

CCB
calcium channel blocker
cancellous cellular bone
conventional core biopsy

CCBV
central circulating blood volume

CCC
calcium cyanamide (carbimide) citrated
cancer care center
care-cure coordination
cathodal-closure contraction (*See also* CaCC)
central counter-adaptive changes
child care clinic
cholangiocellular carcinoma
citrated calcium carbimide
clear cell carcinoma
common carotid compression
comprehensive cancer center
comprehensive care clinic
consecutive case conference
continuing community care
craniocerebellocardiac
critical care complex
cylindrical confronting cisterna

CC&C
colony count and culture

CCCC
centrifugal counter-current chromatography

CC-CKR-5
nonsyncytium-inducing chemokine

CCCL, CCCl
cathodal-closure clonus

CCCP
carbonyl cyanide m-chlorophenylhydrazone

CCCR
closed-chest cardiac resuscitation

CCCS
condom catheter collecting system

CCCT
clomiphene citrate challenge test
closed craniocerebral trauma

CCCU
comprehensive cardiac care unit

CCD
calibration curve data
central collodiaphysial
central core disease
charge-coupled device
childhood celiac disease
choriocapillaris degeneration
cortical collecting duct
countercurrent distribution
crossed cerebellar diaschisis
cumulative cardiotoxic dose

CCDA
calcaneocuboid distraction arthrodesis

ccDNA
closed circle deoxyribonucleic acid

CCDS
color-coded duplex sonography

CCE
carboline-carboxylic (acid) ester
chamois contagious ecthyma
cholesterol crystal embolization
clear-cell endothelioma
clubbing, cyanosis, and edema
countercurrent electrophoresis

CCEI
Crown-Crisp Experimental Index

CCF
cancer coagulation factor
cardiolipin complement fixation
carotid cavernous fistula
centrifuged culture fluid
cephalin-cholesterol flocculation
compound comminuted fracture
congestive cardiac failure
critical corresponding frequency
crystal-induced chemotactic factor

CCFA
cycloserine-cefoxitin-fructose agar

CCFH
cellular cutaneous fibrous histiocytoma

CCG
cationic colloidal gold
cholecystogram
costochondral graft

CCGC
capillary column gas chromatography

CCGG
cytosine-cytosine-guanine-guanine

CCH
chronic cholestatic hepatitis
circumscribed choroidal hemangioma

CCh
carbamylcholine

CCHB
congenital complete heart block

CCHD
cyanotic congenital heart disease

CCHF, C-CHFV
Crimean-Congo hemorrhagic fever

cc/hr
cubic centimeter per hour
ccHRT
continuous-combined hormone
replacement therapy
CCHS
congenital central hypoventilation
syndrome
CCI
chronic coronary insufficiency
College Characteristics Index
corrected count increment
Cronqvist cranial index
CCIC
contrast chromoscopy using indigo
carmine
CCJ
costochondral junction
CCK
cholecystokinin
CCK-4
cholecystokinin tetrapeptide
CCK-8
cholecystokinin octapeptide (*See also*
CCK-OP)
CCK-A and CCK-B
cholecystokinin A and
cholecystokinin B
CCK-GB
cholecystokinin-gallbladder
(cholecystogram)
cc/kg day
cubic centimeters per kilogram per
day
CCK-LI
cholecystokinin-like immunoreactivity
CCKNOW
Crohn and Colitis Knowledge
CCK-OP
cholecystokinin octapeptide (*See also*
CCK-8)
CCK-PZ
cholecystokinin-pancreozymin
CCL
carcinoma cell line
cardiac catheterization laboratory
centrocyte-like (cell)
certified cell line
critical carbohydrate level
critical condition list
c̄cl
with contact lenses

CCLE
chronic cutaneous lupus
erythematosus
CCLI
composite clinical and laboratory
index
CCLO
child-centered literary orientation
CCM
cerebrocostomandibular (syndrome)
congestive cardiomyopathy
contralateral competing message
craniocervical malformation
Crime Classification Manual
critical care medicine
CC/MCL
centrocytic/mantle-cell lymphoma
CCMD-2
Chinese Classification of Mental
Disorders, Second Edition
CCMM
conventional cutaneous malignant
melanoma
CCMS
cerebrocostomandibular syndrome
clean-catch midstream (urine) (*See
also* CCMSU)
clinical care management system
CCMSU
clean-catch midstream urine (*See
also* CCMS)
CCMSUA
clean-catch midstream urinalysis
CCMT
catechol methyltransferase
CCMU
critical care medicine unit
CCN
caudal central nucleus
cervical cord neurapraxia
coronary care nursing
critical care nursing
CCNS
cell-cycle nonspecific (agent)
CCO
continuous cardiac output
CcO$_2$
oxygen concentration in pulmonary
capillary blood
CCOF
chromosomally competent ovarian
failure

NOTES

C-collar
    cervical collar
CCOmbo
    continuous cardiac output with
        SvO_2
CCOT
    clear cell odontogenic tumor
CCP
    chronic calcifying pancreatitis
    ciliocytophthoria
    colitis cystica profunda
    complement control protein
    crippled children's program
    crystalloid cardioplegia
    cytidine cyclic phosphate
CCPD
    continuous cyclic peritoneal dialysis
    crystalline calcium pyrophosphate
        dihydrate
CCPDS
    centralized cancer patient data
        system
CCPQ
    Children's Comprehensive Pain
        Questionnaire
CCPR
    cerebral cortex perfusion rate (*See
        also* CPR)
    crypt cell production rate
CCPT
    chronic calcific pancreatitis of the
        tropics
CCQ
    Chronicle Career Quest
CCR
    cardiac catheterization recovery
    complete continuous remission
    continuous complete remission
    cumulative conception rate
CCR2
    chemokine receptor 2
CCR3
    chemokine receptor 3
CCR5
    chemokine receptor 5
C_{cr}, C/cr/
    creatinine clearance (*See also* CC,
        CrCl, CRC)
CCRC
    continuing care retirement
        community
CCRN
    congenital cartilaginous rest of
        neck
CCRS
    carotid chemoreceptor stimulation

CCRT, CC-RT
    computer-controlled radiotherapy
    concurrent chemoradiotherapy
CCRU
    critical care recovery unit
CCS
    casualty clearing station
    celiac artery compression syndrome
    cell cycle specific (agent)
    central cord syndrome
    Children's Coma Score
    cholecystosonography
    chronic compartment syndrome
    Clinical Classification System
    cloudy-cornea syndrome
    composite cultured skin
    concentration-camp syndrome
    costoclavicular syndrome
    crippled children's services
    critical care services
CC&S
    cornea, conjunctivae, and sclerae
CCSA
    central centrifugal scarring alopecia
    central chemosensitive area
CCSAS
    Canadian Cardiovascular Society
        angina score
CCSC
    Canadian Cardiovascular Society
        classification
    Children's Coping Strategies
        Checklist
CCSCS
    central cervical spinal cord
        syndrome
CCSEQ
    Community College Student
        Experiences Questionnaire
CCSF
    carotid-cavernous sinus fistula
CCSK
    clear cell sarcoma of the kidney
CCSL
    clear cell sarcoma of the liver
CCT
    calcitriol
    carotid compression tomography
    central conduction time
    central corneal thickness
    chocolate-coated tablet
    closed cerebral trauma
    coated compressed tablet
    combined cortical thickness
    composite cyclic therapy
    controlled cord traction
    coronary care team

corrected congenital transposition
(of the great vessels)
cranial computed tomography
crude coal tar
cyclocarbothiamine

cct
circuit

CCTA
coronal computed tomographic
arthrography

CCTDI
California Critical Thinking
Dispositions Inventory

CCTe
cathodal-closure tetanus

CCTET
contact, control, test, evaluate,
treatment

CCTGA
congenitally corrected transposition
of the great arteries

CCT in PET
crude coal tar in petroleum

CCTST
California Critical Thinking Skills
Test

CCTV
closed-circuit television

CCU
cardiac care unit
cardiovascular care unit
Cherry-Crandall unit
community care unit
coronary care unit
critical care unit

CCUA
clean-catch urinalysis

CCUP
colpocystourethropexy

CCV
columnar cell variant
conductivity cell volume

CCVD
chronic cerebrovascular disease

CCVM
congenital cardiovascular
malformation

CCW
childcare worker
counterclockwise

Ccw
chest wall compliance

CCX
complications

CCY
cholecystectomy (See also chole)

CD
cadaver donor
canine distemper
carbohydrate dehydratase
carbon dioxide (See also CO_2)
cardiac disease
cardiac dullness
cardiac dysrrhythmia
cardiovascular deconditioning
cardiovascular disease (See also
CVD)
Carrel-Dakin (fluid)
caudad
caudal (See also caud, cd)
cefaloridine
celiac disease
cell dissociation
central deposition
cervical dystonia
cesarean delivery
channel down
character disorder
chemical dependency
chemotactic difference
childhood disease
circular dichroism
civil defense
Clostridium difficile
cluster of differentiation
collecting duct
colloid droplet
combination drug
common duct
communicable disease
communication deviance
communication disorders
completely denatured
complicated delivery
conduct disorder
conduction defect
consanguineous donor
contact dermatitis
contagious disease
continuous drainage
control diet
convulsive disorder
convulsive dose
copying drawings

NOTES

CD *(continued)*
  corneal dystrophy
  covert dyskinesia
  crossed diagonal
  curative dose
  current diagnosis
  cutdown
  cystic duct
  Czapek-Dox (agar)
  diagonal conjugate diameter of the pelvis [L. *conjugata diagonalis*] with the right hand [L. *colla dextra*]

C-D
  Cotrel-Dubousset

C2D
  C2 deficiency

CD2–72
  cluster of differentiation 2–72

C4D
  C4 deficiency

C7D
  C7 deficiency

CD$_{50}$
  median curative dose

C&D
  curettage and desiccation
  cystoscopy and dilation

C/D
  cigarettes per day
  conjunctiva diagonalis
  cup-to-disc (ratio)

Cd
  cadmium

cd
  candela
  caudal (*See also* caud, CD)
  coccygeal (*See also* COC, coc)
  color denial
  condylion
  cord

CDA
  chenodeoxycholic acid
  ciliary dyskinesia activity
  complement-dependent antibody
  completely denatured alcohol
  congenital dyserythropoietic anemia (types I–III)

2-CDA, 2-CdA
  2-chlorodeoxyadenosine

CdA
  2-chloro-2′-deoxyadenosine

CDAA
  chlorodiallylacetamide (herbicide)

CDAC
  Clostridium difficile-associated colitis (*See also* CDC)

CDAD
  Clostridium difficile-associated diarrhea
  Clostridium difficile-associated disease

CDAI
  Crohn Disease Activity Index

CDAK
  Cordis Dow Artificial Kidney

CDAP
  continuous distending airway pressure

CDB, C&DB
  cough and deep breath

CDBR
  computerized diaphragmatic breathing retraining

CDC
  calculated date of confinement
  cancer detection center
  capillary diffusion capacity
  cardiac diagnostic center
  cell division cycle
  chemical dependency counselor
  chenodeoxycholic (acid) (*See also* CDCA)
  child development clinic
  choledochocholedochostomy
  Clostridium difficile colitis (*See also* CDAC)
  collecting duct carcinoma
  complement-dependent cytotoxicity
  Crohn disease of colon

CDCA
  chenodeoxycholic acid (*See also* CDC)
  choledochocaval anastomosis

CDCF
  Clostridium difficile culture filtrate

CDCR
  conjunctivodacryocystorhinostomy

CDD
  certificate of disability for discharge
  childhood disintegrative disorder
  chronic degenerative disease
  chronic disabling dermatosis
  critical degree of deformation

CDE
  canine distemper encephalitis
  chlordiazepoxide (*See also* CDP, CDX)
  color Doppler energy
  common duct exploration
  cystine dimethylester

CDEIS
  Crohn Disease Endoscopic Index of Severity

CDF
> chondrodystrophia fetalis
> color flow Doppler

CDFI
> color Doppler flow imaging

CDFR
> cumulative duration of the first remission

CDG
> carbohydrate-deficient glycoprotein
> central developmental groove

CDGA
> constitutional delay in growth and adolescence

CDGD
> constitutional delay in growth and development

CDGS
> carbohydrate-deficient glycoprotein syndrome (type I)

CDH
> ceramide dihexoside
> chronic daily headache
> chronic disease hospital
> congenital diaphragmatic hernia
> congenital dislocation of hip
> congenital dysplasia of hip

CDI
> cell-directed inhibitor
> central diabetes insipidus
> Children's Depression Inventory
> chronic diabetes insipidus
> color Doppler imaging
> communicative development inventory
> Cotrel-Dubousset instrumentation (*See also* CDO)

cDICA
> Computerized Diagnostic Interview for Children and Adolescents

CD4-IgG
> cluster of differentiation 4 immunoglobulin G

CDILD
> chronic diffuse interstitial lung disease

CDIS
> continuous distention-irrigation system

CDJ
> choledochojejunostomy

CDK
> climatic droplet keratopathy
> cyclin-dependent kinase (*See also* Cdk)

Cdk
> cyclin-dependent kinase (*See also* CDK)

CDKI
> cyclin-dependent kinase inhibitor

CDL
> chlordeoxylincomycin
> Copying Drawings with Landmarks
> Cornelia de Lange (syndrome) (*See also* BDLS, CLS)

CD 27L
> CD 27 ligand

CD 30L
> CD 30 ligand

CD 40L
> CD 40 ligand

CD62L
> L-selectin molecule

CDLE
> chronic discoid lupus erythematosus

CDM
> Career Decision Making
> change description master
> chemically defined medium
> childhood dermatomyositis
> clinical decision making

cDNA
> complementary deoxyribonucleic acid

CDNF
> ciliary-derived neurotrophic factor receptor

CDNH
> chondrodermatitis nodularis helicis

CDO
> controlled depth osteotomy cutter
> Cotrel-Dubousset Orthopaedic (instrumentation) (*See also* CDI)

CDP
> certified distinct part
> chlordiazepoxide (*See also* CDE, CDX)
> chronic destructive periodontitis
> collagenase-digestible protein
> computerized dynamic posturography
> continuous distending pressure
> cytidine diphosphate
> cytidine 5'-diphosphate

C

NOTES

CDPC, CDP-choline
  cytidine diphosphate choline
CDP-glyceride
  cytidine diphosphoglyceride
CDPP
  computerized dynamic platform posturography
CDPS
  common duct pigment stone
CDP-sugar
  cytidine diphosphosugar
CDQ
  corrected development quotient
CDR
  calcium-dependent regulator
  chronologic drinking record
  Clinical Dementia Rating
  complementarity-determining region
  computed digital radiography
  continuing disability review
CDR3
  third complementarity determining region
CDR(H)
  cup-to-disc ratio horizontal
CDRS-R
  Children's Depression Rating Scale-Revised
CDR(V)
  cup-to-disc ratio vertical
CDS
  caudal dysplasia syndrome
  Chemical Data System
  Children's Depression Scale
  color Doppler sonography
  commercial dialysis solution
  cul-de-sac
  cumulative duration of survival
cd-sr
  candela-steradian
CDSS
  clinical decision support system
CDT
  carbohydrate-deficient transferrin
  carbon dioxide therapy
  combined diphtheria tetanus
CDTA
  cyclohexenediaminetetraacetic acid
CDTe
  cathode-duration tetanus
CDU
  chemical dependency unit
  color Doppler ultrasonography
  cumulative dose unit
CDV
  canine distemper virus

CDX
  chlordiazepoxide (*See also* CDE, CDP)
CDY
  cystoduodenostomy
CDYN, C_{dyn}, Cdyn
  dynamic compliance (of lung in pulmonary function test)
C-E
  chloroform-ether
CE
  California encephalitis
  capillary zone electrophoresis
  capital epiphysis
  cardiac emergency
  cardiac enlargement
  cardioesophageal (junction) (*See also* CEJ)
  carotid endarterectomy
  cataract extraction
  cell extract
  center-edge
  central episiotomy
  chemical energy
  chick embryo
  chloroform-ether
  cholera exotoxin
  cholesterol ester (*See also* chol est, CHE)
  cholinesterase (*See also* CHE, CHS)
  chromatoelectrophoresis
  clinical emphysema
  cocaethylene
  coefficient of error
  columnar epithelium
  community education
  conductive education
  conjugated estrogens
  constant error
  constant estrus
  continuing education
  contractile element
  contrast echocardiology
  converting enzyme
  crude extract
  curettage and electrodesiccation
  cytopathic effect
C&E
  consultation and examination
  cough and exercise
  curettage and electrodesication
Ce
  cerium
CEA
  carcinoembryonic antigen
  carotid endarterectomy
  cholesterol-esterifying activity

cost-effectiveness analysis
crystalline egg albumin

CEA-125, CEA 125
carcinoembryonic antigen-125

CEA-DT
carcinoembryonic antigen doubling time

CEAP
clinical manifestations, etiologic factors, anatomic involvement, pathophysiologic features

CEARP
Continuing Education Approval and Recognition Program

CEB
calcium entry blocker
cotton elastic bandage

CEBD
controlled extrahepatic biliary drainage

C/EBP
CCAAT/enhancer binding protein

CEBV
chronic Epstein-Barr virus

CEC
ciliated epithelial cell
contractile electrical complex

CECD
congenital endothelial corneal dystrophy

CECT
contrast-enhanced computed tomography

CED
chondroectodermal dysplasia
chronic enthusiasm disorder
convection-enhanced delivery
cranioectodermal dysplasia
cultural/ethnic diversity
cystoscopy-endoscopy dilation

CEDIA
cloned enzyme donor immunoassay

CEE
central European encephalitis
chick embryo extract
conjugated equine estrogens

CEEA
circular end-to-end anastomosis

CEEC
calf esophagus epithelial cell

CEEG
computer-analyzed electroencephalography

CEEP
conjugated equine estrogen plus norgestrel

CE-EUS
contrast-enhanced endoscopic ultrasonography

CEEV
central European encephalitis virus

CEF
centrifugation extractable fluid
chick embryo fibroblast
constant electric field

CE/FA
capillary electrophoresis/frontal analysis

c7E3 Fab
chimeric 7E3 Fab

CE-FAST
contrast-enhanced fast sequence
contrast enhanced Fourier-acquired steady state

CEFT
Children's Embedded Figures Test

CEG
chronic erosive gastritis

cEGF
concentration epidermal growth factor

CEH
carboxylic ester hydrolase
cholesterol ester hydrolase

CEHC
calf embryonic heart cell

CEI
character education inquiry
continuous extravascular infusion
converting enzyme inhibitor
corneal epithelial involvement

CEID
crossed electroimmunodiffusion

C1EInh
C1 esterase inhibitor

CEJ
cardioesophageal junction (*See also* CE)
cementoenamel junction

CEK
chick embryo kidney

NOTES

115

CEL
cardiac exercise laboratory
Celsior
chronic eosinophilic leukemia
CELF
Clinical Evaluation of Language
Functions
CELI
Carrow Elicited Language Inventory
CEM
central extensor mechanism
computerized electroencephalographic
map
conventional transmission electron
microscope
CUSA electrosurgical module
cemf
counterelectromotive force
C-EMR
cutting endoscopic mucosal
resection
CEMRA
contrast-enhanced magnetic
resonance angiography
cen
central
centromere
CENP
centromere protein
CENT, cent.
centimeter (*See also* cm)
central (*See also* C)
CEO
chick embryo origin
chloroethylene oxide
CEOT
calcifying epithelial odontogenic
tumor
CEP
centromere enumeration probe
chronic eosinophilic pneumonia
chronic erythropoietic porphyria
congenital erythropoietic porphyria
continuing education program
cortical evoked potential
counterelectrophoresis
CEPA
chloroethane phosphoric acid
CEPB
Carpentier-Edwards porcine
bioprosthesis
CEPH, ceph
cephalic
cephalin
cephalosporin
CEPH FLOC, ceph-floc
cephalin flocculation (test)

CER
capital expenditure review
ceramide
conditioned emotional response
control electrical rhythm
cortical evoked response
CE&R
central episiotomy and repair
CERA
cardiac-evoked response audiometry
CEREC
ceramic reconstruction
CERP
Continuing Education Recognition
Program
CERS
Crisis Evaluation Referral Service
CERT
composite extrarenal rhabdoid
tumor
cert
certificate (*See also* CTF)
certified
CERULO
ceruloplasmin
cerv
cervical
cervix
CES
cardioembolic stroke
cat's-eye syndrome
cauda equina syndrome
central excitatory state
chronic electrophysiologic study
Classroom Environmental Scale
clinical estimation of survival
cognitive environmental stimulation
cranial electrical stimulation
CESD
cholesterol ester storage disease
CES-D
Centers for Epidemiologic Studies
Depression scale
CESI
cervical epidural steroid injection
cESS
circumferential end-systolic stress
CET
capital expenditure threshold
cephalothin
cerebral electrotherapy
congenital eyelid tetrad
controlled environment treatment
CE-TCCS
contrast-enhanced transcranial color-
coded real-time sonography

CETE
central European tick-borne encephalitis
CETP
cholesteryl ester transfer protein
CEU
congenital ectropion uveae
continuing education unit
CEV
California encephalitis virus
CeVD
cerebrovascular disease
CEZ
cefazolin
CF
calcium leucovorin
calf blood flow
calibration factor
cancer free
carbol-fuchsin (stain)
cardiac failure
carotid foramen
carrier-free
cascade filtration
case file
Caucasian female
central fossa
cephalothin
characteristic frequency
chemotactic factor
chest and left leg (lead in electrocardiography)
Chiari-Frommel syndrome
chick fibroblast
choroid fissure
Christmas factor
circumflex
citrovorum factor
clavicular fracture
climbing fiber
clotting factor
clubfoot
colicin factor
collected fluid
colonization factor
colony-forming
color and form
compare [L. *confer*] (*See also* cf., comp)
complement factor
complement fixation (*See also* com fix)

complement-fixing (*See also* C'F)
completely follicular
complex fixation
computed fluoroscopy
constant frequency
contractile force
coronary flow
cough frequency
count fingers (visual acuity test) (*See also* C/F, cf)
counting fingers
coupling factor
cycling fibroblast
cystic fibrosis (*See also* C/F)
CFII
Cohn fraction II
C3F8
perfluoropropane gas
C'F
complement fixing (*See also* CF)
C/F
count fingers (visual acuity test) (*See also* CF, cf)
cystic fibrosis (*See also* CF)
C&F
cell and flare
curettage and fulguration
Cf
californium
252Cf
californium-252
cf
bring together [L. *conferre*]
centrifugal force
count fingers (visual acuity test) (*See also* CF, C/F)
iron carrier [L. *ferrum*]
cf.
compare [L. *confer*] (*See also* CF, comp)
CFA
cerebrofacioarticular syndrome
clofibric acid
colonization factor antigen
colony-forming assay
common femoral artery
complement-fixing antibody
complete Freund adjuvant
cryptogenic fibrosing alveolitis
cystic fibrosis arthropathy

NOTES

CFAC
complement-fixing antibody
consumption

C-factor
cleverness factor

CFA-SFA
common femoral artery-superficial
femoral artery

CFB
central fibrous body

CFBRS
Cooper-Farran Behavioral Rating
Scale

CFC
capillary filtrate collector
capillary filtration coefficient
cardiofaciocutaneous (syndrome)
chlorofluorocarbon
colony-forming capacity
colony-forming cells
continuous-flow centrifugation

CFCL
continuous-flow centrifugation
leukapheresis

CFC-S
colony-forming cells-spleen

CFD
cephalofacial deformity
color-flow Doppler
craniofacial dysostosis

CFDN
cefdinir

CFDS
craniofacial dysostosis

CFE
colony-forming efficiency

CFF
critical flicker frequency
critical flicker fusion (test) (*See
also* cff)
critical fusion frequency (*See also*
cff)
cystic fibrosis factor

cff
critical flicker fusion (test) (*See
also* CFF)
critical fusion frequency (*See also*
CFF)

CFFA
cystic fibrosis factor activity

Cf-Fe
carrier-bound iron [L. *ferrum*]

CFFR
crevicular fluid flow rate

CFI
cardiac function index
chemotactic-factor inactivator
color flow imaging

complement fixation inhibition
confrontation fields intact
contour-facilitating instrument

CFIDS
chronic fatigue immune deficiency
syndrome
chronic fatigue and immune
dysfunction syndrome

CFIT
Culture-Free Intelligence Test

CFL
calcaneofibular ligament

CFLB
carbon fiber lamination braid

CFLP
cleavage fragment length
polymorphism

CFM
cerebral function monitor
chemotactic factor for macrophage
chlorofluoromethane
close-fitting mask
craniofacial microsomia

cfm
cubic feet per minute

CfMNPV
Choristoneura fumiferana
multicapsin nucleopolyhedrovirus

CFND
craniofrontonasal dysostosis
craniofrontonasal dysplasia

CFNG
cross-facial nerve grafting

CFNS
chills, fever, and night sweats

CFP
chronic false-positive
cystic fibrosis protein

CFPD
critical frequency of photic driving

CFQ
Cognitive Failures Questionnaire

CFR
case-fatality ratio
citrovorum-factor rescue
complement-fixation reaction
coronary flow reserve
cyclic flow reduction

CFRD
cystic fibrosis-related diabetes

CFS
call for service
cancer family syndrome
chronic fatigue syndrome
congenital fibrosarcoma
contoured femoral stem
craniofacial stenosis
crush fracture syndrome

cfs
    cubic feet per second
CFSE
    crystal field stabilization energy
CFSEI-2
    Culture-Free Self-Esteem
       Inventories, Second Edition
CFT
    cardiolipin flocculation test
    clinical full-time
    complement-fixation test
    Complex Figure Test
    crystal field theory
    Culture-Free Test
CFTD
    congenital fiber-type disproportion
CFTR
    cystic fibrosis transmembrane
       conductance regulator
CFU
    colony-forming unit
CFUC, CFU-C
    colony-forming unit-culture
CFU-E
    colony-forming unit-erythrocyte
    colony-forming unit-erythroid
CFU$_{EOS}$
    colony-forming unit-eosinophil
CFU-F
    colony-forming unit-fibroblast
    colony-forming unit-fibroblastoid
CFU-GEMM
    colony-forming unit-granulocyte,
       erythrocyte, megakaryocyte,
       macrophage
CFU-GM, CFU$_{GM}$
    colony-forming unit-granulocyte-
       macrophage
CFU$_L$
    colony-forming unit-lymphoid
CFU$_M$, CFU$_{MEG}$, CFU-Meg
    colony-forming unit-megakaryocyte
CFU/mL
    colony-forming units/mL
CFU$_{NM}$
    colony-forming unit-neutrophil-
       monocyte
CFU-S, CFU$_S$
    colony-forming unit-spleen
    colony-forming unit-stem (cell)
CFUV
    Corfou virus

CFVR
    coronary flow velocity reserve
CFW
    calcofluor white stain
    cancer-free white (mouse) (*See also*
       CFWM)
    Carworth farm (mouse), Webster
       strain
CFWM
    cancer-free white mouse (*See also*
       CFW)
CFX
    cefoxitin
    circumflex (coronary artery)
CFZ
    capillary-free zone
    clofazimine
CFZC
    continuous-flow zonal centrifugation
CG
    calcium gluconate
    cardiography
    center of gravity (*See also* cg)
    central gray
    choking gas (phosgene)
    cholecystogram
    cholecystography
    choriogenic gynecomastia
    chorionic gonadotropin (*See also*
       CGT)
    chronic glomerulonephritis (*See also*
       CGN)
    cingulate gyrus
    colloidal gold (*See also* ^{198}Au)
    contact guarding
    control group
    cryoglobulin
    cystine guanine
    phosgene (choking gas)
cg
    center of gravity (*See also* CG)
    centigram
    chemoglobulin
CGA
    catabolite gene activator
    comprehensive geriatric assessment
CgA
    chromogranin A
CGAS
    Children's Global Assessment Scale

NOTES

CGB
chronic gastrointestinal (tract) bleeding
CGCF
central groove of central fossa
CGCG
central giant cell granuloma
CGCL
central giant cell lesion
CGCOT
central granular cell odontogenic tumor
CGCT
combined germ cell tumor
CGD
chromosomal gonadal dysgenesis
chronic granulomatous disease
continuous gastric drip
CGDE
contact glow discharge electrolysis
CGESS
computer-guided endoscopic sinus surgery
CGFH
congenital fibrous histiocytoma
CGH
chorionic gonadotropic hormone
comparative genomic hybridization
CGI
chronic granulomatous inflammation
Clinical Global Impression (Scale)
Clinical Global Improvement
Clinical Global Index
common gateway interface
glycoprotein crystal growth inhibitor
CGIC
Clinical Global Impression of Change
CGI-S
Clinical Global Impression-Severity of Illness Scale
CGL
chronic granulocytic leukemia
correction with glasses (*See also* c gl)
c gl
correction with glasses (*See also* CGL)
CGLV
Changuinola virus
CGM
central gray matter (spinal cord)
coffee-grounds material
cgm
centigram
cGMP
cyclic guanine monophosphate
cyclic guanosine monophosphate
cyclic 3′,5′-guanosine monophosphate
cyclic guanosine 3,′5′-monophosphate
5′-cyclic guanosine monophosphate
CGMS
continuous glucose monitoring system
CGN
chronic glomerulonephritis (*See also* CG)
compressor-generated nebulizer
convalescent growing nursery
CGNB
composite ganglioneuroblastoma
CG/OQ
cerebral glucose oxygen quotient
CGP
choline glycerophosphatide
chorionic growth hormone-prolactin
circulating granulocyte pool
Comparative Guidance and Placement Program
CGPS
Current, Global, Psychiatric-Social Status
CGRH
calcitonin gene-related hormone
CGRP
calcitonin gene-related peptide
CGRS
Clinician's Global Rating Scale
CGS
cardiogenic shock
catgut suture (*See also* CS)
centimeter-gram-second (system, unit) (*See also* cgs)
computer graphic simulation
cgs
centimeter-gram-second (system, unit) (*See also* CGS)
CGT
chorionic gonadotropin (*See also* CG)
cyclodextrin glucanotransferase
CGTT
cortisone-glucose tolerance test
CGV
Chobar Gorge virus
CGVD
chronic graft vascular disease
c-GVHD
chronic graft-versus-host disease
CGY
cystogastrostomy
cGy
centigray

CH

calcium heparin
calcium hydroxide
case history
casein hydrolysate
cervicogenic headache
child (children) (*See also* Ch, ch)
Chinese hamster
chloral hydrate
cholesterol (*See also* C, Ch,
  CHOL, chol, chol.)
Christchurch chromosome
chronic hepatitis
chronic hypertension
cluster headache
common hepatic (duct)
communicating hydrocele
complete healing
congenital hypothyroidism
continuous heparinization
convalescent hospital
coracohumeral
crown-heel (length) (*See also* CHL)
cycloheximide
(wheel)chair (*See also* WC, W/C,
  wh ch)

C-H

carbon-hydrogen

C&H

coarse and harsh (breathing)
cocaine and heroin

CH$_{50}$

(total serum) hemolytic complement

C$_H$

constant domain of H chain

Ch

chest (*See also* ch)
Chido (antibody)
chief (*See also* ch)
child (*See also* CH, ch)
cholesterol (*See also* C, CH,
  CHOL, chol, chol.)
choline
chromosome (*See also* chr)

cH

hydrogen ion concentration

ch

chest (*See also* Ch)
chief (*See also* Ch)
child (*See also* CH, Ch)
chronic

CHA

chronic hemolytic anemia
common hepatic artery
compound hypermetropic
  astigmatism
congenital hypoplasia of adrenal
  glands
congenital hypoplastic anemia
continuous heated aerosols
cyclohexyladenosine
cyclohexylamine

ChA

choline acetylase

ChAc, ChAct

choline acetyltransferase

CHADD

children and adults with attention
  deficit disorder
controlled heat-aided drug delivery

CHAG

coralline hydroxyapatite Goniopora

CHAI

continuous hepatic artery infusion

CHAID

chi-square automatic interaction
  detection

CHAL

chronic haloperidol

CHAMPUS

Civilian Health and Medical
  Programs of Uniformed Services

CHAMPVA

Civilian Health and Medical
  Program of Veterans'
  Administration

CHANDS

curly hair-ankyloblepharon-nail
  dysplasia syndrome

Chang C

Chang conjunctiva (cells)

Chang L

Chang liver (cells)

CHAOS

congenital high airway obstruction
  syndrome

CHAP

Certified Hospital Admission
  Program
Child Health Assessment Program

CHAQ

Childhood Health Assessment
  Questionnaire

NOTES

C

CHAR
continuous hyperfractionated accelerated radiotherapy

CHARGE
coloboma, heart anomaly, choanal atresia, retardation, and genital and ear anomalies
coloboma, heart defects, atresia choanae, retarded growth, genital hypoplasia, and ear anomalies
coloboma, heart disease, atresia choanae, retarded growth and retarded development and/or CNS anomalies, genital hypoplasia, and ear anomalies and/or deafness (syndrome)
coloboma of iris, heart deformities, choanal atresia, retarded growth, genital and ear deformities

CHART
continuous hyperfractionated accelerated radiotherapy
Craig Handicap Assessment and Reporting Technique

CHARTS
Computerized Healthcare And Record Transfer System

CHAT, ChAT, ChaT
choline acetyltransferase

CHB
chronic hepatitis B
complete heart block
congenital heart block

ChBFlow
choroidal blood flow

CHBHA
congenital Heinz body hemolytic anemia

ChBVol
choroidal blood volume

CHC
Canadian Heart Classification
chronic hepatitis C
community health center
concentric hypertrophic cardiomyopathy

CHCP
correctional health-care program

CHCT
caffeine and halothane contracture test

CHD
center hemodialysis
childhood disease
chronic hemodialysis
common hepatic duct
congenital heart defect
congenital heart disease

congenital hip dislocation
congenital hip dysplasia
congestive heart disease
constitutional hepatic dysfunction
coordinate home care
coronary heart disease
cyanotic heart disease

CHE
cholesterol ester (*See also* chol est, CE)
cholinesterase (*See also* CE, CHS)
chronic hepatic encephalopathy

CHEC
community hypertension evaluation clinic

CHEF
Chinese hamster embryo fibroblast
contour-clamped homogeneous electric field (electrophoresis)

chem
chemical
chemistry
chemistry panel
chemistry profile

CHEMLINE
Chemical Dictionary On-Line

chemo
chemotherapy

chem panel
blood chemistry profile

chemrad
chemotherapy and radiotherapy

CHERSS
continuous high-amplitude electroencephalogram rhythmical synchronous slowing

CHESS
chemical shift selective
comprehensive health enhancement support system

CHEST
Chick Embryotoxicity Screening Test

CHF
chick embryo fibroblast
chronic heart failure
congenital hepatic fibrosis
congestive heart failure
Crimean hemorrhagic fever

CHFV
combined high-frequency ventilation

CHG, chg
change
changed

ch gn
chronic glomerulonephritis

CHGV
Chagres virus

CHH
cartilage-hair hypoplasia

chi₂
chi-squared (distribution, test)

chiₑ
electric susceptibility

chiₘ
magnetic susceptibility

CHI
closed head injury
creatinine height index

CHIC
Coping Health Inventory for
Children

CHIKV
Chikungunya virus

CHILD
congenital hemidysplasia with
ichthyosiform erythroderma and
limb defects (syndrome)

CHIME
Collaborative Home Infant
Monitoring Evaluation
coloboma, heart anomaly,
ichthyosis, mental retardation, and
ear abnormality
coloboma, heart defects,
ichthyosiform dermatosis, mental
retardation, ear defects (syndrome)

CHIMV
Chim virus

CHINA
chronic infectious neuropathic agent

CHINS
child in need of service (petition)

CHIP
channel-forming integral protein
comprehensive health insurance
plan
comprehensive hospital infections
project
Coping Health Inventory for
Parents
Coping with Health, Injuries, and
Problems

CHIP-AE
Child Health and Illness Profile,
Adolescent Edition

ChIPS
Children's Interview for Psychiatric
Disorders

CHIV
Chilibre virus

chix
chickenpox (*See also* CHPX, chpx,
Cp)

CHL
Chinese hamster lung
classic Hodgkin lymphoma
conductive hearing loss
crown-heel length (*See also* CH)

chl
chloroform (*See also* chlor)

CHLA
cyclohexyllinoleic acid

CHLD
chronic hypoxic lung disease

chlor
chloroform (*See also* chl)

CHMD
clinical hyaline membrane disease

CHMIS
community health management
information system

CHN
carbon, hydrogen, and nitrogen
central hemorrhagic necrosis
child neurology
Chinese (hamster)
community health network
congenital hypomyelinating
neuropathy

CHO
carbohydrate (*See also* CARB, carb,
carbo)
Chinese hamster ovary
chlorhexidine digluconate
chorea

C_{H2O}
water clearance

choc
chocolate

CHOL, chol, chol.
cholesterol (*See also* C, CH, Ch)

c̄hold
withhold

chole
cholecystectomy (*See also* CCY)

chol est
cholesterol ester (*See also* CHE,
CE)

CHOV
Chaco virus

C

NOTES

CHP

    capillary hydrostatic pressure
    charcoal hemoperfusion
    child psychiatry
    comprehensive health planning
    cutaneous hepatic porphyria
    histiocytic cytophagic panniculitis

ChP

    chest physician

CHPM

    chronic hypertrophic
      pachymeningitis

CHPP

    continuous hyperthermic peritoneal
      perfusion

CHPS

    chronic heel pain syndrome

CHPV

    Chandipura virus

CHPX, chpx

    chickenpox (*See also* chix, Cp)

CHQ

    child health questionnaire
    chlorquinol (topical antiinfective)

CHR

    cerebrohepatorenal (syndrome)
    chromogranin

chr

    chromosome (*See also* Ch)
    chronic (*See also* chron)

ChrA

    chromogranin A

ChRBC

    chicken red blood cell (*See also*
      CRBC)

CHRIS

    Cancer Hazards Ranking and
      Information System

chron

    chronic (*See also* chr)
    chronological

CHRP

    coagulation and hemostatic
      resection of the prostate

CHRPE

    congenital hypertrophy of the
      retinal pigment epithelium

CHRS

    cerebrohepatorenal syndrome
    congenital hereditary retinoschisis

CHS

    central hypoventilation syndrome
    Chediak-Higashi syndrome
    Children's Health Study
    cholinesterase (*See also* CE, CHE)
    chondroitin sulfate
    compression hip screw

    congenital hypoventilation syndrome
    contact hypersensitivity

CHSD

    congenital hyperphosphatasemic
      skeletal dysplasia

CHS/NP

    chronic hyperplastic sinusitis with
      nasal polyposis

CHSS

    cooperative health statistics system

C-H stretch

    carbon-hydrogen stretch

CHT

    closed head trauma
    combined hormone therapy
    contralateral head turning

CHTN

    Cooperative Human Tissue Network

CHU

    closed head unit

CHUK

    conserved helix-loop-helix
      ubiquitous kinase

CHV

    canine herpesvirus

CHVV

    Charleville virus

CHX

    chlorhexidine gluconate

CI

    calcium ionophore
    cardiac index
    cardiac insufficiency
    cell immunity
    cell inhibition
    cell interaction (molecule)
    cephalic index
    cerebral infarction
    cervical incompetence
    cesium implant
    chain initiating
    chemical ionization
    chemoimmunotherapy
    chemotactic index
    chemotherapeutic index
    chronically infected
    chronic inflammation
    clinical investigation
    clinical investigator
    clomipramine
    clonus index
    closure index
    cochlear implant
    cochlear implantation
    coefficient of intelligence
    colloidal iron
    colony inhibition
    complete iridectomy

confidence interval
constraint-induced
contamination index
continuous imaging
continuous infusion
convergence insufficiency
cord insertion
coronary insufficiency
corrected count increment
crystalline insulin
cytotoxic index

C.I.

Colour Index

Ci

curie

CIA

canine inherited ataxia
chemiluminescent immunoassay
chronic idiopathic anhidrosis
chymotrypsin inhibitor activity
collagen-induced arthritis
colony-inhibiting activity
congenital intestinal aganglionosis

CIAA

competitive insulin autoantibodies

CIAC

chronic idiopathic arthritides of
childhood

CIAED

collagen-induced autoimmune ear
disease

cIAPs

cellular inhibitors of apoptosis

CIB, cib

crying-induced bronchospasm
cytomegalic inclusion bodies

CIBD

chronic inflammatory bowel disease

CIBHA

congenital inclusion-body hemolytic
anemia

CIBI

continuous intrathecal baclofen
infusion

CIBP

chronic intractable benign pain

CIC

carbachol inhalation challenge
cardioinhibitor center
chronic inactive cirrhosis
circulating immune complex
clean intermittent catheterization

completely in the canal (hearing
aid)
complex instability of carpus
constant initial concentration
coronary intensive care
crisis intervention center

CICA

cervical internal carotid artery

CICE

combined intracapsular cataract
extraction

CICI

Hymovich Chronicity Impact and
Coping Instrument

CICLP

chronic ischemic colonic lesion
caused by phlebosclerosis

CICU

cardiac intensive care unit
cardiovascular inpatient care unit
coronary intensive care unit

CID

carpal instability dissociation
central integrative deficit
cervical immobilization device
chick infective dose
chronic intestinal dysmotility
combined immunodeficiency
(disease)
cytomegalic inclusion disease (*See
also* CMID)

CIDEP

chemically-induced dynamic electron
polarization

CIDP, CIDPN

chronic inflammatory demyelinating
polyneuropathy
chronic inflammatory demyelinating
polyradiculoneuropathy
chronic inflammatory demyelinating
polyradiculopathy

CIDS

combined immunodeficiency
syndrome
continuous insulin delivery system

CIE

chemotherapy-induced emesis
congenital ichthyosiform
erythroderma
countercurrent immunoelectrophoresis
counterimmunoelectrophoresis
crossed immunoelectrophoresis

NOTES

CIEA
continuous infusion epidural
analgesia

CIE-C
counter
immunoelectrophoresis–colorimetric

CIE-D
counter
immunoelectrophoresis–den-
sitometric

cIEL
crypt intraepithelial lymphocyte

CIES
Correctional Institutions
Environment Scale

CIF

cartilage induction factor
claims inquiry form
clone-inhibiting factor
congenital infantile fibrosarcoma

CIFN
consensus interferon

CIG

cardiointegram
cigarettes
cold-insoluble globulin

CIg
intracytoplasmic immunoglobulin

cIgM
cytoplasmic immunoglobulin M

CIH

carbohydrate-induced
hyperglyceridemia
children in hospital

CIHD
chronic ischemic heart disease

Ci-hr
curie-hour

CIHS
chronic infantile hypotonic
syndrome

CII
Carnegie Interest Inventory

CIIA
common internal iliac artery

CIIPS
chronic idiopathic intestinal pseudoobstruction syndrome

CIIS
Cattell Infant Intelligence Scale

CIL
center for independent living

CILP
cartilage intermediate layer protein

CIM
cardia-intestinal metaplasia
cimetidine

constraint-induced movement
Cumulated Index Medicus

CIMF
chronic idiopathic myelofibrosis

Ci/mL
curies per milliliter

CIMS
chemical ionization mass
spectrometry
clinical information scale
Conflict in Marriage Scale

CIN

cefsulodin-irgasan-novobiocin (agar)
cerebriform intradermal nevus
cervical intraepithelial neoplasia
cervical invasive neoplasia
chemotherapy-induced neutropenia
chromosomal instability
chronic interstitial nephritis
cinoxacin
conjunctival intraepithelial neoplasia

CIN 1–3
cervical intraepithelial neoplasia,
grade 1–3

C_{IN}, C_{in}
inulin clearance

CINCA
chronic infantile neurological,
cutaneous, and articular

CIND
carpal instability nondissociative

CINE
chemotherapy-induced nausea and
emesis
cineangiogram

cine MRI, cine-MRI
cine magnetic resonance imaging

C1INH
first component of complement

CIOP
chromosomally incompetent ovarian
failure

CIP

cellular immunocompetence profile
chronic intestinal pseudoobstruction
comprehensive identification process
critical illness polyneuropathy
critical infrastructure protection

CIPD
chronic intermittent peritoneal
dialysis

CIPF

classic interstitial pneumonitis with
fibrosis
clinical illness promotion factor

CIPO, CIPS, CIPSO
chronic intestinal pseudoobstruction

CIQ
Community Integration
Questionnaire

cir
circuit
circular
circumference (*See also* circ)

circ
circulation
circumcision (*See also* circum)
circumference (*See also* cir)

circ & sen
circulation and sensation

circum
circumcision (*See also* circ)

CIRF
cocaine-induced respiratory failure

CIRP
cold-inducible ribonucleic acid-
binding protein
cooperative institutional research
program

CIRR
cirrhosis

CIS
carcinoma in situ
catheter-induced spasm
central inhibitory state
clinical information system
clinically isolated syndrome
continuous interleaved sampling
coronary implant system

CI-S
Simplified Calculus Index

CiS
cingulate sulcus

CISE
Children's Inventory of Self-Esteem

CISI
Cattell Infant Scale Inventory

CISMD
California Infant Scale for Motor
Development

CISP
chronic intractable shoulder pain

CISS
Campbell Interest and Skill Survey

CIT
citrate (*See also* cit)
cold ischemia time
combined intermittent therapy

conjugated-immunoglobulin technique
conventional immunosuppressive
therapy
conventional insulin therapy
corneal impression test

cit
citrate (*See also* CIT)

CITP
capillary isotachophoresis

CIU
chronic idiopathic urticaria

CIV
Carey Island virus
common iliac vein
continuous intravenous (infusion)
(*See also* CIVI)

CIVI
continuous intravenous infusion
(*See also* CIV)

CIVII
continuous intravenous insulin
infusion

CIVRA
continuous intravenous regional
anesthesia

CIXU
constant infusion excretory urogram

CJ
conjunctivitis

CJD
Creutzfeldt-Jakob disease

CJR
centric jaw relationship

CK
calf kidney
chicken kidney
cholecystokinin
choline kinase
color kinesis
contralateral knee (*See also* ck)
creatine kinase
cyanogen chloride
cytokeratin

CK$_1$, CK$_2$, CK$_3$
isoenzymes of creatine kinase

ck
check
checked
contralateral knee (*See also* CK)

CK-BB
creatine kinase-BB (band)

NOTES

CK-BB *(continued)*
    creatine kinase-BB (isoenzyme)
        (*See also* BB)
    creatine kinase (fraction brain)
CKC
    closed kinetic chain
    cold-knife cone
    cold-knife conization
CKCE
    closed kinetic chain exercise
CKG
    cardiokymograph
    cardiokymography
c/kg
    coulombs per kilogram
CK-ISO
    creatine kinase isoenzyme
CK-MB
    creatine kinase myocardial band
CK-MM
    creatine kinase fraction muscle
        (skeletal)
CKPT
    combined kidney and pancreas
        transplant
CK-PZ
    cholecystokinin-pancreozymin
CKS
    classic form of Kaposi sarcoma
    Continuum knee system
CKW
    clockwise
CL
    capacity of lung
    capillary lumen
    cardinal ligament
    cardiolipin
    cell line
    center line
    centralis lateralis
    cervical line
    chemiluminescence
    chest and left arm
    cholelithiasis
    cholesterol-lecithin
    chronic leukemia
    cirrhosis of liver
    clamp lamp
    clear liquid
    cleft lip
    clinical laboratory
    cloudy (*See also* cl, cldy)
    complex loading
    compliance of the lung (*See also*
        C_L)
    composite lymphoma
    confidence level
    contact lens (*See also* ctl)

    continence line
    corpus luteum (*See also* cl)
    cricoid lamina
    criterion level
    critical list
    current liabilities
    cutaneous leishmaniasis
    cutis laxa
    cycle length
    cytotoxic lymphocyte
C-L
    consultation-liaison (psychiatry)
C_L
    compliance of the lung (*See also*
        CL)
    constant domain of L chain
Cl
    chloride
    clonus
    closure (*See also* cl)
    colistin
cL
    centiliter
cl
    clavicle (*See also* CLAV)
    cleft
    clinic (*See also* clin)
    closure (*See also* Cl)
    cloudy (*See also* CL, cldy)
    corpus luteum (*See also* CL)
CLA
    cervicolinguoaxial
    clarithromycin
    cleft lip and alveolus
    community living arrangements
    conjugated linoleic acid
    contralateral local anesthesia
    cutaneous lymphocyte antigen
    cyclic lysine anhydride
    (X-linked) cerebral ataxia
CLAH
    congenital lipoid adrenal
        hyperplasia
C lam
    cervical laminectomy
CLAMS
    Clinical Linguistic and Auditory
        Milestone Scale
CLAP
    contact laser ablation of prostate
CLARE
    contact lens-induced acute red eye
CLAS
    congenital localized absence of
        skin
class.
    classification

CLASSI
    Cornell Learning and Study Skills Inventory

CLAV, clav
    clavicle (*See also* cl)

CLB
    curvilinear body

CLBBB
    complete left bundle-branch block

CLBP
    chronic low back pain

CLC
    Charcot-Leyden crystal
    Clerc-Levy-Cristeco (syndrome)
    cork, leather, and celastic (orthotic)

CL/CP
    cleft lip and cleft palate

CLCS
    Comprehensive Level of Consciousness Scale

CLD
    central language disorder
    central lung distance
    chronic liver disease
    chronic lung disease
    congenital limb deficiency
    crystal ligand field
    cytoplasmic lipid droplet

cld
    cleared
    colored

CLDH
    choline dehydrogenase

CLDM
    clindamycin

C-LDP
    complete laparoscopic distal pancreatectomy

cldy
    cloudy (*See also* CL, cl)

CLE
    centrilobular emphysema
    columnar-lined esophagus
    continuous lumbar epidural (anesthesia)

CLED
    cystinc-lactose electrolyte-deficient (agar)

CLEF-P
    Clinical Evaluation of Language Function-Preschool

CLEP
    College-Level Examination Program General Examination

cler
    clear (*See also* C)

CLF
    cardiolipin fluorescence (antibody)
    cholesterol-lecithin flocculation

CLH
    chronic lobular hepatitis
    corpus luteum hormone
    cutaneous lymphoid hyperplasia

CLI
    Campbell Leadership Index
    corpus luteum insufficiency
    critical limb ischemia

CLi
    lithium clearance

CLIA
    chemiluminescent immunoassay
    Clinical Laboratory Improvement Act
    Clinical Laboratory Improvement Amendments

CLIA '67
    Clinical Laboratory Improvement Act of 1967

CLIA '88
    Clinical Laboratory Improvement Amendments of 1988

CLIF
    cloning inhibitory factor
    Crithidia luciliae immunofluorescence

CLIFT
    Crithidia luciliae indirect immunofluorescence test

clin
    clinic (*See also* cl)

CLINHAQ
    Clinical Health Assessment Questionnaire

clin path
    clinical pathology

clin proc
    clinical procedure

ClinSeg
    clinoidal segment

CLIP
    cerebral lipidosis (without visceral involvement and with onset of disease past infancy)

NOTES

CLIP *(continued)*
class II invariant chain-derived peptide
corticotropin-like intermediate lobe peptide

CLL
centrocytelike cell
cholesterol-lowering lipid
chronic lymphatic leukemia
chronic lymphocytic leukemia
chronic myelogenous leukemia
cow lung lavage

CLLE
columnar-lined lower esophagus

cl liq
clear liquid

CLM
capillary-lymphatic malformation

CLML
Current List of Medical Literature

CLMN
complete lower motor neuron (lesion)

clmp
clumped

CLN
centrilobar necrosis
computer liaison nurse
neuronal ceroid lipofuscinosis

CLND
complete lymph node dissection

CLO
Campylobacter-like organism
cod liver oil
congenital lobar overinflation

CLOF
clofibrate

C-loop
anatomical position (shape) of duodenum

CLOtest
Campylobacter-like organism test (for *H. pylori*)

CLOT R
clot retraction

CLP
cecal ligation and puncture
chymotrypsin-like protein
cleft lip with cleft palate (*See also* CL&P)
cycle length, paced

CL&P
cleft lip and palate (*See also* CLP)

ClP
clinical pathology

Clpal
cleft palate (*See also* CP)

CLPD
chronic lymphoproliferative disorder

CLQ
cognitive laterality quotient

CLRO
community leave for reorientation

CLRSS
Composite Laryngeal Recurrence Staging System

CLS
capillary leak syndrome
cementless Sportono
confused language syndrome
Cornelia de Lange syndrome (*See also* BDLS, CDL)

CLSE
calf lung surfactant extract

CLSH
corpus luteum stimulating hormone

CLSL
chronic lymphosarcoma (cell) leukemia

CLSM
confocal laser scanning microscopy

CLT
chronic lymphocytic thyroiditis
clot lysis time
clotting time

CLTM
continuous long-term monitoring

CLV
constant linear velocity

CLVM
complex-combined vascular malformation

CL VOID
clean voided specimen (urine)

CLVP
contact laser vaporization of the prostate

CLX
cloxacillin

CM
California mastitis (test)
calmodulin
capreomycin
carboxymethyl (cellulose) (*See also* CMC)
cardiac monitor
cardiac muscle
cardiac myxoma
cardiomyopathy (*See also* CMP)
carpometacarpal
Caucasian male
cell membrane
center of mass
centrum medianum
cerebral malaria

cerebral mantle
cervical mucus
chemotactic migration
Chick-Martin (coefficient)
chloroquine-mepacrine
chondromalacia
chopped meat (medium)
chylomicron
circular muscle
circulating monocyte
clinical medicine
coccidioidal meningitis
cochlear microphonic
combined mechanical
common migraine
community meeting
competing message
complete medium
complications (*See also* cm)
conditioned medium
congenital malformation
congestive myocardiopathy
continuous murmur
contrast medium
copulatory mechanism
costal margin
cow's milk
culture medium
cystic mesothelioma
cytometry
cytoplasmic membrane

C/M

counts per minute (*See also* CPM, cpm)

C&M

cocaine and morphine

C$_m$

maximal clearance

Cm

curium

cM

centimorgan (*See also* cMO)

cm

centimeter (*See also* CENT, cent.)
complications (*See also* CM)
costal margin

cm^2

square centimeter

cm^3

cubic centimeter (*See also* cc, CC, c.c., cu cm)

CMA

Candida metabolic antigen
cerebral microangiopathy
chronic metabolic acidosis
complete maturation arrest
compound myopic astigmatism
Conflict Management Appraisal
cow's milk allergy
cultured macrophages

CMAD

count median aerodynamic diameter

CMAF

centrifuged microaggregate filter

CMAmg

corticomedial amygdaloid (nucleus)

CMAP

compound motor action potential
compound muscle action potential

CMAS

Childhood Myositis Assessment Scale
Children's Manifest Anxiety Scale

C$_{max}$

maximal drug concentration

CMB

carbolic methylene blue
chloromercuribenzoate

CMBBT

cervical mucous basal body temperature

CMC

carboxymethylcellulose (*See also* CM)
care management continuity
carpometacarpal (joint)
cell-mediated cytotoxicity
chronic mucocutaneous candidiasis (*See also* CMCC)
complement-mediated cytotoxicity
corticomedullary contrast
critical micellar concentration (*See also* cmc)
critical micelle concentration (*See also* cmc)

cmc

critical micellar concentration (*See also* CMC)
critical micelle concentration (*See also* CMC)

CMCC

chronic mucocutaneous candidiasis (*See also* CMC)

NOTES

CM-cellulose
carboxymethylcellulose
CMCP
camphorated mono-parachlorophenol
CMCT
central motor conduction time
CMCt
care management continuity (across settings)
CMD
cerebromacular degeneration
congenital muscular dystrophy
corticomedullary differentiation
count median diameter (of particles)
craniomandibular dysfunction
cystoid macular degeneration
cytomegalic disease
CME
cervical mediastinal exploration
cervical mucous extract
continuing medical education
crude marijuana extract
cystoid macular edema
CMEC
central mucoepidermoid carcinoma
CME-MRI
contrast medium-enhanced magnetic resonance imaging
CMER
current medical evidence of record
CM EVA
compression-molded ethylene vinyl acetate
CMF
calcium-magnesium free
catabolite modular factor
chondromyxoid fibroma
cortical magnification factor
craniomandibulofacial
CMFE
calcium and magnesium free plus ethylenediaminetetraacetic acid
CMFTD
congenital muscle fiber-type disproportion
CMG
canine myasthenia gravis
chopped-meat glucose (medium)
congenital myasthenia gravis
cyanmethemoglobin
cystometrogram
cystometrography
CMGN
chronic membranous glomerulonephritis

CMGS
chopped meat-glucose-starch (medium)
CMGT
chromosome-mediated gene transfer
CMH
congenital malformation of heart
CMHC
community mental health center
cm H₂O
centimeters of water (cuff pressure)
CMI
carbohydrate metabolism index
Career Maturity Inventory
care management integration
cell-mediated immunity
cell multiplication inhibition
chronically mentally ill
chronic mesenteric ischemia
circulating microemboli index
clomipramine
computer-managed instruction
Cornell Medical Index
CMID
cytomegalic inclusion disease (*See also* CID)
c/min
cycles per minute (*See also* cpm)
CMIR
cell-mediated immune response
CMIT
current medical information and terminology
CMJ
carpometacarpal joint
CMK
chloromethyl ketone
congenital multicystic kidney
CML
cell-mediated lympholysis
cell-mediated lysis
chronic myelocytic leukemia
chronic myelogenous leukemia
chronic myeloid leukemia
chronic myelomonocytic leukemia
count median length
cross midline
CML AP
chronic myelocytic/myelogenous/myeloid leukemia accelerated phase
CML BC
chronic myelocytic/myelogenous/myeloid leukemia blast crisis

CML CP
chronic myelocytic/myelogenous/myeloid leukemia chronic phase

CMM
cell-mediated mutagenesis
cutaneous malignant melanoma

cmm
cubic millimeter (*See also* cu mm, mm^3)

cm/m²
centimeters per square meter

CMME
chloromethyl methyl ether (carcinogen at technical grade)

CMMHN
cutaneous malignant melanoma of head and neck

CMML, CMMoL
chronic myelomacrocytic leukemia
chronic myelomonocytic leukemia

CMMS
Columbia Mental Maturity Scale

CMN
caudal mediastinal node
congenital melanocytic nevus
congenital mesoblastic nephroma
cranial motor nuclei
cystic medial necrosis

CMN-AA
cystic medial necrosis of ascending aorta

CMO
calculated mean organism
cardiac minute output
card made out
cetylmyristoleate
comfort measures only
corticosterone methyl oxidase

cMO, cMo
centimorgan (*See also* cM)

CMOAT
canicular multispecific organic anion transporter

CMoL
chronic monoblastic leukemia
chronic monocytic leukemia

CMOR
craniomandibular orthopedic repositioning device

CMOS
complementary metal-oxide semiconductor (logic)

CMP
captioned media program
cardiomyopa
cardiomyopathy (*See also* CM)
cervical mucus penetration
chondromalacia patellae
colorimetric microtiter plate
competitive medical plans
complementary medical practice
complexity of mental processes
comprehensive medical plan
cow's milk protein
cross-modal priming
cytidine monophosphate

CMPD
chronic myeloproliferative disorder

CMP/dCMP-K
cytidylate/2′-deoxycytidylate kinase

CMP-FX
complement fixation

CMPGN
chronic membranoproliferative glomerulonephritis

CMP-NANA
cytidine monophospho-*N*-acetylneuraminic acid

CMPS
chronic musculoskeletal pain syndrome

cmps
centimeters per second (*See also* cm/s)

CMPT
cervical mucus penetration test

CMR
cerebral metabolic rate
chief medical resident
common mode rejection
congenital mitral regurgitation
crude mortality ratio

CMRE
California Marriage Readiness Evaluation

CMRG
cerebral metabolic rate of glucose

CMRGI$_c$
cerebral rate of glucose metabolism

CMRL
cerebral metabolic rate of lactate

NOTES

CMRNG
>chromosomally mediated resistant *Neisseria gonorrhoeae*

CMRO, CMRO$_2$
>cerebral metabolic rate of oxygen

CMRP
>cervical magnetic resonance phlebography

CMRR
>common mode rejection ratio (of amplifiers)

CMRT
>chiropractic manipulative reflex technique

CMS
>cardiomediastinal silhouette
>Cardiovascular Measurement system
>central material section
>central material supply
>cervical mucous solution
>Cholesterol Monitoring system
>chromosome modification site
>chronic myelodysplastic syndrome
>circulation, motion, sensation
>clean, midstream (urine)
>click-murmur syndrome
>clofibrate-induced muscular syndrome
>Clyde Mood Scale
>Conflict Management Survey

cm/s
>centimeters per second (*See also* cmps)

CMSE
>cow's milk-sensitive enteropathy

CMSS
>circulation, motor (ability), sensation, and swelling

CMSUA
>clean, midstream urinalysis

CMT
>California mastitis test
>cancer multistep therapy
>catechol methyltransferase
>cervical motion tenderness
>Charcot-Marie-Tooth (disease/syndrome)
>chemotherapy
>chronic motor tic
>circus-movement tachycardia
>combined modality therapy
>Concept Mastery Test
>continuous memory test
>Current Medical Terminology

CMTC
>cutis marmorata telangiectatica congenita

CMU
>cardiac monitoring unit
>chlorophenyldimethylurea
>complex motor unit

CMUA
>continuous motor unit activity

CMV
>Clo Mor virus
>(congenital) cytomegalovirus (infection)
>continuous mechanical ventilation
>controlled mechanical ventilation
>conventional mechanical ventilation
>cool mist vaporizer
>cucumber mosaic virus
>cytomegalic (inclusion) virus
>Cytomegalovirus

CMVIG, CMVIg
>cytomegalovirus immune globulin
>cytomegalovirus immunoglobulin
>cytomegalovirus-specific immune globulin

CMV-IGIV
>cytomegalovirus immune globulin intravenous

CMV-MN
>cytomegaloviral mononucleosis

CMVS
>culture midvoid specimen

CN
>calcaneonavicular
>calcineurin
>caudate nucleus
>cellulose nitrate
>charge nurse
>child nutrition
>clinical nursing
>cochlear nucleus
>congenital nephrosis
>congenital nystagmus
>cranial nerve (*See also* cr nn)
>Crigler-Najjar (syndrome)
>cyanogen
>cyanosis neonatorum

C/N
>carbon-to-nitrogen (ratio)
>carrier-to-noise (ratio)
>contrast-to-noise (ratio) (*See also* CNR)

Cn
>color naming
>cyanide

CNI–XII, CN1–12
>cranial nerves I–XII

CNA
>calcium nutrient agar
>chart not available

CNAF
chronic nonvalvular atrial
fibrillation

CNAG
chronic narrow angle glaucoma

CNAP
compound nerve action potential
continuous negative airway pressure

CNAV
Cananeia virus

CNB
core needle biopsy
cutting needle biopsy

CNBr
cyanogen bromide (poisonous
vapor)

CNC
clear, no creamy (layer)

CNCbl
cyanocobalamin

CND
canned
cannot determine

CNDC
chronic nonspecific diarrhea of
childhood
chronic nonsuppurative destructive
cholangitis

CNDI
congenital nephrogenic diabetes
insipidus

CNE
chronic nervous exhaustion
concentric needle electrode
could not establish

CNEMG
concentric needle electromyography

CNEP
continuous negative extrathoracic
pressure

CNES
chronic nervous exhaustion
syndrome

CNF
chronic nodular fibrositis
congenital nephrotic (syndrome),
Finnish

CNFA
clinically nonfunctioning pituitary
adenoma

CNFS
craniofrontonasal syndrome

CNH
central neurogenic hyperventilation
community nursing home
contract nursing home

CNHC
chronodermatitis nodularis helicis
chronicus

CNHD
congenital nonspherocytic hemolytic
disease

CNK
cortical necrosis of kidneys

CNL
cardiolipin natural lecithin
chronic neutrophilic leukemia

CNLDO
congenital nasolacrimal duct
obstruction

CNM
centronuclear myopathy
computerized nuclear morphometry

CNMD
chronic neuromuscular disease

CNN
congenital nevocytic nevus

CNNA
culture-negative neutrocytic ascites

cNOS
constitutive nitric oxide synthase

CNP
chronic nonbacterial prostatitis
continuous negative pressure
cranial nerve palsy
C-type natriuretic peptide
cyclic nucleotide phosphodiesterase

CNPAS
congenital nasal pyriform aperture
stenosis

CNPase
cyclic nucleotide phosphohydrolase

CNPS
cardiac nuclear probe scan

CNPV
continuous negative-pressure
ventilation

CNQ
Child Neuropsychological
Questionnaire

CNR
contrast-to-noise ratio (*See also*
C/N)

NOTES

CNRS
citrated normal rabbit serum
CNRT
corrected sinus nodal recovery time
CNS
central nervous system
coagulase-negative staphylococcus
  (*See also* CONS, CoNS)
computerized notation system
congenital nephrotic syndrome
cyanide sulfonate (sulfocyanate)
CNSB
coagulase-negative staphulococcus
  bacteremia
CNSD
chronic nonspecific diarrhea
CNSHA
congenital nonspherocytic hemolytic
  anemia
CNS-L
central nervous system leukemia
CNSLD
chronic nonspecific lung disease
CNT
clean needle technique
continuous nebulization therapy
could not test
current night terrors
cutaneous neural tumor
CNTF
ciliary neurotrophic factor
CNTV
Connecticut virus
CNU
chloroethylnitrosourea
CNUV
Chenuda virus
CNV
choroidal neovascularization
conative negative variation
contingent negative variation
cutaneous necrotizing vasculitis
CNVM
choroidal neovascular membrane
CO
calcium oxalate
candidal onychomycosis
carbon monoxide
cardiac output (*See also* Q)
castor oil
casualty officer
centric occlusion
cervical orthosis
choline oxidase
coenzyme
community organization
control

corneal opacity
crossover
Co
cobalt
Co I
coenzyme I
Co II
coenzyme II
co
cutoff
C/O, c/o
in care of
check out
complains of
complaints
under care of
CO_2, Co_2
carbon dioxide (*See also* CD)
CO_3^{2-}
carbonate
57Co, ^{57}Co, Co 57
cobalt-57
cobalt isotope
60Co, ^{60}Co, Co 60
cobalt-60
cobalt isotope
^{58}Co
cobalt-58
COA
calculated opening area
cervicooculoacusticus (syndrome)
child of alcoholic
coagglutination
condition on admission
CoA
aortic arch coarctation
coarctation of the aorta
coenzyme A
COAB
Computer Operator Aptitude Battery
COACH
cerebellar vermis hypo/aplasia,
  oligophrenia, congenital ataxia,
  ocular coloboma, hepatic fibrosis
COAD
chronic obstructive airway disease
COAG
chronic open angle glaucoma
coagulated (*See also* coag)
coagulation (*See also* coag)
coag
coagulated (*See also* COAG)
coagulation (*See also* COAG)
coagulation study
coag pd
coagulation profile–diagnosis
coag pp
coagulation profile–presurgery

coags
    coagulation panel
coagsc
    coagulation screen
coarc
    coarctation (of aorta)
CoASH
    uncombined coenzyme A
CoA-SPC
    coenzyme A-synthesizing protein
      complex
COAT
    Children's Orientation and Amnesia
      Test
    chronic opioid analgesic therapy
COB
    chronic obstructive bronchitis
    coordination of benefits
Coban
    cohesive bandage
COBE
    chronic obstructive bullous
      emphysema
COBOL
    common business-oriented language
COBRA
    Consolidated Omnibus Budget
      Reconciliation Act
COBS
    cesarean (section)-obtained barrier-
      sustained (animals)
    chronic organic brain syndrome
COBT
    chronic obstruction of biliary tract
COC
    calcifying odotogenic cyst
    cathodal-opening clonus (*See also*
      COCL)
    cathodal-opening contraction
    cement-on-crown
    coccygeal (*See also* coc, cd)
    combined oral contraceptive
coc
    coccygeal (*See also* COC, cd)
CO/CI
    cardiac output/cardiac index
COCL, COCl
    cathodal-opening clonus (*See also*
      COC)
COCM
    congestive cardiomyopathy

Co-Cr-Mo
    cobalt-chromium-molybdenum
Co-Cr-W-Ni
    cobalt-chromium-tungsten-nickel
      (alloy metal implant)
COD
    cause of death
    cementoosseous dysplasia
    cerebroocular dysgenesis
    chemical oxygen demand
    codcine (*See also* cod.)
    computerized optical densitometry
    condition on discharge
cod.
    codeine (*See also* COD)
CODAS
    cerebral, ocular, dental, auricular,
      skeletal (syndrome)
COD-MD
    cerebroocular dysplasia-muscular
      dystrophy
COE
    court-ordered examination
coeff
    coefficient
COEPS
    cortical originating extrapyramidal
      system
COF
    cementoossifying fibroma
    cutoff frequency
CoF
    cobra (venom) factor
    cofactor
COFHP
    chronic oral, facial, head pain
COFS
    cerebrooculofacial-skeletal
     (syndrome)
COG
    center of gravity
    clinical obstetrics and gynecology
    cognitive (function tests)
    Cognitive Observation Guide
COGN
    cognition
COGTT
    cortisone-primed oral glucose
      tolerance test
CoHB, COHB
    carboxyhemoglobin (*See also* HbCO)

C

NOTES

COI
    Central Obesity Index
    combination of isotonics
COIB
    Crowley Occupational Interests
      Blank
COIF
    congenital onychodysplasia of the
      index finger
COL, col
    colicin
    colony
    color
    colored
    column
    cost of living
COL2A1
    type II procollagen gene
COLD
    chronic obstructive lung disease
COLD A, cold agg
    cold agglutinin (titer)
COLDER
    character, onset, location, duration,
      exacerbation, remission
COLL, coll
    collect
    collection
    collective
    colloidal
collat
    collateral
collut.
    mouthwash [L. *collutorium*]
coll vol
    collective volume
COLLYR, collyr.
    eyewash [L. *collyrium*]
col/mL
    colonies per milliliter
color
    colorimetry, including
      spectrophotometry and photometry
    let it be colored [L. *coloretur*]
colp, colpo
    colporrhaphy
    colposcopy
COM
    chronic otitis media
    computer output on microfilm
com
    commitment
COMA
    congenital ocular motor apraxia
    congenital ocular motor apraxia
      (type Cogan)

comb.
    combination
    combine
COME
    chronic otitis media with effusion
COMF, comf
    comfortable
com fix
    complement fixation (*See also* CF)
comm
    commission
    commissioner
    committee
    communicable (*See also* commun)
commun
    communicable (*See also* comm)
commun dis
    communicable disease
COMP
    cartilage oligomeric matrix protein
    complication
comp
    comparable
    comparative
    compare (*See also* CF, cf.)
    compensated
    compensation
    complaint
    composition (*See also* compn)
    compound (*See also* CO, compd,
      CP, cpd)
    compounded (*See also* compd)
    compress
    compression
    computer
compd
    compound (*See also* CO, comp,
      CP, cpd)
    compounded (*See also* comp)
compet
    competition
compl
    completed (*See also* cpl)
    completion (*See also* cpl)
    complicated (*See also* complic)
    complication (*See also* complic)
complic
    complicated (*See also* compl)
    complication (*See also* compl)
compn
    composition (*See also* comp)
COMS
    cerebrooculomuscular syndrome
    chronic organic mental syndrome
COMT
    catechol-*O*-methyltransferase
COMTRAC
    computer-based (case) tracing

CON
    certificate of need
Con
    concanavalin
con.
    against [L. *contra*] (*See also* cont.)
Con A, ConA, conA, con A
    concanavalin A
Con A-HRP
    concanavalin A-horseradish
      peroxidase
conc, concentr
    concentrated
    concentration (*See also* C, c)
COND
    cerebroosteonephrodysplasia
cond
    condensation
    condensed
    condition
    conditional
    conditioned
    conductivity (*See also* σ)
cond ref
    conditioned reflex (*See also* CR)
cond resp
    conditioned response (*See also* CR)
conf
    conference
congen, cong
    congenital
congr
    congruent
coniz
    conization (of cervix)
conj
    conjunctiva
    conjunctivae (plural)
    conjunctival
conjug
    conjugated
    conjugation
CONS
    coagulase-negative staphylococcus
      (*See also* CNS, CoNS)
    consultation (*See also* cons)
CoNS
    coagulase-negative staphylococcus
      (*See also* CNS, CONS)
cons
    conservation
    conservative

    conserve
    consultant
    consultation (*See also* CONS)
const
    constant
constit
    constituent
cont
    containing
    contains
    contents
    continuation
    continue
    contusions
cont.
    against [L. *contra*] (*See also* con.)
    bruised [L. *contusus*] (*See also* C)
contag
    contagion
    contagious
contr
    contraction (*See also* C, contrx,
      CTX, CTXN, Cx)
contra
    contraindicated
contralat
    contralateral
contrib
    contributory
contrx
    contraction (*See also* C, contr,
      CTX, CTXN, Cx)
conv
    convalescence
    convalescent
    convalescing
    conventional (rat)
    convergence
    convergent
convergence
    accommodative c.
conv hosp
    convalescent hospital
conv strab
    convergent strabismus
COOD
    chronic obstructive outflow disease
coord
    coordinated
    coordination
CO-oximetry
    carbon monoxide oximetry

C

NOTES

COP

capillary osmotic pressure
change of plaster
cicatricial ocular pemphigoid
circumoval precipitin
coefficient of performance
colloid oncotic pressure
colloid osmotic pressure
cryptogenic organizing pneumonia

COP 1

copolymer 1

COPC

community-oriented primary care

COPD

chronic obstructive pulmonary
disease

COPE

chronic obstructive pulmonary
emphysema
Coping Operations Preference
Enquiry
Coping Orientations to Problems
Experienced

COPES

Community-Oriented Programs
Environment Scale

COPI

California Occupational Preference
Inventory

COP$_i$

colloid osmotic pressure in
interstitial fluid

COP$_p$

colloid osmotic pressure in plasma

COPRO

coproporphyria (*See also* CP)
coproporphyrin (*See also* CP)

COPS

calcinosis cutis, osteoma cutis,
poikiloderma, and skeletal
abnormalities
California Occupational Preference
Survey

CoQ

coenzyme Q (ubiquinone) (*See also*
Q)

CoQ$_{10}$

coenzyme Q10

COR

body [L. *corpus*]
cardiac output recorder
cervicoocular reflex
comprehensive outpatient
rehabilitation (facility)
conditioned orientation reflex
(audiometry)
coroner
corrosion
corrosive
cortisone

CoR

corepressor

Cor

Congo red (*See also* CR)

cor

coronary
corrected (*See also* corr)
correction

CORA

conditioned orientation reflex
audiometry

CORD

chronic obstructive respiratory
disease

Cor Flow

coronary blood flow

corr

corrected (*See also* cor)
correspondence

cort

cortex (*See also* C)
cortical

CORTIS

cortisol

CORV

Corriparta virus

COS

cheirooral syndrome
childhood-onset schizophrenia
clinically observed seizure

cos

change of shift

COSA

child of substance abuser

Cosm

osmolar clearance

COSTAR

computer-stored ambulatory record

COSTART

Coding Symbols for a Thesaurus
of Adverse Reaction Terms

COT

colony overlay test
content of thought
continuous oxygen therapy
contralateral optic tectum
critical off-time

CO$_2$T

total carbon dioxide content

COTD

cardiac output by thermodilution

COTe

cathodal-opening tetanus

COTX

cast off, to x-ray (*See also* COX,
CRTX)

COU
   cardiac observation unit
coul
   coulomb (*See also* Q, C)
COUP
   chicken ovalbumin upstream
      promoter
COUP-TF
   chicken ovalbumin upstream
      promoter-transcription factor
COV
   crossover value
COVESDEM
   costovertebral segmentation defect
      with mesomelia (syndrome)
CoVF
   cobra venom factor
COWAT
   Controlled Oral Word Association
      Test
COWS
   cold-opposite, warm-same (Hallpike
      caloric stimulation response)
COX
   cast-off x-ray (*See also* COTX,
      CRTX)
   coxsackie virus
   cyclooxygenase
   cytochrome c oxidase
COX-1
   cyclooxygenase-1
COX-2
   cyclooxygenase-2
COX mRNA
   cyclooxygenase messenger
      ribonucleoprotein acid
COZ
   cranioorbitozygomatic osteotomy
CP
   candle-power (*See also* cp)
   capillary pressure
   carbamide peroxide
   carbamoyl phosphate
   cardiac pacing
   cardiac performance
   cardiac pool
   cardiopulmonary
   Carr-Purcell (sequence)
   cell passaged
   central pit
   centric position
   cerebellopontine

cerebral palsy
ceruloplasmin
cervical probe
chemically pure (*See also* cp)
chest pain
child psychiatry
child psychology
chloropurine
chloroquine-primaquine
chondrodysplasia punctata
chondromalacia patellae
chronic pain
chronic pancreatitis
chronic polyarthritis
chronic pyelonephritis
cicatricial pemphigoid
circular polarization
classical pathway
cleft palate (*See also* Clpal)
clinical pathology
closing pressure
clottable protein
cochlear potential
Code of Practice
cold pressor
color perception
combination product
combining power
commercially pure
complete physical
compound (*See also* CO, comp,
   compd)
compressed
congenital porphyria
constant pressure
coproporphyria (*See also* COPRO)
coproporphyrin (*See also* COPRO)
coracoid process
cor pulmonale
cortical plate
costal plaque
C peptide
creatine phosphate
creatine phosphokinase
cross-linked protein
crude protein
current practice
cystosarcoma phyllodes
cytosol protein

CPII

   C propeptide of type II collagen

NOTES

141

C/P
cholesterol-phospholipid (ratio)

C&P
compensation and pension
complete and pain-free (range of motion)
cystoscopy and pyelography

C$_p$
constant pressure
phosphate clearance (*See also* Cp)

Cp
ceruloplasmin
chickenpox (*See also* chix, CHPX, chpx)
peak concentration
phosphate clearance (*See also* C$_p$)

cP
centipoise (*See also* cp)

cp
candle-power (*See also* CP)
centipoise (*See also* cP)
chemically pure (*See also* CP)

CPA
calcaneal pitch angle
carboxypeptidase A
cardiophrenic angle
cardiopulmonary arrest
carotid phonoangiography
cerebellopontine angle
chlorophenylalanine
chronic pyrophosphate arthropathy
circulating platelet aggregate
condylar plateau angle
costophrenic angle
cumulative phase advancement
cyproterone acetate

C3PA
complement 3 proactivator (convertase)

CPAB
Computer Programmer Aptitude Battery

C-PAC, CPAC
Clinical Probes of Articulation Consistency

C-PACG
chronic primary angle-closure glaucoma

CPAD
chronic peripheral arterial disease

CPAF
chlorpropamide-alcohol flushing

Cpah, C$_{pah}$
p-aminohippurate clearance
p-aminohippuric acid clearance

CPAI
central principal axis of inertia

CPA/OPG
carotid phonoangiography/oculoplethysmography

CPAP
constant positive airway pressure
continuous positive airway pressure

CPB
cardiopulmonary bypass
competitive protein binding
controlled position brace

CPBA
competitive protein-binding assay

CPBS
cardiopulmonary bypass surgery

CPBV
cardiopulmonary blood volume

CPC
central posterior curve
cerebellar Purkinje cell
cerebral palsy clinic
cetylpyridinium chloride
chest pain center
choroid plexus carcinoma
choroid plexus cyst
chronic passive congestion
circumferential pneumatic compression
clinicopathologic conference
committed progenitor cell
conventional papillary carcinoma

CPCL
congenital pulmonary cystic lymphangiectasia

CP-CML
chronic phase chronic myelogenous leukemia

CPCN
capitated primary care network

CPCP
chronic progressive coccidioidal pneumonitis

CPCR
cardiopulmonary-cerebral resuscitation

cPCR
competitive polymerase chain reaction

CPCS
circumferential pneumatic compression suit
clinical pharmacokinetics consulting service

CPCV
Cacipacore virus

CPD I–IV
cerebelloparenchymal disorder IV

CPD
> calcium pyrophosphate deposition
> calcium pyrophosphate dihydrate
> cephalopelvic disproportion
> childhood polycystic disease
> chorioretinopathy and pituitary
> dysfunction
> chronic peritoneal dialysis
> citrate-phosphate-dextrose
> congenital penile deviation
> congenital polycystic disease
> contact potential difference
> contagious pustular dermatitis
> critical point drying
> cyclopentadiene

cpd
> compound (*See also* CO, comp,
> compd, CP)
> cycles per degree

CPDA, CPD-A, CPD-adenine
> citrate-phosphate-dextrose-adenine

CPDD
> calcium pyrophosphate deposition
> disease
> calcium pyrophosphate dihydrate
> deposition disease (*See also*
> CPPD)

CPDL
> cumulative population doubling
> level

CPDN
> cystic, partially differentiated
> nephroblastoma

CPDV
> contagious pustular dermatitis

CPE
> cardiogenic pulmonary edema
> chronic pulmonary emphysema
> *Clostridium perfringens* enterotoxin
> compensation, pension, and
> education
> complete physical examination (*See
> also* CPX)
> complex partial epilepsy
> corona-penetrating enzyme
> cytopathic effect
> cytopathogenic effect

CPEO
> chronic progressive external
> ophthalmoplegia

CPET
> cardiopulmonary exercise test

CP-EUS
> catheter probe-assisted endoluminal
> ultrasonography

CPF
> clot-promoting factor
> contraction peak force

C-PF
> coronary-pulmonary fistula

CP&FD
> cephalopelvic disproportion and
> fetal distress

CPG
> capillary blood gases
> cardiopneumographic (recording)
> carotid phonoangiogram
> clinical practice guidelines
> computerized pattern generator

CpG
> cytosine phosphate guanine

CPGN
> chronic proliferative
> glomerulonephritis

CpGV
> Cydia pomonella granulovirus

CPH
> chronic paroxysmal hemicrania
> chronic persistent hepatitis
> chronic primary headache

CPHD
> combined pituitary hormone
> deficiency

CPI
> California Personality Inventory
> California Psychological Inventory
> Cancer Potential Index
> chronic pneumonitis of infancy
> congenital palatopharyngeal
> incompetence
> constitutional psychopathic
> inferiority
> conventional planar imaging
> coronary prognostic index
> cysteine proteinase inhibitor

CPIB
> chlorophenoxyisobutyrate

CPID
> chronic pelvic inflammatory disease

CPIP
> chronic pulmonary insufficiency of
> prematurity
> common peak developed
> isovolumetric pressure

C

NOTES

CPIS
clinical pulmonary infection score
CPIT
California Psychological Inventory Test
CPITN
community periodontal index of treatment needs
CPK
creatine phosphokinase
CPK-BB
brain isoenzymes of creatine phosphokinase
CPKD
childhood polycystic kidney disease
CPKI, CPKISO
creatine phosphokinase isoenzyme(s)
CPK-MB (*See also* MB CK)
myocardial band enzymes of creatine phosphokinase
CPK-MM
muscle fraction enzyme of creatine phosphokinase
CPL

caprine placental lactogen
conditioned pitch level
congenital pulmonary lymphangiectasia
C/PL
cholesterol to phospholipid ratio
cpl

complete (*See also* C)
completed (*See also* compl)
cPLA2
cytosol phospholipase A2
CPLM
cysteine-peptone-liver (infusion) medium
CPLS
cleft palate-lateral synechia syndrome
CPM

central pontine myelinolysis
chlorpheniramine maleate
Clinical Practice Model
cognitive-perceptual-motor
Colored Progressive Matrices (*See also* RCPM)
confined placental mosaicism
continue present management
continuous passive motion (device)
counts per minute (*See also* C/M, cpm)
cpm

counts per minute (*See also* C/M, CPM)
cycles per minute (*See also* c/min)

CPmax
peak (maximum) serum concentration
CPMDI
computerized pharmacokinetic model-driven (drug) infusion
CPMG
Carr-Purcell-Meiboom-Gill (sequence, spin-echo technique)
CPMI
central principal moments of inertia
CP min
trough (minimum) serum concentration
CPMM
constant passive-motion machine
CPMP
computer-patient management problems
CPMS
chronic progressive multiple sclerosis
CPN

carboxypeptidase N
celiac plexus neurolysis
chronic polyneuropathy
chronic pyelonephritis
cisplatin nephropathy
cPNET
central primitive neuroectodermal tumor
CPNM
corrected perinatal mortality
CPP

cancer proneness phenotype
canine pancreatic polypeptide
career planning program
central precocious puberty
cerebral perfusion pressure
choroid plexus papilloma
chronic pelvic pain
chronic pigmental purpura
conditioned place preference
cranial perfusion pressure
cryoprecipitate
CPPB

continuous positive-pressure breathing
CPPD

calcium pyrophosphate dihydrate deposition (disease) (*See also* CPDD, CPPDD)
chest percussion and postural drainage (*See also* CP&PD)
CP&PD
chest percussion and postural drainage (*See also* CPPD)

CPPDD
  calcium pyrophosphate deposition
    disease (*See also* CPPD)
CPPS
  chronic pelvic pain syndrome
  chronic prostatitis/pelvic pain
    syndrome
CPPTS
  complete pacemaker patient testing
    system
CPPV
  continuous positive-pressure
    ventilation
CPQ
  Children's Personality Questionnaire
  Conners Parent Questionnaire
CPR
  cardiac and pulmonary rehabilitation
  cardiopulmonary resuscitation
  centripetal rub
  cerebral cortex perfusion rate
  chlorophenyl red
  clinical partial response
  cochleopalpebral reflex
  computer based patient record
  cortisol production rate
  cumulative potency rate
  customary, prevailing, and
    reasonable
CPRAM
  controlled partial rebreathing
    anesthesia method
C protein
  complement protein
CPRS
  Children's Psychiatric Rating Scale
  Comprehensive Psychopathological
    Rating Scale
CPS
  carbamoyl phosphate synthetase
  cardioplegic perfusion solution
  cardiopulmonary support
  central patient station
  characters per second
  Child Personality Scale
  Child Protective Services
  Children's Protective Service
  chloroquine, pyrimethamine, and
    sulfisoxazole
  clinical performance score
  clinical pharmacokinetic service
  coagulase-positive staphylococci

  complex partial seizure
  compliant prestress system
  Comrey Personality Scale
  constitutional psychopathic state
  contagious pustular stomatitis
  C-polysaccharide
  cumulative pain score
  cumulative probability of success
  current population survey
  cycles per second (*See also* cps,
    C/S, c/s, c/sec)
  pneumococcal capsular
    polysaccharide
  pneumococcal C-polysaccharide
cps
  counts per second
  cycles per second (*See also* CPS,
    C/S, c/s, c/sec)
cPSA
  complexed prostate-specific antigen
CPSC
  congenital paucity of secondary
    synaptic clefts (syndrome)
CPSCS
  California Preschool Social
    Competency Scale
CPSI
  Children's Perception of Support
    Inventory
CPSP
  central poststroke pain
CPSR
  chronic paranoid schizophrenic
    reaction
CPT
  carnitine palmitoyltransferase
  carotid pulse tracing
  chest physical therapy
  chest physiotherapy
  child protection team
  choline phosphotransferase
  chromopertubation
  ciliary particle transport
  clinical pharmacokinetics team
  cold pressor test
  collarless, polished, tapered
  combining power test
  conjunctival provocation test
  continuous performance task
  continuous performance test
  current perception threshold
  Current Procedural Terminology

C

NOTES

CPT1, CPTI, CPT I
    carnitine palmitoyltransferase I
        (deficiency)
CPT2, CPT II, CPTII
    carnitine palmitoyltransferase II
        (deficiency)
CPTH
    chronic posttraumatic headache
    C-terminal parathyroid hormone
CPTN
    culture-positive toxin-negative
CPTP
    culture-positive toxin-positive
CPTR
    cyproterone
CPTX
    chronic parathyroidectomy
CPU
    caudate putamen
    central processing unit
CPUE
    chest pain of unknown etiology
CPV
    canine parvovirus
    coastal plains virus
    Cotia virus
    cytoplasmic polyhedrosis virus
CPVD
    congenital polyvalvular disease
cPVL
    cystic periventricular leukomalacia
CPX
    calciphylaxis
    cardiopulmonary exercise
    complete physical examination (*See
        also* CPE)
CPZ
    cefoperazone
    chlorpromazine
    Compazine
CQ
    carboquone
    chloroquine
    circadian quotient
    conceptual quotient
CQA
    concurrent quality assurance
CQIV
    Calchaqui virus
CQM
    chloroquine mustard
CR
    calcification rate
    calorie restricted
    cardiac rehabilitation
    cardiac rhythm
    cardiorespiratory
    cardiorrhexis

caries resistant
cartilage residue
case report
cathode ray
center of rotation
central ray
centric relation
chest and right arm (lead in
    electrocardiography)
chest roentgenogram
chest roentgenography
child-resistant (bottle top)
choice reaction
chromium (*See also* Cr)
chronic rejection
clinical record
clinical research
closed reduction
clot retraction
coefficient (of fat) retention
colon resection
colony-reared (animal)
colorectal
complement receptor
complete remission
complete responders
complete response
computed radiography
computed radiology
conditioned reflex (*See also* cond
    ref)
conditioned response (*See also* cond
    resp)
congenital rubella
Congo red (*See also* Cor)
contact record
continuous reinforcement
controlled release
controlled respiration
controlled response
conversion rate
cooling rate
correct response
correlation
correlation algorithm
corticoresistant
creamed
creatinine (*See also* cre, C, cr)
cremaster ratio
cresyl red
critical ratio
crown
crown-rump (length) (*See also*
    CRL)
cycloplegic refraction
CR0–10
    category ratio 0–10

CR (1–4), CR(1–4)
　complement receptor 1–4
C&R
　cardiac and respiratory
　convalescence and rehabilitation
　cystocopy and retrograde
C/R
　chorioretinal
Cr
　chromium
⁵¹Cr, Cr 51
　chromium isotope
cr
　creatinine (*See also* C, CR, cre)
CRA
　central retinal artery
　chemotherapy-related amenorrhea
　Chinese restaurant asthma
　chronic rheumatoid arthritis
　cis-retinoic acid
　clinical risk assessment
　colorectal adenocarcinoma
　colorectal anastomosis
　coronary rotational atherectomy
13-CRA
　13-*cis*-retinoic acid
CRABP
　cellular retinoic acid-binding protein
CRAC
　compliance related acute
　　complication
　contract relax agonist contract
CRAG
　cerebral radionuclide angiography
CRAI
　continuous regional arterial infusion
CRAMS
　circulation, respiration, abdomen,
　　motor, and speech
cran
　cranial (*See also* CR, Cr)
　cranium (*See also* Cr)
CRAO
　central retinal artery occlusion
CRAS
　Clinician Rated Anxiety Scale
CRASH
　corpus callosum hypoplasia,
　　retardation, adducted thumbs,
　　spastic paraplegia, hydrocephalus
　　(syndrome)

CRB
　chemical, radiological, and
　　biological
　congenital retinitis blindness
CRBBB
　complete right bundle-branch block
CRBC
　chicken red blood cell (*See also*
　　ChRBC)
CRBP
　cellular retinol-binding protein
Cr&Br
　crown and bridge (*See also* C&B)
CRBSI, CR-BSI
　catheter-related bloodstream
　　infection
CRC
　cardiovascular reflex conditioning
　cerebrovascular reserve capacity
　child-resistant container
　clinical research center
　colorectal cancer
　colorectal carcinoma
　concentrated red (blood) cell
　creatinine clearance (urine) (*See
　　also* C$_{cr}$, CrCl, CC)
　crisis resolution center
　cross-reacting cannabinoids
CR&C
　closed reduction and cast
CRCC
　chromophobe renal cell carcinoma
　cystic renal cell carcinoma
CrCl, Crcl
　creatinine clearance (*See also* CC,
　　C$_{cr}$, CRC)
CR/CO
　centric relation-centric occlusion
CRCS
　calciobiotic root canal scaler
　cardiovascular reflex conditioning
　　system
CRCT
　creamatocrit
　volume percent of cream in milk
CRCV
　cerebral red blood cell volume
CRD
　childhood rheumatic disease
　child-restraint device
　chorioretinal degeneration
　chronic renal disease

NOTES

C

CRD *(continued)*
chronic respiratory disease
completely randomized design
complete reaction of degeneration
complex repetitive discharge
cone-rod dystrophy
congenital rubella deafness
crown-rump distance (fetal
measurement)

CR-DIP
chronic relapsing demyelinating
inflammatory polyneuropathy

CRDS
curdlan sulfate

CRE
cAMP-response element
cardiorespiratory endurance
controlled radial expansion
cumulative radiation effect

cre
creatinine (*See also* C, CR, cr)

CREA-S
creatinine urine spot (test)

CREB
cAMP response element-binding

^{51}Cr-EDTA
51-chromium-labeled
ethylenediaminetetraacetate

CREG
cross-reactive (antigen) group

CREM
cAMP-response element modulator

CRENA
crenated (red blood cells)

crep.
crepitation [L. *crepitus*]

CREST
calcinosis cutis, Raynaud
phenomenon, esophageal motility
disorder, sclerodactyly, and
telangiectasia (syndrome)

CRF
cardiac risk factor
case report form
chronic renal failure
chronic respiratory failure
coagulase-reacting factor
continuous reinforcement
coronary reserve flow
corticotropin-releasing factor

CRFK
Crandell feline kidney (cells)

CRG, CR-gram
cardiorespirogram

CRH
corticotropin-releasing hormone

CRH-BP
corticotropin-releasing hormone-
binding protein

CRH-R1
corticotropin-releasing hormone
receptor type 1

CRH-R2
corticotropin-releasing hormone
receptor type 2

CRHV
cottontail rabbit herpesvirus

CRI
Cardiac Risk Index
Caring Relationship Inventory
catheter-related infection
chronic renal insufficiency
chronic respiratory insufficiency
Composite Risk Index
concentrated rust inhibitor
congenital rubella infection
Coping Resources Inventory
cranial rhythmic impulse
cross-reactive idiotype

CRIB
Clinical Risk Index for Babies

CRIE
crossed radioimmunoelectrophoresis

CRIES
crying, requires, increased,
expression, sleepless

CRIS
controlled release infusion
syndrome

crit
critical
hematocrit (*See also* h'crit, HCT)

Crk
cytokinin-regulated kinase

CrkI
cytokinin-regulated kinase I

CrkII
cytokinin-regulated kinase II

CrkL
cytokinin-regulated kinase L

CRL
cell repository line
complement receptor location
complement receptor lymphocyte
crown-rump length (*See also* CR)

CRM
canalith repositioning maneuver
certified raw milk
Certified Reference Materials
contralateral remote masking
cross-reacting material
crown-rump measurement

CRMI
curved, reformatted mandibular image

CRMO
chronic recurrent multifocal osteomyelitis

CR-MVB
Cramer-Rao minimum variance bound

CRN
cerebral radiation necrosis

cRNA
chromosomal ribonucleic acid

CRNF
chronic rheumatoid nodular fibrositis

cr nn
cranial nerves (*See also* CN)

CRO
cathode ray oscilloscope
centric relation occlusion

CROM
cervical range of motion
cervical range-of-motion (instrument)

CROP
compliance, rate, oxygenation, and pressure

CROS
contralateral routing of signals

CR/OV
colorectal/ovarian

CROW
Charcot restraint orthotic walker

CRP
cAMP receptor protein
canalith repositioning procedure
chronic relapsing pancreatitis
confluent, reticulate papillomatosis
corneal-retinal potential
coronary rehabilitation program
C-reactive protein
cross-reactive protein

CrP
creatine phosphate
phosphocreatine

CRPA
C-reactive protein antiserum

CRPD
chronic restrictive pulmonary disease

CRPF
chloroquine-resistant *Plasmodium falciparum*
closed reduction and percutaneous fixation
contralateral renal plasma flow

CRPP
closed reduction and percutaneous pin ring

CRPS
complex regional pain syndrome

CRQ
Chronic Respiratory Questionnaire

CRR
canal resonance response

CRRT
continuous renal replacement therapy

CRS
catheter-related sepsis
caudal regression syndrome
Cell Recovery System
central supply room
cherry-red spot
Chinese restaurant syndrome
Clinical Rating Scale
colorectal surgery
compliance of the respiratory system
congenital rubella syndrome
Conners Rating Scale
Counter Rotation System (brace)

CRSM
cherry-red spot myoclonus
cranial-sacral respiratory mechanism

CRSP
comprehensive renal scintillation procedure

CrSp
craniospinal

CRST
calcinosis cutis, Raynaud phenomenon, sclerodactyly, telangiectasia
cyanosis, redness, scleroderma, telangiectasia

CRT
cadaver renal transplant
cardiac resuscitation team
cathode-ray tube
central reaction time
certified (*See also* C)

C

NOTES

CRT *(continued)*
    chemoradiation therapy
    choice reaction time
    chromium release test
    circuit resistance training
    complex reaction time
    computed renal tomography
    conformal radiation therapy
    copper reduction test
    coronary radiation therapy
    corrected retention time
    cortisone resistant thymocyte
    cranial radiation therapy
    Critical Reasoning Test

cRT-PCR
    competitive reverse transcription-
      polymerase chain reaction

CrTr
    crutch training *(See also* CT)

CRTX
    cast removed, take x-ray *(See also*
      COTX, COX)

CRU
    cardiac rehabilitation unit
    clinical research unit

CRu
    unconfirmed/uncertain complete
      remission

CRV
    central retinal vein
    channel catfish reovirus
    Cowbone Ridge virus

CRVF
    congestive right ventricular failure

CRVO
    central retinal vein occlusion

CRVS
    California Relative Value Studies

CRW
    Cosman-Roberts-Wells (stereotactic
      frame)

CRY-AB
    cryptococcal antibody

CRY-AG
    cryptococcal antigen

cryo
    cryoglobulin
    cryoprecipitate
    cryosurgery
    cryotherapy

crys, cryst
    crystal
    crystalline
    crystallinized

CRYST
    crystal examination screen

crystal meth
    methamphetamine

CS
    calf serum
    camptomelic syndrome
    carcinoid syndrome
    cardiogenic shock
    caries susceptible
    carotid sheath
    carotid sinus
    catgut suture *(See also* CGS)
    cat scratch (disease) *(See also*
      CSD)
    cavernous sinus
    celiac sprue
    central service
    central supply
    cerebrospinal
    cervical spine *(See also* C-S, C-
      spine)
    cervical stimulation
    cesarean section *(See also* C/S, C-
      section, C sect)
    chemical sympathectomy
    chest strap
    cholesterol stone
    chondroitin sulfate
    chorionic somatomammotropin
    chronic schizophrenia
    cigarette smoke
    cigarette smoker
    cigarette smoke (solution)
    citrate synthase
    climacteric syndrome
    clinical (laboratory) scientist
    clinical stage
    close supervision
    Cockayne syndrome
    cold storage
    colistin
    Collet-Sicard (syndrome)
    completed stroke
    completed suicide
    compression syndrome
    concentrated strength (of solution)
    conditioned stimulus
    congenital syphilis
    conjunctivae-sclerae
    conjunctival secretion
    conscious *(See also* cs)
    consciousness *(See also* Cs, cs)
    constant spring
    consultation service
    contact sensitivity
    continue same (treatment)
    continuing smoker
    continuous stripping
    control serum
    convalescence
    convalescent

coronary sclerosis
coronary sinus
corpus striatum
cortical spoking
corticoid sensitive
corticosteroid
corticosteroid (therapy)
crush syndrome
current smoker
current strength
cyclic sedentary
cycloserine
cyclosporin (See also CSP)

C4S

chondroitin 4-sulfate

C-S

cervical spine (See also CS, C-spine)

C&S

conjunctivae and sclerae
cough and sneeze
culture and sensitivity (See also C/S)
culture and susceptibility

C/S

cesarean section (See also CS, C-section, C sect)
Cost-Stirling (antibody)
culture and sensitivity (See also C&S)
cycles per second (See also CPS, cps, c/s, c/sec)

C$_s$

standard clearance (See also Cs)
static (lung) compliance (See also CST)

Cs

case (See also cs)
cell surface antigen
cesium
consciousness (See also CS, cs)
standard clearance (See also C$_s$)

^{132}Cs

radioactive cesium

^{137}Cs

cesium-137

cS

centistoke (See also cSt)

c/s

cycles per second (See also CPS, cps, C/S, c/sec)

cs

case (See also Cs)
conscious (See also CS)
consciousness (See also CS, Cs)

CSA

canavaninosuccinic acid
chondroitin sulfate A
clinically significant arrhythmia
Cognitive Skills Assessment
colon-specific antigen
colony-stimulating activity
compressed spectral assay
Controlled Substance Act
controlled substance analog
corticosteroid sensitive asthma
cross-sectional area

CSAD

cysteine sulfinic acid decarboxylase

CSAP

colon-specific antigen protein
cryosurgical ablation of the prostate

CSAR

conservative subtraction-addition rhinoplasty

CSAS

central sleep apnea syndrome

CSAVP

cerebral subarachnoid venous pressure

CSB

caffeine sodium benzoate
Cheyne-Stokes breathing
contaminated small bowel

CSB I&II

chemistry screening batteries I and II

CSBF

coronary sinus blood flow

CSBI

Child Sexual Behavior Inventory

CSBO

complete small bowel obstruction

CSBS

contaminated small bowel syndrome

CSC

blow on blow (administration of small doses of drugs at short intervals) [Fr. *coup sur coup*]
central serous choroidopathy
cigarette smoke condensate
collagen sponge contraceptive

NOTES

CSC *(continued)*
cornea, sclera, and conjunctiva
cryogenic storage container
cryopreserved stem cell

C/S & CC
culture and sensitivity and colony
count

CSCED
cribriform salivary carcinoma of
excretory duct

CSCI
continuous subcutaneous infusion

CSCR
central serous chorioretinopathy

CSCS
Children's Self-Concept Scale

C1s–C3s
control proteins C1s–C3s

CSCT
central somatosensory conduction
time
comprehensive support care team

CSD
carotid sinus denervation
cat-scratch disease (*See also* CS)
combined system disease
conditionally streptomycin dependent
conduction system disease
congenital sodium diarrhea
cortically spreading depression
craniospinal defect
critical stimulus duration

CS&D
cleaned, sutured, and dressed

CSDD
Cornell Scale for Depression,
Dementia

CSDH
chronic subdural hematoma

CS/DS
chondroitin sulfate/dermatan sulfate

CSE
clinical-symptom/self-evaluation
(questionnaire)
combined spinal/epidural (anesthesia)
complete surgical exploration
conventional silicone elastomer
coping strategy enhancement
cross-sectional echocardiography

CSEA
combined spinal-epidural anesthesia

c/sec
cycles per second (*See also* CPS,
cps, C/S, c/s)

C-section, C sect
cesarean section (*See also* CS, C/S)

CSEP
cortical somatosensory evoked
potential

CSER
cortical somatosensory evoked
response

CSF
cancer family syndrome
cerebrospinal fluid
circumferential shortening fraction
colony-stimulating factor
contoured femoral stem
coronary sinus flow

CSF-1
colony-stimulating factor-1

CSF-FTA-ABS
colony-stimulating factor fluorescent
treponemal antibody-absorption
(test)

CSFH
cerebrospinal fluid hypotension

CSFI
Cholesterol-Saturated Fat Index

CSF-IFE
cerebrospinal fluid immunofixation
electrophoresis

CSF-MHA-TP
colony-stimulating factor
microhemagglutination-*Treponema
pallidum* (test)

CSFP
cerebrospinal fluid pressure

CSFS
coronary slow flow syndrome

CSFs
colony stimulating factor

CSFV
cerebrospinal fluid volume

CSF-VDRL
colony-stimulating factor developed
by Venereal Disease Research
Laboratory

CSF-WR
cerebrospinal fluid–Wassermann
reaction

CSG
chronic superficial gastritis

CSGBM
collagenase soluble glomerular
basement membrane

CSH
capsular synovial-like hyperplasia
carotid sinus hypersensitivity
chronic subdural hematoma
cortical stromal hyperplasia

C-Sh
chair shower

CSHH
congenital self-healing histiocytosis
CSI

Calculus Surface Index
cancer serum index
Caregiver Strain Index
cavernous sinus infiltration
chemical-shift imaging
cholesterol saturation index
continuous subcutaneous infusion
coronary stenosis index
CsI
cesium iodide
CSICU
cardiac surgery intensive care unit
CSII
continuous subcutaneous insulin
infusion
CSIIP
continuous subcutaneous insulin
infusion pump
CSIS
clinical supplies and inventory
system
CSL

cardiolipin synthetic lecithin
central sacral line
computerized speech lab
CSLD
chronic suppurative lung disease
CSLM
confocal scanning microscopy
CSLR
crossed straight leg raising
CSLU
chronic stasis leg ulcer
CSM

carotid sinus massage
central, steady and maintained
fixation
cerebrospinal meningitis
cervical spondylotic myelopathy
circulation, sensation, mobility
Consolidated Standards Manual
cornmeal, soybean, milk
CSMA
chemical shift misregistration
artifact
chronic spinal muscular atrophy
CSME
cotton-spot macular edema

CSMN
chronic sensorimotor neuropathy
CSMT
capillary refill, sensation, motor
function, temperature
CSN

cardiac sympathetic nerve
carotid sinus nerve
cystic suppurative necrosis
CSNG
congenital stationary night blindness
CSNRT, cSNRT
corrected sinus node recovery time
(See also CSRT)
CSNS
carotid sinus nerve stimulation
CSO

common source outbreak
copied standing orders
crescentic shelf osteotomy
CSOM
chronic suppurative otitis media
CSOP
coronary sinus occlusion pressure
CSP

Cancer Surveillance Program
carotid sinus pressure
cavum septum pellucidi
cell surface protein
cellulose sodium phosphate
chemistry screening profile
Cooperative Statistical Program
criminal sexual psychopath
cyclosporin (See also CS)
CSPI

childhood severity of psychiatric
illness
C-spine
cervical spine (See also CS, C-S)
CSPS
continual skin peeling syndrome
CSQ

College Student Questionnaire
Coping Strategies Questionnaire
CSQI
continuous subcutaneous infusion
CSR

central serous retinopathy
central supply room
Cheyne-Stokes respiration
Communicable Disease Surveillance
and Response

NOTES

CSR *(continued)*
    complete subtalar release
    continued-stay review
    corrected sedimentation rate
    corrected survival rate
    corrective septorhinoplasty
    cortisol secretion rate
    cosmetic skin resurfacing
    cumulative survival rate

CSRA
    cementless surface replacement
    arthroplasty

CSRI
    Caregiver's School Readiness
    Inventory

CSRT
    corrected sinus (node) recovery
    time (*See also* CSNRT, cSNRT)

CSS
    Cancer Surveillance System
    carotid sinus stimulation
    carotid sinus syndrome
    cause-specific survival
    cavernous sinus sampling
    chewing, sucking, swallowing
    chronic subclinical scurvy
    coronary sinus stimulation
    cranial sector scan

CSSA
    carotid stent-supported angioplasty

CSSD
    central sterile supply department

CSSEP
    cortical somatosensory evoked
    potential

CSSQ
    College Student Satisfaction
    Questionnaire

CST
    cardiac stress test
    cavernous sinus thrombosis
    Christ-Siemens-Touraine (syndrome)
    Completing Sentence Test
    Compton scatter tomography
    Conceptual Systems Test
    contraction stress test
    convulsive shock therapy
    corticospinal tract
    cosyntropin stimulation test
    craniosacral therapy
    static (lung) compliance (*See also*
    C_s)

cSt
    centistoke (*See also* cS)

CSTR
    complete subtalar release

CSTT
    cold-stimulation time test

CSU
    cardiac surgery unit
    cardiac surveillance unit
    cardiovascular surgery unit
    casualty staging unit
    catheter specimen of urine
    clinical specialty unit

CSUF
    continuous slow ultrafiltration

CSV
    chick syncytial virus

CSVT
    central splanchnic venous
    thrombosis

CSW
    cerebral salt wasting
    current sleepwalker

CSWT
    cardiac shock wave therapy

CT
    calcitonin
    calf testis
    cardiac tamponade
    cardiothoracic (ratio) (*See also*
    CTR)
    carotid tracing
    carpal tunnel
    Category Test
    cationic trypsinogen
    cell therapy
    center thickness
    cerebral thrombosis
    cerebral tumor
    cervical traction (*See also* CXTX)
    chemotaxis (*See also* CTX)
    chemotherapy
    chest tube
    Chlamydia trachomatis
    chloramine T
    chlorothiazide
    cholera toxin
    chordae tendineae
    chronic thyroiditis
    chymotrypsin
    circulation time
    classic technique
    closed thoracotomy
    clotting time
    coagulation time
    coated tablet
    cobra toxin
    cognitive therapy
    coil test
    collecting tubule
    combined tumor
    compressed tablet
    computed tomography
    computerized tomography

connective tissue
continue treatment
continuous-flow tub
contraction time
controlled temperature
Coombs test
corneal thickness
corneal transplant
coronary thrombosis
corrected transposition
correctional transfer
corrective therapy
cortical thickness
cough threshold
cover test
crest time
crutch training (*See also* CrTr)
cystine-tellurite (medium)
cytotechnology
cytotoxic therapy

CT1
primary chemotherapy

CT-1
cardiotropin-1

C3T
clomiphene citrate challenge test

4C-T
four-chamber transverse

5C-T
five-chamber transverse

C$_{T-1824}$
T-1824 (Evans blue) clearance

C&T
color and temperature
counseling and testing

C/T
compression to traction ratio
crossmatch to transfusion ratio

Ct
carboxyl terminal (*See also* C-terminal)

Ct0$_2$
concentration of total oxygen

CTA
chemotactic activity (*See also* CA)
chromotropic acid
clear to auscultation
computed tomographic angiography
computed tomography angiography
congenital trigeminal anesthesia
cyproterone acetate
cystine trypticase agar

cytoplasmic tubular aggregate
cytotoxic assay
menses [L. *catamenia*]

CTAB
cetyltrimethylammonium bromide
(*See also* CTBM)

C-TAB
cyanide tablet

CTAC
Carrow Test for Auditory
Comprehension
cetyltrimethylammonium chloride

CTACK
cutaneous T-cell attracting
chemokine

CTAF, CTAFS
conotruncal anomaly face syndrome

CTAL
cortical thick ascending limb

CTAO
cerebral thromboangiitis obliterans

CTAP
clear to auscultation and percussion
computed tomography arterial
portography
connective tissue-activating peptide

CTAS
colonic transabdominal sonography

CTAT
computerized transaxial tomography

CTB
calciotraumatic band
ceased to breathe
cytotrophoblast

CTBA
cetrimonium bromide

CTBM
cetyltrimethyl-ammonium bromide
(*See also* CTAB)

CTBS
California Test of Basic Skills
Canadian Test of Basic Skills

CTC
Child-Turcotte classification
chlortetracycline
circular tear capsulotomy
clinical transplant coordinator
computed tomographic colonography
contaminating tumor cell
Creativity Tests for Children
cultured T cell

NOTES

155

CTCL
cutaneous T-cell leukemia
cutaneous T-cell lymphoma

ctCO$_2$
concentration of total carbon dioxide

CTD
carpal tunnel decompression
chest tube drainage
chronic tic disorder
clitoral therapy device
congenital thymic dysplasia
connective tissue disease
corrective therapy department
cumulative trauma disorder

CT&DB
cough, turn, and deep breathe (See also TC&DB)

CTDI
computed tomography dose index

CTDW
continues to do well

CTE
calf thymus extract
chronic traumatic encephalopathy
cultured thymic epithelium

CTEI
communal traumatic experiences inventory

CTEM
conventional transmission electron microscopy

CTEPH
chronic thromboembolic pulmonary hypertension

C-terminal
carboxyl terminal (See also Ct)

CTF
cancer therapy facility
certificate (See also cert)
Colorado tick fever
cytotoxic factor

CTFC
corrected TIMI frame count

CTFV
Colorado tick fever virus

CTG
cardiotocography
cervicothoracic ganglion
chymotrypsinogen

C/TG
cholesterol-triglyceride (ratio)

CTGA
complete transposition of great arteries

CTGF
connective tissue growth factor

CTH
ceramide trihexoside
chronic tension headache
clot to hold
computerized tomographic holography

CTHA
computerized tomographic hepatic angiography

CTI
certification of terminal illness

CTICU, CTIU
cardiothoracic intensive care unit

CTL
cervical, thoracic, and lumbar
cytolytic T cell
cytolytic T lymphocyte
cytotoxic lymphocyte
cytotoxic T lymphocyte

ctl
contact lens (See also CL)

CTLA-4
cytotoxic T lymphocyte antigen-4

CTLA4Ig
cytotoxic lymphocyte activation antigen 4 immunoglobulin

CTLD
chlorthalidone (diuretic and antihypertensive agent)

CTLL
cytotoxic T lymphocyte line

CTLM
computed tomography laser mammography

CTLp
cytotoxic T lymphocyte precursor

CTLSO
cervicothoracolumbosacral orthosis

CTLV
cross-table lateral view

CTM
cardiotachometer
cervical tension myositis
Chlamydia transport media
Chlor-Trimeton
computed tomographic myelography
connective tissue massage
continuous tone masking
cricothyroid muscle

CTMM
California Test of Mental Maturity
computed tomographic metrizamide myelography

CTMM-SF
California Test of Mental Maturity-Short Form

CTMP
>contrast threshold for motion
>perception

CT/MPR
>computed tomography with
>multiplanar reconstructions

CTN
>calcitonin
>chronic transplant nephropathy
>computed tomography number

C&TN BLE
>color and temperature normal, both
>lower extremities

cTnI
>cardiac troponin I

cTNM
>clinical (staging) of tumors, nodes,
>and metastases (etc.) as
>determined by noninvasive
>examination

cTnT
>cardiac troponin T

CTO
>cervicothoracic orthosis
>chest tube output
>chronic total occlusion

CTP
>California Test of Personality
>carboxyl terminal peptide
>comprehensive treatment plan
>cytidine triphosphate
>cytidine 5'-triphosphate
>cytosine triphosphate

C-TPN
>cyclic total parenteral nutrition

CTPP
>cerebral tissue perfusion pressure

CTPV
>cavernous transformation of the
>portal vein
>coal tar pitch volatiles

CTPVO
>chronic thrombotic pulmonary
>vascular obstruction

CTQ
>childhood trauma questionnaire
>Conners Teacher Questionnaire

CTR
>cardiothoracic ratio (*See also* CT)
>carpal tunnel release
>carpal tunnel repair
>cricotracheal resection

ctr
>center

CTRS
>carpal tunnel release system

CTRS-28
>Conners Teacher Rating Scale

CT-RT
>chemo- and radiotherapy

CTS
>cardiothoracic surgery
>carpal tunnel syndrome
>Champion Trauma Score
>clitoris tourniquet syndrome
>Collaborative Transplant Study
>composite treatment score
>computed tomographic scan
>computed tomographic scanner
>computed topographic scan
>computed topographic scanner
>contralateral threshold shift
>corneal topography system
>corticosteroid

CTSI
>computed tomography severity
>index

CTSIB
>Clinical Test of Sensory Interaction
>& Balance

CTSNFR
>corrected time of sinoatrial node
>function recovery

CTSP
>called to see patient

CTT
>cefotetan
>central tegmental tract
>compressed tablet triturate
>computed transaxial tomography

cTT
>cerebral transit time

CTU
>cardiac-thoracic unit (*See also*
>CTIU, CTICU)
>centigrade thermal unit
>constitutive transcription unit

CTV
>cervical and thoracic vertebrae
>clinical target volume
>clinical tumor volume

CTVF
>Comprehensive Test of Visual
>Functioning

NOTES

CTW
    central terminal of Wilson
    combined testicular weight

CTX
    cefotaxime (*See also* TAX)
    cerebrotendinous xanthomatosis
    chemotaxis (*See also* CT)
    chemotoxins
    contraction (*See also* C, contr, contrx, CTXN, Cx)

CTx
    cardiac transplantation

CTXN
    contraction (*See also* C, contr, contrx, CTX, Cx)

CTZ
    chemoreceptor trigger zone
    chlorothiazide

CU
    cardiac unit
    casein unit
    cause unknown
    chymotrypsin unit
    clinical unit
    color unit
    contact urticaria
    control unit
    convalescent unit
    copper
    cusp

C_u
    urea clearance

Cu
    copper [L. *cuprum*]

cu
    cubic (*See also* c)

Cu-7
    Copper-7 (intrauterine contraceptive device)

^{62}Cu
    copper-62

^{64}Cu
    copper-64

^{67}Cu
    copper-67

CuB
    copper band

^{13}C-UBT
    carbon-13 urea breath test

^{14}C-UBT
    carbon-14 urea breath test

CUC
    chronic ulcerative colitis

cu cm
    cubic centimeter (*See also* cc, CC, c.c., cm^3)

CUCS
    complex unroofed coronary sinus

CUD
    cause undetermined
    congenital urinary (tract) deformities

CUE
    cumulative urinary excretion

CUES
    College and University Environment Scales

cu ft
    cubic foot

CUG
    cystidine, uridine, and guanidine
    cystourethrogram
    cystourethrography

CuHVL
    copper half-value layer

cu in
    cubic inch

cult.
    culture

CUM
    cumulative report

cu m
    cubic meter (*See also* m^3)

CUMITECH
    Cumulative Techniques and Procedures in Clinical Microbiology

cu mm
    cubic millimeter (*See also* cmm, mm^3)

cUMP
    cyclic uridine 3,′5′-monophosphate

CUP
    cancer of unknown primary
    carcinoma of unknown primary

CUPS
    cancer of unknown primary site
    carcinoma of unknown primary site

CUR
    chronic urinary retention
    curettage
    cystourethrorectal

cur.
    curative
    cure
    current

CUS
    carotid ultrasound examination
    catheterized urine specimen
    chronic undifferentiated schizophrenia
    compression ultrasound
    contact urticaria syndrome

CUSA
    Cavitron ultrasonic aspirator

cusp.
cuspid
CUSUM, cusum
cumulative sum (method)
CUT
chronic undifferentiated type
(schizophrenia)
CuTS
cubital tunnel syndrome
CUX
check-up x-ray
cu yd
cubic yard
Cu/Zn
copper-zinc
Cu/Zn-SOD
copper-zinc superoxide dismutase
CV
cardiac volume
cardiovascular
carotenoid vesicle
cell volume
central venous
cerebrovascular
cervical vertebra
closed vitrectomy
closing volume
coefficient of variation
collateralizing vessel
collecting vein
color vision
concentrated volume
conducting vein
conduction velocity
consonant vowel (syllable)
contrast ventriculography
conventional ventilation
conversational voice
corpuscular volume
costovertebral
craniosacral vault
cresyl violet
critical value
crystal violet
curriculum vitae
cutaneous vasculitis
true conjugate (diameter of pelvic
inlet) [L. *conjugata vera*]
CV4
craniosacral vault four

C/V
cervical/vaginal
coulomb per volt
Cv, C$_v$
specific heat at constant volume
c.v.
coefficient of variation
cv
conceptional vessel
CVA
cardiovascular accident
cerebrovascular accident
cervicovaginal antibody
chronic villous arthritis
costovertebral angle
cresyl violet acetate
CVAD
central venous access device
CVAH
congenital virilizing adrenal
hyperplasia
CVAS
Colored Visual Analogue Scale
C-Vasc
cerebral vascular (profile study)
CVAT
costovertebral angle tenderness
CVB
chorionic villus biopsy
group B coxsackievirus
CVBS
congenital vascular-bone syndrome
CVC
central venous catheter (*See also*
CV cath)
consonant vowel consonant
(syllable)
CV cath
central venous catheter (*See also*
CVC)
CVCT
cardiovascular computed tomography
CVD
cardiovascular disease (*See also*
CD)
cerebrovascular disease
collagen vascular disease
color vision deviant
cvd
curved
CVE
cerebrovascular evaluation

NOTES

CVF
cardiovascular failure
central visual field
cervicovaginal fluid
cobra venom factor

CVG
composite valve graft
contrast ventriculography

CVGV
CSIRO Village virus

CVH
cerebroventricular hemorrhage
cervicovaginal hood
combined ventricular hypertrophy
common variable
hypogammaglobulinemia

CVHD
chronic valvular heart disease

CVI
cardiovascular incident
cardiovascular insufficiency
cerebrovascular incident
cerebrovascular infarction
cerebrovascular insufficiency
Children's Vaccine Initiative
chronic venous insufficiency
common variable immunodeficiency
(See also CVID)
continuous venous infusion
cortical visual impairment

CVID
common variable immunodeficiency
(See also CVI)

CVIR
Cardiovascular Information Registry

CVK
computerized videokeratography

CVL
central venous line
clinical vascular laboratory

CVLP
coronavirus-like particle

CVLT
California Verbal Learning Test

CVM
cardiovascular malformation
cardiovascular monitor
cerebral venous malformation
childhood visceral myopathy
circular vesicomyotomy
congenital vascular malformation

CVMT
Continuous Visual Memory Test

CVN
central venous nutrition
cochleovestibular neurectomy

CVO
central vein occlusion
central venous oxygen
circumventricular organ
obstetric conjugate (of pelvic inlet)
[L. *conjugata vera obstetrica*]

C$_v$O$_2$
mixed venous oxygen content

CVOD
cerebrovascular obstructive disease

CVOR
cardiovascular operating room

CVP
cardiac valve procedure
cardioventricular pacing
cell volume profile
central venous pressure
cerebrovascular profile

CVR
cardiovascular renal (disease) (See
also CVRD)
cardiovascular resistance
cardiovascular-respiratory
cardiovascular review
cephalic vasomotor response
cerebrovascular reactivity
cerebrovascular resistance
coronary flow velocity reserve

CVRD
cardiovascular renal disease (See
also CVR)

CVRI
cardiovascular resistance index
coronary vascular resistance index

CVRR
cardiovascular recovery room

CVRS
California Relative Value Studies

CVS
cardiovascular surgery
cardiovascular system
cerebral vasospasm
challenge virus strain
chorionic villus sampling
clean-voided specimen
collagen vascular sealing
computer vision syndrome
current vital signs
cyclic vomiting syndrome

CVSF
conduction velocity of slower
fibers

CVST
cerebral venous sinus thrombosis

CVSU
cardiovascular specialty unit

CVT
central venous temperature
cerebral venous thrombosis
congenital vertical talus

CVT-ICU, CVTP-ICU
cardiovascular-thoracic intensive care unit
CVTR
charcoal viral transport medium
CVTS
cardiovascular-thoracic surgery
CVUG
cystoscopy and voiding urethrogram
CVV
Cache Valley virus
CVVII
continuous venovenous hemofiltration
CVVHD
continuous venovenous hemodialysis
CVVHDF
continuous venovenous hemodiafiltration
CW
cardiac work
careful watch
case work
case worker
cell wall
chemical warfare
chemical weapon
chest wall
children's ward
circle of Willis
clockwise (See also cw)
clustered waves
compare with
continuous wave (See also cw)
cotton-wool (spots) (See also CWS)
crutch walking
C/W, c/w
compatible with (See also c/w)
consistent with (See also c/w)
cw
clockwise (See also CW)
continuous wave (See also CW)
CWA
carcinoma with adenomatous areas
CWBTS
capillary whole blood true sugar
CWD
cell wall defective
continuous-wave Doppler
CWDF
cell wall-deficient form (bacteria)

CWE
cotton-wool exudates (See also CW)
CWF
Cornell Word Form
CWH
cardiomyopathy and wooly hair-coat (syndrome)
CWI
cardiac work index
CWIF
cold water immersion foot
CWL
cutaneous water loss
CWMS
color, warmth, movement sensation
CWOP
childbirth without pain
CWP
centimeters of water pressure
coal workers' pneumoconiosis
CWS
cell wall skeleton
chest wall stimulation
Child Welfare Service
circumferential wall stress
cold water soluble
comfortable walking speed
cotton-wool spots (See also CW)
CWSN
Children with Special Health Care Needs
CWT
cold water treatment
Cwt, cwt
hundredweight
CWV
Cape Wrath virus
CX
cancel (See also Cx)
cerebral cortex
cervix (See also Cx)
chest x-ray (film) (See also Cx, CXR)
circumflex (See also Cx, CF)
circumflex artery
cloxacillin
controlled expansion
critical experiment
culture
cylinder axis
phosgene oxime

NOTES

Cx
  cancel (*See also* CX)
  cervix (*See also* CX)
  chest x-ray (film) (*See also* CX, CXR)
  circumflex (*See also* CF, CX)
  clearance
  complex
  complication
  contraction (*See also* C, contr, contrx, CTX, CTXN)
  convex

Cx37
  connexin-37

Cx43
  connexin-43

CxBx
  cervical biopsy

CXCR4
  chemokine-related receptor
  macrophage-derived chemokine

CXM
  cefuroxime
  cyclohexamide

CxMT
  cervical motion tenderness

CXR
  chest radiograph
  chest x-ray (film) (*See also* CX, Cx)

C x T
  concentration multiplied by time

CXTX
  cervical traction (*See also* CT)

CY
  calendar year
  cyanogen (*See also* Cy)

Cy
  cyanogen (*See also* CY)
  cyst

cy
  copy

CyA
  cyclosporine

CY-BOCS
  Children's Yale-Brown Obsessive Compulsive Scale

cyc
  cyclazocine
  cycle
  cyclotron

cyclase
  adenylyl c.

cyclic AMP
  adenosine 3′,5′-cyclic monophosphate

Cyclo C
  cyclocytidine hydrochloride

Cyd/dCyd-D
  cytidine/2′deoxycytidine deaminase

CYE
  charcoal yeast extract (medium)

CYL
  casein yeast lactate (medium)

cyl, cyl.
  cylinder (*See also* C)
  cylindrical lens (*See also* C)

CYN
  cyanide

CYNAP
  cytotoxicity negative, absorption positive

CYP
  cyproheptadine
  cytochrome P450 enzyme
  cytochrome pigment
  cytochrome protein

CYP19
  cytochrome P450 enzyme 19

CYP27
  cytochrome P450 enzyme 27

CyP
  cyclophilin

CYP1A1
  cytochrome P450 enzyme 1A1

CYP11A
  cytochrome P450 enzyme 11A

CYP11B1
  cytochrome P450 11-beta-hydroxylase

CYP21B
  cytochrome P450 enzyme 21B

CYP21B1
  cytochrome P450 21-beta-hydroxylase

CYS
  cystoscopy

Cys
  cyclosporin
  cysteine

cys-LT
  cysteinyl leukotriene

CYSTO, cysto
  cystogram
  cystoscopy

CYT
  cytochrome

Cyt
  cytosine

cyt
  cytologic (*See also* cytol)
  cytology (*See also* cytol)
  cytoplasm
  cytoplasmic

cytol
> cytologic (*See also* cyt)
> cytology (*See also* cyt)

cyt ox
> cytochrome oxidase

cyt sys
> cytochrome system

CZ
> cefazolin

Cz
> central midline placement of electrodes in electroencephalography

CZD
> cefazedone

CZE
> capillary zone electrophoresis

CZI
> crystalline zinc insulin

CZP
> clonazepam

NOTES

C

D

cholecalciferol (vitamin D)
coefficient of diffusion
dacryon (*See also* dac)
date (*See also* d)
daughter (*See also* da, dau)
day (*See also* d, da)
dead (*See also* d)
dead air space
debye (unit)
decay
deceased (*See also* d, DEC, dec, decd, dec'd)
deciduous (*See also* DEC, dec)
decimal reduction time
decrease (*See also* d, DC, DEC, dec, DECR, decr)
degree (*See also* d, DEG)
density (*See also* d)
dental
dentin
depression
dermatologic
dermatologist
dermatology
detail response
deuterium (*See also* d)
deuteron (*See also* d)
development(al) (*See also* dev, devel)
deviation (*See also* DEV, dev)
dexter (right, L. *dexter*)
dextro- (*See also* d)
dextrorotatory
dextrose
diagnosis (*See also* DG, Dg, diag, Dx)
diagonal (*See also* diag)
diameter (*See also* d, dia, diam)
diarrhea (*See also* d)
diastole (*See also* dias)
diathermy
didymium (praseodymium)
died (*See also* d)
difference (*See also* DIFF, diff)
diffusing
diffusion (*See also* DIFF, diff)
dihydrouridine (*See also* hU, hu)
dilated
diminished
Dinamap (blood pressure monitor)
diopter (*See also* d, diopt, Dptr)
direct treatment
disease (*See also* dis, DZ, Dz)
distal (*See also* d, dist)

distance
diuresis
diurnal (*See also* d)
diverticulum
divorced (*See also* d, div)
dominant (*See also* DOM, dom)
donor
dorsal
dose [L. *dosis*] (*See also* d, dos)
drive
drug
dual
duodenal
duodenum
duration (*See also* d)
dwarf
(electric) displacement
give [L. *da*] (*See also* DA)
right [L. *dexter*] (*See also* dex.)

D1

day one (first day of treatment)
first diagonal branch (coronary artery)
type 1 deiodinase

1/D

diffusion resistance

1/d

daily, one per day

1D

one-dimensional

D2

second diagonal branch (coronary artery)
$T_4 5'$-deiodinase type 2
type 2 deiodinase

2,4-D

(2,4-dichlorophenoxy) acetic acid
2,4-dichlorophenoxyacetic acid

2D

two dimensional

2/d

twice a day

D3

cholecalciferol
type 3 deiodinase

3D

delayed double diffusion (test)
three dimensional

D/3, $^D/_3$

distal third

4D

four dimensional
4 prism diopters

D5

dextrose 5% injection

165

D5/45
  dextrose 5% in 0.45% sodium chloride injection
D-15
  Farnsworth panel D. color vision test
D50
  50% dextrose injection
D-
  note not dictated, save chart for doctor
  stereochemical structure
Đ
  mean dose
D+
  note has been dictated/look for report
D$_\beta$
  total body bone mineral density
/d
  per day
d
  atomic orbital with angular momentum quantum number 2
  date (*See also* D)
  day [L. *dies*] (*See also* D, da)
  dead (*See also* D)
  deceased (*See also* D, DEC, dec, dec'd, decd)
  deci-
  decigram
  decrease (*See also* D, DC, DEC, dec, DECR, decr)
  degree (*See also* D, DEG)
  density (*See also* D)
  deoxyribose
  deuterium (*See also* D)
  deuteron (*See also* D)
  dextro- (right, clockwise) (*See also* D)
  diameter (*See also* D, dia, diam)
  diarrhea (*See also* D)
  died (*See also* D)
  diopter (*See also* D, diopt, Dptr)
  distal (*See also* D, dist)
  diurnal (*See also* D)
  divorced (*See also* D, div)
  dorsal
  dose (*See also* D, dos)
  doubtful
  duration (*See also* D)
  dyne
  relative to rotation of a beam of polarized light
  right [L. *dexter*] (*See also* D, dex.)
d-
  dextrorotatary

D-
  sterically related to D-glyceraldehyde
D$_5$E$_{48}$
  5% dextrose and electrolyte 48% (solution)
D5E75
  5% dextrose and electrolyte 75 (solution)
D-A
  donor-acceptor
DA
  dark adaptation (test)
  dark agouti (rat)
  daytime asthma
  decubitus angina
  degenerative arthritis
  delayed action
  delivery awareness
  developmental age
  dextroamphetamine
  diabetic acidosis
  diagnostic arthroscopy
  diastolic augmentation
  differentiation antigen
  diphenylchlorarsine
  direct admission
  direct agglutination
  disability assistance
  disaggregated
  dispense as directed (*See also* DAD)
  diversional activity
  dopamine
  drug addict
  drug addiction
  drug aerosol
  ductus arteriosus
  give [L. *da*] (*See also* D)
D4-A
  androstenedione
D/A
  date of accident
  date of admission
  digital-to-analog (converter)
  discharge and advise
D&A
  dilatation and aspiration
Da
  dalton
dA
  day of admission
  deoxyadenosine (*See also* dAdo)
da
  daughter (*See also* D, dau)
  day (*See also* D, d)
  deca-

DAA
- dead after arrival
- dehydroacetic acid
- digital auditory aerobics
- dissection aortic aneurysm
- double aortic arch

DA/A
- drug/alcohol addiction

$D_{A-a}O_2$
- alveolar-to-arterial oxygen difference

DAB
- carcinogenic
- days after birth
- diaminobenzidine
- 3,3'-diaminobenzidine tetrahydrochloride dihydrate
- diaminobutyric acid
- dimethylaminoazobenzene
- dysrhythmic aggressive behavior

DAB-2
- Diagnostic Achievement Battery, Second Edition

DABS
- Derogatis Affects Balance Scale

DAC
- day activity center
- deep abdominal complication
- Depressive Adjective Checklist
- digital-to-analog converter
- disabled adult child
- disaster assistance center

dac
- dacryon (See also D)

DACA
- dissecting aneurysm of the coronary artery
- Drug Abuse Control Amendments

DACL
- Depression Adjective Check List

DACS
- density-adjusted cell sorting

DAD
- delayed afterdepolarization
- diffuse alveolar damage
- diode array detector
- dispense as directed (See also DA)
- drug administration device

DADA
- dichloroacetic acid diisopropylammonium salt

DADAG
- 1,2:5,6-diacetyldianhydrogalactitol

DADDS
- diacetyldiaminodiphenyl sulfone

dAdo
- deoxyadenosine (See also dA)

dADP
- deoxyadenosine diphosphate

DADPS
- diphenylsulfone

DADS
- distal acquired demyelinating symmetrical (neuropathy)

DAdV
- duck adenovirus

DAE
- diphenylanthracene endoperoxide
- diving air embolism

DAEC
- diffusely adherent Escherichia coli

DAF
- decay-accelerating factor
- delayed auditory feedback
- direct amplification fingerprinting
- Draw-A-Family (test)
- dural arteriovenous fistula
- dynamic axial fixator

DAFM
- double aerosol face mask

DAG
- diacylglycerol
- dianhydrogalactitol
- diffuse antral gastritis
- dimeric acidic glycoprotein

DAGT
- direct antiglobulin test

DAGV
- D'Aguilar virus

DAH
- diffuse alveolar hemorrhage
- disordered action of heart

DAI
- diffuse axonal injury

DAL
- diffuse aggressive lymphomas
- drug analysis laboratory

daL
- decaliter

DALA, d-ALA
- delta-aminolevulinic acid

DALE
- Developmental Assessment of Life Experiences
- Drug Abuse Law Enforcement

D

NOTES

DALI
    Dartmouth Assessment of Lifestyle Instrument
DALM
    dysplasia-associated lesion or mass
DALY, DALYs
    disability-adjusted life year(s)
DAM
    degraded amyloid
    diacetylmonoxime
    diacetylmorphine
    discriminant analytic model
dam
    decameter
DAMA
    discharged against medical advice
DAMIA
    direct acute myocardial infarction angioplasty
DAMP
    deficits in attention, motor control, perception
dAMP
    deoxyadenosine monophosphate
    deoxyadenylic acid
DAN
    diabetic autonomic neuropathy
DANA
    designed after natural anatomy
    drug-induced antinuclear antibodies
DAN-PSS
    Danish Prostate Symptom Score
DANS
    1-dimethylamino-naphthalene-5-sulfonic acid
DAO
    diamine oxidase
    duly authorized officer
DAo, Dao
    descending aorta
DAOM
    depressor anguli oris muscle
DAP
    dapsone
    data acquisition processor
    delayed after polarization
    depolarizing afterpotential
    diabetes-associated peptide
    diastolic arterial pressure
    dihydroxyacetone phosphate
    dipeptidyl amino peptidase (*See also* DAT)
    direct (latex) agglutination pregnancy (test) (*See also* DAPT)
    distending airway pressure
    Diversity Awareness Profile
    dose area product
    Draw-A-Person (test)
    dynamic aortic patch
    real-time dose area product
DAPI
    4,6-diamidino-2-phenylindole-2-HCl
DAPP-BQ
    Dimensional Assessment of Personality Pathology-Basic Questionnaire
DAPRE
    Daily Adjusted Progressive Resistance Exercise
DAPRU
    Drug Abuse Prevention Resource Unit
DAPS
    dark-adapted pupil size
    Differentiation of Auditory Perception Skill
DAP:SPED
    Draw-A-Person Screening Procedure for Emotional Disturbance
DAPST
    Denver Auditory Phoneme Sequencing Test
DAPT
    diaminophenyl thiazole
    direct (latex) agglutination pregnancy test (*See also* DAP)
DAQ
    Diagnostic Assessment Questionnaire
DAR
    daily affective rhythm
    data, action, response
    Diagnostic Assessments of Reading
    dual asthmatic reaction
DARE
    data, action, response, and evaluation
    Drug Abuse Resistance Education
DARF
    direct antiglobulin rosette-forming
DARP
    drug abuse reporting program
D/ART
    Depression: Awareness, Recognition, and Treatment
DARTS
    Drug and Alcohol Rehabilitation Testing System
DAS
    data-acquisition system
    day of admission surgery
    dead air space
    dead at scene
    death anxiety scale
    delayed anovulatory syndrome
    developmental apraxia of speech
    dextroamphetamine sulfate

DASA
distal articular set angle
DASE
Denver Articulation Screening
Exam
dobutamine-atropine stress
echocardiography
DASH
Dietary Approaches to Stop
Hypertension (diet)
disabilities of the arm, shoulder,
and hand
Distress Alarm for the Severely
Handicapped
DASI
Developmental Activities Screening
Inventory
Duke Activity Status Index
DASP
double antibody solid phase
DAST
Drug Abuse Screening Test
DAT
definitely abnormal tracing
(electrocardiogram)
delayed-action tablet
dementia of Alzheimer type
dental aptitude test
Developmental Articulation Test
diet as tolerated
differential agglutination test
Differential Aptitude Test
dipeptidyl amino peptidase (See also
DAP)
diphtheria antitoxin
direct agglutination test
direct amplification test
direct antiglobulin (Coombs) test
Disaster Action Team (of Red
Cross)
DATE
dental auxiliary teacher education
DATI
diastolic amplitude time index
dATP
deoxyadenosine triphosphate
DATT
deep anterior tibiotalar
DATTA
Diagnostic and Therapeutic
Technology Assessment

DAU
Dental Auxiliary Utilization
drug abuse urine
dau
daughter (See also D, da)
DAV
Drosophila A virus
DAVM
dural arteriovenous malformation
DAW
dispense as written
DAWG
demucosalized augmentation with
gastric segment
dAXP
total adenine deoxyribonucleotide
DAZ
deleted in azoospermia
DAZH
deleted in azoospermia-homologue
DAZLA
deleted in azoospermia-like
autosomal
DB
Baudelocque diameter
database
date of birth (See also D/B, DOB)
deep breath
demineralized bone
demonstration bath
dense body
dermabrasion
dextran blue
diabetic (See also dia)
diagonal band
diaphragmatic breathing
diet beverage
direct bilirubin (See also DBIL,
DBR)
disability (See also dis)
distobuccal
double-blind (study)
dry bulb
duodenal bulb
Dutch belted (rabbit)
D/B
date of birth (See also DB, DOB)
dB
decibel
db
diabetes

D

NOTES

DBA
  Diamond-Blackfan anemia
  dibenzanthracene
  Dolichos biflorus agglutinin
DBAE
  dihydroxyborylaminoethyl
DBC
  dibencozide
  distance between centers
  distobuccal cusp
  dye-binding capacity
DB&C
  deep breathing and coughing
DBCL
  dilute blood clot lysis (method)
DBCP
  dibromochloropropane
DBCR
  distobuccal cusp ridge
3DBCT
  Three-Dimensional Block
    Construction Test
DBD
  definite brain damage
  DNA-binding domain
DBDC
  distal bile duct carcinoma
DBDG
  distobuccal developmental groove
DBE
  deep breathing exercise
  dibromoethane
DBED
  dibenzylethylenediamine dipenicillin
    (penicillin G benzathine)
dBEMCL
  decibel effective masking
    contralateral
D5BES
  dextrose in balanced electrolyte
    solution
DBF
  disturbed bowel function
DBFF
  distally based fasciocutaneous flap
DBH
  dopamine-beta hydroxylase
dBHL
  decibels hearing level
DBI
  development-at-birth index
  diffuse brain injury
  documented bacterial infection
DBIL, D bili
  direct bilirubin (*See also* DB,
    DBR)
DBIOC
  database input/output control

DBIP
  Discrimination by Identification of
    Pictures
dBk
  decibels above 1 kilowatt
DBKT
  Diabetes: Basic Knowledge Test
DBL
  distance between nasal lines
  double beta-lactam
dbl
  double
DBM
  database management
  decarboxylasebase Moeller
  demineralized bone matrix
  diabetic management
  dibenzoylmethane
  dibromomannitol
  dobutamine
dBm
  decibels above 1 milliwatt
DBMG
  mandelonitrile beta-glucuronide
DBMS
  database management system
DBMT
  displacement bone marrow
    transplantation
dBnHL
  decibels normal hearing level
DBO
  distobuccoocclusal
db/ob
  diabetic obese (mouse)
DBP
  D-binding protein
  demineralized bone powder
  diastolic blood pressure
  di-*tert*-butyl peroxide (*See also*
    DTBP)
  dibutyl phthalate
  distobuccopulpal
  Döhle body panmyelopathy
  vitamin D-binding protein
DBPC
  dual balloon perfusion catheter
DBPCFC
  double-blind placebo-controlled food
    challenge
DBQ
  debrisoquin
DBR
  direct bilirubin (*See also* DB,
    DBIL)
  disordered breathing rate
  distobuccal root

DBS
deep bonding system
deep brain stimulation
Denis Browne splint
desirable body weight
despeciated bovine serum
dibromosalicil
diffuse brain swelling
diminished breath sounds
direct bonding system
direct brain stimulation
dried blood stain

DBSL
dorsal brain stem lipoma

dBSL
decibels sensation level

dBSPL
decibels sound pressure level

DBT
dialectical behavior therapy
disordered breathing time
dry bulb temperature

DBV
Dakar bat virus

DBW
desirable body weight
dry body weight

dBW
decibels above 1 watt

DBZ
dibenzamine

DC
daily census
data communication
daycare
decarboxylase
decrease (*See also* D, d, DEC, dec, DECR, decr)
deep compartment
degenerating cell
dendritic cell
deoxycholate
descending colon
dextran charcoal
dextrocardia
diagnostic center
diagnostic code
diagonal conjugate (diameter)
differentiated carcinoma
differentiated cell
diffuse cortical
digit copying

dilation catheter
dilation and curettage (*See also* D&C)
diphenylarsine cyanide
direct and consensual (*See also* D&C)
direct Coombs (test)
direct current
discharge (*See also* disch)
discharged
discomfort
discontinue (*See also* dc)
discontinued (*See also* D/C'd)
distal colon
distal cusp
distocervical
donor cells
dorsal column
dressing change
dual chamber
duodenal cap
Dupuytren contracture
dynamic compression
dyskeratosis congenita

D&C, D and C
dilation and curettage (*See also* DC)
direct and consensual (*See also* DC)
drugs and cosmetics

D/C
diarrhea/constipation
disconnect

dC
deoxycytidine

dc
discontinue (*See also* DC)

d/c
discharge (vaginal)

DCA
deoxycholate-citrate agar
deoxycholic acid
desoxycorticosterone acetate
dicarboxylic acid
dichloroacetate
directional color angiography
directional coronary angioplasty
directional coronary atherectomy
disk-condyle adhesion
double cup arthroplasty

DCAG
double coronary artery graft

D

NOTES

DCAI
> desmoplastic cerebral astrocytoma of infancy

DC-ART
> disease-controlling antirheumatic therapy

DCB
> dichlorobenzidine
> dilutional cardiopulmonary bypass
> distal communicating branch

DC&B
> dilation, curettage, and biopsy

DCBE
> double-contrast barium enema

DCBF
> dynamic cardiac blood flow

DCBGS
> direct-current bone growth stimulator

DCC
> day care center
> deleted in colorectal carcinoma
> detected in colon cancer
> dextran-coated charcoal
> diabetes care clinic
> dicyclohexylcarbodiimide (*See also* DCCD)
> direct cardiac compression
> direct current cardioversion
> dorsal calcaneocuboid
> dorsal cell column
> double concave (*See also* DCc, DDc)

DCc
> double concave (*See also* DCC, DDc)

DCCD
> dicyclohexylcarbodiimide (*See also* DCC)

DCCF
> dural carotid-cavernous fistula

DC$_{CO2}$
> diffusing capacity for carbon dioxide

DCD
> Dennis Test of Child Development
> developmental coordination disorder

D/C'd
> discontinued (*See also* DC)

DCE
> delayed contrast enhancement
> demosterol-to-cholesterol enzyme
> designated compensable event

DCE-MRI
> dynamic contrast-enhanced magnetic resonance imaging

DCF
> data collection form
> 2'-deoxycoformycin
> direct centrifugal flotation
> dopachrome conversion factor

DCFM
> Doppler color flow mapping

DCG
> dacryocystography
> desoxycorticosterone glucoside
> diagnostic cardiogram
> disodium cromoglycate
> dynamic electrocardiogram

DCGI
> double-contrast barium examination of the upper gastrointestinal tract

DCH
> delayed cutaneous hypersensitivity

DCHA
> dicyclohexylamine

DCHFB
> dichlorohexafluorobutane

DCHN
> dicyclohexylamine nitrate

DCHS
> dysarthria-clumsy hand syndrome

DCI
> delayed cerebral ischemia
> dichloroisoprenaline
> dichloroisoproterenol

DCIA
> deep circumflex iliac artery
> deep circumflex iliac artery (flap)

DCIS
> ductal carcinoma in situ

DCIV
> deep circumflex iliac vein

dCK
> 2'-deoxycytidine kinase

DCL
> dicloxacillin
> diffuse cutaneous leishmaniasis
> digital counter/locator
> disseminated cutaneous leishmaniasis

DCLHb
> diaspirin cross-linked hemoglobin

DCLS
> deoxycholate citrate lactose saccharose (agar)

DCM
> dementia care mapping
> dichloromethane
> dichloromethotrexate
> dilated cardiomyopathy
> dyssynergia cerebellaris myoclonica

DCML
> dorsal column medial lemniscus

DCMO
> dihydrocarboxanilidomethyloxathin

dCMP
deoxycytidine monophosphate
deoxycytidylic acid
dCMP-D
2′-deoxycytidylate deaminase
DCMX
dichloro-*m*-xylenol
DCMXT
dichloromethotrexate
DCN
Data Collection Network (medical
records)
delayed conditioned necrosis
dorsal column nucleus
dorsal cutaneous nerve
D$_{CO}$, DCO
diffusing capacity for carbon
monoxide (*See also* DLCO, D$_{LCO}$,
DL$_{CO}$)
pulmonary diffusion capacity
DCOM
dilated cardiomyopathy
DCP
calcium phosphate, dibasic
des-gamma-carboxy prothrombin
dicalcium phosphate
dichlorophene
discharge planner
dynamic compression plate
DCPC
dichlorodiphenylmethyl carbinol
DCPN
direction-changing positional
nystagmus
DCPU
dorsal caudate putamen
DCR
dacryocystorhinostomy
delayed cutaneous reaction
digitorenocerebral syndrome
direct cortical response
distal cusp ridge
DCRF
data case report forms
3-DCRT, 3DCRT
three-dimensional conformal
radiation therapy
three-dimensional conformal therapy
DCS
decompression sickness
dense canalicular system
department of children's services

diffuse cortical sclerosis
disease control serum
distal coronary sinus
dorsal column stimulation
dorsal column stimulator
dorsal cord stimulation
dyskinetic cilia syndrome
DCSA
double-contrast shoulder
arthrography
1D-CSI
one-dimensional chemical-shift
imaging
DCSU
day care surgical unit
DCT
deceleration time
deep chest therapy
direct Coombs test
distal convoluted tubule
diurnal cortisol test
dynamic computed tomography
3D-CTA
three-dimensional computed
tomographic angiography
DCTD
diffuse connective tissue disease
DCTM
delay computer tomographic
myelography
DCTMA
desoxycorticosterone trimethylacetate
3D-CTP
three-dimensional computed
tomography pancreatography
dCTP
deoxycytidine triphosphate
DCTPA
desoxycorticosterone triphenylacetate
DCU
day care unit
dichloral urea
DCUS
duplex color ultrasonography
DCV
delayed cerebral vasoconstriction
Drosophila C virus
DCW
direct care worker
DCX
double-charge exchange

D

NOTES

DCx
   double convex
dCYD
   2'-deoxycytidine
D-D
   duct-to-duct
DD
   daily [L. *de die*] (*See also* d.d.)
   dangerous drug
   Darier disease
   day of delivery
   degenerative disease
   delayed diarrhea
   delivery date
   delusional disorder
   dependent drainage
   Descemet (membrane) detachment
   detrusor dyssynergia
   developmental disability
   developmentally delayed
   developmentally disabled
   dialysis dementia
   diaper dermatitis
   died of the disease
   differential diagnosis (*See also* D/D,
      DDX, DDx, DIAGNO, diff diag)
   digestive disease
   discharged dead
   discharge diagnosis
   disk diameter
   disk diffusion
   Distortion of Dots
   double diffusion
   double dose
   down drain
   drug dependence
   dry dressing
   dual disorder
   due date
D1–D12
   first through twelfth dorsal
      vertebrae (*See also* T1–T12)
D→D
   discharge to duty
D&D
   debridement and dressing
   diarrhea and dehydration
   drilling and drainage
D/D
   differential diagnosis (*See also* DD,
      DDX, DDx, DIAGNO, diff diag)
Dd
   unusual detail response
dD
   confabulated detail response
d.d.
   daily [L. *de die*] (*See also* DD)

dd
   disc diameter
DDA
   Dangerous Drugs Act
   dideoxyadenosine
   digital differential analyzer
   digital display alarm
   dorsal digital artery
ddAdo
   2',3'-dideoxyadenosine
ddATP
   dideoxyadenosine triphosphate
DDAVP
   desmopressin acetate (generic name)
dDAVP
   deamino-8-D-arginine vasopressin
      (desmopressin acetate)
DDC
   dangerous drug cabinet
   diethyldithiocarbamate
      (diethyldithiocarbamic acid)
   dihydrocollidine
   dihydroxyphenylalanine
      decarboxylase
   direct display console
   diverticular disease of colon
DDc
   double concave (*See also* DCC,
      DCc)
ddC, ddc
   dideoxycytidine
   2'3'-dideoxycytidine (*See also*
      ddCyd)
ddClAdo
   2',3'-dideoxy-2-chloroadenosine
ddCMP
   2'3'-dideoxycytidine 5'-
      monophosphate
ddCyd
   2',3'-dideoxycytidine (*See also* ddC,
      ddc)
DDD
   defined daily dose
   degenerative disk disease
   dense deposit disease
   Denver dialysis disease
   dichlorodiphenyldichloroethane
   dihydroxydinaphthyl disulfide
   double-dose delay
   Dowling Degos disease
   dual-mode, dual-pacing, dual-sensing
      (pacemaker)
DDD CT
   double-dose–delay computed
      tomography
dD/dt
   derived value on apex cardiogram

DDE

dichlorodiphenyldichloroethylene
direct data entry

DDFP

dodecafluoropentane

DDFS

distant-disease-free survival

DDG

deoxy-D-glucose

ddG

dideoxyguanosine

DDGB

double-dose gallbladder
(cholecystogram)

DDGE

denaturing density gradient
electrophoresis

DDH

developmental dysplasia of hip
dissociated double hypertropia

DDI

dideoxyinosine (*See also* ddI,
ddIno)
dressing dry and intact
drug dose intensity

D-Di

D-dimer

ddI

didanosine
dideoxyinosine (*See also* DDI,
ddIno)

DDIB

Disease Detection Information
Bureau

ddIno

dideoxyinosine (*See also* ddI, DDI)

DDIs

drug-drug interactions

DDM

Dyke Davidoff-Masson (syndrome)

DDMC

diabetes disease management clinic

DDMS

degenerative dense microsphere

ddN

2′,3′dideoxynucleoside

dDNA

denatured deoxyribonucleic acid

DDNOS

dissociative disorder not otherwise
specified

DDNS

digestive disease and nutrition
service

DdNTP

2′,3′-dideoxynucleoside-5′-triphosphate

DDP

density-dependent phosphoprotein
difficult-denture patient
distributed data processing
dual drop pelvis

DDR

diastolic descent rate
direct digital radiography
discharged during referral

DD2R

dopamine D2 receptor

DDRA

dead despite resuscitation attempt

DDS

damaged disk syndrome
dendrodendritic synaptosome
dental distress syndrome
Denys-Drash syndrome
depressed DNA synthesis
dialysis disequilibrium syndrome
diaminodiphenylsulfone (dapsone)
(*See also* DDSO)
directional Doppler sonography
disability determination service
disease disability scale
dodecyl sulfate
double decidual sac

DDs

developmental disorders

Dds

detail response to small white
space

DDSO

diaminodiphenylsulfone (dapsone)
(*See also* DDS)

DDST

Denver Developmental Screening
Test

DDT

dichlorodiphenyltrichloroethane
(chlorophenothane)
ductus deferens tumor
dye disappearance test

DDTP

drug dependence treatment program

ddTTP

dideoxythymidine triphosphate

NOTES

175

DDU
> dermodistortive urticaria

DDVP
> dimethyldichlorovinyl phosphate (dichlorvos)

DDW
> double distilled water

D 5% DW
> 5% dextrose in distilled water

D/DW
> dextrose in distilled water

DdW
> detail response elaborating the whole

DDX, DDx
> differential diagnosis (*See also* DD, D/D, DIAGNO, diff diag)

DE
> dendritic expansion
> deprived eye
> dermal epidermal (junction)
> diagnostic error
> dialysis encephalopathy
> diatomaceous earth
> digestive energy
> digitalis effect
> dobutamine echocardiogram
> dobutamine echocardiography
> dose equivalent
> dream elements
> drug evaluation
> duodenal exclusion
> duration of ejection

2DE
> two-dimensional echocardiography

3DE
> three-dimensional echocardiography

D&E
> diet and elimination
> dilatation and evacuation
> dilation and evacuation

de
> edge detail

DEA
> diethanolamine
> diethylamine
> Drug Enforcement Administration
> Drug Enforcement Agency

DEA #
> Drug Enforcement Agency number (physicians' federal narcotic number)

DEA-D, DEAE-D
> diethylaminoethyl dextran

DEAE
> diethylaminoethanol
> diethylaminoethyl (cellulose)

DEAFF
> detection of early antigen fluorescent focus

DEB
> diepoxybutane
> diethylbutanediol
> dystrophic epidermolysis bullosa

deb
> debridement

DEBA
> diethylbarbituric acid

debil
> debility

DEBS
> dominant epidermolysis bullosa simplex

DEC
> deceased (*See also* D, d, dec, decd, dec'd)
> deciduous (*See also* D, dec)
> decimal
> decimeter
> decrease (*See also* D, d, DC, dec, DECR, decr)
> deoxycholate citrate
> Developmental Evaluation Center
> diethylcarbamazine
> dynamic environmental conditioning (cycle)
> pour off [L. *decanta*]

dec
> decant
> deceased (*See also* D, d, DEC, decd, dec'd)
> deciduous (*See also* D, DEC)
> decompose
> decomposition
> decrease (*See also* D, d, DC, DEC, DECR, decr)

DECA
> nandrolone decanoate

decd, dec'd
> deceased (*See also* D, d, DEC, dec)

DECEL, decel
> deceleration

DECO
> decreasing consumption of oxygen

decoct
> decoction

decomp
> decompose
> decomposition

decon
> decontamination

DECR, decr
> decrease (*See also* D, d, DC, DEC, dec)

dec (R)
    decrease, relative
DECUB, decub.
    decubitus position
    lying down [L. *decubitus*]
    pressure ulcer
DED
    date of expected delivery
    defined exposure dose
    delayed erythema dose
    diabetic eye disease
    died in emergency department
DEDLE
    distinctive exudative discoid and
        lichenoid dermatitis
DEEDS
    drugs, exercise, education, diet, and
        self-monitoring
DEEG
    depth electroencephalogram
    depth electroencephalography
    depth electrography
decp gastric-transverse
DEEP-IN
    delirium, dementia, depression,
        drugs; eyes and ears; physical
        performance and "phalls" (falls)-
        incontinence; nutrition
DEET
    diethyltoluamide
    n,n-diethyl-m-toluamide
DEF
    decayed, extracted, filled
        (permanent teeth)
    defecation
    deficiency (*See also* defic)
    deficient (*See also* defic)
    definite, definition
    duck embryo fibroblast
2-DEF
    two-dimensional echo-derived
        ejection fraction
def
    decayed, extracted, filled (deciduous
        teeth)
    deficiency
defib
    defibrillate
    defibrillation
defic
    deficiency (*See also* DEF)

deform.
    deformed
    deformity
DEFS
    detailed evaluation of facial
        symmetry
DEFT
    driven equilibrium Fourier
        transform
DEG, deg
    degeneration (*See also* degen)
    degenerative (*See also* degen)
    degree (*See also* D, d)
    diethylene glycol
degen
    degeneration (*See also* DEG)
    degenerative (*See also* DEG)
DEH
    dysplasia epiphysealis hemimelica
DEHFT
    developmental hand function test
DEHOP
    diethylhomospermine
DEHP
    diethylhexyl phthalate
dehyd
    dehydrated
    dehydration
DEI
    Disease Extent Index
DEJ, dej
    dentinoenamel junction
    dermal-epidermal junction
DEL
    delivered
    deltoid
del
    deletion
    delivery
    delusion
DELFIA
    dissociation-enhanced lanthanide
        fluoroimmunoassay
deliq
    deliquescence
    deliquescent
δ, delta
    delta (fourth letter of Greek
        alphabet), lowercase
    fourth in a series or group
    heavy chain of immunoglobulin D

D

NOTES

Δ, delta
  absence of heat in a reaction
  delta (fourth letter of Greek
    alphabet), uppercase
  delta gap
  difference (mathematics)
  double bond
delta-HCD
  delta-heavy-chain disease
DEM, Dem
  Demerol
  Developmental Eye Movement
  diethylmaleate
  drug evaluation matrix
DEMRI
  dynamic enhanced magnetic
    resonance imaging
DEN
  dengue (fever)
  dermatitis exfoliativa neonatorum
  diethylnitrosamine
denat
  denatured
DENM
  direct eighth nerve monitoring
denom
  denominator
DENS
  direct electrical nerve stimulation
DENT
  Dental Exposure Normalization
    Technique
dent
  dental
  dentist
  dentistry
  dentition
DENV 1–4
  dengue virus 1–4
DEP
  diethylpropanediol
  diethyl pyrocarbonate
  dilution end point
dep
  dependent
  deposit
DEPA
  diethylenephosphoramide
DEPC
  diethylpyrocarbonate
depr
  depressed
  depression
DEPS
  distal effective potassium secretion
DEP ST SEG
  depressed ST segment

dept
  department
DEQ
  Depressive Experiences
    Questionnaire
  digital echo quantification
DER
  disulfiramethanol reaction
  dual-energy radiograph
DeR
  degeneration reaction
  reaction of degeneration
der
  derivative chromosome
  derive
deriv
  derivative
  derived
DERM, Derm, derm
  dermatologic
  dermatologist
  dermatology
DES
  dermal-epidermal separation
  dialysis encephalopathy syndrome
  diethylstilbestrol
  diffuse esophageal spasm
  disequilibrium syndrome
  doctor's emergency service
  dysequilibrium syndrome
DESAT, desat
  desaturated
DESBRS-II
  Devereux Elementary School
    Behavior Rating Scale II
desc
  descendant
  descending
  descent
DESD
  detrusor external sphincter
    dyssynergia
DESF
  desflurane (Suprane)
DESI
  drug efficacy study implementation
DEST
  Denver Eye Screening Test
  dichotic environmental sounds test
DET
  diethyltryptamine
  dipyridamole echocardiography test
Det-6
  detroid-6 (human sternum marrow
    cells)
det
  determine

determ, determin
determination
determined
detn
detention
detox
detoxification
DEUC
direct electronic urethrocystometry
DEV
deviant
deviation (*See also* D)
duck embryo origin vaccine
duck embryo vaccine
duck embryo virus
dev
develop
development(al) (*See also* D, devel)
deviate
deviation (*See also* D)
devel
development
DevPd
developmental pediatrics
DEVR
dominant exudative vitreoretinopathy
DEX
dexamethasone
dexter (right)
dexverapamil
dex
Dextrostix (*See also* D-stix, DSX)
dex.
right [L. *dexter*] (*See also* D)
DEXA
dual-energy x-ray absorptiometry
(scan) (*See also* DXA)
DF
day frequency (of voiding)
decapacitation factor (sperm)
decayed and filled (permanent
teeth)
decontamination factor
deferoxamine
deferred
defibrotide
deficiency factor
defined flora (of an animal)
degree of freedom
dengue fever
dermatofibrosis
desferrioxamine

dexfenfluramine
diabetic father
diabetic fetopathy
diaphragmatic function
diastolic filling
dietary fiber
digital fluoroscopy
discriminant function
disseminated foci
distal fossa
distribution factor
dome fragment
dorsiflexion
drug free
dry (gas) fractional (concentration)
dye free
DF-2
dysgonic fermenter 2
df
decayed and filled (deciduous
teeth)
degrees of freedom
DFA
delayed feedback audiometry
diet for age
difficulty falling asleep
direct fluorescence assay
direct fluorescent antibody (test)
direct fluorescent antigen (test)
direct fluorescent assay
distal forearm
dorsiflexion angle
dorsiflexion assist
hallux dorsiflexion angle
DFA-TP
direct fluorescent antibody (test)
for *Treponema pallidum*
DFAT-TP
direct fluorescent antibody tissue
(test) for *Treponema pallidum*
DFB
dinitrofluorobenzene
dysfunctional (uterine) bleeding
DFC
deletion of final consonants
dry-filled capsule
DFD
defined formula diet
degenerative facet disease
diisopropylphosphorofluoridate
DFDB
demineralized freeze-dried bone

NOTES

D

DFDBA
  decalcified freeze-dried bone
    allograft
  demineralized freeze-dried bone
    allograft
DFDCB
  decalcified freeze-dried cortical
    bone
DFDD
  difluorodiphenyldichloroethane
DFE
  diffuse fasciitis with eosinophilia
  dilated fundus examination
  distal femoral epiphysis
DFECT
  dense fibroelastic connective tissue
DFEN, dFEN
  dexfenfluramine
  D-fenfluramine
d$_{FF}$
  density of the fat mass
d$_{FFM}$
  density of the fat-free mass
DFG
  direct forward gaze
DFI
  deterioration following improvement
  disease-free interval
  dye fluorescence index
D-FISH
  double-fusion fluorescent in situ
    hybridization
DFL
  dense fibrous lamina
DFLE
  disability-free life expectancy
DFM
  decreased fetal movement
  deep friction massage
DFMC
  daily fetal movement count
DFMO
  dl-alpha-difluoromethylornithine
  difluoromethylornithine
DFMR
  daily fetal movement record
DFNA3
  autosomal dominant nonsyndromic
    hearing loss
DFNB1
  autosomal recessive nonsyndromic
    hearing loss
DFNX3
  X-linked progressive mixed
    deafness with perilymphatic
    gusher
DFO, DFOM
  deferoxamine

DFP
  diastolic filling period
  diisopropylfluorophosphonate
DF^{32}P
  radiolabeled diisopropyl
    fluorophosphonate
DFPP
  double filtration plasmapheresis
DFR
  diabetic floor routine
  dialysate filtration rate
2DFr
  two-dimensional Fourier imaging
3DFr
  three-dimensional Fourier imaging
DFRC
  deglycerolized frozen red cells
DFS
  Defensive Functioning Scale
  disease-free survival
  Doppler flow study
  dynamic flow study
DFSP
  dermatofibrosarcoma protuberans
DFT
  defibrillation threshold (*See also*
    XDT)
  discrete Fourier transform
  Doppler flow test
2DFT
  two-dimensional Fourier transform
3DFT
  three-dimensional Fourier transform
DFT$_4$
  dialyzable free thyroxine
DFTT
  Digital Finger Tapping Test
DFU
  dead fetus in utero
  dideoxyfluorouridine
5′-DFUR, 5-dFUR
  5′-deoxy-5-fluorouridine
DFV
  D'Aoust Fineman virus
  dengue fever vaccine
  diarrhea with fever and vomiting
DFW
  Dexide face wash
DFWO
  dorsiflexory wedge osteotomy
DFX
  desferrioxamine
DG
  dark ground
  Davis & Geck (manufacturer)
  dentate gyrus
  deoxyglucose (*See also* 2DG)

diagnosis (*See also* D, Dg, diag, Dx)
diastolic gallop
diglyceride
distogingival
dorsal glides
downward gaze
Duchenne-Griesinger (disease)

2DG
2-deoxy-D-glucose (*See also* DG)

Dg
diagnosis (*See also* D, DG, diag, Dx)

dg
decigram (*See also* dgm)

DGA
DiGeorge anomaly

DGAT
diacylglyceroacyl transferase

DGCI
delayed gamma camera image

DGE
delayed gastric emptying
density gradient electrophoresis

DGER
duodenogastroesophageal reflux

DGF
delayed graft function
digoxin-like factor

DGGE
denaturing gradient gel electrophoresis

DGI
disseminated gonococcal infection

DGJ
deoxygalactonojirimicin

DGKV
Dera Ghazi Khan virus

DGL
deglycyrrhizinated licorice

DG-L
deep gastric-longitudinal

DGLA
dihomogammalinolenic acid

DGM
ductal glandular mastectomy

dgm
decigram (*See also* dg)

dGMP
deoxyguanosine monophosphate
deoxyguanylic acid

DGN
diffuse glomerulonephritis

DGP
deoxyglucose phosphate

DGR
duodenogastric reflux

DGS
developmental Gerstmann syndrome
diabetic glomerulosclerosis
DiGeorge syndrome

DGSX
X-linked dysplasia-gigantism syndrome

DGT
decaffeinated green tea

dGTP
deoxyguanosine triphosphate
2-deoxyguanosine 5'-triphosphate

DGV
dextrose, gelatin, Veronal (solution)

DGVB
dextrose-gelatin-Veronal buffer

DH
daily habits
day hospital
dehydrocholic acid
dehydrogenase
delayed hypersensitivity
deliberate hypotension
dental habits
dermatitis herpetiformis
developmental history
diaphragmatic hernia
diffuse histiocytic (lymphoma)
disseminated histoplasmosis
dominant hand
dorsal horn
drug hypersensitivity
ductal hyperplasia
Dunkin-Hartley (guinea pig)

D-H
Dimon-Hughston (intertrochanteric osteotomy technique)

D+H
delusions and hallucinations

D/H
deuterium/hydrogen (ratio)

DIIA
dehydroalanine
dehydroascorbic acid
dehydroepiandrosterone (*See also* DHEA)

D

DHA *(continued)*
dehydroisoandrosterone
dihydroacetic acid
dihydroxyacetone
district health authority
docosahexaenoic acid

DHAC
dihydro-5-azacytidine

DHAD
dihydroxybis
(hydroxyethylaminoethyl) amino-
anthraquinone dihydrochloride
(mitoxantrone hydrochloride)
mitoxantrone

DHAP
dihydroxyacetone phosphate

DHA-PUVA
dihydroxyacetone-psoralen ultraviolet
A-range

DHB
dihydroxybenzoic acid
duck hepatitis B

DHBP
direct His bundle pacing

DHBS
dihydrobiopterin synthetase

DHBV
duck hepatitis B virus

DHC
dehydrocholate
dehydrocholesterol
11-dehydrocorticosterone

DHCA
deep hypothermic circulatory arrest

DHCC
dihydroxycholecalciferol

DHCP
dental health care provider

DHD
dissociated horizontal deviation
district health department
donor hepatic duct

DHDA
directed heteroduplex analysis

DHE
dihematoporphyrin ether
dihydroergocryptine (*See also*
DHEC, DHK)
dihydroergotamine

DHEA
dehydroepiandrosterone (*See also*
DHA)

DHEA-S, DHEAS
dehydroepiandrosterone sulfate

DHEC
dihydroergocryptine (*See also* DHE,
DHK)

DHE 45(r)
dihydroergotamine mesylate

DHF
dengue hemorrhagic fever
dorsihyperflexion

DHF-DSS
dengue hemorrhagic fever-shock
syndrome

DHFK
Dow Hollow Fiber kidney

DHFR
dihydrofolate reductase

DHFS
dengue hemorrhagic fever shock
(syndrome)

DHFT
developmental hand-function test

DHGA
dihomogammalinolenic acid

DHI
dihydroisocodeine
dihydroxyindole
Dizziness Handicap Inventory
dynamic hyperinflation

DHIC
detrusor hyperactivity with impaired
contractility

DHK
dihydroergocryptine (*See also* DHE,
DHEC)

DHL
diffuse histiocytic lymphoma

DHM
dihydromorphine

DHMA
dihydroxymandelic acid (*See also*
DOMA)

DHO
deuterium hydrogen oxide
dihydroergocornine (*See also* DHO
180)

DHO 180
dihydroergocornine (*See also* DHO)

DHODH
dihydroorotate dehydrogenase

DHP
dehydrogenated polymer
dihydroprogesterone
dihydropyridine
dihydroxyacetone phosphate

DHPc
dorsal hippocampus

DHPG
dihydroxyphenylethylene glycol
dihydroxyphenylglycol
dihydroxypropoxymethyl guanine

DHPLC
denaturing high-performance liquid chromatography

DHPR
dihydropteridine reductase

dhPRL
decidual prolactin

DHPS
dihydopteroate synthase

DHR
delayed hypersensitivity reaction

DHS
delayed hypersensitivity
dihydrostreptomycin (*See also* DHSM, DS, DSM, DST)
duration of hospital stay
dynamic hip screw

D-5-HS
dextrose 5% in Harman solution

DHSM
dihydrostreptomycin (*See also* DHS, DS, DSM, DST)

DHSS
dihydrostreptomycin sulfate

DHST
delayed hypersensitivity test

DHT
dehydrotestosterone
dihydroergotoxine
dihydrotachysterol
dihydrotestosterone
dihydrothymine
dihydroxypropyltheophylline
dissociated hypertropia
Dobhoff tube
domino heart transplantation

DHTF
Dobhoff tube feeding

DHTP
dihydrotestosterone propionate

DHTR
dihydrotestosterone receptor deficiency

DHZ
dihydralazine

DI
(Beck) Depression Inventory
date of injury
Debrix Index
defective interfering
degradation index
dental index

dentinogenesis imperfecta
depression inventory
desorption ionization
deterioration index
detrusor instability
diabetes insipidus
diagnostic imaging
diaphragm (*See also* diaph, DPH)
diaphragmatic (*See also* diaph, DPH)
disability insurance
dispensing information
distal intestine
distoincisal
DNA index
donor insemination
dorsal interosseous
dorsoiliacus
dose intensity
double indemnity
drug information
drug interaction
dyskaryosis index
dyspnea index
Eating Disorders Inventory

D21
dideoxyinosine (*See also* DDI, ddI, ddIno)

DI-S
Debris Index-Simplified

D&I
debridement and irrigation
dilation and irrigation
dry and intact

D$_1$
insulin dialysance

Di
didymium
Diego (blood group)

di
inside detail

DIA
depolarization-induced automaticity
diabetes (*See also* db, dia)
dot immunobinding assay
drug-induced agranulocytosis
drug-induced amenorrhea

DiA
Diego antigen

dia, diab
diabetes (*See also* db, DIA)
diabetic (*See also* DB)

D

NOTES

dia *(continued)*

  diameter (*See also* D, d, diam)

  diathermy (*See also* diath)

DIAC

  diiodothyroacetic acid

diag

  diagnosis (*See also* D, DG, Dg, Dx)

  diagonal (*See also* D)

  diagram

DIAGNO

  differential diagnosis (*See also* DD, D/D, DDX, DDx, diff diag)

DIAL

  Developmental Indicators for Assessment of Learning

DIAL-R

  Developmental Indicators for Assessment of Learning, Revised/AGS Edition

diam

  diameter (*See also* D, d, dia)

diaph

  diaphragm (*See also* DI, DPH)

  diaphragmatic (*See also* DI, DPH)

DIAPPERS

  delirium, infection, atrophic urethritis and vaginitis, pharmaceuticals, psychological disorders, excessive output, restricted mobility, stool impaction

DIAR

  dextran-induced anaphylactoid reaction

dias

  diastole (*See also* D)

  diastolic

DIAS BP

  diastolic blood pressure

diath

  diathermy (*See also* dia)

DIATH SW

  diathermy short wave

DIAZ

  diazepam

DIB

  Diagnostic Interview for Borderlines

  disability insurance benefits

  dot immunobinding

DIBC

  drug-induced blood cytopenias

DIBS

  dead-in-bed syndrome

DIC

  diagnostic imaging center

  differential interference contrast (microscopy)

  diffuse intravascular coagulation

  disseminated intravascular coagulation (*See also* DIVC)

  disseminated intravascular coagulopathy

  drip-infusion cholangiogram

  drip-infusion cholangiography

  drug information center

dic

  dicentric

DICA-C

  Diagnostic Interview for Children and Adolescents-Child Version

DICA-P

  Diagnostic Interview for Children and Adolescents-Parent Version

DICA-R

  Diagnostic Interview for Children and Adolescents-Revised

DICC

  drug-induced cicatricial conjunctivitis

  dynamic infusion cavernosometry and cavernosography

DICD

  dispersion-induced circular dichroism

diclox

  dicloxacillin

DICOM

  Digital Imaging and Communications in Medicine (interface)

DICP

  demyelinated inflammatory chronic polyneuropathy

DICT

  dose-intensive chemotherapy

DID

  dead of intercurrent disease

  delayed ischemic deficit

  dissociative identity disorder

  document image decoding

  double immunodiffusion (technique)

  drug-induced disease

  dystonia-improvement-dystonia

DIDA

  dimethyl iminodiacetic acid

DIDD

  dense intramembranous deposit disease

di-di

  dichorionic-diamniotic (twins)

DIDMO, DIDMOA

  diabetes insipidus, diabetes mellitus, optic atrophy (syndrome)

DIDMOAD

  diabetes insipidus, diabetes mellitus, optic atrophy, and deafness (syndrome)

DIDMOS
    drug-induced delayed multiorgan hypersensitivity syndrome
DIDOX
    dihydroxybenzohydroxamic acid
DIDS
    Dermatology Index of Disease Severity
    4,4'-di-isothiocyanatostilbene-2,2'-disulfonic acid
DIE
    died in emergency (room)
    drug-induced esophagitis
DIEA
    deep inferior epigastric artery
DIEAP
    deep inferior epigastric artery perforator
DIED
    drug-induced esophageal damage
DIEDA
    diethyliminodiacetic acid
DIEP
    deep inferior epigastric perforator
DIF
    differentiation-inducing factor
    diffuse interstitial fibrosis
    diflunisal
    direct immunofluorescence (test)
    dose increase factor
DIFF, diff
    difference (See also D)
    different
    differential (blood count)
    diffusion (See also D)
diff diag
    differential diagnosis (See also DD, D/D, DDX, DDx, DIAGNO)
DIFP
    diffuse interstitial fibrosing pneumonitis
    diisopropyl fluorophosphonate
DIF-test
    direct immunofluorescence test
DIG
    desmoplastic infantile ganglioglioma
    digitalis (See also dig.)
    digitoxin
    digoxin
    digoxin investigators group
    drug-induced galactorrhea

dig.
    digitalis (See also DIG)
DIGS
    Diagnostic Interview for Genetic Study
dig. tox
    digitalis toxicity
DIH
    died in hospital
DIHE
    drug-induced hepatic encephalopathy
DIHPPA
    diiodohydroxyphenylpyruvic acid
DIJOA
    dominantly inherited juvenile optic atrophy
DIL
    daughter-in-law
    dilute (See also dil, dilut)
    diluted (See also dil, dilut)
    dilution (See also dil, diln, dilut)
    drug-induced lupus
    drug information log
Dil
    Dilantin
dil
    dilation (See also dilat)
    dilute (See also DIL, dilut)
    diluted (See also DIL, dilut)
    dilution (See also DIL, diln, dilut)
dilat
    dilation (See also dil)
DILC
    dose-intensity limiting criterion
DILD
    diffuse infiltrative lung disease
    diffuse interstitial lung disease
    drug-induced liver disease
DILE
    drug-induced lupus erythematosus
diln
    dilution (See also DIL, dil, dilut)
DILS
    diffuse infiltrative lymphocytosis syndrome
    drug-induced lupus syndrome
dilut
    dilute (See also DIL, dil)
    diluted (See also DIL, dil)
    dilution (See also DIL, dil, diln)

NOTES

DIM
>   diminish (*See also* dim.)
>   divalent ion metabolism

dim.
>   diminish (*See also* DIM)
>   one-half [L. *dimidus*]

D5IMB
>   Ionosol MB with 5% dextrose
>   injection

DIMD
>   drug-induced movement disorders

DIMIT
>   3,5-dimethyl-3′-isopropyl-L-thyronine

dIMP
>   deoxyinosine monophosphate
>   (deoxyinosinate)

DIMS
>   disorders of initiating and
>   maintaining sleep

DIMSA
>   disseminated intravascular multiple
>   systems activation

DIND
>   delayed ischemic neurologic deficit

3α-diol-G
>   5α-androstane-3α,17β-diol
>   glucuronide

diopt
>   diopter

DIOS
>   distal ileal obstruction syndrome
>   distal intestinal obstruction
>   syndrome

DIP
>   desquamative interstitial pneumonia
>   desquamative interstitial pneumonitis
>   dichlorophenolindophenol
>   diffuse interstitial pneumonia
>   digital imaging processing
>   diisopropyl phosphate
>   diphtheria toxoid vaccine
>   diplopia
>   distal interphalangeal (joint) (*See
>   also* DIPJ)
>   drip-infusion pyelogram
>   drug-induced parkinsonism
>   dual-in-line package (integrated
>   circuits)

dip
>   diploid

DIPA
>   diisopropylamine

DIPant
>   diphtheria antitoxin

DIPC
>   diffuse interstitial pulmonary
>   calcification

>   dynamic infusion
>   pharmacocavemosometry

DIPD
>   daily intermittent peritoneal dialysis

DIPF
>   diffuse interstitial pulmonary
>   fibrosis
>   diisopropylphosphofluoridate

diph
>   diphtheria

diph-tet
>   diphtheria-tetanus (toxoid)

diph-tox
>   diphtheria toxoid

diph-tox AP
>   alum-precipitated diphtheria toxoid

DIPI
>   direct intraperitoneal insemination

DIPJ
>   distal interphalangeal joint (*See also*
>   DIP)

DIR
>   direct
>   director
>   direct treatment
>   disturbed interpersonal relationships
>   double isomorphous replacement

dir.
>   direction [L. *directione*]

DIRD
>   drug-induced renal disease

DIS
>   Diagnostic Interview Schedule
>   digital imaging spectrophotometer
>   disease intervention specialist
>   dislocation (*See also* dis, disl,
>   disloc)

dis
>   disability (*See also* DB)
>   disabled (*See also* DSBL)
>   disease (*See also* D, DZ, Dz)
>   dislocation (*See also* DIS, disl,
>   disloc)
>   distance
>   distribution (*See also* dist)

DISA-SPECT
>   dual-isotope simultaneous acquisition
>   single-photon emission computed
>   tomography

DISC
>   death-inducing signaling complex
>   Diagnostic Interview Schedule for
>   Children
>   disabled infectious single cycle
>   (virus)
>   dynamic integrated stabilization
>   chair

DIS-C
> Diagnostic Interview Schedule for Children

disc
> discontinue (*See also* DC, dc)

disch
> discharge (*See also* DC)

DISC-R
> Diagnostic Interview Schedule for Children-Revised

DISCUS
> Dyskinesia Identification System: Condensed User Scale

DISDA
> diisopropyliminodiacetic acid

DISH
> diffuse idiopathic skeletal hyperostosis

DISI
> dorsal intercalated segment instability
> dorsiflexed intercalated segment instability

DISIDA
> diisopropyl iminodiacetic acid

disinfect.
> disinfection

disl
> dislocation (*See also* DIS, dis, disloc)

disloc
> dislocated
> dislocation (*See also* DIS, dis, disl)

disod
> disodium

D₅ISOM
> dextrose 5% in Isolyte M

D5ISOP
> 5% Dextrose and Isolyte P

DISP, dispo
> disposition

disp
> dispensary
> dispense

DISR
> drug-induced skin reactions

DISS
> Diameter Index Safety system

diss
> dissolve(d)

dissem
> disseminated
> dissemination

dist
> distal (*See also* D, d)
> distillation (*See also* distill.)
> distill(ed)
> distribute (*See also* dis)
> distribution (*See also* dis)
> district

distal/3
> distal third

dist fr
> distinguished from

distill.
> distillation (*See also* dist)

DIT
> diet-induced thermogenesis
> diiodinated tyrosine
> diiodotyrosine
> 3,5-diiodotyrosine
> drug-induced thrombocytopenia

dITP
> deoxyinosine triphosphate

DIU
> death in utero

DiU
> diazolidinyl urea

DIV
> double-inlet ventricle

div
> divergence
> divergent
> divide(d)
> division
> divorced (*See also* D, d)
> double-inlet ventricle

DIVA
> digital intravenous angiography

DIVBC
> disseminated intravascular blood coagulation

DIVC
> disseminated intravascular coagulation (*See also* DIC)

div ex
> divergence excess

DIVP
> dilute intravenous Pitocin

DJD
> degenerative joint disease

D

NOTES

187

DJJ
duodenojejunal junction
DJOA
dominant juvenile optic atrophy
DK
dark (*See also* dk)
decay
degeneration of keratinocytes
diabetic ketoacidosis (*See also* DKA)
diet kitchen
diseased kidney
dog kidney (cells)
dk
dark (*See also* DK)
DKA
diabetic ketoacidosis (*See also* DK)
did keep appointment
DKB
deep knee bend
dideoxykanamycin B
DKC
double knee to chest
dyskeratosis congenita
DKDP
deuterium with potassium dihydrogen phosphate
dkg
decagram
dkL
decaliter
dkm
decameter
DKP
dibasic potassium phosphate
dikalium phosphate
diketopiperazine
DKS
Damus-Kaye-Stansel (procedure)
DKTC
dog kidney tissue culture
DKV
deer kidney virus
DL
danger list
dansyl lysine
deep lobe
developmental level
diagnostic laparoscopy
difference limen (threshold)
diffuse lymphoma
diffusing capacity of lung
directed listening
direct laryngoscopy
disabled list
distolingual
Donath-Landsteiner (antibody) (*See also* D-L Ab)

double lumen
drug level
lethal dose [L. *dosis letalis*]
D$_L$
diffusing capacity of lung (*See also* DL)
DL$_{co}$
diffusing capacity of lung for carbon monoxide
DL-
equal quantities of D and L enantiomorphs (formerly dl-)
dL
deciliter
DLA, DLa
distolabial
D-L Ab
Donath-Landsteiner antibody (*See also* DL)
DLAI, DLaI
distolabioincisal
DLAP, DLaP
distolabiopulpal
DLB
dementia with Lewy bodies
diffuse and lymphoblastic
direct laryngoscopy and bronchoscopy (*See also* DL&B)
DL&B
direct laryngoscopy and bronchoscopy (*See also* DLB)
DLBCL
diffuse large B-cell lymphoma
DLBD
diffuse Lewy body disease
DLC
differential leukocyte count
distolingual cusp
double-lumen catheter
dual-lumen catheter
DLCL
diffuse large cell lymphoma
DLCO, DL$_{CO}$, D$_{LCO}$
diffusing capacity of lung for carbon monoxide (*See also* D$_{CO}$)
DLCO$_2$, D$_{LCO2}$
carbon dioxide diffusing capacity of the lungs
D$_{LCO}$SB
single-breath carbon monoxide diffusing capacity of lungs
D$_{LCO}$SS
steady-state carbon monoxide diffusing capacity of lungs
DLCR
distolingual cusp ridge
DLD
date of last drink

developmental language disorder
disease linkage disequilibrium

DLE

delayed light emission
dialyzable leukocyte extract
discoid lupus erythematosus
disseminated lupus erythematosus

D₁LE

diagonal 1 lower extremity

D₂LE

diagonal 2 lower extremity

DLF

digitalis-like factor
digoxin-like factor
distolingual fossa
dorsolateral funiculus
ductal lavage fluid

DLG

distolingual groove

DLI

distolinguoincisal
donor leukocyte infusion
donor lymphocyte infusion
double label index

DLIF

digoxin-like immunoreactive factor

DLIS

digoxin-like immunoreactive
substance

DLK

deep lamellar keratoplasty

DLLI

dulcitol lysine lactose iron (agar)

DLMP

date of last menstrual period

DLNG

dl-norgestrel

DLNMP

date of last normal menstrual
period

DLO

distolinguoocclusal

DLP

delipidized serum protein
developmental learning problems
direct linear plotting
dislocation of patella
distolinguopulpal
double-limb progression
dysharmonic luteal phase
dyslipoproteinemia

DLPC

dilinoleoylphosphatidylcholine

DLPD

diffuse lymphocytic poorly
differentiated

DLPFC

dorsolateral prefrontal cortex

D₅LR

dextrose 5% in lactated Ringer
(solution)

DLS

daily living skills
digitalis-like substances
ductlike structure
dynamic light scattering

DLSC

double lumen subclavian catheter

DLST

drug-induced lymphocyte stimulation
test

DLT

dihydroepiandrosterone loading test
diode laser trabeculoplasty
dorsolateral tract
dose-limiting toxicity
double lung transplant

DLU

diffused lung uptake

DLV

defective leukemia virus
delavirdine

DLW

doubly labeled water

DLWD

diffuse lymphocytic, well
differentiated

DM

adamsite
dehydrated and malnourished
dermatologist
dermatology
dermatomyositis
Descemet membrane
dextromaltose
dextromethorphan
diabetes mellitus (type 1, 2)
diabetic mother
diastolic murmur
diffuse mixed
diphenylaminechlorarsine
distant metastases
dopamine

D

NOTES

DM *(continued)*
dorsomedial
dose modification
double membrane
double minute (chromosome)
dry matter
duodenal mucosa
membrane diffusing capacity
myotonic dystrophy

DM-1
diabetes mellitus type 1

DM-2
diabetes mellitus type 2

D_M
membrane component of diffusion

dM
decimorgan

dm
decimeter

dm_2
square decimeter

dm_3
cubic decimeter

DMA
dimethoxyamphetamine
dimethyladenosine
dimethylamine
dimethylaniline
dimethylarginine
dimethylarsinic acid
direct memory access (computers)

DMAA
distal metatarsal articular angle

DMAB, DMABA
dimethylaminobenzaldehyde (Ehrlich reagent)

DMAC
dimethylacetamide
disseminated *Mycobacterium avium-intracellulare* complex

DMAE
dimethylaminoethanol

DMAIC
disseminated Mycobacterium avium-intracellulare complex

DMARD
disease-modifying antirheumatic drug

DMAS
deep muscular aponeurotic system
Dementia Mood Assessment Scale
dimethylamine sulfate
Drug Management and Authorization Section

DMAT
disaster medical assistance team

D_{max}
maximum density
maximum depth

DMB
data monitoring board
demineralized bone

DMBA
dimethylbenzanthracene

DMC
demeclocycline
diabetes management center
dichlorodiphenylmethylcarbinol
dimethylcysteine
direct microscopic count
p,p′-dichlorodiphenyl methyl carbinol

DMCC
direct microscopic clump count

DMCM
dimethoxyethylcarboline carboxylate

DMCT, DMCTC
dimethylchlortetracycline

DMD
desmethyldiazepam (*See also* DMDZ)
digital micromirror device
disciform macular degeneration
disease-modifying drug
drowsiness monitoring device
Duchenne (de Boulogne) muscular dystrophy
dystonia musculorum deformans

DMD/BMD
Duchenne (de Boulogne) muscular dystrophy/Becker muscular dystrophy

DMDC
2′-deoxy-2′-methyl-idenecytidine

DMDS
dimethyl disulfide

DMDT
dimethoxydiphenyltrichloroethane

DMD w/SRNM
disciform macular degeneration with subretinal neovascular membrane

DMDZ
desmethyldiazepam (*See also* DMD)

DME
degenerative myoclonus epilepsy
diabetic macular edema
dimethyl ether
diphasic meningoencephalitis
dropping mercury electrode
drug-metabolizing enzyme
Dulbecco modified Eagle (medium)
durable medical equipment

DMF
    decayed, missing, filled (permanent teeth)
    dimethylformamide (*See also* DMFA)
    diphasic milk fever
    Drug Master File

dmf
    decayed, missing, filled (deciduous teeth)

DMFA
    dimethylformamide (*See also* DMF)

DMFC
    demand minimum functional capacity

DMFO
    eflornithine

DMFS
    decayed, missing, filled surfaces (permanent teeth)

dmfs
    decayed, missing, filled surfaces (deciduous teeth)

DMG
    dimethylglycine
    N,N-dimethylglycine

DMGBL
    dimethyl-gamma-butyrolactone

DMGG
    dimethylguanylguanidine

DMH
    diffuse mesangial hypercellularity
    dimethylhydrazine

DMI
    defense mechanism inventory
    desipramine
    desmethylimipramine
    diabetic muscle infarction
    Diagnostic Mathematics Inventory (psychologic testing)
    diaphragmatic myocardial infarct
    Dilamezinsert (prosthesis)
    direct migration inhibition

DM Isch
    diaphragmatic myocardial ischemia

DMKA
    diabetes mellitus ketoacidosis

DML
    diffuse mixed lymphoma
    distal motor latency

DMLO
    dim light melatonin onset

DMM
    desmethylmisonidazole
    diffuse malignant mesothelioma
    dimethylmyleran
    disproportionate micromelia

D0(mm/dd/yy)
    Day zero (treatment start date)

DMN
    dimethylnitrosamine (*See also* DMNA)
    dorsal motor nucleus (of vagus)
    dorsomedial nucleus

DMNA
    dimethylnitrosamine (*See also* DMN)

DMNL
    dorsomedial hypothalamic nucleus lesion

DMO
    dimethyloxazolindinedione

DMOOC
    diabetes mellitus out of control

DMORT
    Disaster Mortuary Team

DMP
    diffuse mesangial proliferation
    dimethylphosphate
    dimethylphthalate
    dura mater prosthesis

DMP-266
    efavirenz

DMPA
    depot medroxyprogesterone acetate

DMPC
    dimyristoyl phosphatidyl choline

DMPE
    dimethoxyphenylethylamine
    ^{99m}Tc-bis-dimethylphosphonoethane

DMPG
    dimyristoyl phosphatidyl glycerol

DMPH
    dysgenetic male pseudohermaphroditism

DMPM
    diffuse malignant pleural mesothelioma

DMPP
    dimethylphenylpiperazinium
    dimethyl-4-phenylpiperazinium

DMPS
    dimercaptopropane-sulfonic acid
    dimethylpolysiloxane
    dysmyelopoietic syndrome

D

NOTES

DMQ
  developmental motor quotient
DMR
  direct myocardial revascularization
  distal marginal ridge
DMRF
  dorsal medullary reticular formation
D-MRI
  dynamic magnetic resonance
    imaging
DMS
  delayed microembolism syndrome
  delayed muscle soreness
  demarcation membrane system
  dense microsphere
  dermatomyositis
  diagnostic medical sonography
  diffuse mesangial sclerosis
  dimethyl sulfate
  dimethyl sulfide
  dysmyelopoietic syndrome
dms
  double minute sphere
DMSA
  dimercaptosuccinic acid
  2,3-dimercaptosuccinic acid
  dimethylsuccinic acid
  disodium monomethanearsonate
  pentavalent dimercaptosuccinate
DMSLT
  daytime multiple sleep latency test
DMSO
  dimethyl sulfoxide
DMT
  dermatophytosis
  dimethyltryptamine
  N,N-dimethyltryptamine
DMTU
  dimethylthiourea
DMU
  dimethanolurea
DMVA
  direct mechanical ventricular
    actuation
D,M,V,P
  disc, macula, vessels, periphery
DMWP
  distal mean wave pressure
DMX
  diathermy, massage, and exercise
DN
  Deiters nucleus
  denuded
  dextrose-nitrogen (ratio)
  diabetic nephropathy
  diabetic neuropathy
  dibucaine number
  dicrotic notch
  down
  dysplastic nevus
D/N
  dextrose/nitrogen (ratio)
D&N
  distance and near (vision)
Dn
  dekanem
dn
  decinem
DNA
  deoxyribonucleic acid
  did not answer
  did not attend
  does not apply
DNA ds
  deoxyribonucleic acid double
    stranded
DNAP
  deoxyribonucleic acid polymerase
DNA-P
  deoxyribonucleic acid phosphorus
DNAse, DNase
  deoxyribonuclease
DNA ss
  deoxyribonucleic acid single
    stranded
DNB
  dinitrobenzene
  dorsal noradrenergic bundle
DNBP
  dinitrobutylphenol
DNBT
  dinitroblue
DNC
  did not come
  dinitrocarbanilide
DNCB
  dinitrochlorobenzene
DND
  died a natural death
DNE
  diabetes nurse educator
DNEPTE
  did not exist prior to enlistment
DNES
  diffuse neuroendocrine system
DNET
  dysembryoplastic neuroepithelial
    tumor
DNFB
  dinitrofluorobenzene (Sanger
    reagent)
DNFC
  does not follow commands
DNH
  diffuse nodular hyperplasia
  do not hospitalize

DNI
 do not intubate

DNIC
 diffuse noxious inhibitory control

DNJ
 N-butyl-deoxynojirimycin

DNKA
 did not keep appointment

DNL
 de novo lipogenesis
 diffuse nodular lymphoma
 disseminated necrotizing
  leukoencephalopathy

DNLL
 dorsal nucleus of lateral lemniscus

DNM
 descending necrotizing mediastinitis
 desmoplastic neurotropic melanoma

DNN
 did not nurse

DNOA
 diabetic neuropathic osteoarthropathy

DNOC
 dinitroorthocresol

DNOCHP
 dinitro-*o*-cyclohexyphenol

DNP
 dendroaspis natriuretic peptide
 deoxyribonucleoprotein (*See also*
  Dnp)
 did not pay
 dinitrophenol
 2,4-dinitrophenol (*See also* Dnp)
 do not publish
 dynamic nuclear polarization

Dnp
 deoxyribonucleoprotein (*See also*
  DNP)
 2,4-dinitrophenol (*See also* DNP)

DNPH
 dinitrophenylhydrazine

DNPM
 dinitrophenolmorphine

DNPT
 diethylnitrophenyl thiophosphate
  (parathion) (*See also* DNTP)

DNR
 did not respond
 do not report
 do not resuscitate
 dorsal nerve root
 dose nonuniformity ratio

DNS
 dansyl (*See also* Dns)
 delayed neuropsychological sequela
 de novo synthesis
 deviated nasal septum
 diaphragmatic nerve stimulation
 did not show
 (doctor) did not see (patient)
 do not show
 do not substitute
 dysplastic nevus syndrome

D5 1/2NS
 dextrose 5% in 0.45% sodium
  chloride injection

D$_5$NS, D$_5$NSS
 dextrose 5% in normal saline
  solution

Dns
 dansyl (*See also* DNS)

DNT
 dermonecrotic toxin
 did not test
 dysembryoplastic neuroepithelial
  tumor

DNTM
 disseminated nontuberculous
  mycobacterial (infection)

DNTP
 diethylnitrophenyl thiophosphate
  (parathion) (*See also* DNPT)

dNTP
 deoxynucleotide triphosphate

DNUA
 distillable nonurea adductable

DNV
 dorsal nucleus of vagus

D-O
 directive-organic

DO
 check doctor's order
 diamine oxidase (histaminase)
 diet order
 digoxin
 dissolved oxygen
 distal-occlusal
 distraction osteogenesis
 doctor's orders
 doxycycline
 drugs only

D/O
 disorder

NOTES

D_1O_2
　　diffusing capacity of lungs for oxygen

D_o
　　oxygen diffusion

d/o
　　died of

do.
　　the same, as before [L. *dicto*]

DO2, Do_2
　　oxygen delivery

DOA
　　date of admission
　　date of arrival
　　dead on arrival
　　diagnostic and operative arthroscopy
　　dominant optic atrophy
　　driver of automobile
　　duration of action

DOAC
　　Dubois oleic albumin complex

DOA-DRA
　　dead on arrival despite resuscitative attempts

DOB
　　dangle out of bed
　　date of birth (*See also* DB, D/B)
　　delta over baseline
　　Dobrava hantavirus
　　dobutamine
　　doctor's order book

DOBI
　　dynamic optical breast imaging system

DOBV
　　double-outlet both ventricles

DOC
　　date of conception
　　death of other cause
　　deoxycholate
　　deoxycorticosterone
　　11-deoxycorticosterone
　　desoxycorticosterone
　　diabetes out of control (*See also* doc, DOOC)
　　died of other causes
　　diet of choice
　　disorder of cornification
　　drug of choice
　　dynamic orthotic cranioplasty

doc
　　diabetes out of control (*See also* DOC, DOOC)
　　document
　　documentation

DOCA
　　deoxycorticosterone acetate

DOCG
　　deoxycorticosterone glucoside

DOCLINE
　　Documents On-Line

DOCP
　　desoxycorticosterone pivalate

DOCS, DOCs
　　deoxycorticoids

DOC-SR
　　deoxycorticosterone secretion rate

DOD
　　date of death
　　date of discharge
　　dead of disease
　　dementia (syndrome) of depression
　　died of disease
　　dissolved oxygen deficit
　　drug overdose

DODD
　　demand oxygen delivery device

DODS
　　demand oxygen delivery system

DOE
　　date of examination
　　desoxyephedrine
　　direct observation evaluation
　　disease-oriented evidence
　　dyspnea on exercise
　　dyspnea on exertion

DOES
　　disorders of excessive sleepiness
　　disorders of excessive somnolence

DOET
　　dimethoxyethylamphetamine

DOF
　　degrees of freedom

DOFOS
　　disturbance of function occlusion syndrome

DOG
　　distal oblique groove

DOHb
　　Döhle bodies

DOI
　　date of implant (pacemaker)
　　date of injury
　　depth of insertion
　　died of injuries

DO2I
　　oxygen delivery index

DOL
　　day of life (followed by number)

dol
　　dolorimetric unit (of pain intensity)

DOLLS
　　(Lee) double-loop locking suture

DOLV
　　double-outlet left ventricle

DOM
deaminated *O*-methyl metabolite
dimethoxy-methylamphetamine
2,5-dimethoxy-4-methylamphetamine
dissolved organic matter
domiciliary
domiciliary care
dominance (*See also* D, dom)
dominant (*See also* D, dom)

dom
domestic
dominance (*See also* D, DOM)
dominant (*See also* D, DOM)

DOMA
dihydroxymandelic acid (*See also* DHMA)

DOMS
delayed-onset muscle soreness

DON
diazooxonorleucine

DONALD
Dortmund Nutritional and Anthropometrical Longitudinally Designed (study)

DOOC
diabetes out of control (*See also* DOC, doc)

DOOR
deafness, onychoosteodystrophy, and mental retardation (syndrome)

DOP
degenerate oligonucleotide primer
dopamine

DOPA, dopa
dihydroxyphenylalanine
3,4-dihydroxyphenylalanine

DOPAC
dihydroxyphenylacetic acid

Dopase
dopamine hydroxylase (*See also* dopa)

DOPC
determined osteogenic precursor cell

DOPE
disease-oriented physician education

DOPP
dihydroxyphenylpyruvate

DOP-PCR
degenerate oligonucleotide primed polymerase chain reaction

DOPS
diffuse obstructive pulmonary syndrome
dihydroxyphenylserine

DOR
date of release

DORC
Direct Optical Research Company

dors
dorsal

DORV
double-outlet right ventricle

DoRx
date of treatment

DOS
day of surgery
deoxystreptamine
disk operating system
doctor's order sheet
dysosteosclerosis

dos
dosage (*See also* D, d)
dose (*See also* D, d)

DOSA
day of surgery admission

DOSC
Dubois oleic serum complex

DOSS
dioctyl sodium sulfosuccinate (docusate sodium)
distal over-shoulder strap

DOST
direct oocyte sperm transfer

DOT
date of transcription
date of transfer
died on (operating) table
directly observed therapy
direct oocyte transfer
Doppler ophthalmic test

DOTA
tetraazacyclododecanetetraacetic acid

DOTC
Dameshek oval target cell

DOTP
tetraazacyclododecanetetraacetic tetramethylene phosphonate

DOTS
directly observed treatment, short course

DOU
direct observation unit

NOTES

DOUV
Douglas virus
DOV
date of visit
discharged on visit
distribution of ventilation
DOX, dox
doxorubicin
doxy
doxycycline
doz
dozen
DP
data processing
debonding pliers
deep pulse
definitive procedure
degradation product
degree of polymerization
deltopectoral
dementia praecox
dementia pugilistica
dense plate
dental prosthesis
developed pressure
dexamethasone pretreatment
diaphragmatic plaque
diastolic pressure
diffuse precipitation
diffusion pressure
digestible protein
diminutive polyp
diphosgene
diphosphate
dipropionate
directional preponderance
disability pension
discharge planning
discriminating power
disopyramide phosphate
displaced person
distal pancreatectomy
distal phalanx
distal pit
distopulpal
donor's plasma
dorsalis pedis
driving pressure
dyspnea (*See also* dysp)
D-penicillamine (*See also* DPA, d-pen)
D-P
dialysis/plasma (urea ratio)
DP-II
Developmental Profile-II
DPA
descending palatine artery

Designed Plan Agencies (medical records)
dextroposition of aorta
diphenolic acid
diphenylamine
dipicolinic acid
dipropylacetate
dual-photon absorptiometry (*See also* DPX)
durable power of attorney
dynamic physical activity
D-penicillamine (*See also* DP, d-pen)
DPAP
diastolic pulmonary artery pressure
D-PAS, dPAS
diastase-periodic acid-Schiff
DPB
days postburn
diffuse panbronchiolitis
dynamic pedobarography
DPBS
Dulbecco phosphate-buffered saline
DPC
delayed primary closure
desaturated phosphatidylcholine
direct patient care
discharge planning coordinator
distal palmar crease
DPCRT
double-blind placebo-controlled randomized clinical trial
DPD
deoxypyridinoline
depression pure disease
desoxypyridoxine hydrochloride
diffuse pulmonary disease
dihydropyrimidine dehydrogenase
diphenamid
dual-photon densitometry
dysgenetic polycystic disease
D-2PD
dynamic two-point discrimination
Dpd
deoxypyridinoline
DPDA
phosphorodiamidic anhydride
DPDL
diffuse poorly differentiated lymphoma
DPDT, dpdt
double-pole double-throw (switch)
dP/dt
upstroke pattern on apex cardiogram

DPE
>   Death Personification Exercise
>   (psychology)
>   dipiperidinoethane

DPEG
>   dual percutaneous endoscopic
>   gastrostomy

d-pen
>   D-penicillamine (*See also* DP, DPA)

DPF
>   Dental Practitioners' Formulary

DPFR
>   diastolic pressure-flow relationship

DPG
>   diphosphoglycerate
>   displacement placentogram

DPGN
>   diffuse proliferative
>   glomerulonephritis

DPGP
>   diphosphoglycerate phosphatase

DPH
>   diaphragm (*See also* DI, diaph)
>   diaphragmatic (*See also* DI, diaph)
>   diphenhydramine
>   diphenylhexatriene
>   diphenylhydantoin

DPHM
>   diphenhydramine

DPI
>   daily permissible intake
>   daily protein intake
>   days postinoculation
>   dietary protein intake
>   diphtheria-pertussis immunization
>   Doppler perfusion index
>   drug-prescribing index
>   dry powder inhaler
>   Dynamic Personality Inventory
>   dynamic pulmonary imaging

DPIF
>   Drug Product Information File

DPIL
>   dextrose (percentage), protein
>   (grams per kilogram) Intralipid
>   (grams per kilogram)

DPJ
>   dementia paralytica juvenilis
>   direct percutaneous jejunostomy

DPL
>   diagnostic peritoneal lavage

dipalmitoyl lecithin
distopulpolingual

DPLa
>   distopulpolabial

D5PLM
>   dextrose 5% and Plasmalyte M
>   injection

DPM
>   digital phase mapping
>   dipyridamole
>   disabling pansclerotic morphea
>   discontinue previous medication
>   disintegrations per minute (*See also*
>   dpm)
>   dopamine
>   drops per minute
>   dual-pedicle dermoparenchymal
>   mastopexy

dpm
>   disintegrations per minute (*See also*
>   DPM)

DPN
>   deep penetrating nevus
>   dermatosis papulosa nigra
>   diabetic peripheral neuropathy
>   diabetic polyneuropathy
>   diphosphopyridine nucleotide (*See
>   also* DPNase, DPNH)
>   disabling pansclerotic morphea

DPNase
>   diphosphopyridine nucleotidase (*See
>   also* DPN, DPNH)

DPNB
>   dorsal penile nerve block

DPNH
>   diphosphopyridine nucleotide
>   (nicotinamide adenine dinucleotide,
>   reduced) (*See also* DPN, DPNase)

DPOA
>   durable power of attorney

DPOAE
>   distortion-product otoacoustic
>   emission

DPOAHC
>   durable power of attorney for
>   health care

DPOC
>   placebo-controlled oral challenge
>   testing

DPP
>   Diabetes Prevention Program
>   differential pulse polarography

NOTES

DPP *(continued)*
  dimethoxyphenylpenicillin
  dorsalis pedal pulse
  Dropout Prediction and Prevention
  duration of positive pressure
DPPC
  dipalmitoylphosphatidylcholine
DPR
  diagnostic procedure room
  doctor/population ratio
  dynamic planar reconstructor
DPRHP
  duodenum-preserving pancreatic
    head resection
DPS
  dimethylpolysiloxane (simethicone-
    antiflatulent)
  disintegration per second
  distal perfusion system
  dysesthetic pain syndrome
dps
  disintegrations per second
DPST, dpst
  double-pole single-throw (switch)
DPT
  dehydration, poisoning, trauma
  Demerol, Phenergan, and Thorazine
  department
  dichotic pitch (discrimination) test
  diphosphothiamine
  diphtheria, pertussis, and tetanus
    (vaccine) (*See also* DTP, DTPa,
    DTPw)
  diphtheric pseudotabes
  dipropyltryptamine
  dumping provocation test
DPTA
  diethylenetriamine pentaacetic (acid)
    (*See also* DTPA)
DPTI
  diastolic pressure-time index
DPTP
  diphtheria, pertussis, tetanus, and
    poliomyelitis (vaccine)
DPTPM
  diphtheria, pertussis, tetanus,
    poliomyelitis, and measles
    (vaccine)
Dptr
  diopter (*See also* D, d, diopt)
DPTS
  delayed pulmonary toxicity
    syndrome
DPTT
  deep posterior tibiotalar
DPU
  delayed pressure urticaria

DPUD
  duodenal peptic ulcer disease
DPV
  disabling positional vertigo
  Drosophila P virus
DPVNS
  diffuse pigmented villonodular
    synovitis
DPVSs
  dilated perivascular spaces
DPW
  distal phalangeal width
DPX
  dextropropoxyphene
  dual-photon absorptiometry (*See also*
    DPA)
DPXA
  dual-photon x-ray absorptiometry
DQ
  developmental quotient
D/Q
  deep quiet
Dq
  curvilinear threshold shoulder
DQE
  detective quantum efficiency
DQOL
  diabetes quality of life
DR
  degeneration reaction
  delivery room
  deoxyribose
  diabetic retinopathy (*See also* dr)
  diagnostic radiology
  diffuse redness
  digital radiography
  dining room
  disposable/reusable
  distal root
  distribution ratio
  diurnal rhythm
  donor-related
  dorsal raphe
  dorsal root (*See also* dr)
  dose ratio
  drug receptor
  drug resistant
  dual-chamber rate-responsive
  reaction of degeneration (muscle
    fibers) (*See also* DeR)
Dr
  rare detail response
dr
  diabetic retinopathy (*See also* DR)
  dorsal root (*See also* DR)
  drachm (apothecary measure)
  drain
  dram

dressing (See also DRSG, drsg, dsg)

(unusual rare) detail response

DRA

despite resuscitation attempts

dextran-reactive antibody

dialysis-related amyloidosis

digital rotational angiography

disease-resistant antigen

distal rectal adenocarcinoma

distal reference axis

drug-related admissions

DRAM

deepithelialized rectus abdominis muscle (graft)

Distress Risk Assessment Method

dynamic random access memory

dr ap

dram, apothecaries' (weight)

DRAPE

drug-related adverse patient event

DRAT

differential rheumatoid agglutination test

DRBC

denatured red blood cell

dog red blood cell (See also DRC)

donkey red blood cell

DRC

damage risk criteria

dendritic reticulum cell

digitorenocerebral (syndrome)

dog red (blood) cell (See also DRBC)

dorsal radiocarpal ligament

dorsal root, cervical

dose-response curve

dynamic range control

dRCA

distal right coronary artery

DRD

dopa-responsive dystonia

dorsal root dilator

dystrophia retinae pigmentosa-dysostosis syndrome

DRE

digital rectal examination

DREAM

downstream regulatory element antagonistic modulator (gene)

DREF

dose reduction effectiveness factor

D reg.

diseased region

DRESS

depth-resolved surface (coil) spectroscopy

drug rash with eosinophilia and systemic symptom

DREZ

dorsal root entry zone

DRF

daily replacement factor (of lymphocytes)

digestive-respiratory fistula

dose-reduction factor

DRFS

distant recurrence-free survival

DRG

diagnosis-related group

dorsal respiratory group

dorsal root ganglion

duodenal-gastric reflux gastropathy

drg, DRGE

drainage (See also drng)

draining (See also drng)

DRI

defibrillation response interval

Dietary Reference Intakes

Discharge Readiness Inventory

dopamine reuptake inhibitor

Doppler Resistive Index

Driver Risk Inventory

dRib

deoxyribose

DRID

double radial immunodiffusion

double radioisotope derivative

DRIFT

drainage, irrigation, fibrinolytic therapy

DRL, DRl

differential reinforcement of low (response rates)

dorsal root, lumbar

dorsoradial ligament

drug-related lupus

D5RL

5% dextrose in Ringer lactate (solution)

DRLST

Del Rio Language Screening Test

DRM

drug-related morbidity

NOTES

DRMS
drug reaction-monitoring system
DRN
dorsal raphe nucleus
drug-related neutropenia
drng
drainage (*See also* drg, DRGE)
draining (*See also* drg, DRGE)
DRnt
diagnostic roentgenology
DRO
differential reinforcement of other
(behavior)
DRP
digoxin reduction product
dorsal root potential
drug-related problem
DRPLA
dentatorubral-pallidoluysian atrophy
DRQ
discomfort relief quotient
DRR
digitally reconstructed radiograph
dorsal root reflex
drug regimen review
DRS, DRs
descending rectal septum
diffuse reflectance spectroscopy
Disability Rating Scale
disease-related symptoms
dorsal root, sacral
drowsiness
Duane retraction syndrome
dynamic renal scintigraphy
Dyskinesia Rating Scale
DRSG, drsg
dressing (*See also* dr, dsg)
DRSI
disease-related symptom
improvement
DRSP
drug-resistant *Streptococcus*
pneumoniae
DRT, DRt
dorsal root, thoracic
drug-related thrombocytopenia
dRTA
distal renal tubular acidosis
DRUB
drug (screen) blood
DRUJ
distal radioulnar joint
DrV
Diplocarpon rosae virus
DRVV
dilute Russell's viper venom
DRVVT
dilute Russell's viper venom time

DS
dead (air) space
deep sedative
deep sleep
defined substrate
delayed sensitivity
dendritic spine
density (optical) standard
dental surgery
deprivation syndrome
dermatan sulfate
dermatology and syphilology (*See
also* D&S)
desynchronized sleep
dextran sulfate
dextrose-saline
dextrose and sodium chloride
dextrose stick
diaphragm stimulation
diastolic murmur
diencephalic syndrome
difference spectroscopy
diffuse scleroderma
digit span
digit symbol
dihydrostreptomycin (*See also* DHS,
DHSM, DSM, DST)
dilute strength
diopter sphere
dioptric strength
discharge summary
discrimination score
discriminative stimulus
disoriented
disseminated sclerosis
dissolved solids
donor's serum
Doppler sonography
double-stranded
double strength
double subordinance
driving signal
drug store
dry swallow
dumping syndrome
duration of systole
D-S
Doerfler-Stewart (test)
D-5-S
dextrose 5% in saline (solution)
D5-1/2S
5% dextrose in 0.45% sodium
chloride (saline) injection
D&S
dermatology and syphilology (*See
also* DS)
diagnostic and surgical
dilation and suction

Ds
associative detail response to white space

ds
double-stranded (DNA, RNA)

DSA
density spectral array
digital subtraction angiography
digital subtraction arteriography
disease-susceptible antigen

DSACT, D-SACT
direct sinoatrial conduction time

DSAP
disseminated superficial actinic porokeratosis

DSAS
dynamic subaortic stenosis

DSB
detachable silicone balloon
drug-seeking behavior

Dsb
single-breath diffusing (capacity)

DSBB
double-sheath bronchial brushing

DSBL
disabled (*See also* dis)

DSBT
donor-specific blood transfusion

DSC
decussation of superior cerebellar (peduncles)
Developing Skills Checklist
differential scanning colorimeter
disodium chromoglycate (*See also* DSCG)
disodium cromoglycate
dobutamine stress echocardiography (*See also* DSE)
Down syndrome child
dynamic susceptibility contrast

DSCF
Doppler-shifted constant frequency

DSCG
disodium cromoglycate (*See also* DSC)

DSCT
dorsal spinocerebellar tract

DSD
degenerative spinal disease
depressed spectrum disease
depression sine depression
depressive spectrum disorder
detrusor sphincter dyssynergia
digital selenium drum (radiology)
discharge summary dictated
dry sterile dressing

DSDB
direct self-destructive behavior

DSDDT
double-sampling dye dilution technique

DS-DNA, dsDNA
double-stranded deoxyribonucleic acid

DSDS
daughter sites of dimer strands

DSE
digital subtraction echocardiogram
digital subtraction echocardiography
dobutamine stress echocardiography (*See also* DSC)

DSEA
deep superior epigastric artery

DSF
disulfiram
dry sterile fluff

DSG
deoxyspergualin (*See also* DSP)
desogestrel
dry sterile gauze

Dsg
desmoglein

Dsg1
desmoglein-1

Dsg3
desmoglein-3

dsg
dressing (*See also* dr, DRSG, drsg)

DSH
deliberate self-harm
dexamethasone-suppressible hyperaldosteronism

DSHR
delayed skin hypersensitivity reaction

DSI
deep shock insulin
Depression Status Inventory
digital subtraction imaging
drug-seeking index

DSIAR
double-stapled ileoanal reservoir

NOTES

DS-ICGA
digital subtraction indocyanine green angiography

DSIP
delta sleep-inducing peptide

DSIS
dynamic stabilizing innersole system

DSL
distal sensory latency

DSL M-U
distal sensory latency–median-ulnar

3D-SLS
three-dimensional superficial liposculpture

dslv
dissolve

DSM
degradable starch microsphere
dextrose solution mixture
Diagnostic and Statistical Manual of Mental Disorders
dihydrostreptomycin (See also DHS, DHSM, DS, DST)
disease state management
dried skim milk

DSM-III
Diagnostic and Statistical Manual of Mental Disorders, 3rd Edition

DSM-III-R
Diagnostic and Statistical Manual of Mental Disorders, Revised Third Edition

DSM-IV
Diagnostic and Statistical Manual of Mental Disorders, 4th Edition

DSM-IV-TR
Diagnostic and Statistical Manual of Mental Disorders, 4th Edition, Text Revision

DSNI
deep space neck infection

DSO
diffuse sclerosing osteomyelitis
distal subungual onychomycosis

DSP
decreased sensory perception
delayed sleep phase
deoxyspergualin (See also DSG)
dexamethasone sodium phosphate
diarrheic shellfish poisoning
dibasic sodium phosphate
digital signal processing
digital sound processing
digital subtraction phlebography

DSp
digit span

DSPC
desaturated phosphatidylcholine

D spine
dorsal spine

DSPN
distal sensory polyneuropathy
distal symmetrical polyneuropathy

DSPS
delayed sleep phase syndrome

DSR
dental stain remover
direct suicide risk
distal splenorenal
double simultaneous recording
dynamic spatial reconstructor

DSRCT
desmoplastic small round-cell tumor

DSRF
drainage subretinal fluid

dsRNA
double-stranded ribonucleic acid

DSRS
distal splenorenal shunt

DSS
dengue shock syndrome
Developmental Sentence Scoring
dextran sodium sulfate
dioctyl sodium sulfosuccinate
Disability Status Scale
discharge summary sheet
discrete subaortic stenosis
disease-specific survival
distal splenorenal shunt
docusate sodium
dosage-sensitive sex (reversal)
double simultaneous stimulation

DSSEP
dermatomal somatosensory-evoked potential

DSSLR
double seated straight leg raise

DSSN
distal symmetric sensory neuropathy

DSSP
distal symmetric sensory polyneuropathy

DSST
digit symbol substitutional test

DST
daylight saving time
desensitization test
dexamethasone suppression test
digit substitution test
dihydrostreptomycin (See also DHS, DHSM, DS, DSM)
disproportionate septal thickening
donor-specific transfusion

double stapling technique
duodenal secretin test

D-stix
　　Dextrostix (*See also* DSX, dex)

DSTR
　　distal soft tissue release

DSU
　　day surgery unit
　　double setup

DSV
　　digital subtraction ventriculography

DSVNI
　　Distress Scale for Ventilated
　　　Newborn Infants

DSVP
　　downstream venous pressure

DSWI
　　deep sternal wound infection

DSX
　　Dextrostix (*See also* D-stix, dex)

DSy
　　digit symbol

DT
　　dental technician
　　depression of transmission
　　dietary thermogenesis
　　dietetic technician
　　differently tested
　　digitoxin
　　diphtheria and tetanus
　　diphtheria-tetanus (immunization)
　　diphtheria toxin
　　diploë thickness
　　dipole tracing
　　discharge tomorrow
　　dispensing tablet
　　distal tubule
　　distance test (hearing)
　　dorsalis tibialis
　　double tachycardia
　　doubling time (of tumor size)
　　duration of tetany (*See also* Dt)
　　dye test

D/T
　　date/time
　　date of treatment
　　deaths/total (ratio)
　　due to

D&T
　　diagnosis and treatment
　　dictated and typed

Dt
　　duration of tetany (*See also* DT)

dT
　　deoxythymidine
　　diphtheria-tetanus toxoid

d4T
　　didehydrodideoxythymidine

DTA
　　descending thoracic aorta
　　differential thermoanalysis

DTaP
　　diphtheria, tetanus toxoids and
　　　acellular pertussis (*See also* DPT,
　　　DTP, DTPa)

DTB
　　dedicated time block

DTBC
　　D-tubocurarine (*See also* DTC, dTc)

DTBN
　　di-*tert*-butyl nitroxide

DTBP
　　di-*tert*-butyl peroxide (*See also*
　　　DBP)

DTC, dTc
　　day treatment center
　　differentiated thyroid carcinoma
　　diticarb (diethyldiothio-carbamate)
　　D-tubocurarine (*See also* DTBC)

2D-TCCS
　　two-dimensional transcranial color-
　　　coded sonography

DTCD
　　Dennis Test of Child Development

DT/CEP
　　Differential Test of Conduct and
　　　Emotional Problems

DTD, dtd
　　delivered total dose
　　diastrophic dystrophia

dTDP
　　deoxythymidine diphosphate
　　thymidine diphosphate
　　thymidine 5′-diphosphate

DTE
　　desiccated thyroid extract

2D TEE
　　two-dimensional transesophageal
　　　echocardiography

DTF
　　deep temporal fascia
　　deep transverse friction
　　desmoid-type fibromatosis

D

NOTES

DTF *(continued)*
    detector transfer function
    distal triangular fossa

D-TGA, d-TGA
    dextro-transposition of great arteries
    D-transposition of great arteries

DTH
    delayed-type hypersensitivity
    (reaction)

dTHd, dThd
    deoxythymidine

DTI
    diffusion-tensor imaging
    Doppler tissue imaging

DTICH
    delayed traumatic intracerebral
    hematoma

D time
    dream time

dTK
    (2′-deoxy) thymidine kinase

DTLA
    Detroit Tests of Learning Aptitude

DTLA-3
    Detroit Tests of Learning Aptitude,
    Third Edition

DTLA-A
    Detroit Tests of Learning Aptitude-
    Adult

DTLA-P:2
    Detroit Tests of Learning Aptitude
    - Primary, Second Edition

DTM
    deep tissue massage
    dermatophyte test media

DTMA
    deoxycorticosterone trimethylacetate

DTMC
    ditrichloromethylcarbinol

DTMP, dTMP
    de novo thymidylate (synthesis)
    deoxythymidylic acid
    thymidine 5′-monophosphate

DTMVmax
    diastolic transmembrane voltage,
    maximum

DTN
    diphtheria toxin normal

DTO
    deodorized tincture of opium

2D TOF
    two-dimensional time-of-flight

DTOGV
    dextral-transposition of great vessels

DTP
    differential time to positivity
    diphtheria, tetanus toxoid, and
    acellular pertussis (vaccine) (*See
    also* DPT, DTPa, DTPw)
    distal tingling on percussion (Tinel
    sign)

DTPA
    diethylenetriamine pentaacetic acid
    (*See also* DPTA)

DTPa
    diphtheria, tetanus toxoids, acellular
    pertussis (vaccine)

DTPT
    dithiopropylthiamine

DTPw, DTwP
    diphtheria, tetanus toxoids, whole-
    cell pertussis (vaccine)

DTR
    deep tendon reflex
    Dietetic Technician Registered

D-transposition
    dextrotransposition

DTRTT
    digital temperature recovery time
    test

DTS
    danger to self
    dense tubular system
    differential temperature sensor
    diphtheria toxin sensitivity
    discrete time sample
    donor transfusion, specific

DTs
    delirium tremens

3D TSE
    three-dimensional turbo-spin echo
    (images)

DTT
    device for transverse traction
    diagnostic and therapeutic team
    diphtheria-tetanus toxoid
    direct transverse reaction
    dithiothreitol

dTTP
    deoxythymidine triphosphate
    2′-deoxythymidine 5′-triphosphate
    thymidine 5′-triphosphate

DTUS
    diathermy, traction, and ultrasound

DTV
    due to void

DT-VAC
    diphtheria-tetanus vaccine

DTVMI
    Developmental Test of Visual
    Motor Integration

DTVP
    Developmental Test of Visual
    Perception

DTVP-2
Developmental Test of Visual Perception, Second Edition

DTwP-HIB
diphtheria, tetanus toxoids, whole-cell pertussis, and *Haemophilus influenzae* type b conjugate

DTX
detoxification

DTZ
diatrizoate

DU
decubitus ulcer
density (optical) unknown
dermal ulcer
developmental unit
diabetic urine
diagnosis undetermined
dialytic ultrafiltration
diazouracil
diffuse and undifferentiated
dog unit
dose unit
duodenal ulcer
duroxide uptake
Dutch (rabbit)

D$_U$
urea dialysance

dU
deoxyuridine

du
dial unit
du mai channel (acupuncture)

DUA
dorsal uterine artery

DUB
Dubowitz (score)
dysfunctional uterine bleeding

DUD
dihydrouracil dehydrogenase

dUDP
deoxyuridine diphosphate

DUE
drug use evaluation

D$_1$UE
diagonal 1 upper extremity

D$_2$UE
diagonal 2 upper extremity

DUF
Doppler ultrasonic flowmeter

DUG
dynamic urinary graciloplasty

DUGV
Dugbe virus

DUI
driving under the influence

DUID
driving under the influence of drugs

DUII
driving under the influence of intoxicants

DUKM
dialysate urea kinetic modeling

DUL
diffuse undifferentiated lymphoma

DUM
dorsal unpaired median (axon, neuron)
drug use monitoring

dUMP
deoxyuridine monophosphate

DUN
dialysate urea nitrogen

duod
duodenal
duodenum

DUP
duodenal ulcer perforation

dup
duplicate
duplication

DUR
Drug Usage Review
drug use review
duration (*See also* D, d, dur)

dur
duration (*See also* D, d, DUR)
hard [L. *duris*]

dURD
2′-deoxyuridine

DUS
digital ultrasound
distal urethral stenosis
Doppler ultrasound stethoscope
dynamic ultrasound of shoulder

3DUS
three-dimensional ultrasound

DUSN
diffuse unilateral subacute neuroretinitis ("wipe-out" syndrome)

dUTP
deoxyuridine triphosphate

NOTES

DUV

damaging ultraviolet
degree of voicelessness

DV

dependent variable
dilute volume (of solution)
distance vision
distemper virus
domestic violence
domiciliary visit
dorsoventral
double vision (*See also* dv)

D&V

diarrhea and vomiting
discs and vessels (ophthalmology)
ductions and versions

dv

double vibrations (unit of
frequency of sound waves)
double vision (*See also* DV)

DVA

developmental venous anomaly
directional vacuum-assisted (biopsy)
distance visual acuity
duration of voluntary apnea (test)
dynamic visual acuity

D/VA

diffusion per unit of alveolar
volume

D value

decimal reduction time

DVB

divinylbenzene

DVC

direct visualization of vocal cords
divanillalcyclohexanone
dorsal vein complex

DVD

dissociated vertical deviation
double-vessel disease

DVE

duck virus enteritis

DVG

double vein graft

DVH

dose-volume histogram

DVI

atrioventricular sequential pacing
deep venous insufficiency
device-independent
digital vascular imaging
documented viral infection
Doppler (systolic) velocity index

DVIS

digital vascular imaging system

DVIU

direct vision internal urethrotomy

DVL

deep vastus lateralis

DVM

digital voltmeter

DVMI

Developmental Test of Visual
Motor Integration

DVN

dorsal vagal nucleus

DVPX

divalproex sodium

DVR

derotational varus osteotomy
digital vascular reactivity
double valve replacement
double vein graft
double ventricular response

DVS

direct vesicoureteral scintigraphy

DVSA

digital venous subtraction
angiography

DVSS

dysfunctional voiding scoring
system

DVT

deep vein thrombosis
deep venous thrombosis

DVTS

deep venous thromboscintigram

DVVC

direct visualization of vocal cords

DVXI

direct vision times one

DW

confabulated whole response
daily weight
deionized water
detention warrant
dextrose in water
diffusion-weighted (imaging)
distilled water
doing well (*See also* D/W)
double wrap
dry weight
whole response to detail

D-W

Danis-Weber (classification for
ankle fractures)

D5W

5% dextrose in water
dextrose 5% in water (solution)

D10W

10% aqueous dextrose solution

D20W

20% dextrose in water

D50W

50% dextrose in water

D70W
> 70% dextrose in water

D/W
> discussed with
> doing well (*See also* DW)
> dry to wet

dw
> dwarf (mouse)

DWA
> died from wounds

DWCL
> daily-wear contact lens

DWD
> died with disease

DWDL
> diffuse well-differentiated
> lymphocytic (lymphoma)

DWI
> diffusion-weighted (magnetic
> resonance) imaging
> driving while impaired
> driving while intoxicated

DWI/MRI
> diffusion-weighted imaging/magnetic
> resonance imaging

DWI/PI
> diffusion-weighted imaging/perfusion
> imaging

DWMHI
> deep white matter hyperintensity

DWMI
> deep white matter infarct

DWML
> deep white matter lesion

DWRT
> delayed work recall test

DWS
> Dandy-Walker syndrome
> Disaster Warning System
> dorsal wrist syndrome

DWSCL
> daily-wear soft contact lens

DWT
> Dichotic Word Test

dwt
> pennyweight

DWW
> dynamic wall walk

DX
> Dextran
> dicloxacillin

Dx, dx
> diagnosis (*See also* D, DG, Dg,
> diag)
> diagnostic therapy

DXA
> dual-energy x-ray absorptiometry
> (*See also* DEXA)

DXD, Dxd
> diagnosed

DXG
> dioxalane guanine

DxLS
> diagnosis responsible for length of
> stay

DXM
> dexamethasone
> dextromethorphan

DXR
> deep x-ray
> delayed xenograft rejection

DXRT
> deep x-ray therapy (*See also* DXT)

DXT
> deep x-ray therapy (*See also*
> DXRT)
> dextrose

dXTP
> deoxyxanthine triphosphate

DXV
> *Drosophila* X virus

D-XYL
> *d*-xylose (in urine)

DY
> dense parenchyma

Dy
> dysprosium

dy
> dystrophia muscularis

DYFS
> Division of Youth and Family
> Services

dyn
> dynamics
> dynamometer
> dyne

DynA
> dynorphin A

dysp
> dyspnea (*See also* DP)

DYTRO
> dynamic tone-reducing orthosis

D

NOTES

DZ
diazepam (*See also* DZP)
disease (*See also* D, dis, Dz)
dizygotic
dizygous
dizziness

Dz, dz
disease (*See also* DZ)

dz
dozen

DZP
diazepam (*See also* DZ)

DZT
dizygotic twins

DZX
dexrazoxane

E

air dose
cortisone (compound E)
East
edema (*See also* ed)
effective
einstein (unit of energy)
elastance
electric affinity (*See also* EA)
electric charge (*See also* e)
electric field vector
electrode potential
electromagnetic force
electron (*See also* e)
eloper
embryo (*See also* emb)
emmetropia
enamel
encephalitis
endangered (animal)
endogenous
endoplasm
enema (*See also* en, cncm)
energy
engorged
enterococcus
entgegen
enzyme
eosinophil
epicondyle
epinephrine (*See also* epi, epineph)
epsilon (fifth letter of Greek alphabet), uppercase
error
erythrocyte (*See also* ERY, eryth)
erythroid
erythromycin (*See also* EM, ETM)
Escherichia (*See also* Esch.)
esophagus (*See also* ES, ESO, eso, esoph)
esophoria (for distance)
ester (*See also* est)
estradiol (*See also* E-diol)
ethanol (*See also* ET, ETH)
ethmoid (sinus)
ethyl (*See also* ET, Et)
etiocholanolone
etiology
evaluation
evening
exa-
examiner
exercise (*See also* EX, exer)
expectancy (wave)

expected frequency in a cell of a contingency table
experiment(al) (*See also* exp, exper, exptl)
expired (air)
expired (died) (*See also* exp)
expired (gas)
extension (*See also* EXT)
extinction (coefficient)
extraction fraction
extraction ratio
extralymphatic
eye
glutamic acid (*See also* Glu)
internal energy
kinetic energy of a particle
mathematical expectation
methylenedioxyme-thamphetamine (MDMA; Extcasy)
opposite (stereo descriptor to indicate configuration at a double bond) [Ger. *entgegen*]
redox potential
vectorcardiography electrode (midsternal)
vitamin E

E_1

estrone

E_2

estradiol
17-β-estradiol

E3

unconjugated estriol

E_3

estriol

4E

four plus edema

E_4

estetrol

E'

esophoria (for near)

E°

standard electrode potential

E*

lesion on erythrocyte cell membrane at the site of complement fixation

E'

elbow

E⁻

negative electron

e

base of natural logarithms
early
egg transfer

e *(continued)*
    electric charge (*See also* E)
    electron (*See also* E)
    elementary charge
    erg
    from [L. *ex*]
e+
    positron (positive electron)
EA
    early amniocentesis
    early antigen
    educational age
    egg albumin
    elbow aspiration
    electric affinity (*See also* E, E_o)
    electroacupuncture (*See also* EAC)
    electroanesthesia
    electrophysiologic abnormality
    embryonic antibody
    embryonic antigen
    emergency area
    endocardiographic amplifier
    endotracheal aspirate
    endotracheal aspiration
    enteral alimentation
    enteroanastomosis
    enzymatic active
    epiandrosterone
    epidural anesthesia
    episodic ataxia
    erythrocyte antibody
    erythrocyte antisera
    esophageal atresia
    esterase activity
    estivoautumnal (malaria)
    ethacrynic acid
EA-2
    episodic ataxia type 2
E&A
    evaluate and advise
E→A
    "E to A" (in pulmonary
    consolidation, all vowels including
    "e" heard as "a" through
    stethoscope)
    E wave to A wave
ea
    each
EAA
    electroacupuncture analgesia
    electrothermal atomic absorption
    essential amino acid
    excitatory amino acid
    excitotoxic amino acid
    extraalveolar air
    extrinsic allergic alveolitis

EAAS
    electrothermal atomic absorption
    spectrophotometry
EAB
    elective abortion
    extraanatomic bypass
EABA
    endogenous avidin-binding activity
EABT
    estrogen add back therapy
EABV
    effective arterial blood volume
EAC
    Ehrlich ascites carcinoma
    electroacupuncture (*See also* EA)
    epithelioma adenoides cysticum
    erythema action (spectrum)
    erythema annulare centrifugum
    erythrocyte, antibody, and
    complement
    esophageal adenocarcinoma
    expandable access catheter
    external auditory canal
EACA
    epsilon-aminocaproic acid
EACD
    eczematous allergic contact
    dermatitis
EACS
    exertional anterior compartment
    syndrome
EAD
    early afterdepolarization
    effective airspace dimension
    extracranial arterial disease
E-ADD
    epileptic attention deficit disorder
eAdHCC
    early advanced hepatocellular
    carcinoma
EADL
    extended activities of daily living
EAE
    effective arterial elastance
    experimental allergic encephalitis
    experimental allergic
    encephalomyelitis
    experimental autoimmune
    encephalitis
    experimental autoimmune
    encephalomyelitis
EAEC
    enteroadherent *Escherichia coli*
EAF
    emergency assistance to families
    eosinophilic angiocentric fibrosis
EAG
    electroantennogram

electroarteriography
electroatriogram
endovascular aortic graft
experimental autoimmune gastritis

EAggEC, EaggEC
enteroaggregative *Escherichia coli*

EAHF
eczema, asthma, and hay fever
(complex)

EAHLG
equine antihuman lymphoblast
globulin

EAHLS
equine antihuman lymphoblast
serum

EAI
Employment and Adaptation Index
erythema ab igne
erythrocyte antibody inhibition

EAL
electronic apex locator
electronic artificial larynx
endoscopic aspiration lumpectomy

EAM
endoscopic aspiration mucosectomy
external auditory meatus

EAMG
experimental autoimmune
myasthenia gravis

EAN
experimental allergic neuritis

EANG
epidemic acute nonbacterial
gastroenteritis

EAO
experimental allergic orchitis

EAP
electroacupuncture
Employee Assistance Program
endoscopic access port
epiallopregnanolone
erythrocyte acid phosphatase
evoked action potential

EAQ
eudismic affinity quotient

e-aq
aqueous electron

EAR
early asthmatic response
electroencephalographic audiometry
(expired air) resuscitation

Ea R
reaction of degeneration [Ger.
Entartungs-Reaktion]

EARD
environmentally associated rheumatic
disorder

EARLY
ergonomic assessment of risk and
liability

ear ox
ear oximetry

EARR
extended aortic root replacement
external apical root resorption

EART
extended abdominal radiation
therapy

EAS
Emotionality Activity Sociability
Scale
endoskeletal alignment system
external anal sphincter

EASI
Eczema Area and Severity Index
extraamniotic saline infusion

EASIC
Evaluating Acquired Skills in
Communication

EAST
elevated-arm stress test
enzyme allergosorbent test
external rotation abduction stress
test

EAST1
enteroaggregative *Escherichia coli*
heat-stable enterotoxin 1

eAST
erythrocyte aspartate
aminotransferase activity

EAT
Eating Attitudes Test
ectopic atrial tachycardia
Edinburgh Articulation Test
Education Appperception Test
Ehrlich ascites tumor
electroaerosol therapy
experimental autoimmune thymitis
experimental autoimmune thyroiditis

EATC
Ehrlich ascites tumor cell

E

NOTES

EATCL, EATL
> enteropathy-associated T-cell lymphoma

EAU
> experimental autoimmune uveitis

EAUS
> endoanal ultrasound

EAV
> electroacupuncture according to Voll
> equine abortion virus
> extraalveolar vessel

EAVC
> enhanced atrioventricular conduction

EAVM
> extramedullary arteriovenous malformation

EAVN
> enhanced atrioventricular nodal (conduction)

EB
> elbow bearing
> elementary body
> endometrial biopsy
> epidermolysis bullosa
> Epstein-Barr (virus)
> esophageal body
> estradiol benzoate (*See also* E_2B)
> ethidium bromide
> Evans blue (dye)

E_2B
> estradiol benzoate (*See also* EB)

EBA
> epidermolysis bullosa acquisita
> epidermolysis bullosa atrophicans
> ethoxybenzoic acid
> extrahepatic biliary atresia

EBAB
> equal breath sounds bilaterally (*See also* EBSB)

EBB
> electron beam boosts
> equal breath bilaterally

EBBS
> equal bilateral breath sounds

EBC
> early (stage) breast cancer
> esophageal balloon catheter

EBCDIC
> extended binary-coded decimal interchange code

EBCT
> electron-beam computed tomography

EBD
> emotional and behavioral difficulties
> endocardial border delineation
> endoscopic balloon dilation
> epidermolysis bullosa dystrophica

> evidence-based decision (making)
> extragenital Bowen disease

EBDA
> effective balloon-dilated area

EBDD
> epidermolysis bullosa dystrophica, dominant

EBDR
> epidermolysis bullosa dystrophica, recessive

EBE
> equal bilateral expansion

EBEA
> Epstein-Barr (virus) early antigen

EBER
> Epstein-Barr early region (protein)
> Epstein-Barr virus-encoded ribonucleic acid

EBER ISH
> Epstein-Barr virus-encoded RNA in situ hybridization

EBF
> erythroblastosis fetalis (*See also* EF)

EBG
> electroblepharogram
> electroblepharography

EBGS
> electrical bone-growth stimulation
> electrical bone-growth stimulator

EBI
> emetine and bismuth iodide
> erythroblastic island
> estradiol-binding index

EBIORT, EB-IORT
> electron-beam intraoperative radiation therapy

EBK
> embryonic bovine kidney

EBL
> endoscopic band ligation
> erythroblastic leukemia
> estimated blood loss

EBL-1
> European bat lyssavirus 1

eBL
> endemic Burkitt lymphoma

EBLL
> elevation of blood lead level

EBL/S
> estimated blood loss/surgery

EBM
> electrophysiologic behavior modification
> epidermolysis bullosa, macular type
> evidence-based medicine (*See also* E-BM)
> expressed breast milk

E-BM

    evidence-based medicine (*See also* EBM)

EBNA

    Epstein-Barr (virus) nuclear antigen

EBNe

    Epstein-Barr nasopharyngeal carcinoma

EBNS

    endoscopic bladder neck suspension

EBO

    evidence-based outcomes

E/BOD

    electrolyte biochemical oxygen demand

EBOV

    Ebola virus

EBP

    epidural blood patch
    estradiol-binding protein

EBPS

    Emotional and Behavior Problem Scale

EBR

    embolus-to-blood ratio
    external beam radiotherapy

EBRs

    evidence-based recommendations

EBRT

    external beam radiation therapy

EBS

    elastic back strap
    electrical brain stimulation
    epidermolysis bullosa simplex
    estrogen binding site

EBSB

    equal breath sounds bilaterally (*See also* EBAB)

EBSD

    endoscopic balloon sphincter dilation

EBSL

    external branch of superior laryngeal

EBSS

    Earle balanced salt solution

EBT

    early bedtime
    electron beam tomography
    erythromycin breath test

    ethylsulfonylbenzaldehyde thiosemicarbazone (subathizone)
    external beam (photon) therapy

EBV

    effective blood volume
    Epstein-Barr virus

EB-VCA

    Epstein-Barr viral capsid antigen

EBZ

    epidermal basement zone

EC

    econazole
    effect of closing (of eyes in electroencephalography)
    effective concentration
    ejection click
    electrochemical
    electron capture
    Ellis-van Creveld (syndrome) (*See also* EVC)
    embryonal carcinoma
    emetic center
    endocervical
    endometrial carcinoma
    endothelial cell
    enteric-coated (tablet) (*See also* ECA, ECT)
    entering complaint
    enterochromaffin cell
    enterochromaffin-cell (hyperplasia)
    entorhinal cortex
    entrance complaint
    environmental complexity
    enzyme-treated cell
    epidermal cell
    epithelial cell
    equalization-cancellation
    Erb-Charcot (syndrome)
    Escherichia coli
    esophageal candidiasis
    esophageal carcinoma
    ether-chloroform (mixture)
    Euro-Collins (solution)
    European Community
    excitation-contraction
    excitatory center
    experimental control
    external carotid
    external conjugate
    extracellular
    extracellular compartment
    extracellular concentration

E

NOTES

EC *(continued)*
    extracranial
    extruded cell
    eye care
    eyes closed

EC50, EC_{50}
    median effective concentration

E/C
    endoscopy/cystoscopy
    estriol/creatinine (ratio)
    estrogen/creatinine (ratio)

ECA
    electric control activity
    electrocardioanalyzer
    enteric-coated aspirin (tablet) (*See also* EC, ECT)
    enterobacterial common antigen
    epidemiologic catchment area
    ethacrynic acid (diuretic)
    ethylcarboxylate adenosine
    external carotid artery

E-CABG
    endoscopic coronary artery bypass grafting

ECAD
    extracranial carotid arterial disease

E-cad
    E-cadherin

ECAF
    extension corner avulsion fracture

ECAO
    enterocytopathogenic avian orphan (virus)

ECASA
    enteric-coated acetylsalicylic acid

ECAT
    emission computer-assisted tomography

ECB
    electric cabinet bath

ECBD
    exploration of common bile duct

ECBI
    Eyberg Child Behavior Inventory

ECBO
    enterocytopathogenic bovine orphan (virus)

ECBV
    effective circulating blood volume

ECC
    early childhood caries
    edema, clubbing, and cyanosis
    electrocorticogram
    embryonal cell carcinoma
    emergency cardiac care
    Emergency Communications Center
    endocervical cone
    endocervical curettage
    enterochromaffin cell
    estimated creatinine clearance
    external cardiac compression
    extracorporeal circulation
    extrusion of cell cytoplasm

ECCE
    extracapsular cataract extraction (*See also* XCCE)

ECCL
    encephalocraniocutaneous lipomatosis

ECCO
    enterocytopathogenic cat orphan (virus)

$ECCO_2R$
    extracorporeal carbon dioxide removal

ECD
    electrochemical detection
    electrochemical detector
    electron capture detector
    endocardial cushion defect
    enzymatic cell dispersion
    equivalent current dipole
    Erdheim-Chester disease
    excision, curettage and drilling
    extended criteria donor
    external cardioverter-defibrillator
    extracellular domain
    extracranial carotid disease
    extracranial Doppler sonography

ECDB
    encourage to cough and deep breathe

ECDEU
    early clinical drug evaluation unit

ECDO
    enterocytopathogenic dog orphan (virus)

ECE
    early childhood education
    endocervical ecchymosis
    equine conjugated estrogen
    extracapsular extension

ECE1
    endothelin-converting enzyme

ECEMG
    evoked compound electromyography

ECEO
    enterocytopathogenic equine orphan (virus)

ECES
    Education and Career Exploration System

ECF
    East Coast fever
    effective capillary flow
    eosinophilic chemotactic factor
    erythroid colony formation

Escherichia coli filtrate
executive cognitive function
executive cognitive functioning
extended care facility
extracellular fluid

ECFA, ECF-A
eosinophil chemotactic factor of anaphylaxis

ECF-C
eosinophilic chemotactic factor-complement

ECFV
extracellular fluid volume (*See also* EFV)

ECG
electrocardiogram (*See also* EKG)
electrocardiograph
electrocardiography

ECGE
extracorporeal gas exchange

ECGF
endothelial cell growth factor

ECGS
endothelial cell growth supplement

ECH
epichlorohydrin
extended care hospital

echino
echinocyte

ECHO
echoencephalography
enterocytopathogenic human orphan (virus)

echo
echocardiogram
echocardiography
echoencephalogram (*See also* echo EG)
echoencephalography (*See also* echo EG)

echo EG
echoencephalogram (*See also* echo)
echoencephalography (*See also* echo)

ECHOG, ECochG
electrocochleography (*See also* ECoG)

ECHO-RV
echocardiography-radionuclide ventriculography

echo-VM
echoventriculometry

ECI
electrocerebral inactivity
eosinophilic cytoplasmic inclusion
extracorporeal irradiation (of blood) (*See also* ECIB)

ECIB
extracorporeal irradiation of blood (*See also* ECI)

ECIC
external carotid and internal carotid
extracranial-intracranial (*See also* EC-IC)

EC-IC (*See also* ECIC)
extracranial-intracranial

ECIDP
intracranial epidural pressure

ECIL
extracorporeal irradiation of lymph

ECIS
endometrial carcinoma in situ

ECK
extracellular kalium (potassium)

ECKI
Escherichia coli K1

ECL
electrochemiluminescence
electrogenerated chemiluminescence
emitter-coupled logic
enhanced chemiluminescence
enterochromaffin-like (type)
euglobulin clot lysis
extent of cerebral lesion
extracapillary lesion

ECLA
excimer laser coronary angioplasty
extracorporeal lung assist

eclec
eclectic

ECLP
extracorporeal liver perfusion

ECLS
extracorporeal life support

ECLT
euglobulin clot lysis time

ECM
embryonic chick muscle
endoscope-controlled microsurgery
erythema chronicum migrans
external cardiac massage
external chemical messenger
extracellular material

E

NOTES

ECM *(continued)*
 extracellular matrix
 extracolonic malignancy
ECM/BCM
 extracellular mass to body cell
  mass ratio
ECMO
 enterocytopathogenic monkey orphan
  (virus)
 extracorporeal membrane
  oxygenation
 extracorporeal membrane oxygenator
ECMP
 enterocoated microspheres of
  pancrelipase
ECN
 epithelioid combined nevi
 extended-care nursery
ECN-DPN
 epithelioid combined nevi deep
  penetrating nevus
EC No.
 Enzyme Commission Number
ecNOS
 endothelial constitutive nitric oxide
  synthase
 endothelial constitutive nitric oxide
  synthetase
ECoG
 electrocochleography *(See also*
  ECHOG)
 electrocorticogram
 electrocorticography
E. coli
 Escherichia coli (See also EC)
ECOM
 endotracheal cardiac output monitor
ECOR
 extracorporeal carbon dioxide
  removal
ECOtox
 Escherichia coli (heat-labile toxin)
  vaccine
ECP
 ectrodactyly-cleft palate (syndrome)
 effective conduction period
 effector cell precursor
 electronic claims processing
 emergency care provider
 emergency contraceptive pill
 endocardial potential
 eosinophil cationic protein
 erythrocyte coproporphyrin
 erythroid committed precursor
 erythropoietic coproporphyria
 Escherichia coli polypeptide
 estradiol cyclopentanepropionate
 external cardiac pressure

 external counterpulsation
 extracorporeal photochemotherapy
 extracorporeal photopheresis
 free cytoporphyrin in erythrocytes
ECPD
 external counterpressure device
ECPL
 endocavitary pelvic
  lymphadenectomy
ECPO
 enterocytopathogenic porcine orphan
  (virus)
ECPOG
 electrochemical potential gradient
ECPP
 extracorporeal photophoresis
ECPR
 external cardiopulmonary
  resuscitation
ECR
 electrocardiographic response
 emergency chemical restraint
 endocervical resection
 evoked cortical response
 extensor carpi radialis
ECRB
 extensor carpi radialis brevis
ECRL
 extensor carpi radialis longus
ECRO
 enterocytopathogenic rodent orphan
  (virus)
ECS
 elective cosmetic surgery
 electrocerebral silence
 electroconvulsive shock
 electronic claims submission
 epileptic confusional state
 extracapsular spread
 extracellular-like, calcium-free
  solution
 extracellular space
E2CS
 Edinburgh 2 Coma Scale
ECSO
 enterocytopathogenic swine orphan
  (virus)
ECSP
 epidermal cell surface protein
ECT
 ectomesenchymal chondromyxoid
  tumor
 electrochemotherapy
 electroconvulsive therapy
 emission computed tomography
 enteric-coated tablet *(See also* EC,
  ECA)
 euglobulin clot test

European compression technique
(bone screw and internal fixation)
extracellular tissue

ECTA
Everyman Contingency Table
Analysis

ECTEOLA
epichlorohydrin and triethanolamine

ECTR
endoscopic carpal tunnel release

ECU
electrocautery unit
environmental control unit
extended care unit
extensor carpi ulnaris
extracorporeal ultrafiltration

ECV
effective circulating volume
emergency center visits
esophageal collateral vein
external cephalic version
extracellular fluid volume
extracellular volume
extracorporeal volume

ECVD
extracellular volume of distribution

ECVE
extracellular volume expansion

ECW
extracellular water

E-D
ego-defense

ED
early differentiation
eating disorder(s)
ectodermal dysplasia
ectopic depolarization
education
effective dose
Ehlers-Danlos (syndrome)
elbow disarticulation
electrodiagnosis (*See also* EDX,
EDx, El Dx)
electrodialysis
electron diffraction
elemental diet
embryonic death
emergency department
emotional defensiveness
emotional disorder
emotional disturbance
emotionally disturbed

end diastole
entering diagnosis
Entner-Doudoroff (metabolic
pathway)
enzyme deficiency
epidural
epileptiform discharge
equilibrium dialysis
equine dermis (cells)
equivalent dose
erectile dysfunction
erythema dose
ethyldichloroarsine
ethylenediamine
ethynodiol diacetate
evidence of disease
exertional dyspnea
extensive disease
extensor digitorum
external diameter
external dyspnea
extra-low dispersion

ED$_{50}$
median effective dose

E$_d$
depth dose

ed
edema (*See also* E)

EDA
elbow disarticulation
electrodermal activity
electrodermal audiometry
electrolyte-deficient agar
electron donor-acceptor (interaction)
end-diastolic area
end-diastolic (cross-sectional) area

EDA+
extradomain A positive

EDAM
edatrexate
electron-dense amorphous material

10-EDAM
10-ethyl-10-diazaaminopterin

EDAMS
encephaloduroarteriomyosynangiosis

EDAP
emergency department approval for
pediatrics

EDAS
encephaloduroarteriosynangiosis

EDAX
energy-dispersive x-ray analysis

NOTES

E

217

EDB

> early dry breakfast
> ethylene dibromide
> extensor digitorum brevis

EDBP

> erect diastolic blood pressure

EDC

> effective dynamic compliance
> electrodesiccation and curettage
> (*See also* ED&C)
> emergency decontamination center
> end-diastolic count
> estimated date of conception
> estimated date of confinement
> expected date of confinement
> expected delivery, cesarean
> extensor digitorum communis

ED&C

> electrodesiccation and curettage
> (*See also* EDC)

EDCF

> endothelium-derived constricting
> factor

EDCI

> energetic dynamic cardiac
> insufficiency

E-DCIS

> endocrine ductal carcinoma in situ

EDCP

> eccentric dynamic compression
> plate
> eccentric dynamic compression
> plating

EDCS

> end-diastolic chamber stiffness
> end-diastolic circumferential stress

EDCT

> early distal proximal tubule

EDD

> effective drug duration
> end-diastolic diameter
> end-diastolic dimension
> enzyme-digested delta (endotoxin)
> esophageal detection device
> estimated discharge date
> estimated due date
> expected date of delivery
> extended daily dialysis

EDDA

> expanded duty dental auxiliary

EDE

> eating disorders examination

EDe

> erosion depth

EDEN

> Evaluation Disposition (toward the)
> Environment

edent

> edentulous

ED-ES

> endolymphatic duct-endolymphatic
> sac

EDF

> elongation, derotation and lateral
> flexion
> end-diastolic flow
> erythroid differentiation factor
> extradural fluid

EDG

> electrodermography
> electrodynogram

EdGr

> Edmondson grade
> Edmondson grading

EDH

> epidural hematoma
> extradural hematoma

EDHF

> endothelium-derived hyperpolarizing
> factor

EDI

> Eating Disorder Inventory
> electrodeionization

EDI-2

> Eating Disorder Inventory, 2nd
> edition

EDIC

> Epidemiology of Diabetes
> Interventions and Complications

EDICP

> electron-dense iron-containing
> particle

EDIE

> extended deep inferior epigastric

EDIM

> epidemic disease of infant mice
> epizootic diarrhea of infant mice

E-diol

> estradiol (*See also* E)

EDit

> electric differential therapy

EDITAR

> extended-duration topical arthropod
> repellent

EDL

> end-diastolic load
> end-diastolic (segment) length
> estimated date of labor
> extensor digitorum longus

ED/LD

> emotionally disturbed and learning
> disabled

EDLF

> endogenous digitalis-like factors

EDLS
    endogenous digitalis-like substance
EDM
    early diastolic murmur
    esophageal Doppler monitor
    extensor digiti minimi
    extramucosal duodenal myotomy
    multiple epiphysial dysplasia
EDMA
    ethylene glycol dimethacrylate
    euclidean distance matrix analysis
EDMD
    Emery-Dreifuss muscular dystrophy
EDN
    electrodesiccation
    eosinophil-derived neurotoxin
EDNO
    endothelium-derived nitric oxide
EDOC
    estimated date of confinement
EDP
    electron-dense particle
    electronic data processing
    emergency department physician
    end-diastolic pressure
    endoscopic digital pancreatography
EDPA
    Erhardt Developmental Prehension
      Assessment
    ethyldiphenylpropenylamine
EDPCS
    exertional deep posterior
      compartment syndrome
EDPS
    esophageal-directed pressure support
EDQ
    extensor digiti quinti
EDR
    early diastolic relaxation
    edrophonium
    effective direct radiation
    electrodermal response (biofeedback)
    electrodialysis with reversed
      (polarity)
    extreme drug resistance
EDRA
    electrodermal response audiometry
EDRF
    endothelium-derived relaxing factor
EDS
    edema disease of swine
    egg drop syndrome

    Ego Development Scale
    Ehlers-Danlos syndrome
    energy-dispersive spectrometer
    epigastric distress syndrome
    excessive daytime sleepiness
    extended data stream
    extradimensional shift
EDSS
    Expanded Disability Status Scale
      (Score)
EDT
    emergency department thoracotomy
    end-diastolic (cardiac wall)
      thickness
    exposure duration threshold
EDTA
    ethylenediaminetetraacetic acid
      (edathamil, edetic acid)
EDTAC
    ethylenediaminetetraacetic acid
      Cetavlon
EDTMP
    ethylenediamine tetramethylene
      phosphoric acid
EDTU
    emergency diagnostic and treatment
      unit
EdU
    eating disorder unit
EDV
    end-diastolic velocity
    end-diastolic volume
    epidermal dysplastic verruciformis
EDVA
    Erhardt Developmental Vision
      Assessment
EDVI
    end-diastolic volume index
EDW
    estimated dry weight
EDWGT
    emergency drinking water
      germicidal tablet
EDWTH
    end-diastolic wall thickness
EDX, EDx
    edatrexate
    electrodiagnosis (*See also* ED, El
      Dx)
EDXA
    energy-dispersed x-ray analysis
    energy-dispersive x-ray analysis

E

NOTES

EDXRF
energy-dispersive x-ray fluorescence

E_{dyn}
respiratory system elastance

E-E
end-to-end (anastomosis) (*See also* EE)
erythema-edema (reaction)

EE
electrosurgical excision
embryo extract
emetic episodes
end-expiration
end-to-end (anastomosis) (*See also* E-E)
end-to-end (bite, occlusion)
energy expenditure
Enterobacteriaceae enrichment (broth)
equine encephalitis
erosive esophagitis
esophageal endoscopy
ethinyl estradiol
ethynyl estradiol
exercise echocardiogram
expressed emotion
external ear
eyes and ears (*See also* E&E)

E&E
eyes and ears (*See also* EE)

EEA
electroencephalic audiometry
elemental enteral alimentation
end-to-end anastomosis
energy expended with activity

EEC
ectrodactyly, ectodermal (dysplasia), clefting (syndrome)
endogenous erythroid colony
enteropathogenic *Escherichia coli*
enterovirulent *Escherichia coli*

EECD
endothelial-epithelial corneal dystrophy

EECG
electroencephalogram (*See also* EEG)
electroencephalography (*See also* EEG)

EECP
enhanced external counterpulsation

EECS
extraembryonic celomic space

EED
erythema elevatum diutinum

EEDQ
ethoxycarbonylethoxydihydroquinoline

EEE
eastern equine encephalitis
eastern equine encephalomyelitis
edema, erythema, and exudate
experimental enterococcal endocarditis
external eye examination

EEEP
end-expiratory esophageal pressure

EEEV
eastern equine encephalitis virus
eastern equine encephalomyelitis virus

EEG
electroencephalogram
electroencephalograph
electroencephalography

EEGA
electroencephalographic audiometry

EEGF
esophageal epidermal growth factor

EEJ
electroejaculation

EEL
external elastic lamina

EELS
electron energy loss spectroscopy

EELV
end-expiratory lung volume

EEM
ectodermal dysplasia, ectrodactyly, macular dystrophy (syndrome)
erythema exudativum multiforme
external elastic membrane
Test for Examining Expressive Morphology

EEME
ethynylestradiol methyl ether

EEMG
evoked electromyogram
evoked electromyography

EEN
estimated energy needs

EENT
eyes, ears, nose, throat

EEO
electroendoosmosis

EEP
end-expiratory phase
end-expiratory pressure
equivalent effective photon

E-EPE
established extraprostatic extension

EEPI
extraretinal eye position information

EEPLND
extraperitoneal endoscopic pelvic lymph node dissection

EER
   electroencephalographic response
   extended endocardial resection
EERP
   extended endocardial resection
      procedure
EES
   endometrial stromal sarcoma
   erythromycin ethylsuccinate
   ethyl ethanesulfate
   expandable esophageal stent
EESG
   evoked electrospinogram
EET
   early exercise testing
   epoxyeicosatrienoic (acid)
EEU
   environmental exposure unit
EEV
   elastic equilibrium volume
   encircling endocardial
      ventriculotomy
EF
   eccentric fixation
   ectopic focus
   edema factor
   ejection fraction
   elastic fiber
   elastic fibril
   electric field
   elongation factor
   embryo fetal
   embryo fibroblast
   emergency facility
   emotional factor
   encephalitogenic factor
   endothoracic fascia
   endurance factor
   eosinophilic fasciitis
   epithelial focus
   equivalent focus
   erythroblastosis fetalis (See also
      EBF)
   erythrocytic fragmentation
   essential findings
   exophthalmic factor
   exposure factor
   extended field (radiation therapy)
   extrafine
   extra food
   extrinsic factor

EF-4
   eugonic fermenter 4
EFA
   essential fatty acid
   extrafamily adoptee
EFAD
   essential fatty acid deficiency
EFAS
   embryofetal alcohol syndrome
EFBW
   estimated fetal body weight
EFC
   elastin fragment concentration
   endogenous fecal calcium
EFD
   episode free day
EFDA
   expanded function dental assistant
EFE
   endocardial fibroelastosis
   epidemic fatal encephalopathy
EFF
   electromagnetic focusing field
      (probe)
eff
   effect
   efferent (See also effer)
   efficient
   effusion
effect.
   effective
effer
   efferent (See also eff)
EFFU
   epithelial focus-forming unit
EF-G
   elongation factor G
EFH
   explosive follicular hyperplasia
EFHBM
   eosinophilic fibrohistiocytic (lesion
      of) bone marrow
EFL
   effective focal length
   external fluid loss
EFM
   elderly fibromyalgia
   electronic fetal monitoring
   external fetal monitoring
EFMM
   external fetal maternal monitor

NOTES

E

EFMT
electric field mediated transfer
EFP
effective filtration pressure
endoneural fluid pressure
EFPS
epicardial fat pad sign
EFR
effective filtration rate
extended field radiation
E FRAG
erythrocyte fragility (test)
EFS
electric field stimulation
event-free survival
EFT
Embedded Figures Test
extended family therapy
EFV
efavirenz
extracellular fluid volume (*See also* ECFV)
EFVC
expiratory flow-volume curve
EFW
estimated fetal weight
EF/WM
ejection fraction/wall motion
EG
enteroglucagon
eosinophilic gastroenteritis
eosinophilic granuloma
Erb-Goldflam (syndrome)
esophagogastrectomy
esophagogastric
external genitalia
e.g.
for example [L. *exempli gratia*]
EGA
esophageal gastric (tube) airway
estimated gestational age
EGAT
Educational Goal Attainment Test
EGb
extract of *Ginkgo biloba*
EGBPS
equilibrium-gated blood pool study
EGBT
esophagogastric balloon tamponade
EGBUS, EG/BUS
external genitalia, Bartholin,
urethral, and Skene (glands) (*See
also* EXGBUS)
EGC
early gastric carcinoma
endocrine granule constituent
epithelioid-globoid cell

EGCG
epigallocatechin gallate
EGCUS
early gastric cancer of the upper
stomach
EGD
esophagogastroduodenoscopy
EGDF
embryonic growth and development
factor
EGDT
esophagogastric devascularization
and transection
EGE
eosinophilic gastroenteritis
EGF
endothelial growth factor
epidermal growth factor
eGFP
enhanced green fluorescent protein
EGFR
epidermal growth factor receptor
EGG
electrogastrogram
electrogastrography
electroglottography
EGH
equine growth hormone
EGI
endogenous GAD inhibitor
EGJ
esophagogastric junction
EGL
eosinophilic granuloma of lung
EGLT
euglobulin lysis time
EGM
electrogram
extracellular granular material
extraglandular manifestation
extraglomerular mesangium
EGN
experimental glomerulonephritis
EGNB
enteric gram-negative bacillary
EGOT
erythrocyte glutamic oxaloacetic
transaminase
erythrocytic glutamic oxaloacetic
transaminase
EGP
endogenous glucose production
EGP-2
epithelial glycoprotein-2
EGR
erythrocyte glutathione reductase

EGRA

    equilibrium-gated radionuclide angiography

EGS

    electrogalvanic stimulation
    ethylene glycol succinate
    extragonadal seminoma

EGT

    ethanol gelation test
    exuberant granulation tissue

EGTA

    esophageal gastric tube airway
    esophagogastric tube airway
    ethyleneglycoltetraacetic acid
    ethylene glycol tetraacetic acid

EH

    early healed
    eccentric hypertrophy
    educationally handicapped
    emotional handicap
    emotionally handicapped
    endometrial hyperplasia
    enlarged heart
    enteral hyperalimentation
    environment and heredity (*See also* E&H)
    epidermolytic hyperkeratosis
    epithelioid hemangioendothelioma
    epoxide hydratase
    essential hypertension
    extramedullary hematopoiesis

E&H

    environment and heredity (*See also* EH)

E_h, eH

    oxidation-reduction potential (*See also* ORP)

EHAA

    epidemic hepatitis-associated antigen

EHB

    elevate head of bed
    extensor hallucis brevis

EHBA

    extrahepatic biliary atresia

EHBD

    extrahepatic bile duct

EHBDA

    extrahepatic bile duct atresia

EHBF

    estimated hepatic blood flow
    exercise hyperemia blood flow
    extrahepatic blood flow (clearance)

EHC

    enterohepatic circulation
    enterohepatic clearance
    essential hypercholesterolemia
    extended health care
    extrahepatic cholestasis

eHCC

    early hepatocellular carcinoma

EH-CF

    Entamoeba histolytica-complement fixation

EHD

    electrohemodynamic
    epizootic hemorrhagic disease

EHDA, EHDP

    ethanehydroxydiphosphonic acid (etidronate sodium)

EHDV

    epizootic hemorrhagic disease virus 1–8

EHE

    epithelioid hemangioendothelioma

EHEC

    enterohemorrhagic *Escherichia coli*

EHF

    electrohydraulic fragmentation
    epidemic hemorrhagic fever
    exophthalmos-hyperthyroid factor
    extremely high factor
    extremely high frequency

EHH

    esophageal hiatal hernia

EHI

    Edinburgh Handedness Inventory
    exertional heat illness

EHL

    effective half-life (of radioactive substance)
    electrohydraulic lithotripsy
    endogenous hyperlipidemia
    endoscopic hemorrhoid ligation
    Environmental Health Laboratory
    essential hyperlipidemia
    extensor hallucis longus

EHLL

    epithelial hyperplastic laryngeal lesion

EHM

    embryonic heart motion
    extrahepatic metastasis

E

NOTES

EHME
Employee Health Maintenance Examination

EHMS
electrohydrodynamic ionization mass spectrometry

EHN
ethotoin

EHO
extrahepatic obstruction

EHP
Environmental Health Perspectives
excessive heat production
extra high potency

EHPH
extrahepatic portal hypertension

EHPO
extrahepatic portal vein obstruction

EHPT
Eddy hot plate test

EHPVO
extrahepatic portal vein obstruction

EHS
employee health service
exertional heat stroke

EHSDS
Experimental Health Services Delivery System

EHT
electrohydrothermal
essential hypertension

EHV
Edge Hill virus
equine herpesvirus

EI
electrolyte imbalance
electron impact
electron ionization
emotionally impaired
endovascular irradiation
environmental illness
enzyme immunoassay
enzyme inhibitor
eosinophilic index
erythema infectiosum
excretory index
extensor indicis
external ilium
external intervention

E of I
evidence of insurability

E/I
expiration/inspiration (ratio)

E&I
endocrine and infertility

EIA
electroimmunoassay
enteroinsular axis
enzymatic immunoassay
enzyme immunosorbent assay
equine infectious anemia
exercise-induced anaphylaxis
exercise-induced asthma

EIA-2
second-generation enzyme immunoassay

EIAB
extracranial-intracranial arterial bypass

EIB
electrophoretic immunoblotting
erythema induration of Bazin
exercise-induced bronchoconstriction
exercise-induced bronchospasm

EIC
elastase inhibition capacity
electrical impedance cardiography
endometrial intraepithelial carcinoma
enzyme inhibition complex
epidermal inclusion cyst
extensive intraductal carcinoma
extensive intraductal component

EICDT
Ego-Ideal and Conscience Development Test

EICL
Eldercare Initiative in Consumer Law

EICT
external isovolumic contraction time

EID
egg-infectious dose
electroimmunodiffusion
electronic induction desorption
electronic infusion device
emergency infusion device

EIDC
extreme intervertebral disk collapse

EIDCR
endoscopic intranasal dacryocystorhinostomy

EIEC
enteroinvasive *Escherichia coli*

EIEE
early infantile epileptic encephalopathy

EIF, eIF
erythrocyte initiation factor
eukaryotic initiation factor

EIFT
embryo intrafallopian transfer

EIL
elective induction of labor

EILV
end-inspiratory lung volume

EIM
    excitability-inducing material
    extraintestinal manifestation
EIMS
    electron ionization mass
      spectrometry
EI/MV
    endotracheal intubation and
      mechanical ventilation
EIN
    endometrial intraepithelial neoplasia
EIO
    exploratory insight-oriented
      psychotherapy
EIOA
    excessive intake of alcohol
EIP
    early intervention program
    elective interruption of pregnancy
    end-inspiratory pause
    extensor indicis proprius
EIPS
    endogenous inhibitor of
      prostaglandin synthase
EIPV, eIPV
    enhanced inactivated polio vaccine
EIR
    early ischemic recurrence
    entomological inoculation rate
EIRDS
    exercise-induced respiratory distress
      syndrome
EIRnv
    extra-incidence rate in
      nonvaccinated (groups)
EIRP
    effective isotropic radiated power
EIRv
    extra incidence rate in vaccinated
      (groups)
EIS
    endoscopic injection sclerotherapy
    Environmental Impact Statement
Eis
    Eisenmenger syndrome
EISA
    electroencephalogram interval
      spectrum analysis
EIT
    electrical impedance tomography
    erythroid iron turnover

EITB
    enzyme-linked immunotransfer blot
EI.U
    ELISA unit
EIV
    external iliac vein
EJ
    ejection (fraction)
    elbow jerk
    external jugular
EJB
    ectopic junctional beat
EJN
    extended jaundice of newborn
EJP
    excitatory junction potential
EJV
    external jugular vein
EK
    electrophoretic karyotyping
    enterokinase
    erythrokinase
EKC
    epidemic keratoconjunctivitis
EKG
    electrocardiogram (*See also* ECG)
    electrocardiograph
    electrocardiography (*See also* ECG)
EKO
    echoencephalogram
eKru
    equivalent residual renal urea
      clearance
EKV
    erythrokeratodermia variabilis
EKY
    electrokymogram
    electrokymography
E-L
    external lids
EL
    early latent
    egg lecithin
    elastic limit
    electrolarynx
    electroluminescence
    elixir (*See also* elix)
    elopement
    erythroleukemia
    exercise limit
    external lamina

E

NOTES

El
    elastase
ELA
    endotoxin-like activity
    excimer laser-assisted angioplasty
ELAD
    extracorporeal liver assist device
ELAFF
    extended lateral arm free flap
E-LAM, ELAM
    endothelial-leukocyte adhesion
        molecule
ELAM-1
    endothelial-leukocyte adhesion
        molecule-1
ELAS
    extended lymphadenopathy
        syndrome
ELAT
    enzyme-linked antiglobulin test
ELB
    early light breakfast
elb
    elbow
ELBF
    estimated liver blood flow
ELBNS
    extraperitoneal laparoscopic bladder
        neck suspension
ELBW
    extremely low birth weight
ELBWI
    extremely low birth weight infant
ELC
    earlobe crease
ELCA
    excimer laser coronary angioplasty
ELD
    egg lethal dose
ELDH
    extraforaminal lumbar disc
        herniation
El Dx
    electrodiagnosis (*See also* ED,
        EDX, EDx)
ELEC
    elective
elec, elect.
    electric
    electricity
    electuary (confection)
elem
    elementary
elev
    elevated
    elevation
    elevator

ELF
    elective low forceps (delivery)
    endoscopic laser foraminotomy
    epithelial lining fluid
    extremely low frequency
ELFA
    enzyme-linked fluorescent
        immunoassay
ELG
    eligible
    endolumenal gastroplication
    endoluminal graft
elgon
    electrogoniometer
ELH
    egg-laying hormone
    endolymphatic hydrops
ELI
    endomyocardial lymphocytic
        infiltrates
    Environmental Language Inventory
    exercise lability index
ELIA
    enzyme-labeled immunoassay
ELICT
    enzyme-linked immunocytochemical
        technique
ELIEDA
    enzyme-linked
        immunoelectrodiffusion assay
ELIFA
    enzyme-linked immunofiltration
        assay
ELIG
    eligible
ELISA
    enzyme-linked immunoabsorbent
        assay
ELISPOT
    enzyme-linked immunospot assay
    (solid-phase) enzyme-linked
        immunospot
ELITT
    endometrial laser intrauterine
        thermal therapy
elix
    elixir (*See also* EL)
ELLIP
    elliptocyte
ELM
    early language milestone
    Early Language Milestone (Scale)
    epiluminescence microscopy
    epiluminescent microscopy
    external limiting membrane
    extravascular lung mass
ELMS
    epithelioid leiomyosarcoma

ELMT
> elements (on urinalysis)

ELN
> elastin

ELND
> elective lymph node dissection

ELOP
> estimated length of program

ELOS
> estimated length of stay
> extralymphatic organ site

ELP
> early labeled peak
> elastase-like protein
> electrophoresis
> endogenous limbic potential
> Estimated Learning Potential
> exogenous lipoid pneumonia
> extracorporeal liver perfusion

ELPS
> excessive lateral pressure syndrome

ELR
> Equal Listener Response (scale)

ELS
> electron loss spectroscopy
> endolymphatic sac
> endolymphatic sac (surgery)
> extracorporeal life support
> extralobar sequestration

ELSI
> ethical, legal, and social
>   implications

ELSS
> emergency life support system

ELT
> endless loop tachycardia
> endoscopic laser therapy
> euglobulin lysis test
> euglobulin lysis time

ELU
> extended length of utterance

ELUS
> endoluminal rectal ultrasonography

ELV
> erythroid leukemia virus

EM
> early memory
> effective masking
> ejection murmur
> electromagnetic (*See also* em)
> electromechanical
> electron micrograph

electron microscope
electron microscopy (*See also* EMC, E-MICR)
electrophoretic mobility
emergency medicine
emmetropia (normal vision)
emotional (disorder)
emotionally (disturbed)
emphysema (*See also* emph)
ergonovine maleate
erythema migrans
erythema multiforme
erythrocyte mass
erythromycin (*See also* E, ETM)
esophageal manometry
esophageal motility
excreted mass
extensive metabolizers
external monitor
extraordinary meridian

E-M
> Embden-Meyerhof (glycolytic pathway)

E of M
> error of measurement

E&M
> endocrine and metabolic

e/m
> ratio of (electron) charge to mass

em
> electromagnetic (*See also* EM)

EMA
> early morning awakening
> electronic microanalyzer
> emergency assistance
> emergency assistant
> emergency medical attendant
> endomysial antibody
> epithelial membrane antigen

E-Mac
> English MacIntosh (system)

EMAD
> equivalent mean age at death

EMAG
> environmental metaplastic atrophic gastritis

EMAP
> evoked muscle action potential

EMAP II
> endothelial-monocyte activating polypeptide II

E

NOTES

EMAS
Endler Multidimensional Anxiety Scale

Emax
maximum ventricular elastance

EMB
embryology (*See also* emb, embryol)
endometrial biopsy
endomyocardial biopsy
engineering in medicine and biology
eosin-methylene blue (Levine agar)
ethambutol
Explanation of Medicare Benefits

emb
embolus
embryo (*See also* E)
embryology (*See also* EMB, embryol)

EMBASE
Excerpta Medica Database

EMBP
estramustine binding protein

embryol
embryology (*See also* emb, EMB)

EMBT
endocervical mucinous borderline tumor

EMC
electron microscopy (*See also* EM, E-MICR)
emergency medical care
encephalomyocarditis
endometrial curettage
essential mixed cryoglobulinemia
extraskeletal myxoid chondrosarcoma

E&M codes
evaluation and management codes

EMC&R
emergency medical care and rescue

EMCV
encephalomyocarditis virus

EMD
electromechanical dissociation
Emery-Dreifuss muscular dystrophy
esophageal motility disorder

EMDA
electromotive drug administration
intravesical electromotive drug administration

EMDR
eye movement desensitization and reprocessing

EME
epithelial-myoepithelial (carcinoma)
extreme medical emergency

EMEG
electromagnetoencephalograph

EMEM
Eagle minimal essential medium

EMER
electromagnetic molecular electronic resonance

emer, emerg
emergency (*See also* EMG)

EMF
elective midforceps
electromagnetic field(s)
electromagnetic flowmeter
electromotive force (*See also* emf)
endomyocardial fibrosis
erythrocyte maturation factor
evaporated milk formula

emf
electromotive force (*See also* EMF)

EMG
electromyelogram
electromyelography
electromyogram
electromyograph
electromyographic
electromyography
emergency (*See also* emer, emerg)
essential monoclonal gammopathy
exomphalos, macroglossia, and gigantism (syndrome)
eye movement gauge

EMGN
extramembranous glomerulonephritis

EMGORS
electromyogram sensors

EMH
educationally mentally handicapped
extramedullary hematopoiesis

EMI
elderly and mentally infirm
electromagnetic interference
electromechanical impactor
emergency medical information

EMIC
emergency maternal and infant care

E-MICR
electron microscopy (*See also* EM, EMC)

EMI/RFI
electromagnetic interference/radiofrequency interference

EMIT
enzyme-multiplied immunoassay technique
enzyme-multiplied immunoassay test

EMJH
Ellinghausen-McCullough-Johnson-Harris (medium)

EML
effective mandibular length

EMLA
eutectic mixture of local anesthetics

EMLB
erythromycin lactobionate

EMLD
external muscle layer damaged

EMM
erythema multiforme major

EMMA
eye movement measuring apparatus

EMMM
epidermotropic metastatic malignant melanoma

EMMPRIN
extracellular matrix metalloproteinase inducer

EMMV
extended mandatory minute ventilation

EMO
Epstein-Macintosh-Oxford (inhaler)
exophthalmos, myxedema circumscriptum praetibiale, and osteoarthropathia hypertrophicans (syndrome)

EMo
ear mold

emot
emotion
emotional

EMP
electrical membrane property
electromagnetic pulse
electromolecular propulsion
Embden-Meyerhof pathway
epimacular proliferation
epiretinal membrane proliferation
external membrane protein
extramedullary plasmacytoma
extramedullary solitary plasmacytoma

EMPD
extramammary Paget disease

EMPEP
electrophoretic pattern
erythrocyte membrane protein

emph
emphysema (*See also* EM)

EMPP
ethylmethylpiperidinopropiophenone

EMR
educable mentally retarded
electrical muscle stimulation
electromagnetic radiation
electronic medical record
emergency mechanical restraint
empty, measure, and record
endomyometrial resection
endoscopic magnetic resonance
endoscopic mucosal resection
essential metabolism ratio
ethanol metabolic rate
eye movement recording

EMRC
endoscopic mucosal resection, cap method

E-MRI
extremity MRI

EMRL
endoscopic mucosal resection with ligation

EMRN
encephalomyeloradiculoneuropathy

EMRSA
epidemic methicillin-resistant *Staphylococcus aureus*

EMRT
endoscopic mucosal resection, tube method

EMS
early morning stiffness
electrical muscle stimulation
emergency medical services
emergency medical system
encephalomyosynangiosis
endometriosis
eosinophilia-myalgia syndrome
esophageal manometric sequence
ethyl methanesulfonate
extramedullary site

EMSA
electrophoretic mobility shift analysis
electrophoretic mobility shift assay

EMS-C
emergency medical services for children

E

NOTES

EMSU
    early morning specimen of urine
EMT
    emergency medical tag
    emergency medical team
    emergency medical treatment
EMTC
    emergency medical trauma center
EM/TEN
    erythema multiforme/toxic epidermal
      necrolysis
EMU
    early morning urine
    electromagnetic unit (*See also* emu)
    epilepsy monitoring unit
emu
    electromagnetic unit (*See also*
      EMU)
emul
    emulsion
EMV
    equine morbilli virus
    eye, motor, voice (Glasgow coma
      scale)
    eyes, motor, verbal
EMVC
    early mitral valve closure
EMW
    electromagnetic waves
EN
    easy normal
    electronarcosis
    endocardial (*See also* ENDO)
    enema (*See also* E, en)
    enteral nutrition
    erythema nodosum
E 50% N
    extension 50% of normal
En, en
    enema (*See also* E, enem, EN)
ENA
    extractable nuclear antigen
ENaC
    epithelial sodium channel
ENANB
    enterically transmitted non-A, non-B
      (hepatitis)
ENB
    esthesioneuroblastoma
ENBD
    endoscopic nasobiliary drainage
ENC
    encourage
END
    early neonatal death
    elective neck dissection
    endocrinology

    endorphin
    enhancement Newcastle disease
end, end.
    endoreduplication
ENDO, Endo
    endocardial (*See also* EN)
    endocardium
    endocrine
    endocrinology
    endodontia
    endodontics
    endoscopy
    endotracheal (*See also* ET)
EndoCAB
    plasma antiendotoxin core antibody
endocr
    endocrine
    endocrinology
endo-ECG
    endocoronary electrocardiography
ENDOR
    electron nuclear double resonance
endos
    endosteal
ENDRB
    endothelin-receptor-B
ENE
    ethylnorepinephrine
ENeG
    electroneurography
enem
    enema (*See also* E, en)
ENF
    Enfamil
ENFcFE
    Enfamil with iron
ENG
    electroneurography
    electronystagmogram
    electronystagmograph
    electronystagmography
    engorged
ENI
    elective neck irradiation
ENK
    enkephalin
1-ENK
    leucine-enkephalin
ENL
    easy normal left
    erythema nodosum leprosum
enl
    enlarged
    enlargement
ENL-DCR
    endonasal laser
      dacryocystorhinostomy

ENMG
electroneuromyography
ENNAS
Einstein Neonatal Neurobehavioral Assessment Scale
ENNS
Early Neonatal Neurobehavior Scale
Eno
enolase
eNO
exhaled nitric oxide
ENog
electroneurogram
electroneuronography
eNOS
endothelial nitric oxide synthase
ENP
extractable nucleoprotein
ENR
easy normal right
eosinophilic nonallergic rhinitis
extrathyroidal neck radioactivity
ENS
enteral nutritional support
enteral nutrition solution
enteric nervous system
ethylnorsuprarenin
exogenous natural surfactant
ENSV
Enseada virus
ENT
ears, nose, and throat
enzootic nasal tumor
extranodular tissue
ENTOM
entomology
ENTV
Entebbe bat virus
ENV
ethylnitrosourea
env
envelope (of cell)
ENVD
elevated new vessels on the disk
ENVE
elevated new vessels elsewhere
environ
environment
environmental
ENVT
environment

enz, enz.
enzymatic
enzyme
EO
effect of opening (eyes)
elbow orthosis
embolic occlusion
eosinophil (*See also* EOS, eos, eosin)
eosinophilia
ethylene oxide (*See also* ETOX)
eyes open
E&O
evaluation and observation
E_o
electric affinity (*See also* E, EA)
skin (epidermis) dose (radiation) (*See also* E, EA)
E_o+, E^o
oxidation-reduction potential (*See also* E_h, eH, ORP)
EOA
effective orifice area
erosive osteoarthritis
esophageal obturator airway
examination, opinion, and advice
external oblique aponeurosis
EOAE
evoked otoacoustic emission
EOB
edge of bed
emergency observation bed
explanation of benefits
EOC
electrooptical characteristic
Emergency Operations Center
enema of choice
epithelial ovarian cancer
EO CT
eosinophil count
EOD
electrical organ discharge
end of day
end organ damage
entry on duty
every other day
extent of disease
EOE
ethiodized oil emulsion
extraosseous Ewing sarcoma

E

NOTES

231

EOF
> end of field
> end of file

EOFAD
> early-onset form of familial
> Alzheimer disease

EOG
> electrooculogram
> electrooculograph
> electrooculography
> electroolfactogram
> electroolfactography
> eosinophilic gastroenteritis
> Ethrane, oxygen, and gas (nitrous
> oxide)

EOIT
> ego-oriented individual therapy

EOJ
> extrahepatic obstructive jaundice

EOL
> end of life

EOM
> end of message
> equal ocular movement
> error of measurement
> external otitis media
> extraocular motion
> extraocular movement
> extraocular muscle

EOMA
> emergency oxygen mask assembly

EOM F & Conj
> extraocular movements full and
> conjugate

EOMI
> extraocular movements intact
> extraocular muscles intact

EOM NL
> extraocular eye movements normal

EOO
> external oculomotor ophthalmoplegia

EOP
> emergency outpatient
> endogenous opioid peptide
> equivalent oxygen performance

EOP1
> end-of-phase 1

EOP2
> end-of-phase 2

EOR
> emergency operating room
> end of range
> exclusive OR (binary logic)

EORA
> elderly-onset rheumatoid arthritis

EOS
> early-onset schizophrenia
> eligibility on-site

> end of study
> eosinophil (*See also* EO, eos,
> eosin)
> Extra Oral System

eos, eosin
> eosinophil (*See also* EO, EOS)

EOSB
> end of saturated bombardment

EOT
> effective oxygen transport

EOU
> epidemic observation unit

EOWPVT
> Expressive One-Word Picture
> Vocabulary Test

EP
> ectopic pregnancy
> edible portion
> electrophoresis
> electrophoretic
> electrophysiologic
> electrophysiology
> electroprecipitin
> elopement precaution
> emergency physician
> emergency procedure
> endogenous pyrogen
> endoperoxide
> endorphin
> end point
> enteropeptidase
> environmental protection
> enzyme product
> eosinophilic pneumonia
> ependymal (cell)
> epicardial
> Episcopalian
> epithelial (*See also* EPITH)
> epithelium (*See also* EPITH)
> erythrocyte protoporphyrin
> erythrophagocytosis
> erythropoietic porphyria
> esophageal pressure
> esophoria
> evoked potential
> excretory phase
> extreme pressure

E&P
> estrogen and progesterone

EPA
> eicosapentaenoic acid
> erect posterior-anterior (projection)
> ethylphenacemide
> exophthalmos-producing activity
> extrinsic plasminogen activator

EPAB
> extracorporeal pneumoperititoneal
> access bubble

E-panel
  electrolyte panel
EPAP
  expiratory positive airway pressure
EPAQ
  Extended Personal Attributes
    Questionnaire
EPAS1
  endothelial PAS-domain protein-1
EPB
  Environmental Pre-Language Battery
  extensor pollicis brevis
EPBD
  endoscopic papillary balloon
    dilation
EPBF
  effective pulmonary blood flow
EPC
  electronic pain control
  end-plate current
  epilepsia partialis continua
  erosive prephloric changes
  extent of pleural carcinomatosis
    score
  external pneumatic calf compression
  external pneumatic compression
EPCA
  external pressure circulatory
    assistance
EPCG
  endoscopic pancreatocholangiography
EPCL
  Everyday Problem Checklist
EPD
  effective pressor dose
  electrode placement device
  endoscopic papillary balloon
    dilation
  enzyme potentiated desensitization
  equilibrium peritoneal dialysis
  extramammary Paget dise
EPDML
  epidemiologic
  epidemiology
EpDRF
  epithelium-derived relaxation factor
EPDS
  Edinburgh Postnatal Depression
    Scale
EPE
  erythropoietin-producing enzyme

  extraprostatic extension
  extrapyramidal effect
EPEA
  expense-per-equivalent admission
EPEC
  enteropathogenic *Escherichia coli*
EPEM
  Emory Pain Estimate Model
EPF
  early pregnancy factor
  endocarditis parietalis fibroplastica
  endoscopic plantar fasciotomy
  endothelial proliferating factor
  Enfamil premature formula
  eosinophilic pustular folliculitis
  exophthalmos-producing factor
  exposed protruding form
EPG
  eggs per gram
  electronic pupillography
  electropneumogram
  electropneumography
  Episodic Payment Group
  ethanolamine phosphoglyceride
EPH
  edema, proteinuria, hypertension
  episodic paroxysmal hemicrania
  extensor proprius hallucis
EpHM
  intraesophageal pH monitoring
EPI
  echo-planar imaging
  Emotions Profile Index
  epileptic (*See also* epil)
  epitheloid cell
  epitympanic
  evoked-potential index
  exercise pressure index
  exocrine pancreatic insufficiency
  extrapyramidal involvement
  extremely premature infant
  Eysenck Personality Inventory
epi
  epicardium
  epiglottis
  epinephrine (*See also* E, epineph)
EPIC
  evaluation, prediction, intervention,
    and control
EPID
  epidural

NOTES

E

233

epid
epidemic
epig
epigastric
epil
epilepsy
epileptic (*See also* EPI)
epineph
epinephrine (*See also* E, epi)
EPIS, epis
epileptic postictal sleep
episiotomy
episode
epistaxis
EPITH, epith
epithelial (*See also* EP)
epithelium (*See also* EP)
EPK
early prenatal karyotype
EPL
effective path length
effective patient life
essential phospholipid
extensor pollicis longus
external plexiform layer
extracorporeal piezoelectric
lithotripsy
EPM
electronic pacemaker
electron-probe microanalysis
electrophoretic mobility
energy-protein malnutrition
extraosseous plasmacytoma of the
mediastinum
EPMR
electronic patient medical record
EPN
emphysematous pyelonephritis
estimated protein needs
EPO
epoetin alfa
erythropoietin
evening primrose oil
exclusive provider organization
EPP
endplate potential
equal-pressure point
erythropoietic porphyria
erythropoietic protoporphyria
extrapleural pneumonectomy
extrapulmonary pneumocystosis
EPPB
end positive-pressure breathing
EPPER
eosinophilic, polymorphic, and
pruritic eruption associated with
radiotherapy

EPPS
Edwards Personal Preference
Schedule
EPQ
Eysenck Personality Questionnaire
EPR
early-phase reaction
early progressive resistance
electron paramagnetic resonance
electrophrenic respiration
emergency physical restraint
estimated protein requirement
estradiol production rate
evoked potential response
extraparenchymal resistance
EPROM
erasable programmable read-only
memory
EPS
early progressing stroke
ear, patella, short stature
(syndrome)
elastosis perforans serpiginosa
electrophysiologic study
endoscopic pancreatic
sphincterotomy
endoscopic pancreatic stenting
enzymatic pancreatic secretion
exhaustion syndrome
exophthalmos-producing substance
expressed prostatic secretions
extrapyramidal side effect (*See also*
EPSE)
extrapyramidal symptom
extrapyramidal syndrome
EPSA
early postoperative suture
adjustment
evoked potential signal averaging
EPSCCA
extrapulmonary small cell
carcinoma
EPSD
E-point to septal distance
EPSDT
Early and Periodic Screening,
Diagnosis, and Treatment
(program)
EPSE
extrapyramidal side effect (*See also*
EPS)
EPSEM
equal probability of selection
method
ε, epsilon
chain of hemoglobin
dielectric constant

ε
epsilon (fifth letter of Greek alphabet), lowercase
extinction coefficient
fifth in a series or group
heavy chain of immunoglobulin E
molar absorption coefficient
molar absorptivity
molar extinction coefficient
permittivity
specific absorptivity

EPSP
excitatory postsynaptic potential

EPSS
E-point to septal separation

EPT
early pregnancy test
Eidetic Parents Test
endoscopic papillotomy

EPTE
existed prior to enlistment

EPTFE, E-PTFE, e-PTFE
expanded polytetrafluoroethylene

EPTS
existed prior to service

EPWF
epidural pressure waveform

EPX
eosinophil protein X

EPXMA
electron probe x-ray microanalyzer

EQ
education quotient
encephalization quotient
energy quotient
equal to
equilibrium (See also eq)

Eq
equation (See also eqn)
equivalency (See also eq, equiv)
equivalent (See also eq, equiv)

eq
equal
equilibrium (See also EQ)
equival
equivalency (See also Eq, equiv)
equivalent (See also Eq)

EQA
external quality assessment

eqn
equation (See also Eq)

EQP
extensor quinti proprius

equip.
equipment

equiv
equivalency (See also Eq, eq)
equivalent (See also Eq, eq)
equivocal

ER
early repolarization
early reticulocyte
efficacy ratio
ejection rate
electroresection
emergency room
endoplasmic reticulum
end range
enhanced reactivation
enhancement ratio
environmental resistance
epigastric region
equine rhinopneumonia
equivalent roentgen (unit)
erythrocyte receptor
esophageal rupture
estradiol receptor
estrogen receptor
evoked response
expiratory reserve
extended external rotation
extended release (tablet)
extended resistance
external reduction
external resistance
external rotation
extraction ratio
eye research

ERα, ER alpha
estrogen receptor alpha

ERβ, ER beta
estrogen receptor beta (See also ER beta)

ER−
decreased estrogen receptor
estrogen receptor-negative

ER+
estrogen receptor-positive
increased estrogen receptor

E&R
equal and reactive
examination and report

Er
erbium

NOTES

235

ERA
    echo record access
    electrical response activity
    electric response audiometry
    endometrial resection and ablation
    estradiol receptor assay
    estrogen receptor assay
    evoked-response audiometry

%ERAD
    eradication rates

ERAS
    Electronic Residency Application
    Service

ERB
    ethnic relational behavior

ERBAC
    excimer laser, rotational
    atherectomy, and balloon
    angioplasty

ERBD
    endoscopic retrograde biliary
    drainage

ERBF
    effective renal blood flow

ERC
    endoscopic retrograde cholangiogram
    endoscopic retrograde
    cholangiography
    enterocytopathogenic human orphan-
    rhinocoryza (virus)
    erythropoietin-responsive cell
    (pupils) equal, reactive, and
    contracting

ERCCE
    endoscopic retrograde
    cholecystoendoprosthesis

ERCP
    endoscopic retrograde
    cholangiopancreatogram
    endoscopic retrograde
    cholangiopancreatography

ERCT
    emergency room computerized
    tomography

ERD
    early retirement with disability
    event-related desynchronization
    evoked-response detector

ERE
    estrogen-response element
    external rotation in extension

ERF
    edge response function
    esophagorespiratory fistula
    external rotation in flexion

erf
    error function

ERFC, E-RFC
    erythrocyte rosette-forming cell

ERG
    electrolyte replacement with glucose
    electron radiography
    electroretinogram
    electroretinograph
    electroretinography

erg
    energy unit

ERH
    egg-laying release hormone

ERHD
    exposure-related hypothermia death

ERI
    elective replacement indicator
    Employee Reliability Inventory
    Environmental Response Inventory
    erythrocyte rosette inhibitor

ERIA
    electroradioimmunoassay

ER by ICA (*See also* ERβ)
    estrogen receptor
    immunocytochemistry assay

ER/IR
    external rotation/internal rotation

ERISA
    Employee Retirement Income
    Security Act

ERK
    extracellular regulated kinase

ERL
    effective refractory length

ERLND
    elective regional lymph node
    dissection

ERM
    electrochemical relaxation method
    epiretinal membrane
    extended radical mastectomy

ERMBT
    erythromycin breath test

ERMS
    embryonal rhabdomyosarcoma
    exacerbating-remitting multiple
    sclerosis

ERNA
    equilibrium radionuclide angiography

ERO
    effective regurgitant orifice

ERP
    early receptor potential
    effective refractory period
    emergency room physician
    endocardial resection procedure
    endoscopic retrograde pancreatogram
    endoscopic retrograde
    pancreatography

endoscopic retrograde
parenchymography
equine rhinopneumonitis
estrogen-receptor protein
event-related (brain) potential

ERPC

evacuation of retained products of
conception

ERP-CT

computed tomography under
endoscopic retrograde
pancreatography

ERPF

effective renal plasma flow

ERPLV

effective refractory period of the
left ventricle

ERPM

early receptor potential mottling

ERPP

endoscopic retrograde
parenchymography of pancreas

ER/PR

estrogen receptor/progesterone
receptor

ERR, err.

error

ERRT

extrarenal rhabdoid tumor

ERS

endoscopic retrograde
sphincterotomy
evacuation of retained secundines
(afterbirth)
extended, rotated, sidebent

ERSL

extended, rotated, sidebent left

ERSNA

efferent renal sympathetic nerve
activity

ERSP

event-related slow-brain potential

ERSR

Electronic Regulatory Submission
and Review
extended, rotated, sidebent right

ERSS

Edinburgh Rehabilitation Status
Scale

ERT

emergency response to terrorism
esophageal radionuclide transit

estrogen replacement therapy
external radiation therapy
pancreatic enzyme replacement
therapy

ERTD

ElectroRegenesis therapy device
emergency room triage
documentation

ERUS

endorectal ultrasound

ERV

equine rhinopneumonitis virus
Estero Real virus
expiratory reserve volume

e-RX

electronic prescription

ERY

erysipelas
erythrocyte (*See also* E, eryth)

Er:YAG

erbium:yttrium-aluminum-garnet
(laser)

ERYTH

erythromycin

eryth

erythema
erythrocyte (*See also* E, ERY)

erythro-AZT

3'-alpha-azido-2',3'-dideoxythymidine

ES

Ego Strength (test)
ejection sound
elastic suspensor
electrical stimulation
electrophilic stress
electroshock
electrospray
electrotherapy system
Elejalde syndrome
Eleutherococcus senticosus (Siberian
Ginseng)
elopement status (psychology)
embryonic stem (cells)
emergency service
emission spectrometry
endometritis-salpingitis
endoscopic sclerosis
endoscopic sclerotherapy
endoscopic sphincterotomy
end stage
end systole

E

NOTES

237

ES *(continued)*
  end-to-side (anastomosis) (*See also* E-S, ETS)
  environmental stimulation
  enzyme substrate
  epileptic syndrome
  epithelioid sarcoma
  esophageal scintigraphy
  esophagus (*See also* E, ESO, eso, esoph)
  esophoria
  esterase (*See also* EST)
  Ewing sarcoma
  excretory-secretory
  exfoliation syndrome
  Expectation Score
  experimental study
  ex-smoker
  exterior surface
  extracapsular spread
  extra strength
  extrasystole

E-S
  end-to-side (anastomosis) (*See also* ES, ETS)

Es
  einsteinium

²⁵⁵Es
  einsteinium-255

ESA
  Early School Assessment
  early systolic acceleration
  end-to-side anastomosis
  epididymal sperm aspiration
  ethmoid sinus adenocarcinoma

ESADDI
  estimated safe and adequate daily dietary intake

ESAF
  endothelial cell-stimulating angiogenesis factor

ESAP
  evoked sensory (nerve) action potential

ESAS
  Edmonton Symptom Assessment Scale

ESAT
  extrasystolic atrial tachycardia

ESB
  Effective School Battery
  electric stimulation of the brain

ESBL
  extended-spectrum beta-lactamase

ESBLPE
  extended-spectrum beta-lactamase-producing Enterobacteriaceae

ES/BS
  erosion surface per bone surface

ESC
  electromechanical slope computer
  end-systolic count
  erythropoietin-sensitive stem cell

ESCA
  electron spectroscopy for chemical analysis

ESCC
  electrolyte steroid cardiopathy by calcification
  epidural spinal cord compression
  esophageal squamous cell carcinoma

ESCH
  electrolyte steroid-produced cardiopathy (characterized by) hyalinization

Esch.
  Escherichia (*See also* E)

ESCN
  electrolyte and steroid cardiopathy with necrosis

ESCS
  Early Social Communication Scale
  electrical spinal cord stimulation

ESD
  electronic summation device
  electron-stimulated desorption
  emergency services department
  emission spectrometric detector
  end-systolic diameter
  end-systolic dimension
  environmental sex determination
  esophagus, stomach, and duodenum
  esterase D
  exoskeletal device

ESE
  electrostatic unit [Ger. *electrostatische Einheit*]

ESEP
  elbow sensory potential
  extreme somatosensory evoked potential

ESF
  electrosurgical filter
  erythropoiesis-stimulating factor
  erythropoietic-stimulating factor
  external skeletal fixation

ES-FISH
  extra ABL signal fluorescent in situ hybridization

ESFL
  end-systolic force-length (relationship)

ESFT
  Ewing sarcoma family of tumors

ESG
electrospinogram
estrogen
exfoliation syndrome glaucoma

ESI
Ego State Inventory
Electro-Surgical Instrument
enamel surface index
enzyme substrate inhibitor
epidural steroid injection
extent of skin involvement

ESIMS
electrospray ionization mass
spectrometry

ES-IMV
expiration-synchronized intermittent
mandatory ventilation

ESIN
elastic stable intramedullary nailing

ESL
end-systolic (segment) length
English as a second language
extracorporeal shockwave lithotripsy

ESLD
end-stage liver disease
end-stage lung disease

ESLF
end-stage liver failure

ESM
ejection systolic murmur
endolymphatic stromal myosis
endothelial specular microscope
ethosuximide

ESN
educationally subnormal
estrogen-stimulated neurophysin

ESN(M)
educationally subnormal-moderate

ESN(S)
educationally subnormal-severe

ESO, eso
electrospinal orthosis
esophagoscopy (*See also* esoph)
esophagus (*See also* E, ES, eso,
esoph)

ESO/D
esotropia at distance

ESO/N
estropia at near

esoph
esophagoscopy (*See also* ESO)
esophagus (*See also* E, ES, ESO)

esoph steth
esophageal stethoscope

ESP
Early Speech Perception Test
early systolic paradox
effective sensory projection
effective systolic pressure
electrosensitive point
electrosurgical pencil
endometritis-salpingitis-peritonitis
end-systolic pressure
eosinophil stimulation promoter
epidermal soluble protein
especially (*See also* esp)
evoked synaptic potential
extended supraplatysmal plane
extramedullary solitary
plasmacytoma
extrasensory perception

esp
especially (*See also* ESP)

ESPA
electrical stimulation-produced
analgesia

ESPI
electronic speckle pattern
interferometry

ESPLR
end-systolic pressure-length
relationship

ES/PNET
Ewing sarcoma/peripheral
neuroectodermal tumor

ESPQ
Early School Personality
Questionnaire

ESR
electric skin resistance
electron spin resonance
erythrocyte sedimentation rate

ESRD
end-stage renal disease

ESRF
end-stage renal failure

ESRRL
extension, sidebent right, rotated
left

ESRS
extrapyramidal symptom rating
scale

ESS
emotional, spiritual, and social

NOTES

ESS (*continued*)
  empty sella (turcica) syndrome
  endometrial stromal sarcoma
  endoscopic sinus surgery
  endostreptosin
  end-systolic stress
  ENtec surgery system
  Epworth Sleepiness Scale
  Epworth Sleepiness Score
  erythrocyte-sensitizing substance
  European Stroke Scale
  euthyroid sick syndrome
  excited skin syndrome

ess
  essence
  essential

ESSF
  external spinal skeletal fixator

ess neg
  essentially negative

EST
  Eastern Standard Time
  electric shock therapy
  electric shock treatment
  electroshock therapy
  electroshock treatment
  electrostimulation therapy
  endodermal sinus tumor
  endoscopic sphincterotomy
  Erhard Seminar Training
  established patient
  esterase (*See also* ES)
  exercise stress test
  expression sequence tagged

E$_{st}$
  static elastance

est
  ester (*See also* E)
  estimated
  estimation

esth
  esthetic

E-stim
  electrical stimulation

estn
  epithelioid soft-tissue neoplasm

ESU, esu
  electrostatic unit
  electrosurgical unit

E-sub
  excitor substance

ESV
  end-systolic (ventricular) volume
  end-systolic volume
  esophageal valve

ESVI
  end-systolic volume index

ESVS
  epiurethral suprapubic vaginal
    suspension

ESWI
  end-systolic wall index

ESWL
  electrohydraulic shock wave
    lithotripsy
  extracorporeal shock wave
    lithotripsy

ESWS
  end-systolic wall stress

ESWT
  end-systolic wall thickness
  extracorporeal shock wave therapy

ESY
  expressed sequence tag

ET
  Ebbinghaus test
  edge thickness
  educational therapy
  effective temperature
  ejection time
  electroneurodiagnostic technologist
  embryo transfer
  endometrial thickness
  endothelin
  endotoxin
  endotracheal (*See also* ENDO)
  endotracheal tube (*See also* ETT)
  end-tidal
  endurance time
  enterostomal therapist
  enterostomal therapy
  epithelial tumor
  esotropia
  esotropic
  essential thrombocythemia
  essential tremor
  ethanol (*See also* E, ETH, EtOH)
  ethyl (*See also* E, Et)
  etiocholanolone test
  etiology (*See also* et [L.], etio,
    etiol)
  eustachian tube
  Ewing tumor
  exchange transfusion
  exercise test
  exercise treadmill
  expiration time
  extracellular tachyzoite

ET′, ET−, ET$_1$
  esotropia at near
  esotropia for near
  near esotropia

E/T
  effector to target ratio

E(T)
    intermittent esotropia
ET@20'
    esotropia at 6 meters (infinity)
E(T')
    intermittent esotropia at near
ET$_3$
    erythrocyte triiodothyronine
ET$_4$
    effective thyroxine (test)
Et
    ethyl (*See also* E, ET)
η, eta
    absolute viscosity
    eta (seventh letter of Greek
      alphabet), lowercase
ETA
    eicosatetraenoic acid
    electron-transfer agent
    endotracheal aspirate
    estimated time of arrival
    ethionamide
EtA
    endothelin A
ETAB
    extrathoracic-assisted breathing
ETAC
    electrothermally assisted
      capsulorrhaphy
et al.
    and others [L. *et alii*]
EtB
    endothelin B
ETBD
    etiology to be determined
E$_2$TBG
    estradiol-testosterone-binding globulin
ETC
    emergency and trauma center
    endoscopic tissue culture
    esophagotracheal combination tube
    esophagotracheal Combitube
    estimated time of conception
ETc
    corrected ejection time
etc.
    and so forth [L. *et cetera*]
ETCD
    endoscopic transpapillary cyst
     drainage
    external tachyarrhythmia control
     device

ETCG
    endoscopic transpapillary
     catheterization of gallbladder
ETCL
    enteropathy-associated T-cell
     lymphoma
ETCO$_2$
    end-tidal carbon dioxide
     (concentration)
ETD
    endoscopic transformational
     diskectomy
    eustachian tube dysfunction
    eye-tracking dysfunction
ETDLA
    esophageal-tracheal double lumen
     airway
ETE
    end-to-end (anastomosis)
ETEC
    enterotoxigenic *Escherichia coli*
E-test
    epsilometer test
ET-1–ET-3
    endothelin-1–endothelin-3
ETF
    electron transfer flavoprotein
    eustachian tube function
    extension teardrop fracture
ETF-DH
    electron transfer flavoprotein
     dehydrogenase
ETFE
    ethylene tetrafluor ethylene
ETFVL
    exercise tidal flow-volume loop
ETG
    episodic treatment group
ETH
    elixir terpin hydrate
    ethanol (*See also* E, ET, EtOH)
    ethionamide
    ethmoid
    Ethrane (enflurane)
eth
    ether (*See also* Et$_2$O)
ETHC, ETH/C
    elixir terpin hydrate with codeine
ETI
    ejective time index
    endotracheal intubation

E

NOTES

ETIO
  etiocholanolone
etio, etiol
  etiology (*See also* ET, et [L.])
ETK
  erythrocyte transketolase
ETKTM
  every test known to mankind
ETL
  echo-train length
  expiratory threshold load
et [L.]
  and
  etiology (*See also* ET, etio, etiol)
ETLE
  extratemporal lobe epilepsy
ETM
  erythromycin (*See also* E, EM)
ETN
  ethanol-induced tumor necrosis
Et₃N
  triethylamine
ET-NANBH
  enterically transmitted non-A, non-B
    hepatitis
ETO
  estimated time of ovulation
  ethylene oxide (gas)
  eustachian tube obstruction
EtO
  ethylene oxide
Et₂O
  ether (*See also* eth)
E-TOF
  electron time-of-flight
EtOH
  ethyl alcohol (consumption,
    dependency)
ETOP
  elective termination of pregnancy
    (*See also* ETP)
ETOX
  ethylene oxide (*See also* EO)
ETP
  elective termination of pregnancy
    (*See also* ETOP)
  electron transport particle
  entire treatment period
  ephedrine, theophylline, and
    phenobarbital
  eustachian tube pressure
ETPS
  electrotherapeutic point stimulation
ETR
  effective thyroxine ratio
  epitympanic recess
  estimated thyroid ratio

ETS
  educational testing service
  electrical transcranial stimulation
  electrosleep therapy
  elevated toilet seat
  endoscopic transthoracic
    symphathectomy
  endotracheal suction
  end-to-side (anastomosis) (*See also*
    ES, E-S)
  environmental tobacco smoke
  erythromycin topical solution
ETT
  endotracheal tube (*See also* ET)
  epinephrine tolerance test
  esophageal transit time
  exercise tolerance test
  exercise treadmill test
  extrathyroidal thyroxine
ETTH
  episodic tension-type headache
ETTN
  ethyltrimethyloltrimethane trinitrate
ETT-TI
  exercise treadmill test with
    thallium
ETU
  emergency and trauma unit
  emergency treatment unit
ETV
  educational television
  extravascular thermal volume
ETX
  edatrexate
  ethosuximide
ETYA
  eicosatetroenoic acid
EU
  Ehrlich unit
  emergency unit
  endotoxin unit
  entropy unit
  enzyme unit
  equivalent unit
  esophageal ulcer
  esterase unit
  etiology unknown
  excretory urography (*See also* EXU)
  expected utility
Eu
  europium
  euryon
EUA
  examination under anesthesia
EUAL
  external ultrasound-assisted
    lipoplasty

EUBV
Eubenangee virus
EUCD
emotionally unstable character disorder
EUD
external urinary device
EUG
extrauterine gestation
EUL
expected upper limit
extra uterine life
EUM
external urethral meatus
EUP
extrauterine pregnancy
EUS
echoendoscopy
endorectal ultrasonography
endoscopic ultrasonography
endoscopic ultrasound
external urethral sphincter
EUs
esophageal ultrasound
EUS-FNA
endoscopic ultrasound-guided fine-needle aspiration
eust
eustachian
EUV
extreme ultraviolet (laser)
EV
emergency vehicle
enterovirus
epidermodysplasia verruciformis
esophageal varices
estradiol valerate
eversion (*See also* ever.)
evoked (response)
excessive ventilation
expected value
extravascular
EV71
enterovirus-71
eV
electron volt
EVA
American eel virus
enlarged vestibular aqueduct syndrome
Entry and Validation Application

ethylene vinyl acetate
ethyl violet azide (broth)
EVAC, evac
evacuate
evacuated
evacuation
EVAc
ethylene-vinyl acetate copolymer
eval
evaluate
evaluated
evaluation
EVAN
ergonomic vascular access needle
evap
evaporated
evaporation
EVB
esophageal variceal bleeding
EVC
Ellis-van Creveld (syndrome) (*See also* EC)
EVCI
expected value of clinical information
EVD
external ventricular drainage
extravascular (lung) density
eve
evening
ever.
eversion (*See also* EV)
everted
EVEV
Everglades virus
EVF
ethanol volume fraction
EVG
electroventriculogram
electroventriculography
electrovomerogram
endovascular grafting
EVH
esophageal variceal hemorrhage
EVI
endocardium, vascular (structures), interstitium (of striated muscle)
EVL
endoscopic variceal ligation
EVLW
extravascular lung water

E

NOTES

EVM
electronic voltmeter
extravascular mass
eye, motor, voice

evol
evolution

EVP
episcleral venous pressure
evoked visual potential

EVR
endocardial viability ratio
endovascular repair
evoked visual response

EVRS
early ventricular repolarization
syndrome

EVS
endoscopic variceal sclerosis
endoscopic variceal sclerotherapy
esophageal variceal sclerotherapy

EVSD
Eisenmenger ventricular septal
defect

EVTV
extravascular thermal volume

EVUS
endovaginal ultrasound

EW
Edinger-Westphal (nucleus)
emergency ward
expiratory wheeze

ew
elsewhere

EWB
emotional well-being
estrogen withdrawal bleeding

EWBH
extracorporeal whole body
hyperthermia

EWCL
extended-wear contact lens

EWE
Eastern and Western
encephalomyelitis vaccine

EWHO
elbow-wrist-hand orthosis

EWI
Experiential World Inventory

EWL
egg-white lysozyme
estimated weight loss
evaporation water loss

EWSCL
extended-wear soft contact lens

EWS-PNET
Ewing sarcoma-primitive
neuroectodermal tumor

EWT
erupted wisdom teeth
esophageal wall thickness

EX, ex
exacerbation
exaggerated (*See also* exag)
examination (*See also* exam)
examined
example
excision (*See also* exc)
exercise (*See also* E, exer)
exophthalmos
exposure
external movement
extraction (*See also* EXT)
extra point

E(X)
expected value of the random
variable X

EXAFS
extended x-ray absorption fine
structure (spectroscopy)

exag
exaggerated (*See also* EX)

exam
examination (*See also* EX)
examine
examined (*See also* EX)

Ex-B
extra point on the back of the
trunk (acupuncture)

EXBF
exercise hyperemia blood flow

exc
except
excision (*See also* EX)

Ex-CA
extra point on the chest and
abdomen (acupuncture)

EXD
ethylxanthic disulfide

EXEC 22
executive 22 chemistry profile

exec
executive

Ex-ECG
exercise stress electrocardiography

Ex-Echo
exercise stress echocardiography

ExEF
ejection fraction during exercise

EXELFS
extended electron-loss line fine
structure

exer
exercise (*See also* E, EX)

EXGBUS
  external genitalia, Bartholin, urethral, and Skene (glands) (*See also* EGBUS)
Ex-HN
  extra point on the head and neck (acupuncture)
EXH VT
  exhaled tidal volume
exist.
  existing
EXIT
  ex utero intrapartum tracheloplasty
  ex utero intrapartum treatment
EXL
  elixir
ex lap
  exploratory laparotomy
Ex-LE
  extra point on the lower extremity (acupuncture)
EXO
  exonuclease
  exophoria
EXOPH
  exophthalmos
EXP
  experienced
  exploration
  expose
exp
  expected
  expectorant (*See also* expec)
  experiment(al) (*See also* E, exper, exptl)
  expiration (*See also* expir)
  expiratory (*See also* expir)
  expire (*See also* expir)
  expired (*See also* expir)
  exploration
  exploratory
  exponent
  exponential (function)
  exposed
  exposure
expec, expect.
  expectorant (*See also* exp)
exper
  experiment(al) (*See also* E, exptl)
ExPGN
  extracapillary proliferative glomerulonephritis

expir
  expiration (*See also* exp)
  expiratory (*See also* exp)
  expired (*See also* exp)
expn
  expression
exptl
  experimental (*See also* E, exp, exper)
EXREM
  external radiation-emission-man (radiation dose)
EXS
  externally supported
  extrinsically supported
EXT, ext
  exchange transfusion
  extension (*See also* E)
  external
  extract (*See also* EX)
  extraction (*See also* EX)
  extremity (*See also* extr)
ext aud
  external auditory
extd
  extended
  extracted
EXT-DCR
  external dacryocystorhinostomy
ext fd
  fluid extract
ext FHR
  external fetal heart rate (monitoring)
ext mon
  external monitor
extr
  extremity (*See also* EXT)
extrap
  extrapolate
  extrapolation
extrav
  extravasation
ext rot
  external rotation
EXTUB
  extubation
EXU
  excretory urogram
  excretory urography (*See also* EU)

E

NOTES

Ex-UE
extra point on the upper extremity (acupuncture)

EY
egg yolk
epidemiology year

EYA
egg yolk agar

EYAV
Eyach virus

EYCAT
egg yolk-cobalamin absorption test

EYES
Early Years Easy Screen

EZ
Edmonston-Zagreb (vaccine)

Ez
eczema

EZ-HT
Edmonston-Zagreb high-titer (vaccine)

F

bioavailability
brother [L. *frater*]
conjugative plasmid in F+ bacterial cells
cortisol
degree of fineness of abrasive particles
facial
facies
factor (*See also* Fac)
Fahrenheit
failure
fair
false
family (*See also* fam)
farad (*See also* f, far.)
Faraday (constant)
fascia
fasting (test)
fat (dietary)
father (*See also* FR)
fecal
feces
Fellow
female (*See also* fe, FEM, fem)
fermentative
fermi (energy)
fertility (factor)
fetal
fibroblast
fibrous (protein)
Ficol
field of vision
filament (*See also* fil)
filial generation
fine
finger
firm
fissure
flexed
flexion (*See also* f)
flow (of blood)
fluid (*See also* f, Fl, fl, FLD, fld)
fluoride
fluorine
flutter wave
focal length
focus
foil
fontanelle
foot (*See also* f, ft)
foramen
force
form (*See also* f)

forma (*See also* f)
form response
formula
formulary
fossa
fractional (composition of gas in gas phase)
fragment of antibody
free
free energy
French
frequency (*See also* f, freq)
frontal
frontal electrode placement in electroencephalography
full (diet)
function (*See also* fn, FXN)
fundi (plural)
fundus
fusion beat
gilbert (unit of magnetomotive force)
Helmholtz free energy
hydrocortisone (compound F)
inbreeding coefficient
(luminous) flux
make (*See also* f)
phenylalanine (*See also* Phe)
son [L. *filius*]
variance ratio
vectorcardiography electrode (left foot)
visual field (*See also* VF, Vf, VFD)

F0, F₀

fundamental frequency

F1.2

prothrombin fragment 1.2

F₁

first filial generation

F₃

TFT—trifluorothymidine

F344

Fischer 344 (rat)

F7

factor VII

F8

factor VIII

14F

14-hour fast required

F-18

fluorine-18

F′

hybrid F plasmid
secondary focal point (of lens)

F

247

°F
degree Fahrenheit

FI–FXIII
factor I through XIII (blood)

F₂
second filial generation

/F
full lower denture (*See also* FLD)

F/
full upper denture (*See also* FUD)

F+
good form response

(F)
final

F⁺
bacterial cell with an F plasmid
good form response

F⁻
bacterial cell lacking an F plasmid
fluoride
poor form response

f
atomic orbital with angular
  momentum quantum number 3
farad (*See also* F, far.)
femto-
fingerbreadth (*See also* FB, fb)
fission
flexion (*See also* F)
fluid (*See also* F, Fl, fl, FLD, fld)
focal
following (*See also* ff)
foot (*See also* F, ft)
form (*See also* F)
forma (*See also* F)
formyl
fostered (experimental animal)
frequency (*See also* F, freq)
frequently
fugacity
make (*See also* f)
respiratory frequency

f.
let it be made [L. *fiat*]

FIX
factor IX (nine)

FXI
Factor XI

F XIIIa
factor XIIIa

F=
firm and equal

FA
failure analysis
false aneurysm
Fanconi anemia
far advanced
fatty acid
febrile antigen
femoral anteversion
femoral artery
fertilization antigen
fetal age
fetus active
fibrinolytic activity
fibroadenoma
fibrosing alveolitis
field ambulance
filterable agent
filterable air
filtered air
first aid
fluorescein angiography
fluorescent antibody
fluorescent antibody (stain)
fluorescent assay
fluoroalanine
folic acid
follicular area
foramen
forearm
fortified aqueous (solution)
free acid
Freund adjuvant
Friedreich ataxia
functional activities
fusaric acid
fusidic acid

FA-1
fertilization antigen-1

F/A
fetus active

fa
fatty (rat)

FAA
febrile antigen agglutination
flavone acetic acid
folic acid antagonist
formaldehyde, acetic acid, and
  alcohol (solution)

FAAD
fetal activity acceleration
  determination

FAAH
fatty acid amide hydrolase

FAAP
family assessment adjustment pass

FAASOL
formalin, acetic, and alcohol
  solution

FAB
digoxin immune Fab
fast atom bombardment
formalin ammonium bromide

fragment (of immunoglobulin G involved in) antigen binding (*See also* Fab)

French-American-British (leukemia classification system)

functional arm brace

Fab

fragment antigen binding

fragment (of immunoglobulin G involved in) antigen binding (*See also* FAB)

F(ab′)₂

fragment (of immunoglobulin G) after digestion with the enzyme pepsin

FABER, faber

flexion, abduction, external rotation

FABERE, fabere

flexion, abduction, external rotation, extension

FABF

femoral artery blood flow

FAB L1

acute lymphoblastic leukemia in children

FAB L2

acute lymphoblastic leukemia in older children

FAB L3

acute lymphoblastic leukemia secondary to Burkitt lymphoma

FAB M1

acute myelogenous leuke

FAB M3

acute promyelocytic leukemia (*See also* APL, AProL)

FAB M4

acute myelomonocytic leukemia

FAB M5

acute monocytic leukemia

FAB M6

erythroleukemia

FAB/MS

fast atom bombardment mass spectrometry

FABP

fatty acid-binding protein

finger arterial blood pressure

folic acid-binding protein

FABP2

fatty acid-binding protein 2

FABP_{pm}

plasma membrane fatty acid binding protein

FABQ

Fear Avoidance Beliefs Quest

FAC

femoral arterial cannulation

ferric ammonium citrate

fetal abdominal circumference

fractional area change

fractional area concentration

free available chlorine

functional aerobic capacity

Functional Ambulation Categories

Fac

factor (*See also* F)

Facb

fragment, antigen, and complement binding

FACE

fluorophore-assisted carbohydrate electrophoresis

FACES

Family Adaptability and Cohesion Evaluation Scale

(unique) facies, anorexia, cachexia, and eye and skin (syndrome)

FACES-III, FACES III

Family Adaptability and Cohesion Scale-III

FACH

forceps to aftercoming head

FACO₂

fraction of alveolar carbon dioxide

FACS

Facial Action Coding System

fluorescence-activated cell sorter (*See also* FACScan)

fluorescence-activated cell sorting

fluorescent-activated cell sorting

FACScan

fluorescence-activated cell sorter

fluorescence-activated cell sorter scan (*See also* FACS)

FACT

Flanagan Aptitude Classification Test

focused appendix computed tomography

Functional Acuity Contrast Test

Functional Assessment of Cancer Therapy

F

NOTES

FACT-22
Focus Angioplasty Catheter Technology
FACT-B
Functional Assessment of Cancer Therapy-Breast
FACT-F
Functional Assessment of Cancer Therapy-Fatigue
FACT-G
Functional Assessment of Cancer Therapy-General
FACT-HN
Functional Assessment of Cancer Therapy–Head and Neck
F-actin
filamentous actin
FACT-L
Functional Assessment of Cancer Therapy-Lung
FACT-P
Functional Assessment of Cancer Therapy-Prostate
FACWA
familial amyotrophic chorea with acanthocytosis
FAD
familial Alzheimer dementia
familial Alzheimer disease
familial autoimmunity in diabetes
familial autonomic dysfunction
Family Assessment Device
fetal abdominal diameter
fetal activity-acceleration determination
flavin adenine dinucleotide (*See also* FADN)
FADD
Fas-associating protein with death domain
FADF
fluorescent antibody dark-field
FADH$_2$
flavin adenine dinucleotide (reduced form)
FADIR, fadir
flexion, adduction, internal rotation
FADIRE, fadire
flexion, adduction, internal rotation, and extension
FADN
flavin adenine dinucleotide (*See also* FAD)
FADS
fetal akinesia deformation sequence
FADU
fluorometric analysis of DNA unwinding

FAE
fetal alcohol effect
Fogarty arterial embolectomy
FAF
fatty acid free
fibroblast-activating factor
FAG
fundic atrophic gastritis
FAGA
full-term appropriate for gestational age
FAH
fumarylacetoacetase hydrolase
fumarylacetoacetate hydrolase
FAHI
functional assessment of human immunodeficiency
FAI
first aid instruction
functional aerobic impairment
functional assessment inventory
FAIDS
feline AIDS
FAJ
fused apophyseal joints
FAK
focal adhesion kinase
FAL
femoral arterial line
functional and anatomic loading
FALG
fowl antimouse lymphocyte globulin
FALL
fallopian
FALP
fluoroscopic-assisted lumbar puncture
FALS
familial amyotrophic lateral sclerosis
FAM
full allosteric modulators
functional assessment measure
Fam, fam
familial
family (*See also* F)
FAMA
fluorescence antimembrane antibody
fluorescent antibody to membrane antigen (test)
fluorescent antimembrane antibody (test)
fam doc
family doctor (*See also* FD, FMD)
FAME
fast acquisition multiple excitation
fatty acid methyl ester
finger-assisted malar elevation

fam hist
  family history (*See also* FH, FH$_x$)
FAM-M
  familial atypical mole and
    melanoma
FAMM
  facial artery musculomucosal
  facial artery myomucosal
  familial atypical multiple melanoma
FAMMM
  familial atypical mole malignant
    melanoma
  familial atypical multiple-mole
    melanoma (syndrome)
fam per par
  familial periodic paralysis
fam phys
  family physician (*See also* FP)
FAN
  finger tension
  fuchsin, amido black, and naphthol
    yellow
FANA
  fluorescent antinuclear antibody
    (assay)
FANCAP
  fluids, aeration, nutrition,
    communication, activity, and pain
    (nursing)
FANCAS
  fluids, aeration, nutrition,
    communication, activity, and
    stimulation (nursing)
FANG
  fluorescent angiography
FANPT
  Freeman Anxiety Neurosis and
    Psychosomatic Test
FANSS&M
  fundus anterior, normal size and
    shape, and mobile
FAO
  fatty acid oxidation
FAP
  familial adenomatous polyposis
  familial amyloidotic polyneuropathy
  familial amyloid polyneuropathy
  fatty acid poor
  fatty acids polyunsaturated
  femoral artery pressure
  fibrillating action potential

  fixed action pattern
  frozen animal procedure
fap-1
  fas-associated phosphatase-1
FAPD
  fibrosing alopecia in a pattern
    distribution
FAQ
  Family Attitudes Questionnaire
  frequently asked question(s)
FAR
  flight aptitude rating
  fractional albuminuria rate
F^{AR}
  immediate good function followed
    by accelerated rejection
far.
  farad (*See also* F, f)
  faradic
FARI
  filtered atrial rate interval
FARS
  Fatal Accident Reporting System
FARV
  Farallon virus
FAS
  fatty acid synthetase
  femoral access stabilization
  fetal alcohol syndrome
  fluorescent actin staining
FASC
  free-standing ambulatory surgical
    center
fasc
  fasciculation
  fasciculus
  fasicle
FASE
  fast asymmetric spin echo
FASF
  Factor Analyzed Short Form
FASIAR
  follicle aspiration, sperm injection,
    and assisted rupture
FasL, Fas-L
  Fas ligand
FASPS
  familial advanced sleep-phase
    syndrome
FASS
  foot and ankle severity scale

F

NOTES

FAST
Fein Articulation Screening Test
fetal acoustic stimulation testing
Filtered Audiometer Speech Test
flow-assisted short-term (balloon catheter)
Flowers Auditory Screening Test
fluorescent allergosorbent test
fluorescent antibody staining technique
fluoroallergosorbent test
focused assessment by sonography for trauma
Fourier-acquired steady-state technique
Frenchay Aphasia Screening Test
Functional Assessment Staging

FAT
Family Apperception Test
family attitudes test
fast axoplasmic transport
fatty acid translocase
female athlete triad
Fetal Activity Test
fluorescent antibody technique
fluorescent antibody test
food awareness training
function, appearance, time

FATG
fat globules

FATP
fatty acid transport protein

F₁ATPase
F_1 adenosine triphosphatase

FATS
fast adiabatic trajectory in steady state

FATSA
Flowers Auditory Test of Selective Attention

FATWO
female adnexal tumor of probable wolffian origin

FAV
facioauriculovertebral
feline ataxia virus
floppy aortic valve
fowl adenovirus

FAVS
facioauriculovertebral spectrum

FAZ
foveal avascular zone

FB
factor B
fasting blood (sugar) (*See also* FBS)
feedback
fiberoptic bronchoscopy (*See also* fib. bronc, FOB)
fingerbreadth (*See also* f, fb)
flexible bronchoscope
foreign body
Fusobacterium

F/B
followed by
forward/backward
forward bending

fb
fingerbreadth (*See also* f, FB)

f-b
face-bow

FBA
fecal bile acid

FBC
full blood count
functional bactericidal concentration

FBCOD
foreign body of the cornea, oculus dexter (right eye)

FBCOS
foreign body of the cornea, oculus sinister (left eye)

FBCP
familial benign chronic pemphigus

FBD
familial British dementia
fibrocystic breast disease
functional bowel disease
functional bowel disorder
functional bowel distress

FbDP
fibrin degradation product (*See also* FDP, fdp)

FBDSI
Functional Bowel Disorder Severity Index

FBE
full blood examination

FBEC
fetal bovine endothelial cell

FBEP
Fort Bragg evaluation project

FBF
forearm blood flow

FBG
fasting blood glucose
fibrinogen (*See also* fbg, FG, FGN, FI, FIB, fib.)
foreign body-type granuloma

fbg
fibrinogen (*See also* FBG, FG, FGN, FI, FIB, fib.)

FBH
familial benign hypercalcemia
hydroxybutyric dehydrogenase

FBHH
familial benign hypocalciuric hypercalcemia

FBI
fat-blood interface
flossing, brushing, and irrigation
food-borne illness
full bony impaction

FBL
fecal blood loss
focal brain lesion
follicular basal lamina

FBM
felbamate
fetal bone marrow
fetal breathing movement
foreign body, metallic

FBP
femoral blood pressure
fibrin breakdown product
fibrinogen breakdown product
fructose-bisphosphatase

FBR
fresh-blood reaction [Ger. *Frischblut*]

FBRCM
fingerbreadth below right costal margin

FBS
failed back syndrome
fasting blood glucose
fasting blood sugar (*See also* FB)
feedback signal
feedback system
fetal bovine serum
foreign body sensation (eye)

FBSS
failed back surgery syndrome

FBU
fingers below umbilicus (measurement) (*See also* F↓U)

FBV
fiber bundle volume

FBW
fasting blood work

FC
family conference
fasciculus cuneatus
fast component (of neuron)
febrile convulsion
fecal coli (broth)
feline conjunctivitis
female child
ferric citrate
fever, chills
fibrocystic
fibrocyte
financial class
finger clubbing
finger counting
flexion contracture
flow compensation
flow cytometry
foam cuffed (tracheal or endotrachael tube)
Foley catheter (*See also* F cath)
follows commands
formed response of colored area
form (response determined by) color
foster care
free cholesterol
frontal cortex
functional capacity
functional class

F&C
flare and cell (*See also* F/C, F+C)
foam and condom

F/C
facilitated communication
fever and chills
flare and cell (*See also* F&C, F+C)

F+C
flare and cells (*See also* F/C)

Fc
centroid frequency
fragment, crystallizable (of immunoglobulin)
shading response to black areas
shading response to gray areas

Fc′
fragment crystallized in minute quantities (immunoglobulin)
shade response to light gray area

fc
footcandle

FCA
Federal False Claims Act
ferritin-conjugated antibody
fracture, complete, angulated
Freund complete adjuvant

F cath
Foley catheter (*See also* FC)

NOTES

FCBD, FCDB
fibrocystic breast disease
fibrocystic disease of breast

FCC
familial cerebral cavernoma
familial colon cancer
familial colonic cancer
family centered care
femoral cerebral catheter
follicular center cell
fracture complete and compound
fracture compound and comminuted

fcc
face-centered-cubic

f/cc
fibers per cubic centimeter (of air)

FCCA
Final Comprehensive Consensus
Assessment

FCCC
fracture complete, compound, and
comminuted

FCCL
follicular center cell lymphoma

FCCU
family centered care unit

FCD
fecal containment device
feces collection device
fibrocystic disease
fibrocystic dysplasia
final consonant deletion
focal cytoplasmic degradation
fracture complete and deviated

FCE
fibrocartilaginous embolism
functional capacity evaluation

FCF
fetal cardiac frequency
fibroblast chemotactic factor

FCFC
fibroblast colony-forming cells

FCFD
fluorescence capillary-fill device

FCG
fifth cusp groove
French catheter gauge

FCH, FCHL
familial combined hyperlipidemia
fibrosing cholestatic hepatitis
folliculosebaceous cystic hamartoma

FCHL
familial combined hyperlipidemia

FCI
fixed cell immunofluorescence
food-chemical intolerance

FCIS
Flint Colon Injury Scale

FCL
fibular collateral ligament
follicle center lymphoma (cell)

fcly
face lying (position)

FCM
fetal cardiac motion
fibroblast-conditioned medium
flow cytometric
flow cytometry

FCMC
family-centered maternity care

FCMD
Fukuyama congenital muscular
dystrophy

FCMN
family-centered maternity nursing

F/C/N/V
fever, cough, nausea, and vomiting

FCOD
focal cementoosseous dysplasia

FCOU
finger count, both eyes

FCP
fasting chemistry profile
final common pathway
florid cutaneous papillomatosis
flow cytometric platelet
formocresol pulpotomy
Functional Communication Profile
(of aphasic adults)
functional conduction period

FCPD
fibrocalculous pancreatic diabetes

FCR
flexor carpi radialis (muscle)
fractional catabolic rate

FcR
Fc receptor

FCRA
fecal collection receptacle assembly

FCRB
flexor carpi radialis brevis

FCRT
fetal cardiac reactivity test
focal cranial radiation therapy

FCS
faciocutaneoskeletal
fecal containment system
feedback control system
fetal calf serum
fever, chills, and sweating
fluorescence correlation spectroscopy
foot compartment syndrome
full cervical spine

FCSNVD
fever, chills, sweating, nausea,
vomiting, and diarrhea

FCT
  fluorescein clearance test
  food composition table
FCU
  flexor carpi ulnaris
FCV
  feline calicivirus
FCVD
  fracture complete and varus
    deformity
FCx
  frontal cortex
FCXM
  flow cytometry crossmatch
FD
  failure to descend
  familial dysautonomia
  family doctor (*See also* fam doc,
    FMD)
  fan douche
  fatal dose
  fetal danger
  fetal demise
  fetal distress
  fibrinogen derivative
  fibrous dysplasia
  field desorption
  fixed and dilated (*See also* F&D)
  fluorescence depolarization
  fluphenazine decanoate
  focal disease
  focal distance
  Folin-Denis (assay)
  follicular diameter
  foot drape
  forceps delivery
  freedom from distractability
  free drain
  freeze-dried
  frequency deviation
  full denture
  fully dilated
F/D
  fracture/dislocation (*See also* fx-dis)
F&D
  fixed and dilated (*See also* FD)
FD$_{50}$
  median fatal dose
Fd
  animo-terminal portion of heavy
    chain of immunoglobulin

  ferredoxin
  fundus
FDA
  Frenchay Dysarthria Assessment
  frontodextra anterior (position)
  right frontal anterior (position of
    fetus) [L. *frontodextra anterior*]
FDACL
  first definite apical clearance lens
FDB
  first-degree burn
  flexor digitorum brevis
FDBL
  fecal daily blood loss
FDC
  flexor digitorum communis
  follicular dendritic cell
  frequency dependence of
    compliance
  perfluorodecalin (blood substitute)
FDCT
  Franck Drawing Completion Test
FddA
  2′β-fluoro-2′,3′-dideoxyadenosine
FddaraA
  2′,3′-dideoxy-2′-fluoro-9-beta-D-
    arabinofuranosyladenine
FDDB
  freeze-dried demineralized bone
FDDC
  ferric dimethyldithiocarbonate
FDDQ
  Freedom from Distractibility
    Deviation Quotient
FDDS
  Family Drawing Depression Scale
FDE
  female day equivalent
  final drug evaluation
  fixed drug eruption
FDF
  fast death factor
  flexor digitorum profundus (tendon)
  further differentiated fibroblast
FDFG
  free dermal-fat graft
FDFQ
  Food/Drink Frequency Questionnaire
FDG
  feeding (*See also* fdg)
  [^{18}F]fluoro-2-deoxy-D-glucose
  [^{13}F]fluorodeoxyglucose

F

NOTES

FDG *(continued)*
　　fluorodeoxyglucose
　　18-fluorodeoxyglucose
fdg
　　feeding (*See also* FDG)
FDGF
　　fibroblast-derived growth factor
FDG-F-18
　　^{18}F-labeled fluorodeoxyglucose
FDG-PET
　　fluorine-18 2-fluoro-2-deoxy-D-
　　glucose-positron emission
　　tomography
FDGS
　　feedings
FDH
　　familial dysalbuminemic
　　hyperthyroxinemia
　　focal dermal hypoplasia
FDI
　　Facial Disability Index
　　first digital interosseous (muscle)
　　first dorsal interosseus
　　food-drug interaction
　　frequency domain imaging
　　(ultrasound)
　　frequency-duration index
　　Functional Disability Index
FDICT
　　frequency-difference interferential
　　current therapy
FDIP
　　Facial Disability Index Physical
FDIS
　　Facial Disability Index Social
FDIU
　　fetal death in utero
FDL
　　flexor digitorum longus
　　fluorescein dilaurate
FDLMP
　　first day of last menstrual period
FDLV
　　fer-de-lance virus
FDM
　　fetus of diabetic mother
　　fibrous dysplasia of the mandible
　　flexor digiti minimi (muscle)
　　flexor digiti quinti (muscle)
FDMA
　　first dorsal metatarsal artery
FDNB
　　fluoro-2,4-dinitrobenzene
　　fluorodinitrobenzene (Sanger
　　reagent)
FDNS
　　familial dysplastic nevus syndrome

FDP
　　factitious disorder by proxy
　　fibrin degradation product (*See also*
　　FbDP, fdp)
　　fibrin/fibrinogen degradation
　　products
　　fixed-dose procedure
　　flexor digitorum profundus (muscle)
　　frontodextra posterior (position)
　　fructose diphosphate
　　right frontal posterior (position of
　　fetus) [L. *frontodextra posterior*]
fdp
　　fibrin degradation product (*See also*
　　FbDP, FDP)
　　fibrinogen degradation product (*See
　　also* FDP)
FDPALD
　　fructose diphosphate aldolase
FDPase
　　fructose diphosphatase
FDPCA
　　fixed-dose patient-controlled
　　analgesia
FD-PET
　　fluorodopa-positron emission
　　tomography
^{18}FDP PET
　　^{18}fluoro-deoxy-D-glucose positron
　　emission tomography
FDQB
　　flexor digiti quinti brevis
　　flexor digitorum quinti brevis
FDR
　　first-dose reaction
　　fractional disappearance rate
　　frequency dependence of resistance
FDS
　　for duration of stay
　　fiberduodenoscope
　　flexor digitorum sublimis
　　flexor digitorum superficialis
FDT
　　right frontal transverse (position of
　　fetus) [L. *frontodextra transversa*]
F$_3$dTMP
　　trifluorothymidylate
FDTVMP
　　Frostig Developmental Test of
　　Visual Motor Perception
FDTVP
　　Frostig Developmental Test of
　　Visual Perception
FdUMP
　　fluorodeoxyuridylate
5-FdUMP
　　5-fluorodeoxyuridylate

FDV
 Fiji disease virus
 Friend disease virus

FDZ
 fetal danger zone

FE
 fatty ester
 fecal emesis
 fetal erythroblastosis
 fluid extract
 fluorescing erythrocyte
 forced expiratory
 formalin and ethanol
 freely eating

Fe
 iron [L. *ferrum*]

^{52}Fe
 iron-52

^{55}Fe
 iron-55

^{59}Fe
 iron-59

fe
 female (*See also* F, FEM, fem)

feb
 febrile

FEBP
 fetal estrogen-binding protein

FEC
 forced expiratory capacity
 free erythrocyte coproporphyrin
  (*See also* FECP)
 free-standing emergency center
 Friend erythroleukemia cell

FECG
 fetal electrocardiogram

FeCh
 ferrochelatase

$FECO_2$, F_{ECO2}
 fractional concentration of carbon
  dioxide in expired gas
 fraction of expired carbon dioxide

FECP
 free erythrocyte coproporphyrin
  (*See also* FEC)

FECT
 fibroelastic connective tissue

FECV
 functional extracellular (fluid)
  volume

FED
 fish eye disease

FeD, Fe def
 iron (ferrum) deficiency

FEE
 forced equilibrating expiration

FEEG
 fetal electroencephalogram

Fe-EHPG
 Fe-ethylenehydroxyphenylglycine

FEER
 field-echo sequence with even-echo
  rephasing

FEES
 fiberoptic endoscopic evaluation of
  swallowing
 fiberoptic endoscopic examination
  of swallowing
 flexible endoscopic evaluation of
  swallowing

FEESST
 fiberoptic endoscopic evaluation of
  swallowing with sensory testing
 flexible endoscopic evaluation of
  swallowing with sensory testing

FEF
 Family Evaluation Form
 forced expiratory flow
 frontal eye field

$FEF_{25-75\%}$
 mean forced expiratory flow during
  the middle of FVC
 mean midexpiratory flow rate

FEF_{50}
 forced expiratory flow after 50%
  of vital capacity has been
  expelled

FEFEK
 fractional excretion of potassium

FEF_{50}/FIF_{50}
 ratio of expiratory flow to
  inspiratory flow at 50% of
  forced vital capacity

FEFmax
 maximal forced expiratory flow

FEFV
 forced expiratory flow volume

FEH
 focal epithelial hyperplasia

FEIA
 fluorescent enzyme immunoassay

FEIBA
 factor VIII inhibitor bypassing
  activity

F

NOTES

FEKG
> fetal electrocardiogram

FEL
> familial erythrophagocytic
> lymphohistiocytosis

FELC
> Friend erythroleukemia cell

FELI
> fractional excretion of lithium

FEM
> femoral (*See also* fem)
> femur (*See also* fem)
> finite element method
> fluid-electrolyte malnutrition

fem
> female (*See also* F, fe)
> feminine
> femoral (*See also* FEM)
> femur (*See also* FEM)

***fem* factor**
> factor essential for resistance to
> methicillin

FEM-FEM
> femoral femoral (bypass)

FEM-POP
> femoral-popliteal (bypass) (*See also*
> F-P)

FEM-TIB
> femoral tibial (bypass)

FEN
> fluids, electrolytes, nutrition

FENa, FE_Na
> fractional excretion of sodium

FENF
> fenfluramine

FEN-PHEN
> fenfluramine and phentermine

FENS
> field-electrical neural stimulation

FEO
> familial expansile osteolysis

Fe_3O_4
> magnetite

F_{EO2}
> fractional concentration of oxygen
> in expired gas

FEOM
> full extraocular motion
> full extraocular movement

FEOT
> fecal occult blood test

FEP
> fluorinated ethylene-propylene
> (polymer)
> free erythrocyte porphyrin
> free erythrocyte protoporphyrin (*See
> also* FEPP)
> functional exercise program

FEPB
> functional electronic peroneal brace

F-EPE
> focal extraprostatic extension

FEPP
> free erythrocyte protoporphyrin (*See
> also* FEP)

FER
> flexion, extension, and rotation
> fractional esterification rate
> frozen embryo replacement

FERG
> focal electroretinogram

fert
> fertility
> fertilized

FES
> Falls Efficacy Scale
> Family Environment Scale
> fat embolism syndrome
> flame emission spectroscopy
> forced expiratory spirogram
> functional electrical stimulation
> functional endoscopic sinus (*See
> also* FESS)

FESA
> finite element stress analysis

FESE
> flexible endoscopic swallowing
> examination

FESEM
> field emission scanning electron
> microscopy

$FeSO_4$
> ferrous sulfate

FESS
> functional endoscopic sinus surgery
> (*See also* FES)

FET
> field-effect transistor
> finger extension test
> Fisher exact test
> fixed erythrocyte turnover
> forced expiratory time

fet
> fetus

FETE
> Far Eastern tick-borne encephalitis

FETENDO
> fetal endoscopic

FETI
> fluorescence energy transfer
> immunoassay
> fluorescence excitation transfer
> immunoassay

Fe/TIBC
> iron saturation of serum transferrin

FETs
    forced expiratory time in seconds

FEU
    fibrinogen equivalent unit

FEUO
    for external use only

Fe-UR
    iron in urine

FEV-1, FEV$_1$
    forced expiratory volume at one
    second

FEV$_{1\%VC}$
    forced expiratory volume in one
    second as percent of FVC

fev
    fever

FEVB
    frequency ectopic ventricular beat

FEV/FVC
    forced expiratory volume timed to
    forced vital capacity ratio

FEV$_1$/FVC
    forced expiratory volume in one
    second to forced vital capacity
    ratio

FEVR
    familial exudative vitreoretinopathy

FEV$_t$
    forced expiratory volume timed

FEV$_1$/VC
    ratio of one-second forced
    expiratory volume to vital
    capacity

FEXE
    formalin, ethanol, xylol, and
    ethanol

FeZ
    iron zone

FF
    degree of fineness of abrasive
    particles
    fat free
    father factor
    fear of failure
    fecal frequency
    femorofemoral
    fertility factor
    fibrillation-flutter
    fibrofolliculoma
    fibrotic focus
    fields of Forel
    filtration factor

    filtration fraction
    fine fiber
    fine fraction
    finger flexion
    finger-to-finger (*See also* FTF, f-f,
      f→f)
    five-minute format
    fixation fluid
    fixing fluid
    flat feet
    flatfoot
    flip-flop (electronic logic circuitry)
    fluorescent focus
    follicular fluid
    force fluids (*See also* ff)
    forearm flow
    forward flexion
    foster father
    free fraction
    fresh frozen
    fundus firm (*See also* ff)
    further flexion

F&F
    filiform (bougie) and follower
    filiform and follower
    fixes and follows

F/F
    face to face

fF
    ultrafine fiber
    ultrafine fraction

ff
    following (*See also* f)
    force fluids (*See also* FF)
    fundus firm (*See also* FF)

f-f, f→f
    finger-to-finger (*See also* FF, FTF)

FFA
    female-female adaptor
    free fatty acid
    frontal fibrosing alopecia
    fundus fluorescein angiogram
    (unesterified) free fatty acid (*See
    also* UFA)

FFAP
    free fatty-acid phase

FFAT
    Free-Floating Anxiety Test

FFB
    fast feedback
    flexible fiberoptic bronchoscopy

F

NOTES

FFC
fixed flexion contracture
free from chlorine
FFCS
forearm flexion control strap
FFD
fat-free diet
focal film distance
focus film distance
FFDCA
Federal Food, Drug, and Cosmetic Act
FFDD II
focal facial dermal dysplasia II
F-18 FDG
fluorine-18 fluorodeoxyglucose
FFDM
freedom from distant metastases
free from distant metastases
FFDR
full florid diabetic retinopathy
FFDW
fat-free dry weight
FFE
fast-field echo
fecal fat excretion
flexible fiberoptic endoscope
free flow electrophoresis
FFEM
freeze fracture electron microscopy
FFF
degree of fineness of abrasive particles
field-flow fractionation
flicker fusion frequency (test)
Fuzzy Functional Form
FFG
free fat graft
FFI
fast food intake
fatal familial insomnia
Foot Function Index
free from infection
fundamental frequency indicator
FFIT
fluorescent focus inhibition test
FFL
fetal foot length
floral variant of follicular lymphoma
FFM
fat and fat-free mass
fat-free (body) mass
five-finger movement
freedom from metastases
FFN
fetal fibronectin

FFP
flexible fluoropolymer
freedom from progression
free from progression
fresh frozen plasma
FFPB
flexible fiberoptic bronchoscopy with protected brush
FFPE
formalin-fixed paraffin-embedded
FFR
fixed frequency response
fractional flow reserve
freedom from relapse
frequency-following response
FFR$_{myo}$
myocardial fractional flow reserve
FFROM
full, free range of motion
FFr-TMS
fast-frequency repetitive transcranial magnetic stimulation
FFS
failure of fixation suppression
failure-free survival
fat-free solid
fat-free supper
fee for service
five-factor score
flexible fiberoptic sigmoidoscopy
FFT
flicker fusion test
flicker fusion threshold
free-floating thrombus
FFTP
first full-term pregnancy
FFU
femur-fibula-ulna (syndrome)
focus-forming unit
FF1/U
fundus firm 1 cm above umbilicus
FF2/U
fundus firm 2 cm above umbilicus
FFU/1
fundus firm 1 cm below umbilicus
FFU/2
fundus firm 2 cm below umbilicus
FF@u
fundus firm at umbilicus
FFW
fat-free weight
FFWC
fractional free-water clearance
FFWW
fat-free wet weight
FG
fasciculus gracilis
fast-glycolytic (muscle fiber)

fast green
Feeley-Gorman (agar)
fibrin glue
fibrinogen (*See also* FBG, fbg, FGN, FI, FIB, fib.)
field gain
Flemish giant (rabbit)
French gauge

fg
femtogram

FGAR
formylglycinamide ribonucleotide
N-formylglycinamide ribotide

FGB
fully granulated basophil

FGC
familial gigantiform cementoma
fibrinogen gel chromatography
full gold crown

FGD
familial glucocorticoid deficiency
fatal granulomatous disease

FGDS
fibrogastroduodenoscopy

FGF
father's grandfather
fibroblast growth factor
fibroblastic growth factor
fresh gas flow

FGFa
(acidic) fibroblast growth factor (*See also* aFGF)
fibroblast growth factor, acidic

FGFR, FGF-R
fibroblast growth factor receptor

FGFR2
fibroblast growth factor receptor 2

FGG
focal global glomerulosclerosis
fowl gamma globulin
free gingival groove

FGID
functional gastrointestinal disorder

FGL
fasting gastrin level

FGLU
fasting glucose

FGM
father's grandmother
female genital mutilation (*See also* FGTM)

FGN
fibrinogen (*See also* FBG, fbg, FG)
focal glomerulonephritis

FGP
fundic gland polyp

FGR
fetal growth restriction

FGRN
finely granular

FGS
Facial Grading System
fibrogastroscopy
focal glomerular sclerosis

FGT
female genital tract
fluorescent gonorrhea test

FGTCS
female genital tract carcinosarcoma

FGTM
female genital tract mutilation (*See also* FGM)

FH
facial hemihyperplasia
familial hypercholesterolemia (*See also* FHC)
family history (*See also* fam hist, FH_x)
fasting hyperbilirubinemia
favorable histology
femoral hypoplasia
fetal head
fetal heart
fibromuscular hyperplasia (*See also* FMH)
Ficoll-Hypaque (technique)
floating hospital
follicular hyperplasia
Frankfort horizontal (plane of skull)
fundal height

FH⁻
family history negative (*See also* FHN)

FH⁺
family history positive (*See also* FHP)

FH₄
folacin
tetrahydrofolic acid

fh
fostered by hand (experimental animal)

NOTES

FHA
    familial hypoplastic anemia
    filamentous hemagglutinin
    filterable hemolytic anemia
    fimbrial hemagglutinin
    functional hypothalamic amenorrhea

FHB
    flexor hallucis brevis (muscle)

FHBL
    familial hypobetalipoproteinemia

FHC
    familial hypercholesterolemia (See also FH)
    familial hypertrophic cardiomyopathy
    familial hypertrophy
    family health center
    Ficoll-Hypaque centrifugation
    Fuchs heterochromic cyclitis

FHCH
    fortified hexachlorocyclohexane

FHCIC
    Fuchs heterochromic iridocyclitis (See also FHI)

FHD
    familial histiocytic dermatoarthritis
    family history of diabetes

FHF
    familial Hibernian fever
    fetal heart frequency
    fulminant hepatic failure

FHH
    familial hypercalcemia with hypocalciuria
    familial hypocalciuric hypercalcemia
    family history of hirsutism
    fetal heart heard

FHI
    frontal horn index
    Fuchs heterochromic iridocyclitis (See also FHCIC)

FHIP
    family health insurance plan

FHIT
    fragile histidine triad

FHL
    familial hemophagocytic lymphohistiocytosis
    femoral head line
    flexor hallucis longus
    focal hypoechoic lesion
    functional hearing loss

FHLD
    flexor hallucis longus dysfunction

FHLDL
    familial hypercholesterolemia, low-density lipoprotein

FHLH
    familial hemophagocytic lymphohistiocytosis

FHM
    familial hemiplegic migraine
    fat head minnow (cells)
    fetal heart motion

FH-M
    fumarate hydratase, mitochondrial

FHMI
    family history of mental illness

FHN
    family history negative

FHNH
    fetal heart not heard

FHO
    family history of obesity

FHP
    family history positive (See also FH$^+$)

FHR
    familial hypophosphatemia
    familial hypophosphatemic rickets
    fetal heart rate
    fetal heart rhythm

FHRB
    fetal heart rate baseline

FH-RDC, FHRDC
    family history research diagnostic criteria

FHR-NST
    fetal heart rate nonstress test

FHRV
    fetal heart rate variability

FHS
    fetal heart sound
    fetal hydantoin syndrome
    floating harbor syndrome

FH-S
    fumarate hydratase, soluble

FHT
    fetal heart tone

FHTG
    familial hypertriglyceridemia

FHUF, FH-UFS
    femoral hypoplasia unusual facies (syndrome)

FHVP
    free hepatic venous pressure

FH$_x$
    family history (See also fam hist, FH)

FI
    fasciculus interfascicularis
    fever caused by infection
    fibrinogen (See also FBG, fbg, FG, FGN, FIB, fib.)
    fiscal intermediary

fixateur interne
fixed interval
fixed interval (schedule)
flame ionization
forced inspiration
frontoiliacus
functional inquiry
Functional Integration (test)
fundamental imaging
fungal infection
fusion inhibitor

FI$_{O2}$

forced inspiratory oxygen
fraction of inspired oxygen

FIA

familial intracranial aneurysms
feline infectious anemia
fluorescent immunoassay
fluoroimmunoassay
focal immunoassay
Freund incomplete adjuvant

FIAC

fiacitabine

FIAU

fialuridine

FIB

fibrin
fibrinogen (*See also* FBG, fbg, FG,
  FGN, FI, fib.)
fibrositis
fibula

fib.

fiber
fibrillation (*See also* fibrill)
fibrinogen (*See also* FBG, fbg, FG,
  FGN, FI, FIB)

fib. bronc

fiberoptic bronchoscopy (*See also*
  FB, FOB)

fibrill

fibrillation (*See also* fib.)

FIC

fasting intestinal contents
forced inspiratory capacity
fractional inhibitory concentration
functional inhibitory concentration
growth factor-inducible chemokine

FICA

food immune complex assay

FICO$_2$, FiCO$_2$

fraction of inspired carbon dioxide

FICU

fetal intensive care unit

FID

father in delivery
flame ionization detector
free-induction decay
free induction decay
fungal immunodiffusion

FIDD

fetal iodine deficiency disorder

FIF

feedback inhibition factor
forced inspiratory flow
formaldehyde-induced fluorescence
Functional Intact Fibrinogen (test)
(human) fibroblast interferon (*See
  also* FIFN)

FIFN

(human) fibroflast interferon (*See
  also* FIF)

FIFR

fasting intestinal flow rate

fig.

figure

FIGD

familial idiopathic gonadotropin
  deficiency

FIGE

Field inversion gel electrophoresis

FIGLU

formiminoglutamic acid (test)

FIGLU-uria

formiminoglutamicaciduria

FIH

familial isolated hypoparathyroidism
fat-induced hyperglycemia

FIHP

familial isolated primary
  hyperparathyroidism

FIL

father-in-law

fil

filament (*See also* F)

FILAR

filariasin

FILE

Family Index of Life Events
Family Inventory of Life Events
  and Changes

filt

filter
filtration

F

NOTES

FIM
field ion microscopy
functional independence measure
FIN
fine intestinal needle
flexible intramedullary nail
FINCC
familial idiopathic nonarteriosclerotic
cerebral calcification
FIND
follow up intervention for normal
development
F-insulin
fibrous insulin
FIO₂, FiO2, FiO₂
fractional concentration of inspired
oxygen
fractional inspired oxygen
concentration
fractional percentage of inspired
oxygen
fraction of inspired oxygen
FIP
feline infectious peritonitis
flatus in progress
FIPH
full scan with interpolation
projection
FIPT
periarteriolar transudate
FIPV
feline infectious peritonitis virus
FIQ
Fibromyalgia Impact Questionnaire
full scale intelligence quotient
FIR
far infrared
fold increase in resistance
FIRDA
frontal irregular rhythmic delta
activity (electroencephalography)
FIRI
fasting insulin resistance index
FIRM
Family Inventory of Resources for
Management
FIRO-B
Fundamental Interpersonal Relations
Orientation-Behavior
FIRO-F
Fundamental Interpersonal Relations
Orientation-Feelings
FIS
fiberoptic injection sclerotherapy
forced inspiratory spirogram
FISC
Facial Impairment Scales for
Children

FISCA
Functional Impairment Scale for
Children and Adolescents
FISH
fluorescent in situ hybridization
FISP
fast imaging with steady precession
fast imaging with steady-state free
precession
FISP-3D MRI
fast-imaging steady precession
sequence three-dimensional
magnetic resonance imaging
FISS
Flint Infant Security Scale
fiss
fissure
fist.
fistula
FIT
fibrous intimal thickening
Flanagan Industrial Test
Fracture Intervention Trial
fusion-inferred threshold (test)
FITC
fluorescein isothiocyanate
FITT
frequency, intensity, time, and type
(exercise)
FIUO
for internal use only
FIV
feline immunodeficiency virus
forced inspiratory volume
FIV₁
forced inspiratory volume in one
second
FIVC
forced inspiratory vital capacity
F-J
Fisher-John (melting point method)
F-JAS
Fleishman Job Analysis Survey
FJB
facet joint block
FJD
facet joint disease
FJN
familial juvenile nephrophthisis
FJN-MCD
familial juvenile nephrophthisis-
medullary cystic disease
FJP
familial juvenile polyp
familial juvenile polyposis
FJRM, FJROM
full joint range of motion
full joint range of movement

FJS
　finger joint size
FJV
　first jejunal vein
FK
　feline kidney
　functioning kasai (Belgian Congo anemia)
FK506, FK-506
　tacrolimus
　tacrolimus (Prograf)
FKA
　formally known as
FKBP
　FK-binding protein
FKBP12
　FK-binding protein 12
FKD
　Kinetic Family Drawing
FKE
　full knee extension
FL
　factor level
　fatty liver
　feline leukemia
　femoral length
　femur length
　fetal length
　fibers of Luschka
　fibroblast-like
　filtered load (See also Fl, fl)
　flavomycin
　flow limitation
　fluorescein
　flutamide andleuprolide acetate
　focal length
　follicular lymphoma
　frontal lobe
　full liquids (dict)
　functional length
FL-2
　feline lung (cell)
F/L
　father-in-law
Fl
　filtered load (See also FL, fl)
　fluid (See also F, f, fl, FLD, fld)
　fluorescence (See also fl, fluores)
　follicle lysis (See also fl)
fL
　femtoliter

fl
　filtered load (See also FL, Fl)
　flank
　flexible
　flexion
　fluid (See also F, f, Fl, FLD, fld)
　fluorescence (See also Fl, fluores)
　flutter
　follicle lysis (See also Fl)
FLA
　fluorescent-labeled antibody
　free-living amebic (ameba)
　left frontal anterior (position of fetus) [L. frontolaeva anterior]
　low-friction arthroplasty
FL/AC
　femur length to abdominal circumference ratio
flac
　flaccid
　flaccidity
FLACC
　face, legs, activity, cry, consolability
FLAIR
　fluid attenuated inversion recovery
　fluid attenuation inversion recovery
FLAK
　flow artifact killer
Fl Ang
　fluorescein angiography
FLAP
　5-lipoxygenase-activating protein
FLASH
　fast low-angle shot
FLAV
　Flanders virus
FLAVO
　flavopiridol
FLB
　four-layer bandage
　funny-looking beat (heart)
FLC
　fatty liver cell
　fetal liver cell
　follicular large cell lymphoma
　Friend leukemia cell
FLCOD
　florid local cementoosseous dysplasia
FLD
　fatty liver disease

F

NOTES

FLD *(continued)*
fibrotic lung disease
fluid (*See also* F, f, Fl, fl, fld)
flutamide and leuprolide acetate depot
full lower denture (*See also* /F)

fld
field
fluid (*See also* F, f, Fl, fl, FLD)

fld ext
fluid extract (*See also* fldxt)

fl dr
fluid dram

fld rest.
fluid restriction

fl drs
fluff dressing

fldxt
fluid extract (*See also* fld ext)

FLE
frontal lobe epilepsy

FLES
Fairview Language Evaluation Scale

FLET
Fairview Language Evaluation Test

FLEV
Flexal virus

FLEX
Federation Licensing Examination

flex.
flexion
flexor

flex sig
flexible sigmoidoscopy

FLGA
full-term, large for gestational age

FLH
focal lymphoid hyperplasia

FL-HCC
fibrolamellar hepatocellular carcinoma

FLI
fluorescent light intensity

FLIC
Functional Living Index-Cancer

FLIE
Functional Living Index-Emesis

FLIT
Figurative Language Interpretation Test

FLK
funny-looking kid

FLKS
fatty liver and kidney syndrome

FLM
fasciculus longitudinalis medialis
fetal lung maturity

FLN
fluorescence-lactose-denitrification medium

floc, flocc
flocculation

flor.
flowers (mineral substance in powdery state after sublimation) [L. *flores*]

fl oz
fluid ounce

FLP
fasting lipid profile
Functional Limitation Profile
left frontal posterior (position of fetus) [L. *frontolaeva posterior*]

FLPD
flashlamp pulsed dye laser (*See also* FPDL)

FLPR
flurbiprofen

FLR
funny-looking rash

FL REST
fluid restriction

FLS
fatty liver syndrome
fibroblast-like synoviocyte
fibrous long-spacing (collagen)
flashing lights and/or scotoma
flow-limiting segment
Functional Life Scale

FLSA
follicular lymphosarcoma

FLSP
fluorescein-labeled serum protein

FLT
3′fluoro-2′,3′-dideoxythymidine
fluorothymidine
left frontal transverse (position of fetus) [L. *frontolaeva transversa*]

FLTA
Fullerton Language Test for Adolescents

FLTAC
Fisher-Logemann Test of Articulation Competence

FLU
fluconazole
fludarabine
flunisolide
flunisolide
fluoxetine
fluphenazine (*See also* FPZ)
fluticasone propionate

flu
influenza

flu A
    influenza A
FLUO
    Fluothane
fluores
    fluorescence (*See also* Fl, fl)
    fluorescent
fluoro
    fluoroscopy
FLUP
    front-loading ultrasound probe
fl up
    flareup
    follow up
flut
    flutamide
FLV
    feline leukemia virus
    Friend leukemia virus
FLW
    fasting laboratory work
FLZ
    flurazepam
FM
    face mask
    facilities management
    fathom
    fat mass
    feedback mechanism
    fetal movement
    fibrin monomer
    fibromuscular
    fibromyalgia
    filtered mass
    fine motor
    flavin mononucleotide
    floor manager
    flowmeter
    fluid movement
    fluorescent microscopy
    foramen magnum
    forensic medicine
    formerly married
    foster mother
    fragrance mix
    frequency modulation
    Friend-Moloney (antigen)
    functional movement
    fusobacteria microorganisms
F&M
    firm and midline (uterus)

Fm
    fermium
^{255}Fm
    fermium-255
fm
    femtometer
    from (*See also* fr)
FMA
    Frankfort mandibular (plane) angle
FMAC
    fetal movement acceleration test
FMAIT
    fetomaternal alloimmune
      thrombocytopenia
FMAP
    feeding mean arterial pressure
FMB
    full maternal behavior
FMC
    family medicine center
    fetal movement count
    flight medicine clinic
    focal macular choroidopathy
FMD
    family medical doctor (*See also*
      fam doc, FD)
    fibromuscular dysplasia
    flow-mediated dilation
    flow-mediated vasodilation
    foot-and-mouth disease
    foramen magnum decompression
    frontometaphyseal dysplasia
FMDV
    foot-and-mouth disease virus
FME
    full-mouth extraction
FMEL
    Friend murine erythroleukemia
FMEN
    familial multiple endocrine
      neoplasia
FMET, F-met, fMet
    formylmethionine
FMF
    familial Mediterranean fever
    fetal movement felt
    flow microfluorometry
    forced midexpiratory flow
FMFD1
    familial multiple factor deficiency
      1

NOTES

F

FMG
fibrin matrix gel
fine mesh gauze
foreign medical graduate

FMH
familial hemiplegic migraine
family medical history
fat-mobilizing hormone
fetomaternal hemorrhage
fibromuscular hyperplasia (See also
FH)
first metatarsal head

FMI
fixed mandibular implant
Foods and Moods Inventory

FMIA
Frankfort mandibular incisor angle

FMISO
F-misonidazole

FMIV
forced mandatory intermittent
ventilation

FML
flail mitral leaflet
fluorometholone

FMLA
Family Medical Leave Act
Family and Medical Leave Act of
1993

FMLH
familial hemophagocytic
lymphohistiocytosis

FML-Neo
fluorometholone and neomycin
sulfate

FMLP, fMLP
N-formyl-1-methionyl-1-leucyl-1-
phenylalamine
N-formyl-methyonyl-leucyl-
phenylalanine

FMN
first malignant neoplasm
flavin mononucleotide
frontomaxillonasal (suture)

FMNH, FMNH$_2$
reduced form of flavin
mononucleotide

FMO
flavin-containing mono-oxygenase
metabolic system

fmol
femtomole

fmoles/mg
femtomoles per milligram

FMP
family member presence
fasting metabolic panel
first menstrual period
functional maintenance program

FMPA
full-mouth periapicals

FMPSPGR imaging
fast multiplanar spoiled gradient-
recalled imaging

FMR
fetal movement record
focused medical review
Friend-Moloney-Rauscher (antigen)
functional magnetic resonance
(imaging)

FMR1
fragile (site) mental retardation 1
(See also FRAXE1)

FMR2
fragile (site) mental retardation 2
(See also FRAXE2)

fMRA
functional magnetic resonance
angiography

FMRD
full-mouth restorative dentistry

fMRI
functional magnetic resonance
imaging
functional MRI

FMRP
fragile X mental retardation protein

FMS
fat-mobilizing substance
fatty meal sonogram
fibromyalgia syndrome (See also
FS)
full-mouth series (dental x-ray
films)

FMSTB
Frostig Movement Skills Test
Battery

FMT
fetal mesencephalic tissue
floating mass transducer
functional muscle test

FMTC
familial medullary thyroid cancer
familial medullary thyroid
carcinoma

FMU
first morning urine

FMULC
free monoclonal urinary light chain

FMV
floppy mitral valve
Fort Morgan virus

FMX
full-mouth x-ray

FMZ
flumazenil
F-N, F to N, F→N
finger-to-nose (coordination test)
(*See also* FN, FTN)
FN
facial nerve
false negative (*See also* Fneg)
false-negative
fastigial nucleus
febrile neutropenia
femoral neck
fibronectin
final nitrogen
finger-to-nose (coordination test)
(*See also* F-N, F→N, FTN)
flight nurse
fluoride number
F/N
fluids and nutrition
fn
function (*See also* F, FXN)
FNA
fine-needle aspiration
Functional Needs Assessment
FNa
filtered sodium
FNAB
fine-needle aspiration biopsy
FNAC
fine-needle aspiration cytology
FNB
femoral nerve block
FNC
fatty nutritional cirrhosis
FNCJ
fine-needle catheter jejunostomy
FND
febrile neutrophilic dermatosis
focal neurological deficit
frontonasal dysplasia
functional neck dissection
Fneg
false negative (*See also* FN)
FNF
false-negative fraction
femoral neck fracture
finger-nose-finger (coordination test)
FNH
focal nodular hyperplasia
follicular nodular hyperplasia

FNHL
follicular non-Hodgkin lymphoma
FNHTR
febrile nonhemolytic transfusion
react
FNI
facial nerve injury
FNIC
Food and Nutrition Information
Center
FN-MCD
familial nephronophthisis-medullary
cystic disease
FNMTC
familial nonmedullary thyroid
carcinoma
fn p
fusion point
FNR
false-negative rate
FNS
food and nutrition services
functional neuromuscular stimulation
F/NS
fever and night sweats
FNSD
face-near-straight-down (infant sleep
position)
FNT
false neurochemical transmitter
finger-to-nose test
FNTC, FNTHC
fine-needle transhepatic
cholangiogram
fine-needle transhepatic
cholangiography
FO
fast oxidative
fiberoptic
focus out
foot orthosis
foramen ovale
forced oscillation
foreign object
frontooccipital (fetal position)
Fo
fomentation
fomenting
phonation
FOAM
fluorescence overlay antigen
mapping

F

NOTES

FOAR
  faciooculoacousticorenal (syndrome)
FOAVF
  failure of all vital forces
FOB
  father of baby
  fecal occult blood
  feet out of bed
  fiberoptic bronchoscope
  fiberoptic bronchoscopy (*See also* FB)
  foot of bed
  foreign object/body
FOBT
  fecal occult blood test
FOC
  father of child
  fluid of choice
  frequency of contact (scale)
  frontooccipital circumference
FOCAL
  formula calculation (computer language)
FOCALCROS
  focal contralateral routing of signals
FOCMA
  feline oncornavirus-associated cell membrane antigen
FOD
  fixing right eye
  focus object distance
  free of disease
FOEB
  feet over edge of bed
FOG
  fast-oxidative-glycolytic (fiber)
  Fluothane, oxygen, and gas (nitrous oxide)
  full-on gain
FOH
  family ocular history
FOI
  flight of ideas
FOIA
  Freedom of Information Act
FOID
  fear of impending doom
FOL
  fiberoptic laryngoscopy
  fiberoptic light
fol
  following
FOM
  figure of merit (measure of diagnostic value per radionuclide radiation dose)
  floor of mouth

FOMV
  Fomede virus
FONAR
  field focused nuclear magnetic resonance
FONSI
  finding of no significant impact
FOOB
  fell out of bed
FOOSH
  fall on outstretched hand
FOP
  fibrodysplasia ossificans progressiva
  forensic pathology
FOPR
  full outpatient rate
FOPS
  fiberoptic proctosigmoidoscopy
FO-PT
  fiberoptic phototherapy
FOPT
  fibroosseous pseudotumor
FOR, for
  forensic
for.
  foreign
  formula (*See also* form.)
form.
  formula (*See also* for.)
FORMIL
  foreign military
FORTRAN, Fortran
  formula translation (computer language)
FORV
  Forecariah virus
FOS
  fiberoptic sigmoidoscope
  fiberoptic sigmoidoscopy
  fissura orbitalis superior
  fixing left eye
  fosphenytoin
  fractional osteoid surface
  fructooligosaccharide
  full of stool
  future order screen
FOSC
  freestanding outpatient surgery center
FOSQ
  Functional Outcomes of Sleep Questionnaire
FOT
  Finger Oscillation Test
  forced oscillation technique
  form of thought
  frontal outflow tract

found.
    foundation
four Rs
    remove, replace, reinoculate, repair
FOV
    field of view
FOVI
    field of vision intact
FOW
    fenestration open window
    fenestration of oval window
FOZR
    front optic zone radius
FP
    fall precautions
    false-positive
    familial porencephaly
    family physician (*See also* fam phys)
    family planning
    family practice
    family practitioner
    family presence
    fibrinolytic potential
    fibrinopeptide
    fibrous proliferation
    filling pressure
    filter paper
    final pressure
    first pass
    fixation protein
    flat plate
    flavin phosphate
    flavoprotein
    flexor profundus
    fluid pressure
    fluorescence polarization
    fluticasone propionate
    food poisoning
    foot process
    forearm pronated (*See also* fp)
    freezing point (*See also* fp)
    frontoparietal
    frontopolar
    frozen plasma
    full period
    fundal pressure
    fundus photo
    fusion point
F-P
    femoral-popliteal (*See also* FEM-POP)

F-6-P
    fructose-6-phosphate
F/P
    fluid-plasma (ratio)
    fluorescein to protein (ratio)
Fp
    filtered phosphate
    frontal polar electrode placement in electroencephalography
fp
    flexor pollicis
    forearm pronated (*See also* FP)
    freezing point
FPA
    fibrinopeptide A (*See also* fpA)
    filter paper activity
    fluorophenylalanine
    foot-progression angle
    frontopolar artery
fpA
    fibrinopeptide A (*See also* FPA)
fpa
    far point of accommodation
FPAA
    female pattern androgenetic alopecia
FPAL
    full-term (deliveries), premature (deliveries), abortion(s), living (children)
FPB
    femoral-popliteal bypass
    fibrinopeptide B
    flexor pollicis brevis
FPC
    familial polyposis coli
    family planning clinic
    family practice center
    fish protein concentrate
    forced pair copulation
    frozen packed cells
FPCL
    fibroblast-populated collagen lattice
FPD
    fetopelvic disproportion
    fixed partial denture
    flame photometric detector
FPDD
    familial pure depressive disease
FPDL
    flashlamp-pumped pulsed-dye laser (*See also* FLPD)

F

NOTES

FPDVP
Frostig Program for the Development of Visual Perception
FPE
first-pass effect
F-18-PET
fluoride ion positron emission tomography
FPF
false-positive fraction
fibroblast pneumocyte factor
FPG
fasting plasma glucose
fluorescence plus Giemsa (stain)
focal proliferative glomerulonephritis (*See also* FPGN)
FPGN
focal proliferative glomerulonephritis (*See also* FPG)
FPH
familial progressive hyperpigmentation
FPH_2
flavin phosphate, reduced
FPHA
family planning health assistant
FPHE
formaldehyde-treated pyruvaldehyde-stabilized human erythrocytes
formalin-treated pyruvaldehyde-stabilized human erythrocytes
FPHx
family psychiatric history
FPI
femoral pulsatility index
formula protein intolerance
Freiburger Personality Inventory
FPIA
fluorescence-polarization immunoassay
fluorescent polarization immunoassay
FPIR
first-phase insulin response
FPK
fructose-6-phosphokinase
FPL
fasting plasma lipid
final printed labeling
flexor pollicis longus
FPLA
fibrin plate lysis area
FPLV
feline panleukopenia virus
FPM
filter paper microscopic (test)
first-pass metabolism
full passive movements
fpm
feet per minute
FPMA
first plantar metatarsal artery
FPN
ferric chloride, perchloric acid, and nitric acid (solution)
FPNA
first-pass nuclear angiocardiography
FPO
faciopalatoosseous
freezing point osmometer
FPOR
follicle puncture for oocyte retrieval
FPP
familial paroxysmal polyserositis
ferriprotoporphyrin
free portal pressure
FPPDL
flashlamp-pumped pulsed dye laser
FPPH
familial primary pulmonary hypertension
FPR
facilitated positional release
fastigial pressor response
fluorescence photobleaching recovery
fractional proximal resorption
Functional Performance Record
FPRA
first-pass radionuclide angiogram
FPS
fetal PCB (polychlorinated biphenyl) syndrome
footpad swelling
fps
feet per second
foot-pound-second (system, unit)
frames per second
FP/Salm Combo
fluticasone propionate/salmeterol
FPSLT
Fluharty Preschool Speech and Language Screening Test
FPT
fixed parenchymal turnover
FPU
family participation unit
fetoplacental unit
FPV
Facey's Paddock virus
feline panleukopenia virus
fowl plague virus
FPVB
femoral-popliteal vein bypass

FPZ
    fluphenazine (*See also* FLU)
FPZ-D
    fluphenazine decanoate
FQ
    fluoroquinolones
FR
    failure rate (contraception)
    fair
    father (*See also* F)
    Federal Register
    feedback regulation
    fibrinogen related
    first responder
    Fisher-Race (notation)
    fixed ratio
    flocculation reaction
    flow rate
    fluid restriction
    fluid retention
    fractional reabsorption
    free radical
    frequency of respiration
    frequent relapses
    frothy
    full range
    functional reach
    functional residual (capacity)
    reticular formation [L. *formatio reticularis*]
FR3
    third framework region
F/R
    fire/rescue
F&R, F and R
    force and rhythm (of pulse)
Fr
    francium
    franklin (unit charge)
    French scale
fr
    fried
    from (*See also* fm)
FRA
    fall risk assessment
    fibrinogen-related antigen
    fibrin-related antigen
    fluorescent rabies antibody
    fragile
    fragile chromosome site
    fragile gene

fra
    fragile
    fragile chromosome site
    fragile gene
    fragile site (chromosome in cytogenetics)
frac
    fracture (*See also* fract, frx, fx, FXR)
fract
    fraction (*See also* FX)
    fracture (*See also* Fr, frac, frx, fx, FXR)
FRACTS
    fractional urines
frag
    fragile
    fragility
    fragment
FRAP
    family risk assessment program
    FK-binding protein rapamycin-associated protein
    fluorescence recovery after photobleaching
FRAST
    Free Running Asthma Test
FRAT
    free radical assay technique
FRAX, fra(X)
    fragile X (chromosome, syndrome)
    fragile X gene
FRAXA
    fragile X type A
    X-linked first site of fragility
FRAXE
    fragile X-E
    X-linked second site of fragility
FRAXE1
    X-linked mental retardation-fragile site 1 (*See also* FMR1)
FRAXE2
    X-linked mental retardation-fragile site 2 (*See also* FMR2)
FRBB, Fr BB
    fracture of both bones (*See also* Fx BB)
FRBS
    fast red B salt
FRC
    feedback reduction circuit
    frozen red cell

F

NOTES

FRC *(continued)*
    functional reserve capacity (of lungs)
    functional residual capacity (of lungs)

FRCD
    fixed ratio combination drugs

FRD
    flexion-rotation-drawer

FRE
    Fischer rat embryo
    flow-related enhancement

FRED
    fog reduction elimination device

frem.
    vocal fremitus [L. *fremitus vocalis*]

freq
    frequency (*See also* F, f)

FRET
    fluorescence resonance energy transfer
    fluorescent resonance energy transfer

FRF
    fasciculus retroflexus
    filtration replacement fluid
    follicle-stimulating hormone-releasing factor (*See also* FSH-RF)

FRFC
    functional renal failure of cirrhosis

FRG
    Functional Related Groups

FRH
    follicle-stimulating hormone-releasing hormone (*See also* FSH-RH)

FRHS
    fast-repeating high sequence

frict
    friction (rub)

Fried
    Friedman (test for pregnancy)

FRIV
    Frijoles virus

FRJM
    full range joint motion
    full range joint movement

FRM
    full range of motion (*See also* FROM)

FRN
    fetal rhabdomyomatous nephroblastoma
    fully resonant nucleus

FRNS
    frequently relapsing nephrotic syndrome

FRNT
    focus-reduction neutralization test

FROA
    full range of affect

FROM
    full range of motion (*See also* FRM)

FROMAJE
    functioning, reasoning, orientation, memory, arithmetic, judgment, and emotion (mental status evaluation)

FROS
    front routing of signal

FRP
    follicle regulatory protein
    formaldehyde-releasing preservative
    functional refractory period

FRPS
    functional resting position splint

FR r, fr r
    friction rub

FRS
    ferredoxin-reducing substance
    first rank symptom
    first rank symptoms
    flexed, rotated, sidebent
    fluid retention syndrome
    furosemide (*See also* FSM, FUR)

FRSL
    flexed, rotated, sidebent left

FRSR
    flexed, rotated, sidebent right

FRT
    Family Relations Test
    full recovery time

FRTL-5
    Fischer rat thyroid line-5

Fru
    fructose

FRV
    functional residual volume

frx
    fracture (*See also* frac, fract, fx, FXR)

FS
    factor of safety
    fetoscope
    fibromyalgia syndrome (*See also* FMS)
    fibrosarcoma
    fibrous synovium
    field stimulation
    fine structure
    fingerstick
    fire setter (psychology)
    flexible sigmoidoscopy
    focal spot
    fogo selvagem
    food service
    forearm supination

Fourier series
fractional shortening
fracture, simple
fracture site
fragile site
Friesinger score
frozen section (*See also* FZ)
full-scale (IQ)
full and soft (diet) (*See also* F&S)
full strength
functional shortening
functional status
function study
(human) foreskin (cells)

F/S

female, spayed (animal)

F&S

full and soft (diet) (*See also* FS)

FSA

fetal sulfoglycoprotein antigen
frozen section assay

FSAD

female sexual arousal disorder

FSALO

Fletcher-Suit afterloading ovoids
(gynecologic cancer treatment)

FSALT

Fletcher-Suit afterloading tandem
(gynecologic cancer treatment)

FSB

fetal scalp blood
Fokes sentence builder
full spine board

FSBG

fingerstick blood gas
fingerstick blood glucose

FSBM

full-strength breast milk

FSBP

finger systolic blood pressure

FSBS

fingerstick blood sugar

FSBT

Fowler single breath test

FSC

Fatigue Symptom Checklist
flexible sigmoidoscopy
Forer Sentence Completion (Test)
fracture simple and comminuted
fracture simple and complete
free secretory component
free-standing clinic

FSCC

fracture simple complete and
comminuted

FSCR

flexible surface-coil-type resonator

FSD

face-straight-down (infant sleep
position)
female sexual dysfunction
Fletcher-Suit-Delclos (applicator)
focus-skin distance
fracture simple and depressed
full-scale deflection

FS-DFSP

fibrosarcomatous variant of
dermatofibrosarcoma protuberans

FSDQ

Frost Self-Description Questionnaire

FSE

fast spin echo
fetal scalp electrode
filtered smoke exposure

FSF

fibrin-stabilization factor

FSG

fasting serum glucose
focal sclerosing glomerulonephritis
(*See also* FSGN)
focal segmental glomerulosclerosis

FSGA

full-term, small for gestational age

FSGHS

focal segmental glomerular
hyalinosis and sclerosis

FSGN

focal sclerosing glomerulonephritis
(*See also* FSG)

FSGO

floating spherical gaussian orbital

FSGS

focal segmental glomerular sclerosis
focal segmental glomerulosclerosis

FSGSH

focal segmental glomerular sclerosis
and hyalinosis

FSH

facioscapulohumeral
fascioscapulohumeral
focal and segmental hyalinosis
follicle-stimulating hormone
follicular stimulating hormone
follitropin

F

NOTES

FSHD
facioscapulohumeral (muscular) dystrophy

FSH/LR-RH
follicle-stimulating hormone and luteinizing hormone-releasing hormone

FSHMD
facioscapulohumeral muscular dystrophy

FSH-RF
follicle-stimulating hormone-releasing factor (*See also* FRF)

FSH-RH
follicle-stimulating hormone-releasing hormone (*See also* FRH)

FSI
foam stability index
Functional Status Index

FSIA
foot shock-induced analgesia

FSIQ
Full-Scale Intelligence Quotient

FSL
fasting serum level
fixed slit lamp

FSM
functional status measures
furosemide (*See also* FRS, FUR)

F-SM/C
fungus, smear, and culture

FSME
Frühsommer meningoencephalitis

FSO
for screws only (prosthetic cups)

FS$_p$O$_2$
fetal arterial oxygen saturation

F-SP
special form (taxonomy) [L. *forma specialis*]

FSP
familial spastic paraplegia
fibrinogen split product
fibrinolytic split product
fibrin split product
fine suspended particulate
free secretory piece

FS projection
full-scan projection

FSQ
Functional Status Questionnaire

FSR
film screen radiography
fractionated stereotactic radiosurgery
fragmented sarcoplasmic reticulum
fusiform skin revision

FSRRL
flexion, sidebent right, rotated left

FSRT
fractionated stereotactic radiotherapy

FSS
Familiar Sensory Stimulation
Fear Survey Schedule
fetal scalp sampling
focal segmental sclerosis
French steel sound
frequency-selective saturation
front support strap
full-scale score
functional systems scale

FSSE
fat-suppressed spin-echo

FSST
Full-Scale Score Total

FST
foam stability test

FSU
family service unit
functional spinal unit
functional subunit

FSUM
focused segmented ultrasound machine

FSV
feline fibrosarcoma virus
Fort Sherman virus
forward stroke volume

FSW
feet of sea water (pressure)
field service worker
flexible spiral wire

fsw
feet of sea water

FT
false transmitter
family therapy
fast twitch
feeding tube
ferritin (*See also* F$_t$)
ferromagnetic tamponade
fetal tonsil
fibrous tissue
filling time
finger tapping
fingertip
flexor tendon
fluidotherapy
followthrough (after barium meal)
formol toxoid
Fourier transform
free testosterone
free thyroxine
frontotemporal
full term
function test

FT₃
  free triiodothyronine
F3T
  trifluridine
FT4
  free thyroxine
FT₄
  free thyroxine
  free (unbound) thyroxine
Fₜ
  ferritin (*See also* FT)
ft
  feet
  foot (*See also* F, f)
  foot/feet (*See also* F, f)
FTA
  femorotibial angle
  fluorescein treponemal antibody
    (test)
  fluorescent titer antibody
  fluorescent treponemal antibody
    (test) (*See also* FTAT)
FTA-ABS, FTA-Abs
  fluorescence treponemal antibody
    absorption
  fluorescent treponemal antibody
    absorption (test)
FTA-ABS-DS
  fluorescent treponemal antibody
    absorption doublestaining
F-TAG
  fast-binding target-attaching globulin
FTAT
  fluorescent treponemal antibody test
    (*See also* FTA)
FTB
  fingertip blood
FTBD
  fit to be detained
  full term, born dead
FTBE
  focal tick-borne encephalitis
FTBI
  fractionated total body irradiation
FTBS
  Family Therapist Behavioral Scale
FTC
  fibulotalocalcaneal
  frames to come (optometry)
  frequency threshold curve
  full to confrontation

fTCD
  functional transcranial Doppler
    sonography
FTD
  failure to descend
  femoral total density
  frontotemporal dementia
  full-term delivery
FTE
  failure to engraft
  full-time equivalent (resident)
FTEQ
  Functional Time Estimation
    Questionnaire
FTF
  finger-to-finger (test)
  free thyroxine fraction
FTFTN
  finger-to-finger-to-nose (test)
FTG
  full-thickness graft
FTI
  farnesyltransferase inhibitor
  force-time integral
FT₃I
  free triiodothyronine index
FT4I, FT₄I
  free thyroxine index
  free T₄ index
FTIR
  Fourier transform infrared
    (spectroscopy)
  functional terminal innervation ratio
FTIUP
  full-term intrauterine pregnancy
FTJ
  femorotibial joint
FTKA
  failed to keep appointment
FTLB
  full-term live birth
ft·lbf
  foot pound-force
FTLD
  frontotemporal lobar degeneration
FTLE
  full-thickness local excision
FTLFC
  full-term living female child
FTLMC
  full-term living male child

F

NOTES

FTM
> fluid thioglycolate medium
> fractional test meal

FTN
> finger-to-nose (coordination test)
> (*See also* FN, F-N, F→N)
> full-term nursery

FTNB
> full-term newborn

FTND
> Fagerstrom Test for Nicotine
> Dependence
> full-term normal delivery

FTNS
> functional transcutaneous nerve
> stimulation

FTNSD
> full-term, normal, spontaneous
> delivery

FTO
> fructose-terminated oligosaccharide
> fulltime occlusion (eye patch)

FTOC
> fetal thymus organ culture

FTP
> failure to progress (in labor)
> full-term pregnancy

FTPA
> perfluorotripropylamine (blood
> substitute)

ft·pdl
> foot poundal

FTPSA, F:T PSA
> free to total prostate-specific
> antigen

FTQ
> Fagerstrom tolerance questionnaire

FTR
> failed to report
> failed to respond
> father
> force translation
> fractional turnover rate
> for the record

FTRAM
> free transverse rectus abdominis
> myocutaneous (flap)

FTS
> face-to-side
> Family Tracking System
> feminizing testis syndrome
> fetal tobacco syndrome
> fingertips
> fissured tongue syndrome
> serum thymic factor [Fr. *facteur
> thymique sérique*]

FTSD
> full-term spontaneous delivery

FTSG
> full-thickness skin graft

FTSP
> fallopian tube sperm perfusion

FTT
> failure to thrive
> fat tolerance test
> fetal tissue transplant
> Finger-Tapping Test
> fraternal twins raised together
> fructose tolerance test

FTU
> fingertip unit
> fluorescence thiourea

Ftube
> feeding tube

FTUPLD
> full-term uncomplicated pregnancy,
> labor, and delivery

FTV
> fetal thrombotic vasculopathy
> Fortovase
> functional trial visit

FTW
> failure to wean

FTX
> field training exercise

FU
> fecal urobilinogen
> Finsen unit (*See also* Fu)
> followup (*See also* F/U)
> fractional urinalysis
> fraction unbound
> fundus (at umbilicus) (*See also*
> F/U)

F/U
> followup (*See also* FU)
> fundus at umbilicus (*See also* FU)

F↑U
> fingers above umbilicus
> (measurement)

F↓U
> fingers below umbilicus
> (measurement) (*See also* FBU)

F&U
> flanks and upper quadrants

FU-I
> first set of followup data

FU-II
> second set of followup data

Fu
> Finsen unit (*See also* FU)

FUB
> found under bridge
> functional uterine bleeding

FUC
> fucosidase

Fuc
    fucose
FUCA
    alpha-L-fucosidase
FU$_{CO}$
    functional uptake of carbon
      monoxide
FUD
    fear, uncertainty, and doubt
    full upper denture (*See also* F/)
FUdR
    circadian-modified floxuridine
    fluorodeoxyuridine
    5-fluoro-2-deoxyuridine
5-FUdR
    floxuridine
FUDS
    fluorourodynamic study
FUDT
    forensic urine drug testing
FU Dtr
    full upper denture
FUE
    fever of unknown etiology
FUFA
    free volatile fatty acid
FU/FL
    full upper, full lower (denture)
FUL
    federal upper limit (price list)
    functional urethral length
fulg
    fulguration
FU/LP
    full upper denture, partial lower
      denture
FUM
    fumarase
    fumarate
    fumigation
FUMP
    fluorouridine monophosphate
FUN
    followup note
func, funct
    function
    functional
FUNG-C
    fungus culture
FUNG-S
    fungus smear

FUO
    fever of undetermined origin
    fever of unknown origin
FUOV
    followup office visit
FUP
    followup
    follow up
    follow-up
fu p
    fusion point
FUR
    fluorouridine
    furosemide (*See also* FRS, FSM)
FUS
    feline urologic syndrome
    first-use syndrome
    fusion
FUT
    fibrinogen uptake test
FUTP
    fluorouridine triphosphate
FUV
    follow-up visit
FV
    femoral vein
    flow velocity
    flow volume
    fluid volume
    formaldehyde vapors
F(v)
    velocity distribution function
f/V$_t$
    frequency to tidal volume
FVA
    Friend virus anemia
FVC
    false vocal cord
    filled voiding flow rate (*See also*
      FVFR)
    forced vital capacity
FVCA
    forced vital capacity analysis
FVD
    fibrovascular tissue on disk
FVE
    fibrovascular tissue elsewhere
    forced volume, expiratory
FVFR
    filled voiding flow rate (*See also*
      FVC)

F

NOTES

FVH
focal vascular headache
fulminant viral hepatitis

F VIII
factor VIII

FVL
femoral vein ligation
flexible video laparoscope
flow-volume loop
force, velocity, length

FVM
familial visceral myopathy

FVN
familial visceral neuropathy

FVOP
finger venous opening pressure

FVP
Friend virus polycythemia

FVPTC
follicular variant of papillary
thyroid carcinoma

FVR
feline viral rhinotracheitis
forearm vascular resistance
fractional velocity reserve

FVS
fetal valproate syndrome
fetal varicella syndrome

FVU
first-void urine

FVWs
flow-velocity waveforms (umbilical
artery Doppler)

FW
fetal weight
Folin and Wu (method)
forced whisper
fracturing wall
fragment wound

F/W
followed with

Fw
F wave (fibrillatory wave, flutter
wave)

fw
fresh water

FWB
full weightbearing
functional well-being

FWCA
functional work capacity assessment

FWD
fairly well developed

FWHM
full width at half maximum
full width (of line-spread function)
half maximal height

full width (of photopeak measured
at) half maximal (count)
(tomography)

FWM
Folin-Wu method (*See also* FW)

FWR
Felix-Weil reaction
Folin-Wu reaction

FWS
fetal warfarin syndrome

FWW
front wheel walker

FX
fluoroscopy
fornix
fractional (*See also* F, fract, fx)

FX
factor X

fx
fractional (*See also* F, fract, FX)
fracture (*See also* frac, fract, frx,
FXR)
friction

Fx BB
fracture of both bones (*See also*
FRBB)

fx-dis
fracture-dislocation (*See also* F/D)

FXN
function (*See also* F, fn)

FXR
fracture (*See also* frac, fract, frx,
fx)

FXS
fragile X syndrome

FY
fiscal year
full year

FYA
Duffy antigen A positive
phenotype

FYAN
Duffy antigen A negative
phenotype

FYB
Duffy antigen B positive phenotype

FYBN
Duffy antigen B negative
phenotype

FYC
facultative yeast carrier

FYI
for your information

F-Y test
fibrinogen qualitative test

FZ
flutamide and goserelin acetate
focal zone

frontozygomatic
frozen section (*See also* FS)
furazolidone

Fz

frontal midline placement of
electrodes in
electroencephalography

FZD

fozivudine tidoxil

FZRC

frozen section red (blood) cell

NOTES

F

G

conductance
force (pull of gravity) (*See also* g)
gallop (heart sound)
ganglion
gap (in cell cycle)
gas (*See also* g)
gastrin
gastrostomy
gauss
gavage feeding
gender (*See also* GEN)
general factor (single variance common to different intelligence tests)
geometric efficiency
Gibbs free energy
Giemsa (banding stain)
giga-
gingiva
gingival
glabella
globular (protein)
globulin
glucose (*See also* Glc, GLU, gluc)
glycogen
gold inlay
gonidial (colony)
good
goose
grade (*See also* gr)
Grafenberg spot
Gram (stain)
gravida (pregnant)
gravitational (constant)
gravitational (unit)
gravity (unit)
Greek
green (*See also* GRN, Grn)
Gross (leukemia antigen)
guaiac
guanidine
guanine
gynecology
immunoglobulin G.
Newtonian constant of gravitation
unit of force of acceleration

G₀

gap₀
quiescent phase of cells leaving the mitotic cycle

G1, G₁

first pregnancy
gap 1

gap₁
grid 1 (in electroencephalography)
presynthetic gap (phase of cells prior to DNA synthesis)

G1–G6

grade 1–6 (heart murmur)

G_{II}

hexachlorophene

G2, G₂, G-II

gap 2
gap₂
grid 2 (in electroencephalography)
postsynthetic gap (phase of cells following DNA synthesis)
second pregnancy
secundigravida

GII

Generation II (orthotic)

G3

tertigravida
third pregnancy

G₄

dichlorophen

G+

guaiac positive

G⁺

gram-positive (*See also* GM+, GP, gr⁺, GrP)

G˙

guaiac negative

G⁻

gram-negative (*See also* GM–, GN, gr⁻, GrN)

G°

standard free energy

GΩ

gigaohm (one billion ohms)

g

acceleration (force)
gas (*See also* G)
gauge (of needle) (*See also* ga)
grain (*See also* GR, gr)
gram
gravity
group (*See also* GP, gp, grp)
ratio of magnetic moment of a particle to Bohr magneton
standard acceleration due to gravity, 9.80665 m/s^2

g%

gram percent (*See also* g/dL)

g

relative centrifugal force

G

GA
  gastric analysis
  gastric antrum
  general anesthesia (*See also* gen-an)
  general appearance
  genetic algorithm
  gentisic acid
  gestational age
  Getting Along (psychologic test)
  ginger ale (*See also* G'ale)
  gingivoaxial
  glucoamylase
  glucose/acetone
  glucuronic acid
  glycyrrhetinic acid
  Golgi apparatus
  gramicidin A
  granulocyte adherence
  granulocyte agglutination
  granuloma annulare
  guessed average
  gut-associated
  gyrate atrophy
G/A
  globulin/albumin (ratio)
  G/A recombinant
Ga
  gallium
Ga-67, ^{67}Ga
  gallium-67
  gallium citrate
^{68}Ga
  gallium-68
ga
  gauge (of needle) (*See also* g)
GAA
  gossypol acetic acid
GAAS
  Goldberg Anorectic Attitude Scale
GABA
  gamma-aminobutyric acid
  gamma-aminobutyric acidemia
GABA/BZD
  gamma-aminobutyric
    acid/benzodiazepine
GABA-T
  GABA transaminase
  gamma-aminobutyric acid
    transaminase
GABEB
  generalized atrophic benign
    epidermolysis bullosa
GABHS
  group A beta hemolytic
    streptococcus (*See also* GABS)
  group A β-hemolytic streptococcus
GABOA, GABOB
  gamma-amino-beta-hydroxybutyric

  gamma-amino-beta-hydroxybutyric
    acid
  hydroxyl derivative of GABA
GABS
  group A beta hemolytic
    streptococcus (*See also* GABHS)
GAD
  generalized anxiety disorder
  glutamate decarboxylase
  glutamic acid decarboxylase
GADH
  gastric alcohol dehydrogenase
gadolinium-DTPA
  gadolinium-diethylenetriamine
    pentaacetic acid
GADS
  gas atomized dispersion
    strengthened
  gonococcal arthritis/dermatitis
    syndrome
GAE
  granulomatous amebic encephalitis
GAEL
  Grammatical Analysis of Elicited
    Language
GAF
  geographic adjustment factors
  giant axon formation
  glia-activating factor
  global assessment of functioning
GAGUA
  glycosaminoglycan uronate
GAHS
  galactorrhea amenorrhea
    hyperprolactinemia syndrome
GAI
  guided affective imagery
GAIPAS
  General Audit Inpatient Psychiatric
    Assessment Scale
GAIT
  great toe arthroplasty implant
    technique
GAL
  galactose
  galactosemia
  galactosyl
  galanthamine hydrobromide
  gallus adenolike (virus)
  glucuronic acid lactone
gal
  gallon [L. *congius*]
gal 1–2
  Galius adenovirus 1–2
gal.
  gallon
GA LAW
  glucose, age, LDH, AST, WBC

G-ALB
　　globulin-albumin
GALC
　　galactocerebrosidase deficiency
GALE
　　uridine diphosphate-galactose-4-
　　　epimerase deficiency
G'ale
　　ginger ale (*See also* GA)
GALF
　　glycyrrhetinic acid like factor
GALK
　　galactokinase
gal/min
　　gallons per minute
GalN
　　galactosamine
GalNAc
　　N-acetyl-D-galactosamine
GALOP
　　gait disorder, autoantibody, late-age
　　　onset, polyneuropathy
gal-1-P
　　galactose-1-phosphate
GALS
　　Gait, Arms, Legs, and Spine
GALT
　　galactose-1-phosphate
　　　uridyltransfcrase
　　gastrointestinal-associated lymphoid
　　　tissue
　　gut-associated lymphoid tissue
GalTase
　　4-galactosyltransferase
GAL TT
　　galactose tolerance test
GALV
　　gibbon ape leukemia virus
GaLV
　　gibbon ape lymphosarcoma virus
Galv, galv
　　galvanic
　　galvanism
　　galvanized
GAMA
　　General Ability Measure for Adults
GAMG
　　goat antimouse immunoglobulin G
γ, gamma
　　activity coefficient
　　carbon separated from the carboxyl
　　　group by two other carbon atoms

chain of fetal hemoglobin
constituent of gamma protein
　plasma fraction
gamma (third letter of Greek
　alphabet), lowercase
10^{-4} gauss
heavy chain of immunoglobulin G
monomer in fetal hemoglobin
photon (gamma ray) (*See also* hv)
plasma protein (globulin)
Γ, gamma
　　gamma (third letter of Greek
　　　alphabet), uppercase
gamma-BHC
　　gamma-benzenc hexachloride
　　　(lindane) (*See also* GBH)
gamma-GTP
　　gamma-glutamyl transpeptidase
gamma-HCD
　　gamma-heavy-chain disease
gamma-HCH
　　hexachlorocyclohexane (lindane)
　　　(*See also* HCC, HCH)
gamma-MSH
　　gamma-melanocyte-stimulating
　　　hormone
gamma-T
　　gamma-tocopherol
γ-T
　　gamma-tocopherol
GAMT
　　guanidinoacetate methyltransferase
GAMV
　　Gamboa virus
GAN
　　giant axonal neuropathy
gang, gangl
　　ganglion
　　ganglionic
GANS
　　granulomatous angiitis of the
　　　central nervous system
GANT
　　gastrointestinal autonomic nerve
　　　tumor
GAP

Gardner Analysis of Personality
　(Survey)
general all purpose
glans approximation procedure
glyceraldehyde phosphate
GnRH-associated peptide

G

NOTES

285

GAP *(continued)*
gonadotropin-releasing hormone-
associated peptide
growth-associated protein
GTPase-activating protein
guanosine triphosphate-activating
protein

GAP-43
growth-associated protein-43

GAPD, GAPDH
glyceraldehyde phosphate
dehydrogenase
glyceraldehyde-3-phosphate
dehydrogenase

GAPO
growth retardation, alopecia,
pseudoanodontia, and optic
atrophy (syndrome)

GAPS
Guidelines for Adolescent
Preventive Services

GAR
genitoanorectal (syndrome)
goat antirabbit gamma globulin
(*See also* GARGG)
gonococcal antibody reaction

GARF
Global Assessment of Relational
Functioning

GARFT
glycinamide ribonucleotide formyl
transferase

garg
gargle

GARGG
goat antirabbit gamma globulin
(*See also* GAR)

GARS
Gait Abnormality Rating Scale

GARS-M
Gait Abnormality Rating Scale
Modified

GART
genotypic antiretroviral resistance
testing

GAS
galactorrhea-amenorrhea syndrome
gastric acid secretion
gastroenterology
gene-activating sequence
general adaptation syndrome
generalized arteriosclerosis
Glasgow Assessment Schedule
Goal Attainment Scale
group A *Streptococcus*

GASA
growth-adjusted sonographic age

Gas Anal F&T
gastric analysis, free and total

Ga scan
gallium scan

GASP
gastric augment and single pedicle
tube

GAST, gastroc
gastrocnemius (muscle)
gonadotropin agonist stimulation
test

gastro
gastroenterology
gastrointestinal

GAT
gas antitoxin
gelatin agglutination test
geriatric assessment team
Gerontological Apperception Test
group adjustment therapy

GATase
6-alkyl guanine alkyl transferase

GATB
General Aptitude Test Battery

GAU
geriatric assessment unit

GAV
Grand Arbaud virus

gav
gavage

GAVE
gastric antral vascular ectasia

Gaw
airway conductance (*See also* C_{AW},
C_{aw})

GAX
glutaraldehyde cross-linked collagen

GAZT
glucuronide derivative of
azidothymidine

GB
gallbladder
Ginkgo biloba
glass bead
glial bundle
goofball (barbiturate pill)
Guillain-Barré (syndrome)

G&B
good and bad (days)

gb
gallbladder channel (acupuncture)

GBA
ganglionic blocking agent
gingivobuccoaxial

GBCE
Grassi Basic Cognitive Evaluation

GBD
gallbladder disease

gender behavior disorder
glassblower's disease
granulomatous bowel disease

GBE

Ginkgo biloba extract

GBEF

gallbladder ejection fraction

GBER

gallbladder ejection rate

GBF

gingival blood flow

GBG

glycine-rich beta-glycoprotein
gonadal steroid-binding globulin

GBH

gamma-benzene hexachloride
(lindane) (*See also* gamma-BHC)
graphite, benzalkonium, heparin

GBI

gingival bleeding index
globulin-bound insulin

GBIA

Guthrie bacterial inhibition assay

GBL

gamma-butyrolactone
glomerular basal lamina

GBM

glioblastoma multiforme
glomerular basement membrane

GBMI

guilty but mentally ill

GBO

gastric bacterial overgrowth

GBP

gabapentin (*See also* GP)
galactose-binding protein
gastric bypass
gastric bypass procedure
gated blood pool

GBPS

gallbladder pigment stones
gated blood-pool study

GBq

gigabecquerel

GBR

gamma band response (audiology)
good blood return
guided bone regeneration

GBS

gallbladder series
gastric bypass surgery
glycerine-buffered saline

group B (beta-hemolytic)
streptococcus
group B streptococcal sepsis
group B streptococcus
Guillain-Barré syndrome (*See also*
GB)

GBSS

Grey balanced saline solution

GBT

gastric bleeding time

GBV

GB virus

GBV-C

GB virus C

GBV-C/HGV

GB virus C/hepatitis G virus

GBV-C/HGV-RNA

hepatitis G virus RNA

GBW

generalized body weakness

GBX

gall bladder extraction
(cholecystectomy)

GC

ganglion cell
gas chromatography
gastric cancer
gel chromatography
general circulation
general closure
general condition
geriatric care
geriatric chair
germinal center
gingival crevice
gingival curettage
glucocorticoid
glycocholate
goblet cell
Golgi complex
goniocurettage
gonococcal (infection)
gonococcus (*See also* GN)
gonorrhea culture
good condition
graham cracker
granular cast
granular cyst
granule cell
granulocyte cytotoxic
granulomatous colitis
granulosa cell

NOTES

G

GC (*continued*)
    group-specific component
    guanine cytosine
    guanylcyclase

G-C
    gram-negative cocci (*See also* GMC)

G+C
    gram-positive cocci (*See also* GPC)

Gc
    gigacycle
    group-specific component

GCA
    gastric cancerous area
    germinal cell aplasia
    ghost cell ameloblastoma
    giant cell arteritis

g-cal
    gram calorie (small calorie) (*See also* gm cal)

GCB
    gonococcal base

GCBM
    glomerular capillary basement

GCBP
    gated cardiac blood pool

GCC
    giant cell collagenoma
    goblet cell carcinoid
    guanylyl cyclase C

GCD
    giant colonic diverticulum

GCDAS
    Gesell Child Development Age Scale

GCDFP
    gross cystic disease fluid protein

GCDP
    gross cystic disease protein

GCE
    general conditioning exercise

GCF
    giant cell fibroblastoma
    gingival crevicular fluid
    greatest common factor

GCFT
    gonococcal complement-fixation test
    gonorrhea complement-fixation test

G-CFU
    granulocyte colony-forming unit

GCH
    giant cell hepatitis

GCI
    General Cognitive Index
    gestational carbohydrate intolerance

GCII
    glucose-controlled insulin infusion

GCIS
    isolated gland carcinoma in situ

GCKD
    glomerulocystic kidney disease

GCM
    geriatric care manager
    good control maintained

g-cm
    gram-centimeter

GCMN
    giant congenital melanocytic nevus

GC-MS, GC/MS
    gas chromatographic-mass spectrometry
    gas chromatography-mass spectrometry

GCP
    gentamicin, clindamycin, and polymyxin topical preparation
    good clinical practices

GCPS
    Greig cephalopolysyndactyly syndrome

GCR
    gastrocolonic response
    glucocerebrosidase
    glucocorticoid receptor
    Group Conformity Rating

GCRH
    glucose counterregulatory hormone

GCRS
    gynecological chylous reflux syndrome

GCS
    general clinical service
    Generalized Contentment Scale
    Glasgow Coma Scale
    Glasgow Coma Score
    glucocorticosteroid
    glutamylcysteine synthetase
    graduated compression stockings

Gc/s
    gigacycles per second

GCSA
    Gross cell surface antigen

GCSF, G-CSF
    granulocyte colony-stimulating factor

G-CSF-R
    granulocyte colony-stimulating factor receptor

GCST
    Gibson-Cooke sweat test

GCT
    general care and treatment
    General Clerical Test
    germ-cell tumor
    giant-cell thyroiditis
    giant-cell transformation

giant-cell tumor
granular cell tumor
granulosa cell tumor
GCT-LMP
giant-cell tumor of low malignant potential
GCTSPS
germ-cell tumor with synchronous lesions in pineal and suprasellar region
GCTTS
giant-cell tumor of tendon sheath
GCU
gonococcal urethritis
GCV
ganciclovir
great cardiac vein
GCVF
great cardiac vein flow
GCW
glomerular capillary wall
GCY
gastroscopy
GD
gastric distension
gastroduodenal
Gaucher disease
general diagnostics
general dispensary
general duties
generalized delays
gestational day
gestational diabetes
glare disability
gonadal dysgenesis
gravely disabled
Graves disease
growth and development (*See also* G&D)
G&D
growth and development (*See also* GD)
Gd
gadolinium
gd
good
GDA
gastroduodenal artery
germine diacetate
GDB
gas-density balance

Gd-BOPTA
gadolinium benzylopropionic tetracetate
GDC
giant dopamine-containing cell
Guglielmi detachable coil
Gd-CDTA
gadolinium cyclohexanediaminetetraacetic acid
GDD
glaucoma drainage device
Gd-DOTA
gadolinium tetraazacyclododecanetetraacetic acid
Gd-DTPA
gadolinium-diethylenetriamine pentaacetic acid
Gd-DTPA-BMA
gadolinium-diethylenetriamine pentaacetic acid-bismethylamide
Gd-EDTA
gadolinium in chelated form
gadolinium ethylenediaminetetraacetic acid
gadolinium ethylenediamine tetraacetic acid
Gd-EOB-DTPA
gadolinium EOB-DTPA
GDF
growth differentiation factor
GDF-9
growth differentiation factor-9
GD FA
grandfather (*See also* GF, GR-FR)
GDH
glucose dehydrogenase
glutamate dehydrogenase
glutamic acid dehydrogenase
glycerophosphate dehydrogenase
gonadotropic hormone
growth and differentiation hormone (in insects)
Gd-HP-DO3A
gadoteridol
GDID
genetically determined immunodeficiency disease
g/dL
grams per deciliter (*See also* g%)
GDM
gestational diabetes mellitus

NOTES

G

GDM A-1
gestational diabetes mellitus, insulin controlled, type 1

GDM A-2
gestational diabetes mellitus, diet controlled, type 2

Gd-MRI
gadolinium-enhanced magnetic resonance imaging

GDN
glyceryl dinitrate

gdn
guardian

GDNF
glial cell line-derived neurotropic factor
glial-derived neurotrophic factor

GDP
gastroduodenal pylorus
gel diffusion precipitin
guanosine diphosphate
guanosine 5′-diphosphate
guanyldiphosphate

GDR
glucose disposal rate

GDS
Geriatric Depression Scale
Gesell Developmental Scale
Gesell Developmental Schedules
Global Deterioration Scale
Gordon diagnostic system
gradual dosage schedule

GDSS
Glasgow Dyspepsia Severity Score

GDT
gel development time

Gd-Tex
gadolinium texaphyrin

GDW
glass-distilled water

GE
gainfully employed
gastric emptying
gastroemotional
gastroenteritis
gastroenterology
gastroenterostomy
gastroesophageal
gastrointestinal endoscopy
gel electrophoresis
generalized epilepsy
generator of excitation
genome equivalent
glandular epithelium

G/E
granulocyte/erythroid (ratio)

Ge
Gerbich red cell antigen
germanium

GEA
gastroepiploic artery

GEC
galactose elimination capacity
glomerular epithelial cell

GED
General Education Development (high school equivalency)
graduated electronic decelerator

GEE
Global Evaluation of Efficacy
glycine ethyl ester
graft enteric erosion

GEF
gastroesophageal fundoplication
glossoepiglottic fold
gonadotropin-enhancing factor
graft enteric fistula

GEFT
Group Embedded Figures Test

GEH
glycerol ester hydrolase

GEI
Grief Experience Inventory

GEIN
gradual elongation intramedullary nailing

GEJ
gastroesophageal junction

gel.
gelatin

GELS
gravity extension locking system

GEM
gemfibrozil
generalized erythema multiforme

GEM 91
25-mer phosphorothioate oligomer

GEMS
good emergency mother substitute

GEMU
geriatric evaluation and management unit

GEN
gender (*See also* G)
generation
genetics (*See also* gen, genet)
genital (*See also* gen, genit)
gradual elongation nailing

gen
general (*See also* gen'l)
genetics (*See also* GEN, genet)
genital (*See also* GEN, genit)
genus

gen-an
general anesthesia (*See also* GA)
gen-endo
general anesthesia with endotracheal intubation
genet
genetic
genetics (*See also* GEN, gen)
gen. et sp. nov.
new genus and species [L. *genus et species nova*]
genit
genital (*See also* GEN, gen)
genitalia
gen'l
general (*See also* gen)
gen. nov.
new genus [L. *genus novum*]
gen proc
general procedure
GENPS
genital neoplasm-papilloma syndrome
gent.
gentamicin (*See also* GM)
genta/P
gentamicin peak (level)
genta/T
gentamicin trough (level)
GEP
gastric emptying procedure
gastroenteropancreatic
GEPG
gastroesophageal pressure gradient
GEQ
generic equivalent
GER
gastroesophageal reflux
geriatrics (*See also* geriat)
granular endoplasmic reticulum
Ger
German
GERD
gastroesophageal reflux disease
geriat
geriatric
geriatrics (*See also* GER)
GERL
Golgi endoplasmic reticulum lysosome
Geront
gerontologic

gerontologist
gerontology
GERV
Germiston virus
GES
Gifted Evaluation Scale
glucose-electrolyte solution
Group Encounter Scale
Group Encounter Survey
Group Environment Scale
GE SPECT
gradient-echo single-photon emission computed tomography
GEST, gest
gestation
GET
gastric emptying time
graded (treadmill) exercise test
GET1/2, GET½
gastric emptying half-time
GETA
general endotracheal anesthesia
GETV
gadolinium-enhancing tumor volume
Getah virus
GEU
geriatric evaluation unit
gestation, extrauterine
GeV
gigaelectron volt
GEX
gas exchange
GF
gastric fistula
gastric fluid
germ-free
glass factor (tissue culture)
globule fibril
glomerular filtrate
glomerular filtration
gluten-free
grandfather (*See also* GR-FR, GD FA)
griseofulvin
growth factor
growth failure
growth fraction
G-F
globular-fibrous (protein)
gf
gram-force

NOTES

G

GFA
> glial fibrillary acidic (protein)
> global force applicator

GFAP
> glial fibrillary acidic protein

GF-BAO
> gastric fluid, basal acid output

GFCL
> Goldmann fundus contact lens

GFD
> gluten-free diet
> Goodenough Figure Drawing

GFFF
> gravitational field-flow fractionation

GFFS
> glycogen- and fat-free solid

GFH
> glucose-free Hanks (solution)

GFI
> glucagon-free insulin
> ground-fault interrupter

GFJ
> grapefruit juice (*See also* GJ)

GFL
> giant follicular lymphoma

GFM
> good fetal movement

GFP
> gamma-fetoprotein
> gel-filtered platelet
> glomerular-filtered phosphate
> green fluorescent protein

GFPM
> gastric first-pass metabolism (of ethanol)

GFR
> glomerular filtration rate
> grunting, flaring, and retracting (breathing)

GFS
> glaucoma filtering surgery
> global focal sclerosis

GFT
> gradient field transform

GFTA
> Goldman-Fristoe Test of Articulation

GFV
> Gabek Forest virus

G-F-W
> Goldman-Fristoe-Woodcock (Auditory Skills Test Battery)

GFX
> grepafloxacin

GG
> gamma globulin
> genioglossus
> glyceryl guaiacolate
> glycylglycine
> guar gum

G=G
> grips equal and good

GGA
> general gonadotropic activity
> ground-glass attenuation

GGCT
> ground-glass clotting time

GGE
> Gastrografin enema
> generalized glandular enlargement
> gradient gel electrophoresis

ggELISA
> glycoprotein-based enzyme-linked immunosorbent assay

GGFC
> gamma globulin-free calf (serum)

GGG
> gambodium
> glycine-rich gamma-glycoprotein

GGM
> glucose-galactose malabsorption

GGO
> ground-glass opacification
> ground-glass opacity

GGPNA
> gamma-glutamyl-*p*-nitroanilide

GGPP
> geranylgeranylpyrophosphate

GGS, GG or S
> glands, goiter, or stiffness (of neck)
> group G streptococcus

GGT
> gamma-glutamyltransferase
> gamma-glutamyl transpeptidase (*See also* GGTP)

GGTP
> gamma-glutamyl transpeptidase (*See also* GGT)

GGU
> giant gastric ulcer

GGV
> Gan Gan virus

GgV-019/6A
> *Gaeumannomyces graminis* virus 019/6-A

GGVB
> gelatin, glucose, and Veronal buffer
> glucose-gelatin Veronal buffer

GgV-87-1-H
> *Gaeumannomyces graminis* virus 87-1-H

GgV-T1-A
> *Gaeumannomyces graminis* virus T1-A

GGYV
    Gadget's Gully virus
GH
    Gee-Herter (disease)
    general health
    general hospital
    genetically hypertensive (rat)
    genetic hemochromatosis
    genetic hypertension
    geniohyoid
    gingival hyperplasia
    glenohumeral
    good health
    growth hormone
GH3
    Gerovital
GHA
    glucoheptanoic acid
GHAQ
    General High Altitude
        Questionnaire
GHB
    gamma hydroxybutyrate
GHb
    glycosylated hemoglobin
GHBA
    gamma-hydroxybutyric acid
GHBP
    growth hormone-binding protein
GHBSS
    gelatin Hank buffered salt solution
GHCH
    giant hepatic cavernous
        hemangioma
GHD
    growth hormone deficiency
GHDA
    growth hormone deficiency
        (syndrome) in adults
GHDT
    Goodenough-Harris Drawing Test
GHI
    growth hormone insensitivity
    growth hormone insufficiency
GHIH, GH-IH
    growth hormone-inhibiting hormone
    growth hormone inhibitory hormone
GHJ, G-H jt
    glenohumeral joint
GHK
    Goldman-Hodgkin-Katz (equation)

GHL
    glenohumeral ligament
GH-N
    growth hormone (normal)
GHPP
    Genetically Handicapped Persons
        Program
GHPQ
    General Health Perception
        Questionnaire
GHQ
    General Health Questionnaire
GHR
    granulomatous hypersensitivity
        reaction
    growth hormone receptor
GHRD
    growth hormone receptor deficiency
GHRF, GH-RF
    growth hormone-releasing factor
        (*See also* GRF)
GHRH, GH-RH
    growth hormone-releasing hormone
        (*See also* GRH)
GHRH-R
    growth hormone-releasing hormone
        receptor
GHRIF, GH-RIF
    growth hormone release-inhibiting
        factor (*See also* GRIF)
    growth hormone-release inhibiting
        factor
GHRIH, GH-RIH
    growth hormone release-inhibiting
        hormone
GHRP
    growth hormone-releasing peptide
GHS
    growth hormone secretagogue
GHSR
    growth hormone secretagogue
        receptor
GHST
    growth hormone stimulation test
GHT
    geniculohypothalamic tract
GH-V
    growth hormone (variant)
GHV
    goose hepatitis virus
GHz
    gigahertz

G

NOTES

293

GI
gastrointestinal
gelatin infusion (medium)
General Inquiry
Gingival Index
globin insulin
glomerular index
glucose intolerance
granuloma inguinale
growth inhibiting
growth inhibition

Gi
good impression (California Psychological Inventory)

gi
gill (¼ pint) (*See also* gl)

G$_i$
G inhibiting protein

GIA
gastrointestinal anastomosis
gastrointestinal anisakiasis
gastrointestinal assistant
Global Institute for Asthma

GIB
gastric ileal bypass
gastrointestinal bleeding

GIBF
gastrointestinal bacterial flora

GIC
gastric interdigestive contraction
general immunocompetence

GICA
gastrointestinal cancer antigen
gastrointestinal cancer-associated antigen

GID
gastrointestinal distress
gender identity disorder

GIDA
gastrointestinal diagnostic area

GIF
glycosylation-inhibiting factor
gonadotropin-inhibitory factor (somatostatin)
growth hormone-inhibiting factor

GIFT
gamete intrafallopian transfer
gamete intrafallopian tube transfer
granulocyte immunofluorescence test

GIGO
garbage in, garbage out (computers)

GIH
gastric-inhibitory hormone
gastrointestinal hemorrhage
gastrointestinal hormone
growth hormone-inhibiting hormone
growth-inhibiting hormone

GIK
glucose-insulin-potassium
glucose, insulin, and potassium
glucose-insulin-potassium (solution)

GIL
gastrointestinal (tract) lymphoma

GILCU
gradual increase in length and complexity of utterance

GIM
gonadotropin-inhibiting material
gonadotropin-inhibitory material

GING
gingivectomy

ging
gingiva
gingival

g-ion
gram-ion

GIOP
glucocorticoid (steroid)-induced osteoporosis

GIP
gastric inhibitory peptide
gastric inhibitory polypeptide
gastrointestinal polyposis
giant (cell) interstitial pneumonia
giant (cell) interstitial pneumonitis
glucose-dependent insulin-releasing peptide
glucose insulinotropic peptide
gonorrheal invasive peritonitis

GIPACT
gastrointestinal pacemaker cell tumor

GIPU
gastrointestinal procedure unit

GIQLI
Gastrointestinal Quality of Life Index

GIR
Global Improvement Rating

GIRMS
gas isotope ratio mass spectrometry

GIS
gas in stomach
gastrointestinal series
gastrointestinal symptom
gastrointestinal system
Gender Identity Service

GISA
glycopeptide-insensitive *Staphylococcus aureus*
glycopeptide intermediate-resistant *Staphylococcus aureus*
glycopeptide-intermediate *Staphylococcus aureus*

GIST
 gastrointestinal smooth muscle tumor
 gastrointestinal stromal tumor

GIT
 gastrointestinal tract
 glutathione-insulin transhydrogenase

GITS
 gastrointestinal therapeutic system
 gut-derived infectious toxic shock

GITT
 gastrointestinal transit time
 glucose insulin tolerance test

GITUP
 glanduloplasty and in situ tubularization of urethral plate
 glansplasty and in situ tubularization of urethral plate
 glanuloplasty and in situ tubularization of urethral plate

GIV
 gastrointestinal virus
 Great Island virus

giv
 give
 given

GIWU
 gastrointestinal workup

GJ
 gap junction
 gastric juice
 gastrojejunostomy
 grapefruit juice (See also GFJ)

GJAV
 Guajara virus

GJIC
 gap junction intercellular communication

GJT
 gastrojejunostomy tube

GK
 galactokinase
 glomerulocystic kidney
 glucokinase
 glycerol kinase

GKA
 guinea pig keratocyte

GKD
 glycerol kinase deficiency

GKI
 glucose potassium insulin

GKMDT
 Graham-Kendall Memory for Designs Test

GKN
 glucose-potassium-sodium

GL
 gastric lavage
 germline
 gland (See also gl)
 glaucoma
 glomerular layer
 glucagon
 glycolipid
 glycosphingolipoid
 granular layer
 greatest length (fetus)
 gustatory lacrimation

Gl
 glabella

g/L
 grams per liter

gl
 gill (¼ pint) (See also gi)
 gland (See also GL)
 glandular (See also gland.)

GLA
 alpha-galactosidase
 gamma-carboxyglutamic acid
 gamma linolenic acid
 gene-linkage analysis
 giant left atrium
 gingivolinguoaxial
 D-glucaric acid
 glucose-lowering agents

Gla
 4-carboxyglutamic acid
 gamma-carboxyglutamic acid

glac
 glacial

GLAD
 gold-labeled antigen detection (technique)

gland.
 glandular (See also gl)

GLAT
 galactose (enzyme) activator

glau
 glaucoma (See also glc)

GLB
 gay, lesbian, bisexual

GLB-1
 beta-galactosidase-1

NOTES

G

GLC
gas-liquid chromatography
Glc
d-glucose
glucose (*See also* G, GLU, gluc)
glc
glaucoma (*See also* glau)
GlcA
gluconic acid
GLC/MS
gas-liquid chromatography/mass spectrometry
GlcN
glucosamine
GlcNAc
N-acetylglucosamine
GlcUA
glucuronic acid
GLD
glanders (*Actinobacillus mallei*) vaccine
globoid leukodystrophy
glutamate dehydrogenase (*See also* GLDH)
GLDH
glutamate dehydrogenase (*See also* GLD)
GLH
germinal layer hemorrhage
giant lymph node hyperplasia
GLI
glicentin
glucagon-like immunoreactivity
GLIM
generalized linear interactive model
generalized linear interactive modeling
GLIO
glioblastoma
glio
glioma
GLIP
glucagonlike insulinotropic peptide
GLL
glabellolambda line (craniometric point)
GLM
general linear model
GLMA
gastric laryngeal mask airway
GLN
glomerulonephritis
Gln
glucagon
glutamine (*See also* Q)
GLNH
giant lymph node hyperplasia

GLNS
gay lymph node syndrome (obsolete)
GLO, glo
glyoxalase
glob.
globular
globulin
GLOC
gravity induced loss of consciousness
GLOF
global level of functioning
GLORIA
gold-labeled optical rapid immunoassay
GLOV
Gray Lodge virus
GLP
glucagon-like peptide
glucose-L-phosphate
glycolipoprotein
good laboratory practice
grid laser photocoagulation
group-living program
GLP-1
glucagon-like peptide-1
Glp
5-oxoproline
GLPC
gas-liquid phase chromatography
GLPD
granular lymphocyte-proliferative disorder
GLPP, GL-PP
glucose, postprandial
GLPT
glutamate pyruvate transaminase
GLR
graphic level recorder
gravity lumbar reduction
GLS
gait lock splint
generalized lymphadenopathy syndrome
guinea (pig) lung strip
GLSH
glucose, lactalbumin, serum, and hemoglobin
GLTN
glomerulotubulonephritis
GLTT
glucose-lactate tolerance test
GLU, glu
glucose (*See also* G, Glc, gluc)
glucuronidase
glutamic acid
glutamine

GLU-5
 five-hour glucose tolerance test
Glu
 glutamic acid (*See also* E)
GluA
 glucuronic acid
GLUC
 glucosidase
gluc
 glucose (*See also* G, Glc, GLU)
GLUC-S
 urine glucose spot (test)
glucur
 glucuronide
glu ox.
 glucose oxidase
GluR1
 glutamide receptor subunit
GLUS
 granulomatous lesions of unknown
  significance
GLUT
 glucose transporter
GLUT-1, GLUT1
 glucose-transport protein 1
GLUT-2, GLUT2
 glucose-transport protein 2
GLUT-3, GLUT3
 glucose-transport protein 3
GLUT-4, GLUT4
 glucose-transport protein 4
GLUT-5, GLUT5
 glucose-transport protein 5
GLUT-6, GLUT6
 glucose-transport protein 6
GLUT-7, GLUT7
 glucose-transport protein 7
GLV
 Gross leukemia virus
 Gumbo Limbo virus
Glx
 glutamic acid
 glutaminyl and/or glutamyl
  (indicates uncertainty between Glu
  and Gln)
GLY, gly
 glycerite (*See also* glyc)
 glycerol (*See also* glyc)
 glycyl
Gly
 glycine (*See also* G)

glyc
 glyceride
 glycerin
 glycerite (*See also* GLY)
 glycerol (*See also* GLY)
GM
 gastric mucosa
 Geiger-Müller (counter)
 general medical
 general medicine
 genetically modified
 genetic manipulation
 gentamicin (*See also* gent.)
 geometric mean
 giant melanosome
 gingival margin
 grand mal
 grandmother (*See also* GR-MO)
 grand multiparity
 granulocyte-macrophage
 granulocyte-monocyte
 gray matter
 growth medium
 monosialoganglioside (genetic
  marker)
GM+
 gram-positive (*See also* G$^+$, GP,
  gr$^-$, GrP)
GM−
 gram-negative (*See also* G$^-$, GN,
  gr$^-$, GrN)
Gm
 gamma (allotype marker on heavy
  chains of immunoglobins)
g/m
 gallons per minute
g-m
 gram-meter
GMA
 glyceral methacrylate
 glycol methacrylate
 gross motor activity
GMAV
 Guama virus
GMB
 gastric mucosal barrier
 granulomembranous body
GMBF
 gastric mucosal blood flow
GMC
 general medical clinic
 general medical condition

G

NOTES

GMC *(continued)*
> geometric mean concentration
> giant migrating contraction
> grivet monkey cell

gm cal
> gram calorie (small calorie) (*See also* g-cal)

gm/cc
> grams per cubic centimeter

GMCD
> grand mal convulsive disorder

GM-CFU
> granulocyte-macrophage colony-forming unit

GM-CSA
> granulocyte-macrophage colony-stimulating activity

GM-CSF
> granulocyte-macrophage colony-stimulating factor

GMCU
> gracilis myocutaneous unit

GMD
> geometric mean diameter
> glycopeptide moiety (modified) derivative

GMDS
> Griffiths Mental Developmental Scale

GME
> gaseous microembolus
> graduate medical education

GMEPP
> giant miniature endplate potential

GMER
> gastric mucosal ectopia in rectum

GMF
> general medical floor
> glia maturation factor

GMFM
> Gross Motor Function Measure

GMH
> germinal matrix hemorrhage

GMK
> green monkey kidney (cells)

GML
> glabellomeatal line
> gut mucosal lymphocyte

g/mL
> grams per milliliter

GMLOS
> geometric mean length of stay

GMM
> Goldberg-Maxwell-Morris (syndrome)

GMN
> gradient moment nulling

g-mol
> gram-molecule

GMOs
> genetically modified organisms

G-MP
> G-myeloma protein

GMP
> general medical panel
> Good Manufacturing Practices
> guanosine monophosphate
> guanosine 5′-monophosphate
> guanylic acid (reductase, synthetase)

3′,5′-GMP
> guanosine 3′,5′-cyclic phosphate

GMP-K
> guanylate kinase

GMR
> gallops, murmurs, or rubs
> gradient moment reduction
> gradient moment rephasing
> gradient motion rephasing

GMS
> Galloway-Mowat syndrome
> galvanic muscle stimulation
> general medicine and surgery (*See also* GM&S)
> glyceryl monostearate
> Gomori methenamine silver (stain)
> goniodysgenesis, mental retardation, short stature
> Grocott-Gomori methenamine silver nitrate
> Grocott methenamine silver (stain)

GM&S
> general medicine and surgery (*See also* GMS)

GMSPS
> Glasgow Meningococcal Septicemia Prognostic Score

GMT
> geometric mean (antibody) titer
> geometric mean titer
> gingival margin trimmer
> Greenwich Mean Time

GMV
> gram-molecular volume

GMW
> gram-molecular weight

GN
> ganglioneuroma
> gaze nystagmus
> glomerulonephritis
> glucagon
> glucose/nitrogen (ratio in water)
> gnotobiote
> gonococcus (*See also* GC)
> gram-negative (*See also* G⁻, GM–, gr⁻, GrN)

G/N
glucose/nitrogen (ratio in urine)
(*See also* GN, G/Nr)

Gn
gnathion
gonadotropin

GNA
Galanthus nivalis agglutinin
general nursing assistance

GNB
ganglioneuroblastoma
gram-negative bacillus
gram-negative bacteremia

GNBL
ganglioneuroblastoma

GNBM
gram-negative bacillary meningitis

GNC
general nursing care
glandular neck cell
gram-negative cocci (*See also* G-C)

GNCA
gastric noncancerous area

GND
gram-negative diplococcus

gnd
ground

GNG
generalized nephrographic

GNID
gram-negative intracellular
diplococcus

GNR
gram-negative rod (*See also* G-R)

G/Nr
glucose/nitrogen ratio (in urine)
(*See also* GN, G/N)

GNRF
guanine nucleotide-releasing factor

GnRF
gonadotropin-releasing factor (*See
also* GRF)

GnRH, Gn-RH
gonadotropin-releasing hormone (*See
also* GRH)

GnRHa
gonadotropin-releasing hormone
agonist

GnRH-R
gonadotropin-releasing hormone
receptor

GNRP
guanine nucleotide regulatory
protein

GNS
gram-negative sepsis

G/NS
glucose in normal saline

GnSAF
gonadotropin surge attenuating
factor

GO
glucose oxidase (*See also* GOD)
gonorrhea
Graves ophthalmopathy
Greek Orthodox

G&O
gas and oxygen

Go
Golgi
gonion

GOA
generalized osteoarthritis

GOAT
Galveston Orientation and Amnesia
Test
Galveston Orientation and
Awareness Test

GOBAB
gamma-hydroxy-beta-aminobutyric
acid

GOBI
growth monitoring, oral rehydration,
breast feeding, and immunization

GOCL-II
Gordon Occupational Checklist-II

GOCS
Global Obsessive-Compulsive Scale

GOD
generation of diversity
glucose oxidase (*See also* GO)

GOD/POD
glucose oxidase-perioxidase
(method)

GOE
gas, oxygen, and ether (anesthesia)

GOH
geroderma osteodysplastica
hereditaria

GOL
glabelloopisthion line

NOTES

G

GOLPH
Giannetti Online Psychosocial History

GOM
granular osmiophilic material

GOMBO
growth retardation, ocular abnormalities, microcephaly, brachydactyly, oligophrenia

GOMV
Gomoka virus

GON
gonococcal ophthalmia neonatorum
greater occipital neuritis

GONA
glaucomatous optic nerve atrophy

GOND
glaucomatous optic nerve damage

gonio
gonioscopy

GOO
gastric outlet obstruction

GO-POG
gonion to pogonion (craniometric)

GOQ
glucose oxidation quotient

GOR
gastroesophageal reflux
general operating room

GORD
gastro-oesophageal reflux disease (United Kingdom)

GORT
Gilmore Oral Reading Test
Gray Oral Reading Test

GORT-3
Gray Oral Reading Test, Third Edition

GORT-R
Gray Oral Reading Test-Revised

GORV
Gordil virus

GOS
Glasgow Outcome Scale
Glasgow Outcome Score

GOSV
Gossas virus

GOT
glucose oxidase test
glutamic-oxaloacetic transaminase (aspartate aminotransferase)
goals of treatment

GOTM, GOT-M
glutamic-oxaloacetic transaminase, mitochondrial

GOT-S
glutamic-oxaloacetic transaminase, soluble

govt
government

GP
gabapentin (*See also* GBP)
gastroplasty
general paralysis
general paresis
general practice
general practitioner
general proprioception
general purpose
genetic prediabetes
geometric progression
globus pallidus
glucose phosphate
glucose polymer
glucose production
glutathione peroxidase
glycerophosphate
glycopeptide
glycoprotein
gram-positive (*See also* G$^+$, GM+, gr$^+$, GrP)
group (*See also* g, gp, grp)
guinea pig
gutta-percha

G6P
glucose-6-phosphate

G/P
gravida/para

G-1,6-P
glucose-1,6-phosphate

G3P, G-3-P
glyceraldehyde 3-phosphate

gp
gene product
glycoprotein
group (*See also* g, GP, grp)

gp 41
glycosylated protein spanning viral envelope

GPA
glutaraldehyde, picric acid, acetic acid
grade point average
gravida, para, abortus
guinea pig albumin

GPAC
gram-positive anaerobic coccus

GPAIS
guinea pig antiinsulin serum

G6PASE, G-6-Pase
glucose-6-phosphatase

GPB
glossopharyngeal breathing
gram-positive bacillus
gram-positive bacteremia

GPBB
>glycogen phosphorylase isoenzyme BB

GPBP
>guinea pig myelin-basic protein

GPC
>gastric parietal cell
>gel permeation chromatography
>giant papillary conjunctivitis
>glycerolphosphorylcholine
>glycerophosphorylcholine
>G-protein coupled
>gram-positive cocci (*See also* G+C)
>granular progenitor cell
>guinea pig complement

GPCL
>gas permeable contact lens

GPCR
>G protein-coupled receptor

GPC/TP
>glycerophosphorylcholine to total phosphate (ratio)

GPD
>glycerophosphate dehydrogenase
>guinea pig dander

G6PD, G-6-PD
>glucose-6-phosphatase deficiency
>glucose-6-phosphate dehydrogenase
>glucose-6-phosphate dehydrogenase (deficiency)

G6PDA
>glucose-6-phosphate dehydrogenase, variant A

GPE
>glycerylphosphorylethanolamine
>guinea pig embryo

gpELISA
>glycoprotein-based enzyme-linked immunosorbent assay

GPF
>glomerular plasma flow
>granulocytosis-promoting factor

GPGG
>guinea pig gamma globulin

GPGL
>gamma probe guided lymphoscintigraphy

GPH
>giant papillary hypertrophy

GPHN
>giant pigmented hairy nevus

GPI
>general paralysis of the insane
>general paresis of insane
>Gingival-Periodontal Index
>glucose phosphate isomerase
>glycosylphosphatidylinositol
>Gordon Personal Inventory
>gram-positive identification
>guinea pig ileum

GPi
>globus pallidus interna

GPIIa
>glycoprotein IIa

GPIIb
>glycoprotein IIb

GPIIbIIIa
>glycoprotein IIb-IIIa

GPJ
>glossopalatal junction

GPK
>guinea pig kidney (antigen)

GPKA
>guinea pig kidney absorption (test)

G-PLT
>giant platelets

Gply
>gingivoplasty

GPM
>general preventive medicine
>giant pigment melanosome

GPMAL
>gravida, para, multiple births, abortions, live births

GPMT
>guinea pig maximization test

GPN
>glossopharyngeal neuralgia

GPO
>group purchasing organization

GPP
>Gordon Personal Profile

GPPI
>Gordon Personal Profile Inventory

GPPQ
>General Purpose Psychiatric Questionnaire

GPR
>glucose production rate
>good partial response
>gram-positive rod (*See also* G+R)
>Grenoble-Paris-Rennes (epilepsy)

G

NOTES

GPRBC
  guinea-pig red blood cell
GPRL
  gamma probe radiolocalization
GPRVS
  giant prosthetic reinforcement of
    the visceral sac
GPS
  gray platelet syndrome
  guinea pig serum
  guinea pig spleen
GP-ST
  group A streptococcus direct test
GPT
  glutamic-pyruvic transaminase
  guinea pig trachea
GpTh
  group therapy (*See also* GT)
GPTSM
  guinea pig tracheal smooth muscle
GPU
  guinea pig unit
GPUT
  galactose phosphate uridyl
    transferase
GPx
  glutathione peroxidase
GQAP
  general question-asking program
GR
  gamma-ray
  gamma roentgen (*See also* gr)
  gastric resection
  generalized rash
  general relief
  general research
  glucocorticoid receptor
  glucose response
  gluthathione reductase (*See also*
    GSR, GSSG-R)
  good recovery
  grain (*See also* g, gr)
  granulocyte
  gravid (*See also* gr)
  growth rate
  pulse generated runoff
G-R
  gram-negative rod (*See also* GNR)
G+R
  gram-positive rod (*See also* GPR)
Gr
  Greek
gr
  gamma roentgen (*See also* GR)
  grade (*See also* G)
  graft
  grain (*See also* g, GR)
  gravid (*See also* GR)
  gray
  great
  gross (*See also* GRS)
gr⁻
  gram-negative (*See also* G⁻, GM–,
    GN, GrN)
gr⁺
  gram-positive (*See also* G⁺, GM+,
    GP, GrP)
GRA
  gated radionuclide angiography
  glucocorticoid-remediable
    aldosteronism
  gonadotropin-releasing agent
  granisetron (Kytril)
grad., grad
  gradient
  gradually
  graduate
GRAE
  generally regarded as effective
gran
  granulated
  granule
GRAS
  Generally Recognized As Safe
GRASE
  Generally Recognized as Safe and
    Effective
GRASS
  gradient-recalled acquisition in
    steady state
  gradient-refocused acquisition in a
    steady state
GRB
  general reading backwardness
GRBAS
  grade, rough, breathy, asthenic,
    strained
GRC
  gastric remnant cancer
GRD
  beta-glucuronidase (*See also* GRS,
    GUSB)
  gastroesophageal reflux disease
  gender role definition
grd
  ground
GRE
  glucocorticoid response element
  glucocorticoid-responsive element
  glycopeptide-resistant enterococcus
  graded resistive exercise
  gradient-echo
  gradient-recalled echo (technique)
  gradient-refocused echo
  Graduate Record Examination

GREAT
  Graduate Record Examination Aptitude Test

GRF
  gelatin, resorcinol, formaldehyde
  GH-releasing factor
  gonadotropin-releasing factor (*See also* GnRF)
  growth hormone-releasing factor (*See also* GHRF, GH-RF)

GRFoma
  growth hormone-releasing factor tumor

GR-FR
  grandfather (*See also* GF, GD FA)

GRG
  glycine-rich glycoprotein

GRH
  glucocorticoid-remediable hyperaldosteronism
  gonadotropin-releasing hormone (*See also* GnRH)
  growth hormone-releasing hormone (*See also* GHRH, GH-RH)

GRID
  gay-related immunodeficiency disease (obsolete)

GRIF
  growth hormone release-inhibiting factor (*See also* GHRIF, GH-RIF)

GRIMS
  Golombok-Rust Inventory of Marital State

GRIP 1
  glucocorticoid receptor-interacting protein 1

GRL
  granular layer

GR-MO
  grandmother (*See also* GM)

GRN
  granules
  green (*See also* G, Grn)

GrN
  gram-negative (*See also* G−, GM−, GN, gr−)

Grn
  glycerone
  green (*See also* G, GRN)

GRO
  growth-related oncogene

gros
  coarse [L. *grossus*]

GROV
  Guaroa virus

GRP
  gastrin-releasing peptide
  glycine-rich RNA-binding protein

GrP
  gram-positive (*See also* G+, GM+, GP, gr+)

grp
  group (*See also* g, GP, gp)

GRPP
  glicentin-related pancreatic polypeptide

GRPS
  glucose-Ringer-phosphate solution

GRS
  beta-glucuronidase (*See also* GRD, GUSB)
  Golabi-Rosen syndrome
  Graphic Rating Scale
  gross (*See also* gr)

GRSA
  glycopeptide-resistant *Staphylococcus aureus*

GRS&MIC
  gross and microscopic

GRT
  gastric residence time
  giant retinal tear
  glandular replacement therapy
  Group Reading Test

GRTH
  generalized resistance to thyroid hormone

GrTr
  graphite treatment

GRV
  gastric residual volume

GRW
  giant ragweed (test)

GRWR
  graft-to-recipient weight ratio

gr wt
  gross weight

GS
  gallstone
  gastric shield
  gastrocnemius (and) soleus (muscles)
  generalized seizure

NOTES

G

GS *(continued)*
  general surgery
  gestational sac
  Gleason score
  glomerular sclerosis
  glucagon secretion
  glucosamine
  glucosamine sulfate
  glutamine synthetase
  gluteal sets
  goat serum
  graft survival
  Gram stain
  granulocyte substance
  granulocytic sarcoma
  grip strength
  Griscelli syndrome
  group section
  group specific *(See also* gs)
  Guérin-Stern (syndrome)

G/S
  glucose and saline

G$_s$
  G-stimulating protein

gs
  group specific *(See also* GS)

g/s
  gallons per second

GSA
  general somatic afferent (nerve)
  Gross (sarcoma) virus antigen
  Gross virus antigen
  group-specific amplification
  group-specific antigen
  guanidinosuccinic acid

GSA65
  Giardia-specific antigen 65

GSAP
  greatest single allergen present

GSB
  graduated spinal block

GSBG
  gonadal steroid-binding globulin

G-SC
  guanosine-coupled spleen cell

GSC
  gas-solid chromatography
  gravity settling culture (plate)

GSCN
  giant serotonin-containing neuron

GSCU
  geriatric skilled care unit

GSD
  genetically significant dose (of mutagenic radiation)
  glutathione synthetase deficiency
  glycogen storage disease (type Ia, Ib, II–VII) *(See also* GT1-GT10)
  glycogen storage disorder

GSE
  general somatic efferent (nerve)
  genital self-examination
  gluten-sensitive enteropathy
  grips strong and equal

GSF
  galactosemic fibroblast
  genital skin fibroblast

GSH
  glomerulus-stimulating hormone
  glutathione
  golden Syrian hamster
  Green-Seligson-Henry (orthopedic nail)
  growth-stimulating hormone
  reduced glutathione

GSHP
  reduced glutathione peroxidase

GSI
  genuine stress incontinence
  Global Severity Index
  Group Styles Inventory

GSI-BSI
  Global Severity Index of Brief Symptom Inventory

GSIS
  glucose-stimulated insulin secretion

GSK
  glycogen synthetase kinase

GSK3
  glycogen synthase kinase-3

GSL
  goniosynechialysis

GSM
  gray-scale median

GSMD
  gestational sac and maternal date

GSMS
  Great Smoky Mountains Study of Youth

GSN
  giant serotonin-containing neuron

GSNO
  S-nitrosoglutathione

GSP
  galvanic skin potential
  generalized social phobia
  general survey panel
  glycogen synthetase phosphatase
  glycosylated serum protein

GSPECT
  gated single-photon emission computed tomography

GSPN
> greater superficial petrosal neurectomy

GSR
> galvanic skin resistance
> galvanic skin response
> gastrosalivary reflex
> generalized Shwartzman reaction
> glutathione reductase (*See also* GR, GSSG-R)

GSRA
> galvanic skin response audiometry

GSRS
> Gastrointestinal Symptom Rating Scale

GSS
> gamete-shedding substance
> Gerstmann-Straüssler-Scheinker (disease, syndrome)
> gestational sac size
> gloves and socks syndrome

GSSG
> glutathionc
> oxidized gluthathione

GSSG-R
> glutathione reductase (*See also* GR, GSR)

GSSI
> Global Sexual Satisfaction Index

GSSR
> generalized Sanarelli-Shwartzman reaction

GST
> glutathione-*S*-transferase
> gold salt therapy
> gold sodium thiomalate (*See also* GSTM)
> graphic stress telethermometry
> graphic stress thermography
> group striction

GSTG
> gold sodium thioglucose

GSTM
> gold sodium thiomalate (*See also* GST)

GSUI
> genuine stress urinary incontinence

GSV
> golden shiner virus

GSW
> gunshot wound

GSWA
> gunshot wound to abdomen

GSWH
> gunshot wound to head

GT
> gait
> gait training
> galactosyl transferase
> gamma-glutamyl transferase
> Gamow-Teller (strength)
> gastrostomy
> gastrostomy tube (*See also* G-tube)
> generation time (*See also* Tg)
> genetic therapy
> gingiva treatment
> Glanzmann thrombasthenia (*See also* GTA)
> glucagon test
> glucose tolerance
> glucose transport
> glucuronyl transferase
> glutamyl transpeptidase
> glycityrosine
> grand total
> granulation tissue (*See also* g/t)
> greater trochanter
> great toe
> green tea
> group tension
> group therapy (*See also* GpTh)

GT1-GT10
> glycogen storage disease, types 1 to 10

G&T
> gowns and towels

gt.
> gutta (drop)

g/t
> granulation time
> granulation tissue (*See also* GT)

GTA
> Glanzmann thrombasthenia (*See also* GT)
> glutaraldehyde

GTAM
> Gore-Tex augmentation material
> Gore-Tex augmentation membrane

GTB
> gastrointestinal tract bleeding

GTC, GTCS
> generalized tonic clonic
> generalized tonic-clonic seizure

NOTES

GTD
gestational trophoblastic disease

GTE
general therapeutic exercise
green tea extract

GTF
gastrostomy tube feeding
glucose tolerance factor
glucosyltransferase

GTG
gold thioglucose

GTH
gonadotropic hormone

GTHR
generalized thyroid hormone
resistance

GTL
glomerular tip lesion

GTN
gestational trophoblastic neoplasm
glomerulotubulonephritis
glyceryl trinitrate (nitroglycerin)

GTO
Golgi tendon organ

GTP
deoxyguanosine triphosphate
glutamyl transpeptidase
green tea polyphenol
guanosine triphosphate
guanosine 5'-triphosphate
guanyltriphosphate

GTPase
guanosine triphosphatase

GTR
galvanic tetanus ratio
generalized time reflex
granulocyte turnover rate
gross total resection
guided tissue regeneration

GTS
Gilles de la Tourette syndrome
glucose transport system
guided trephine system

GTSTD
Grid Test of Schizophrenic
Thought Disorder

GTT
gelatin-tellurite-taurocholate (agar)
gestational transient thyrotoxicosis
gestational trophoblastic tumor
glucose tolerance test

gtt.
drops [L. *guttae*]

GTT3H
glucose tolerance test 3 hours
(oral)

G-tube
gastrostomy tube (*See also* GT)

GTV
gross tumor volume

GU
gastric ulcer
genitourinary
glucose uptake
glycogenic unit
gonococcal urethritis
gravitational ulcer

GUA
group of units of analysis

GUAR
guarantor

GUD
genital ulcer disease

GUI
genitourinary infection

guid
guidance

GUK
guanylate kinase

GULHEMP
general (physique), upper
(extremity), lower (extremity),
hearing, eyesight, mentality,
personality

Guo
guanosine

GURV
Gurupi virus

GUS
genitourinary sphincter
genitourinary system

GUSB
beta-glucuronidase (*See also* GRD,
GRS)

GV
gastric volume
gentian violet
germinal vesicle
granulosis virus
griseoviridin
growth velocity

gv
governing vessel

GVA
general visceral afferent (nerve)

GVB
gelatin-veronal buffer

GVBD
germinal vesicle breakdown

GVD
graft vessel disease

GVE
gastric vascular ectasia
general visceral efferent (nerve)

GVF
Goldman visual fields
good visual fields
GVG
vigabatrin (gamma-vinyl GABA)
GVH
generalized visceral hypersensitivity
graft versus host
GVHD, GvHD
graft-versus-host disease, grade 1–4
GVHR
graft-versus-host reaction
graft-versus-host response
GVL
graft-versus-leukemia (effect)
GVN
gentamicin, vancomycin, and
nystatin
GVS
gastric vertical stapling
GVTY
gingivectomy
GW
gastric wrap
general ward
germ warfare
gigawatt
glycerin in water
gradual withdrawal
group work
G&W
glycerin and water
G/W
glucose in water
GWAFD
Genée-Wiedemann acrofacial
dysostosis
GWBI
General Well-Being Index

GWBS
global ward behavior scale
GWD
Guinea worm disease
GWE
glycerin and water enema
GWS
Gulf War syndrome
GWX
guide wire exchange
GXM
glucuronoxylomannan
GXP
graded exercise program
GXT
graded exercise test
GXT EKG
graded exercise electrocardiogram
Gy, Gy rad
gray (unit of absorbed dose of
ionizing radiation)
GYN, gyn
gynecologic
gynecologist
gynecology
GYS
guaranteed yield strength
GZAS
Guilford-Zimmerman Aptitude
Survey
GZII
Guilford-Zimmerman Interest
Inventory
GZPT
Guilford-Zimmerman Personality
Test
GZTS
Guilford-Zimmerman Temperament
Survey

NOTES

G

307

H

bacterial antigen in serologic classification of bacteria [Ger. *Hauch* flagellum]

deflection in His bundle in electrogram (spike)

draft, drink [L. *haustus*] (*See also* haust., ht.)

electrically induced spinal reflex

enthalpy (physics)

eta (seventh letter of Greek alphabet), uppercase

Haemophilus

Hauch (motile with flagellum)

head

heart (*See also* He, HT, ht)

heavy

heelstick

Helicobacter

hemagglutination

hemisphcrc

hemolysis (*See also* HEM)

hemolytic (*See also* HEM)

henry

heparin (*See also* HEP, HP)

hernia (*See also* her., hern)

herniated (*See also* hcr., hern)

herniation (*See also* her., hern)

heroin

hetacillin

high

Hispanic

histidine (*See also* His)

history (*See also* hist, Hx, Hy)

Hoffmann (reflex)

Holzknecht (unit)

homosexual

horizontal (*See also* h, hor, horiz)

hormone

horse (slang for heroin) (*See also* Ho)

hospital (*See also* hosp, HX)

hospitalization (*See also* hosp, HX)

hot

Hounsfield (unit) (*See also* HU)

hour (*See also* h, HR, hr)

human (*See also* h, hu)

husband (*See also* husb, HSB)

hydrogen

hydrolysis

hygiene (*See also* hyg)

hygienic (*See also* hyg)

hyoscine (scopolamine)

hypermetropia (*See also* h, Hy)

hyperopia (*See also* h, Hy)

hyperopic (*See also* h, Hy)

hyperphoria

hyperplasia

hypothalamus (*See also* HT, Ht, Hth, hyp)

magnetic field

magnetization

mustard gas (dichlorodiethyl sulfide)

objective angle

per hypodermic

region of sarcomere containing only myosin filaments [Ger. *heller* lighter]

vectorcardiography electrode (neck)

H₀

null hypothesis

H1, ¹H, H¹

hydrogen-1

protium (light hydrogen)

H₁

alternative hypothesis

histamine receptor type 1

H2, ²H, H²

deuterium (heavy hydrogen)

hydrogen-2

H₂

histamine 2

H3, ³H, H³

hydrogen-3

tritium

H₃

procaine hydrochloride

H'

hip

(H)

hip

hypodermic (*See also* h, hypo)

H⁺

hydrogen ion

[H⁺]

hydrogen ion concentration

h

coefficient of heat transfer

hand-rearing (of experimental animals)

hecto-

heteromorphic (region)

high

horizontal (*See also* H, hor, horiz)

hour (*See also* H, HR, hr)

human (*See also* H, hu)

human response

hundred

hypermetropia (*See also* H, Hy)

h *(continued)*
    hyperopia (*See also* H, Hy)
    hyperopic (*See also* H, Hy)
    hypodermic (*See also* (H), hypo)
    negatively staining region of chromosome
    Planck constant
    specific enthalpy

hν
    photon (*See also* γ)

HA
    hallux abductus
    halothane anesthesia
    H antigen
    Hartley (guinea pig)
    headache
    hearing aid
    heart attack
    heated
    heated aerosol (*See also* ht aer)
    height age
    hemadsorbent
    hemadsorption (test)
    hemagglutinating activity
    hemagglutinating antibody
    hemagglutinating antigen
    hemagglutination
    hemolytic anemia
    hemophiliac with adenopathy
    hepatic adenoma
    hepatic artery
    hepatitis A
    hepatitis-associated (virus)
    herpangina
    heterophil antibody
    Heyden antibiotic
    high anxiety
    hippuric acid
    Hispanic American
    histamine
    histidine ammonialyase
    histocompatibility antigen
    Horton arteritis
    hospital acquired
    hospital administration (*See also* HAD, HAd)
    hospital admission
    hospital apprentice
    household activity
    hyaluronan
    hyaluronic acid
    hydroxyanisole
    hydroxyapatite
    hydroxylapatite
    hyperalimentation
    hyperandrogenic anovulation
    hyperandrogenism
    hypermetropic astigmatism

    hyperopia, absolute
    hypersensitivity alveolitis
    hypoplastic aorta
    hypothalmic amenorrhea

H/A
    headache
    head-to-abdomen (ratio)
    holding area

Ha
    absolute hypermetropia
    hahnium
    hamster

H/a
    home with advice

HAA
    hearing aid amplifier
    hemolytic anemia antigen
    hepatitis A antibody (*See also* HAAb)
    hepatitis A antigen (*See also* HAAg)
    hepatitis-associated antigen
    heterocyclic aromatic amine
    hospital activity analysis

HAAb
    hepatitis A antibody (*See also* HAA)

HAAg
    hepatitis A antigen (*See also* HAA)

HAAP
    HTLV-1-associated arthropathy

HAART
    highly active antiretroviral therapy
    highly active antiretroviral treatment

HABA
    hydroxyazobenzoic acid
    hydroxybenzeneazobenzoic acid

HABF
    hepatic artery blood flow

HAb/HAd
    horizontal abduction/adduction

HAC
    human artificial chromosome

HAc
    acetic acid

HACA
    human antichimeric antibodies

HACCP
    Hazard Analysis Critical Control Point(s)

HACE
    hepatic artery chemoembolization
    high-altitude cerebral edema

HACEK
    Haemophilus aphrophilus, Actinobacillus actinomycetemcomitans, Cardiobacterium hominis,

Eikenella corrodens, and *Kingella kingae*

HAChT
high-affinity choline transport

HACR
hereditary adenomatosis of colon and rectum

HAD
hearing aid dispenser
hemadsorption (*See also* HAd)
HIV (human immunodeficiency virus)-associated dementia
hospital administration (*See also* HA, HAd)
Hospital Anxiety and Depression
human adjuvant disease
hypertonic acetate dextran
hypophysectomized alloxan diabetic

HAd
hemadsorption (*See also* HAD)
hospital administration (*See also* HA, HAD)

HADD
hydroxyapatite deposition disease

HAd-I
hemadsorption inhibition

HADS
Hospital Anxiety and Depression Scale

HAD test
hemadsorption test

HAdV 1–47
human adenovirus 1–47

HAE
health appraisal examination
hearing aid evaluation
hepatic artery embolization
herb-related adverse event
hereditary angioedema
hereditary angioneurotic edema

HAEC
Hirschsprung-associated enterocolitis
human aortic endothelial cell

HAEM
herpes-associated erythema multiforme
herpes (simplex)-associated erythema multiforme

HAF
hepatic arterial flow
hyperalimentation fluid

HaF
Hageman factor

HAFM
hospital-acquired *Plasmodium falciparum* malaria

HAFOE
high air flow with oxygen entrainment

HAFP
human alpha-fetoprotein

HAG
heat-aggregated globulin
Histoplasma capsulatum antigen

HAGG
hyperimmune antivariola gamma globulin

HAGL
humeral avulsion of the glenohumeral ligament

HAH
high-altitude headache

HAHTG
horse antihuman thymus globulin

HAI
hemagglutination inhibition (titer) (*See also* HI)
hepatic arterial infusion
hepatitis activity index
histologic activity index
history activity index

HAIC
hepatic arterial infusional chemotherapy

H&A Ins
health and accident insurance

HAIR-AN, HAIRAN
hirsutism, androgen excess, insulin resistance, acanthosis nigricans (syndrome)
hyperandrogenism, insulin resistance, and acanthosis nigricans (syndrome)

HAI test
hemagglutination inhibition test

HAK
hyperalimentation kit

HaK
hamster kidney

HAL
haloperidol
halothane (*See also* hal, HALO)
hand-assisted laparoscopy

NOTES

311

HAL *(continued)*
  hemorrhoidal artery ligation
  hepatic artery ligation
  hyperalimentation
  hypoplastic acute leukemia
Hal
  halogen
hal
  halothane *(See also* HAL, HALO)
HALF
  hyperacute liver failure
HALK
  hyperopic automated lamellar
    keratoplasty
halluc
  hallucination
HALN
  hand-assisted laparoscopic (radical)
    nephrectomy
HALNU
  hand-assisted laparoscopic
    nephroureterectomy
HALO
  halothane *(See also* HAL, hal)
  hemorrhage, abruption, labor,
    placenta previa with mild
    bleeding
  hours after light onset
halo
  hypoechoic band
HALP
  hyperalphalipoproteinemia
HALRI
  hospital-acquired lower respiratory
    infections
HALS
  hand-assisted laparoscopic surgery
  Health and Activity Limitation
    Survey
HALT-C
  hepatitis C antiviral long-term
    treatment to prevent cirrhosis
HaLV
  hamster leukemia virus
HAM
  hearing aid microphone
  helical axis of motion
  hexazomacrocycle
  human albumin microsphere
  human alveolar macrophage
  human T-cell lymphotropic virus-1-
    associated myelopathy
  human T-cell lymphotropic virus
    type I associated myelopathy
  hypoparathyroidism, Addison
    disease, and mucocutaneous
    candidiasis (syndrome)

hypoparathyroidism, adrenal
    insufficiency, mucocutaneous
    candidiasis (syndrome)
HAM-56
  human alveolar macrophage-56
HAMA
  Hamilton Anxiety (Scale)
  human antimouse antibody
HAMD
  Hamilton Depression (Scale)
HAMM
  human albumin minimicrosphere
hams.
  hamstrings *(See also* HS)
HaMSV
  Harvey murine sarcoma virus
HAM/TSP
  HTLV-1-associated myelopathy or
    tropical spastic paraparesis
HAN
  heroin-associated nephropathy
  hyperplastic alveolar nodule
HANA
  hemagglutinin neuraminidase
handicp
  handicapped
HANE
  hereditary angioneurotic edema
HANES
  health and nutrition examination
    survey
hANP
  human atrial natriuretic peptide
H antigens
  flagella antigens of motile bacteria
    [Ger. *Hauch*]
HAO
  hearing aid orientation
HAODM
  hypoplasia of anguli oris depressor
    muscle
HA-P
  hemagglutinin-protease
HAP
  hearing aid problem
  held after positioning
  hepatic arterial-dominant phase
  hepatic arterial phase
  heredopathia atactica
    polyneuritiformis
  high-amplitude peristalsis
  histamine acid phosphate
  hospital-acquired pneumonia
  humoral antibody production
  hydrolyzed animal protein
  hydroxyapatite (fractionation
    procedure)
  hyperthermic antiblastic perfusion

HAPA
> hemagglutinating antipenicillin antibody

HAPC
> high-amplitude contraction
> hospital-acquired penetration contact

HAPD
> home-automated peritoneal dialysis

HAPE
> high-altitude pulmonary edema

HA-PI
> hepatic arterial pulsatility index

HAPO
> high-altitude pulmonary (o)edema

HAPS
> hepatic arterial perfusion scintigraphy

HAPTO
> haptoglobin (*See also* HP, Hp, Hpt)

HAQ
> Headache Assessment Questionnaire
> Health Assessment Questionnaire
> Stanford Health Assessment Questionnaire

HAQ DI
> Health Assessment Questionnaire Disability Index

HAR
> high-altitude retinopathy
> hyperacute rejection

Har
> homoarginine

HARD
> hydrocephalus, agyria, retinal dysplasia (syndrome)

HARD+/-E
> hydrocephalus, agyria, retinal dysplasia with or without encephalocele (syndrome)

HAREM
> heparin assay rapid easy method

HARH
> high-altitude retinal hemorrhage

HARM
> heparin assay rapid method

harm.
> harmonic

HARP
> harmonic phase
> Hospital Admission Risk Profile
> hypobetalipoproteinemia, acanthocytosis, retinitis

pigmentosa, and pallidal degeneration (syndrome)

HARPPS
> heat, absence of use, redness, pain, pus, swelling (symptoms of infection)

HARS
> Hamilton Anxiety Rating Scale

HART
> hyperfractionated accelerated radiation therapy

HARTS
> heat-activated recoverable temporary stent

HAS
> Hamilton Anxiety Scale
> health advisory service
> high-amplitude sucking (technique)
> highest asymptomatic (dose)
> home assessment service
> hospital administrative service
> hospital advisory service
> hospitalized attempted suicide
> hyperalimentation solution
> hypertensive arteriosclerotic

HASCHD, HASIID
> hypertensive arteriosclerotic heart disease (*See also* HASHD)

HASCI
> head and spinal cord injury

HASCVD
> hypertensive arteriosclerotic cardiovascular disease

HASMC
> human aortic smooth muscle cell

HAsP
> health aspects of pesticides

HAST
> high-altitude simulation test

HASTE
> half-Fourier acquisition single-shot turbo spin-echo

HAstV-1–7
> human astrovirus serotype 1–7

HAT
> Halstead Aphasia Test
> handgrip apexcardiographic test
> harmonic attenuation table
> harmonic attenuation test
> head, arms, and trunk
> heparin-associated thrombocytopenia
> hepatic artery thrombosis

NOTES

H

313

HAT (*continued*)
    heterophil antibody titer
    histone acetyltransferase
    hospital arrival time
    human African trypanosomiasis
    (sleeping sickness)
    hypoxanthine, aminopterin,
    thymidine
    hypoxanthine, azaserine, and
    thymidine

HATG
    horse antihuman thymocyte globulin

HATH
    Heterosexual Attitudes Toward
    Homosexuality (scale)

H$^+$-ATPase
    hydrogen adenosine triphosphatase

HATT
    hemagglutination treponemal test
    heparin-associated thrombocytopenia
    and thrombosis

HATTS
    hemagglutination treponemal test
    for syphilis

HAU
    hemagglutinating unit

haust.
    draft, drink [L. *haustus*] (*See also*
    H, ht.)

HAV
    hallux abductovalgus
    hemadsorption virus
    hepatitis A vaccine
    hepatitis A virus

HAVAB
    hepatitis A virus antibody

HAV-HBV
    hepatitis A virus and hepatitis B
    virus vaccine

HAWIC
    Hamburg-Wechsler Intelligence Test
    for Children

HAZV
    Hazara virus

HAZWOPER
    Hazardous Waste Operations and
    Emergency Response

HB
    head backward
    health board
    heart-beating (donor)
    heart block (*See also* hb)
    heel to buttock
    held backward
    hemoglobin (*See also* Hb, Hbg,
    hemo, HG, hg, HGB, hgb)
    hemolysis blocking
    hepatitis B

    high calorie
    His bundle
    hold breakfast
    hospital bed
    housebound
    Hutchinson-Boeck (disease)
    hybridoma bank
    hydrocodone bitartrate
    hyoid body

HB1°
    first-degree heart block

HB2°
    second-degree heart block

HB3°
    third-degree heart block

Hb
    hemoglobin (*See also* HB, Hbg,
    hemo, HG, hg, HGB, hgb)

hb
    heart block (*See also* HB)

HbA, Hb A
    adult hemoglobin
    hemoglobin A
    hemoglobin α-chain

HbA°
    hemoglobin determination

HbA$_1$
    major component of adult
    hemoglobin

HbA$_{1c}$, HbA1C, HbA1c
    glycosylated hemoglobin
    hemoglobin A$_{1c}$

HbA$_2$
    minor fraction of adult hemoglobin

HBAb
    hepatitis B antibody

HBAC
    hyperdynamic beta-adrenergic
    circulatory

HBAg, HbAg
    hepatitis B antigen

HbAS
    heterozygosity for hemoglobin A
    and hemoglobin S (sickle-cell
    trait)

HBB
    hemoglobin b (chain)
    hospital blood bank
    hydroxybenzylbenzimidazole

HbBC
    hemoglobin-binding capacity

HBBW
    hold breakfast for blood work

HBC
    hereditary breast cancer
    hit by car

HB$_c$, HB core
    hepatitis B$_c$

hepatitis B core (antibody, antigen) (*See also* HB core, HB$_c$Ab, AHBC)

hepatitis B core (antigen)

HbC, Hb C
hemoglobin C

HB$_c$Ab, HBCAB, HB$_{cAb}$, HBcAb
antibody to hepatitis B core antigen
hepatitis B core antibody (*See also* HB$_c$, HB core, AHBC)

HB$_c$Ag, HBCAG, HB$_{cAg}$, IIBcAg
hepatitis B core antigen

HBCG
heat-aggregated bacille Calmette-Guérin

Hb$_{Chesapeake}$
hemoglobin Chesapeake

HbCO
carbon monoxide hemoglobin
carboxyhemoglobin (*See also* CoHB)

HbCS
hemoglobin Constant Spring

HBCT
helical biphasic contrast-enhanced CT

HbCV
Haemophilus b conjugate vaccine

HBD
has been drinking
heart-beating donor
hemoglobin delta chain
hormone-binding domain
hydroxybutyrate dehydrogenase (*See also* HBDH)
hydroxybutyric dehydrogenase (*See also* HBDH)
hypophosphatemic bone disease

HbD
hemoglobin D

HBDH
hydroxybutyrate dehydrogenase (*See also* HBD)

HBDT
human basophil degranulation test

HBE, HbE
hemoglobin ε chain
hemoglobin E
His bundle electrogram
human bronchial epithelial (cells)
hypopharyngoscopy, bronchoscopy, and esophagoscopy

HBE$_1$
His bundle electrogram, distal

HBE$_2$
His bundle electrogram, proximal

HB$_e$, HBe
hepatitis B$_e$
hepatitis B$_e$ antigen
hepatitis B e antigen

HB$_e$Ab, HB$_{eAb}$
antibody to hepatitis B e antigen
hepatitis B e antibody
hepatitis B early antibody

HB$_e$Ag, HBEAG, HBeAg
hepatitis B e antigen (*See also* HBeAg, HB$_e$Ab, IIBc)
hepatitis B early antigen

HBED
hydroxybenzylethylene-diamine diacetic acid

HB-EGF
heparin-binding epidermal growth factor
heparin-binding epidermal growth factorlike growth factor

HBF
fetal hemoglobin (*See also* HbF)
hand blood flow
hemispheric blood flow
hemoglobinuric bilious fever
hepatic blood flow
hypothalamic blood flow

HbF, Hb F
fetal hemoglobin (*See also* IIBF)
hemoglobin F

HBG1
hemoglobin γ chain A

HBG2
hemoglobin γ chain G

Hbg
hemoglobin (*See also* HB, Hb, hemo, HG, hg, HGB, hgb)

HBGA
had it before, got it again

HBGF
heparin-binding growth factor

HBGF-1
heparin-binding growth factor-1

HBGF-2
heparin-binding growth factor-2

HBGM
home blood glucose monitoring

NOTES

H

315

HBGS
House-Brackmann Grading Scale
HbH
hemoglobin H
HBHC
home-based hospital care
Hb-Hp
hemoglobin-haptoglobin (complex)
HBI
Harvey-Bradshaw Index
hemibody irradiation
hepatobiliary imaging
high serum-bound iron
high (serum)-bound iron
Hutchins Behavior Inventory
HBID
hereditary benign intraepithelial
dyskeratosis
HBIG, H-BIG, HBIg
hepatitis B immune globulin
hepatitis B immunoglobulin
hepatitis B virus immunoglobulin
hyperimmune serum globulin
HBIR
Hering-Breuer inflation reflex
Hb$_{Kansas}$
mutant hemoglobin with low
affinity for oxygen
HBL
hepatoblastoma
HBLA
human B-lymphocyte antigen
Hb$_{Lepore}$
hemoglobin Lepore
HBLLSB
heard best at left lower sternal
border
HBLP
hyperbetalipoproteinemia
HBLUSB
heard best at left upper sternal
border
HBLV
human B lymphotropic virus
HBM
Health Belief Model
human bone marrow
hypertonic buffered medium
HbM
hemoglobin M
HBME-1
human mesothelial cell membrane
HbMet
methemoglobin (See also Met-Hb,
MHB, MHb, MHGB)
HBNK
heparin-binding neurotrophic factor

HBO
hyperbaric oxygenation
hyperbaric oxygen (therapy) (See
also HBOT)
oxygenated hemoglobin (See also
HbO$_2$)
HbO$_2$, HBO2
hyperbaric oxygen
oxygenated hemoglobin (See also
HBO)
oxyhemoglobin
HBOC
hemoglobin-based oxygen carrier
hereditary breast and ovarian
cancer
HbOC
hepatitis B oligosaccharide-CRM197
vaccine
HBOT
hyperbaric oxygen therapy (See also
HBO)
HBP
helix-bundle peptide
hepatic binding protein
high blood pressure
HbP
primitive (fetal) hemoglobin
HBPM
home blood pressure monitoring
HBQ
human health and behavior
questionnaire
HBr
hydrobromic acid
HbR
methemoglobin reductase
HBS
Health Behavior Scale
hepatitis B surface
hyperkinetic behavior syndrome
HB$_s$
hepatitis B surface (antibody,
antigen)
HB$_s$
hepatitis B surface antigen
HbS
hemoglobin S
sickle cell hemoglobin
sulfhemoglobin (See also SHB,
SHb, SULFHB)
Hb$_s$, Hb S
sickle cell hemoglobin
HB$_s$A
hepatitis B surface associated
HB$_s$Ab, HB$_{sAb}$, HBsAb
antibody to hepatitis B surface
antigen
hepatitis B surface antibody

HB$_s$Ag, HB$_{sAg}$, HBsAg
  hepatitis B surface antigen (*See also* HBsAg, HB$_{sAg}$)

HBsAg/adr
  hepatitis B surface antigen manifesting group-specific determinant *a* and subtype-specific determinants *d* and *r*

HBSC
  hemopoietic blood stem cell

HbSC, HbsC
  sickle cell hemoglobin C

HBSS
  Hanks balanced salt solution

HbSS
  homozygosity for hemoglobin S

HBSSG
  Hanks balanced salt solution plus glucose

HbS-Thal
  hemoglobin S-thalassemia
  sickle thalassemia

HBT
  home-based telemetry
  human (blood) bilayer Tween
  human brain thromboplastin
  human breast tumor
  hydrogen breath test

HBV
  hepatitis B vaccine
  hepatitis B virus
  honey-bee venom

HBV DNA
  hepatitis B DNA detection

HBVP
  high biological value protein

HBVV
  hepatitis B virus vaccine

HBW
  high birth weight

H/BW
  heart-to-body weight (ratio)
  height-to-body weight (ratio)

HbZ
  hemoglobin ξ chain
  hemoglobin Z
  hemoglobin zeta
  hemoglobin Zürich

HC
  hair cell
  hairy cell
  handicapped (*See also* HCAP, HCP)

head check
head circumference
head compression
healthy control
heart catheterization
heart cycle
heat conservation
heavy chain
heel cord
hemochromatosis
hemoglobin concentration
hemorrhage, cerebral
heparin cofactor
hepatic catalase
hepatitis C
hepatocellular cancer
hereditary coproporphyria (*See also* HCP)
Hickman catheter
high calorie (*See also* hg-cal)
hippocampus
histamine challenge
histochemistry
home call
home care
home collection
homocystinuria
hospital course
hospitalized controls
hot compress
house call
Huntington chorea
hyaline cast
hydranencephaly
hydraulic concussion
hydrocarbon
hydrocephalus
hydrocodone
hydrocortisone (*See also* HCT, Hyd)
hydroxycorticoid (*See also* HOC)
hyoid cornu
hypercholesterolemia
hypertrophic cardiomyopathy

4-HC, 4HC
4-hydroperoxycyclophosphamide

H&C
hot and cold

Hc
hydrocolloid

HCII
heparin cofactor II

NOTES

H

HCA
> health care aide
> heart cell aggregate
> heel cord advancement
> hepatocellular adenoma
> heterocyclic antidepressant
> home-care aide
> hybrid capture assay
> hydrocortisone acetate
> hypercalcemia
> hypothermic circulatory arrest

HCAP
> handicapped (*See also* HC, HCP)

HCB
> hexachlorobenzene

HCC
> heat conservation center
> hepatitis contagiosa canis (virus)
> hepatocellular carcinoma
> hepatoma carcinoma cell
> hexachlorocyclohexane (lindane)
> (*See also* HCH, gamma-HCH)
> history of chief complaint
> hydroxycholecalciferol

25-HCC
> 25-hydroxycholecalciferol

HCCC
> hyalinizing clear cell carcinoma

HCC-CC
> clear cell hepatocellular carcinoma

HCD
> h-caldesmon (antibody)
> health care delivery
> heavy-chain disease (protein)
> herniated cervical disk
> high caloric density
> high carbohydrate diet (*See also* HICHO)
> higher cerebral dysfunction
> homologous canine distemper (antiserum)
> hydrocolloid dressing

HCE
> hypoglossal carotid entrapment

H(c)ELISA
> hemagglutinin enzyme-linked immunosorbent assay

HCF
> hereditary capillary fragility
> high-carbohydrate, high-fiber (diet)
> highest common factor
> Horsley-Clarke stereotactic frame
> hypocaloric carbohydrate feeding

HCFC
> hydrochlorofluorocarbon

HCFSH
> human chorionic follicle-stimulating hormone

HCFU
> hexylcarbamoylfluorouracil (carmofur-antineoplastic)

hCG
> human chorionic gonadotropin

HCGN
> hypocomplementemic glomerulonephritis

HCH
> hexachlorocyclohexane (lindane)
> (*See also* HCC, gamma-HCH)
> Hygroscopic Condenser Humidifier

hch
> hemochromatosis

HCHO
> formaldehyde

HCHWA
> hereditary cerebral hemorrhage with amyloidosis

HCHWA-D
> hereditary cerebral hemorrhage with amyloidosis, Dutch type

HCI
> home care instructions

HcImp
> hydrocolloid impression

HCL
> hairy cell leukemia
> hard contact lens
> hemacytology index
> hemicentral, lateral
> human cultured lymphoblast

HCl
> hydrochloric (acid)
> hydrochloride

HCLF
> high carbohydrate, low fiber (diet)

HCLV
> hairy cell leukemia variant

HCM
> health care maintenance
> health care management
> heterogeneous cation-exchange membrane
> hypercalcemia of malignancy
> hypertrophic cardiomyopathy

HCMA
> hyperchloremic metabolic acidosis

HCMM
> hereditary cutaneous malignant melanoma

HCMV
> human cytomegalovirus (infection)

HCN
> hereditary chronic nephritis
> high calorie and nitrogen
> hydrocyanic acid
> hydrogen cyanide

HCO$_3$
    bicarbonate (*See also* bicarb)

HCP
    handicapped (*See also* HC, HCAP)
    healthcare provider
    hearing conservation programs
    hepatocatalase peroxidase
    hereditary coproporphyria (*See also* HC)
    hexachlorophene
    high cell passage
    home chemotherapy program
    hospital chemistry profile

H&CP
    hospital and community psychiatry

HCPCS
    HCFA (Health Care Financing Administration) Common Procedure Coding System

HCPS
    hantavirus cardiopulmonary syndrome

HCQ
    hydroxychloroquine

HCR
    health care review
    heme-controlled repressor
    host-cell reactivation
    human-controlled repressor
    hydrochloric acid
    hysterical conversion reaction

HCr
    hemoglobin content of reticulocyte

HCRC
    hereditary clear cell renal carcinoma

hCRH
    human corticotropin-releasing hormone

h'crit
    hematocrit (*See also* crit, HCT)

HCRM
    home cardiorespiratory monitor

HCS
    health care support
    heel-cord stretches
    hematocystic spot
    holocarboxylase synthetase
    hourglass contraction of stomach
    human cord serum
    hydroxycorticosteroid (*See also* OH, OHCS)

hCS
    human chorionic somatomammotropin (human placental lactogen) (*See also* hCSM)
    human chorionic somatotropin

HCSE
    horse chestnut seed extract

hCSM
    human chorionic somatomammotropin (human placental lactogen) (*See also* hCS)

HCSS
    hypersensitive carotid sinus syndrome

HCT
    head computerized (axial) tomography
    Health Check Test
    heart-circulation training
    hematocrit (*See also* crit, h'crit, HCT)
    hematopoietic stem cell transplantation
    histamine challenge test
    historic control trial
    homocytotrophic
    human calcitonin (*See also* hCT)
    hydrocortisone (*See also* HC, Hyd)
    hydroxycortisone

hCT
    human calcitonin (*See also* HCT)
    human chorionic thyrotropin (*See also* HCT)

hct
    hundred count

HCTA
    helical computed tomographic angiography

HCTD
    hepatic computed tomographic density
    high cholesterol and tocopherol deficient

HCTS
    high cholesterol and tocopherol supplemented

HCTU
    home cervical traction unit

HCTZ
    hydrochlorothiazide

NOTES

H

HCTZ-TA
>hydrochlorothiazide-triamterene

HCU
>homocystinuria
>hyperplasia cystica uteri

HCV
>hepatitis C vaccine
>hepatitis C virus
>human coronary virus

HCVD
>hypertensive cardiovascular disease
>(*See also* HTCVD)

HCV EIA 20 test
>hepatitis C virus enzyme
>immunoassay

HCVR
>hypercapnic ventilatory response

HCV RNA
>hepatitis C virus RNA

HCVS
>human corona virus sensitivity

HCW
>health care worker

Hcy
>homocysteine

HD
>Hajna-Damon (broth)
>haloperidol decanoate (*See also* HLD, HL-D)
>hard corn [L. *heloma durum*]
>Harris design
>hearing distance
>heart disease
>helium dilution
>Heller-Dor (procedure)
>heloma durum (hard corn)
>hemidiaphragm
>hemodialysis
>hemolysing dose
>hemolytic disease
>hepatitis D
>herniated disk
>high density
>high dosage
>high dose
>hip disarticulation
>histidine decarboxylase
>hormone dependent
>hospital day (*See also* HOD)
>hospital discharge
>house dust
>human diploid (cell)
>hydatid disease
>hydroxydopamine (*See also* HDA)
>hypnotic dosage
>mustard gas

H and D, H-D, H&D
>Hunter-Driffield
>Hunter and Driffield (curve)

HD#
>hospital day number

HD$_{50}$
>hemolyzing dose of complement that lyses 50% of sensitized erythrocytes

Hd
>human figure parts response

HDA
>heteroduplex analysis
>high-dose arm
>hydroxydopamine (*See also* HD)

HDAg
>hepatitis D antigen

HDBD
>hydroxybutyric dehydrogenase

HDBQ
>Hilton Drinking Behavior Questionnaire

HDC
>habilitative day care
>high-dose chemotherapy
>histamine dihydrochloride
>histidine decarboxylase
>human diploid cell
>hyperdiploid cell
>hypodermoclysis

HDCS
>human diploid cell strain
>human diploid cell system

HDC-SCR, HDC/SCR
>high-dose chemotherapy and stem cell rescue

HDCT
>high-dose chemotherapy

HDCV
>human diploid cell (culture rabies) vaccine
>human diploid cell (rabies) vaccine
>human diploid cell vaccine

HDD
>half-dose depth
>high-dose depth

HDE
>higher-dose therapy with epinephrine
>humanitarian device exemption

HDF
>hemodiafiltration
>high dry field
>host defensive factor
>human diploid fibroblast

HDFL
>human development and family life

HDFP
Hypertension Detection and Followup Program

HDG
high-dose group
hydrogel (dressing)

HDH
heart disease history
high density humidity
Hostility and Direction of Hostility (questionnaire) (*See also* HDHQ)

HD-HIV
Hodgkin disease and HIV infection

HDHQ
Hostility and Direction of Hostility Questionnaire (*See also* HDH)

HDI
hemorrhagic disease of infants
high-definition image
high-definition imaging
histologically detectable iron

HDIC
hepatodiaphragmatic interposition of colon

HDIT
high-dose immunosuppressive therapy

HDL
high-density lipoprotein

HDL-C
high-density lipoprotein C
high-density lipoprotein-cholesterol

HDL-c
high-density lipoprotein-cell surface (receptor)

HDLS
hereditary diffuse leukoencephalopathy with spheroids

HDLW
hearing distance, left, watch (distance from which watch ticking is heard by left ear)

HDM
hexadimethrine
high-dose morphine
home-delivered meals
house dust mite

HDMEC
human dermal microvascular endothelial cell

HDMP
high-dose methylprednisolone

HDN
hemolytic disease of newborn
hemorrhagic disease of newborn
heparin dosing nomogram
high-density nebulizer

hDNA
deoxyribonucleic acid, histone

HDNS
Hodgkin disease, nodular sclerosis

HDoov
Humpty Doo virus

HDP
hexose diphosphate
high definition power
high-density polyethylene
hydroxydimethylpyrimidine

HDPAA
heparin-dependent platelet-associated antibody

HDPC
handpiece

HDR
heparin dose response
high dose rate
husband to delivery room

HDRA
histoculture drug response assay

HDRB
high dose rate brachytherapy

HDRS
Hamilton Depression Rating Scale

HDRV
human diploid (cell strain) rabies vaccine

HDRW
hearing distance, right, watch (distance from which watch ticking is heard by right ear)

HDS
Hamilton Depression (Rating) Scale
healthcare data systems
health data services
health delivery system
hematuria-dysuria syndrome
herniated disk syndrome
HIV Dementia Scale
hospital discharge survey

HDSCR
health deviation self-care requisite

NOTES

H

HDT
- habilitative day treatment
- Hand Dynamometer Test
- hearing distraction test
- high-dose therapy

HDU
- head-drop unit (curare standard)
- hemodialysis unit
- high-dependency unit (an intensive care unit)

HDV
- hepatitis delta virus
- hepatitis D virus

HDVD
- high-definition video display

HDW
- hearing distance (with) watch
- reticulocyte hemoglobin distribution width

HDYF
- how do you feel

HDZ
- hydralazine

H-E
- heat exchanger

HE
- half-scan with extrapolation
- hard exudate
- health educator
- Hektoen enteric (agar)
- hemagglutinating encephalomyelitis
- hematoxylin and eosin (*See also* H&E)
- hemoglobin electrophoresis
- hepatic encephalopathy
- hepatitis E
- hereditary elliptocyto
- hereditary elliptocytosis
- hollow enzyme
- human ehrlichiosis
- human enteric (virus)
- hyperextension
- hypogonadotropic eunuchoidism
- hypophysectomy
- hypoxemic episode

H&E
- hematoxylin and eosin (stain) (*See also* HE)
- hemorrhage and exudate
- heredity and environment

He
- heart (*See also* H, HT, ht)
- Hedstrom number
- helium

³He
- helium-3

⁴He
- helium-4

he
- heart channel (acupuncture)

HEA
- health
- hexone-extracted acetone
- human erythrocyte antigen

HEADSS
- home (life), education (level), activities, drug (use), sexual (activity), suicide (ideation/attempts) (adolescent medical history)

HEAL
- Health Education Assistance Loan

HEAR
- hospital emergency ambulance radio

HEAT
- human erythrocyte agglutination test

HEB
- hematoencephalic barrier (blood-brain barrier)
- hydrophilic emollient base

HEC
- hamster embryo cell
- health education center
- health evaluation center
- human endothelial cell
- hydroxyergocalciferol

HED
- hydrotropic electron donor
- hydroxyephedrine
- hypohidrotic ectodermal dysplasia
- skin erythema dose [Ger. *Haut-Erythem-Dosis*]
- unit skin dose (of x-rays) [Ger. *Haut-Einheits-Dosis*]

HeD
- helper determinant

HEDH
- hypohidrotic ectodermal dysplasia with hypothyroidism

HEDIS
- Health (Plan) Employer Data and Information Set

HEDSPA
- ^{99m}Tc-etidronate (bone-imaging agent)

HEENT
- head, ears, eyes, nose, throat

HEEP
- health effects of environmental pollutants

HEF
- hamster embryo fibroblast
- human embryo fibroblast

HEG
- hemorrhagic erosive gastritis

hEGF, h-EGF
    human epidermal growth factor
HEHR
    highest equivalent heart rate
HEI
    high-energy intermediate
    homogeneous enzyme immunoassay
    human embryonic intestine (cell)
HEIR
    health effects of ionizing radiation
    high-energy ionizing radiation
HEIS
    high-energy ion scattering
HEK
    human embryo kidney (cell)
    human embryonic kidney
HEL
    Helicobacter pylori vaccine
    hen egg lysozyme
    hen egg-white lysozyme
    human embryo lung (cell culture)
    human erythroleukemia line
HeLa
    continuously cultured carcinoma cell line used for tissue cultures (named for patient, Henrietta Lacks)
    Henrietta Lacks (cells)
HELF
    human embryoic lung fibroblast
heliox
    helium and oxygen
    helium-oxygen mixture
HELLP
    hemolysis, elevated liver enzymes, and low platelet (count)
    hemolysis, elevated liver enzymes, low platelets
HELM
    helmet cell
HELP
    Hawaii Early Learning Profile
    Health Education Library Program
    Health Emergency Loan Program
    Health Evaluation and Learning Program
    heat escape lessening posture
    heparin-induced extracorporeal low-density lipoprotein precipitation
    Heroin Emergency Life Project
    Hospital Equipment Loan Project

HEM, hem
    hematologist
    hematology (*See also* hemat)
    hematuria
    hemolysis (*See also* H)
    hemolytic (*See also* H)
    hemorrhage
    hemorrhoid
HEMA
    hydroxyethylmethacrylate
    2-hydroxyethyl methacrylate
hemat
    hematology (*See also* HEM, hem)
hematem
    hematemesis
hemi
    hemiparalysis
    hemiparesis
    hemiplegia
    hemisphere
hemo
    hemoglobin (*See also* HB, Hb, Hbg, HG, hg, HGB, hgb)
    hemophilia
hemocyt, hemocyt.
    hemocytometer
hemorr
    hemorrhage
HEMOSID
    hemosiderin
HEMPAS
    hereditary erythroblastic multinuclearity with positive acidified serum
HEMRI
    hereditary multifocal relapsing inflammation
HEMS
    helicopter emergency medical services
HEN
    hemorrhages, exudates, and/or nicking
    home enteral nutrition
He-Ne, HeNe
    helium-neon
HEP
    hemoglobin electrophoresis
    hemolysis end point
    heparin (*See also* H, HP)
    hepatic
    hepatoerythrocytic porphyria

NOTES

H

HEP *(continued)*
hepatoerythropoietic porphyria
hepatoma
high egg passage (virus)
high-energy phosphate
histamine equivalent prick
home exercise program
human epithelial (cell) (*See also* HEp)

HEp
human epithelial (cell) (*See also* HEP)

HEp-1
human cervical carcinoma cells

HEp-2
human laryngeal tumor cells

hEP
human endorphin

hep
hepatitis

HEPA
hamster egg penetration assay
high-efficiency particulate air (filter)
high-efficiency particulate arresting

HEP-AC
hepatitis battery-acute

Hep B
hepatitis B

hep cap
heparin cap

Hep/Clav
hepatoclavicular

HEPES
4-(2-hydroxyethyl)-1-piperazineethanesulfonic acid
N-[2-hydroxyethyl]piperazine N′-[2-ethanesulfonic acid]

hep lock
heparin lock (*See also* HL, H/L)

HEPM
human embryonic palatal mesenchymal (cell)

HER
hemorrhagic encephalopathy of rats

HER-2
human epidermal growth receptor 2

her.
hernia (*See also* H, hern)
herniated (*See also* H, hern)
herniation (*See also* H, hern)

hered
hereditary
heredity

HERG
human ether-a-go-go-related gene

hern
hernia (*See also* H, her.)

herniated (*See also* H, her.)
herniation (*See also* H, her.)

HERP
human exposure (dose)/rodent potency

HERS
Health Evaluation and Referral Service

HES
(acute) hypereosinophilic syndrome
health examination survey
hematoxylin-eosin stain
hetastarch (hydroxyethyl starch; Hespan)
human embryonic skin
human embryonic spleen
hydroxyethyl starch (solution)
hypereosinophilic syndrome

HEs
hypertensive emergencies

HESX1
homeobox gene expressed in ES cells

HET
Health Education Telecommunications
helium equilibration time

het
heterophil (antibody)
heterozygous

HETE
hydroxyeicosatetraenoic (acid)

12-HETE
12-hydroxyeicosatetraenoic acid

20-HETE
20-hydroxyeicosatetraenoic acid

HETF
home enteral tube feeding

HETP
height equivalent to a theoretical plate (gas chromatography)

HE-TUMT
high-energy transurethral microwave thermotherapy

HEV
health and environment
hemagglutination encephalomyelitis virus
hemorrhagic endovasculitis
hemorrhagic endovasculopathy
hepatitis E vaccine
hepatitis E virus
hepatoencephalomyelitis virus
high-endothelial venule
human enteric virus

HEV1, HEVI
hibernal epidemic viral infection

HEX
> hexosaminidase

HEx
> hard exudate

HEX A
> hexosaminidase A (α-subunit)

HEX B
> hexosaminidase B (β-subunit)

HF
> Hageman factor
> half (*See also* hf, S, sem., semi,
> ss)
> haplotype frequency
> hard feces
> hard filled (capsule)
> harvest fluid
> hay fever
> head of fetus
> head forward
> heart failure
> helper factor
> hemofiltration
> hemorrhagic factor
> hemorrhagic fever
> hepatocyte function
> Hertz frequency
> high-fat (diet)
> high flow
> high frequency (*See also* hf)
> Hispanic female
> hollow filter (dialyzer)
> hot flashes
> hot fomentation
> house formula
> human fibroblast
> hydrogen fluoride (catalyst)
> hyperflexion

H/F
> HeLa/fibroblast (hybrid)

Hf
> hafnium

hf
> half (*See also* HF, S, sem., semi,
> ss)
> high frequency (*See also* HF, Hfr)

HFA
> health facility administrator
> high-functioning autism
> hydrofluoroalkane-134a

H-FABP
> heart fatty acid binding protein

HFAK
> hollow-fiber artificial kidney

HFAS
> hereditary flat adenoma syndrome

HFB
> high frequency band

HFBA
> heptafluorobutyric anhydride

HFC
> hand-filled capsule
> high-frequency current
> histamine-forming capacity
> hydrofluorocarbon

HFCB
> horizontal flow clean bench

HFCC
> high-frequency chest compression
> high-frequency chest wall
> compression (*See also* HFCWC)

HFCS
> high-fructose corn syrup

HFCWC
> high-frequency chest wall
> compression (*See also* HFCC)

HFCWO
> high-frequency chest wall
> oscillation

HFD
> hemorrhagic fever of deer
> high-fiber diet
> high forceps delivery
> high-frequency discharges
> high-frequency Doppler
> hospital field director
> Human Figure Drawing

HF dialyzer
> hollow filter dialyzer

HFDK
> human fetal diploid kidney (cell)

HFDL
> human fetal diploid lung (cell)

HFEA
> Human Fertilization and
> Embryology Authority

HFEC
> human foreskin epithelial cell

HFEE
> high-frequency epicardial
> echocardiography

HFF
> high-filter frequency
> human foreskin fibroblast

NOTES

H

HFFI
high-frequency flow interruption
HFG
hand-foot-genital (syndrome)
hFGF
Kaposi sarcoma human growth factor
HFH
hemifacial hyperplasia
homozygous familial hypercholesterolemia
hFH
heterozygous familial hypercholesterolemia
HFHL
high-frequency hearing loss
HFI
half-Fourier imaging
Hand Functional Index
hereditary fructose intolerance
human fibroblast interferon (*See also* HFIF)
HFIF
human fibroblast interferon (*See also* HFI)
HFIP
hexafluoroisopropranolol
HFJ
high-frequency jet
HFJV
high-frequency jet ventilation
HFL
human fetal lung (fibroblast)
HFLL
hemosiderotic fibrohistiocytic lipomatous lesion
H flu
Haemophilus influenzae (*See also* HI, HIF)
HFM
hand-foot-and-mouth (disease) (*See also* HFMD)
hemifacial microsomia (*See also* HM)
HFMD
hand-foot-and-mouth disease (*See also* HFM)
HFO
hard food orientation
high-frequency oscillation
high-frequency oscillatory
HFOC
high-flow oxygen conserver
HFOV
high-frequency oscillatory ventilation
HFP
hepatic functional panel

Hoffa fat pad
hypofibrinogenic plasma
HFPP
high-frequency positive pressure
HFPPV
high-frequency positive-pressure ventilation
HFPV
high-frequency percussive ventilation
HFR
heart frequency
Hfr
high frequency
high frequency of recombination
high-frequency recombination
HFRS
hemorrhagic fever with renal symptoms
hemorrhagic fever with renal syndrome
HFS
hand-foot syndrome
hemifacial spasm
hfs
hyperfine structure
hFSH
human follicle-stimulating hormone
HFST
hearing-for-speech test
HFT
hemofiltration therapy
high-frequency transduction
high-frequency transfer
HFU
hand-foot-uterus (syndrome)
high-intensity focused ultrasound
HFUPR
hourly fetal urine production rate
HFUPS
high-frequency ultrasound probe sonography
HFV
hepatitis F virus
high-frequency ventilation
high-fruit/vegetable (diet)
HFX RT
hyperfractionated radiation therapy
HG
handgrasp
hand grip (exercise)
hemoglobin (*See also* HB, Hb, Hbg, hemo, hg, HGB, hgb)
herpes genitalis
herpes gestationis
Heschl gyrus
high glucose
high grade
human gonadotropin

human growth (factor)
hypoglycemia

H/G

H. recombinant

Hg

mercury [L. *hydrargyrum* silver water] (*See also* hydrarg.)

^{195m}Hg

mercury-195m

hg

hectogram
hemoglobin (*See also* HB, Hb, Hbg, HG, HGB, hgb)

HGA

high-grade astrocytomas
homogentisate (homogentisic acid oxidase)
homogentisic acid

HGA$_{1c}$

glycosylated hemoglobin

HGB, hgb

hemoglobin (*See also* HB, Hb, Hbg, hemo, HG, hg)

Hgb ELECT

hemoglobin electrophoresis

Hgb F, Hg-F

fetal hemoglobin

Hgb S

sickle cell hemoglobin

HGBV

hepatitis GB virus

HGC

hard gel capsule

hg-cal

high caloric (*See also* HC)

HgCl2

mercury chloride

HGD

high-grade dysplasia

HGE

human granulocytic ehrlichiosis
hyperglycemic-glycogenolytic factor

HGES

handgrasp equal and strong

HGF

hepatocyte growth factor (*See also* HPG)
hyperglycemic-glucogenolytic factor (glucagon)
hyperglycemic-glycogenolytic factor

HGG

herpetic geniculate ganglionitis

hGG

human gamma globulin

hGH

human growth hormone
human (pituitary) growth hormone
somatotropin

HGI

Human Genome Initiative

HGM

hog gastric mucin
human glucose monitoring

HGMCR

human genetic mutant cell repository

HGN

hypogastric nerve

HGO

hepatic glucose output
hip guidance orthosis
human glucose output

HGP

hepatic glucose production
Human Genome Project
hyperglobulinemia purpura

HGPRT, HG-PRTase

hypoxanthine guanine phosphoribosyltransferase

HGSHS

Harvard Group Scale of Hypnotic Susceptibility

HGSHS:A

Harvard Group Scale of Hypnotic Susceptibility, Form A

HGSIL

high-grade squamous intraepithelial lesion

Hgt

height (*See also* HT, ht)

HGV

hepatitis G vaccine
hepatitis G virus

HH

halothane hepatitis
hand held
hard of hearing (*See also* HOH)
head hood
healthy hemophiliac
hereditary hemochromatosis
hiatal hernia
holistic health
home health
home help

NOTES

H

HH *(continued)*
homonymous hemiopia
household
hydroxyhexamide
hypergastrinemic hyperchlorhydria
hyperhidrosis
hypogonadotropic hypogonadism
hyporeninemic hypoaldosteronism

H-H
head-to-head sperm agglutination

H/H, H&H
hemoglobin and hematocrit

Hh
hemopoietic histocompatibility

HHA
health hazard appraisal
hereditary hemolytic anemia
hypogonadotropic hypogonadism-
anosmia syndrome
hypothalamic-hypophyseal-adrenal
(system)

HHAA
hypothalamo-hypophyseo-adrenal axis

HH Assist
hand-held assistance

HHAV
human hepatitis A virus

HHB, HHb
hypohemoglobinemia
nonionized hemoglobin
reduced hemoglobin

HHb
hypohemoglobin
reduced hemoglobin

HHC
home health care

HHCA
hypothermic hypokalemic
cardioplegic arrest

HHCS
high-altitude hypertrophic
cardiomyopathy syndrome

HHD
Hailey-Hailey disease
handheld dynamometer
hand-held dynamometer
high heparin dose
home hemodialysis
hypertensive heart disease (*See also*
HTHD)

HHE
health hazard evaluation
hemiconvulsion-hemiplegia-epilepsy
(syndrome)

HHF-35
muscle-specific actin (*See also*
MSA)

HHFM
high-humidity face mask

HHG
hypertrophic hypersecretory
gastropathy

HHH
hyperammonemia, hyperornithinemia,
homocitrullinuria (syndrome)

HHHO
hypotonia, hyperphagia,
hypogonadism, obesity
hypotonia, hypomentia,
hypogonadism, and obesity
(syndrome)

HHIE, HHIE-S
Hearing Handicap Inventory for the
Elderly

HHLL
histocytoid hemangioma-like lesion

HHM
hemohydrometry
high-humidity mask
humoral hypercalcemia of
malignancy

H-Hm
compound hypermetropic
astigmatism

HHN
hand-held nebulizer
hyperosmolar hyperglycemic
nonketotic (syndrome)

HHNC, HHNK
hyperosmolar hyperglycemic
nonketotic (coma)

HHNKS
hyperglycemic hyperosmolar
nonketotic syndrome

HHPC
hyperoxic-hypercapnic

HHPS
hypothalamohypophysial portal
system

HHRH
hereditary hypophosphatemic rickets
with hypercalciuria (syndrome)
hypothalamic hypophysiotropic-
releasing hormone

HHS
Harris hip score
Hearing Handicap Scale
hereditary hemolytic syndrome
Hoyeraal-Heidarsson syndrome
human hypopituitary serum
hyperglycemic hyperosmolar
syndrome
hyperkinetic heart syndrome

HHT
>head halter traction (*See also* HHTx)
>hereditary hemolytic telangiectasia
>hereditary hemorrhagic telangiectasia
>heterotopic heart transplant
>heterotopic heart transplantation
>hydroxyheptadecatrienoic (acid)
>hypertensive hypervolemic therapy

HHTA
>hypothalamohypophyseothyroidal axis

HHTC
>high-humidity tracheostomy collar

HHTM
>high-humidity tracheostomy mask

HHTS
>high-humidity tracheostomy shield

HHTx
>head halter traction (*See also* HHT)

HHV, HHV 1–7
>human herpesvirus 1–8

HHV-6A
>human herpesvirus 6Λ

HHV-6B
>human herpesvirus 6B

HHV-8/KSHV
>human herpesvirus 8/Kaposi sarcoma herpesvirus

HHW
>hand-held weight

HI
>*Haemophilus influenzae* (*See also* H flu, HIF)
>harmonic imaging
>head injury
>health insurance
>hearing impaired
>heart infusion
>heat inactivated
>heat input
>hemagglutination inhibition (titer) (*See also* HAI)
>hemorrhagic infarction
>hepatic insufficiency
>hepatobiliary imaging
>high impulsiveness
>homicidal ideation
>hormone dependent
>hormone insensitive
>hospital induced
>hospital insurance

>human insulin
>humoral immunity
>hydrogen iodide
>hydroxyindole
>hyperglycemic index
>hypoglycemic index
>hypomelanosis of Ito
>hypothermic ischemia

HI-30
>bikunin (protease inhibitor)
>human inhibitor 30 (inter-alpha-trypsin inhibitor)

Hi
>histamine

HIA
>heat infusion agar
>hemagglutinating inhibition antibody
>hemagglutination inhibition antibody
>hemagglutination inhibition assay
>hyperventilation-induced asthma

HIAA
>hydroxyindoleacetic acid (*See also* OH-IAA)

5-HIAA
>5-hydroxyindoleacetic acid

21-HIAA
>21-hydroxyindoleacetic acid

HIAD
>high-impact aerobic dance

HIAP
>human intracisternal A-type particle

HIB
>*Haemophilus influenzae* type b (vaccine) (*See also* HITB, Hib)
>heart infusion broth
>hemolytic immune body
>hyperpnea-induced bronchoconstriction
>hypoxia, intussusception, brain mass

Hib
>*Haemophilus influenzae* type b

HIB-C, HIBcn
>*Haemophilus influenzae* type b conjugate vaccine

HIBHbOC
>*Haemophilus influenzae* type vaccine oligosaccharide-CRM197 vaccine conjugate

HIBPRP-D
>*Haemophilus influenzae* type b vaccine, PRP-D conjugate vaccine

NOTES

H

HIBPRP-OMP
Haemophilus influenzae type b vaccine, PRP-OMP conjugate vaccine

HIBPRP-T
Haemophilus influenzae type b vaccine, PRP-T conjugate vaccine

HIBps
Haemophilus influenzae type b polysaccharide vaccine

HIC
hepatic iron concentration
Human Investigation Committee

hi-cal
high caloric

H-ICD-A
International Classification of Diseases, Adopted Code for Hospitals

HICHO
high carbohydrate (diet) (*See also* HCD)

HiCn
cyanmethemoglobin

HICROS
high-frequency contralateral routing of offside signals
high-frequency contralateral routing of signals

HID
headache, insomnia, and depression (syndrome)
herniated intervertebral disk
human infectious dose
hyperimmunoglobulinemia syndrome
hyperkinetic impulse disorder

HIDA
dimethyl iminodiacetic acid
hepatic 2,6-dimethyliminodiacetic acid
hepatoiminodiacetic acid

HID/AB
high-iron diamine/Alcian blue

HIDS
hyperimmunoglobulinemia D syndrome

HIE
human intestinal epithelium
hyper-IgE
hyperimmunoglobulin E
hypoxic-ischemic encephalopathy

HIER
heat-induced epitope retrieval

HIES
hyperimmunoglobulin E syndrome

HIF
Haemophilus influenzae (*See also* HI, H flu)
higher integrative function
higher intellectual function
histoplasma (tissue) inhibitory factor
Historical Information Form
HIV-inducing factor

HIF-1alpha
hypoxia-inducible factor-1-alpha

HIFBS
heat-inactivated fetal bovine serum

HIFC
hog intrinsic factor concentrate

HIFCS
heat-inactivated fetal calf serum

HIFT
high-frequency ventilation trial

HIFU
high-intensity focused ultrasonography
high-intensity focused ultrasound

HIg
hyperimmunoglobulin

hIG
human immunoglobulin

HIH
hypertensive intracerebral hemorrhage

HIHA
high impulsiveness high anxiety

HIHARS
hyperventilation-induced high-amplitude rhythmic slowing

HII
hemagglutination inhibition immunoassay
hepatic iron index

HIIC
heated intraoperative intraperitoneal chemotherapy

HIL
hypoxic-ischemic lesion

HILA
high impulsiveness low anxiety

HILP
hyperthermic isolated limb perfusion

HIM
health information management
hemopoietic inductive microenvironment
hepatitis-infectious mononucleosis
hexosephosphateisomerase
Hill Interaction Matrix (psychologic test)
hyper-IgM syndrome

HIMC
hepatic intramitochondrial crystalloid

HIMP
high-dose intravenous
methylprednisolone
HIMT
hemagglutination inhibition
morphine test
Hind II, Hind III
restriction endonucleases from
Haemophilus influenzae
H inf
hypodermoclysis infusion
HINI
hypoxic-ischemic neuronal injury
HINT
Harris Infant Neuromotor Test
Hint.
Hinton (flocculation test for
syphilis)
HIO
health insuring organization
hepatic iron overload
hole-in-one (technique)
hypoiodism
hypoiodite (salt of hypoiodous
acid)
HIOMT
hydroxyindole-*O*-methyltransferase
HIOS
high index of suspicion
HIP
health illness profile
health insurance plan
homograft incus prosthesis
hospital insurance program
humoral immunocompetence profile
hydrostatic indifference point
Hypnotic Induction Profile
HIPAA
Health Insurance Portability and
Accountability Act
Health Insurance Portability and
Accountability Act of 1996
HIPC
hormone independent prostate
cancer
HiPIP
high-potential iron protein
HIPO
hemihypertrophy, intestinal web,
preauricular skin tag, and
congenital corneal opacity
(syndrome)

Hospital Indicator for Physicians'
Orders
HIPPS
Health Insurance Prospective
Payment System
HiPro, HiProt
high protein (diet) (*See also* HP)
HIR
head injury routine
hepatic ischemia and reperfusion
high irradiance response
HIRF
histamine inhibitory releasing factor
HIS
Hanover Intensive Score
Haptic Intelligence Scale
health information system
Health Intention Scale
Health Interview Survey
high intermittent suction
Home Incapacity Scale
hospital information system
hyperimmune serum
hyperimmunized suppressed
His
histidine (*See also* H)
His-
histidyl
-His
histidino
HISG
human immune serum globulin
HISMS
How I See Myself Scale
(psychologic test)
His-Pro-DKP
histidyl-proline-diketopiperazine
HISS
human immune status survey
HIST
hospital in-service training
hist
histidinemia
history (*See also* H, Hx, Hy)
HISTLINE
History of Medicine On-Line
(obsolete)
HISTO
histoplasmosis
histo
histology
histoplasmin skin test

NOTES

H

331

Histo-Dx
> histologic diagnosis

histol
> histologic
> histologist
> histology

HIT
> hemagglutination inhibition test
> heparin-induced thrombocytopenia
> histamine inhalation test
> histamine ion transfer
> Holtzman Inkblot Technique
> home infusion therapy
> hypertrophic infiltrative tendinitis
> hypertrophied inferior turbinate

HITB, HiTb
> *Haemophilus influenzae* type b
> (*See also* HIB)

HITES
> hydrocortisone, insulin, transferrin, estradiol, and selenium

HITS
> high-intensity transient signal

HITT, HITTS
> heparin-induced thrombocytopenia-thrombosis
> heparin-induced thrombosis-thrombocytopenia syndrome

HiTT
> high-dose thrombin time

HIU
> head injury unit
> hyperplasia interstitialis uteri

HIV
> human immunodeficiency virus

HIV-1
> human immunodeficiency virus type 1

HIV-2
> human immunodeficiency virus type 2

HIV-Ab
> human immunodeficiency virus antibody

HIVAN
> human immunodeficiency virus-associated nephropathy

HIVAT
> home intravenous antibiotic therapy

HIV-1C
> human immunodeficiency virus-1 subtype C

HIV-D
> human immunodeficiency virus dementia

HIVD
> herniated interverterbral disk

HIV-G
> human immunodeficiency virus gingivitis

HIVIg
> anti-human immunodeficiency virus immune serum globulin
> HIV immunoglobulin
> human immunodeficiency virus immunoglobulin

HiVit
> high vitamin

HIVMP
> high-dose intravenous methylprednisolone

HIV-NHL
> human immunodeficiency virus-associated non-Hodgkin lymphoma

HIV-P
> human immunodeficiency virus-associated periodontitis

HIV-PARSE
> human immunodeficiency virus-patient-reported status and experience

HIV-QAM
> human immunodeficiency virus quality audit marker

HIV-QOL
> human immunodeficiency virus quality-of-life question

HIV-SGD
> human immunodeficiency virus-associated salivary gland disease

HIZ
> high-intensity zone

HJA
> hip joint angle

HJB
> high jugular bulb
> Howell-Jolly bodies

HJR
> hepatojugular reflux

HJV
> Highlands J virus

HK
> heat killed
> heel-to-knee (test) (*See also* H-K, HTK)
> hexokinase
> human kidney (cell) (*See also* HKC)

H-K, H→K
> hand-to-knee (coordination)
> heel-to-knee (test) (*See also* HK, HTK)

HK1
> hexokinase 1

hK2
human kallikrein-2
hK3
human kallikrein-3
HKAFO
hip-knee-ankle-foot orthosis
HKAO
hip-knee-ankle orthosis
HKC
human kidney cell (*See also* HK)
hKGK1
human kidney glandular kallikrein-1 gene
HKH
hyperkinetic heart syndrome
HKLM
heat-killed *Listeria monocytogenes*
HKMN
Hickman (catheter)
HKO
hip-knee orthosis (splint)
HKS
heel-knee-shin (test)
hyperkinesis syndrome
HKT
heterotopic kidney transplant
HL
hairline
hairy leukoplakia
half-life (element, pharmaceutical)
hallux limitus
haloperidol
harelip
hearing level
hearing loss
heart disease, low risk
heart and lungs (*See also* H&L)
heavy lifting
heel lance
hemilaryngectomy
hemolysis
heparin lock (*See also* H/L, hep lock)
hepatic lipase
Hickman line
histiocytic lymphoma
histocompatibility locus
Hodgkin lymphoma
human leukocyte
human lymphocyte
humerus length
hygienic laboratory

hyperlipidemia
hyperlipoproteinemia
hypermetropia, latent
hypertrichosis lanuginosa
lateral habenular (nucleus)
H/L
heparin lock (*See also* HL, hep lock)
hydrophil/lipophil (ratio)
H&L
heart and lungs (*See also* HL)
HL7
health level seven
hL
hectoliter
HLA
heart, lungs, and abdomen
histocompatibility leukocyte antigen
homologous leukocyte antibody
horizontal long axial
human leukocyte antibody
human leukocyte antigen (system)
hypoplastic left atrium
HLA-A, HLA-B, HLA-C, HLA-D, HLA-DR
varieties of human leukocyte antigen
HLA-A24
human leukocyte antigen-A24
HLA allele
human leukocyte antigen allele
HLA-B57
human leukocyte antigen restriction element
HLA-LD
human lymphocyte antigen-lymphocyte defined
HLALD
horse liver alcohol dehydrogenase
HLA-SD
human lymphocyte antigen-serologically defined
HLB
head, limbs, and body
hydrophilic-lipophilic balance
hypotonic lysis buffer
HLBI
human lymphoblastoid interferon
HLC
heat loss center
HLCL
human lymphoblastoid cell line

NOTES

H

HLD
> haloperidol decanoate (*See also* HD, HL-D)
> hepatolenticular degeneration
> herniated lumbar disk
> high-level disinfection
> hypersensitivity lung disease

HL-D
> haloperidol decanoate (*See also* HD, HLD)

HLDH
> heat-stable lactic dehydrogenase

HLDP
> hypoglossia-limb deficiency phenotype

HLE
> human leukocyte elastase

HLEG
> hydrolysate lactalbumin Earle glucose

HLF
> heat-labile factor
> human lung fibroblast

hLF
> human lung field
> human lung fluid

HLFCB
> horizontal laminar flow clean benches

HLG
> hypertrophic lymphocytic gastritis

HLGR
> high-level gentamicin resistance

HLH
> helix-loop-helix
> hemophagocytic lymphohistiocytosis
> human luteinizing hormone (*See also* hLH)
> hypoplastic left heart (syndrome) (*See also* HLHS)

hLH
> heterodimeric luteinizing hormone
> human luteinizing hormone (*See also* HLH)

HLHS
> hypoplastic left heart syndrome (*See also* HLH)

HLI
> hemolysis inhibition

hLI
> human leukocyte interferon
> human lymphocyte interferon

HLK, H-L-K
> heart, liver, and kidneys

HLL
> hypoplasia of left heart

HLM
> hemosiderin-laden macrophages

HLN
> hilar lymph node
> hyperplastic liver nodule

hLN
> human Lesch-Nyhan (cell)

H&L OK
> heart and lungs normal

HLP
> hepatic lipoperoxidation
> hind leg paralysis
> hyperkeratosis lenticularis perstans
> hyperlipoproteinemia

HLR
> heart-lung resuscitation
> heart-lung resuscitator
> heart-to-lung ratio

HLS
> Health Learning System

hLS
> human lung surfactant

HLT
> heart-lung transplant
> heart-lung transplantation
> high lateral tension

hLT
> human lipotropin
> human lymphocyte transformation

hlth
> health

HLV
> herpeslike virus
> hypoplastic left ventricle

HLVS
> hypoplastic left ventricular syndrome

HM
> hand motion
> hand movement
> harmonic mean
> head movement
> health maintenance
> heart murmur
> heavily muscled
> heloma molle (soft corn)
> hemifacial microsomia (*See also* HFM)
> hepatic metabolism
> high-magnification
> Hispanic male
> Holter monitor
> home management
> homosexual male
> hospital management
> human milk
> human semisynthetic insulin
> humidity mask
> hydatidiform mole
> hyperimmune mouse

hyperopia, manifest (hypermetropia)
(*See also* Hm)
hypoxic-metabolic

Hm

hyperopia, manifest (hypermetropia)
(*See also* HM)
manifest hyperopia

hm

hectometer

HMA

hemorrhage and microaneurysm
heteroduplex mobility assay

hMAM RNA

human mammaglobin RNA

HMAS

hyperimmune mouse ascites (fluid)

HMB

beta-hydroxy-beta methylbutyrate (a
leucine metabolite)
hydroxy beta methylbutyrate

HMB45, HMB 45

homatropine methylbromide

HMBA

hexamethylene bisacetamide

HMC

hand-mirror cell
health maintenance cooperative
heroin, morphine, and cocaine
hospital management committee
hydroxymethyl cytosine
hyoscine-morphine-codeine
hypertelorism-microtia-clefting
(syndrome)
minor histocompatibility complex

hMCAF

human macrophage-monocyte
chemotactic and activating factor

HMCAS

hyperdense middle cerebral artery
sign

HMCCMP

human mammary carcinoma cell
membrane proteinase

HMCK

high molecular weight cytokeratin

HMD

head-mounted display
hyaline membrane disease

HMDP

hydroxymethylene diphosphonate

HMDS

hexamethyldislazane

HME

Health Media Education
heat, massage, and exercise (*See
also* HMX)
heat/moisture exchanger
hereditary multiple exostosis
home medical equipment
human monocytic ehrlichiosis

HMEF

heat and moisture exchanging filter

HMETSC

heavy metal screen

HMF

human milk fortifier
hydroxymethylfurfural

HMFG

human milk fat globule

HM/3ft

hand motion at 3 feet (vision test)

HMG

high mobility group
hydroxymethylglutaric (acid)
hydroxymethylglutaryl

hMG

human menopausal gonadotropin

HMG CoA, HMG-CoA

beta-hydroxy-beta-methylglutaryl-
coenzyme A
beta-hydroxy-β-methylglutaryl-CoA

HMI

healed myocardial infarction
history of medical illness

HMIS

hallux metatarsophalangeal
interphalangeal scale
hospital medical information system

HMK

high molecular weight kininogen
(*See also* HMWK)
homemaking

hML

human milk lysozyme

HM & LP

hand motion and light perception
(vision test)

HMM

heavy meromyosin (of muscle)

HMMA

4-hydroxy-3-methoxymandelic acid

HMO

health maintenance organization

NOTES

H

HMO *(continued)*
    heart minute output
    hypothetical mean organism
HMP
    health maintenance plan
    hexose monophosphate
    hexose monophosphate pathway
    hot moist pack
    hydromotive pressure
HMPA
    hexamethylphosphoramide
HMPAO
    hexametazime
    hexamethylpropyleneamine oxime
    hexamethyl-propyleneamine oxime
^{99mTc}**-HMPAO**
    ^{99mTc}-hexamethylpropyleneamine
    oxime
HMPAO-SPECT
    technetium-99m hexamethylpropylene
    amine oxime single-photon
    emission computed tomography
HMPG
    hydroxymethoxyphenylglycol
HMPS
    hexose monophosphate shunt *(See
    also* HMS)
HMPT
    hexamethylphosphoric triamide
HMR
    histiocytic medullary reticulosis
    Hoechst Marion Roussel (stain)
H-mRNA
    H-chain messenger ribonucleic acid
1H-MRS
    proton magnetic resonance
    spectroscopy
HMRTE
    human milk reverse transcriptase
    enzyme
HMRU
    Hazardous Materials Response Unit
HMS
    hexose monophosphate shunt *(See
    also* HMPS)
    high methacholine sensitivity
    hyperactive malarial splenomegaly
    hypermobility syndrome
    hypodermic morphine sulfate
    hypothetical mean strain
HMSAS
    hypertrophic muscular subaortic
    stenosis
hMSC
    human mesenchymal stem cell
HMSN
    hereditary motor-sensory neuropathy
    (type IA, II, III–VII)

HMSR
    high medical-social risk
HMSS
    hyperactive malarial splenomegaly
    syndrome
HMT
    hexamethylenetetramine
    (methenamine) *(See also* HMTA)
    histamine methyltransferase
    Hodkinson Mental Test
    hospital management team
hMT
    human molar thyrotropin
HMTA
    hexamethylenetetramine
    (methenamine) *(See also* HMT)
HMTV
    human mammary tumor virus
HMW
    high molecular weight
HMWC
    high molecular weight component
HMW-CK
    high molecular weight cytokeratin
HMWGP
    high molecular weight glycoprotein
HMWK
    high molecular weight kininogen
    (See also HMK)
HMW-MAA
    high molecular weight-melanoma-
    associated antigen
HMWPE
    high molecular weight polyethylene
HMX
    heat, massage, and exercise *(See
    also* HME)
HN
    head and neck *(See also* H&N)
    head nurse
    hemagglutinin neuraminidase
    hematemesis neonatorum
    hemorrhage of newborn
    hereditary nephritis
    high nitrogen
    hilar node
    histamine-containing neuron
    home nursing
    hospital man
    hypertensive nephrosclerosis
    hypertrophic neuropathy
H&N
    head and neck *(See also* HN)
HN$_2$, HN2
    nitrogen mustard
HNA
    heparin-neutralizing activity
    hypothalamoneurohypophysial axis

HNAC
Heymann nephritis antigenic complex

HNB
human neuroblastoma
hydroxynitrobenzylbromide

HNC
hypernephroma cell
hyperosmolar nonketotic coma
hyperoxic normocapnic
hypothalamoneurohypophyseal complex

hNC
human neutrophil collagenase

HNE
human neutrophil elastase

HNF
hepatocyte nuclear factor

HNF3
hepatocyte nuclear factor-3

HNF4
hepatocyte nuclear factor-4

HNF4a
hepatocyte nuclear factor-4a

HNHL
hepatic non-Hodgkin lymphoma

HNI
hospitalization not indicated

HNID
Haemophilus-Neisseria identification

HNK
human natural killer (cell)

HNKDC
hyperosmolar nonketotic diabetic coma

HNKDS
hyperosmolar nonketotic diabetic state

HNL
histiocytic necrotizing lymphadenitis
human neutrophil lipocalin

HNLN
hospitalization no longer necessary

H&N mot
head and neck motion

HNN
hybrid neural network

HNP
hereditary nephritic protein
herniated nucleus pulposus (*See also* HPN)
human neurophysin

HNP-4
human neutrophil peptide-4

HNPCC
hereditary nonpolyposis colon cancer
hereditary nonpolyposis colon carcinoma
hereditary nonpolyposis colorectal cancer
hereditary nonpolyposis colorectal carcinoma

HNPP
hereditary neuropathy (with susceptibility to) pressure palsy

HNR
head-neck replacement

hnRNA
heterogeneous nuclear ribonucleic acid

hnRNP
heterogeneous nuclear ribonucleoprotein

HNS
head, neck, and shaft (of bone)
head and neck surgery
home nursing supervisor
0.45% sodium chloride injection (half-normal saline)

HNSCC
head and neck squamous cell carcinoma

HNSHA
hereditary nonspherocytic hemolytic anemia

HNSN
home, no services needed

HNT
Hantaan (hantavirus) vaccine

HNTD
highest nontoxic dose

HNTLA
Hiskey-Nebraska Test of Learning Aptitude

HnTT
heparin neutralized thrombin time

HNU
human *neu* unit

HNV
has not voided

HNWG
has not worn glasses

NOTES

H

337

HO

hand orthosis
hematology-oncology
heme oxygenase
heterotopic ossification
high oxygen
hip orthosis
house officer
hyperbaric oxygen
hypertrophic ossification

H2O

water

H2O2

hydrogen peroxide

H/O, h/o

history of

Ho

holmium
horse (slang for heroin) (*See also* H)
horse (veterinary)

HOA

hip osteoarthritis
hypertrophic osteoarthritis
hypertrophic osteoarthropathy
hypertrophic osteoarthroscopy

Ho antigen

low-frequency blood group antigen

HoaRhLG

horse anti-Rhesus lymphocyte globulin

HoaTTG

horse antitetanus toxoid globulin

HOB

head of bed

HOBT

hyperbaric oxygen therapy

HOB UPSOB

head of bed up for shortness of breath

HOC

human ovarian cancer
hydroxycorticoid (*See also* HC)
hypertrophic obstructive cardiomyopathy

HOCA

high-osmolar contrast agent

HOCM

high-osmolar contrast medium (*See also* HOM)
high-osmolarity contrast medium
hypertrophic obstructive cardiomyopathy

HOD

hereditary opalescent dentin
hospital day (*See also* HD)
hyperbaric oxygen drenching

13-HODE

13-hydroxyoctadecadienoic acid

HOF, hof

height of fundus
hepatic outflow
human oviduct fluid

Hoff

Hoffmann (reflex)

HOG

halothane, oxygen, and gas (nitrous oxide)

HOGA

hyperornithinemia with gyrate atrophy

HOH

hard of hearing (*See also* HH)

HOI

hospital onset of infection
hypoiodous acid

HoIg

horse immunoglobulin

HOLD

hemostatic occlusive leverage device

HoLRP

holmium laser resection of the prostate

HOM

high-osmolar (contrast) medium (*See also* HOCM)

HOME

Home Observation for Measurement of the Environment
Home-Oriented Maternity Experience

Homeo, Homeop

homeopathy

HOMO

highest occupied molecular orbital

homolat

homolateral

HONK

hyperosmolar nonketotic (coma)

HOOD, HOODS

hereditary onychoosteodysplasia syndrome
hereditary osteoonychodysplasia

HOOI

Hall Occupational Orientation Inventory

HOP

high oxygen pressure
hourly output
hypothalamic-pituitary-ovarian
hypothyroxinemia of prematurity

HOPD

hospital outpatient department

HOPE
> health-oriented physical education
> high oxygen percentage
> holistic orthogonal parameter
> estimation

HOPE-ROP
> high oxygen percentage in
> retinopathy of prematurity

HOPES
> human immunodeficiency virus
> overview of problems evaluation
> system

HOPI
> history of present illness (*See also*
> HPI)

HOPP
> hepatic-occluded portal pressure

HOPT
> hamster oocyte penetration test

hor, horiz
> horizontal (*See also* H, h)

HORF
> high-output renal failure

HORS
> Hemiballism/Hemichorea Outcome
> Rating Score

HOS
> human osteogenic sarcoma
> human osteosarcoma
> hypoosmotic swelling

HoS
> horse serum (*See also* HS)

hosp
> hospital (*See also* H, HX)
> hospitalization (*See also* H, HX)

HOST
> hypoosmotic shock treatment

HOT
> human old tuberculin
> hyperbaric oxygen therapy
> hypertension optimal treatment

HOTC
> heterozygous ornithine
> transcarbamylase

HOTS
> hypercalcemia-osteolysis-T-cell
> syndrome

HOW
> hypothermia oxygen warmer

HOX
> homeobox (gene)

Ho:YAG, Ho:YAG laser
> holmium:yttrium-aluminum-garnet
> holmium yttrium aluminum garnet
> laser
> holmium:yttrium-argon-garnet

HP
> *Haemophilus pleuropneumoniae*
> halogen phosphorus
> handicapped person
> haptoglobin (*See also* HAPTO, Hp,
> Hpt)
> Harding-Passey (melanoma)
> hard palate
> Harvard pump
> hastening phenomenon
> health professional
> heater probe
> heat production
> heel-to-patella (*See also* H→P)
> *Helicobacter pylori*
> hemiparesis
> hemipelvectomy
> hemiplegia (*See also* Hp)
> hemoperfusion
> heparin (*See also* H, HEP)
> hereditary pancreatitis
> herpetiform pemphigus
> highly purified
> high potency
> high power
> high pressure
> high protein
> high protein (diet) (*See also* HiPro)
> Hodgen and Pearson (suspension
> traction) (*See also* H&P)
> horizontal plane
> horsepower
> hospital participation
> hot pack
> hot pad
> human pituitary
> hybridoma product
> Hydrocollator pack
> hydrogen peroxide
> hydrophilic petrolatum
> hydrophobic protein
> hydrostatic pressure
> hydroxyproline (*See also* HYP, hyp,
> hypro)
> hydroxypyruvate
> hyperparathyroidism (*See also* HPT,
> HPTH, hyperpara)

NOTES

H

HP *(continued)*
    hyperphoria
    hyperplastic polyp
    hypersensitivity pneumonitis
    hypertension plus proteinuria
    hypoparathyroidism
    hypopharynx

H&P
    history and physical (examination)
      (*See also* HPE)
    Hodgen and Pearson (suspension
      traction) (*See also* HP)

H→P
    heel-to-patella (*See also* HP)

Hp
    haptoglobin (*See also* HAPTO, HP,
      Hpt)
    hematoporphyrin
    hemiplegia (*See also* HP)

hp
    heaping
    horsepower

HPA
    alpha-haptoglobin
    Helix pomatia agglutinin
    hemagglutinating penicillin antibody
    Hereford Parental Attitude (Survey)
    Histoplasma capsulatum
      polysaccharide antigen
    human pancreatic amylase
    human papillomavirus
    human platelet antigen
    hypothalamic-pituitary-adrenal (axis)
    hypothalamic-pituitary axis
    hypothalamopituitary adrenal
    hypothalmo-pituitary-adrenocortical
      (system) (*See also* HPAC)

HPA-23
    antimoniotungstate (French HIV
      drug)

HPAA
    hydroperoxyarachidonic acid
    hydroxyphenylacetic acid
    hydroxyphenylpyruvic acid
    hypothalamic-pituitary-adrenal axis

HPAC
    hypothalamic-pituitary-adrenocortical
      (system) (*See also* HPA)

HPAEPAD
    high-pH anion exchange
      chromatography coupled with
      pulsed amperometric detection

hPASP
    human pancreas-specific protein

HPAT
    home parenteral antibiotic therapy

HPBC
    hyperpolarizing bipolar cell

HPBF
    hepatotropic portal blood factor

HPBL
    human peripheral blood leukocyte

HPC
    hemangiopericytoma
    hematopoietic progenitor cell
    heterotopic plate count (bacteria)
    hippocampal pyramidal cell
    history of present complaint
    hydrophilic coated
    hydrophilic-coated (guidewire)
    hydroxyphenylcinchoninic (acid)
    hydroxypropylcellulose
    hyperplastic-like mucosal change

HPC-1
    hereditary prostate cancer 1 locus

HPCD
    hemostatic puncture closure device

HPCE
    high-performance capillary
      electrophoresis

HPCF
    high-performance chromatofocusing

HPD
    hearing protection device
    hematoporphyrin derivative (*See also*
      HpD)
    highly probably drunk
    high-protein diet
    home peritoneal dialysis

HP-D
    Hough-Powell digitizer

HpD
    hematoporphyrin derivative (*See also*
      HPD)

HPE
    hemorrhage, papilledema, exudate
    hepatic portoenterostomy
    high permeability edema
    history and physical examination
      (*See also* H&P)
    holoprosencephaly
    hydrostatic pulmonary edema

HPET
    Helicobacter pylori eradication
      therapy

HPETE
    hydroperoxyeicosatetraenoic acid

5-HPETE
    5-hydroperoxyeicosatetraenoic acid

12-HPETE
    12-hydroperoxyeicosatetraenoic acid

HPF
    heparin-precipitable fraction
    hepatic plasma flow
    high-pass filter
    high-power field

high-power field (microscope) (*See also* hpf)
hypocaloric protein feeding

hpf

high-power field (microscope) (*See also* HPF)

HPFH

hereditary persistence of fetal hemoglobin

hPFSH, HPFSH

human pituitary follicle-stimulating hormone

HPG

hepatocyte growth factor (*See also* HGF)
hypothalamic-pituitary-gonadal

hPG

human pituitary gonadotropin (*See also* HPG)

HPGe

high-purity germanium

HPH

halothane-percent-hour
hypoxia-induced pulmonary hypertension

HPI

Haemophilus parainfluenzae
hepatic perfusion index
hepatocyte proliferation inhibitor
Heston Personality Index
Heston Personality Inventory (Test)
history of present illness (*See also* HOPI)

HPIEC

high-performance ion exchange chromatography

HPIP

history, physical, impression, and plan

HPL

human parotid lysozyme
human peripheral lymphocyte
human placental lactogen (*See also* hPL)
hyperplexia

hPL

human placental lactogen (*See also* HPL)

HPLA

hydroxyphenyllactic acid

HPLAC

high-pressure liquid affinity chromatography

HPLC

high-performance liquid chromatography
high-pressure liquid chromatography

HPLO

Helicobacter pylori-like organism

HPM

Harding-Passey melanoma
hemiplegic migraine

HPMC

high-performance membrane chromatography
human peripheral mononuclear cell
hydroxypropyl methylcellulose

HPN

home parenteral nutrition
hypertension (*See also* HT, HTN, hypn)

HP-NAP

neutrophil-activating protein of *Helicobacter pylori*

HPNI

hemodialysis prognostic nutrition index

HPNS

high-pressure neurologic syndrome

HPNT

Hundred Pictures Naming Test

HPO

high-pressure oxygen
hydroperoxide
hydrophilic ointment
hypertrophic pulmonary osteoarthritis
hypertrophic pulmonary osteoarthropathy (*See also* HPOA)
hypothalamic-pituitary-ovarian

HPOA

hypertrophic pulmonary osteoarthropathy (*See also* HPO)

HPP

hereditary pyropoikilocytosis
history (of) presenting problems
hydroxyphenylpyruvate
hydroxypyrazolopyrimidine

2HPP

two-hour postprandial (blood sugar)

hPP

human pancreatic polypeptide

NOTES

H

HPPA
    hydroxyphenylpyruvic acid
HPPH
    hydroxyphenylphenylhydantoin
HPPM
    hyperplastic persistent pupillary
        membrane
HPPO
    high partial pressure of oxygen
    hydroxyphenylpyruvate oxidase
HPP/SQ
    Hilson Personnel Profile/Success
        Quotient
HPr, hPrL
    human prolactin
hPr
    hospital peer review
HPRC
    hereditary papillary renal cancer
    hereditary papillary renal carcinoma
    hereditary papillary renal (cell)
        carcinoma
hPRP
    human platelet-rich plasma
HPRT
    hot plate reaction time
    hypoxanthine-guanine
        phosphoribosyltransferase
    hypoxanthinephospho-
        ribosyltransferase
    hypoxanthine
        phosphoribosyltransferase
HPS
    hantavirus pulmonary syndrome
    hematoxylin-phloxine-saffron (stain)
    hemophagocytic syndrome
    hepatopulmonary syndrome
    high-protein supplement
    His-Purkinje system
    human platelet suspension
    hypertrophic pyloric stenosis
    hypothalamic pubertal syndrome
HpSA
    Helicobacter pylori stool antigen
HPSEC
    high-performance size-exclusion
        chromatography
HPT
    heparin protamine titration
    histamine provocation test
    home pregnancy test
    hot plate test
    hyperparathyroid
    hyperparathyroidism (*See also* HP,
        HPTH, hyperpara)
    hypothalamic-pituitary-thyroid

Hpt
    haptoglobin (*See also* HAPTO, HP,
        Hp)
hPT
    human placental thyrotropin
    human proximal tubule
HPTD
    highly permeable transparent
        dressing
HPTH
    hyperparathyroidism (*See also* HP,
        HPT, hyperpara)
hPTH
    human parathyroid hormone
hPTIN
    human pancreatic trypsin inhibitor
HPTM
    home prothrombin time monitoring
HPTX
    hemopneumothorax
HPU
    heater probe unit
HPUS
    hydrogen peroxide ultrasound
hPUTH
    human placental uterotropic
        hormone
HPV
    Haemophilus pertussis vaccine
    Hart Park virus
    hepatic portal vein
    human papillomavirus
    human parvovirus
    hypoxic pulmonary vasoconstriction
HPV-16, HPV 16
    human papillomavirus type 16
HPVD
    hypertensive pulmonary vascular
        disease
HPV-DE
    high-passage virus-duck embryo
        (cell)
HPV-DK
    high-passage virus-dog kidney (cell)
HPVG
    hepatic portal venous gas
HPX
    high peroxide-containing (cell)
    hypophysectomized (*See also* HX,
        hypox)
    partial hepatectomy
Hpx
    hemopexin (serum protein)
***H. pylori*, H-pylori**
    Helicobacter pylori
HPZ
    high-pressure zone

H₂Q
ubiquinol (*See also* Q-H₂)

HQC
hydroquinone cream

HQL
health-related quality of life

H&R
hysterectomy and radiation

HR
hallux rigidus
Halstead-Reitan (battery) (*See also* HRB)
Harrington rod
hazard ratio
heart rate (*See also* HRT)
hemirectococcygeus
hemorrhagic retinopathy
heterosexual relations (scale)
higher rate
high resolution
high-risk
hormonal response
hospital record
hospital report
hour (*See also* H, h, hr)
human resources
hydroxyethylrutosides (treatment for venous disorders)
hyperimmune reaction
hypertensive retinopathy
hypoxic responder

2HR
two-hour pregnancy test

H₂R
histamine-2 receptor

Hr -2
minus two hours (two hours prior to treatment)

hr
hour (*See also* H, h, HR)

Hr 0
zero hour (when treatment starts)

HRA
health risk appraisal
health risk assessment
heart rate audiometry
high right atrium
histamine-releasing activity

H2RA
histamine-2 receptor antagonist
histamine₂ receptor antagonist

HRAE
high right atrium electrocardiogram

HRANA
histone-reactive antinuclear antibody

HRARE
hybrid rapid acquisition with relaxation enhancement

HRB
Halstead-Reitan Battery (*See also* HR)
histamine release from basophils

HRBC
high-risk breast cancer
horse red blood cell

HRC
help-rejecting complainer
high-resolution chromatography
histidine-rich calcium-binding protein
horse red cell
human rights committee

HRCT
high-resolution computed tomography

HRD
human retroviral disease

HRE
hair removal efficiency
high-resolution electrocardiography
high-resolution protein electrophoresis
hormone-receptor enzyme
hormone response element

HREC
hepatic reticuloendothelial cell

HREH
high-renin essential hypertension

HREM
high-resolution electron microscopy

HRES
high-resolution endoluminal sonography

HRF
Harris return flow
health-related facility
high-resolution fingerprint
histamine-releasing factor
hypertensive renal failure

HRH
hypothalamic-releasing hormone

HRHS
hypoplastic right heart syndrome

NOTES

H

343

HRI
>Harrington rod instrumentation
>high-resolution infrared (imaging)

3H-RIA
>3H-radioimmunoassay
>tritium radioimmunoassay

HRIF
>histamine inhibitory releasing factor
>histamine release inhibitory factor

HRIG
>human rabies immune globulin
>human rabies immunoglobulin

HRL
>head rotation to left

HRLA
>human reovirus-like agent

HRLM
>high-resolution light microscopy

hRLX-2
>synthetic human relaxin

HRMPC
>hormone-refractory metastatic
>   prostate cancer

HRMS
>high-resolution multisweep

HRMTP
>high-risk model of threat
>   perception

hRNA
>heterogeneous ribonucleic acid

HRNB, HRNTB
>Halstead-Reitan Neuropsychological
>   Battery
>Halstead-Reitan Neuropsychological
>   Test Battery

HRNES
>Halstead Russell Neuropsychological
>   Evaluation System

HRP
>high right parasternal (view)
>high-risk pregnancy
>histidine-rich protein
>horseradish peroxidase

HRPBC
>high-risk primary breast cancer

HRPC
>hormone-refractory prostate cancer
>hormone-resistant prostate cancer

HRPD
>Hamburg Rating Scale for
>   Psychiatric Disorders

HRP-II
>histidine-rich protein-II

HRQL, HRQOL
>health-related quality of life

HRR
>haplotype relative risk

>Hardy-Rand-Ritter (color vision test
>   kit)
>head rotation to right
>heart rate range
>heart rate reserve
>high-risk recipient
>high-risk register

HRS
>Hamilton Rating Scale
>Hamman-Rich syndrome
>Haw River syndrome
>hepatorenal syndrome
>Hodgkin-Reed-Sternberg (cells)
>hormone receptor site
>humeroradial synostosis

HRSA
>heart rate power spectral analysis

HRS-D
>Hamilton Rating Scale for
>   Depression

HRST
>heat, reddening, swelling, or
>   tenderness
>heavy resistance strength training

HRSV
>human respiratory syncytial virus

HRT
>half relaxation time
>heart rate (*See also* HR)
>Heidelberg retina tomograph
>heparin response test
>high-risk transfer
>hormone replacement therapy
>hyperfractioned radiation (therapy)

HRTE
>human reverse transcriptase enzyme

HRTEM
>high-resolution transmission electron
>   microscopy

HRU
>hormone response unit

HRV
>heart rate variability
>heterogeneous resistance to
>   vancomycin
>human rotavirus

HRVL
>human reovirus-like

H/S
>helper-suppressor (ratio)
>hysterosalpingogram (*See also* HSG)
>hysterosalpingography (*See also* HS,
>   HSG, HSP)

HS
>at bedtime [L. *hora somni hour
>   of sleep*] (*See also* h.s., HS,
>   QHS, q.h.s.)
>half-scan

half strength
hamstrings (*See also* hams.)
hamstring sets
hand surgery
Hartmann solution
head sign
head sling
healthy subject
heart size
heart sound
heat stable
heavy smoker
heel spur
heelstick
heme synthetase
heparin sulfate
hereditary spherocytosis
herpes simplex
hidradenitis suppurativa
high school
hippocampal sclerosis
homologous serum
Hopelessness Scale
horizontally selective (visual cell)
horse serum (*See also* HoS)
hospital ship
hospital staff
hospital stay
hour of sleep
house surgeon
human serum
hypereosinophilic syndrome
hyperplastic synovium
hypersensitivity
hypertonic saline
hypertrophic scar
hysterosalpingography (*See also* HSG, IISP, H/S)

H&S

hearing and speech
hemorrhage and shock
hysterectomy and sterilization

H→S

heel-to-shin (test) (*See also* HTS)

H₂S

Hering law-EOM innervation, both eyes
Sherrington law-EOM innervation, one eye

Hs

hypochondriasis
hypochondriasis scale

h.s.

at bedtime [L. *hora somni hour of sleep*] (*See also* HS)

HSA

Hazardous Substances Act
health service area
human serum albumin (*See also* HuSA)
hypersomnia-sleep apnea (syndrome)

HSAG

hydroxyethylpiperazine ethanesulfonic acid-saline-albumin-gelatin

HSAN

hereditary sensory and autonomic neuropathy (types I-IV)

HSAP

heat-stable alkaline phosphatase

HSAS

hydrocephalus due to congenital stenosis of aqueduct of Sylvius
hypertrophic subaortic stenosis (*See also* HSS)

HSB

husband (*See also* H, husb)

HSBG

heel-stick blood gas

HSBS

evening blood sugar

HSC

health sciences center
health screening center
hematopoietic stem cell
hepatic stellate cell
horizontal semicircular canal
human skin collagenase

HSCCP

High School Career-Course Planner

HSCL

Hopkins Symptom Checklist

HSCL-90

Hopkins Symptom Checklist-90

HSCL-90 T

Hopkins Symptom Checklist-90 Total Score

HS-CoA

reduced coenzyme A

HSCT

hematopoietic stem cell transplantation

HSD

honest significance difference

NOTES

H

HSD *(continued)*
  hydroxysteroid dehydrogenase
  hypoactive sexual desire (disorder)
HSD2
  hydroxysteroid dehydrogenase type
  2
17β-HSD
  17-beta-hydroxysteroid
  dehydrogenase
HSDA
  high single dose alternate day
HSDI
  Health Self-Determination Index
HSE
  health and safety executive
  hemorrhagic shock and
  encephalopathy
  herpes simplex encephalitis
  human serum esterase
  human skin equivalent
  hypertonic saline-epinephrine
  (solution)
Hse
  homoserine
HSES
  hemorrhagic shock-encephalopathy
  syndrome
HSF
  heated soybean flower
  histamine-induced suppressor factor
  histamine-sensitizing factor
  hypothalamic secretory factor
HSG
  herpes simplex genitalis
  hysterosalpingogram (*See also* H/S)
  hysterosalpingography (*See also* HS,
  HSP, H/S)
  hysterosonography
hSGF
  human skeletal growth factor
hSGP
  human sialoglycoprotein
HSGYV
  heat, steam, gum, yawn, and
  Valsalvas maneuver
HSHC
  hemisuccinate of hydrocortisone
HSI
  heat stress index
  human seminal (plasma) inhibitor
H-SIL, HSIL
  high-grade squamous intraepithelial
  lesion
  high-grade squamous intraepithelial
  lesions
HSK
  herpes simplex keratitis
  herpetic stromal keratitis

HSL
  herpes simplex labialis
  hormone sensitive lipase
H-SLAP
  human stromelysin aggregated
  proteoglycan
HSLC
  high-speed liquid chromatography
HSM
  heparin surface-modified intraocular
  lens
  hepatosplenomegaly
  holosystolic murmur
HSMN
  hereditary sensorimotor neuropathy
HSMN I–III
  hereditary sensory motor neuropathy
  (type I–III)
HSN
  Hansen-Street nail
  heart sounds normal
  hereditary sensory neuropathy
  herpes simplex neonatorum
HSNC
  human skin nurse cell
hSOD
  human superoxide dismutase
HSP
  health systems plan
  heat shock protein (*See also* hsp)
  hemostatic screening profile
  Henoch-Schönlein purpura
  hereditary sclerosing poikiloderma
  hereditary spastic paraplegia
  human serum prealbumin
  human serum protein
  hypersensitivity pneumonitis panel
  hysterosalpingography (*See also* HS,
  HSG, H/S)
HSP47
  heat shock protein 47
HSP70
  heat shock protein 70
hsp
  heat shock protein (*See also* HSP)
HSPC
  hydrogenated soy phosphatidyl
  choline
HSPE
  high-strength pancreatic enzymes
HSPG
  (glycosylphosphatidylinositol-
  anchored) heparan sulfate
  proteoglycan
  heparan sulfate proteoglycan
H spike
  His bundle electrogram deflection

HSPM

hippocampal synaptic plasma membrane

HSPN

Henoch-Schönlein purpura nephritis

HSPQ

High School Personality Questionnaire

HSQ

Health Status Questionnaire

HSR

Harleco synthetic resin
heated serum reagent
homogeneously staining region
homogeneous staining region (of chromosome)
hypersensitivity reaction
hypofractionated stereotactic radiotherapy

HSRA

high-speed rotational atherectomy

HSRCCT

high-spatial-resolution cine computed tomography

HSRD

hypertension secondary to renal disease

HSRS

Health-Sickness Rating Scale
Hess School Readiness Scale

HSS

half-strength saline (0.45% sodium chloride)
hepatic stimulatory substance
high-speed supernatant
hyperstimulation syndrome
hypertrophic subaortic stenosis (*See also* HSAS)

HSSCC

hereditary site-specific colon cancer

HSSE

high soapsuds enema

HSSG

hysterosalpingosonography

HST

health screening test
Hemoccult slide test
horseshoe tear

hst-1

human stomach cancer-transforming factor-1

hst-2

human stomach cancer-transforming factor-2

HSTF

human serum thymus factor

HSTS

human-specific thyroid stimulator

HSV

herpes simplex virus
highly selective vagotomy
hyperviscosity syndrome

HSV-1, HSV1, HSV-I

herpes simplex virus 1

HSV-2, HSV2, HSV-II

herpes simplex virus 2

HSVE

herpes simplex virus encephalitis

HSV-TK, HSVtk, HSV-tk

herpes simplex virus thymidine kinase

HSyn

heme synthase

HT

hammertoe
hand test
Hand Test (psychologic test)
Hashimoto thyroiditis
hearing test
hearing threshold
heart (*See also* H, He, ht)
heart test
heart tone (*See also* ht)
heart transplant
heart transplantation
height (*See also* Hgt, ht)
hemagglutination titer
hemorrhagic transformation
high temperature
high tension (*See also* ht)
histotechnology
home treatment
hormonotherapy
hospital treatment
Hough transform
House-Tree (Test)
Hubbard tank
Huhner test
human thrombin
hydrocortisone test
hydrotherapy (*See also* hydro)
5-hydroxytryptamine (serotonin) (*See also* 5-HT, 5HT, HTA)

NOTES

H

HT *(continued)*
   hyperopia, total (hypermetropia)
      (See also Ht)
   hypertension *(See also* HPN, HTN,
      hypn)
   hyperthermia
   hyperthyroid
   hyperthyroidism
   hypertransfusion
   hypertropia
   hypodermic tablet
   hypothalamus *(See also* H, Ht, Hth,
      hyp)

H-T
   head-to-tail sperm agglutination

3-HT
   3-hydroxytyramine (dopamine)

5-HT, 5HT
   5-hydroxytryptamine (serotonin) *(See
      also* HT, HTA)
   monoamine serotonin
   serotonin

H&T
   hospitalization and treatment

H/T
   heel and toe (walking)

H(T)
   intermittent hypertropia

Ht
   height of heart
   heterozygote
   hypermetropia, total
   hyperopia, total *(See also* HT)
   hypothalamus *(See also* H, HT,
      Hth, hyp)
   total hyperopia

ht
   heart *(See also* H, He, HT)
   heart tone *(See also* HT)
   heat
   height *(See also* Hgt, HT)
   high tension *(See also* HT)

ht.
   draft, drink [L. *haustas*] *(See also*
      H, haust.)

5-HT$_{2A}$
   5-hydroxytryptamine 2A

HTA
   heterophil transplantation antigen
   human thymocyte antigen
   5-hydroxytryptamine (serotonin) *(See
      also* HT, 5-HT, 5HT)
   hypertension (French)
   hypophysiotropic area (of
      hypothalamus)

HTACS
   human thyroid adenylcyclase
      stimulator

ht aer
   heated aerosol *(See also* HA)

HTAT
   human tetanus antitoxin

HTB
   hot tub bath
   house tube (feeding) *(See also*
      HTF)
   human tumor bank

HTC
   heated tracheostomy collar
   hepatoma cell
   hepatoma tissue culture
   homozygous typing cell
   hypertensive crisis

HTCA
   human tumor colony assay

HTCP
   Hendler Test for Chronic Pain

HTCVD
   hypertensive cardiovascular disease
      (See also HCVD)

HTD
   human therapeutic dose

HTDW
   heterosexual development of women

hTERT
   human telomerase reverse
      transcriptase

HTF
   heterothyrotropic factor
   house tube feeding *(See also* HTB)

HTG
   high-tension glaucoma
   hypertriglyceridemia

hTg
   human thyroglobulin

HTGL
   hepatic triglyceride lipase

HTH
   helix-turn-helix
   homeostatic thymus hormone

Hth
   hypothalamus *(See also* H, HT, Ht,
      hyp)

HTHD
   hypertensive heart disease *(See also*
      HHD)

HTI
   hemisphere thrombotic infarction
   hepatic tumor index
   human tetanus immunoglobulin

HTIG, hTIg
   homologous tetanus immune
      globulin
   human tetanus immune globulin
   human tetanus immunoglobulin

HTK
> heel-to-knee (test) (*See also* HK, H-K, H→K)

HTL
> hamster tumor line
> hearing threshold level
> histologic technologist
> histotechnologist
> honey-thick liquid (diet consistency)
> human T-cell leukemia
> human T-cell lymphoma
> human thymic leukemia

HTLA
> high titer, low acidity
> human T-lymphocyte antigen

HTLV
> human T-cell leukemia-lymphoma virus
> human T-cell leukemia virus
> human T-cell lymphoma virus
> human T-cell lymphotropic virus

HTLV-1, HTLV-I, HTLV I
> human T-cell leukemia virus I
> human T-lymphotropic virus 1

HTLV-2, HTLV-II
> human T-cell leukemia virus type II
> human T-cell lymphotropic virus II
> human T-lymphotropic virus 2

HTLV-3, HTLV III
> human T-cell leukemia virus type III
> human T-cell lymphotropic virus III

HTLV-III/LAV
> human T-lymphotrophic virus/lymphadenopathy associated virus

IITLV-MA
> human T-cell leukemia virus-associated membrane antigen

HTM
> *Haemophilus* test medium
> high threshold mechanoceptors

HTML
> hypertext markup language

HTN
> hypertension (*See also* HPN, HT, hypn)

HTNV
> Hantaan virus (*See also* HV)

HTO
> heterotropic ossification
> high tibial osteotomy
> hospital transfer order

HTOH
> hydroxytryptophol

HTP
> House-Tree-Person (Projective Technique psychologic test)
> hydroxytryptophan
> hypothalamic, pituitary, thyroid
> hypothromboplastinemia

5-HTP, 5HTP
> 5-hydroxytryptophan
> 5-hydroxy-L tryptophan

HTPN
> home total parenteral nutrition

HTR
> hard tissue replacement
> hemolytic transfusion react
> hypermetropia, right

hTR
> human thyroid hormone receptor

HTRCCT
> high-temporal-resolution cine computed tomography

HTR-MFI
> hard tissue replacement-malleable facial implant

hTRT
> human telomerase reverse transcriptase

IITS
> hammertoc syndrome
> head trauma syndrome
> heel-to-shin (test) (*See also* H→S)
> hcmangioma-thrombocytopenia syndrome
> Hematest stools
> high-throughput screening
> human thyroid-stimulating (hormone) (*See also* hTSH)

hTSAb
> human thyroid-stimulating antibody

HTSCA
> human tumor stem cell assay

hTSH
> human thyroid-stimulating hormone (*See also* HTS)

HTST
> high temperature-short time (pasteurization)

NOTES

H

HTT
hand thrust test
HT/TCP
hydroxyapatite/tricalcium phosphate
HTV
heat temperature vulcanized
herpes-type virus
HTVD
hypertensive vascular disease (*See also* HVD)
HTX
heart transplantation (*See also* HT, HTx)
hemothorax
HTx
heart transplant (*See also* HT, HTX)
HU
head unit
heat unit
hemagglutinating unit
hemagglutinin unit
hemolytic unit
Hounsfield unit (*See also* Hu)
human urinary
human urine
hydroxyurea (*See also* HUR, HYD)
hyperemia unit
hypertensive urgencies
H.U.
heat unit
Hu
Hounsfield unit (*See also* H, HU)
human (*See also* H, h)
hU, hu
dihydrouridine (*See also* D)
HUAEC
human umbilical endothelial cell
HUAM
home uterine activity monitor
home uterine activity monitoring
HUAV
Huacho virus
HUC
hypouricemia
HUCB
human umbilical cord blood
HU-CSF
human urinary CSF
HuCV
human calicivirus
huEPO
human erythropoietin
hu-FSH, HU-FSH
human urinary follicle-stimulating hormone
HuGe
Human Genome

HuGe index
Human Gene Expression
HuGE Net
Human Genome Epidemiology Network
HUGV
Hughes virus
HUI
Harris uterine injector
headache unit index
Health Utilities Index
HUI2
Health Utilities Index Mark 2
HUIFM
human leukocyte interferon Meloy
HuIFN
human interferon
HUIS
high-dose urea in invert sugar
HUK
human urinary kallikrein
HUM
heat (or hot packs), ultrasound, and massage
hematourimetry
home uterine monitoring
HUM 70/30
(Humulin 70/30 insulin)
hum.
humerus
HUMARA
human androgen receptor assay
human androgen receptor gene
X-linked human androgen receptor
HUMI
Harris-Kronner uterine manipulator-injector
HUP
Hospital Utilization Project
HUR
hydroxyurea (*See also* HU, HYD)
HURA
health in underserved rural areas
HURT
hospital utilization review team
HUS
hemolytic uremic syndrome
hyaluronidase unit for semen
HuSA
human serum albumin (*See also* HSA)
husb
husband (*See also* H, HSB)
HUS/TTP
hemoglobinuria and glomerular thrombosis

hemolytic uremic syndrome/thrombotic thrombocytopenia purpura

HUT
head-up tilt

HUTHAS
human thymus antiserum

HUTTT
head-up tilt-table test

HUV
human umbilical vein

HUVEC
human umbilical vein endothelial cell

HUVS
hypocomplementemic urticarial vasculitis syndrome

HV
hallux valgus
Hantaan virus (*See also* HTNV)
has voided
heart volume
height velocity
Hemovac
hepatic vein
herpesvirus
herpes virus
high vacuum
high voltage
high volume
home visit
hospital visit
hyperventilation
hypervolemic

H&V
hemigastrectomy and vagotomy

HVA
hallux valgus angle
homovanillic acid

HVAC
heating, ventilating, and air conditioning

HVC
hepatitis C virus
high voltage can

HVc
hyperstriatum ventrale, pars caudale

HVD
hantavirus disease
hypertensive vascular disease (*See also* HTVD)
hypoxic ventilatory drive

HVDO
hypovitaminosis D osteopathy

HVE
hepatic vascular exclusion
hepatic venous effluence
high-voltage electrophoresis
high-volume evacuator

HVEM
high voltage electron microscope

HVF
hepatocycle volume fraction
Humphrey visual field

HVFP
hepatic vein free pressure

HVG
hematoxylin and van Gieson (stain)
host-versus-graft (disease, response)

HVGS
high-voltage galvanic stimulation (physical therapy)

HVH
Herpesvirus hominis

HVHMA
Herpesvirus hominis membrane antigen

HVI
hepatic vascular isolation
hollow viscus injury

HVID
horizontal visible iris diameter

HVI-DHP
hepatic venous isolation by direct hemoperfusion

HVII
hypervariable segment II

HVJ
hemagglutinating virus of Japan

HVL, hvl
half-value layer
hippocampal volume loss

HVLA
high-velocity low-amplitude

HVLP
high-volume, low-pressure

HVLT
high-velocity lead therapy

HVM
high-velocity missile
hypothalamic ventromedial (nucleus)

HVO
hallux valgus orthosis

NOTES

H

HVOD
hepatic venoocclusive disease

HVOO
hepatic venous outflow obstruction

HVOT
Hooper Visual Organization Test

HVPC
high-voltage pulsed current

HVPE
high-voltage paper electrophoresis

HVPG
hepatic venous pressure gradient

HVPGS
high-voltage pulsed galvanic
  stimulation

HVPS
high-voltage pulsed stimulation

HVPT
hyperventilation provocation test

HVR
hypoxic ventilatory response

HVR1
hypervariable region 1

HVS
herpesvirus saimiri
herpesvirus sensitivity
hyperventilation syndrome
hyperviscosity syndrome

HVSA
high-voltage slow activity

H vs A
home versus (against) advice

HVSD
hydrogen-detected ventricular septal
  defect

HVT
half-value thickness
herpesvirus of turkeys
high-voltage therapy

HVTEM
high-voltage transmission electron
  microscopy

HVUS
hypocomplementemic vasculitis
  urticaria syndrome

HW
healing well
heart weight
hemisphere width
hemodynamically-weighted MRI
heparin well
homework
housewife (*See also* HWFE)

HWB, hwb
hot water bottle

HWE
hot water extract

HWFE
housewife (*See also* HW)

HWG
has worn glasses

HWH
halfway house

HWOK
heel walking normal (OK)

HWP
hepatic wedge pressure
hot wet pack

HWPG
has worn prescription glasses

HWS
hot water soluble

HWY
hundred woman years (of
  exposure)

HX
histiocytosis X
hospital (*See also* H, hosp)
hospitalization (*See also* H, hosp)
hydrogen exchange
hypophysectomized (*See also* HPX,
  hypox)

Hx
history (*See also* H, hist, Hy)
hypoxanthine (*See also* hyp)

2-HxG
di(hydroxyethyl)glycine

HxGPRT
hypoxanthine-guanine phosphoribosyl
  transferase

HXIS
hard x-ray imaging spectrometer

HXR
hypoxanthine riboside

HY
hypophysis (*See also* hyp)

Hy
history (*See also* H, hist, Hx)
hydraulics
hydrostatics
hypermetropia (*See also* H, h)
hyperopia (*See also* H, h)
hyperopic (*See also* H, h)
hypothenar

hy
hysteria (*See also* hys, hyst)

HYCX
hydrocephalus due to congenital
  stenosis of aqueduct of Sylvius

HYD
hydralazine
hydrated to hydration
hydroxyurea (*See also* HU, HUR)

Hyd
hydrocortisone (*See also* HC, HCT)
hydrostatics
hydr
hydraulic
hydrarg.
mercury [L. *hydrargyrum* silver water] (*See also* Hg)
HYDRO
hydronephrosis
hydro
hydrotherapy (*See also* HT)
hydrox
hydroxyline
hyd and tur
hydration and turgor
hyg
hygiene (*See also* H)
hygienic (*See also* H)
HYL, Hyl
hydroxylysine
5Hyl
5-hydroxylysine
HYLL
healthy years of life lost
HYLO
hyaline
HYP
hydroxyproline (*See also* HP, hypro)
hypnosis (*See also* hypno)
3Hyp
3-hydroxyproline
hyp
hydroxyproline (*See also* HP, HYP, hypro)
hypalgesia
hyperresonance
hypertrophy
hypophysectomy (*See also* HE)
hypophysis (*See also* HY)
hypothalamus (*See also* H, HT, Ht, Hth)
hypoxanthine (*See also* Hx)
HYPER
above
higher than
hyperal, hyper-al
hyperalimentation
hyper-IgE
hyperimmunoglobulin E
hyperimmunoglobulinemia E

hyper K
hyperkalemia
hyperpara
hyperparathyroidism (*See also* HP, HPT, HPTH)
hyper T&A
hypertrophy of tonsils and adenoids
hypes
hypesthesia
hypn
hypertension (*See also* HPN, HT, HTN)
hypno
hypnosis (*See also* HYP)
HYPO
below
lower than
%HYPO
percentage of hypochromic red cell
hypo
hypochromasia
hypochromia
hypodermic (*See also* (H), h)
hypo A
hypoactive
hypo K
hypokalemia
hypopit
hypopituitarism
hypox
hypophysectomized (*See also* HPX, HX)
HYPP
hypersegmented neutrophil
HypRF
hypothalamic-releasing factor
hypro
hydroxyproline (*See also* HP, HYP)
HYPT
hyperventilation provocation test
HYs
healthy years of life
hys, hyst
hysterectomy
hysteria (*See also* hy)
hysterical
HZ
herpes zoster
hypertrophic zone
Hz
hertz

NOTES

H

HZD
    herpes zoster dermatitis
HZFO
    hamster zona-free ovum (test)
HZI
    hemizona assay index

HZO
    herpes zoster ophthalmicus
HZV
    herpes zoster virus

I

electric current
implantation
impression (*See also* IMP, imp)
inactive (*See also* inac)
incisal
incisor (deciduous, permanent)
incontinent
increased
independent (*See also* ind)
index (*See also* ind)
indicated
indirect treatment
induction (*See also* ind)
inhalation (*See also* INH, inhal)
inhibiting (*See also* inhib)
inhibition (*See also* inhib)
inhibitor
initial
insoluble (*See also* insol)
inspiration (*See also* insp, inspir)
inspired (gas)
insulin (*See also* IN, In, INS)
intact (bag of waters)
intake
intensity
intensity of magnetism
intermediate (*See also* INT, int, intmd)
intestine
iodide
iodine
ionic strength
iota (ninth letter of Greek alphabet), uppercase
iris
isochromosome
isoleucine
isotope
isotropic (band, disk)
luminous intensity
moment of inertia
one (Roman numeral)
optically inactive (chemical)
radiant intensity
resultant current
vector cardiography electrode (right midaxillary line)

I-125

iodine-125

^{123}I, I-123

iodine-123

^{125}I

iodine-125

^{127}I

iodine-127

^{131}I

iodine-131
radioactive iodine

I-131

iodine-131

^{132}I

iodine-132

I_{Cl}

chloride current

I_F

pacemaker current

IA

ibotenic acid (*See also* ibo)
ideational apraxia
image amplification
immune adherence
immunobiologic activity
impedance angle
inactive alcoholic
incidental appendectomy
incurred accidentally
Indian American (Native American)
indolaminergic-accumulating (cells)
indulin agar
infantile apnea
infantile autism
infected area
inferior angle
inferior apical
inhibitory antigen
internal auditory
intraalveolar
intraamniotic (*See also* iam)
intraaortic
intraarterial
intraarticular
intraatrial
intrinsic activity
invasive aspergillosis
isonicotinic acid

I/A, I&A

irrigating and aspirating
irrigation and aspiration

Ia

immune (region)-associated antigen

Ia+

immune-associated antigen-positive

IAA

ileoanal anastomosis
indoleacetic acid
infectious agent, arthritis
inhibitory amino acid
insulin autoantibody

IAA *(continued)*
  interrupted aortic arch
  interruption of aortic arch
  iodoacetic acid

I-3-AA
  indole-3-acetic acid

IA-A-F
  idiopathic anaphylaxis-angioedema-
  frequent

IA-A-I
  idiopathic anaphylaxis-angioedema-
  infrequent

IAAR
  imidazoleacetic acid ribonucleotide

IAAT
  Iowa Algebra Aptitude Test

IAB
  incomplete abortion
  induced abortion
  intermittent androgen blockade
  intraabdominal
  intraaortic balloon

IABA
  intraaortic balloon assistance

IABC
  intraaortic balloon catheter
  intraaortic balloon counterpulsation
  (*See also* IABCP)

IABCP
  intraaortic balloon counterpulsation
  (*See also* IABC)

IABM
  idiopathic aplastic bone marrow

IABP
  intraaortic balloon pulsation
  intraaortic balloon pump (*See also*
  IBP)
  intraaortic balloon pumping
  intraarterial blood pressure

IABPA
  intraaortic balloon pumping
  assistance

IAC
  indwelling arterial catheter
  ineffective airway clearance
  interatrial communication
  internal auditory canal
  interposed abdominal compression
  intraarterial chemotherapy
  Inventory of Anger
  Communications
  isolated angiitis of the CNS

IACB
  intraaortic counterpulsation balloon

IAC-CPR
  interposed abdominal compressions-
  cardiopulmonary resuscitation

IACD
  implantable automatic cardioverter-
  defibrillator
  intraatrial conduction defect

IACG
  intermittent angle closure glaucoma

IACH
  immediate active cutaneous
  anaphylaxis

IACNS
  isolated angiitis of central nervous
  system

IACOV
  Iaco virus

IACP
  intraaortic counterpulsation

IAD
  implantable atrial defibrillator
  inactivating dose
  inhibiting antibiotic dose
  intermittent androgen deprivation
  internal absorbed dose
  intracranial atherosclerotic disease
  intractable atopic dermatitis

IADH
  inappropriate antidiuretic hormone

IADHS
  inappropriate antidiuretic hormone
  syndrome

IADL
  impairment of activities of daily
  living
  Instrumental Activities of Daily
  Living

IAds
  immunoadsorption

IADSA
  intraarterial digital subtraction
  angiogram
  intraarterial digital subtraction
  angiography

IAE
  intraarterial electrocardiogram
  intraatrial electrocardiogram

IAF
  idiopathic alveolar fibrosis

IAFI
  infantile amaurotic familial idiocy

IA-G-F
  idiopathic anaphylaxis-generalized-
  frequent

IA-G-I
  idiopathic anaphylaxis-generalized-
  infrequent

IAGT
  indirect antiglobulin test (*See also*
  IAT, IDAT)

IAH
    idiopathic adrenal hyperplasia
    idiopathic adrenocortical hyperplasia
    implantable artificial heart

IAHA
    idiopathic autoimmune hemolytic
      anemia
    immune adherence hemagglutination
      assay

IAHC
    intraarterial hepatic chemotherapy

IAHD
    idiopathic acquired hemolytic
      disease

IAHIA
    immune adherence immunosorbent
      assay (*See also* IAIA)

IAHS
    infection-associated hemophagocytic
      syndrome

IAI
    intraabdominal infection
    intraabdominal injury
    intraamniotic infection

IAIA
    immune adherence immunosorbent
      assay (*See also* IAHIA)

IAIS
    intraamniotic infection syndrome

IALD
    instrumental activities of daily
      living

IAM
    internal acoustic meatus
    internal auditory meatus

iam
    intraamniotic (*See also* IA)

IAN
    idiopathic aseptic necrosis
    inferior alveolar nerve
    intern admission note

IAO
    immediately after onset
    intermittent aortic occlusion

IAP
    immunosuppressive acidic protein
    independent adjudicating panel
    innervated antral pouch
    inosinic acid pyrophosphorylase
    intermittent acute porphyria
    intraabdominal pressure
    intracarotid amobarbital procedure

    intrapartum antibiotic prophylaxis
    islet-activating protein

IAPG
    interatrial pressure gradient

IAPP
    islet amyloid polypeptide

IAQ
    indoor air quality

IA-Q
    idiopathic anaphylaxis-questionable

IAR
    immediate asthmatic reaction
    inhibitory anal reflex
    iodine-azide reaction

IARF
    ischemic acute renal failure

IARP
    Integrated Auricular Reconstruction
      Protocol

IARSA
    idiopathic acquired refractory
      sideroblastic anemia

IART
    intraatrial reentrant tachycardia
    intraatrial reentry tachycardia

IAS
    idiopathic ankylosing spondylitis
    illness attitude scale
    immunosuppressive acidic substance
    infant apnea syndrome
    Integrated Assessment System
    interatrial septum
    interatrial shunting
    intermittent androgen suppression
    internal anal sphincter
    intraabdominal sepsis
    intraamniotic saline (infusion)
    intraarterial secretin

IASA
    idiopathic acquired sideroblastic
      anemia
    interatrial septal aneurysm

IASD
    interatrial septal defect (*See also*
      ISD)

IASH
    isolated asymmetric septal
      hypertrophy

IAT
    immunoaugmentative therapy
    indirect antiglobulin test (*See also*
      IAGT, IDAT)

NOTES

IAT *(continued)*
  instillation abortion time
  intraoperative autologous transfusion
  invasive activity test
  iodine azide test
  Iowa Achievement Test
IATT
  intra-arterial thrombolytic therapy
IA-V
  idiopathic anaphylaxis-variant
IAV
  interactive video
  intermittent assisted ventilation
  intraarterial vasopressin
IAVB
  incomplete atrioventricular block
IAVM
  intramedullary arteriovenous
    malformation
IB
  idiopathic blepharospasm
  ileal bypass
  immune balance
  immune body
  inclusion body (*See also* IncB)
  index of body build
  infantile botulism
  infectious bronchitis
  inferior basal
  insulin receptor binding test
  irradiated bone
  isolation bed
I-B
  interbody (vertebral)
IBA
  isobutyric acid
IB1A
  interferon beta-1a (Avonex)
IBAM
  idiopathic bile acid malabsorption
I band
  isotropic band (striated muscle
    fiber) (*See also* I disk)
IBAT
  intravascular bronchoalveolar tumor
IBAV
  Ibaraki virus
IBB
  intestinal brush border
IBBB
  intra-blood-brain barrier
IBBBB
  incomplete bilateral bundle branch
    block
IBC
  Illness Behavior Checklist
  inflammatory breast cancer
  invasive bladder cancer
  iodine-binding capacity
  iron-binding capacity
  isobutyl cyanoacrylate (*See also*
    IBCA)
IBCA
  isobutyl cyanoacrylate (*See also*
    IBC)
IBD
  identical by descent
  infectious bowel disease
  infectious bursal disease
  inflammatory bowel disease
  ischemic bowel disease
IBDQ
  Inflammatory Bowel Disease
    Questionnaire
IBDV
  infectious bursal disease virus
IB-EP
  immunoreactive beta endomorphin
IBF
  immature brown fat (cell)
  immunoglobulin-binding factor
  Insall-Burstein-Freeman (total knee
    instrumentation)
IBG
  iliac bone graft
  insoluble bone gelatin
IBI
  intermittent bladder irrigation
  internal borderzone infarct
  ischemic brain infarction
ibid.
  in the same place [L. *ibidem*]
IBIDS
  ichthyosis, brittle (hair), (impaired)
    intelligence, decreased (fertility),
    short (stature) (syndrome)
IBILI
  indirect bilirubin
IBK
  infectious bovine keratoconjunctivitis
IBL
  immunoblastic lymphadenopathy
  immunoblastic lymphoma
IBM
  ideal body mass
  inclusion body myositis
  isotonic-isometric brief maximum
IBMI
  initial body mass index
IBNR
  incurred but not reported
ibo
  ibotenic acid (*See also* IA)
IBOW
  intact bag of waters

IBP
  intraaortic balloon pump (*See also* IABP)
  iron-binding protein
IBPMS
  indirect blood pressure measuring system
IBPS
  Insall-Burstein posterior stabilizer
IBQ
  Illness Behavior Questionnaire
IBR
  immediate breast reconstruction
  Infant Behavior Record
  infectious bovine rhinotracheitis
IBRS
  Inpatient Behavior Rating Scale
IBRV
  infectious bovine rhinotracheitis virus
IBS
  ichthyosis bullosa of Siemens
  imidazole-buffered saline
  inside bathing solution
  Interpersonal Behavior Study
  Interpersonal Behavior Survey
  irritable bowel syndrome
  isobaric solution
IBSA, iBSA
  immunoreactive bovine serum albumin
  iodinated bovine serum albumin
IBSN
  infantile bilateral striatal necrosis (syndrome)
IBT
  immune-based therapy
  immunobead test
  ink blot test (Rorschach test)
  interblinking time
  intracavitary brachytherapy
IBTR
  ipsilateral breast tumor recurrence
IBU
  ibuprofen
  international benzoate unit
IBV
  (avian) infectious bronchitis virus
  infectious bronchitis vaccine
  infectious bronchitis virus
IBW
  ideal body weight

IC
  between meals [L. *inter cibos*] (*See also* i.c.)
  icteric (*See also* ICT)
  ileocecal
  iliac crest
  iliococcygeal
  iliorostral
  immune complex
  immune cytotoxicity
  immunocompromised
  immunocytochemistry (*See also* ICC)
  impedance cardiogram
  incipient cataract (grade 11 to 41)
  incomplete (diagnosis)
  indeterminate colitis
  indirect calorimetry
  indirect Coombs (test)
  individual counseling
  infection control
  inferior colliculus
  information content
  informed consent
  inhibitory concentration
  inner canthal (distance)
  inorganic carbon
  inspiratory capacity
  inspiratory center
  institutional care
  integrated care
  integrated circuit
  integrated concentration
  intensive care
  intercarpal
  intercostal (space) (*See also* ICS, IS)
  intercourse
  intermediate care
  intermittent catheterization
  intermittent claudication
  internal capsule
  internal carotid
  internal cerebral
  internal cholecystectomy
  internal conjugate (diameter)
  internal connection
  International Classification
  interstitial cell
  interstitial change
  interstitial cystitis
  intracameral

NOTES

IC *(continued)*
intracapsular
intracardiac
intracarotid
intracavitary
intracellular (concentration)
intracerebral
intracisternal *(See also* ICI)
intracoronary
intracranial
intracutaneous
intraincisional
intrapleural catheter
invasive cancer
irritable colon
Isaacson classification
islet cell (of pancreas)
isovolumic contraction

I/C
imipenem-cilastatin (Primaxin)
invalid chair

IC$_{50}$
concentration that inhibits 50%

i.c.
between meals [L. *inter cibos*]
(See also IC)

ICA
ileocolic anastomosis
immunocytochemical assay
intercountry adoption
intermediate care area
internal carotid artery
intracranial abscess
intracranial anatomy
intracranial aneurysm
islet cell antibody *(See also* ICAb)
islet cell antigen

I$_{Ca}$
calcium current

iCa
ionized calcium

ICAb
islet cell antibody *(See also* ICA)

ICAF
internal carotid artery flow

ICAM
intercellular adhesion molecule

ICAM-1
intercellular adhesion molecule-1

ICAM-2
intercellular adhesion molecule-2

ICAM-3
intercellular adhesion molecule-3

ICAO
internal carotid artery occlusion

ICAP
intracisternal A particle

ICAS
intermediate coronary artery
syndrome

ICAT
infant cardiac arrest tray
intracoronary aspiration
thrombectomy

ICAV
intracavitary

ICB
intracranial bleeding

ICBF
inner cortical blood flow
intramyocardial coronary blood flow

ICBG
iliac crest bone graft

ICBP
intracellular binding protein

ICBT
intercostobronchial trunk

ICC
immunocompetent cell
immunocytochemistry *(See also* IC)
Indian childhood cirrhosis
intensive coronary care
interchromosomal crossing-over
intermediate cell column
intermittent clean catheterization
internal conversion coefficient
interstitial cells of Cajal
intraclass correlation coefficient
intracluster correlation coefficient
intrahepatic cholangiocarcinoma
invasive cervical cancer
islet cell carcinoma

ICCD
intensified charge-coupled device

ICCE
intracapsular cataract extraction

ICCEc̄PI
intracapsular cataract extraction
with peripheral iridectomy

ICCM
idiopathic congestive
cardiomyopathy

ICCU
intensive coronary care unit
intermediate coronary care unit

ICD
I-cell disease
immune complex disease
immune complex dissociation
implantable cardioverter-defibrillator
impulse control disorder
inclusion cell disease
indigocarmine dye
induced circular dichroism
informed consent document

initial consonant deletion
inner canthal distance
instantaneous cardiac death
intercanthal distance
internal cardioverter-defibrillator
internal cervical device
International Classification of
  Diseases (of World Health
  Organization)
intracervical device
intrauterine contraceptive device
  (*See also* IUCD, IUD)
Inventory for Counseling and
  Development
irritant contact dermatitis
ischemic coronary disease
isocitrate dehydrogenase (*See also*
  ICDH)
isolated conduction defect

ICD-9
International Classification of
  Diseases, 9th Edition

ICD-10
International Classification of
  Diseases (and Related Health
  Problems), 10th Edition

ICDA
International Classification of
  Diseases, Adapted (for use in
  United States)

ICD-ATP
implantable cardioverter-
  defibrillator/atrial tachycardia
  pacing

ICDB
incomplete database

ICDC
implantable cardioverter/defibrillator
  catheter

ICDCD
International Classification of
  Diseases and Causes of Death

ICD-CM
International Classification of
  Diseases–Clinical Modification

ICD-9-CM
International Classification of
  Diseases, 9th Edition, Clinical
  Modification

ICDH
isocitrate dehydrogenase (*See also*
  ICD)

isocitric acid dehydrogenase (*See
  also* IDH)

ICD-O
International Classification of
  Diseases for Oncology

ICD p24
immune complex-dissociated p24
  antigen

ICDS
Integrated Child Development
  Scheme

ICE
ice, compression, and elevation
ichthyosis-cheek-eyebrow (syndrome)
immunoglobulin-complexed enzyme
individual career exploration
interleukin-1 alpha converting
  enzyme
interleukin-1 beta converting
  enzyme
intracardiac echocardiography
iridocorneal endothelial (syndrome)

+ice
add ice

ICEDP
intracranial epidural pressure

ICEEG
intracranial electroencephalography

I-cell
inclusion cell

ICER
inducible cAMP early repressor
inducible cyclic adenosine
  monophosphate early repressor

ICES
ice, compression, elevation, and
  support

ICET
(Forty-Eight) Item Counseling
  Evaluation Test

ICEUS
intracaval endovascular
  ultrasonography
intracaval endovascular ultrasound

ICF
immunodeficiency, centromeric
  instability, facial anomalies
  (syndrome)
indirect centrifugal flotation
intensive care facility
intercellular fluorescence
interciliary fluid

NOTES

ICF *(continued)*
    intermediate care facility
    intracellular fluid
    intravascular coagulation and
      fibrinolysis (syndrome)

ICFA
    incomplete Freund adjuvant (*See
      also* IFA)
    induced complement-fixing antigen

ICFM
    isolated congenital folate
      malabsorption

ICF-MR
    intermediate-care facility for
      mentally retarded

IC fx
    intracapsular fracture

ICG
    indocyanine green (dye)
    isotope cisternography

ICGA
    indocyanine green angiography

ICGN, IC-GN
    ICR strain-derived glomerular
      nephritis
    immune complex glomerulonephritis

ICH
    idiopathic cortical hyperostosis
    immunocompromised host
    infectious canine hepatitis
    intracerebral hematoma
    intracerebral hemorrhage
    intracerebral hypertension
    intracranial hemorrhage
    intracranial hypertension

ICHD
    ischemic coronary heart disease

ICI
    Interpersonal Communication
      Inventory
    intracardiac injection
    intracisternal (*See also* IC)
    intracranial injury

IC-IC
    intracranial to intracranial
      (anastomosis)

ICIDH
    International Classification of
      Impairments, Disabilities, and
      Handicaps

ICIS
    imaging center information system

ICISS
    International Classification of
      Diseases (9th Ed.) Injury Severity
      Score

ICIT
    intensified conventional insulin
      therapy
    intracavernosal injection therapy

ICJ
    ileocecal junction

ICK
    infectious crystalline keratopathy

ICL
    idiopathic CD4+ lymphocytopenia
    idiopathic CD4 T-cell
      lymphocytopenia
    implantable contact lens
    intracorneal lens
    intracorporeal laser lithotripsy
    iris-clip lens
    isocitrate lyase

ICLE
    intracapsular lens extraction

ICM
    (DNA) image cytometry
    infracostal margin
    inner cell mass
    intercostal margin
    intercostal muscle
    interference-contrast microscopy
    intracytoplasmic membrane
    ion conductance modulator
    ipsilateral competing message
    isolated cardiovascular malformation

ICMA
    immunochemiluminescence assay
    immunochemiluminescent assay
    immunochemiluminometric assay

ICMI
    Inventory of Childhood Memories
      and Imaginings

ICN
    inferior calcaneonavicular ligament
    intensive care neonatal
    intensive care nursery
    intermediate care nursery

ICNC
    intracerebellar nuclear cell

ICO
    idiopathic cyclic oedema (edema)
    impedance cardiac output
    intracellular organism

ICOV
    Icoaraci virus

ICP
    incubation period (*See also* IP)
    inductively coupled plasma
    infection control professional
    infectious cell protein
    inflammatory cloacogenic polyp
    intercostal position (for chest lead)
    intermittent catheterization protocol

intracranial pressure
intracytoplasmic
intrahepatic cholestasia of
pregnancy
intrahepatic cholestasis of
pregnancy

↑**ICP**

increased intracranial pressure (*See
also* IICP)

ICPC

intracranial pressure catheter

ICPMM

incisors, canines, premolars, and
molars (permanent dentition
formula)

ICP-MS

inductively-coupled plasma-mass
spectrometer

ICP-OES

inductively-coupled plasma-optical
emission spectrometry

ICPP

intubated continuous positive-
pressure

ICPS

Interpersonal Cognitive Problem
Solving

ICR

(distance between) iliac crests
intercostal retractions
intermittent catheter routine
international calibrated ratio
intracardiac catheter recording
intracavitary radium
intracranial reinforcement
intrastromal corneal ring
ion cyclotron resonance

ICRF

bispiperazinedione

I-CRF

immunoreactive corticotropin-
releasing factor

ICrH

intracranial hemorrhage

ICRS

intrastromal corneal ring segments

ICRT

Individualized Criterion Referenced
Testing
intracoronary radiation therapy

ICRTM

Individualized Criterion Reference
Testing Mathematics

ICRTR

Individualized Criterion Reference
Testing Reading

ICRU

International Commission on
Radiation Units (and
Measurements)

ICS

ileocecal sphincter
immotile cilia syndrome
impulse-conducting system
inferior capsular shift
inhaled corticosteroid
intensive care, surgical
intercellular space (*See also* IS)
intercostal space (*See also* IC, IS)
International compression system
intracellular-like, calcium-bearing
crystalloid solution
intracranial stimulation
irritable colon syndrome

ICSA

islet cell surface antibody

ICSC

idiopathic central serous
chorioretinopathy

ICSD

International Classification of Sleep
Disorders: (Diagnostic and
Coding Manual)

ICSF

idiopathic calcium (renal) stone
formation

ICSH

interstitial cell-stimulating hormone

ICSHI

intracytoplasmic sperm head
injection

ICSI

intracytoplasmic sperm injection

ICSR

Individual Case Safety Reports
intercostal space retractions

ICSS

intracranial self-stimulation

ICT

icteric (*See also* IC)
icterus (*See also* ict)
immunoglobulin consumption test

NOTES

ICT *(continued)*
  indirect Coombs test
  indirect Coombs titer
  inflammation of connective tissue
  insulin coma therapy
  insulin convulsive therapy
  intensive conventional therapy
  intermittent cervical traction (*See also* ICTX)
  interstitial cell tumor
  intracardiac thrombus
  intracranial tumor
  intracutaneous test
  intradermal cancer test
  intraoral cariogenicity test
  islet cell transplant
  isolated cortical tubule
  isovolumic contraction time (*See also* IVCT)

iCT
  immunoreactive calcitonin

ict
  icterus (*See also* ICT)

ict ind
  icterus index (*See also* II)

ICTP
  carboxyterminal cross-linked telopeptide of type I collagen
  carboxy terminal telopeptide of type 1 collagen

ICTS
  idiopathic carpal tunnel syndrome

ICTX
  intermittent cervical traction (*See also* ICT)

ICU
  immunological contact urticaria
  immunologic contact urticaria
  infant care unit
  intensive care unit
  intermediate care unit

ICUS
  intracoronary ultrasound

ICV
  internal cerebral vein
  intracellular volume
  intracerebroventricular (*See also* icv)

icv
  into cerebral ventricles
  intracerebroventricular (*See also* ICV)

ICVH
  ischemic cerebrovascular headache

ICVM
  intracerebroventricular administration of morphine

ICW
  in connection with
  intact canal wall
  intensive care ward
  intercellular water
  intracellular water

ICX
  immune complex

ICXA
  intermediate circumflex artery

ID
  identification
  identify
  iditol dehydrogenase
  ill-defined
  immune deficiency
  immunodeficiency
  immunodiffusion (test)
  immunoglobulin deficiency
  inappropriate disability
  inclusion disease
  index of discrimination
  individual dose
  induction delivery
  infant death
  infecting dose
  infectious disease (*See also* inf dis)
  infective dose
  inhibitory dose
  inhomogeneous deposition
  initial diagnosis
  initial dose
  initial dyskinesia
  injected dose
  inner diameter
  inside diameter
  insufficient data
  interdigitating (cells)
  internal derangement
  internal diameter
  interstitial disease
  intradermal (*See also* i.d.)
  intraduodenal
  isosorbide dinitrate (*See also* ISD, ISDN)

I-D
  intensity-duration (curve)

I&D
  incision and drainage
  irrigation and debridement
  irrigation and drainage

ID$_{50}$
  median infective dose

Id
  idiotypic
  infradentale
  interdentale

i.d.
  intradermal (*See also* ID)

id.
the same [L. *idem*]

IDA
alpha-L-iduronidase
idiopathic destructive arthritis
image display and analysis
iminodiacetic acid
insulin-degrading activity
iron-deficiency anemia

IDAM
infant of drug abusing mother

IDAT
indirect antiglobulin test (*See also* IAGT, IAT)

IDAV
immunodeficiency-associated virus

IDB
incomplete database

IDBR
indirect bilirubin

IDBS
infantile diffuse brain sclerosis

IDC
idiopathic dilated cardiomyopathy
infiltrating ductal carcinoma
interdigitating cells
interdigitating dendritic cell
intervertebral disk calcification
intraductal carcinoma
invasive ductal carcinoma

IDCF
immunodiffusion complement fixation
immunodiffusion complement-fixing

IDCI
intradiplochromatid interchange

IDCM
idiopathic dilated cardiomyopathy

IDCN
intermediate dorsal cutaneous nerve

IDCS
diffuse cutaneous scleroderma
interdigitating dendritic cell sarcoma

IDD
excess incidence
intraluminal duodenal diverticulum
iodine-deficiency disorder

IDDF
investigational drug data form

IDDM
insulin-dependent diabetes mellitus

IDDS
implantable drug delivery system
investigational drug data sheet

IDDT
immunodouble diffusion test

IDE
inner dental epithelium
insulin-degrading enzyme
Investigational Device Exemption

IDEA
Individuals with Disabilities Education Act

IDEAS
Interest Determination, Exploration and Assessment System
Interest Determination, Exploration and Assessment System, (Enhanced Version)

ID/ED
internal diameter to external diameter (cardiac valve replacement ratio)

IDEM
ischemic, drug, electrolyte, metabolic (effect)

IDET
intradiskal electrothermal therapy

IDFC
immature dead female child

IDG
interdental groove
interdisciplinary group
intermediate dose group

IDGH
ischemic disease of the growing hip

IDH
intradialytic hypotension
intramural duodenal hematoma
isocitric acid dehydrogenase (*See also* ICDH)

IDH1, IDH-S
isocitrate dehydrogenase, soluble

IDH2, IDH-M
isocitrate dehydrogenase, mitochondrial

IDI
immunologically detectable insulin
induction-delivery interval
Interpersonal Dependency Inventory
intractable diarrhea of infancy
intrathecal drug infusion

NOTES

365

IDIS
intraoperative digital subtraction (angiography)

I disk
isotropic disk (striated muscle fiber) (*See also* I band)

IDK
internal derangement of knee (joint)

IDL
Index to Dental Literature
intensity difference limen
intermediate-density lipoprotein

IDM
idiopathic disease of myocardium
immune defense mechanism
indirect method
infant of diabetic mother
intensive diabetes management
intermediate dose methotrexate

IDMC
immature dead male child
interdigestive motility complex
interdigestive motor complex

IDMEC
interdigestive myoelectric complex (*See also* IMC)

ID-MS
isotope dilution-mass spectrometry

IDMS
isolated diffuse mesangial sclerosis

IDMTX
intermediate-dose methotrexate

IDN
interdigital neuroma

IDNA
iron-deficient, not anemic

iDNA
intercalary deoxyribonucleic acid

IDO
indoleamine 2,3-dioxygenase

IDP
imidodiphosphonate
immunodiffusion procedure
initial dose period
initiate discharge planning
inosine diphosphate (*See also* IDPase)
inosine 5'-diphosphate (*See also* IDPase)
instantaneous diastolic pressure

IDPase
inosine diphosphatase (*See also* IDP)

IDPH
idiopathic pulmonary hemosiderosis (*See also* IPH)

IDPN
(beta)-iminodipropionitrile
intradialytic parenteral nutrition

IDR
idiosyncratic drug reaction
intradermal reaction

IDS
iduronate sulfatase (deficiency)
immunity deficiency state
infectious disease service
inhibitor of DNA synthesis
integrated delivery system
intraduodenal stimulation
intrinsic sphincter deficiency (*See also* ISD)
investigational drug service

IDSA
intraoperative digital subtraction angiography

IDST
intraductal secretin test

IDT
immune diffusion test
instillation delivery time
intensive diabetes treatment
interdisciplinary team
interdivision time
intradermal test
intradermal typhoid (and paratyphoid vaccine)

IDTP
immunodiffusion tube precipitin

IDU
idoxuridine (*See also* IDUR, IdUrd, IUDR)
infectious disease unit
injecting drug user
injection drug user
intravenous drug use
iododeoxyuridine (*See also* IUDR)
5-iodo-2'-deoxyuridine
Ivy dog unit

IdUA
iduronic acid

IDUR, IdUrd
idoxuridine (*See also* IDU, IUDR)

IDUS
intraductal ultrasonography
intraductal ultrasound

IDV
indinavir
intermittent demand ventilation

IDVC
indwelling venous catheter

IDWG
interdialytic weight gain

IDX
4'-iodo-4'-deoxydoxorubicin

Idx
cross-reactive idiotype

IE
immediate early
immunizing unit [Ger. *immunitäts Einheit*] (*See also* IU, ImmU)
immunoelectrophoresis (*See also* IEP)
induced emesis
infectious endocarditis
infective endocarditis
inner ear
intake energy (unit of food)
internal ear
internal elastica
international unit (European abbreviation)
intraepithelial
Introversion-Extroversion (scale)

I-E
internal versus external

I&E
internal and external

I/E, I:E
inspiratory to expiratory ratio

i.e.
that is [L. *id est*]

IEA
immediate early antigen
immunoelectroadsorption
immunoelectrophoretic analysis
infectious equine anemia
inferior epigastric artery
intravascular erythrocyte aggregation

IEBD
intraesophageal balloon distention

IEC
injection electrode catheter
inpatient exercise center
intestinal epithelial cell
intradiskal electrothermal coagulation
intraepithelial carcinoma
ion-exchange chromatography

IE Ca cx
intraepithelial carcinoma of cervix

IECRT
intraoperative endoscopic Congo red test

IED
immune-enhancing diet
inherited epidermal dysplasia

IEE
inner enamel epithelium

IEF
isoelectric focusing (electrophoresis)

IEF-PAGE
isoelectric focusing electrophoresis in polyacrylamide gel

IEHL
intracorporeal electrohydraulic lithotripsy

IEI
idiopathic environmental intolerance
isoelectric interval

IEL
intestinal epithelial cell
intimal elastic lamina
intraepithelial leukocyte
intraepithelial lymphocyte

IEM
immune electron microscopy
immunoelectron microscopy
inborn error of metabolism
ineffective esophageal motility
internal elastic membrane

IEMG
integrated electromyogram

IEOP
immunoelectroosmophoresis

IEP
electroimmunoassay
immunoelectrophoresis (*See also* IE)
individualized education program
isoelectric point (*See also* IP, i.p., pH_i, PI, pI, pIs)

IEPA
immunoelectrophoresis analysis

IERIV
Ieri virus

IERM
idiopathic epiretinal membrane

IES
Impact of Events Scale
inferior esophageal sphincter
ingressive-egressive sequence
introversion-extroversion scale

IET
infantile estropia

IEU
idiopathic esophageal ulcer

IF
idiopathic fibroplasia
idiopathic flushing

NOTES

IF *(continued)*
    immersion foot
    immunofluorescence *(See also* IFL)
    immunofluorescent
    indirect fluorescence
    inferior facet
    infrared *(See also* IFR, infra., IR)
    inhibiting factor
    initiation factor
    injury factor
    inspiratory force
    interferon *(See also* IFN, INF, ITF)
    interfollicular
    interfrontal
    intermaxillary fixation *(See also* IMF)
    intermediate filament *(See also* IMF)
    intermediate frequency
    internal fixation
    internal friction
    interstitial fluid *(See also* ISF)
    intracellular fluid
    intrinsic factor
    involved field
    screen-intensifying factor

IFA
    idiopathic fibrosing alveolitis
    immune fluorescent antibody
    immunofluorescence antibody
    immunofluorescence assay
    immunofluorescent antibody (assay)
    immunofluorescent assay
    incomplete Freund adjuvant *(See also* ICFA)
    indirect fluorescent antibody
    indirect fluorescent assay
    indirect immunofluorescent antibody
    silver stain

IF-A
    inflammatory factor of anaphylaxis

I-FABP
    intestinal fatty acid-binding protein

IFAP
    ichthyosis, follicularis, atrichia (or alopecia), photophobia syndrome

IFAT
    indirect fluorescent antibody test

IFC
    inspiratory flow cartridge
    interferential current
    interferential stimulation
    intermittent flow centrifugation
    intrinsic factor concentrate

IFCL
    intermittent flow centrifugation leukapheresis

IFCS
    inactivated fetal calf serum

IFDC
    infiltrating ductal carcinoma

IFDS
    isolated follicle-(stimulating hormone) deficiency syndrome

IFE
    immunofixation electrophoresis
    in-flight emergency
    interfollicular epidermis

IFEV
    Ife virus

IFF
    inner fracture face

IFG
    impaired fasting glucose
    inferior frontal gyrus

IFGS
    interstitial fluids and ground substance

IFI
    indirect immunofluorescence
    Institutional Functioning Inventory (psychologic test)
    intrafollicular insemination

IFIX
    immunofixation

IFL
    immunofluorescence *(See also* IF)
    indolent follicular lymphoma
    inferior frontal lobe

IFLrA
    recombinant human leukocyte interferon A

IFM
    internal fetal monitoring
    intrafusal muscle

IFN
    immunoreactive fibronectin
    interferon *(See also* IF, INF, ITF)

IFN-ε
    interferon-epsilon

IFN-ω
    interferon-omega

IFN-α$_1$
    interferon alpha$_1$

IFN-alpha
    (human leukocyte) interferon
    interferon alfa
    interferon alpha

IFN-alpha 2-alpha
    interferon alpha 2-alpha

IFNB
    interferon beta-1 b (Betaseron)

IFN-B1a
    interferon-β 1a
    interferon beta 1a

IFN-B1b
> interferon-β 1b
> interferon beta 1b

IFN-beta
> (human fibroblast) interferon
> interferon beta

IFN-C
> partially pure human leukocyte
> interferon

If nec
> if necessary

IFN-G, IFN-γ, IFN-gamma
> gamma interferon
> interferon gamma

IFO
> in front of

IFOBT
> immunological fecal occult blood
> test

IFP
> inflammatory fibroid polyp
> insulin, Kendall compound F
> (hydrocortisone), and prolactin
> intermediate filament protein
> intrapatellar fat pad

IFR
> infrared (light) (*See also* IF, infra.,
> IR)
> inspiratory flow rate

IFRA
> indirect fluorescent rabies antibody
> (test)

IFROS
> ipsilateral frontal routing of signals

IFS
> interstitial fluid space

IFSA
> individualized functional status
> assessment

IFSAC
> Inventory of Functional Status
> After Childbirth

IFSE
> internal fetal scalp electrode

IFSP
> Individualized Family Service Plan

IFT
> immunofluorescence technique
> immunofluorescence test
> International Frequency Tables
> inverse Fourier transform

IFU
> interferon unit

IFV
> interstitial fluid volume (*See also*
> ISFV)
> intracellular fluid volume

IG
> image guide
> immature granule
> immunoglobulin (*See also* Ig)
> intragastric (*See also* ig)

I-G
> insulin-glucagon

Ig
> immunoglobulin (*See also* IG)

iG
> immunoreactive human gastrin

ig
> intragastric (*See also* IG)

IGA
> infantile genetic agranulocytosis

IgA
> immunoglobulin A

IgA1
> immunoglobulin A1
> immunoglobulin A subclass 1

IgA2
> immunoglobulin A2
> immunoglobulin A subclass 2

IgA-IFA
> IgA immunofluorescent antibody

IgA tTG
> immunoglobulin A transglutaminase
> antibody

IGBB
> image-guided breast biopsy

IGC
> intragastric cannula

IGCN
> intratubular germ cell neoplasia

IGCNU
> intratubular germ cell neoplasia,
> unclassified type

IGCS
> inpatient geriatric consultation
> services

IGD
> idiopathic growth hormone
> deficiency
> interglobal distance
> isolated gonadotropin deficiency

NOTES

IgD
immunoglobulin D
IgD1
immunoglobulin D subclass 1
IgD2
immunoglobulin D subclass 2
IGDE
idiopathic gait disorders of elderly
IGDM
infant of mother with gestational diabetes mellitus
IGE
impaired gas exchange
IgE
immunoglobulin E
IgE1
subclass of immunoglobulin E
IGF
insulinlike growth factor (*See also* ILGF)
IGF-1, IGF1, IGF-I
insulinlike growth factor-1
IGF-2, IGF2
insulinlike growth factor-2
IgF
immunoglobulin F
IGFA
indocyanine-green fundus angiography
IGFBP
IGF-binding protein
insulinlike growth factor-binding protein
IGFBP-1
insulinlike growth factor-binding protein-1
IGFBP-2
insulinlike growth factor-binding protein-2
IGFBP-3
insulinlike growth factor-binding protein-3
IGFBP-4
insulinlike growth factor-binding protein-4
IGFBP-5
insulinlike growth factor-binding protein-5
IGFBP-6
insulinlike growth factor-binding protein-6
IG-FESS
image-guided functional endoscopic sinus surgery
IGFET
insulated gate field effect transistor
IGF-2R
insulinlike growth factor-II receptor

IgG
immunoglobulin G
IgG1
immunoglobin G1
IgG2
immunoglobulin G2
IgG4
immunoglobulin G4
IgG2a
immunoglobulin G2a
IgG AGA
immunoglobulin G antigliadin antibody
IGGNU
intratubular germ cell neoplasia of the unclassified type
IgG RF
immunoglobulin G rheumatoid factor
IGH
idiopathic growth hormone
immunoreactive growth hormone (*See also* IRGH)
IGHD
isolated growth hormone deficiency
IGHD-IB
isolated growth hormone deficiency type IB
IGHD-II
isolated growth hormone deficiency type II
IGHD-III
isolated growth hormone deficiency type III
IGHL
inferior glenohumeral ligament
IGI
Institutional Goals Inventory
IgIM
immunoglobulin, intramuscular
IgIV
immunoglobulin, intravenous
IGLLC
inferior glenohumeral ligament labral complex
IgM
immunoglobulin M
IgM1
subclass of immunoglobulin M
IgM-IFA
IgM immunofluorescent antibody
IgM-RF, IgM RF
immunoglobin M-rheumatoid factor
IGP
injection gold probe
intestinal glycoprotein
IGPA
infragenicular popliteal artery

IGPD
    inherited giant platelet disorder
IgQ
    immunoglobulin quantitation
IGR
    immediate generalized reaction
    integrated gastrin response
    intrauterine growth retardation
IGS
    image-guided surgery
    inappropriate gonadotropin secretion
IgSC
    immunoglobulin-secreting cell
IGSS
    immunogold-silver staining
IGT
    impaired glucose tolerance
    interpersonal group therapy
    intragastric titration
IGTN
    ingrown toenail
IGTT
    intravenous glucose tolerance test
IGV
    idiopathic genu valgum
    intrathoracic gas volume (*See also* ITGV)
    isolated gastric varices (type 1, 2)
IH
    in hospital
    ichthyosis hystrix
    idiopathic hirsutism
    idiopathic hypercalciuria
    immediate hypersensitivity
    incomplete healing
    indirect hemagglutination
    industrial hygiene
    infantile hydrocephalus
    infectious hepatitis
    inguinal hernia
    inhibiting hormone
    in-house
    inner half
    inpatient hospital
    intermittent heparinization
    intimal hyperplasia
    intracerebral hematoma
    intracranial hypertension
    intramural hematoma
    intraretinal hemorrhage
    iris hamartoma
    iron hematoxylin

IHA
    idiopathic hyperaldosteronism
    immune hemolytic anemia
    indirect hemagglutination antibody (test)
    indirect hemagglutination assay
    indirect hemagglutinin assay
    infusion hepatic arteriography
    intrahepatic atresia
IHAS
    idiopathic hypertrophic aortic stenosis
IHB
    incomplete heart block
IHb
    hemoglobin content index
    hemoglobin content indices
IHBT
    incompatible hemolytic blood transfusion
IHBTD
    incompatible hemolytic blood transfusion disease
IHC
    idiopathic hemochromatosis
    idiopathic hypercalciuria
    immobilization hypercalcemia
    immunohistochemical
    immunohistochemistry
    inner hair cell (of cochlea)
    intrahepatic cholestasis (*See also* IHPC)
IHCA
    isocapnic hyperventilation with cold air
IHCM
    ichthyosis hystrix Curth-Macklin (type)
IHD
    in-center hemodialysis
    intermittent hemodialysis
    intraheptic duct(ule)
    ischemic heart disease
IHDN
    integrated health delivery network
IHES
    idiopathic hypereosinophilic syndrome
IHF
    interhemispheric fissure
IHG
    ichthyosis hystrix gravior

NOTES

IHGD
isolated human growth deficiency

IHH
idiopathic hypogonadotropic hypogonadism
idiopathic hypothalamic hypogonadism
infectious human hepatitis
isolated hypogonadotropic hypogonadism

IHHS
idiopathic hyperkinetic heart syndrome

IHMS
(sodium) isonicotinylhydrazide methanesulfonate

IHNV
infectious hematopoietic necrosis virus

IHO
idiopathic hypertrophic osteoarthropathy

IHP
idiopathic hypoparathyroidism
idiopathic hypopituitarism
inferior hypogastric plexus
interhospitalization period
inverted hand position
isolated hepatic perfusion
isolated hepatic portal and arterial perfusion

IHPC
intrahepatic cholestasis (*See also* IHC)

IHPH
intrahepatic portal hypertension

IHPS
infantile hypertrophic pyloric stenosis

IHR
inguinal hernia repair
intrahepatic resistance
intrinsic heart rate

IHRA
isocapnic hyperventilation with room air

IHS
Idiopathic Headache Score
idiopathic hypereosinophilic syndrome
inactivated horse serum
infrahyoid strap (*See also* IS)
integrated healthcare system

IHSA
iodinated human serum albumin

IHSC
immunoreactive human skin collagenase

IHSS
idiopathic hypertrophic subaortic sclerosis
idiopathic hypertrophic subaortic stenosis

IHT
insulin hypoglycemia test
intravenous histamine test
ipsilateral head turning

I5HT
intraplatelet serotonin

IHU
inpatient hospice unit

IHW
inner heel wedge

II
icterus index (*See also* ict ind)
image intensifier
insurance index
irradiated iodine

I or I
illness or injuries

IIA
internal iliac artery

IIBD
idiopathic inflammatory bowel disease

IIC
integrated ion current

IICP
increased intracranial pressure (*See also* ↑ICP)

IICU
infant intensive care unit

IID
insulin-independent diabetes

IIDM
insulin-independent diabetes mellitus

IIE
idiopathic ineffective erythropoiesis

IIEF
International Index of Erectile Function

IIF
immune interferon
indirect immunofluorescence
indirect immunofluorescent

IIFT
intraoperative intraarterial fibrinolytic therapy

IIGR
ipsilateral instinctive grasp reaction

IIH
idiopathic infantile hypercalcemia
idiopathic intracranial hypertension
iodine-induced hyperthyroidism

IIIVC
 infrahepatic interruption of inferior vena cava

IIM
 idiopathic inflammatory myopathy
 intracortical interaction mapping

[¹²³I]IMP
 iodoamphetamine

IINB
 iliohypogastric nerve block
 ilioinguinal iliohypogastric nerve block
 ilioinguinal nerve block

IIP
 idiopathic interstitial pneumonia
 idiopathic intestinal pseudo-obstruction
 indirect immunoperoxidase
 Intra- and Interpersonal (Relations Scale)

IIPF
 idiopathic interstitial pulmonary fibrosis

IIQ-R
 Incontinence Impact Questionnaire-Revised

IIS
 intensive immunosuppression
 intermittent infusion set

IIT
 ineffective iron turnover
 integrated isometric tension

I-J
 ileojejunal (*See also* IJ)

IJ
 ileojejunal (*See also* I-J)
 internal jugular (vein)
 intrajejunal

IJC
 internal jugular catheter

IJD
 inflammatory joint disease

IJO
 idiopathic juvenile osteoporosis

IJP
 inhibitory junction potential
 internal jugular pressure

IJR
 idiojunctional rhythm

IJT
 idiojunctional tachycardia

IJV
 internal jugular vein

IK
 immobilized knee
 immune body [Ger. *Immunekörper*]
 immunoconglutinin
 infusoria killing (unit) (*See also* IKU)
 interstitial keratitis

IKE
 ion kinetic energy

IKI
 iodine potassium iodide (Lugol solution)

IKU
 infusoria killing unit (*See also* IK)

IL
 ileum (bowel)
 iliolumbar
 ilium (bone)
 immature lung
 incisolingual
 independent laboratory
 insensible loss
 inspiratory loading
 intensity level
 interleukin
 intermediary letter
 intestinal lymphocyte
 intralipid
 intralumbar
 intraocular lens

IL-1–IL-18
 interleukin-1–18

I-L
 intensity-latency

Il
 illinium (promethium)

il
 intralesional

ILA
 inferior lateral angle
 insulin-like activity
 insulinlike activity

IL-1A, IL-1 alpha, IL-1-alpha
 interleukin-1A
 interleukin-1-alpha

ILa
 incisolabial

¹³¹I-labeled MIBG
 ¹³¹I-labeled metaiodobenzylguanidine

NOTES

ILAP
    interstitial laser ablation of the prostate

ILB
    incidental Lewy body
    infant, low birth (weight) (*See also* ILBW)

IL-1B, IL-1 beta, IL-1-beta
    interleukin-1B
    interleukin-1-beta

ILBBB
    incomplete left bundle-branch block

ILBW
    infant, low birth weight (*See also* ILB)

ILC
    ichthyosis linearis circumflexa
    incipient lethal concentration
    infiltrating lobular carcinoma
    Integrated Light Control
    interstitial laser coagulation
    invasive lobular cancer

Ilc
    isoleucine (*See also* ILE, Ile, Ileu, ISL)

ILCP
    interstitial laser coagulation of the prostate

ILD
    immature lung disease
    indentation load deflection
    intermediate density lipoproteins
    interstitial lung disease
    ischemic leg disease
    ischemic limb disease
    isolated lactase deficiency

ILDCSI
    Individual Learning Disabilities Classroom Screening Instrument

ILDL
    intermediate low-density lipoprotein

ILE, Ile, Ileu
    infantile lobar emphysema
    isoleucine (*See also* Ilc, ISL)

ILEAD
    Instructional Leadership Evaluation and Development Program

ILEV
    Ilesha virus

ILFC
    immature living female child

ILGF
    insulin-like growth factor (*See also* IGF)

ILHDL
    isolated low high-density lipoprotein

ILHP
    ipsilateral hemidiaphragmatic paresis

ILHV
    Ilheus virus

ILI
    influenza-like illness

ILL
    inequality in leg length
    intermediate lymphocytic lymphoma
    intracorporeal laser lithotripsy

ILM
    insulin-like material
    internal limiting membrane

ILMC
    immature living male child

ILMI
    inferolateral myocardial infarct (ion)

ILNR
    intralobar nephrogenic rest

ILo
    iodine lotion

ILP
    inadequate luteal phase
    interstitial laser photocoagulation
    interstitial lymphocytic pneumonia
    intralesional laser photocoagulation
    isolated limb perfusion

ILQTS
    idiopathic long QT (interval) syndrome

ILR
    irreversible loss rate

IL-2R
    interleukin-2 receptor

IL-4R
    interleukin-4R

IL-1RA
    interleukin-1 receptor antagonist

IL-3Ra[bright]
    interleukin-3Ra[bright]

ILS
    idiopathic leucine sensitivity
    idiopathic lymphadenopathy syndrome
    increase in life span
    infrared liver scanner
    intralabyrinthine schwannomas
    intralobular sequestration
    intraluminal stapler

ILSA
    Interpersonal Language Skills and Assessment

ILSS
    integrated life support system
    intraluminal somatostatin

ILUS
    intraluminal ultrasound

ILVEN
    inflamed linear verrucous epidermal nevus

inflammatory linear verrucous
epidermal nevus

IM

ice massage
idiopathic myelofibrosis (*See also*
IMF)
immunosuppression method
Index Medicus (*See also* Ind Med)
indomethacin (*See also* IMT, IND,
INDO)
industrial medicine (*See also* Ind-
Med)
infection medium
infectious mononucleosis (*See also*
INFM)
inner membrane
innocent murmur
inspiratory muscle
intermediate megaloblast
intermetatarsal
intermuscular
internal malleolus
internal mammary (artery)
internal medicine (*See also* Int Med)
internal monitor
intestinal malrotation
intestinal mesenchyme
intracellular macroadenoma
intramedullary
intramuscular
intramuscular (injection) (*See also*
i.m.)
invasive mole

i.m.

intramuscular (*See also* IM)

IMA

immunometric assay
inferior mesenteric artery
intermetatarsal angle
internal mammary artery

IMAA

iodinated macroaggregated albumin

IMAB

internal mammary artery bypass

IMAC

immobilized metal affinity
chromatography

IMAG

internal mammary artery graft

IMAI

internal mammary artery implant

IMARD

immunomodulating antirheumatic
drug

IMAX

internal maxillary artery

IMB

intermenstrual bleeding

IMBC

indirect maximal breathing capacity

IMBP

immobilized mismatch binding
protein

IMBT

intestinal mucinous borderline
tumor

IMC

immunohistochemical
index of marrow conversion
information memory concentration
interdigestive migrating complex
interdigestive migrating contraction
interdigestive myoelectric complex
(*See also* IDMEC)
intermittent catheterization
intestinal (mucosal) mast cell
intramedullary catheter

IMCD

inner medullary collecting duct

IMCI

Integrated Management of
Childhood Illness

IMCU

intermediate medical care unit

IMD

immune-mediated diabetes
immunologically mediated disease
inherited metabolic disorder
intramammary distance

ImD$_{50}$

immunizing dose sufficient to
protect 50% of subjects

IMDC

intramedullary metatarsal
decompression

IMDD

idiopathic midline destructive
disease

IME

important medical event
independent medical examination
indirect medical education

NOTES

IMEHD
implantable middle ear hearing device

IMEM
improved minimal essential medium

IMEM-HS
improved minimal essential medium, hormone supplemented

IMET
isometric endurance time

IMF
idiopathic myelofibrosis (*See also* IM)
immobilization mandibular fracture
inframammary fold
intermaxillary fixation (*See also* IF)
intermediate filament (*See also* IF)

IMG
inferior mesenteric ganglion
internal mammary graft
internal medicine group (practice)
international medical graduate

IMGG
intramuscular gamma globulin

IMGU
insulin-mediated glucose uptake

IMH
idiopathic myocardial hypertrophy
indirect microhemagglutination (test) (*See also* IMHT)
intramural hemorrhage

IMHT
indirect microhemagglutination test (*See also* IMH)

IMI
imipramine
immunologically measurable insulin
Impact Message Inventory
impending myocardial infarction
indirect membrane immunofluorescence
inferior myocardial infarct
inferior myocardial infarction
intermeal interval
intramuscular injection

I-123-MIBG
iodine-123 metaiodobenzylguanidine

I-125 MIBG
iodine-125 metaiodobenzylguanidine

131I-MIBG
iodine 131-metaiodobenzylguanidine

131I-mIBG
monoiodobenzylguanidine

IMIG
intramuscular immunoglobulin

IML
intermetacarpal ligament
internal mammary lymphoscintigraphy

IMLA, IMLAD
intramural left anterior descending (artery)

IMLC
incomplete mitral leaflet closure

IMLNS
idiopathic minimal lesion nephrotic syndrome

ImLy
immune lysis

IMM
immune modulating nutrition (immunonutrition)
immunizations
inhibitor-containing minimal medium
internal medial malleolus

immat
immature
immaturity

IMMC
interdigestive migrating motor complex

immed
immediately

immobil
immobilization
immobilize

ImmU
immunizing unit (*See also* IE, IU)

immun
immune
immunity
immunization

immunol
immunology

IMN
internal mammary (lymph) node
intramedullary nailing

IMP
iatrogenic multiple pregnancy
idiopathic myeloid proliferation
impacted (*See also* imp, Impx)
important (*See also* imp)
impression (*See also* I, imp)
improved (*See also* imp)
incomplete male pseudohermaphroditism
Innovative Medical Products
inosine 5'-monophosphate
inosine monophosphate (inosinic acid)
Inpatient Multidimensional Psychiatric (scale)
intramembranous particle
intramuscular (compartment) pressure

imp

impacted (*See also* IMP, Impx)
important (*See also* IMP)
impression (*See also* I, IMP)
improved (*See also* IMP)

IMPA

incisal mandibular plane angle

IMPDH

inosine monophosphate
dehydrogenase

imperf

imperfect
imperforate

IMPEX

immediate postexercise

IMPL

impulse

IMPS

Inpatient Multidimensional
Psychiatric Scale

IMPT

intensity-modulated proton therapy

Impvt

improvement

Impx

impacted (*See also* IMP, imp)

IMR

individual medical record
infant mortality rate
infectious mononucleosis receptor

IMRA

immunoradiometric assay

IMRAD, IMRD

introduction, materials and methods,
results, and discussion (formal
structure of scientific article)

Imreg-1, Imreg-2

immunomodulator 1–2

IMRT

intensity-modulated radiation therapy

IMS

immunosuppressants
incurred in military service
industrial methylated spirit
integrated medical services

IMSC

intramedullary supracondylar

IMSS

in-flight medical support system

IMT

indomethacin (*See also* IM, IND,
INDO)

induced muscular tension
inflammatory myofibroblastic tumor
inspiratory muscle training
intimal-medial thickness

IMU

intermediate medicine unit

ImU

international milliunit

IMV

inferior mesenteric vein
intermittent mandatory ventilation
intermittent mechanical ventilation

IMVC, IMViC, imvic

indole, methyl red, Voges-
Proskauer, and citrate (test)

IMVP

idiopathic mitral valve prolapse

IMX

whole-body antibody technique

IN

icterus neonatorum
impetigo neonatorum
incidence
incompatibility number
infantile nephrotic (syndrome)
infundibular nucleus
insulin (*See also* I, In, INS)
intermediate nucleus
interneuron
internist (*See also* INT, int)
interstitial nephritis
intranasal

In

indium
inion
insulin (*See also* I, IN, INS)
internal
inulin

in.

inch

in^2

square inch

in^3

cubic inch

^{111}In

indium-111

^{113m}In

indium-113m

INA

infectious nucleic acid
inferior nasal artery

NOTES

I_{Na}
sodium current
INAA
instrumental neutron activation analysis
inac
inactive (*See also* I)
INAD
infantile neuroaxonal dystrophy
investigational new animal drug
in no apparent distress
INAH
isonicotinic acid hydrazide
INB
intercostal nerve blockade
internuclear bridging
ischemic necrosis of bone
inbr
inbreeding
INC
illuminated near card
incisal
incision
incomplete (*See also* inc)
inconclusive
incontinent (*See also* inc)
increase (*See also* inc, incr)
inside-the-needle catheter
interstitial nucleus of Cajal
Inc.
incorporated
inc
incisional
including (*See also* incl)
incompatibility
incomplete (*See also* INC)
inconclusive
incontinent (*See also* INC)
increase (*See also* INC, incr)
increment (*See also* incr)
incurred
INCA
infant nasal cannula assembly
Inc Ab
incomplete abortion
IncB
inclusion body (*See also* IB)
INCD
infantile nuclear cerebral degeneration
incl
including (*See also* inc)
incomp, incompl
incomplete
incont
incontinent

incr
increase (*See also* INC, inc)
increment (*See also* inc)
inc (R)
increase (relative)
INCS
incomplete resolution, scan (to) follow
incur
incurable
IND
indapamide
indinavir
indirect treatment
indomethacin (*See also* IM, IMT, INDO)
induced
industrial (medicine) (*See also* indust)
internodal distance
intestinal neuronal dysplasia
investigational new drug
ind
independent (*See also* I)
index (*See also* I)
indicate
indigent
indigo
indirect
induction (*See also* I)
INDA
Investigational New Drug Application
INDEP
independent
indic
indicated
indication
indig
indigestion
INDIV
individual
INDM
infant of nondiabetic mother
Ind Med
Index Medicus (*See also* IM)
Ind-Med
industrial medicine (*See also* IM)
INDO
indomethacin (*See also* IM, IMT, IND)
¹¹¹In-DTPA
indium pentate
indust
industrial (medicine) (*See also* IND)
INE
infantile necrotizing encephalomyelopathy

I

INEX
   inexperienced
INF
   infant (*See also* inf)
   infantile (*See also* inf)
   infarction
   infected (*See also* inf, infect., infx)
   infection (*See also* inf, infect., infx)
   infectious (disease)
   infective (*See also* inf, infect.)
   inferior (*See also* inf, infer.)
   infirmary (*See also* inf)
   information
   infundibulum (of neurohypophysis)
   infused
   infusion (*See also* inf)
   interferon (*See also* IF, IFN, ITF)
   intravenous nutritional fluid
   pour in [L. *infunde*] (*See also* inf.)
inf
   infancy
   infant (*See also* INF)
   infantile (*See also* INF)
   infarct
   infect
   infected (*See also* INF, infect.)
   infection (*See also* INF, infect., infx)
   inferior (*See also* INF, infcr.)
   infirmary (*See also* INF)
   infus
   infusion (*See also* INF)
inf.
   pour in [L. *infunde*] (*See also* INF)
INFa
   influenza virus, attenuated live vaccine
INFC
   infected
   infection
InfCM
   inflammatory cardiomyopathy
inf dis
   infectious disease (*See also* ID)
infect.
   infected (*See also* INF, inf)
   infection (*See also* INF, inf, infx)
   infective (*See also* INF, inf)
infer.
   inferior (*See also* INF, inf)

INFH
   ischemic necrosis of femoral head
INFi
   influenza virus inactivated vaccine
infl
   inflamed
   inflammation (*See also* inflamm)
   inflammatory (*See also* inflamm)
   influence
   influx
inflamm
   inflammation (*See also* infl)
   inflammatory (*See also* infl)
infl proc
   inflammatory process
INFM, inf mono
   infectious mononucleosis (*See also* IM)
Inf MI
   inferior (wall) myocardial infarction
info
   information
infra.
   infrared (*See also* IF, IFR, IR)
INFs
   influenza virion vaccine, split virion
INFs-AB3
   influenza virus inactivated vaccine, split virion, types A and B, trivalent
INFw
   influenza virion vaccine, whole virion
infx
   infection (*See also* INF, inf, infect.)
ING
   inguinal (*See also* ing)
   isotope nephrogram
ing
   inguinal (*See also* ING)
INGV
   Ingwavuma virus
INH
   inhalation (*See also* I, inhal)
   isoniazid
   isonicotine hydrazine (isoniazid)
   isonicotinic acid hydrazide (isoniazid)
inh
   inhaler

NOTES

inhal
inhalation (*See also* I, INH)
INH-G
isonicotinoylhydrazone of D-glucuronic acid lactone (glyconiazide)
inhib
inhibiting (*See also* I)
inhibition (*See also* I)
INI
intranasal insulin
intranuclear inclusion (agent)
INIV
Inini virus
inj
injection (*See also* inject.)
injured
injurious
injury
inject.
injection (*See also* inj)
INK
injury not known
INKV
Inkoo virus
inl
inlay
INLSD
ichthyosis and neutral lipid storage disease
INN
International Nonproprietary Name
innerv
innervated
innervation
INO
infantile nephrotic (syndrome), other (types)
inhaled nitrous oxide
internuclear ophthalmoplegia
Ino
inosine
iNO
inhaled nitric oxide
INOC, inoc
inoculate
inoculation
INOH
instantaneous orthostatic hypotension
INOP
internodal ophthalmoplegia
inop
inoperable
inorg
inorganic
iNOS
induced nitric oxide synthase

inducible nitric oxide synthase
inducible nitric oxide synthetase
Inox
inosine, oxidized
INP
idiopathic neutropenia
INPAV
intermittent negative pressure-assisted ventilation (*See also* INPV)
INPEA
isopropylnitrophenylethanolamine (β-adrenergic blocker)
INPH
iproniazid phosphate
INPRCNS, INPRONS
information processing in central nervous system
IN-PT
inpatient
INPV
intermittent negative pressure-(assisted) ventilation (*See also* INPAV)
INQ
inferior nasal quadrant
Inquiry Mode Questionnaire: A Measure of How You Think and Make Decisions
INR
international normalized ratio
INREM
internal roentgen equivalent, man (radiation dose)
INS
idiopathic nephrotic syndrome
inspection
insulin (*See also* I, IN, In)
insurance (*See also* ins)
ins
insertion
insurance (*See also* INS)
insured
INS Ab
insulin antibody
insem
insemination
insid
insidious
insol
insoluble (*See also* I)
insp
inspect
inspection
inspiration (*See also* I, inspir)
inspir
inspiration (*See also* I, insp)

INSS
> International Neuroblastoma Staging System
> International Staging System

INST
> instrumental (delivery)

inst
> institute
> instrument

insuf, insuff
> insufficiency
> insufficient
> insufflation

INT
> intermediate (*See also* I, int, intmd)
> intermittent (*See also* int, INTR)
> intermittent needle therapy
> intern (*See also* int)
> internal (*See also* int, intern.)
> internist (*See also* IN, int)
> *p*-iodonitrotetrazolium

int
> intact
> integral
> interest
> intermediate (*See also* I, INT, intmd)
> intermittent (*See also* INT, INTR)
> intern (*See also* INT)
> internal (*See also* INT, intern.)
> internist (*See also* IN, INT)
> interval
> intestinal (*See also* intest)

int2
> integration gene 2

INTEG
> integument

intern.
> internal (*See also* INT, int)

internat
> international

INTERP
> interpretation

intertroch
> intertrochanteric

intest
> intestinal (*See also* int)
> intestine (*See also* int)

int/ext
> internal/external (rotation)

INTH
> intrathecal (anesthesia injection) (*See also* IT, ITh, i-thec)

int hist
> interval history

intmd
> intermediate (*See also* I, INT, int)

Int Med
> internal medicine (*See also* IM)

int mon
> internal monitor

int obst
> intestinal obstruction (*See also* IO)

intol
> intolerance

INTOX
> intoxication

INTR
> intermittent (*See also* INT, int)

int-rot
> internal rotation (*See also* IR)

int trx
> intermittent traction (*See also* IT)

intub
> intubation

INV
> inferior nasal vein

inv
> invalid
> inverse
> inversion (*See also* inver)
> involuntary (*See also* invol)

inver
> inversion (*See also* inv)
> inverted

invest.
> investigation

invet
> inveterate

inv/ev
> inversion/eversion

inv ins
> inverted insertion

INVM
> isolated noncompaction of the ventricular myocardium

invol
> involuntary (*See also* inv)

involv
> involved
> involvement

NOTES

INVOS
in vivo optical spectroscopy

IO
incisal opening
inferior oblique
inferior oblique (eye muscle)
inferior olive
initial opening (pressure)
inside-out (vesicle)
intensive observation
internal os (cervix)
intestinal obstruction (*See also* int obst)
intraocular (pressure)
intra-Ommaya (reservoir)
intraoperative
intraosseous

I&O, I and O, I/O
input/output
intake and output (*See also* I and O)
in and out

Io
ionium (slope of thorium)

IOA
inner optic anlage
intact on admission

IOC
intern on call
intraoperative cholangiogram (*See also* IOCG)
intraoperative cholangiography
in our culture

IOCG
intraoperative cholangiogram (*See also* IOC)

IOCM
isosmolar contrast medium

IOD
injured on duty
integrated optical density
interorbital distance

IODM
infant of diabetic mother

IOE
intraoperative echocardiography
intraoperative endoscopy
intraoperative enteroscopy

IOEBT
intraoperative electron beam therapy

IOECS
intraoperative electrical cortical stimulation

IOF
intraocular fluid
intraoperative fentanyl

IOFB
intraocular foreign body

IOFNA
intraoperative fine-needle aspiration

IOH
idiopathic orthostatic hypotension

IOHDR
intraoperative high dose rate

IOI
intraosseous infusion

IOIS
idiopathic orbital inflammatory syndrome

IOL
intraocular lens

IOLI
intraocular lens implantation

IOLP
intraocular lens power

IOM
infraorbital margin
interosseous membrane
intraocular muscle
intraoperative neurophysiologic monitoring

IOML
infraorbitomeatal line

ION
ischemic optic neuropathy

IONIS
indirect optic nerve injury syndrome

IONTO
iontophoresis

IOOA
inferior oblique overaction

IOP
intraocular pressure

IOPN
intraductal oncocytic papillary neoplasm

IOR
ideas of reference
immature oocyte retrieval
index of response
inferior oblique recession
information outflow rate

IO-RB
intraocular retinoblastoma

IORT
intraoperative (electron beam) radiotherapy
intraoperative radiation therapy

IOS
intraoperative sonography

IOT
intraocular tension
intraocular transfer
ipsilateral optic tectum

ι, iota
> iota (ninth letter of Greek alphabet), lowercase

IOTA
> information overload testing aid

IOTEE
> intraoperative transesophageal echocardiography

IOU
> intensive (therapy) observation unit
> international opacity unit

IOUS
> intraocular ultrasound
> intraoperative ultrasonography
> intraoperative ultrasound

IOV
> initial office visit

IOVP
> intraesophageal variceal pressure

IOWA
> inattention-overactivity with aggression

IP
> ice pack
> icterus praecox
> ileoproctostomy
> iliopsoas (muscle)
> immune precipitate
> immunoblastic plasma
> immunoperoxidase
> implantation
> inactivated pepsin
> incisoproximal
> incisopulpal
> incontinentia pigmenti
> incubation period (*See also* ICP)
> individualized plan
> induced potential
> induction period
> industrial population
> infection prevention
> infrapatellar
> infundibular process
> infundibulopelvic (ligament)
> infusion pump
> initial pressure
> inlet pouch
> inorganic phosphate
> inosine phosphorylase
> inpatient
> instantaneous pressure
> International Pharmacopoeia

> interpeduncular (nucleus)
> interphalangeal (joint) (*See also* IPH, IPJ)
> interpharyngeal
> interpositus (nucleus)
> interpupillary
> interstitial pneumonia
> intervening peptide
> intestinal permeability
> intestinal pseudoobstruction
> intracellular proteolysis
> intraperitoneal (*See also* i.p.)
> invasive procedure
> ionization potential
> isoelectric point (*See also* IEP, i.p., pH_i, PI, pI, pIs)
> isoproterenol (*See also* IPT, IS, ISO, ISP)
> in plaster

IP3, IP$_3$
> inositol triphosphate
> inositol 1,4,5-triphosphate

IP-10
> interferon-inducible protein 10

I/P
> iris and pupil

i.p.
> intraperitoneal (*See also* IP)
> isoelectric point (*See also* pI, IEP, pH_i, PI, pIs)

IPA
> idiopathic pulmonary arteriosclerosis
> incontinentia pigmenti achromians
> independent practice association
> indole pyruvic acid
> International Phonetic Alphabet
> interpleural analgesia
> intrapulmonary artery
> invasive pulmonary aspergillosis
> isopropyl alcohol

IPAA
> ileal pouch anal anastomosis

IPAO
> insulin-induced peak acid output

IPAP
> inspiratory positive airway pressure

IPAT
> (Cattell's) Institute for Personality and Ability Testing (Anxiety Scale)
> Iowa Pressure Articulation Test

NOTES

IPB

infrapopliteal bypass

IPC

intermediate posterior curve
intermittent pneumatic compression
interpeduncular cistern
intraductal papillary carcinoma
intraperitoneal chemotherapy
ion-pair chromatography
ischemic preconditioning
isopropyl chlorophenyl
isopropyl phenylcarbamate
(propham)

IPCD

idiopathic paroxysmal cerebral
dysrhythmia
infantile polycystic (kidney) disease
(*See also* IPCK)

IPCK

infantile polycystic kidney (disease)
(*See also* IPCD)

IPCS

infrapatellar contracture syndrome
intrauterine progesterone
contraceptive system

IPCT

intraperitoneal chemotherapy

IPCV

idiopathic polypoidal choroidal
vasculopathy

IPD

idiopathic Parkinson disease
idiopathic protracted diarrhea
immediate pigment darkening
incomplete pancreas divisum
increase in pupillary diameter
incurable problem drinker
inflammatory pelvic disease
intermittent peritoneal dialysis
intermittent pigment darkening
interpupillary distance
Inventory of Psychosocial
Development

IPE

infectious porcine encephalomyelitis
initial psychiatric development
injury pulmonary edema
interstitial pulmonary emphysema
iris pigment epithelium

IPEC

intragastral provocation under
endoscopy

IPEH

intravascular papillary endothelial
hyperplasia

IPEUS

intraportal endovascular
ultrasonography

IPF

idiopathic pulmonary fibrosis
infection-potentiating factor
International Primary Factors (Test
Battery)
interstitial pulmonary fibrosis
intramural protruding form

IPF-1

insulin promoter factor-1

IPFD

intrapartum fetal distress

IPG

impedance phlebograph
impedance plethysmography
implantable pulse generator
individually polymerized grass
inspiratory phase gas

iPGE

immunoreactive prostaglandin E

IPGTT

intraperitoneal glucose tolerance test

IPH

idiopathic portal hypertension
idiopathic pulmonary hemorrhage
idiopathic pulmonary hemosiderosis
(*See also* IDPH)
infant passive hand
inflammatory papillary hyperplasia
intraparenchymal hemorrhage
intraperitoneal hemorrhage
intraplaque hemorrhage
isolated postchallenge hyperglycemia

IPHC

intraperitoneal hyperthermic
chemotherapy

IPHEP

independent progressive home
exercise program

IPHP

inflammatory papillary hyperplasia
of the palate
intraperitoneal hyperthermic
perfusion

IPHR

inverted polypoid hamartoma of
rectum

IPI

Imagined Process Inventory
infertility perceptions inventory
International Prognostic Index
interphonemic interval
interpulse interval
intraperitoneal insemination
Inwald Personality Inventory

IPIA

immunoperoxidase infectivity assay

IPITx
isolated pancreatic islet transplantation

IPJ
interphalangeal joint (*See also* IP)

IPK
indurated plantar keratoma
interphalangeal keratosis
intractable plantar keratosis

IPKD
infantile polycystic kidney disease

IPL
inner plexiform layer
intense pulsed light
interpupillary line
intrapleural

IPLS
intense pulsed light source

IPLVAS
implantable left ventricular assist system

IPM
impulses per minute
inches per minute
infant passive mitt (slang for hand)
interventional pain management
intrapulmonary metastasis
intrauterine pressure monitor

IPMI
inferoposterior myocardial infarction

IPMN
intraductal papillary mucinous neoplasm

IPMT
intraductal papillary mucinous tumor

IPN
infantile periarteritis nodosa
infantile polyarteritis nodosa
infected pancreatic necrosis
interim progress note
intern's progress note
interpeduncular nucleus
interpenetrating polymer network

IPn
interstitial pneumonitis

IPNA
isopropylnoradrenaline (isoproterenol)

IPNM
intraductal papillary mucinous neoplasm

IPNP
intraductal papillary neoplasm of the pancreas

IPNV
infectious pancreatic necrosis virus

IPO
improved pregnancy outcome
initial planning option

IPOF
immediate postoperative fitting

IPOM
intraperitoneal onlay mesh (hernia repair)

IPOP
immediate postoperative prosthesis

IPP
independent practice plan
inferior point of pubic (bone)
inflatable penile prosthesis
inorganic pyrophosphate (*See also* PPi, PP$_i$)
inosine, pyruvate, and (inorganic) phosphate
intermittent positive pressure
intrahepatic portal pressure
intrapleural pressure
isolated pelvic perfusion

IPPA
inspection, palpation, percussion, and auscultation

IPPB
intermittent positive-pressure breathing

IPPB/I
intermittent positive-pressure breathing/inspiratory

IP-PDT
intraperitoneal photodynamic therapy

IPPF
immediate postoperative prosthetic fitting

IPPI
interruption of pregnancy for psychiatric indication

IPPO
intermittent positive-pressure (inflation with) oxygen

IPPR
integrated pancreatic polypeptide response
intermittent positive-pressure respiration

NOTES

IPPT
Inter-Person Perception Test
IPPUAD
immediate postprandial upper abdominal distress
IPPV
intermittent positive-pressure ventilation
IPPYV
Ippy virus
IPQ
Intermediate Personality Questionnaire (for Indian Pupils)
intimacy potential quotient
IPR
immediate phase reaction
independent professional review
insulin production rate
interval patency rate
intraparenchymal resistance
iproniazid
i-Pr
isopropyl- (prefix denoting 1-methylethyl group)
IPRL
isolated perfused rabbit lung
isolated perfused rat liver
IPRT
interpersonal reaction test
IPS
idiopathic postprandial syndrome
immediate postoperative stability
impulse per second
inches per second
infundibular pulmonary stenosis
initial prognostic score
intermittent photic stimulation (electroencephalography)
Interpersonal Perception Scale
intraparietal sulcus
intraperitoneal shock
intraurethral prostaglandin suppository
Inventory of Perceptual Skills
ischiopubic synchondrosis
Ips
iodophenylsulfonyl
ips
inches per second
IPSB
intrapartum stillbirth
IPSC
inhibitory postsynaptic current
IPSC-E
Inventory of Psychic and Somatic Complaints in the Elderly

IPSF
immediate postsurgical fitting (of prosthesis)
IPSI
Iowa Structured Psychiatric Interview
IPSID
immunoproliferative small intestine disease
IPSP
inhibitory postsynaptic potential
intrapixel sequential processing
IPSS
inferior petrosal sinus sampling
International Prostate Symptom Score
IPSTL
inferior parietal and superior temporal lobe
IPSY
intermediate psychiatry
IPT
immunoperoxidase technique
immunoprecipitation
industrial physical therapist
inflammatory pseudotumor
intermittent pelvic traction (*See also* IPTX)
interpersonal psychotherapy
interpersonal therapy
intraductal papillary tumor
ipratropium
isoproterenol (*See also* IP, IS, ISO, ISP)
IPTA
Illinois Test of Psycholinguistic Abilities
IPTG, iPrSGal
isopropylthiogalactoside
iPTH
immunoreactive parathyroid hormone
intact parathyroid hormone
IPTX
intermittent pelvic traction (*See also* IPT)
IPU
inpatient unit
IPV
inactivated poliomyelitis (virus) vaccine
inactivated poliovirus vaccine
incompetent perforator vein
infectious pustular vaginitis
infectious pustular vulvovaginitis (of cattle)
intermittent percussive ventilation
intrapulmonary percussive ventilation

intrapulmonary vein
polio vaccine

IPVC

interpolated premature ventricular
contraction

IPVD

index of pulmonary vascular
disease

IPW

interphalangeal width

IPZ

insulin-protamine zinc

IQ

intelligence quotient

IQR

interquartile range

IQ&S

iron, quinine, and strychnine

I-R

Ito-Reenstierna (reaction, test)

IR

ileal resection
immediate-release (tablets)
immune response (genes) (*See also*
Ir)
immunization rate
immunologic response
immunoreactive (*See also* ir)
immunoreagent
incisal ridge
index of response
individual reaction
inferior rectus (muscle)
infrared (light) (*See also* IFR)
inside radius
insoluble residue
inspiratory reserve
inspiratory resistance
insulin receptor
insulin requirement
insulin resistance
insulin response
integer ratio
intelligence ratio
internal reduction
internal resistance
internal rotation (*See also* int-rot)
intrastent restenosis
inversion recovery
inverted repeats
ionizing radiation
irritant reaction

isotonic reversal
isovolumetric relaxation

I&R

insertion and removal

I/R

ischemia and reperfusion

Ir

immune response
immune response (genes) (*See also*
IR)
iridium

^{192}Ir

iridium-192

^{194}Ir

iridium-194

ir

immunoreactive (*See also* IR)
intrarectal
intrarenal

IRA

ileorectal anastomosis
immunoradioassay
immunoregulatory α-globulin
inactive renin activity
infarct-related artery

IR-ACTH

immunoreactive adrenocorticotropic
hormone

IRA-EEA

ileorectal anastomosis with end-to-
end anastomosis

IRAK

integrated reference air-kerma

IRAP

interleukin-1 receptor antagonist
protein

IRB

institutional review board

IRBBB

incomplete right bundle-branch
block

IRBC

immature red blood cell (*See also*
iRBC)
infected red blood cell
irradiated red blood cells

iRBC

immature red blood cell (*See also*
IRBC)

IRBP

interphotoreceptor retinoid-binding
protein

NOTES

IRC
    implant related complications
    indirect radionuclide cystography
    infrared coagulator
    infrared photocoagulation
    inspiratory reserve capacity
    instantaneous resonance curve
    instrument recirculation center

IRCA
    intravascular red cell aggregation

IRCS
    International Research
      Communications System

IRCU
    intensive respiratory care unit

IRD
    immune renal disease
    infantile Refsum syndrome
    isorhythmic dissociation

IRDA
    intermittent rhythmic delta activity

IRDM
    insulin-resistant diabetes mellitus

IRDS
    idiopathic respiratory distress
      syndrome
    infant respiratory distress syndrome

IRE
    inhibitory response element
    internal rotation in extension

I-receptor
    imidazoline receptor

IRED
    infrared emission detection

IRES
    internal ribosome entry site

IRF
    idiopathic retroperitoneal fibrosis
    interferon regulatory factor
    internal rotation in flexion

IRF-1
    interferon regulatory factor-1

IRF-2
    interferon regulatory factor-2

IRG
    immunoreactive gastrin
    immunoreactive glucagon (*See also*
      IRGl)
    immunoreactive glucose

IRGH
    immunoreactive growth hormone
      (*See also* IGH)

IRGl
    immunoreactive glucagon (*See also*
      IRG)

IRH
    intraretinal hemorrhage

IRHC, IRHCS
    immunoradioassayable human
      chorionic somatomammotropin
    immunoradioassayable human
      chorionic (somatomammotropin)

IRhCG
    immunoreactive human chorionic
      gonadotropin

IRhCS
    immunoreactive human chorionic
      somatomammotropin

IRhGH
    immunoreactive human growth
      hormone

IRhPL
    immunoreactive human placental
      lactogen

IRI
    immunoreactive insulin
    insulin radioimmunoassay
    insulin resistance index

IRIA
    indirect radioimmunoassay

irid
    iridescent

IRI/G
    immunoreactive insulin to serum or
      plasma glucose (ratio)

IRIg
    insulin-reactive immunoglobulin

IRIS
    intensified radiographic imaging
      system
    interleukin regulation of immune
      system

IRIV
    immunopotentiating reconstituted
      influenza virosomes
    Irituia virus

IRKO
    insulin receptor knockout

IRLT
    intravascular red light therapy

IRM
    idiopathic retractile mesenteritis
    inherited releasing mechanism
    innate releasing mechanism
    intermediate restorative material
    magnetic resonance imaging
      (French)

IRMA
    Immediate Response Mobile
      Analysis
    immunoradiometric analysis
    immunoradiometric assay
    intraretinal microangiopathy
    intraretinal microvascular
      abnormality

IRME
immunoreactive methionine-enkephalin

IRMP
intersegmental range of motion palpation

IRMS
isotope ratio mass spectrometry

iRNA
immune ribonucleic acid
informational ribonucleic acid

IROS
ipsilateral routing of signal

IRP
idiopathic recurrent pancreatitis
immunoreactive plasma
immunoreactive proinsulin
incus replacement prosthesis
inhibitor of radical processes
insulin-releasing polypeptide
International Reference Preparation
interstitial radiation pneumonitis

IR-PCR
inter-repeat PCR

IR-PEP
inspiratory resistance and positive expiratory pressure

IRPGN
idiopathic rapidly progressive glomerulonephritis

IRR
infrared radiation
infrared refractometry
insulin receptor-related receptor
intrarenal reflux
irregular rate and rhythm
irritation (*See also* irr)

irr
irradiation
irritation (*See also* IRR)

irreg
irregular
irregularity

IRR HYDRO
irreversible hydrocolloid

IRRIG, IRRG
irrigate
irrigation

IRS
idiopathic recurring stupor
immunoreactive secretin
impaired regeneration syndrome
infrared spectrophotometry
insulin receptor species
insulin receptor substrate
insulin-resistance syndrome

IRS-1
insulin receptor substrate-1

IRS-2
insulin receptor substrate-2

IRSA
idiopathic refractory sideroblastic anemia
iodinated rat serum albumin

IRSB
intravenous regional sympathetic block

IRSE
inversion recovery spin-echo sequence

IRT
immunoreactive trypsin
immunoreactive trypsinogen
instrument retrieval container
interresponse time
interstitial radiation therapy
intracoronary radiation therapy
isometric relaxation time
item response theory (psychologic testing)

IRTO
immunoreactive trypsin output

IRTU
integrating regulatory transcription unit

IRU
industrial rehabilitation unit
interferon reference unit

IRV
inferior radicular vein
inspiratory reserve volume
inverse-ratio ventilation

IS
ileal segment (intestine)
ilial segment (bone)
iliosacral
immediate sensitivity
immune serum
immune suppressor
immunosuppression
incentive spirometer
index of saponification
index of sexuality
induced sputum

NOTES

IS *(continued)*
infant size
information system
infrahyoid strap *(See also* IHS)
initial segment
insertion sequence
insufficient signal
insulin secretion
intercellular space *(See also* ICS)
intercostal space *(See also* IC, ICS)
interictal spike (in electroencephalography)
internal standard
international standard
interspace *(See also* i.s., ISP)
interstitial space
interventricular septum *(See also* IVS)
intracardial shunt
intraspinal
intrasplenic
intrastriatal
invalided from service
inventory of systems
Ionescu-Shiley (artificial cardiac valve) *(See also* I-S)
ipecac syrup
Irvine syndrome
ischemic score
island *(See also* is.)
isoproterenol *(See also* IP, IPT, ISO, ISP)
in situ (in original place) [L. *in situ*] *(See also* i.s.)

I-10-S
invert sugar (10%) in saline

I-S
Ionescu-Shiley (artificial cardiac valve) *(See also* IS)

I/S
instruct/supervise

is.
island *(See also* IS)
islet
isolation

i.s.
interspace *(See also* IS, ISP)
in situ *(See also* IS)

ISA
ileosigmoid anastomosis
induced sputum analysis
intraoperative suture adjustment
intrinsic stimulating activity
intrinsic sympathomimetic activity
iodinated serum albumin
irregular spiking activity (in electroencephalography)

ISA₅
internal surface area (of lung at volume of) five (liters)

ISADH
inappropriate secretion of antidiuretic hormone

ISAGA
immunosorbent agglutination assay

ISAM
infant of substance-abusing mother

ISB
incentive spirometry breathing

ISBP
interscalene brachial plexus

ISC
immunoglobulin-secreting cell
indwelling subclavian catheter
infant servo-control
infant skin control
insoluble collagen
intensive supportive care
intermittent self-catheterization
intermittent straight catheterization
International Statistical Classification
intershift coordination
interstitial cell
intersystem crossing
irreversible sickle cell
irreversibly sickled cell
Isolette Servo control

ISCA
Interview Schedule for Children and Adolescents

ISCCO
intersternocostoclavicular ossification

ISCF
interstitial cell fluid

ISCM
intramedullary spinal cord metastasis

ISCN
intensive special care nursery
International System for (Human) Cytogenetic Nomenclature

ISCOM
immunostimulating complex

ISCP
infection surveillance and control program

ISCU
infant special care unit
intensive special care unit

ISD
immunosuppressive drug
inhibited sexual desire
initial sleep disturbance
intensity (of service), severity (of illness), discharge (screens)

interatrial septal defect (*See also* IASD)

interventricular septal defect (*See also* IVSD)

intrinsic sphincter deficiency (*See also* IDS)

intrinsic sphincter dysfunction

isosorbide dinitrate (*See also* ID, ISDN)

ISDB

indirect self-destructive behavior

ISDN

isosorbide dinitrate (*See also* ID, ISD)

ISE

inhibited sexual excitement

integrated square error

ion-selective electrode

ion-sensitive electrode

ISED

Interview Schedule for Events and Difficulties

ISEDP

intraspinal epidural pressure

ISEL

Interpersonal Support Evaluation List

in situ end labeling

ISF

interstitial fluid (*See also* IF)

ISFET

ion-specific field effect transducer

ISFV

interstitial fluid volume (*See also* IFV)

Isfahan virus

ISG

immune serum globulin

ISH

icteric serum hepatitis

isocapnic hyperventilation

isolated septal hypertrophy

isolated systolic hypertension

in situ hybridization

ISHH

in situ hybridization histochemistry

ISHT

isolated systolic hypertension

ISI

infarct size index

initial slope index

injection scan interval

injury severity index

International Sensitivity Index

International Slope Index

interstimulus interval

ISIH

interspike interval histogram

ISIS

integrated shape and imaging system

ISK

immune stromal keratitis

isokinetic

ISKD

intramedullary skeletal kinetic distractor

ISKV

Issyk-Kul virus

ISL

interscapular line

interspinous ligament

isoleucine (*See also* Ilc, ILE, Ile, Ileu)

Is of Lang

islets of Langerhans

ISM

intersegmental muscle

ISMA

infantile spinal muscular atrophy

ISMLCSA

intrastent minimal lumen cross-sectional area

IS-5-MN, Is-5-Mn

isosorbide-5-mononitrate

ISNA

iron-sufficient, not anemic

ISO

isodose

Isolette (*See also* Isol)

isoproterenol (*See also* IP, IPT, IS, ISP)

isotropic

ISO2, ISO$_2$

oxygen saturation indices

ISO-30

Inventory of Suicide Orientation-30

iso

isoproterenol (*See also* IP, IPT, IS, ISO, ISP)

isotropic (*See also* ISO)

ISOE

isoetharine

NOTES

ISOF
isoflurane (Florane)
ISOK
isokinetic
Isol
Isolette (*See also* ISO)
isol
isolated
isolation
isom
isometric
isometropic
isoPAG
phenylacetylisoglutamine
8-iso-PGF$_{2alpha}$
8-iso-prostaglandin F$_{2alpha}$
IsoRAS
isorenin-angiotensin system
isox
isoxsuprine
ISP
distance between iliac spines
immunoreactive substance P
immunosuppressed protocol
inferior spermatic plexus
input signal processor
interspace (*See also* IS, i.s.)
interspinal
intraspinal
isoproterenol (*See also* IP, IPT, IS, ISO)
IS-PCR
in situ polymerase chain reaction
ISPT
interspecies (ovum) penetration test
isp-Tx
intrasplenic transplantation
ISPX
Ionescu-Shiley pericardial xenograft
ISR
information storage (and) retrieval (*See also* IS and R)
injection site reaction
in-stent restenosis
insulin secretion rate
insulin secretory response
integrated secretory response
IS and R
information storage and retrieval (*See also* ISR)
ISS
idiopathic short stature
immunostimulatory DNA sequence
Individual Self-Rating Scale
inferior sagittal sinus
Injury Severity Scale
Injury Severity Score
Integrated Summary of Safety

invasive surgical staging
ion-scattering spectroscopy
ion surface scattering
irritable stomach syndrome
IS10S
10% invert sugar in 0.9% sodium chloride (saline) injection
ISSD
infantile sialic acid storage disorder
ISSHL
idiopathic sudden sensory hearing loss
ISSI
interspinous segmental spinal instrument
interspinous segmental spinal instrumentation (technique)
ISSLC
International Staging System for Lung Cancer
ISSNHL
idiopathic sudden sensorineural hearing loss
ISS-ODN
immunostimulatory oligodeoxynucleotide
ISSP
Infant Support Services Program
IST
immunosuppressive therapy
injection sclerotherapy
insulin sensitivity test
insulin shock therapy
interstitiospinal tract
isometric systolic tension
ISTD
insulin standard
ISU
intermediate surgical unit
ISUB
immunosubtraction
I-sub
inhibitor substance
ISW
interstitial water
IS10W
10% invert sugar injection (in water)
ISWI
incisional surgical wound infection
ISY
intrasynovial
IT
iliotibial
immunity test
immunologic test
immunotherapy
immunotoxin therapy

implantation test
incentive therapy
individual therapy
inferior temporal
inferior turbinate
information technology
inhalation test
inhalation therapist
inhalation therapy
inner table thickness
inspiratory time (*See also* I-time)
insulin treatment
intact
intensive therapy
intentional tremor
intermittent traction (*See also* int trx)
internal thoracic
interpreted
interstitial tissue
intertrochanteric
intertuberous (pelvic diameter)
intimal thickening
intolerance and toxicity
intracellular tachyzoite
intradermal test
intratesticular
intrathecal
intrathecal (anesthesia injection) (*See also* INTH, ITh, i-thec)
intrathoracic
intratracheal (tube) (*See also* ITR)
intratumoral (*See also* i-tumor)
ischial tuberosity
isomeric transition (of radioactive isotopes)

I/T
intensity/duration (contractions)
intensity/time (duration of contractions)

ITA
individual treatment assessment
inferior temporal artery
internal thoracic artery
itaconic acid
itasetron

ITAG
internal thoracic artery graft

ITAL
intrathoracic artificial lung

ITAM
immunoreceptor tyrosine-based activation motif

ITAQ
Insight and Treatment Attitudes Questionnaire

ITAS
internal telomerase standard

ITAV
Itaituba virus

ITB
iliotibial band
intrathecal baclofen

ITBC
intraluminal typical bronchial carcinoid

ITBFS
iliotibial band friction syndrome

ITBS
iliotibial band syndrome
Iowa Tests of Basic Skills

^{131}I-TBS
iodine-131 total body scan

ITBV
intrathoracic blood volume

ITC
incontinence treatment center
inferior temporal cortex
infrared thermographic calorimetry
Interventional Therapeutics Corporation
in-the-canal (hearing aid)
isothermal titration calorimetry

ITc
International Table calorie

ITCL
interosseous talocalcaneal ligament

ITCM
integral traditional Chinese medicine

ITCP
idiopathic thrombocytopenic purpura (*See also* ITP)

ITCU
intensive thoracic cardiovascular unit

ITCVD
ischemic thrombotic cerebrovascular disease

ITD
insulin-treated diabetic

NOTES

ITE
in the ear (hearing aid)
insufficient therapeutic effect
in-the-ear
intrapulmonary interstitial
emphysema
ITERS
Infant/Toddler Environment Rating
Scale
ITET
isotonic endurance test
ITF
inpatient treatment facility
interferon (*See also* IF, IFN, INF)
ITFF
intertrochanteric femoral fracture
ITFS
iliotibial tract friction syndrome
incomplete testicular feminization
syndrome
ITGCN
intratubular germ cell neoplasia
ITGP
immunotactoid glomerulopathy
ITGV
intrathoracic gas volume (*See also*
IGV)
ITH
immediate-type hypersensitivity
ITh, i-thec
intrathecal (anesthesia injection)
(*See also* INTH, IT)
ITI
inter-alpha-trypsin inhibitor
intertrial interval
intratubal insemination
I-time
inspiration time
inspiratory time (*See also* IT)
ITIV
Itimirim virus
ITL
inspiratory threshold load
ITLC
instant thin-layer chromatography
ITLC-SG
instant thin-layer chromatography-
silica gel
ITM
improved Thayer-Martin (medium)
ITMg
intratracheal magnesium
ITN
idiopathic trigeminal neuralgia
ITOC
intratracheal oxygen catheter
ITOP
intentional termination of pregnancy

ITOU
intensive therapy observation unit
ITP
idiopathic thrombocytopenic purpura
(*See also* ITCP)
immune thrombocytopenic purpura
inosine triphosphate
inosine 5'-triphosphate
interim treatment plan
inverse treatment planning
islet-cell tumor of the pancreas
ITPA
Illinois Test of Psycholinguistic
Abilities
inosine triphosphatase (*See also*
ITPase)
intrathecal *Treponema pallidum*
antibody
ITPase
inosine triphosphatase (*See also*
ITPA)
ITPV
intratracheal pulmonary ventilation
Itaporanga virus
ITQ
Infant Temperament Questionnaire
inferior temporal quadrant
ITQV
Itaqui virus
ITR
intraocular tension recorder
intratracheal (*See also* IT)
isotretinoin
ITRA
itraconazole
I tracing
interrupted tracing
ITS
internal transcribed spacer
isometric trunk stabilization
ITSC
It Scale for Children (psychologic
test)
ITSCU
infant-toddler special care unit
ITSHD
isolated thyroid-stimulating hormone
deficiency
ITT
identical twins (raised) together
iliotibial tract
insulin tolerance test
intention-to-treat (analysis)
internal tibial torsion
iron tolerance test
ITTP
idiopathic thrombocytopenic purpura

ITU
   infant-toddler unit
   intensive therapy unit
   intensive treatment unit
i-tumor
   intratumoral (*See also* IT)
ITUV
   Itupiranga virus
ITV
   impedance threshold valve
   infantile tibia vara
   inferior temporal vein
ITVAD
   indwelling transcutaneous vascular
     access device
ITW
   idiopathic toe-walker
   idiopathic toe-walking
ITX
   immunotoxin(s)
   intertriginous xanthoma
ITZ
   itraconazole (Sporanox)
IU
   immunizing unit (*See also* IE,
     ImmU)
   International Unit
   intrauterine
   in utero
[I]U
   concentration of insulin in urine
iu
   infectious unit
IUA
   intrauterine adhesion
IUC
   idiopathic ulcerative colitis
   intrauterine catheter
IUCD
   intrauterine contraceptive device
     (*See also* ICD, IUD)
IUD
   intrauterine (contraceptive) device
     (*See also* ICD, IUCD)
   intrauterine death
IUDE
   in utero drug exposure
IUDR
   iododeoxyuridine (*See also* IDU)
IUF
   isolated ultrafiltration

IUFB
   intrauterine foreign body
IUFD
   intrauterine fetal death
   intrauterine fetal demise
   intrauterine fetal distress
IUFGR
   intrauterine fetal growth retardation
IUFT
   intrauterine fetal transfusion
IUG
   infusion urogram
   intrauterine gas
   intrauterine gestation
   intrauterine growth
IUGR
   intrauterine growth rate
   intrauterine growth restriction
   intrauterine growth retardation
IUI
   intrauterine infection
   intrauterine insemination (catheter)
IU/L
   International Unit per liter
IUM
   internal urethral meatus
   intrauterine (fetally) malnourished
   intrauterine malnourishment
   intrauterine membrane
IU/min
   International Unit per minute
IUP
   intrauterine pregnancy
   intrauterine pressure
IUPC
   intrauterine pressure catheter
IUPD
   intrauterine pregnancy, delivered
IUPM
   infectious units per million
IUPTB
   intrauterine pregnancy, term birth
IUP,TBCS
   intrauterine pregnancy, term birth,
     cesarean section
IUP,TBLC
   intrauterine pregnancy, term birth,
     living child
IUP,TBLI
   intrauterine pregnancy, term birth,
     living infant

NOTES

IUR
    intrauterine retardation
IUT
    intrauterine transfusion
IUTD
    immunizations up-to-date
IV
    ichthyosis vulgaris
    interventricular
    intervertebral
    interview
    intravascular
    intravenous (*See also* i.v.)
    intraventricular (*See also* IVT)
    intravertebral
    invasive
    inversion
    iodine value
    in vitro
    in vivo
i.v.
    intravenous (*See also* IV)
IVA
    integrated visual and auditory
    Intervir-A
    intraoperative vascular angiography
IVAC
    intravenous accurate control (device)
IVAD
    implantable vascular access device
    implantable venous access device
IVag
    intravaginal
IVAP
    in vitro antibody production (assay)
    in vivo adhesive platelet
IVAR
    insulin variable
IVB
    intravitreal blood
IVBAT
    intravascular bronchioalveolar tumor
    intravascular (sclerosing) bronchioloalveolar tumor
IVBC
    intravascular blood coagulation
IVC
    individually viable cell
    indwelling venous catheter
    inferior vena cava
    inferior venacavogram (*See also* IVCV)
    inferior venacavography (*See also* IVCV)
    inspiratory vital capacity
    inspired vital capacity
    integrated vector control

    intravascular coagulation
    intravenous chemotherapy
    intravenous cholangiogram (*See also* IVCh)
    intravenous cholangiography (*See also* IVCh)
    intraventricular catheter
    intraventricular conduction
    isovolumic contraction
IVc-2
    intravascular catheter-2
IVCC
    intravascular consumption coagulopathy
IVCD
    intraventricular conduction defect
    intraventricular conduction delay
IVCh
    intravenous cholangiogram (*See also* IVC)
    intravenous cholangiography (*See also* IVC)
IVCP
    inferior vena cava pressure
IVCR
    inferior vena cava reconstruction
IVCT
    inferior vena cava thrombosis
    intravenously (enhanced) computed tomography
    isovolumic contraction time (*See also* ICT)
IVCU
    isotope voiding cystourethrography
IVCV
    inferior venacavogram (*See also* IVC)
    inferior venacavography (*See also* IVC)
IVD
    intervertebral disk
    intravenous drip
IVDA
    intravenous drug abuse
IVDSA
    intravenous digital subtraction angiography
IVDSI
    intervertebral disc space infection
IVDU
    intravenous drug use
    intravenous drug user
IVET
    in vivo expression technology
IVF
    interventricular foramen
    intravascular fluid
    intravenous fluid

intravenous fluorescein
intravertebral foramen
in vitro fertilization
in vivo fertilization

IVFA
intravenous fluorescein angiography

IVFE
intravenous fat emulsion

IVF-ET
in vitro fertilization-embryo transfer

IVFT
intravenous fetal transfusion

IVG
isotopic ventriculogram

IVGG
intravenous gamma globulin

IVGTT
intravenous glucose tolerance test

IVH
intravenous hyperalimentation
intraventricular hemorrhage (Grade 1–4)
intraventricular hemorrhage (Grade I–IV)

IVH2RA
intravenous H2 receptor antagonist

IVI
intravaginal insemination

IVIG, IVIg
intravenous immune (serum) globulin
intravenous immunoglobulin

IVJC
intervertebral joint complex

IVL
indwelling venous line
intravenous leiomyomatosis
intravenous lock

IVLBW
infant of very low birth weight

IVM
immediate visual memory
intracranial venous malformation
intravascular mass

IVMP
intravenous methylprednisolone

IVN
intravenous nutrition

IVNC
isolated ventricular noncompaction

IVNF
intravitreal neovascular frond

IVO
intraoral vertical osteotomy

IVOTTS
Irvine viable organ-tissue transport system

IVOX
intravascular oxygenator

IVP
intravenous push (dose) (*See also* IVp, IVPU)
intravenous pyelogram
intravenous pyelography
intraventricular pressure
intravesical pressure

IVp, IVPU
intravenous push (dose) (*See also* IVP, IVPU)

IVPB
intravenous piggyback (drug administration)

IVPD
in vitro protein digestibility

IVPF
isovolume pressure flow (curve)

IVR
idioventricular rhythm
interactive voice-response (system)
internal visual reference
intravaginal ring
intravenous retrograde
intravenous rider
isolated volume responder
isovolumic relaxation (time) (*See also* IVRT)

IVRA
intravenous regional anesthesia

IVRAP
intravenous retrograde access port

IVRF
incomplete vertical root fracture

IVRG
intravenous retrograde

IV-RNV
intravenous radionuclide venography

IVRO
intraoral vertical ramus osteotomy

IVRP
isovolumetric relaxation period

IVRT
isovolumic relaxation time (*See also* IVR)

NOTES

IVS

inappropriate vasopressin secretion
intact ventricular septum
intervening sequence
interventricular septal thickness
interventricular septum (*See also* IS)
intervillous space
irritable voiding syndrome

IVSD

interventricular septal defect (*See also* ISD)

IVSE

interventricular septal excursion

IVSO

intraoral vertical segmental osteotomy

IVSS

intravenous Soluset

IVST

interventricular septal thickness

IVT

idiopathic ventricular tachycardia
index of vertical transmission
interactive video technology
intrauterine fetal transfusion
intravenous transfusion
intraventricular (*See also* IV)
isovolumic time

IVTTT

intravenous tolbutamide tolerance test

IVU

intravenous urogram
intravenous urography

IVUC

intravenous ultrasound catheter

IVUS

intracoronary vascular ultrasound
intravascular ultrasound

IVV

influenza virus vaccine
intravenous vasopressin

IW

inner wall
inspiratory wheeze

I-5-W

invert sugar 5% in water

IWB

Index of Well-Being

IWD

individual with a disability

IWI

inferior wall infarction
interwave interval

IWL

insensible water loss

IWMI

inferior wall myocardial infarction

IWML

idiopathic white matter lesion

IWP

ischial weightbearing prosthesis

IWS

Index of Work Satisfaction

IWT

ice water test
impacted wisdom teeth

IYS

inverted Y-suspensor

IZ

infarction zone

IZS

insulin zinc suspension

J
- dynamic movement of inertia
- electric current density
- jejunostomy
- Jewish
- joint (*See also* jnt, jt)
- joule
- joule equivalent
- juice (*See also* j, jc)
- juvenile (*See also* juv)
- juxtapulmonary-capillary (receptor)
- magnetic polarization
- polypeptide chain in polymeric immunoglobulins
- reference point following QRS complex, at beginning of ST segment
- sound intensity

J1–J3
- Jaeger test type number 1–3

J
- flux (density)

j
- jaundice (*See also* jaund, JD)
- juice (*See also* J, jc)

JA
- jet area
- joint aspiration
- juvenile arthritis
- juvenile atrophy
- juxtaarticular

Jack
- jacknife position

JACV
- Jacareacanga virus

JAFAR
- Juvenile Arthritis Functional Assessment Report

JAG1
- human jagged-1 gene

JAI
- juvenile amaurotic idiocy

JAK, Jak
- Janus family tyrosine kinase
- Janus kinase

JAK1, Jak1
- Janus kinase 1

JAK2, Jak2
- Janus kinase 2

Jak/Stat
- Janus kinase/signal transducer and activator of transcription

JAM
- joint alignment and motion

JAMG
- juvenile autoimmune myasthenia gravis

JAMV
- Jamanxi virus

JAN
- Japanese Accepted Name

JAPV
- Japanaut virus

JARAN
- junior assistant resident admission note

JARIV
- Jari virus

JAS
- Jenkins Activity Survey (psychologic test)
- Job Attitude Scale
- joint activated system
- juvenile ankylosing spondylitis

jaund
- jaundice (*See also* j, JD)

JBC
- Jesness Behavior Checklist

JBE
- Japanese B encephalitis

JBS
- Johanson Blizzard syndrome

JC
- Jakob-Creutzfeldt (disease)
- Jamestown Canyon
- joint contracture
- junior clinician

J/C
- joule per coulomb

jc
- juice (*See also* J, j)

JCA
- juvenile chronic arthritis

JCE
- job capacity evaluation

JCF
- juvenile calcaneal fracture

JCGC
- Japanese Classification for Gastric Carcinoma

JCL
- job control language (computers)

J/cm
- joules per centimeter

J/cm^2
- joules per centimeter squared

JCML
- juvenile chronic myelocytic leukemia

JCML *(continued)*
juvenile chronic myelogenous leukemia

JCP
juvenile chronic polyarthritis

JCQ
Job Content Questionnaire

JCT
juxtaglomerular cell tumor

jct
junction

JD
jaundice (*See also* j, jaund)
jejunal diverticulitis
jugulodigastric (node)
juvenile delinquent
juvenile-onset diabetes (*See also* JDM, JOD, JODM)

JDI
Job Description Index

JDM
juvenile dermatomyositis
juvenile diabetes mellitus
juvenile-onset diabetes mellitus (*See also* JD, JOD, JODM)

JDMS
juvenile dermatomyositis

JDMS/PM
juvenile dermatomyositis/polymyositis

JDV
Juan Diaz virus

JE
Japanese encephalitis
junctional escape

JEB
junctional epidermolysis bullosa
junctional escape beat

JEE
Japanese equine encephalitis

JEJ, jej
jejunum

JEMBEC
agar plates for transporting cultures of gonococci

JEN
Japanese encephalitis vaccine

JEPI
Junior Eysenck Personality Inventory

JER
Japanese erection ring
junctional escape rhythm

JET
jejunal extension tube
junctional ectopic tachycardia

JETPEG
jejunal tube through percutaneous endoscopic gastrostomy

JE-VAX
Japanese encephalitis virus vaccine

JF
joint fluid
jugular foramen
junctional fold

JFET
junction field-effect transistor

JFS
jugular foramen syndrome

JG
June grass (test)
juxtaglomerular (*See also* jg, j-g)
juxtaglomerular cell

jg, j-g
juxtaglomerular (*See also* JG)

JGA
juxtaglomerular apparatus

JGC
juxtaglomerular cell

JGCT
juvenile granulosa cell tumor
juxtaglomerular cell tumor

JGI
jejunogastric intussusception
juxtaglomerular granulation index
juxtaglomerular index

JGP
juvenile general paralysis

JH
Jarisch-Herxheimer (reaction) (*See also* JHR)
juvenile hormone (of insects)

j_H
heat transfer factor

JHA
juvenile hormone analog

JHMV
J. Howard Mueller virus

JHR
Jarisch-Herxheimer reaction (*See also* JH)

JI
jejunoileal (bypass)
jejunoileitis
jejunoileostomy
Jesness Inventory

JIA
juvenile idiopathic arthritis

JIB
jejunoileal bypass

JIDC
juvenile intervertebral disk calcification

J

juvenile intervertebral disk calcifications

JIH
joint interval histogram

JIRI
Johnston Informal Reading Inventory

JIS
juvenile idiopathic scoliosis

JJ
jaw jerk
jejunojejunostomy

J&J, J & J
Johnson & Johnson

J/kg
joule per kilogram

JKST
Johnson-Kenney Screening Test (psychologic test)

JL
jet length
Judkins left (catheter)

JL4
Judkins left 4 (catheter)

JL5
Judkins left 5 (catheter)

JLO
Judgment of Line orientation

JLP
junvenile laryngeal papillomatosis
juvenile laryngeal papilloma

JM
josamycin
jugomaxillary
juxtamembrane

j_M
mass transfer factor (in heat transfer)

JMC
Jansen metaphyseal chondrodysplasia

JMD
juvenile macular degeneration

JME
juvenile myoclonic epilepsy

JMH
John Milton Hagen (antibody)

JMML
juvenile myelomonocytic leukemia

JMR
Jones-Mote reactivity

JMS
Juberg-Marsidi syndrome

JNA
juvenile nasopharyngeal angiofibroma

JNB
jaundice of newborn

JNCL
juvenile-onset neuronal ceroid lipofuscinosis

JND
just noticeable difference

JNK
c-*Jun* N-terminal kinase
Jun kinase

JNP
Jadassohn nevus phakomatosis

JNPA
juvenile nasopharyngeal angiofibroma

jnt
joint (*See also* J, jt)

JNVD
jugular neck vein distention

JOAG
juvenile open-angle glaucoma

JOD, JODM
juvenile-onset diabetes (*See also* JD, JDM)

JODM
juvenile-onset diabetes mellitus

JOIV
Joinjakaka virus

JOMAC
judgment, orientation, memory, abstraction, and calculation

JOMID
juvenile-onset multisystem inflammatory disease

JOR
jaw-opening reflex

jour
journal (*See also* jrnl)

JP
Jackson-Pratt (drain)
Jobst pump
joint protection (*See also* JTP)
juvenile periodontitis
juvenile polyposis

JPA
juvenile pilocytic astrocytoma

JPB
junctional premature beat

NOTES

JPBS
Jackson-Pratt to bulb suction

JPC
junctional premature contraction

JPD
juvenile plantar dermatitis
juvenile plantar dermatosis
juxtapapillary diverticulum

JPI
Jackson Personality Inventory

JPS
joint position sense
juvenile polyposis syndrome

JR
jaw reflex
Jolly reaction
Judkins right (catheter)
junctional rhythm

JR4
Judkins right 4 (catheter)

JR5
Judkins right 5 (catheter)

JRA
juvenile rheumatoid arthritis (type I, II)

JRAN
junior resident admission note

Jr BF
junior baby food

JRC
joint replacement center

jrnl, jrl
journal (*See also* jour)

JROM
joint range of motion

JS
jejunal segment
junctional slowing
Junkman-Schoeller (unit of thyrotropin) (*See also* JSU, JS unit)

J/s
joule per second

JSF
Japanese spotted fever

JSI
Jansky Screening Index (psychologic test)

JSU, JS unit
Junkman-Schoeller unit (of thyrotropin) (*See also* JS)

JSV
Jerry-Slough virus

JT
jejunostomy tube
junctional tachycardia

J/T
joule per tesla

jt
joint (*See also* J, jnt)

JTA
job task analysis

jt asp
joint aspiration

JTF
jejunostomy tube feeding

JTJ
jaw-to-jaw (position)

JTP
joint protection (*See also* JP)

JTPS
juvenile tropical pancreatitis syndrome

J-tube
jejunostomy tube

Ju
jugale (craniometric point)

jug.
jugular

jug. comp.
jugular compression (test)

JUGV
Jugra virus

junct
junction (*See also* Jx)

JUNV
Junin virus

JURV
Jurona virus

JUTV
Jutiapa virus

juv
juvenile (*See also* J)

juxt.
near [L. *juxta*]

JV
jugular vein
jugular venous (pressure, pulse)

JVBF
Jan van Breemen Function Questionnaire

JVC
jugular venous catheter

JVD
jugular venous distention
jugulovenous distention

JVIS
Jackson Vocational Interest Survey

JVP
jugular venous pressure
jugular venous pulsation
jugular venous pulse

JVPT
jugular venous pulse tracing

JW
jump walker

JWHS
Juvenile Wellness and Health Survey

JWS
Jackson-Weiss syndrome

Jx
joint
junction (*See also* junct)

JXG
juvenile xanthogranuloma

NOTES

J

K

burst of diphasic slow waves in response to stimuli during sleep (in electroencephalography)

calix [Gr. *kalyx* cup]

capsular antigen [Ger. *Kapsel* capsule]

carrying capacity (genetics)

cathode (*See also* C, CA, C, cath)

coefficient of heat transfer

coefficient of scleral rigidity

cornea

cornea curvature

cretaceous

dissociation constant (*See also* K_d)

electron capture

electrostatic capacity

equilibrium constant

ionization constant

kalium (potassium)

kallikrein inhibiting unit

kanamycin (*See also* KM)

kappa (10th letter of Greek alphabet), uppercase

Kell blood group

Kell blood system

Kell factor

kelvin (SI fundamental unit of temperature)

keratometer

keratometric power

kerma

ketamine (Super K)

ketotifen

kidney

killer (cell)

kilo- (*See also* k)

kilodalton (*See also* kD)

kilopermeability coefficient

kinetic energy (*See also* KE)

knee (*See also* Kn, kn)

kosher

Küntscher (nail)

lysine (*See also* LYS)

modulus of compression

motor coordination (in General Aptitude Test Battery)

1024 (number of bytes in kilobyte)

one thousand (*See also* kilo)

phylloquinone (*See also* K_1)

potassium [L. *kalium*] (*See also* kal, pot., potass)

ratio of curvature of flattest meridian of apical cornea (in fitting of contact lens)

thousand

vitamin K.

K1

phytonadione

K_1

phylloquinone (*See also* K)

K2

menatetrenone

K_3

menadione

K_4

menadiol sodium diphosphate

^{39}K

potassium-39

^{40}K

potassium-40

^{42}K

potassium-42

^{43}K

potassium-43

$°K$

degree on the Kelvin scale (obsolete, now K)

K^+

potassium ion

k

Boltzmann constant

constant

kilo- (*See also* K)

magnetic susceptibility

rate constants

rate of velocity constant

reaction rate constant

velocity constants

K-A

King-Armstrong (unit) (*See also* KA, KAU)

KA

alkaline phosphatase (*See also* AKP, ALK-P, alk phos, alk p'tase, ALP, AlPase, AP, P'ase)

kainic acid

keratoacanthoma

ketoacidosis

King-Armstrong (unit) (*See also* K-A, KAU)

kynurenic acid

K/A

ketogenic/antiketogenic (ratio)

K_a

acid ionization (dissociation) constant

equilibrium association constant

K_a
dissociation constant of an acid (*See also* K_d)

Ka
kallikrein

kA
kiloampere

KAAD
kerosene, alcohol, acetic acid, and dioxane (mixture)

KAB
knowledge, attitude, behavior

KABC
Kaufman Assessment Battery for Children

KABINS
knowledge, attitude, behavior, and improvement in nutritional status

KACT
kaolin-activated clotting time

KADV
Kadam virus

KAF
conglutinogen-activating factor
killer-assisting factor
kinase-activating factor

KAFO
knee-ankle-foot orthosis

KAIT
Kaufman Adolescent and Adult Intelligence Test

KAIV
Kaikalur virus

kal
potassium [L. *kalium*] (*See also* K, pot., potass)

KALIG-1
Kallmann syndrome interval gene 1

KAMV
Kamese virus

KANV
Kannamangalam virus

KAO
knee-ankle orthosis

KAP
knowledge, aptitudes, (and) practices (fertility)

κ
kappa (10th letter of Greek alphabet), lowercase
magnetic susceptibility
one of two immunoglobulin light chains

KAR
killer-activating receptor

KAS
Katz Adjustment Scales (psychologic test)

KASH
knowledge, abilities, skills, (and) habits

KASS
Kaneda anterior spinal/scoliosis system

KAST
Kindergarten Auditory Screening Test

KASV
Kasba virus

KAT
kanamycin acetyltransferase
kinesthetic ability trainer

kat
katal (enzyme unit of measurement)

kat/L
katal per liter

KAU
King-Armstrong unit (*See also* KA, K-A)

KB
human oral epidermoid carcinoma cells
ketone body
kilobyte
knee-bearing
knee brace
knuckle-bender (splint)

K-B
Kleihauer-Betke (test)

K_b, K_b
base ionization constant
dissociation constant of a base

kb
kilobase

K-BIT
Kaufman Brief Intelligence Test

kbp
kilobase pair (nucleic acid molecules)

kBq
kilobecquerel

KBR
ketone body ratio

KBr
potassium bromide

KC
cathodal (kathodal) closing
katacalcin
keratoconjunctivitis
keratoconus
knees to chest
knuckle cracking
Korean conflict
Kupffer cell

kC
kilocoulomb
kc
kilocycle
kcal
kilocalorie
kilogram calorie
k$_{cat}$
turnover number
KCC
cathodal (kathodal) closing
contraction [Ger. *Kathodenschlie
βungs-Kontraktion*] (*See also* KSK)
Kulchitsky cell carcinoma
KCCT
kaolin-cephalin clotting time
KCD
kinestatic charge detector
K cell
killer cell
KCG
kinetocardiogram
KChIPs
potassium channel-interacting
proteins
KCI
Kolbe Conative Index
kCi
kilocurie
KCl
potassium chloride
KCNJ1
potassium inwardly-rectifying
channel, subfamily J, member 1
K complex
slow waves related to sleep
arousal (in electroencephalography)
KCS
keratoconjunctivitis sicca
kc/sec, kc/s
kilocycle per second
KCV
Kern Canyon virus
KCZ
ketoconazole
KD
cathodal (kathodal) duration
ketogenic diet
kidney donor
killed
knee disarticulation
knitted Dacron

knowledge deficit
Krabbe disease
K$_d$
dissociation constant (*See also* K)
dissociation constant of an acid
(*See also* K$_a$)
distribution coefficient
equilibrium dissociation constant
partition coefficient
kD, kDa
kilodalton (*See also* K)
KDA
known drug allergies
kDNA
kinetoplast deoxyribonucleic acid
KDO
ketodeoxyoctonic (acid)
KDP
potassium dihydrogen phosphate
KDS
Kaufman Development Scale
KDSS
Kurtzke Disability Status Scale
KDU
Kidney Dialysis Unit
kdyn
kilodyne
KE
first order elimination rate constant
in hr.-1
Kendall compound E (cortisone)
kinetic energy (*See also* K)
K$_e$
exchangeable body potassium
KEAT
Kaprelian easy-access tweezers
KED
Kendrick extrication device
K3 EDTA
tripotassium
ethylenediaminetetraacetate
kel
elimination rate constant
kemo Tx
chemical therapy (chemotherapy)
KEMV
Kemerovo virus
K$_{eq}$
equilibrium constant
KER
keratin

K

NOTES

kera
keratitis
kerma
kinetic energy released in the medium
KET
ketoconazole
ketones
KETO
ketoconazole
KETV
Ketapang virus
KEUV
Keuraliba virus
keV
kiloelectron volt
KEVD
Krupin eye valve with disk
KEYV
Keystone virus
KF
Kayser-Fleischer (ring)
Kenner-fecal (medium)
kidney function
Klippel-Feil (syndrome)
kf
flocculation rate in antigen-antibody reaction
KFA
kinetic fibrinogen assay
KFAB, KFAb
kidney-fixing antibody
K factor
gamma-ray dose (roentgens per hour at 1 cm from 1-mCi point source of radiation)
KFAO
knee-foot-ankle orthosis
KFD
Kikuchi-Fujimoto disease
Kinetic Family Drawings
KFR
Kayser-Fleischer ring
KG
ketoglutarate
K-G
Kimray-Greenfield (filter)
KG-1
Koeffler Golde-1 (cell line)
kG
kilogauss
kg
kilogram (*See also* kilo)
KGC
Keflin (cephalothin), gentamicin, and carbenicillin
kg-cal
kilogram-calorie

kg/cm²
kilogram per square centimeter
KGDH
ketoglutarate dehydrogenase
KGDHC
ketoglutarate dehydrogenase complex
KGF
keratinocyte growth factor
KGF-2
keratinocyte growth factor-2
kgf
kilogram-force
KGFR
keratinocyte growth factor receptor
kg/L
kilogram per liter
kg-m
kilogram-meter
kg/m²
kilogram per meter squared
kg-m/s²
kilogram-meter per second squared
Kgn
kininogen
KGS
ketogenic steroid
17-KGS
17-ketogenic steroid
kg/s
kilogram per second
KGTI
Kinetik great toe implant
KGy
kiloGray
KH
Krebs-Henseleit (cycle)
K24H
potassium in 24-hour (urine)
KHB
Krebs-Henseleit bicarbonate (buffer)
KHb
potassium hemoglobinate
KHC
kinetic hemolysis curve
knot holding capacity
KHD
kinky-hair disease
KHE
kaposiform hemangioendothelioma
KHF
Korean hemorrhagic fever
KHM
keratoderma hereditaria mutilans
KHN
Knoop hardness number (of solids)
KHS
kinky hair syndrome
Krebs-Henseleit solution

K

kHz
    kilohertz
KI
    karyopyknotic index (*See also* KPI)
    knee immobilizer
    Krönig isthmus
    potassium iodide
K_I
    dissociation of enzyme-inhibitor
      complex
    inhibition constant
kI
    kidney channel (acupuncture)
KIA
    Kligler iron agar (medium)
KIC
    ketoisocaproic (acid)
KICB
    killed intracellular bacteria
KID
    keratitis, ichthyosis, and deafness
      (syndrome)
    kidney
KIDDIE-SADS
    Schedule for Affective Disorders
      and Schizophrenia for School-Age
      Children
KIDS
    Kent Infant Development Scale
kilo
    kilogram (*See also* kg)
    kilometer (*See also* km)
    one thousand (*See also* K)
KIMV
    Kimberley virus
KIN
    kinetic
KIP
    key intermediary protein
    kinase inhibitory protein
KIPS
    knowledge information processing
      system
KIR
    killer cell inhibitory receptor
K_{ir}6.2
    inward-rectifying K^+-channel 6.2
KIR-HLA
    killer inhibitor receptors-human
      leukocyte antigen
KISS
    key integrative social system

    kidney internal splint/stent
    potassium iodide, saturated solution
KISV
    Kismayo virus
KIT
    Kahn intelligence test
    kinase tyrosine
KIU
    kallikrein inactivating unit
    kallikrein inactivation unit
    kallikrein-inhibiting unit
KJ, kj
    knee jerk
kJ
    kilojoule
KJR
    knee jerk reflex
KK
    kallikrein-kinin
    knee kick
    knock-knee
kkat
    kilokatal
KKV
    Kaeng Khoi virus
KL
    kidney lobe
    kit ligand
    Klebs-Löffler (bacillus)
kL
    kiloliter
kl
    musical overtone (ringing, in
      acoustics) [Ger. *Klang*]
KLA
    keratolimbal allograft
KLAV
    Klamath virus
KLB
    Klebsiella vaccine
KL-BET
    Kleihauer-Betke (test) (*See also* K-
      B)
Kleb
    Klebsiella
K level
    lowest level (of x-rays)
KLH
    keyhole-limpet hemocyanin
KLK1
    kallikrein 1

NOTES

KLS
kidneys, liver, spleen

KLST
Kindergarten Language Screening Test

KM
κ-immunoglobulin (light chain)
kanamycin (*See also* K)
keratomileusis

Km, K$_m$
Michaelis constant
Michaelis-Menten dissociation constant

km
kilometer (*See also* kilo)

km^2
square kilometer

kMc
kilomegacycle

K-MCM
potassium-containing minimal capacitation medium

kMc/s, kMcps
kilomegacycle per second

KMDAT
Key Math Diagnostic Arithmetic Test

KMEF
keratin, myosin, epidermin, and fibrin (class of proteins)

KMFTR
Kotz modular femur and tibia resection

KMG
kangaroo-mother care

KmnO4
potassium permanganate

KMO
Kaiser-Meyer-Olkin (measure of statistical sampling adequacy)

kmps, km/s
kilometer per second

KMPV
Kammavanpettai virus

KMS
Kabuki makeup syndrome
kwashiorkor-marasmus syndrome

KMV
killed measles virus (vaccine)

Kn
knee (*See also* K, kn)
Knudsen number (low-pressure gas flow)

kN
kilonewton

kn
knee (*See also* K, Kn)

KNF model
Koshland-Némethy-Filmer model

KNO
keep needle open

knork
knife and fork (physical medicine)

KNRK
Kirsten sarcoma virus in normal rat kidney (cell)

KNSA
Kron Nutritive Sucking Apparatus

KO
keep on (continue) (*See also* K/O)
keep open (*See also* K/O)
killed organism
knee orthosis
knocked out (*See also* KO'd)

K/O
keep on (continue) (*See also* KO)
keep open (*See also* KO)

KOC
cathodal (kathodal-obsolete) opening contraction

KO'd
knocked out (*See also* KO)

KOH
potassium hydroxide (stain)

KOIS
Kuder Occupational Interest Survey

KOKV
Kokobera virus

KOLV
Kolongo virus

KOOV
Koongol virus

KOR
keep open rate

KOT
Knowledge of Occupations Test

KOTV
Kotonkan virus

KOUV
Koutango virus

KOWV
Kowanyama virus

KP
hot pack
Kaufmann-Peterson (base)
keratitic precipitate
keratitis punctata
keratoprecipitate
keratotic patch
kidney protein
kidney punch (trauma)
killed parenteral (vaccine)
kinetic perimetry
knowledge of performance
Köbner phenomenon

K-P
Kaiser Permanente (diet)
kPa
kilopascal
kPas/L
kilopascal-second per liter
KPB
kalium (potassium) phosphate buffer
ketophenylbutazone (kebuzone)
KPE
Kelman phacoemulsification
KP-e
experimentally induced Köbner
phenomenon
KPG
potassium penicillin G
KP-h
Köbner phenomenon by history
KPI
karyopyknotic index (*See also* KI)
KPM
kilopound meter
kilopounds per minute
KPR
key pulse rate
Kuder Preference Record
KPR-V
Kuder Preference
Record—Vocational
KPS
Karnofsky performance score
Karnofsky performance status
KPT
kidney punch test (physical exam)
Kuder Performance Test
KPTI
Kunitz pancreatic trypsin inhibitor
KPTT
kaolin partial thromboplastin time
KPV
killed parenteral vaccine
killed polio vaccine
KR
knowledge of result
Kopper Reppart (medium)
17-KR
17-ketosteroid reductase
Kr
krypton
81mKr
krypton-81m

kR
kiloroentgen
KRB, KRBB
Krebs-Ringer bicarbonate (buffer)
KRBG
Krebs-Ringer bicarbonate (buffer)
with glucose
KRBS
Krebs-Ringer bicarbonate solution
KRD
kinetic rehab device
K readings
keratometric readings
KRIV
Kairi virus
K-rod
Küntscher rod
KRP
Kolmer (test with) Reiter protein
(antigen)
Krebs-Ringer phosphate
KRPS
Krebs-Ringer phosphate solution
KRT
Kindergarten Readiness Test
KS
Kabuki syndrome
Kaposi sarcoma
keratan sulfate
ketosteroid
kidney stone
Kveim-Siltzbach (test)
17-KS
17-ketosteroid
ks
kilosecond
KSA
knowledge, skills, and abilities
K-SADS
Schedule for Affective Disorders
and Schizophrenia for School-Age
Children
K-SADS-E
Schedule for Affective Disorders
and Schizophrenia for School-Age
Children-Epidemiologic Version
K-SADS-P
Schedule for Affective Disorders
and Schizophrenia for School-Age
Children-Present Episode

K

NOTES

KSBOP
Kaderavek-Sulzby Bookreading Observational Protocol

KSCC
keratinizing squamous cell carcinoma

KSE
knee sling exercises

K-SEALS
Kaufman Survey of Early Academic and Language Skills

KSHV
Kaposi sarcoma herpesvirus

KSIV
Karshi virus

KSK
cathodal closing contraction [Ger. *Kathodenschlie βungs-Kontraktion*] (*See also* KCC)

KS/OI
Kaposi sarcoma and opportunistic infections

KSOV
Kaisodi virus

KSP
Karolinska Scale of Personality
kidney-specific protein

K$_{sp}$
potassium solubility product

KSR
potassium chloride sustained release (tablets)

KSU
Kent State University (Speech Discrimination Test)

KSV
Kao Shuan virus

KSW
knife stab wound

KT
kidney transplant
kidney transplantation
kidney treatment
kinesiotherapy
known to
Kuder test

KTC
knee-to-chest

K-TEA
Kaufman Test of Educational Achievement

KTI
kallikrein-trypsin inhibitor

KTP
potassium titanyl phosphate

KTP laser
potassium titanyl phosphate laser

KTS
kethoxal thiosemicarbazone

KTSA
Kahn Test of Symbol Arrangement

KTU
kidney transplant unit
known to us

KTVS
Keystone Telebinocular Visual Survey

KTx
kidney transplantation

KTZ
ketoconazole

KU
kallikrein unit
Karmen unit
Kimbrel unit

Ku
kurchatovium

KUB
kidneys, ureters, bladder (x-ray)
kidneys and urinary bladder
kidney ultrasound biopsy

KUNV
Kunjin virus

KUS
kidneys, ureters, and spleen (x-ray)

KV
kanamycin-vancomycin
kanamycin and vancomycin
killed vaccine

kV
kilovolt
kilovoltage

kVA
kilovolt-ampere

KVBA
kanamycin-vancomycin blood agar

kVcp
kilovolt constant potential

KVE
Kaposi varicelliform eruption

KVLB
kanamycin-vancomycin laked blood

KVLBA
kanamycin-vancomycin laked blood agar

KVO
keep vein open (IV lines)

KVO C D5W
keep vein open with 5% dextrose in water

kVp
kilovoltage peak
kilovoltage potential

KW
    Keith-Wagener (classification of eye
    ground findings) (*See also* KWB)
    kidney weight
    Kimmelstiel-Wilson (disease)
    Kruskal-Wallis (test)
K$_w$
    dissociation constant of water
kW
    kilowatt
KWAV
    Kwatta virus
KWB
    Keith-Wagener-Barker (classification
    of eye ground findings) (*See also*
    KW)

kWh, kW-hr
    kilowatt-hour
KWIC
    keyword in context (computers)
K wire, K-wire
    Kirschner wire
KWOC
    keyword out of context
        (computers)
kyph
    kyphosis
KYZV
    Kyzylagach virus

NOTES

K

L

angular momentum
Avogadro constant/number *(See also* Λ, NA)
boundary [L. *limes*] *(See also* LIM)
coefficient of induction
diffusion length
fifty (Roman numeral)
inductance
lambert (unit of luminance) *(See also* La)
latent (heat)
latex *(See also* LX, Lx)
Latin
left *(See also* (L), l, lf, LT, lt)
length *(See also* l)
Lente (insulin)
lesser
let
lethal (Erlich's symbol for fatal) *(See also* l)
leucine *(See also* Leu)
levorotatory
lewisite
licensed (to practice)
lidocaine *(See also* LIDO)
ligament, ligamentum *(See also* Lgt, lgt, lig)
light (chain of protein molecules) *(See also* LT, lt)
light sense
lilac (indicator color)
limes
lincomycin
lingual *(See also* ling)
linking number
linking (number)
liquor
Listeria
liter
liver *(See also* LIV)
living *(See also* liv)
longitudinal (section)
low *(See also* LO)
lower *(See also* LO)
lowest *(See also* LO)
lumbar
lumbar vertebra
lumen *(See also* lm)
luminance
lung *(See also* LU, Lu)
lymph
lymphocyte
lymphogranuloma
lysosome

radiance
self-inductance
syphilis (lues)
threshold

L1–L5, L_1–L_5
first through fifth lumbar vertebrae or lumbar nerve

L-I, L-II, L-III
stages of lues (syphilis)

L_0
limes zero (neutralized toxin-antitoxin mixture) [L. *limes nul*]

L/3
lower third (of leg bone)

(L)
left *(See also* L, l, lf, LT, lt)
lunch

L_+
limes tod (toxin-antitoxin mixture that contains one fatal dose in excess)

l
left *(See also* L, (L), lf, LT, lt)
length *(See also* L)
lethal (Erlich's symbol for fatal) *(See also* L)
line
liter *(See also* L)
long
longitudinal
radioactive constant
specific latent heat

l-
levorotatory

L-
sterically related to L-glyceraldehyde

LA
lactic acid
language age
laparoscopic adrenalectomy
laparoscopic appendectomy
large amount
late abortion
late antigen
lateral apical
latex agglutination
Latin American
left angle
left angulation
left arm
left atrial (pressure)
left atrium
left atrium (echocardiography image)
left auricle

LA *(continued)*
leucine aminopeptidase *(See also*
LAP)
leukemia antigen
leukoagglutinating
leukoaraiosis
leuprolide acetate
levator ani (muscle)
lichen amyloidosis
light adaptation
linguoaxial
linoleic acid
lobuloalveolar
local anesthesia
long acting
long-acting (drug)
long arm (cast)
Los Angeles
low anxiety
Ludwig angina
lupus anticoagulant
lymphocyte antibody

LA50
total body surface area of burn
that will kill 50% of patients
(lethal area)

L&A, L+A, l&a
light and accommodation
living and active (family history)

La
labial
lambert *(See also* L)
lanthanum

LAA
left atrial abnormality
left atrial appendage
left auricular appendage
leukemia-associated antigen
leukocyte ascorbic acid

LA:A
left atrial to aortic (ratio)

La:A
left atrial to aortic

LAAH
laparoscopic-assisted abdominal
hysterectomy

LAAL
lower anterior axillary line

LAAM
levomethadyl acetate

L-AAM
L-alpha-acetylmethadiol 3

LAAO
L-amino acid oxidase

LA:Ao
left atrial to aortic

LAARD
long-acting antirheumatic drug

LAB
left abdomen
Leisure Activities Blank
(psychology)

lab
laboratory *(See also* LB)
rennet ferment coagulating milk
[Ger. *Lab* chymosin]

LABA
laser-assisted balloon angioplasty

LABBB
left anterior bundle branch block

LABC
locally advanced breast cancer

LABD
linear IgA bullous dermatosis

LABS
laboratory admission baseline
studies

LABV
left atrial ball valve

LABVT
left atrial ball-valve thrombus

LAC
laceration *(See also* lac)
La Crosse
Lactobacillus acidophilus vaccine
lactose
left antecubital
left atrial contraction
linguoaxiocervical
locally advanced cancer
long arm cast
low amplitude contraction
lung adenocarcinoma cell
lupus anticoagulant

LaC
labiocervical

lac
laceration *(See also* LAC)
lactate *(See also* lact)
lactation *(See also* lact)

LACC
Life After Cancer Care
locally advanced cervical carcinoma

lac & cont
laceration and contusion

LACD
left apexcardiogram, calibrated
displacement

LACI
lacunar circulation infarct
lipoprotein-associated coagulation
inhibitor

LACN
local area communications network

lacr
lacrimal

LACS
  lacunar syndrome
LACT
  Lindamood Auditory
    Conceptualization Test
    (psychology)
LAC T
  lactose tolerance
lact
  lactate (*See also* lac)
  lactating
  lactation (*See also* lac)
  lactic
LACT-ART
  lactate arterial
lact hyd
  lactalbumin hydrolysate
LACV
  La Crosse virus
LAD
  lactic acid dehydrogenase (*See also*
    LADH)
  language acquisition device
  left anterior descending (coronary
    artery) (*See also* LADA, LADCA)
  left atrial diameter
  left atrial dimension
  left axis deviation
  leukocyte adhesion deficiency
  ligament augmentation device
  ligamentous anterior dislocation
  linoleic acid depression
  lipoamide dehydrogenase
  lymphocyte-activating determinant
LAD-1, LAD1
  leukocyte adhesion deficiency type
    1
LAD-2, LAD2
  leukocyte adhesion deficiency type
    2
LAD-3, LAD3
  leukocyte adhesion deficiency type
    3
LAD-4, LAD4
  leukocyte adhesion deficiency type
    4
LADA
  laboratory animal dander allergy
  latent autoimmune diabetes of
    adults
  left acromiodorsoanterior (position
    of fetus)

LADCA
  left anterior descending coronary
    artery (*See also* LAD, LADA)
LADD
  lacrimoauriculodentodigital
    (syndrome)
  left anterior descending diagonal
    (branch of coronary artery)
LADH
  lactic acid dehydrogenase (*See also*
    LAD)
  liver alcohol dehydrogenase
LADME
  liberation, absorption, distribution,
    metabolism, and excretion
LAD-MIN
  left axis deviation, minimal
LADP
  left acromiodorsoposterior (position
    of fetus)
LADPG
  laparoscopically assisted distal
    partial gastrectomy
LADu
  lobuloalveolar-ductal
LAE
  left atrial enlargement
  long above-elbow (cast)
LAEC
  locally advanced esophageal cancer
LAEDV
  left atrial end-diastolic volume
LAEI
  left atrial emptying index
LAER
  late auditory evoked response
LAESV
  left atrial end-systolic volume
LAF
  laminar air flow
  Latin American female
  left atrial enlargement
  leukocyte-activating factor
  low animal fat
  lymphocyte-activating factor
LAF-3
  leukocyte antigen factor-3
LAFB
  left anterior fascicular block
LAFR
  laminar air flow room

L

NOTES

LAFS
> long-axis fractional shortening

LAFU
> laminar air flow unit

LAG
> labiogingival (*See also* LaG)
> linguoaxiogingival
> lymphangiogram
> lymphangiography

LaG
> labiogingival (*See also* LAG)

LAGB
> Lap-Band adjustable gastric banding
> system

LAH
> lactalbumin hydrolysate
> laparoscopic-assisted hepatectomy
> left anterior hemiblock (*See also*
> LAHB)
> left atrial hypertrophy
> lithium-aluminum hydride

LAHB
> left anterior hemiblock (*See also*
> LAH)

LA-HFOV
> liquid-assisted high-frequency
> oscillatory ventilation

LAI
> labioincisal (*See also* LaI)
> laboratory-acquired infection
> latex (particle) agglutination
> inhibition
> left atrial involvement
> left atrial isomerism
> leukocyte adherence inhibition
> (assay)
> leukocyte adhesion inhibitor

LaI
> labioincisal (*See also* LAI)

LAID
> left anterior internal diameter

LAIF
> leukocyte adherence inhibition
> factor

LAIT
> latex agglutination-inhibition test

LAK
> lymphokine-activated killer (cell)

LAL
> left axillary line
> limulus amebocyte lysate
> low air loss

LaL
> labiolingual

L-Ala
> L-alanine

LALI
> lymphocyte antibody
> lymphocytolytic interaction

LALLS
> low-angle laser light scattering

LALT
> larynx-associated lymphoid tissue
> low air loss therapy (mattress)

LAM
> lactation amenorrhea method (birth
> control)
> laminar air flow
> laminectomy (*See also* lam)
> laser-assisted myringotomy
> late ambulatory monitoring
> Latin American male
> left anterior measurement
> left atrial myxoma
> limb accurate measurement
> lymphangioleiomyomatosis
> lymphangiomyomatosis

LAM-1
> leukocyte adhesion molecule-1

lam
> lamina
> laminectomy (*See also* LAM)
> laminogram

LAMA
> laser-assisted microanastomosis

LA–MAX
> maximal left atrial (dimension)

LAMB
> lentigines, atrial myxomas,
> cutaneous papular myxomas, blue
> nevi

L AmB, L-AmB
> liposomal amphotericin B

Λ
> Avogadro number (*See also* NA, L,
> Λ)
> lambda (11th letter of Greek
> alphabet), uppercase
> Ostwald solubility coefficient
> radioactive constant
> wavelength

λ
> craniometric point (lambda)
> decay constant
> junction of lambdoid and sagittal
> sutures (craniotomy)
> lambda (11th letter of Greek
> alphabet), lowercase
> mean free path
> microliter (*See also* μL)
> one of two forms of
> immunoglobulin light chain
> thermal conductivity (*See also* TC)
> wavelength (*See also* WL)

lam & fus
 laminectomy and fusion
lami
 laminotomy
LAMM
 L-a-acetylmethadol
 levo-alpha-acetylmethadol
LAMMA
 laser microprobe mass analyzer
LAMP-1
 lysosomal membrane glycoprotein-1
LAMP-2
 lysosomal membrane glycoprotein-2
LAN
 local area network
 long-acting neuroleptic
 lymphadenopathy
LANA
 latency-associated nuclear antigen
LANC
 long arm navicular cast
lang
 language
L ANT
 left anterior
LANV
 left atrial neovascularization
LAO
 left anterior oblique
 left anterior occipital
 left atrial overloading
LAP
 laparoscopy (*See also* lap.)
 laparotomy (*See also* lap.)
 laser-assisted palatoplasty
 latency-associated peptide
 left abdominal pain
 left atrial pressure
 leucine aminopeptidase (*See also* LA)
 leukocyte alkaline phosphatase (stain)
 liver-enriched activating protein
 low atmospheric pressure
 lower abdominal pain
 lymphangiomatous polyp
 lyophilized anterior pituitary
 lyophilized anterior pituitary (tissue)
LAP-1
 Los Angeles preservation solution 1

lap.
 laparoscopy (*See also* LAP)
 laparotomy (*See also* LAP)
LAPA
 leukocyte alkaline phosphatase activity
 locally-advanced pancreatic adenocarcinoma
LAP-APPY
 laparoscopic appendectomy
LAPC
 locally advanced prostate cancer
LAP CHOLE
 laparoscopic cholecystectomy
LAPF
 low-affinity platelet factor
LAPMS
 long arm posterior-molded splint
lap Nissen
 laparoscopic Nissen fundoplication
LAP test
 leucine aminopeptidase test
LAPW
 left atrial posterior wall
LAQ
 long arc quad
LAR
 laryngeal adductor reflex
 laryngology (*See also* Laryngol)
 late asthmatic response
 left arm, reclining (blood pressure, pulse measurement)
 left arm, recumbent (blood pressure, pulse measurement)
 long-acting release
 low anterior resection
lar
 larynx (*See also* lx)
LARC
 leukocyte automatic recognition computer
LAR/CAA
 low anterior resection in combination with coloanal anastomosis
LARD
 lacrimoauriculoradiodental (syndrome)
LARM
 left arm

NOTES

LARS
> Language-Structured Auditory Retention Span (Test)
> laparoscopic antireflux surgery
> leucyl-transfer ribonucleic acid synthetase

LARSI
> lumbar anterior-root stimulator implant

laryn
> laryngeal
> laryngitis
> laryngoscopy

Laryngol
> laryngology (*See also* LAR)

LAS
> laboratory automation system
> lateral amyotrophic sclerosis
> laxative abuse syndrome
> left anterior superior
> left arm, sitting (blood pressure, pulse measurement)
> leucine acetylsalicylate
> linear alkyl sulfonate
> local adaptation syndrome
> long arm splint
> low-amplitude signal
> lower abdominal surgery
> lymphadenopathy syndrome
> lymphangioscintigraphy
> lysine acetylsalicylate

LASA
> left anterior spinal artery
> Linear Analogue Self-Assessment (scales)
> lipid-associated sialic acid
> Lisfranc articular set angle

LASE
> laser-assisted spinal endoscopy

LASEC
> left atrial spontaneous echo contrast

laser
> light activation by stimulated emission of radiation

LASFB
> left anterior-superior fascicular block

LASGB
> laser adjustable silicone gastric banding

LASH
> left anterior-superior hemiblock
> left anterosuperior hemiblock

LASIK
> laser-assisted intrastromal keratomileusis
> laser-assisted in situ keratomileusis

LASS
> labile aggregation stimulating substance
> Linguistic Analysis of Speech Samples

LASSI
> Learning and Study Strategies Inventory

LASSI-HS
> Learning and Study Strategies Inventory-High School Version

LAST
> left anterior small thoracotomy
> leukocyte-antigen sensitivity testing
> limited anterior small thoracotomy

LASV
> Lassa virus

LAT
> lactic acidosis threshold
> latency-associated transcript
> latent
> lateral (*See also* lat)
> lateral atrial tunnel
> latex agglutination test
> left anterior thigh
> left atrial thrombus
> lidocaine, adrenaline, tetracaine
> limbal autograft transplantation
> linker for activation of T cell

lat
> lateral (*See also* LAT)
> latissimus (dorsi)
> latitude

LAT-A
> latrunculin A

LAT-B
> latrunculin B

LATC
> lateral talocalcaneal
> lateral talocalcaneal angle

LATCH
> literature attached to charts

lat & loc
> lateralizing and localizing

l·atm
> liter-atmosphere

lat men
> lateral meniscectomy

LATP
> left atrial transmural pressure

LATPT
> left atrial transesophageal pacing test

lat Rin
> lactated Ringer (solution) (*See also* LR)

LATS
>long-acting thyroid-stimulating (hormone)
>long-acting transmural stimulator

lats
>latissimus dorsi (muscle)

LATS-P
>long-acting thyroid stimulator-protector

LATu
>lobuloalveolar tumor

LATV
>Latino virus

LAUP
>laser-assisted uvulopalatoplasty

LAV
>lymphadenopathy-associated virus
>lymphocyte-associated virus

LAVA
>laser-assisted vasal anastomosis

LAVH
>laparoscopic-assisted vaginal hysterectomy
>laparoscopic-assisted vaginal hysteroscopy

LAW
>LDH, AST, WBC (blood tests)
>left atrial wall

LAWER
>life-terminating acts without the explicit request

LAX
>long axis

lax.
>laxative
>laxity

LB
>laboratory (data) (*See also* lab)
>lamellar body
>large bowel
>lateral basal
>lateral bending
>left breast
>left bundle
>left buttock
>leiomyoblastoma (*See also* LMB)
>lipid body
>live birth
>liver biopsy
>living bank
>loose body
>low back (pain) (*See also* LBP)

>low breakage
>lung biopsy
>lymphoid body

L-B
>Liebermann-Burchard (test for cholesterol)

L&B
>left and below

lb.
>pound (*See also* pnd.)
>pound [L. *libra*] (*See also* L, pnd.)

LBA
>laser balloon angioplasty
>left basal artery

LBA$_4$
>leukotriene B$_4$

LBAll
>Leader Behavior Analysis II

lb avdp
>avoirdupois pound [L. *libra avoirdupois*]

LBB
>left breast biopsy
>left bundle branch
>long back board
>low back bend

LBBB
>left bundle-branch block

LBBsB
>left bundle branch system block

LBBX
>left breast biopsy examination

LBC
>lamellar body count
>lidocaine blood concentration
>locoregional breast cancer
>lymphadenosis benigna cutis

LBCD
>left border of cardiac dullness

LBCF
>Laboratory Branch Complement Fixation (test)

LBCL
>large B-cell lymphoma

L/B/Cr
>electrolytes, blood urea nitrogen, and serum creatinine

LBD
>lamellar body density
>large bile duct
>left border dullness (of heart to percussion)

NOTES

LBD *(continued)*
 left brain damage
 Lewy body dementia
 low back disability
LBDQ
 Leader Behavior Description
  Questionnaire
LBE
 line bisection error
 long below-elbow (cast)
LBF

 Lactobacillus bulgaricus factor
  (pantetheine)
 limb blood flow
 liver blood flow
lbf
 pound-force
lbf-ft
 pound-force foot
lb-ft
 pound-feet
LBG
 Landry-Guillain-Barré (syndrome)
LBH
 length, breadth, height
LBI
 low serum-bound iron
lb/in^2
 pounds per square inch (*See also*
  PSI)
LBL
 labeled lymphoblast
 lymphoblastic lymphoma (*See also*
  LL)
LBM
 last bowel movement
 lean body mass
 little brown mushroom
 loose bowel movement
 lung basement membrane
LBMI
 last body mass index
LBNA
 lysis bladder neck adhesions
LBNP
 lower body negative pressure
LBO
 large bowel obstruction
LBP
 lipopolysaccharide binding protein
 low back pain (*See also* LB)
 low blood pressure
LBPQ
 Low Back Pain Questionnaire
LBQC
 large base quad cane
LBRF
 louse-borne relapsing fever

LBS
 lactobacillus selector (agar)
 low back syndrome
LBSA
 lipid-bound sialic acid (*See also*
  LSA)
lbs. (plural)
 pounds [L. *librae*]
LBT
 loaded breathing test
 low back tenderness
 low back trouble
 lupus band test
LBTI
 lima bean trypsin inhibitor
LBV
 Lagos bat virus
 left brachial vein
 low biological value
 lung blood volume
LBVO
 left brachial vein occlusion
LBW
 lean body weight
 low birth weight
LBWC
 limb-body wall complex
LBWI
 low birth weight infant
LBWR
 lung-body weight ratio
LC
 inductance-capacitance
 lactation consultant
 Laënnec cirrhosis
 lamina cortex
 Langerhans cell
 laparoscopic cholecystectomy
 large cell
 large chromophobe
 large cleaved (cell)
 late clamped (umbilical cord)
 lateral compression
 lateral projection
 lecithin cholesterol (acyltransferase)
 left circumflex (coronary artery)
  (*See also* LCCA, LCF, LCX,
  LCx)
 left (ear), cold (stimulus)
 leisure counseling
 lethal concentration
 level of consciousness
 life care
 light chain
 light coagulation
 lingual cusp
 linguocervical
 lining cell

lipid cytosome
liquid chromatography
liquid crystal
lithocolic (acid)
live clinic
liver cirrhosis
liver clinic
living children
locus ceruleus
long-chain (triglycerides)
longus capitis
low calorie (*See also* lo cal)
lung cancer
lung cell
lymphangitic carcinomatosis
lymph capillary
lymphocyte count
lymphocytic colitis
lymphocytotoxin (*See also* LCT, LT)
lymphoma culture

3LC

triple-lumen catheter

LCA

latent class analysis
lateral cricoarytenoid
Leber congenital amaurosis
left carotid artery
left circumflex artery
left coronary angiography
left coronary artery
leukocyte common antigen
light contact assist
lithocholic acid
lithocolic acid
liver cell adenoma
lymphocyte chemoattractant activity
lymphocytotoxic antibody (*See also* LCTA)

LCAD

long-chain acyl-coenzyme A dehydrogenase

LCA-DCA

lithocolic acid-deoxycholic acid (ratio)

LCAD/MCAD

long- and medium-chain fatty acid coenzyme-A dehydrogenase deficiency

LCAD/VLCAD

long- and very-long-chain acyl-CoA dehydrogenase

LCAH

life-care at home

LCAL

large cell anaplastic lymphoma

LCAO

linear combination of atomic orbitals

LCAO-MO

linear combination of atomic orbital-molecular orbital

LCAR

late cutaneous anaphylactic reaction

LCAT

lecithin-cholesterol acyltransferase

LCB

left costal border
lymphomatosis cutis benigna

LCBF

local cerebral blood flow

LCC

lactose coliform count
large cell change
left coronary cusp
liver cell carcinoma
long calcaneocuboid

LCCA

late cortical cerebellar atrophy
left circumflex coronary artery (*See also* LC, LCX, LCx)
left common carotid artery
leukoclastic angiitis
leukocytoclastic angiitis

LCCE

length contraction compensation element

LCCP

limited channel-capacity process

LCCS

lower cervical cesarean section

LCCSCT

large-cell calcifying Sertoli cell tumor

LCD

lipochondral degeneration
liquid crystal display
liquor carbonis detergens (coal tar solution)
localized collagen dystrophy
low-calcium diet

LC-DCP, LCDCP

low-contact dynamic compression plate

NOTES

L

LCDD
> light-chain deposition disease

LCDE
> laparoscopic common duct exploration

LCE
> laparoscopic cholecystectomy
> left carotid endarterectomy
> lower completely edentulous

LCED
> liquid chromatography with electrochemical detection

LC-EMR
> lift-and-cut endoscopic mucosal resection

LCF
> least common factor
> left circumflex (coronary artery) (*See also* LC, LCCA, LCX, LCx)
> left common femoral (artery)
> linear correction factor
> low-frequency current field
> lymphocyte chemoattractant factor
> lymphocyte culture fluid

LCFA
> long-chain fatty acid

LCFA-CoA
> long chain fatty acyl-coenzyme A

LCFAO
> long-chain fatty acid oxidation

LCFC
> linear combination of fragment configuration

LCFM
> laser cell and flare meter
> left circumflex marginal

LCFU
> leukocyte colony-forming unit

LCG
> Langerhans cell granule
> Langerhans cell granulomatosis
> liquid chemical germicide

LCGU
> local cerebral glucose utilization

LCH
> Langerhans cell histiocytosis
> local city hospital

LCHAD
> long-chain-3-hydroxyacyl-CoA dehydrogenase
> long-chain 3-hydroxyacyl coenzyme A dehydrogenase

L chain
> light chain (polypeptides with low molecular weight)

LCI
> length complexity index
> lung clearance index

LCIS
> lobular carcinoma in situ

LCL
> large cell lymphoma
> lateral collateral ligament
> Levinthal-Coles-Lillie
> Levinthal-Coles-Lillie (bodies)
> Levinthal-Coles-Lillie (cytoplasmic inclusion body)
> localized cutaneous leishmaniasis
> lower confidence limit
> lymphoblastoid cell line
> lymphocytic leukemia (*See also* LL)
> lymphocytic lymphosarcoma
> lymphoid cell line

LCLC
> large cell lung carcinoma

LCM
> laser-capture microdissection
> latent cardiomyopathy
> left costal margin
> leukocyte-conditioned medium
> lower costal margin
> lowest common multiple
> lymphatic choriomeningitis
> lymphocytic choriomeningitis

LCMG
> long-chain monoglyceride

l/cm H₂O

l/cm H_2O
> liters per centimeter of water

LCMI
> left ventricular mass index

LC-MS-MS
> liquid chromatography coupled to tandem mass spectrometry

LCMV
> lymphocytic choriomeningitis virus

LCN
> lateral cervical nucleus
> left caudate nucleus
> lidocaine

LCNB
> large-core needle biopsy

LCNEC
> large-cell neuroendocrine carcinoma

LCNHL
> large-cell non-Hodgkin lymphoma

LCNST
> late central nervous system toxicity

LCO
> low cardiac output

LCOS
> low cardiac output syndrome

LCP
> Legg-Calvé-Perthes (disease) (*See also* LCPD)
> leukocytapheresis

long-chain polysaturated (fatty acid)
long, closed, posterior (cervix)
LCPD
Legg-Calvé-Perthes disease (*See also* LCP)
LCPUFA
long-chain polyunsaturated fatty acid
LCQG
left caudal quarter ganglion
LCR
laryngeal cough reflex test
late cortical response
late cutaneous reaction
ligamentous and capsular repair
ligase chain reaction
LCRS
Living Conditions Rating Scale
LCS
LaparoSonic coagulating shears
laser correlational spectroscopy
lateral crural steal
left coronary sinus
Leydig cell stimulation
lichen chronicus simplex
life care service
liquor cerebrospinalis
low constant suction
low-contact stress
low continuous suction
LCSG
left cardiac sympathetic ganglionectomy
LCSS
Lung Cancer Symptom Score
LCSW
low continuous wall suction
LCT
Leydig cell tumor
liquid crystal thermography
Listening Comprehension Test
liver cell tumor
long-chain triglyceride
low cervical transverse
lung capillary time
Luscher Color Test
lymphocytotoxicity test
lymphocytotoxin (*See also* LC, LT)
LCTA
lungs clear to auscultation
lymphocytotoxic antibody (*See also* LCA)

LCTCS
low cervical transverse cesarean section
LCTD
low-calcium test diet
LCU
laparoscopic contact ultrasonography
life change unit
LCV
Lake Clarendon virus
lecithovitellin
leukocytoclastic vasculitis
low cervical vertical (incision)
LCVA
left hemisphere stroke
LCVP
laser coagulation vaporization procedure
LCX, LCx
left circumflex (coronary artery) (*See also* LC, LCCA, LCF)
LD
L-dopa
laboratory data
labor and delivery (*See also* L&D)
labyrinthine defect
lactate dehydrogenase (*See also* LDG, LDH, LHD)
lactic (acid) dehydrogenase (*See also* LDG, LDH)
lactic dehydrogenase
last dose
learning disability
learning disabled
learning disorder
left deltoid
Legionnaire disease
Leishman-Donovan (body) (*See also* L-D)
lethal dose
levodopa (*See also* L-DOPA, L-dopa)
lichenoid dysplasia
light-dark
light difference
light differentiation
light duty
limited disease
linear dichroism
linguodistal
lipodystrophy
lithium diluent

L

NOTES

LD *(continued)*
　　lithium discontinuation
　　liver disease
　　living donor
　　loading dose
　　Lombard-Dowell (agar)
　　longitudinal diameter (of heart)
　　long (time) dialysis
　　low density
　　low dose
　　lung destruction
　　Lyme disease
　　lymphocyte defined
　　lymphocyte depletion
　　lymphocytically determined

L-D
　　Leishman-Donovan
　　Leishman-Donovan (body) *(See also*
　　　LD)

L/D
　　light/dark (ratio)

L&D
　　labor and delivery *(See also* LD)
　　light and distance (in
　　　ophthalmology)

LD$_{100}$
　　lethal dose in all exposed subjects

LD$_{50}$
　　median lethal dose (lethal for 50%
　　　of test subjects)

LD$_{50/30}$
　　dose that is lethal dose for 50%
　　　of test subjects within 30 days

LD$_1$–LD$_5$
　　lactate dehydrogenase fraction 1
　　　through 5 *(See also* LDH$_1$–LDH$_5$)

LDA
　　laser Doppler anemometry
　　lateral disk attachment
　　left dorsoanterior (fetal position)
　　limiting dilution analysis
　　linear discriminant analysis
　　linear displacement analysis
　　low density area
　　low-dose arm
　　lymphocyte-dependent antibody

LDAR
　　latex direct agglutination reaction

LDB
　　lamb dysentery bacillus
　　Legionnaire disease bacillus
　　ligand-binding domain

LDC
　　leukocyte differential count
　　lymphoid dendritic cell

L-DC
　　Langerhans-dendritic cell

LDCC
　　lectin-dependent cellular cytotoxicity

LDCI
　　low-dose continuous infusion

LDCOC
　　low-dose combination oral
　　　contraceptive

LDCT
　　late distal cortical tubule

LDD
　　laser disk decompression
　　late dedifferentiation
　　lead locking device
　　Lee and Desus D (test)
　　light-dark discrimination
　　low drain (class) D

LDDS
　　local dentist

LDE
　　Lateral Dominance Examination
　　lauric diethamide

LDEA
　　left deviation of electrical axis

LDER
　　lateral-view dual-energy radiography

LDES
　　Learning Disability Evaluation
　　　Scale

LD-EYA
　　Lombard-Dowell egg yolk agar

LDF
　　laser Doppler flowmetry
　　laser Doppler flux
　　limit dilution factor
　　lumbodorsal fascia

LDG
　　lactate dehydrogenase *(See also* LD,
　　　LDH, LHD)
　　lactic (acid) dehydrogenase *(See
　　　also* LD, LDH)
　　lingual developmental groove
　　long-distance group
　　low-dose group

LDH
　　lactate dehydrogenase *(See also* LD,
　　　LDG, LHD)
　　lactic (acid) dehydrogenase *(See
　　　also* LD, LDG)
　　low-dose heparin

LDH$_1$–LDH$_5$
　　lactate dehydrogenase fraction 1
　　　through 5 *(See also* LD$_1$–LD$_5$)

LDHA
　　lactate dehydrogenase A

LDHB
　　lactate dehydrogenase B

LDHD
  lymphocyte-depleted Hodgkin
  disease
LDHI
  lactate dehydrogenase isoenzyme
  (*See also* LDISO)
LDHV
  lactic dehydrogenase virus
LDIH
  left direct inguinal hernia
LDIR
  low-dose of ionizing radiation
LDISO
  lactate dehydrogenase isoenzyme
  (*See also* LDHI)
LDI-TOF-MS
  laser desorption/ionization time-of-
  flight-mass spectrometer
LDL
  loudness discomfort level
  low-density lipoprotein (*See also*
  LDLP)
  low-density lymphocyte
LDLA
  low-density lipoprotein apheresis
LDL-C
  low-density lipoprotein-cholesterol
LDLC, LDL-C
  low-density lipoprotein cholesterol
LDLP
  low-density lipoprotein (*See also*
  LDL)
LDLT
  living donor liver transplantation
LDM
  lactate dehydrogenase, muscle
  lorazepam, dexamethasone, and
  metoclopramide
LDMA
  lymphocyte detected membrane
  antigen
LDMCF, LDMF
  latissimus dorsi myocutaneous flap
LDMRT
  low-dose mediastinal radiation
  therapy
LDN
  laparoscopic donor nephrectomy
LD-NEYA
  Lombard-Dowell neomycin egg
  yolk agar

LDNF
  lung-derived neurotrophic factor
L-DOPA, l-dopa, L-dopa
  levodopa
  levodopamine
LDP
  late diastolic potential
  left dorsoposterior (fetal position)
  lumbodorsal pain
LD-PCR
  limiting dilution polymerase chain
  reaction
LDR
  labor, delivery, and recovery
  length-to-diameter ratio
  long-duration response
  low-dose rate
L/D ratio
  light/dark amplitude ratio
LDRP
  labor, delivery, recovery,
  postpartum
LDS
  late dumping syndrome
  ligate-divide-staple
  ligating and dividing stapler
LDSST
  low-dose short synacthen test
LDT
  left dorsotransverse (fetal position)
LD-T
  lactic dehydrogenase total
LDU, LDUB
  long double upright (brace)
LDUH
  low-dose unfractionated heparin
LDV
  lactate dehydrogenase elevating
  virus
  lactic dehydrogenase virus
  large dense-cored vesicle
  laser Doppler velocimetry
  lateral distant view
  Le Dantec virus
LE
  left ear
  left eye (*See also* O.L., O.S.)
  lens extraction
  leucine enkephalin
  leukocyte esterase (*See also*
  LKESTR)
  leukoerythrogenetic

NOTES

LE *(continued)*
    leukoerythrogenic
    live embryo
    Long Evans (rat)
    lower extremity (*See also* L ext, l/ext, LX, Lx, lx)
    lupus erythematosus
    lupus erythematosus (cell)

Le
    Leonard (cathode ray unit)
    Lewis antibody
    Lewis (number, diffusivity:diffusion coefficient of a fluid)

Le^a
    Lewis a antibody

Le^b
    Lewis b antibody

LEA
    language experience approach
    local education agency
    lower extremity amputation
    lower extremity arterial
    lumbar epidural anesthesia

LEAD
    lower extremity arterial disease

LEADS
    Leadership Evaluation and Development Scale

LEAP
    latex ELISA for antigen protein
    Lewis expandable adjustable prosthesis

LEB
    lumbar epidural block
    lupus erythematosus body

LEBV
    Lebombo virus

LEC
    lens epithelial cell
    leukoencephalitis
    life events checklist
    Life Experiences Checklist
    low-energy charged (particle)
    lymphoepithelioma-like carcinoma

LECBD
    laparoscopic exploration of the common bile duct

LECP
    low-energy charged particle

LED
    light-emitting diode
    lowest effective dose
    lupus erythematosus disseminatus

LEDC
    low energy direct current

LEDS
    life events and difficulties schedule

LEDV
    Lednice virus

LEED
    low-energy electron diffraction

LEEDS
    low-energy electron diffraction spectroscopy

LEEP
    left end-expiratory pressure
    loop electrocautery excision procedure
    loop electrosurgical excision procedure

LEER
    lower extremity equipment related

LEE W
    Lee White tritium (clotting time) (*See also* L&W, L/W, LWCT)

LEF
    leukokinesis-enhancing factor
    lower extremity fracture
    lupus erythematosus factor

LEFS
    Lower Extremity Functional Scale

leg.
    legal
    legislation
    legislative

leg com
    legal commitment
    legally committed

LEH
    liposome-encapsulated hemoglobin

LEHPZ
    lower esophageal high-pressure zone

LeIF
    leukocyte interferon

leio
    leiomyoma

LEIS
    low-energy ion scattering

LEJ
    ligation of esophagogastric junction

LEL
    low-energy laser
    lowest effect level (of toxicity)
    lymphoepithelial lesion

LELC
    lymphoepithelioma-like carcinoma

LEM
    lateral eye movement
    Leibovitz-Emory medium
    leukocyte endogenous mediator
    light electron microscope

LEMG
    laryngeal electromyography

LEMO
  lowest empty molecular orbital
LEMS
  Lambert-Eaton myasthenic syndrome
LENI
  lower extremity noninvasive
lenit
  lenitive
lenit.
  gently [L. *leniter*]
LENT
  late effects normal tissue
  late effects of normal tissue
LEOD
  lens extraction, oculus dexter
LEOPARD
  lentigines, electrocardiographic
    (conduction abnormalities), ocular
    (hypertelorism), pulmonary
    (stenosis), abnormal (genitalia),
    retardation (of growth), and
    deafness (syndrome)
LEOS
  lens extraction, oculus sinister
LEP
  leptospirosis
  lethal effective phase (leptospirosis)
  lipoprotein electrophoresis (*See also*
    LPE)
  liposome-encapsulated paclitaxel
  longitudinal epiphyseal bracket
  low egg passage (strain of virus)
  lower esophageal pressure
LEP2
  leptospirosis 2
L$_{EPN}$
  effective perceived noise level
LE$_{prep}$
  lupus erythematosus preparation
LEPT
  leptocyte
LEPTOS
  leptospirosis agglutinins
Leq
  loudness equivalent
LER
  lysozymal enzyme release
LERG
  local electroretinogram
L-ERX
  leukoerythroblastic reaction

LES
  Lawrence Experimental Station
    (agar)
  lesser esophageal sphincter
  Life Experience Survey
  Liquid Embolic System
  local excitatory state
  Locke egg serum (medium)
  lower esophageal segment
  lower esophageal sphincter
  lower esophageal stricture
  lumbar epidural steroids
  lupus erythematosus, systemic
les
  lesion
  low excitatory state
LESA
  liposomally entrapped second
    antibody
LESEP
  lower extremity somatosensory
    evoked potential
LESI
  lumbar epidural steroid injection
LESP
  lower esophageal sphincter pressure
LESR
  lower esophageal sphincter
    relaxation
LESS
  lateral electrical spine stimulation
  lateral electrical surface stimulation
LET
  language enrichment therapy
  left esotropia
  leukocyte esterase test
  lidocaine, epinephrine, tetracaine
  linear energy transfer
  liposome-encapsulated tetracaine
  low energy transfer
LETC
  lymphoepithelioma-like thymic
    carcinoma
LETD
  lowest effective toxic dose
LET-II
  Learning Efficiency Test-II
LETS
  large external transformation-
    sensitive (fibronectin)

L

NOTES

429

LE-TUMT
　　low-energy transurethral microwave thermotherapy
LETZ
　　loop excision of the transformation zone
LEU
　　leukocyte equivalent unit
Leu
　　leucine (*See also* L)
leu-CAM
　　leukocyte cell adhesion molecule
leuk, leuko
　　leukocyte
LEUKAP
　　leukocyte alkaline phosphatase
LEV
　　levamisole
　　lower extremity venous
lev
　　levator (muscle)
levit.
　　lightly [L. *leviter*]
LEW
　　Lewis (rat)
LEX
　　lactate extraction
L ext, l/ext
　　lower extremity (*See also* LE, LX, Lx, lx)
LF
　　labile factor
　　laparoscopic fundoplication
　　laryngofissure
　　Lassa fever
　　latex fixation
　　lavage fluid
　　leaflet
　　left foot
　　left forearm
　　lethal factor
　　leucine flux
　　ligamentum flavum
　　limit of flocculation (*See also* Lf)
　　lingual fossa
　　living female
　　low-fat (diet)
　　low forceps (delivery) (*See also* LFD)
　　low frequency (*See also* lf)
Lf
　　limes flocculation (unit, dose of toxin per mL)
　　limit of flocculation (*See also* LF)
lf
　　left (*See also* L, (L), l, LT, lt)
　　low frequency (*See also* LF)

LFA
　　left femoral artery
　　left forearm
　　left frontoanterior (fetal position)
　　leukocyte function-associated antigen
　　leukotactic factor activity
　　low friction arthroplasty
　　lymphocyte function-associated antigen
LFA-1
　　leukocyte factor antigen-1
　　lymphocyte function antigen-1
　　lymphocyte function-associated antigen-1
LFA-2
　　lymphocyte function-associated antibody-2
LFA-3
　　lymphocyte function-associated antigen-3
LFAC
　　low frequency alternating current
LFB
　　lingual-facial-buccal
　　liver, iron, and B complex
　　low-flow cardiopulmonary bypass
　　low frequency band
LFBW
　　lateral frontal bone window
LFC
　　lateral femoral cutaneous
　　left frontal craniotomy
　　living female child
　　low fat and cholesterol (diet)
LFCS
　　low flap cesarean section
LFCT
　　lung-to-finger circulation time
LFD
　　lactose-free diet
　　large for date
　　late fetal death
　　lateral facial dysplasia
　　least fatal dose
　　low-fat diet
　　low-fiber diet
　　low forceps delivery (*See also* LF)
　　lunate fossa depression
LFECT
　　loose fibroelastic connective tissue
LFER
　　linear free-energy relationship
LFF
　　low-filter frequency
LFGNR
　　lactose fermenting gram-negative rod

LFH
 left femoral hernia
LFIT
 low-friction ion treatment
LFL
 left frontolateral
 leukocyte feeder layer
LFLA
 lactoferrin latex bead agglutination
LFM
 laser flare meter
 lateral force microscopy
 leflunomide
LFN
 lactoferrin
L-form
 Lister-form
LFOV
 large field of view
LFP
 left frontoposterior position (fetal)
LFPPV
 low-frequency positive pressure
  ventilation
LFR
 lymphoid follicular reticulosis
LF-RF
 local-regional failure
LFS
 lateral facet syndrome
 leukemia-free survival
 limbic forebrain structure
 liver function series
LFT
 lateral femoral torsion
 latex fixation test
 latex flocculation test
 left frontotransverse (fetal position)
 liver function test
 localized fibrous tumor
 low flap transverse
 low-frequency tetanic (stimulation)
 low-frequency tetanus
 low-frequency transduction
 low-frequency transfer
LFTSW
 left foot switch
LFU
 limit flocculation unit
 lipid fluidity unit
 lost to follow-up

LFV
 large field of view
 Lassa fever virus
 low-frequency ventilation
L fx
 linear fracture
LG
 lactoglobulin
 lamellar granule
 large (*See also* lg, lge)
 laryngectomy
 lateral ground
 left gluteal
 left gluteus
 light guide
 lingual groove
 linguogingival
 lipoglycopeptide
 liver graft
 low glucose
 lymph gland
 lymphocytic gastritis
 lymphography
L-G
 Lich-Gregoire (ureteroneocystostomy)
lg
 large (*See also* LG, lge)
 leg
 long
LGA
 large for gestational age
 left gastric artery
 low-grade astrocytoma
LGB
 Landry-Guillain-Barré (syndrome)
 lateral geniculate body
LGC
 left giant cell
LGD
 Leaderless Group Discussion
  (situational test)
 low-grade dysplasia
LGd
 dorsal lateral geniculate (nucleus)
LGE
 Langat encephalitis (*See also* LGT)
 linear gingival erythema
lge
 large (*See also* LG, lg)
LGF
 lateral giant fiber

L

NOTES

431

LGG

    Lactobacillus GG
    low-grade glioma

L-GG

    Lactobacillus rhamnosus strain GG

LGH

    lactogenic hormone (*See also* LTH)
    little growth hormone

LGI

    large glucagon immunoreactivity
    lower gastrointestinal

LGIB

    lower gastrointestinal bleeding

LGIOS

    low-grade intraosseous-type
      osteosarcoma

LGL, LGLS

    large granular leukocyte
    large granular lymphocyte
    lobular glomerulonephritis
    low grade lymphoma
    Lown-Ganong-Levine syndrome
    Lown-Ganong-Levine (syndrome)

LGM

    left gluteus medius

LGMD

    limb-girdle muscular dystrophy

LGN

    lateral geniculate nucleus
    lobular glomerulonephritis

LG-NHL, lg-NHL

    low-grade non-Hodgkins lymphoma

LGP

    labioglossopharyngeal

LGS

    Langer-Giedion syndrome
    large green soft (stool)
    Lennox-Gastaut syndrome (*See also*
      LG)
    limb-girdle syndrome
    low Gomco suction

LGSIL

    low-grade squamous intraepithelial
      lesion

LGT

    Langat encephalitis (*See also* LGE)
    late generalized tuberculosis

Lgt, lgt

    ligament, ligamentum (*See also* L,
      lig)

LGTV

    Langat virus

LGV

    large granular vesicle
    lymphogranuloma venereum (*See
     also* LVG)

LGV-CFT

    lymphogranuloma venereum
      complement fixation test

LGVHD

    lethal graft-versus-host disease

LGV-TRIC

    lymphogranuloma venereum-trachoma
      inclusion conjunctivitis

LgX

    lymphogranulomatosis X

LH

    late healed
    lateral hypothalamic (syndrome)
    lateral hypothalamus
    learning handicap
    left hand
    left hemisphere
    left hyperphoria
    liver homogenate
    loop of Henle
    lower half
    lues hereditaria (hereditary syphilis)
    lung homogenate
    luteinizing hormone
    luteotropic hormone (*See also* LTH)
    lutropin

LH-β

    luteinizing hormone-beta

L/H

    lymphocytic/histiocytic (cell)

LHA

    lateral hypothalamic area
    left hepatic artery

LHB

    long head of biceps

LHb

    lateral habenular

LHBT

    lactose hydrogen breath testing
    lactulose hydrogen breath test

LHBV

    left heart blood volume

LHC

    Langerhans cell histiocytosis
    left heart catheterization
    left hypochondrium

L/H cell

    lymphocytic-histiocytic

LHCG

    luteinizing hormone-chorionic
      gonadotropin (hormone)

LH/CG

    luteinizing hormone/human chorionic
      gonadotropin

LHD

    lactate dehydrogenase (*See also* LD,
      LDG, LDH)
    lateral head displacement

left-hand dominant
left hemisphere brain damage
left hemisphere damage
left hepatic duct

LHF
left heart failure
ligament of head of femur

LHFA
lung Hageman factor activator

LH-FSH
luteinizing hormone-follicle-
stimulating hormone

LH/FSH-RF
luteinizing hormone/follicle-
stimulating hormone-releasing
factor

LHG
left-hand grip
localized hemolysis in gel

LHH
left homonymous hemianopia

LHI
lipid hydrocarbon inclusion

LHL
left hemisphere lesion
left hepatic lobe

LHM
lisuride hydrogen maleate
lymphohistiocytoid mesothelioma

LHMP
Life Health Monitoring Program

LHMT
low-range heparin management test

LIIN
lateral hypothalamic nucleus

LHON
Leber hereditary optic neuropathy

LHP
left hemiparesis
left hemiplegia

LHPC
lipomatous hemangiopericytoma

LHPZ
lower (esophageal) high-pressure
zone

LHR
leukocyte histamine release (test)
liquid holding recovery
right lung-to-head circumference
ratio

l-hr
lumen-hour (unit quantity of light)

LH-RF, LHRF
luteinizing hormone-releasing factor
(*See also* LRF)

LHRH, LH-RH
LH-releasing hormone
luteinizing hormone-releasing
hormone (*See also* LRH)

LHRH-A
luteinizing hormone-releasing
hormone analogue

LHRT
leukocyte histamine release test

LHS
left-hand side
left heart strain
left heel strike
long-handled sponge
lymphatic and hematopoietic system

LHSH
long-handled shoe horn

LHT
left hypertropia

LHV
left hepatic vein

LI
labeling index
lactose intolerance
lacunar infarction
lamellar ichthyosis
language impairment
large intestine
laser iridotomy
laterality index
learning impaired
left injured
left involved
life island
linguoincisal
lithogenic index
liver involvement
loop ileostomy
low impulsiveness

L&I
liver and iron

Li
labrale inferius
lithium

li
large intestine channel
(acupuncture)

LIA
laser interference acuity

NOTES

L

LIA *(continued)*
    left iliac artery
    leukemia-associated inhibitory
        activity
    local infiltrative anesthesia
    lock-in amplifier
    lymphocyte-induced angiogenesis
    lysine-iron agar
LIAC
    light-induced absorbance change
LIAD
    low-impact aerobic dance
LIAF
    laser-induced arterial fluorescence
    lymphocyte-induced angiogenesis
        factor
LIAFI
    late infantile amaurotic familial
        idiocy
LIB
    left in bottle
LIBC
    latent iron-binding capacity
LIBR
    Librium
LIC
    left iliac crest
    left internal carotid
    leisure-interest class
    limiting isorrheic concentration
LICA
    laser image custom arthroplasty
    left internal carotid artery
LICC
    lectin-induced cellular cytotoxicity
LICD
    lower intestinal Crohn disease
LICM
    left intercostal margin
Li2CO3
    lithium carbonate
LICS
    left intercostal space (*See also* LIS)
LICU
    laparoscopic intracorporal ultrasound
    laparoscopic intracorporeal
        ultrasonography
LID
    late immunoglobulin deficiency
    lymphocytic infiltrative disease
LIDC
    low-intensity direct current
LIDO
    lidocaine (*See also* L)
LIE
    labioincisal edge
    linguoincisal edge

LIF
    laser-induced fluorescence
    left iliac fossa
    left index finger
    leukemia-inhibiting factor
    leukocyte infiltration factor
    leukocyte inhibitory factor
    leukocytosis-inducing factor
    liver (migration) inhibitory factor
    local intra-arterial fibrinolysis
LiF
    lithium fluoride
LIFE
    laser-induced fluorescence emission
    light-induced fluorescence
        endoscopic
    lung imaging fluorescence
        endoscope
    lung imaging fluorescent endoscopy
LIFEC
    lumbar intersomatic fusion
        expandable cage
LIFE-GI
    light induced fluorescence
        endoscopy system
L-IFN
    human lymphoblastoid interferon
LIFO
    last in, first out (re: computer
        data)
LIFS
    laser-induced fluorescence
        spectroscopy
LIFT
    laser-assisted internal fabrication
        technique
    lymphocyte immunofluorescence test
LIG
    leukemia inhibitory factor
    lymphocyte immune globulin
lig
    ligament, ligamentum (*See also* L,
        Lgt, lgt)
    ligate
    ligation
    ligature (*See also* ligg)
ligg
    ligamenta (plural)
    ligaments (plural)
    ligature (*See also* lig)
LIGHT
    homologous to lymphotoxin, shows
        inducible expression and competes
        with herpes simplex virus
        glycoprotein D for h
    virus entry mediator, a receptor
        expressed by T lymphocyte

LIGHTS
  phototherapy lights
LIH
  laparoscopic inguinal herniorrhaphy
  left inguinal hernia
LIHA
  low impulsiveness, high anxiety
LII
  Leisure Interest Inventory
LiI
  lithium iodine
LIJ
  left internal jugular
LIKE
  Learning Inventory of Kindergarten
    Experiences
LILA
  low impulsiveness, low anxiety
LILI
  low-intensity laser irradiation
LIM
  boundary [L. *limes*] (*See also* L)
  limited toxicology screening
lim
  limit
  limitation
LIMA
  left internal mammary artery
  left internal mammary artery (graft)
LIMS
  laboratory information management
    system(s)
LIN
  laryngeal intraepithelial neoplasia
lin
  linear
  liniment (*See also* Linim)
LINAC
  linear accelerator (system)
LINCL
  late infantile neural ceroid
    lipofuscinosis
LINDI
  lithium-induced nephrogenic diabetes
    insipidus
LINES
  long interspersed elements
ling
  lingual (*See also* L)
  lingular
Linim
  liniment (*See also* lin)

LIO
  laser-indirect ophthalmoscope
  left inferior oblique (muscle)
LIOU
  laparoscopic intraoperative
    ultrasound
LIP
  lipoid interstitial pneumonitis
  lithium-induced polydipsia
  liver-enriched inhibiting protein
  lymphocytic interstitial pneumonia
  lymphocytic interstitial pneumonitis
  lymphoid interstitial pneumonia
  lymphoid interstitial pneumonitis
lip
  lipoate (lipoic acid)
LIPA
  line probe assay
  lysosomal acid lipase A
LiPA
  line probe assay
LIPB
  lysosomal acid lipase B
LIPHE
  Life Interpersonal History Enquiry
lipoMM
  lipomyelomeningocele
LIP   P
  lipid profile
LIPS
  Leiter International Performance
    Scale
LIPT
  Leiter International Performance
    Test
LIPV
  left inferior pulmonary vein
  Lipovnik virus
LIQ
  low inner quadrant
liq.
  liquid [L. *liquor*]
  liquor [L. *liquor*]
liq dr
  liquid dram
liq oz
  liquid ounce
liq pt
  liquid pint
liq qt
  liquid quart

L

NOTES

LIR
  left iliac region
  left inferior rectus
LIRBM
  liver, iron, red bone marrow
LIS
  laboratory information system
  lateral intercellular space
  left intercostal space (*See also* LICS)
  lithium salicylate
  lobular in situ (carcinoma)
  locked-in syndrome
  low intermittent suction
  low ionic strength
  lung injury score
LISL
  laser-induced intracorporeal shock wave lithotripsy
LISP
  List Processing Language
LISS
  low ionic strength solution (medium test)
LIT
  literature
  liver injury test
LITA
  left internal thoracic artery
LITH
  lithotomy
litho
  lithotripsy
LITT
  laser-induced thermography
  laser-induced thermotherapy
LITx
  liver and intestinal transplantation
LIV
  law of initial value
  left innominate vein
  liver (*See also* L)
  louping ill virus
liv
  live
  liver channel (acupuncture)
  living (*See also* L)
LIVB
  live birth
LIV-BP
  leucine, isoleucine, and valine-binding protein
LIVC
  left inferior vena cava
LIVEN
  linear inflammatory verrucous epidermal nevus

LIVIM
  lethal intestinal virus of infant mice
L-IVP
  limited intravenous pyelogram
LIVPRO
  liver profile
LIWS
  low intermittent wall suction
LJ
  left jugular
  Löwenstein-Jensen (medium) (*See also* LJM)
LJAV
  Landjia virus
LJL
  lateral joint line
LJM
  limited joint mobility
  Löwenstein-Jensen medium (*See also* LJ)
LJP
  localized juvenile periodontitis
LJV
  La Joya virus
LK
  lamellar keratoplasty (*See also* LKP)
  left kidney (*See also* LKID)
  lichenoid keratosis
LK⁺
  low potassium ion
LKA
  Lazare-Klerman-Armour (Personality Inventory)
LKESTR
  leukocyte esterase (*See also* LE)
LKID
  left kidney (*See also* LK)
LKKS
  liver, kidneys, and spleen (*See also* LKS)
LKM
  liver-kidney microsome
LKM-1
  liver-kidney-microsomal
LKP
  lamellar keratoplasty (*See also* LK)
LKPD
  Lillehei-Kaster pivoting disk
LKS
  Landau-Kleffner syndrome
  liver, kidneys, and spleen (*See also* LKKS)
  liver, kidneys, spleen
LKSB
  liver, kidneys, spleen, and bladder

LKS non. pal.
  liver, kidneys, and spleen not palpable
LKT
  liver and kidney transplantation
LKV
  laked kanamycin vancomycin (agar)
  Lengyeh-Kerman-Vargar (rating)
LL
  large local
  large lymphocyte
  laser lithotripsy
  late latent
  lateral lemniscus
  left lateral (*See also* LLAT, L lat, lt lat)
  left leg
  left lower
  left lung
  lepromatous leprosy
  lesion length
  Lewandowski-Lutz (syndrome)
  lid lag
  lines
  lingual lipase
  lipoprotein lipase (*See also* LPL)
  long leg
  loudness level
  lower (eye)lid
  lower lid
  lower limb
  lower lip
  lower lobe
  lumbar laminectomy
  lumbar length
  lung length
  lymphoblastic lymphoma (*See also* LBL)
  lymphocytic leukemia (*See also* LCL)
  lymphocytic lymphoma
  lymphoid leukemia
  lysolecithin (*See also* LLT)
LL2
  limb lead two
L&L
  lids and lashes
LLA
  lids, lashes, and adnexa
  limulus lysate assay
  lupus-like anticoagulant

L lam
  lumbar laminectomy
LLAT
  left lateral (*See also* LL, L lat, lt lat)
  lysolecithin acyltransferase
  lysolecithin-lecithin acyltransferase
L lat
  left lateral (*See also* LL, LLAT, lt lat)
LLB
  last living breath
  left lateral bending
  left lateral border
  left lower border
  long leg brace
  lower lobe bronchus
LLBCD
  left lower border of cardiac dullness
LLBP
  long leg brace with pelvic (band)
LLC
  labrum-ligament complex
  laparoscopic laser cholecystectomy
  laser laparoscopic cholecystectomy
  Lewis lung carcinoma
  liquid-liquid chromatography
  long leg cast
  lower level of care
  lymphocytic leukemia, chronic
LLCC
  long leg cylinder cast
LLD
  Lactobacillus lactis, Dorner (factor)
  left lateral decubitus (muscle)
  leg length discrepancy
  limb-length discrepancy
  liquid-liquid distribution
  long-lasting depolarization
LLDA
  labial-lingual double articulation
LLDF
  Lactobacillus lactis Dorner factor (vitamin B$_{12}$)
LLDH
  liver lactate dehydrogenase
LLDP
  left lateral decubitus position

NOTES

LLE
> left lower extremity (*See also* LLX)
> little league elbow

LLETZ
> large loop excision of transformation zone
> large loop excision of transition zone

LLETZ/LEEP
> large loop excision of transformation zone/loop electrosurgical excision procedure

LLF
> Laki-Lorand factor (factor XIII)
> left lateral femoral (site of injection)
> left lateral flexion

LLFG
> long leg fiberglass (cast)

LLG
> left lateral gaze

LL-GXT
> low-level graded exercise test

LLI
> leg length inequality

LLL
> left liver lobe
> left long leg (brace)
> left lower (eye)lid
> left lower leg
> left lower limb
> left lower lobe (of lung)
> left lower lung
> localized *Leishmania* lymphadenitis
> lower fossa active, lateral knee pain, and long leg on the side ipsilateral to the weak fossa

LLLE
> lower lid, left eye (*See also* LLOS)

LLLL
> lids, lashes, lacrimals, lymphatics

LLLM
> low liquid level monitor

LLLNR
> left lower lobe, no rales

LLLT
> low-level laser therapy

LLM
> localized leukocyte mobilization

LLNA
> local lymph-node assay

LLO
> *Legionella*-like organism
> lower limb orthosis

LLOD
> lower lid, oculus dexter (right eye) (*See also* LLRE)
> lower limit of detection

LLOS
> lower lid, oculus sinister (left eye) (*See also* LLLE)

LLP
> late luteal phase
> long-lasting potentiation
> long leg plaster (cast)
> lower limb prosthesis

LLPDD
> late luteal phase dysphoric disorder

LLPMS
> long leg posterior molded splint

LLPS
> low-load prolonged stress
> low-load prolonged stretch
> low-pressure plasma spray

LLQ
> Leatherman Leadership Questionnaire
> left lower quadrant

LLR
> large local reaction
> left lateral rectus (eye muscle)
> left lumbar region

LLRE
> lower lid, right eye (*See also* LLOD)

LLS
> lateral loop suspensor
> lazy leukocyte syndrome
> long leg splint

LLSB
> left lower scapular border
> left lower sternal border

LLSV
> Llano Seco virus

LLT
> left lateral thigh
> lowest level term
> lysolecithin (*See also* LL)

LLV
> lymphatic leukemia virus
> lymphoid leukosis virus

LLV-F
> lymphatic leukemia virus, Friend (virus associated)

LLVP
> left lateral ventricular pre-excitation

LLW
> low-level waste

LLWBC
> long leg weightbearing cast

LLWC
> long leg walking cast

LLX
 left lower extremity (*See also* LLE)
LM
 labiomental
 lactic (acid) mineral (medium)
 lactose malabsorption
 laryngeal melanosis
 laryngeal muscle
 lateral malleolus
 left main
 left median
 legal medicine
 lemniscus medialis
 leptomeningeal
 leptomeningeal metastasis
 light microscope
 light microscopy
 light minimum
 lincomycin
 lingual margin
 linguomesial
 lipid mobilization
 liquid membrane
 living male
 longitudinal muscle
 lower motor (neuron) (*See also* LMN)
 lung metastases
 lymphatic malformation
L/M
 liters per minute (*See also* L/min, Lpm)
lm
 lumen (*See also* L)
LMA
 lactose malabsorption
 laryngeal mask airway
 left mentoanterior (fetal position)
 left mentoanterior position
 limbic midbrain area
 liver (cell) membrane autoantibody
 liver membrane antibody
LMB
 Laurence-Moon-Biedl (syndrome) (*See also* LMBBS)
 left main stem bronchus
 leiomyoblastoma (*See also* LB)
LMBBS
 Laurence-Moon-Biedl-Bardet syndrome (*See also* LMB)
LMBD
 lingular mandibular bony defect

LMC
 large motile cell
 lateral motor column
 left main coronary (artery)
 left main coronary disease
 left middle cerebral (artery)
 living male child
 lymphocyte-mediated cytolysis
 lymphocyte-mediated cytotoxic
 lymphocyte-mediated cytotoxicity
 lymphocyte microcytotoxicity
 lymphomyeloid complex
LMCA
 left main coronary artery
 left middle cerebral artery
LMCAD
 left main coronary artery disease
LMCAT
 left middle cerebral artery thrombosis
LMCL
 left midclavicular line
 lower midclavicular line
LMCT
 ligand-to-metal charge transfer
LMD
 left main disease
 left main disease (cardiology)
 lipid-moiety modified derivative
 local medical doctor
 low molecular weight dextran
 low molecular (weight) dextran (*See also* LMDX, LMWD)
LMDF
 lupus miliaris disseminatus faciei
LMDX
 low molecular (weight) dextran (*See also* LMD, LMWD)
LME
 left mediolateral episiotomy (*See also* LMLE)
 leukocyte migration enhancement
LMEE
 left middle ear exploration
LMF
 left middle finger
 leukocyte mitogenic factor
 lymphocyte mitogenic factor
lm/ft²
 lumen per square foot

L

NOTES

LMG
  lethal midline granuloma
  low mobility group
LMH
  lipid-mobilizing hormone
lm·h
  lumen hour
LMI
  lateral medullary infarction
  leukocyte migration inhibition
    (assay)
LMIF
  leukocyte migration inhibition factor
L/min
  liters per minute (*See also* L/M,
    LPM)
L/min/m²
  liter per minute per square meter
LMIR
  leukocyte migration inhibition
    reaction
LMIS
  AOFAS Lesser Metatarsophalangeal-
    Interphalangeal Scale
LMIT
  leukocyte migration inhibition test
LMJA
  longitudinal midtarsal joint axis
LML
  large and medium lymphocytes
  left mediolateral (episiotomy)
  left middle lobe
  lower midline
LMLE
  left mediolateral episiotomy (*See
    also* LME)
LML scar w/h
  lower midline scar with hernia
LMM
  Lactobacillus maintenance medium
  lentigo maligna melanoma
  light molecular (weight)
    meromyosin
lm/m²
  lumen per square meter
LMN
  lower motor neuron (*See also* LM)
LMNL
  lower motor neuron lesion
LMO
  localized molecular orbital
LMP
  last menstrual period
  left mentoposterior (fetal position)
    (*See also* MLP)
  low malignant potential
  lumbar puncture (*See also* LP)

LMP-1
  latent membrane protein-1
  latent membrane protein-1
    (expression)
LMR
  left medial rectus (eye muscle)
  linguomandibular reflex
  localized magnetic resonance
  log magnitude ratio
LMRM
  left modified radical mastectomy
LMRP
  local medical review policy
LMS
  lateral medullary syndrome
  leiomyosarc
  leiomyosarcoma (*See also* LS)
lm·s
  lumen-second
LMS-CAD
  left main stem coronary artery
    disease
LMSV
  left maximal spatial voltage
LMT
  left main trunk
  left mentotransverse (fetal position)
  leukocyte migration technique
  light moving touch
  luteomammotrophic (hormone)
LMTA
  Language Modalities Test for
    Aphasia
LMV
  larva migrans visceralis
LMW
  low molecular weight
lm/W
  lumen per watt (*See also* lpw)
LMWD
  low molecular weight dextran (*See
    also* LMD, LMDX)
LMWH
  low molecular weight heparin
LN
  labionasal
  laminin
  latent nystagmus
  later (onset) nephrotic (syndrome)
  left nostril (naris)
  lipoid nephro
  lipoid nephrosis
  lobular neoplasia
  lupus nephritis
  lymph node
L/N
  letter/numerical (system)

LN₂
    liquid nitrogen
ln
    logarithm, natural
LNA
    alpha linolenic acid (*See also* ALA)
    latent nuclear antigen
    linolenic acid
LNa
    low sodium (*See also* LoNa, LS)
LNAA
    large neutral amino acid
LNAB
    large-needle aspiration biopsy (*See also* LNB)
LNaCl
    low salt
L-NAME
    N^G-nitro-L-arginine methyl ester
LNB
    large-needle aspiration biopsy (*See also* LNAB)
    Lyme neuroborreliosis
    lymph node biopsy
LNC
    large noncleaved
    lymph node cell
LND
    light-near dissociation
    lonidamine
    lymph node dissection
LNE
    lymph node enlargement
    lymph node excision
LNF
    laparoscopic Nissen fundoplication
LNG
    levonorgestrel
    liquified natural gas
LNH
    large number hypothesis
LNI
    logarithm neutralization index
LNKS
    low natural killer syndrome
LNL
    lower normal limit
    lymph node lymphocyte
LNLS
    linear-nonlinear least squares

LNM
    lymph node metastasis
LNMC
    lymph node mononuclear cells
LN-met
    lymph node metastasis
L-NMMA
    N^G-monomethyl-L-arginine
LNMP
    last normal menstrual period
LNNB
    Luria-Nebraska Neuropsychological Battery
LNP
    large neuronal polypeptide
LNPF
    lymph node permeability factor
LNR
    lymph node region
LNRS
    lymph node revealing solution
LNS
    lateral nuclear stratum
    localized nodular synovitis
    lymph node sampling
    lymph node seeking (equivalent)
LNT
    late neurological toxicity
LNV
    last normal vertebra
LO
    lateral oblique (x-ray view)
    leucine oxidation
    linguo-occlusal
    low (*See also* L)
    lower (*See also* L)
    lowest (*See also* L)
    lumbar orthosis
5-LO
    5-lipoxygenase
LOA
    late-onset agammaglobulinemia
    leave of absence
    Leber optic atrophy
    left occipitoanterior (fetal position)
    looseness of associations
    loosening of associations
    lysis of adhesions
LOAD
    late-onset Alzheimer disease

NOTES

441

LOAEL
> lowest observed adverse effect level

LOB
> loss of balance

LOBC
> large operable breast cancer

LOC
> laxative of choice (*See also* LXC)
> left main disease
> level of care
> level of comfort
> level of concern
> level of consciousness
> liquid organic compound
> local (*See also* loc)
> locus of control
> loss of consciousness

loc
> local (*See also* LOC)
> localized
> location

LOCA
> low-osmolality contrast agent
> low-osmolar contrast agent

LoCa, lo calc
> low calcium (diet) (*See also* lo calc)
> low-calcium (diet)

lo cal
> low-calorie (diet)

LOC-C
> Locus of Control-Chance

loc. cit.
> in the place cited [L. *loco citato*]

LOCD
> local cementoosseous dysphasia

LOC-E
> Locus of Control-External

LOCF
> last-observation-carried-forward

LoCHO
> low carbohydrate

LoChol
> low cholesterol

LOC-I
> Locus of Control-Internal

LOCM
> low osmolality contrast material
> low osmolality contrast media
> low-osmolar contrast medium

LOC-PO
> Locus of Control-Powerful Others

LOCS
> Lens Opacification Classification System

LOCS II
> Lens Opacities Classification System II

LOD
> limit of detection
> line of duty
> logarithm of odds (method of genetics linkage analysis) (*See also* lod)

lod
> logarithm of odds (*See also* LOD)

LOE
> left otitis externa

LOF
> leaking of fluid
> leave on floor
> low outlet forceps

LOFD
> low outlet forceps delivery

log.
> logarithm

logMAR
> logarithmic Minimum Angle of Resolution

LOH
> loop of Henle
> loss of heterogeneity
> loss of heterozygosity

LOHF
> late onset hepatic failure

LOI
> level of incompetence
> level of injury
> Leyton Obsessive Inventory
> limit of impurities
> loss of imprinting

LOIH
> left oblique inguinal hernia

LOINC
> Logical Observation Identifier Names and Codes

LoK
> low kalium (potassium)

LOKV
> Lokern virus

LOL
> laughing out loud
> left occipitolateral (fetal position)

Lol p
> Lolium perenne (perennial rye grass)

LOM
> left otitis media
> limitation of motion
> limitation of movement
> loss of motion
> loss of movement
> low-osmolar (contrast) medium

LOMPT
Lincoln-Oseretsky Motor
Performance Test
LOMSA
left otitis media, suppurative, acute
LOMSC, LOMSCH
left otitis media, suppurative,
chronic
LoNa
low sodium (*See also* LNa, LS)
long.
longitudinal
LOO
length of operation
LOP
laparoscopic orchiopexy
leave on pass
left occipitoposterior position
left occiput posterior (fetal
position)
level of pain
LoPro
low protein (*See also* LP)
LOPS
length of patient stay
loss of protective sensation
LOQ
Leadership Opinion Questionnaire
limit(s) of quantitation
lower outer quadrant
LOR
lorazepam (*See also* LRZ, LZP)
lorcainide
loss of resistance
loss of righting (reflex)
lord
lordosis
lordotic
LORS-1
Level of Rehabilitation Scale 1
LOS
length of stay
lipooligosaccharide
loss of sight
low (cardiac) output syndrome
lower (o)esophageal sphincter
(pressure)
LOT
lateral olfactory tract
left occipitotransverse (fetal
position)

left occipitotransverse position
Lengthened-Off-Time
lot.
lotion
LOU
lower obstructive uropathy
LOV
large opaque vesicle
loss of vision
LOVA
loss of visual acuity
LOVE
laser office ventilation of ears
LOVE IT
laser office ventilation of ears with
insertion of tubes
LOWBI
low-birth-weight infant
lox.
liquid oxygen
LOZ
lozenge
LP
labile peptide
labile protein
laboratory procedure
lactic peroxidase
lamina propria
laryngopharyngeal
latency period
latent period
lateral plantar
lateral pylorus
latex particle
leading pole
leukocyte poor
leukocytic pyrogen
levator palati
lichen planus
ligamentum patellae
lightly padded
light perception (*See also* LPerc)
linear programming
linguopulpal
lipid panel
lipoprotein
lost privileges
low potency
low power (microscopy)
low pressure
low protein (*See also* LoPro)
lumbar puncture (*See also* LMP)

L

NOTES

LP *(continued)*
    lumboperitoneal
    lung parenchyma
    lung perfusion
    lymphocyte predominant
    lymphoid plasma
    lymphoid predominance
    lymphomatoid papulosis
    lymphomatous polyposis
    (nucleus) lateralis posterior

L/P
    lactate/pyruvate (ratio)
    liver/plasma (concentration ratio)
    lymphocyte/polymorph (ratio)
    lymph/plasma (ratio)

LPA
    larval photoreceptor axon
    latex particle agglutination
    left pulmonary artery
    lymphocyte proliferation assay
    lymphocytic proliferation assay
    lysophosphatidic acid

LPA%
    left pulmonary artery oxygen
    saturation

Lp(a)
    lipoprotein(a)

LPAM, L-PAM, *l*-PAM
    L-phenylalanine mustard

LPB
    lipoprotein B
    low-profile bioprosthesis (*See also* LPBP)

LPBP
    low-profile bioprosthesis (*See also* LPB)

LPC
    laser photocoagulation
    late positive component
    leukocyte-poor cell
    licensed professional counselor
    limiting precursor cell
    lysophosphatidyl choline

LPCB
    lactophenol cotton blue

LPCh
    lateral posterior choroidal

LPC-L
    lymphoplasmacytoid lymphoma

LPCM
    low-placed conus medullaris

LPc̄P
    light perception with projection

LPCR
    late-phase cutaneous reaction

LPCT
    late proximal cortical tubule

LPCV
    laser photocoagulation of the communicating vessel

LPD
    leiomyomatosis peritonealis disseminata
    low potassium dextran
    low-protein diet
    luteal phase defect
    luteal phase deficiency
    lymphoproliferative disease

LPDA
    left posterior descending artery

LPDF
    lipoprotein-deficient fraction

LPE
    lipoprotein electrophoresis (*See also* LEP)
    lower partially edentulous

LPEP
    left pre-ejection period

LPerc
    light perception (*See also* LP)

LPF
    leg protection factor
    leukocytosis-promoting factor
    leukopenia factor
    lipopolysaccharide factor
    liver plasma flow
    localized plaque formation
    low-power field (*See also* lpf)
    lymphocytosis-promoting factor

lpf
    low-powered field
    low-power field (*See also* LPF)

LPFB
    left posterior fascicular block

LPFN
    low–pass-filtered noise

LPFS
    low–pass-filtered signal

LPG
    lipophosphoglycan
    liquified petroleum gas

LPH
    lactase-phlorizin hydrolase
    left posterior hemiblock (*See also* LPHB)
    lipotropic hormone
    lipotropic pituitary hormone (lipotropin)
    lipotropin

LPHB
    left posterior hemiblock (*See also* LPH)

LPHC
    low probability, high consequence event

LPHD
> lymphocyte predominance Hodgkin disease
> lymphocyte-predominant Hodgkin disease

LPHR
> laparoscopic paraesophageal hernia repair

LPHS
> loin pain hematuria syndrome

LPI
> laser iridotomy
> laser peripheral iridectomy
> Laser Photonics, Inc.
> Leadership Practices Inventory
> left posterior-inferior
> leukotriene pathway inhibitor
> long process of incus
> lysinuric protein intolerance

LPICA
> left posterior internal carotid artery

LPIFB
> left posterior-inferior fascicular block

LPIH
> left posterior inferior hemiblock

LPI/LRI
> lymphocyte proliferation/regression index

LPK
> liver pyruvate kinase

LPL
> lamina propria lymphocyte
> laparoscopic pelvic lymphadenectomy
> left posterolateral
> lichen planus-like lesion
> lipoprotein lipase (See also LL)
> long plantar ligament
> lymphoplasmacytoid lymphoma

LPLA
> lipoprotein lipase activity

LPLC
> low-pressure liquid chromatography

LPLND
> laparoscopic pelvic lymph node dissection

LPM
> latent primary malignancy
> lateral pterygoid muscle
> left posterior measurement
> liver plasma membrane

> localized pretibial myxedema
> lymphoproliferative malignancy

Lpm
> liters per minute (See also L/M, L/min)

lpm
> lines (printed) per minute

Lpm/m²
> liters per minute per meter squared

LPO
> lateral preoptic (area)
> left posterior oblique
> left posterior occipital
> light perception only
> lobus parolfactorius

LPOA
> lateral preoptic area

L POST
> left posterior

LPP
> lateral pterygoid plate
> leak point pressure
> lichen planopilaris

LP&P
> light perception and projection

LPPC
> leukocyte-poor packed cells

LPPH
> late postpartum hemorrhage

LPPS
> low-pressure plasma-sprayed

LPR
> lactate pyruvate ratio
> late-phase reaction
> late-phase response
> leprosy (Hansens disease) vaccine

LPRBC
> leukocyte-poor red blood cell

LProj
> light projection

LPS
> last Pap smear
> late progressing stroke
> lateral pharyngeal space
> levator palpebrae superioris (muscle)
> linear profile scan
> lipase
> lipopolysaccharide
> London Psychogeriatric Scale

lps
> liter per second

NOTES

LPSA
late postoperative suture adjustment
LP SHUNT
lumboperitoneal shunt
LPSP
light perception without projection
LPSR
lipopolysaccharide receptor
LPSS
laryngopharyngeal sensory stimulation
LPT
Language Proficiency Test
lateral position test
leptospirosis (Leptospira) vaccine
lipotropin
lymphocyte-predominant thymoma
LPV
left portal view
left pulmonary vein
lymphopathia venereum
lymphotropic papovavirus
LPVP
left posterior ventricular pre-excitation
LPW
lateral pharyngeal wall
lpw
lumen per watt (*See also* lm/W)
LPX, Lp-X
lipoprotein-X
LQ
linear-quadratic
longevity quotient
lordosis quotient
lower quadrant
lowest quadrant
LQTS
long QT syndrome
LR
labeled release (experiment)
laboratory reference
laboratory report
labor room
lactated Ringer (solution) (*See also* lat Rin)
large reticulocyte
laser resection
latency reaction
latency relaxation
lateral rectus
lateral rectus (eye muscle)
lateral rotation
left rotation
leishmaniasis recidivans
ligand receptor
light reaction
light reflex
likelihood ratios
limit of reaction
lingual ridge
lingual root
livedo reticularis
local recurrence
lymphatic reconstruction
lymphocyte recruitment
L-R, L R, L→R, L/R
left to right
L&R
left and right
L/R
left-to-right ratio
Lr
lawrencium
limes reacting (dose of diphtheria toxin)
LRA
left radial artery
left renal artery
low right atrium
LRC
locomotor-respiratory coupling
lower rib cage
LRCH
lymphocyte-rich classic Hodgkin
LRCM
longitudinal random coefficient model
LRD
limb reduction defects
limb reduction deformity
living related donor
living renal donor
LRDT
living related donor transplant
LRE
lamina rara externa
least restrictive environment
leukemic reticuloendotheliosis
localization-related epilepsy
lymphoreticuloendothelial
LREH
low renin essential hypertension
LRF
latex and resorcinol formaldehyde
left rectus femoris
left ring finger
leukoreduction filter
liver residue factor
local-regional failure
luteinizing hormone-releasing factor (*See also* LH-RF)
LRFS
local recurrence-free survival

LRH
luteinizing hormone-releasing hormone (*See also* LHRH, LH-RH)

LRHT
living related hepatic transplantation

LRI
lamina rara interna
lower respiratory (tract) illness (*See also* LRTI)
lower respiratory (tract) infection (*See also* LRTI)
lymphocyte reactivity index

LRL
long radiolunate

LRLT
living related donor transplantation

LRM
left radical mastectomy
local regional metastases

LRMP
last regular menstrual period

LRN
laparoscopic radical nephrectomy
lateral reticular nucleus

LRNA
low renin, normal aldosterone

LRND
left radical neck dissection

LRO
long range objective

LROP
lower radicular obstetrical paralysis

Lrot
left rotation

LROU
lateral rectus, both eyes

LRP
laparoscopic radical prostatectomy
LDL receptor-related protein
lichen ruber planus
lipoprotein receptor-related protein
locking reconstruction plate
long-range planning
low-density lipoprotein receptor-related protein
lung-resistance protein
lung resistance-related protein

LRPH
laparoscopic repair of paraesophageal hernia

LRQ
lower right quadrant

LRQG
left rostral quarter ganglion

LRR
labyrinthine righting reflex
leucine rich repeat
light reflection rheography
lymphatic return rate

LRRFS
locoregional recurrence-free survival

LRRT
locoregional radiotherapy

LRS
lactated Ringer solution
lateral recess stenosis
lateral recess syndrome
lumboradicular syndrome
lymphoreticular system

LRSF
lactating rat serum factor
liver regenerating serum factor

LR-SH
left-right shunt

LRSP
long-range systems planning

LRSS
late respiratory systemic syndrome

LRT
living related liver transplantation
living related transplant
living renal transplant
local radiation therapy
lower respiratory tract
low-risk tumor

LRTD
living relative transplant donor

LRTI
ligament reconstruction with tendon interposition
living related transplant donor
lower respiratory tract illness (*See also* LRI)
lower respiratory tract infection (*See also* LRI)

LRUT
locally made rapid urease test

LRV
left renal vein
log reduction value

LRZ
lorazepam (*See also* LOR, LZP)

L

NOTES

LS

Laron syndrome
lateral septal
lateral suspensor (ligament)
least squares
left sacrum
left septum
left side
legally separated
leiomyosarcoma (*See also* LMS)
length of stay
lesser sac
lichen sclerosus et atrophicus (*See also* LSA, LS&A)
life science
light sensitive
light sensitivity
light sleep
Likert scale
liminal sensation
liminal sensitivity
linear scleroderma
lipid synthesis
liver scan
liver and spleen (*See also* L&S)
long seal
long stem
lower segment
Lowe syndrome
low-sodium (diet) (*See also* LNa, LoNa)
lumbar spine
lumbosacral (*See also* L/S)
lung sounds
lung strip
lymphosarcoma (*See also* LSA, Lyp)

L5-S1

lumbar fifth vertebra to sacral first vertebra

L-S

lipid-saccharide

L/S

lactase/sucrase (ratio)
lecithin-sphingomyelin
lecithin to sphingomyelin
lecithin/sphingomyelin
lecithin/sphingomyelin (ratio) (*See also* l/s)
liver/spleen (ratio)
lumbosacral (*See also* LS)

L&S

ligation and stripping
liver and spleen (*See also* LS)

l/s

lecithin/sphingomyelin
lecithin/sphingomyelin (ratio) (*See also* L/S)

LSA

Language Sampling Analysis
left sacroanterior (fetal position)
left sacroanterior position
left subclavian artery
leukocyte-specific activity
lichen sclerosus (et) atrophicus (*See also* LS&A, LS)
lipid-bound sialic acid (*See also* LBSA)
lymphosarcoma (*See also* LS, Lyp)

LS&A

lichen sclerosus et atrophicus (*See also* LSA, LS)

LSAB

labeled streptavidin biotin

LSANA

leukocyte-specific antinuclear antibody

LSAR

lymphosarcoma cell

LSA/RCS

lymphosarcoma-reticulum cell sarcoma

LSAT

low oxyhemoglobin saturation

LSB

least significant bit (binary numbers)
left scapular border
left sternal border
local standby
long spike burst
lower sternal border
lumbar spinal block
lumbar sympathetic block

LSBE

long-segment Barrett esophagus

LSBM

lumbar spine bone mineral density

LS BPS

laparoscopic bilateral partial salpingectomy

LSC

last sexual contact
late systolic click
least significant change
left-sided colon (cancer)
left subclavian (artery)
lichen simplex chronicus
liquid scintillation counting
liquid-solid chromatography
lower segment cesarean (section) (*See also* LSCS)

LSCA, LScA

left scapuloanterior (fetal position)
left subclavian artery

LSCC
　　laryngeal squamous cell carcinoma
LSCCB
　　limited-state small-cell cancer of
　　　the bladder
LSCL
　　lymphosarcoma cell leukemia
LSCM
　　laser-scanning confocal microscopy
LSCP, LScP
　　left scapuloposterior (fetal position)
LSCS
　　lower segment cesarean
　　lower segment cesarean section
　　　(*See also* LSC)
LSCTS
　　long-segment congenital tracheal
　　　stenosis
LSCV
　　left subclavian vein
LSCVP
　　left subclavian central venous
　　　pressure
LSD
　　least significant difference
　　least significant digit (computers)
　　low-salt diet
　　low-sodium diet
　　lysergic acid diethylamide (*See also*
　　　LSD-25)
LSD-25
　　lysergic acid diethylamide (*See also*
　　　LSD)
LSE
　　left sternal edge
　　lifestyle education
　　living skin equivalent
　　local side effect
L/sec
　　liters per second
LSed
　　level of sedation
LSEP
　　left somatosensory evoked potential
LSES
　　Salamon-Conte Life Satisfaction in
　　　the Elderly Scale
LSESR
　　lipidosterolic extract of *Serosa
　　　repens*
LSF
　　line spread function

line-spread function
Lisofylline
low saturated fat
lymphocyte-stimulating factor
LSFA
　　low-saturated fatty acid (diet)
LSG
　　labial salivary gland
　　lymphoscintigraphy
LSGB
　　left stellate ganglionic blockade
LSH
　　laparoscopic supracervical
　　　hysterectomy
　　leishmaniasis vaccine
　　low-grade squamous intraepithelial
　　　lesion
　　lutein-stimulating hormone
　　lymphocyte-stimulating hormone
LSI
　　large-scale integration
　　levonorgestrel subdermal implant
　　Life Satisfaction Index
　　light scattering index
　　Limb Salvage Index
　　lumbar spine index
LSIA
　　Life Satisfaction Index A
LSIB
　　Life Satisfaction Index B
LSIL, L-SIL
　　low-grade squamous intraepithelial
　　　lesion
LSK
　　liver, spleen, and kidneys
LSKM
　　liver-spleen-kidney megaly
LSL
　　left sacrolateral (fetal position)
　　left short leg (brace)
　　lymphosarcoma (cell) leukemia
LSLF
　　low sodium, low fat (diet)
LSM
　　laser scanning microscope
　　late systolic murmur
　　least squares mean
　　lifestyle modification
　　limited sampling model
　　liver, spleen masses
　　lymphocyte separation medium

NOTES

LSMB
    lumbar spine bone mineral density

LSMFT
    liposclerosing myxofibrous tumor

LSMT
    life-sustaining medical treatment

LSN
    left substantia nigra
    left sympathetic nerve

LSNRC
    lower sacral nerve root
      compression

LSO
    lateral superior olive (of brain)
    left salpingo-oophorectomy
    left superior oblique
    lumbosacral orthosis

LSP
    Learning Style Profile
    left sacroposterior (fetal position)
    left sacroposterior position
    liver-specific membrane lipoprotein
    liver-specific protein

LSp
    life span

L-spine
    lumbar spine

LSQ
    least square
    Life Situation Questionnaire

LSR
    lanthanide shift reagent (in
      magnetic resonance imaging)
    laser skin resurfacing
    left superior rectus
    Life Satisfaction Rating

LSRA
    low septal right atrium

LSRT
    lens-sparing external beam radiation
      therapy

LSS
    lexical-syntactic syndrome
    Life Span Study
    Life Study Sample
    life support station
    limb sparing surgery
    liver-spleen scan
    lumbar spinal stenosis
    lumbosacral spine
    scapholunate ligament

LSSA
    lipid-soluble secondary antioxidant

LSSS
    Liverpool Seizure Severity Scale

LST
    laser tomography scanner
    lateral sinus thrombophlebitis
    lateral spinothalamic tract
    left sacrotransverse (fetal position)
    lysis, storage, and transportation

LSTC
    laparoscopic tubal cautery
    laparoscopic tubal coagulation

LSTL
    laparoscopic tubal ligation (*See also*
      LTL)

Ls & Ts
    lines and tubes

LSU
    lactose-saccharose-urea (agar)
    life support unit

LSV
    lateral sacral vein
    left subclavian vein
    Lone Star virus

LSV2
    Vocational Learning Styles

LSVC
    left superior vena cava

LSW
    left-sided weakness

LSWA
    large amplitude, slow wave activity
      (in electroencephalography)

LT
    (heat-)labile toxin
    lactate threshold
    laminar tomography
    left (*See also* L, (L), l, lf, lt)
    left thigh
    left triceps
    length-tension curve
    less than
    lethal time
    leukotriene
    Levin tube
    levothyroxine
    light (*See also* L, lt)
    light touch
    long term
    low temperature
    low transverse
    L-tryptophan
    lues test
    lumbar traction
    lung transplant
    lung transplantation
    lunotriquetral
    lymphocyte transformation
    lymphocyte transitional
    lymphocytic thyroiditis
    lymphocytotoxin (*See also* LC,
      LCT)
    lymphotoxin

LT4, LT$_4$
    levothyroxine
    l-thyroxine

L-T$_3$
    liothyronine

lt
    left (*See also* L, (L), l, lf, LT)
    light (*See also* L, LT)
    low tension

LTA
    laryngeal tracheal anesthesia
    laryngotracheal applicator
    lateral thoracic arteries
    leukotriene A
    lipoate transacetylase
    lipoteichoic acid
    local tracheal anesthesia
    lymphocyte-transforming activity

LTA$_4$
    leukotriene A$_4$

LTAC
    long-term acute care

LTAF
    local tissue advancement flap

LTAR
    low-temperature antigen retrieval

LTAS
    lead tetraacetate Schiff
    left transatrial septal

LTB
    laparoscopic tubal banding
    laryngotracheobronchitis
    leukotriene B
    life-threatening behavior

LTB4, LTB$_4$
    leukotriene B4

LTC
    large transformed cell
    lateral talocalcaneal ligament
    left to count
    leukotriene C
    lidocaine tissue concentration
    long-term care
    long thick closed
    low transverse cesarean
    lysed tumor cell

LTC4, LTC$_4$
    leukotriene C4

LTC-101
    long-term care form-101

LTCBDE
    laparoscopic transcystic common bile duct exploration

LTC-1C
    long-term culture-initiating cells

LTCCS
    low transverse cervical cesarean section

LTCF
    long-term care facility

LTCL
    laparoscopic transcystic lithotripsy

LTCP
    levo-tryptophan-containing product
    L-tryptophan-containing product

LTCS
    low transverse cervical (cesarean) section

LTD
    largest tumor dimension
    Laron-type dwarfism
    leg transfer device
    leukotriene D
    limited (*See also* ltd)
    long-term disability

LTD4, LTD$_4$
    leukotriene D4

ltd
    limited (*See also* LTD)

LTDA
    limited quantity (test performed on small specimen)

LTE
    laryngotracheoesophageal
    less than effective
    leukotriene E

LTE4, LTE$_4$
    leukotriene E4

LT-ECG
    long-term electrocardiography

LTED
    long-term estrogen deprivation

LTF
    lipotropic factor
    lost to followup
    lymphocyte-transforming factor

LTFU
    long-term follow-up

LTG
    lamotrigine
    long-term goal
    low-tension glaucoma

L

NOTES

LTGA
> left transposition of great artery

LTH
> lactogenic hormone (*See also* LGH)
> local tumor hyperthermia
> low-temperature holding
> (pasteurization)
> luteotropic hormone (*See also* LH)

LtH
> left-handed

LTHMAR
> low-temperature, heat-mediated
> antigen retrieval

LTI
> low temperature isotropic
> lupus-type inclusion

LTK
> laser thermal keratoplasty

LTL
> laparoscopic tubal ligation (*See also*
> LSTL)

lt lat
> left lateral (*See also* LL, LLAT, L
> lat)

LTM
> long-term memory
> long-term monitoring

LTNP
> long-term nonprogressor

LTO
> laparoscopic total occlusion

LTOM
> low turnover osteomalacia

LTOT
> long-term oxygen therapy

LTP
> laryngotracheoplasty
> laser trabeculoplasty
> leukocyte thromboplastin
> long-term plan
> long-term potentiation
> L-tryptophan

LTPP
> lipothiamide pyrophosphate

LTR
> laryngotracheal reconstruction
> local twitch response
> long terminal repeat (sequence)
> lower trunk rotation
> lymphocyte transfer reaction

LTRA
> leukotriene receptor antagonist

L-transposition
> levotransposition

LTS
> laparoscopic tubal sterilization
> laryngotracheal stenosis
> long-term storage

> long-term surviving
> long tract sign (neurology)

LTT
> lactose tolerance test
> lateral tibial torsion
> leucine tolerance test
> limited treadmill test
> lymphoblastic transformation test
> lymphocyte transformation test

LTUI
> low transverse uterine incision

LTV
> long-term variability
> Lucké tumor virus
> lung thermal volume

LTV0
> long-term variability-absent

LTV+
> long-term variability-average to
> moderate

LTVC
> long-term venous catheter

LTW
> Leydig-cell tumor in Wistar (rat)

LTWN
> long-term low-level white noise

LTX
> lophotoxin

LTx
> lung transplant

LTZ
> letrozole

LU
> left uninjured
> left uninvolved
> left upper (limb)
> left ureteral
> living unit
> loudness unit
> lung (*See also* L, Lu)
> Lutheran
> lytic unit

L&U
> lower and upper (extremities)

Lu
> lung (*See also* L, LU)
> lutetium

^{177}Lu
> lutetium-177

lu
> lung channel (acupuncture)

LUA
> left upper arm
> Legionella urinary antigen

LUC
> large unstained cell

LUCL
> lateral ulnar collateral ligament

LUD
    left uterine displacement device
LUE
    left upper extremity (*See also* LUX)
Lues I
    primary syphilis
Lues II
    secondary syphilis
Lues III
    tertiary syphilis
LUF
    luteinized unruptured follicle
LUFS
    luteinized unruptured follicle syndrome
LUIS
    low-dose urea in invert sugar
LUKV
    Lukuni virus
LUL
    left upper (eye)lid
    left upper limb
    left upper lobe (lung)
    left upper lung
lum, lumb
    lumbar
LUMO
    lowest unoccupied molecular orbital
LUNA
    laser uterosacral nerve ablation
LUO
    left ureteral orifice
LUOB
    left upper outer buttock
LUOQ
    left upper outer quadrant
LUP
    left ureteropelvic (junction)
    low urethral pressure
LUPP
    laser uvulopalatoplasty
LUQ
    left upper quadrant
LURD
    living unrelated donor
LUS
    laparoscopic ultrasonography
    laparoscopic ultrasound
    lower uterine segment

LUSB
    left upper scapular border
    left upper sternal border
LUSLR
    laparoscopic resection of the ureterosacral ligament
LUST
    lower uterine segment transverse (cesarean section)
LUT
    lower urinary tract
LUTD
    lower urinary tract dysfunction
LUTS
    lower urinary tract symptom
LUTT
    lower urinary tract tumor
LUV
    large unilamellar vesicle
LUW
    lungworm vaccine
LUX
    left upper extremity (*See also* LUE)
LV
    Lactobacillus viridescens
    lactoovovegetarian
    laryngeal vestibule
    lateral ventricle
    left ventricle
    left ventricular (echocardiography images)
    leukemia virus
    liquid ventilation
    live vaccine
    live virus
    low vertical
    low volume
    lumbar vertebra
    lung volume
lv
    leave
LVA
    left ventricular aneurysm
    left ventricular aneurysmectomy
    left vertebral artery
    low vision aid
LVAD
    left ventricular assist device
LV Angio
    left ventricular angiogram

L

NOTES

LVAS
> left ventricular assist system

LVAT
> left ventricular activation time

LVBBB
> left ventricular bundle branch block

LVBP
> left ventricle bypass pump

LVC
> laser vision correction
> low-viscosity cement
> low vision clinic

LVCS
> low vertical cesarean section

LVD, LVDI, LVEDD
> left ventricular dimension (*See also* LVDI)
> left ventricular dysfunction
> left ventricular end-diastolic diameter
> left ventricular end-diastolic dimension

LV_D, LVd
> left ventricular (end-)diastolic (pressure)

LVDd, LVdd
> left ventricular diastolic dimension
> left ventricular dimension (in end)-diastole

LVDP
> left ventricular diastolic pressure

LVDs
> left ventricular systolic diameter

LVDT
> linear variable differential transformer

LVDV
> left ventricular diastolic volume

LVE
> left ventricular ejection
> left ventricular enlargement

LVECoG
> low-voltage electrocortical activity

LVED
> left ventricular end diastole

LVEDa
> left ventricular end-diastolic area

LVEDC
> left ventricular end-diastolic circumference

LVEDI
> left ventricular end-diastolic volume index

LVEDV
> left ventricular end-diastolic volume

LVEF
> left ventricular ejection fraction

LVEndo
> left ventricular endocardial (half)

LVEP, LVEDP
> left ventricular end-diastolic pressure

LVER
> liver fraction elevated

LVESa
> left ventricular end-systolic area

LVESD
> left ventricular end-systolic dimension

LVESV
> left ventricular end-systolic volume

LVESVI
> left ventricular end-systolic volume index

LVET
> left ventricular ejection time

LVETI
> left ventricular ejection time index

LVF
> left ventricular failure
> left ventricular function
> left visual field
> low-voltage fast
> low-voltage foci

LVFA
> low-voltage fast activity

LVFP
> left ventricular filling pressure

LVFS
> left ventricular functional shortening

$LVFT_2$
> left ventricular slow filling time

LVFW
> left ventricular free wall

LVG
> left ventriculogram
> left ventrogluteal
> lymphogranuloma venereum (*See also* LGV)

LVH
> large vessel hematocrit
> left ventricular hypertrophy

LV-HRSEM
> low-voltage-high-resolution scanning electron microscopy

LVI
> large-vessel infarction
> left ventricular insufficiency
> left ventricular ischemia
> lymphatic vessel invasion
> lymph vessel invasion

LVID
> left ventricular internal diameter
> left ventricular internal diastolic
> left ventricular internal dimension

LVIDD, LVIDd
  left ventricular internal diastolic diameter
  left ventricular internal diastolic dimension
  left ventricular internal dimension diastole

LVID(ed)
  left ventricular internal diameter (end diastole)

LVID(es)
  left ventricular internal diameter (end systole)

LVIDP
  left ventricular initial diastolic pressure

LVIDs
  left ventricular internal dimension at end systole
  left ventricular internal dimension systole

LVIV
  left ventricular infarct volume
  left ventricular inflow volume

LVL
  large volume leukapheresis
  left vastus lateralis (muscle)

LVLG
  left ventrolateral gluteal (injection site)

LVM
  lateral ventromedial (nucleus)
  left ventricular mass
  lymphaticovenous malformation
  lymphatic-venous malformation

LVMF
  left ventricular minute flow

LVMI
  left ventricular mass index

LVMM
  left ventricular muscle mass

LVN
  lateral ventricular nerve
  lateral vestibular nucleus
  limiting viscosity number

LVO, LVOA
  left ventricular outflow
  left ventricular overactivity

LVOT
  left ventricular outflow tract

LVOTO
  left ventricular outflow tract obstruction

LVOV
  left ventricular outflow volume

LVP
  large-volume paracentesis
  large-volume parenteral (infusion)
  left ventricular pressure
  levator veli palatini (muscle)
  lysine-vasopressin

LVPC
  localized vulvar pemphigoid of childhood

LVPEP
  left ventricular preejection period

LVPFR
  left ventricular peak filling rate

LVPSP
  left ventricular peak systolic pressure

LVPW
  left ventricular posterior wall

LVPWT
  left ventricular posterior wall thickness

LVR
  left ventricular reduction
  limb vascular resistance
  lung volume reduction

L$_2$VR
  second lumbar ventral (nerve) root

L$_1$VR
  first lumbar ventral (nerve) root

LVRS
  lung volume reduction surgery

LVRT
  liver volume replaced by tumor

LVS
  lateral venous sinus
  left ventricular strain
  live vaccine strain

LVs
  (mean) left ventricular systolic (pressure)

LVSB
  leftward ventricular septal bowing

LVSD
  left ventricular systolic dimension
  left ventricular systolic dysfunction

L

NOTES

455

LVSEMI
>left ventricular subendocardial myocardial ischemia

LVSI
>left ventricular systolic index
>lymphovascular space invasion
>lymphvascular involvement

LVSO
>left ventricular systolic output

LVSP
>left ventricular systolic pressure

LVST
>lateral vestibulospinal tract

LVSV
>left ventricular stroke volume

LVSVI
>left ventricular stroke volume index

LVSW
>left ventricular septal wall
>left ventricular stroke work

LVSWI
>left ventricular stroke work index

LVT
>left ventricular tension
>levetiracetam
>lysine vasotonin

LVT$_1$
>left ventricular fast filling time

LVV
>left ventricular volume
>LeVeen valve
>live varicella vaccine

LVW
>lateral vaginal wall
>lateral ventricular width
>left ventricular wall
>left ventricular work

LVW/HW
>lateral ventricular width to hemispheric width

LVWI
>left ventricular work index

LVWM
>left ventricular wall motion

LVWMA
>left ventricular wall motion abnormality

LVWMI
>left ventricular wall motion index

LVWT
>left ventricular wall thickness

LW
>laboratory worker
>lacerating wound
>lateral wall
>Lee-White (blood clotting method) (*See also* L&W, L/W, LWCT)
>left (ear), warm (stimulus)
>Léri-Weill (syndrome)
>living will
>lung weight
>lung width

L-10-W
>levulose (10%) in water

L/W, L&W
>Lee and White (clotting time) (*See also* LW, LWCT)
>living and well

LWAQ
>Living with Asthma Questionnaire

LWBS
>left without being seen

LWC
>leave without consent

LWCT
>Lachar-Wrobel Critical Items
>Lee-White clotting time (*See also* LW, L&W, L/W)
>left without completing treatment

LWD
>living with disease

LWK
>large white kidney

LWOP
>leave without pay

LWOT
>left without treatment

LWP
>large whirlpool
>lateral wall pressure

LWS
>Lowry-Wood syndrome

LX, Lx
>latex (*See also* L)
>local irradiation
>lower extremity (*See also* LE, L ext, l/ext, lx)
>lux (*See also* lx)

lx
>larynx (*See also* lar)
>lower extremity (*See also* LE, L ext, l/ext, LX, Lx)
>lux (*See also* LX, Lx)

LXC
>laxative of choice (*See also* LOC)

LXT
>left exotropia

LY
>lyophilization

LYCD
>live yeast cell derivative

LYDMA
>lymphocyte-detected membrane antigen

LYEL
>lost years of expected life

LYG
lymphomatoid granulomatosis
LYM
Lyme disease vaccine
lymph
LYMPH%
percentage of lymphocytes (in differential count)
lymph
lymphocyte
lymphocytic
LyNeF
lytic nephritic factor
lyo
lyophilized
LYP
lactose, yeast, and peptone (agar)
lower yield point
LyP
lymphomatoid papulosis
Lyp
lymphosarcoma (*See also* LS, LSA)
LYS, Lys
large yellow soft (stools)

lysine (*See also* K)
lysosome
Lys
lys
LySLk
lymphoma syndrome leukemia
LYST
lysosomal trafficking regulator protein
lysosome trafficking regulator
lytes
electrolyte panel
electrolytes
LZ
landing zone
LZM, lzm
lysozyme
LZP
lorazepam (*See also* LOR, LRZ)
LZRS
Lazarus
LZT
lead/zirconium/titanium

NOTES

L

μ, micro

micro-
micron

M

blood factor in the MNS blood group system
cardiac murmur (*See also* m, (m))
chin [L. *mentum*]
concentration in moles per liter
death [L. *mors*]
dullness (of sound) [L. *mutitas*]
dumbness [L. *mutitas*]
handful [L. *manipulus*] (*See also* man., manip.)
macerated [L. *macerare*] (*See also* m)
macerate [L. *macerare*] (*See also* m.)
macroglobulin
magnetization
male
malignant (*See also* MAL, mal, malig)
manual
marital
married
masculine
masked (audiology)
mass
massage (*See also* mass, MSS, mss)
maternal contribution
matrix
matte (dull, slightly granular, bacterial colonies)
mature (*See also* MAT, mat.)
maximum
mean (*See also* m, μ)
meatus
media
medial
median (*See also* m, md)
mediator (chemical released in the tissues)
medical
medicine
medium
mega-
melts at (*See also* m)
membrane
memory (associative)
mental
mesial (*See also* m, MES)
meta-
metabolite

metal
metastasis (*See also* MET, met)
meter
methionine (*See also* Met)
method
mexiletine
microfold
mild
million
minim (*See also* m)
minimum (*See also* MIN, min)
minute (*See also* m, MIN, min)
mitochondria
mitosis
mitoxantrone
mitral
mix
mixed
mixture
molarity
molar (permanent tooth)
molar (solution)
mole
molecular
molecular weight
moment of force
Monday
monkey
monoclonal
monocyte
month (*See also* MO, mo, mon)
morgan (unit of gene separation)
morphine
mother (*See also* MO, MOM, MTR)
motile
mouse
mouth
movement (response to human figure)
mucoid (colony)
mucous (adjective)
mucus (noun)
multipara
murmur (*See also* m, (m))
muscle
muscular (response to electrical stimulation of motor nerve)
mu (12th letter of Greek alphabet), uppercase
Mycobacterium
Mycoplasma
myeloma or macroglobulinemia (component)
myopia

M

459

M *(continued)*
  myopic
  myosin
  noon [L. *meridies*] *(See also* N)
  soften [L. *macerare*] *(See also* mac.)
  strength of pole
  thousand [L. *mille*]

M1, M₁
  left mastoid
  mitral first sound (slight dullness)
  myeloblast
  tropicamide 1% ophthalmic solution (Mydriacyl)

M2
  right mastoid

M-2
  medical student 2nd year

M²
  square meter (body surface) *(See also* m²)

M₂
  mitral second sound (marked dullness)
  promyelocyte

M-3
  medical student 3rd year

M/3
  middle third (long bones)

M₃
  mitral third sound (absolute dullness)
  myelocyte at third stage of maturation

M-4
  medical student 4th year

M₄
  myelocyte at fourth stage of maturation

M₅
  metamyelocyte

M₆
  band form in sixth stage of myelocyte maturation

M₇
  polymorphonuclear neutrophil *(See also* PMN)

M₈
  spin quantum number

M/10
  tenth molar solution

M/100
  hundredth molar solution

(m)
  by mouth *(See also* m, OS, per os, PO, p.o.)
  murmur *(See also* M, m)

m
  by mouth *(See also* (m), PO, p.o., OS, per os)
  electromagnetic moment
  electron rest mass
  in the morning [L. *mane*]
  magnetic moment *(See also* μ)
  magnetic quantum number
  mass
  mean *(See also* M, μ)
  median *(See also* M)
  melts at *(See also* M)
  mesial *(See also* M, MES)
  meter
  milli-
  minim *(See also* M)
  minute *(See also* M, min, MIN)
  modulus
  molality
  molar (deciduous tooth)
  moles (per liter)
  morphine
  motile
  mucoid
  murmur *(See also* M, (m))
  sample mean

m.
  mix [L. *misce*]
  mixture [L. *mistura*]
  send [L. *mitte*]

m²
  meters squared *(See also* MSQ)
  square meter (body surface) *(See also* M²)

m³
  cubic meter *(See also* cu m)

m-
  meta-

MA
  machine
  mafenide acetate
  main arteriole
  mandelic acid
  manifest achievement
  Martin-Albright (syndrome)
  masseter
  maternal aunt
  matrix
  mean arterial
  mechanically assisted
  medical abbreviation
  medical assistance
  medical audit
  medical authorization
  mega ampere
  megaloblastic anemia
  megestrol acetate
  membrane antigen

menstrual age
mental age
mentum anterior (fetal position)
metabolic acidosis
metastatic adenocarcinoma
metatarsus adductus
meter angle
Mexican American
microagglutination
microalbuminuria
microaneurysm
microcytotoxicity assay
microscopic agglutination
migraine with aura
Miller-Abbott (tube)
milliampere
mitochondrial antibody
mitogen activation
mitotic apparatus
mixed agglutination
mixed apnea
moderately advanced
monoamine
monoarthritis
monoclonal antibody (*See also*
  MAB, MAb, MCA, MCAB,
  MoAb)
monomorphic adenoma
motorcycle accident (*See also*
  MCA)
multiple action
muscle actin
muscle activity
mutagenic activity
mycophenolic acid
myelinated axon

M/A
male, altered (animal) (*See also*
  MALT)
mood and/or affect

MA–1
mechanically assisted (Bennett
  brand of respirator)

Ma
mass of atom
masurium (technetium)

mA
meter-angle
microampere
milliamp
milliamperage

milliampere (*See also* ma)
milliangstrom

ma
milliampere (*See also* mA)

MAA
macroaggregated albumin (*See also*
  MIAA)
macroaggregated albumin (*See also*
  ^{99mTc}-MAA)
mandibular advancement appliance
Medical Assistance for the Aged
melanoma-associated antigen
microphthalmia or anophthalmos
  (with associated anomalies)
monoarticular arthritis

^{99mTc}-MAA
technetium-99m macroaggregated
  albumin (*See also* MAA)

MAAAP
macroaggregated albumin arterial
  perfusion

MAACL
Multiple Affect Adjective Check
  List

MAAP
multiple arbitrary amplicon profiling

MAAS
MAAS-R
Maastricht History and Advice
  Checklist-Revised

MAB, MAb
management of assaultive behavior
maximal androgen blockade
monoclonal antibody (*See also* MA,
  MCA, MCAB, MoAb)

MABI
Mother's Assessment of the
  Behavior of Her Infant

MAb-LA
monoclonal antibody-based latex
  agglutination

MABP
maltose-binding protein
mean arterial blood pressure

MAC
MacConkey (agar)
MacIntosh (blade) (*See also* Mac)
macrocytic erythrocyte
macrophage
macule
malignancy-associated change
maximal acid concentration

M

NOTES

461

MAC (*continued*)
maximal allowable concentration
maximal allowable cost
maximum allowable cost
McAndrews Alcoholism Scale
medical alert center
membrane attack complex
membranolytic attack complex
Mental Adjustment to Cancer
(scale)
microcystic adnexal carcinoma
midarm circumference
minimal alveolar concentration
minimal anesthetic concentration
minimal antibiotic concentration
minimum alveolar anesthetic
concentration
minimum alveolar concentration
Minimum Auditory Capabilities
Test
mitral annular calcium
mitral annulus calcification
modulator of adenylate cyclase
monitored anesthesia care
monitored anesthesia control
multiaccess catheter
multidimensional actuarial
classification
Mycobacterium avium-intracellulare
complex

1-MAC
1-minimum alveolar concentration

Mac
MacIntosh (laryngoscope blade)
(*See also* MAC)
macula

mac.
maceration (*See also* macer)
soften [L. *macerare*] (*See also* M)

MAC AWAKE
minimal alveolar (anesthetic)
concentration (patient recovering
from general anesthesia able to
respond to instructions)

MACC
macroovalocyte

MACE
major adverse cardiac event
Malon antegrade continence enema
methylchloroform chloroacetophenone

MAC EIA
immunoglobulin M antibody capture

macer
maceration (*See also* mac.)

MACH1
metronidazole, amoxicillin,
clarithromycin, *H. pylori*, one-
week therapy

mAChR
muscarinic acetylcholine receptor

MACI
Millon Adolescent Clinical
Inventory

MACIS
metastasis, age, completeness of
resection, local invasion, and
tumor size

MACR
macrocytosin
mean axillary count rate

macro
macrocyte
macrocytic
macroscopic

macro-EMG
macroelectromyography

MACS
magnetically activated cell sorter

MACTAR
McMaster-Toronto Arthritis Patient
Reference (Disability
Questionnaire)

MACV
Machupo virus

MAD
major affective disorder
mandibular advancement device
maximal allowable dose
maximum accumulated dose
maximum acid output
methandriol
methylandrostenediol
mind-altering drug
minimal average dose
moderate atopic dermatitis
myoadenylate deaminase

mAD, MADA
muscle adenylate deaminase

MadCAM-1
mucosal addresin cell adhesion
molecule-1

MADD
mixed anxiety depression disorder
multiple acyl-coenzyme A
dehydrogenase deficiency

MADL
mobility activities of daily living

MADRS
Montgomery-Asberg Depression
Rating Scale
Montgomery-Åsberg Depression
Rating Scale

MADV
Madrid virus

MAE
medical air evacuation

moves all extremities
Multilingual Aphasia Examination

mAECA
monoclonal antiendothelial cell
antibody

MAEEW
moves all extremities equally well

MAES
moves all extremities slowly

MAEW
moves all extremities well

MAF
macrophage-activating factor
macrophage activation factor
macrophage-agglutinating factor
malignant ascites fluid
master apical file
metabolic activity factor
metanephric adenofibroma
Mexican American female
minimal audible field
minimum acceptable field
minimum audible field
mouse amniotic fluid
movement after effect

MAFA
midarm fat area
movement-associated fetal (heart
rate) accelerations

MAFH
macroaggregated ferrous hydroxide

MAFO
molded ankle-foot orthosis

MAFP
maternal alpha fetoprotein

MAG
medication administration guideline
(record)
mercaptoacetyltriglycerine
Minnesota antilymphocyte globulin
multifocal atrophic gastritis
myelin-associated glycoprotein

MAG-3
mercaptotriglycine
mercaptotriglycylglycine

mag
large [L. *magnus*]
magnification
magnify

mag cit
magnesium citrate

MAGE
mean amplitude of glycerine
excursion
melanoma-associated gene

MAGF
male accessory gland fluid

MAggF
macrophage agglutination factor

MAGIC
microprobe analysis generalized
intensity correction

MAGP
meatal advancement glans-
phalloplasty
microfil-associated glycoprotein

MAGPI
meatal advancement and glansplasty
meatal advancement, glansplasty,
penoscrotal junction meatotomy

MAGS
microscopic angiogenesis grading
system
Multidimensional Assessment of
Gains in School (psychologic
test)

mag sulf
magnesium sulfate

MAGV
Maguari virus

MAH
minimal acceptable height

mAH
milliampere-hours

MAHA
microangiopathic hemolytic anemia
(*See also* MHA)

MAHH
malignancy-associated humoral
hypercalcemia

MAI
Marriage Adjustment Inventory
maximal aggregation index
microscopic aggregation index
minor acute illness
morbid anxiety inventory
movement arousal index
movement assessment of infants
Mycobacterium avium

mAi
milliampere impulse

M

NOTES

463

MAIC
> *Mycobacterium avium-intracellulare* complex

MAIDS
> murine-acquired immunodeficiency syndrome

MAII
> Milwaukee Academic Interest Inventory

MAK-4
> Maharishi Amrit Kalash-4

MAK-5
> Maharishi Amrit Kalash-5

MAK-6
> Maharishi Amrit Kalash-6

MAKA
> major karyotypic abnormality

MAL
> malaria vaccine
> malfunction
> malignant (*See also* M, mal, malig)
> midaxillary line

mal
> ill [L. *malum*]
> maleate
> malfunction (*See also* MAL)
> malignant (*See also* M, MAL, malig)

MALA
> malarial parasites

MALAR
> malaria

Mal-BSA
> maleated bovine serum albumin

MALDI
> matrix-assisted laser desorption ionization

MALDIMS
> matrix-assisted laser desorption and ionization mass spectrometry

MALDI-TOF
> matrix-assisted laser desorption ionization-time of flight

MALDI-TOFMS
> matrix-assisted laser desorption ionization-time-of-flight mass spectrometry

MALG
> Minnesota antilymphoblast globulin

malig
> malignant (*See also* M, MAL, mal)

MALIMET
> Master List of Medical (Indexing) Terms

MALL
> massive all layer liposuction

MALT
> male, altered (animal) (*See also* M/A)
> mucosa-associated lymphoid tissue

MALToma
> mucosa-associated lymphoid tissue lymphoma

MALV
> Malakal virus

MAM
> mammogram
> methylazoxymethanol
> Mexican American male
> monitored administration of medication
> *Mycoplasma arthritidis* mitogen

M-Am
> compound myopic astigmatism

mam
> milliampere-minute (*See also* MA min, ma-min)

MAMA
> midarm muscle area
> monoclonal antimalignin antibody

MAM Ac
> methylazoxymethanol acetate

MAMC
> mean arm muscle circumference
> midarm muscle circumference

MAmg
> medial amygdaloid (nucleus)

MA min, ma-min
> milliampere-minute (*See also* mam)

mammo
> mammogram
> mammography

MAMP
> milliampere

MAMSA, mAMSA, m-AMSA
> amsacrine

MaMT
> Maudsley Mentation Test

MAMTT
> minimal active muscle tendon tension

MAN
> magnocellular nucleus (of anterior neostratum)
> malignancy associated neutropenia
> mannose

Man
> mannose

man.
> handful [L. *manipulus*] (*See also* M, manip.)
> manipulate
> morning [L. *mane*]

MANCOVA
multivariate analysis of covariance
mand
mandible
mandibular
MANE
Morrow Assessment of Nausea and Emesis
manip.
handful [L. *manipulus*] (*See also* M, m)
manipulation
MANOVA
multivariate analysis of variance
MAO
maximal acid output
medical ankle orthosis
monoamine oxidase
MAO-A, MAOA
monoamine oxidase type A
MAO-B
monoamine oxidase type B
MAOI
monoamine oxidase inhibitor
MAP
magnesium, ammonium, and phosphate (Struvite stones)
malignant atrophic papulosis
maximal aerobic power
mean airway pressure
mean aortic pressure
mean arterial pressure
megaloblastic anemia of pregnancy
mercapturic acid pathway
methyl acceptor protein
methylacetoxyprogesterone
methylaminopurine
microlithiasis alveolarum pulmonum
microtubule-associated protein
Miller Assessment for Preschoolers (test for developmental delays)
minimal audible pressure
minimum audible pressure
mitogen-activated protein
mitogen-activating protein
monophasic action potential
morning after pill (oral contraceptives)
mouse antibody production (test)
multiantigenic peptide
Multiaxial Assessment of Pain

Muma Assessment Program (student assessment)
muscle-action potential
Musical Aptitude Profile
MAPA
muscle adenosine phosphoric acid
MAPC
migrating action potential complex
MAPCA
major aortopulmonary collateral artery
MAPD
monophasic action potential duration
MAPE
Multidimensional Assessment of Philosophy of Education
MAPF
microatomized protein food
MAPI
microbial alkaline protease inhibitor
Millon Adolescent Personality Inventory
MAPK
mitogen-activated protein kinase
MAPS
Make A Picture Story (test)
MAPSS
multiangle polarized scatter separation
MAPV
Mapputta virus
MAR
main admitting room
marasmus
marital
marrow
maximal aggregation ratio
mean atrial rate
medication administration record
microanalytical reagent
mineral apposition rate
minimal angle resolution
mixed agglutination reaction
mixed antiglobulin reaction
mar22
marker 22
mar.
margin (*See also* marg, MG)
marker (chromosome)

NOTES

M

465

MARC
multifocal and recurrent choroidopathy

MARE
manual active-resistive exercise

marg
margin (*See also* mar., MG)

MARIA
macroaggregated radioiodinated albumin

MARS
Mathematics Anxiety Rating Scale
mixed antiinflammatory syndrome
Modular Acetabular Revision System
molecular adsorbent recirculating system
motion artifact rejection system
mouse antirat serum

MARS-A
Mathematics Anxiety Rating Scale-Adolescents

MARSA
methicillin-aminoglycoside-resistant *Staphylococcus aureus*

MART, MART-1
melanoma antigen reacting to T cell
melanoma antigen recognized by T cell

MARTI
mobile advanced real-time image

MARV
Marburg virus
Marrakai virus

marX
marker X

MAS
MacAndrew Addiction Scale
macrophage activation syndrome
mammary aspiration specimen
Management Appraisal Survey
Manifest Anxiety Scale
Maternal Attitude Scale
mean allograft survival
meconium aspiration syndrome
medical advisory service
Memory Assessment Scale
mesoatrial shunt
milk-alkali syndrome
minimum-access surgery
minor axis shortening (of left ventricle)
mobile arm support
motion analysis system
Motor Assessment Scale
multiple anal sphincterotomies
mycobacteria antibiotic supplement

mAs, mA-s
milliampere second

MASA
mutant allele-specific amplification

masc
masculine
mass concentration (*See also* massc)

MASCT
mammary aspiration specimen cytology test

MASDASM
multiple-allele-specific diagnostic assay

MASE
microsurgical extraction of sperm from epididymis

MASER
microwave amplification by stimulated emission of radiation

MASF
Melcher acid-soluble fraction

MASH
multiple automated sample harvester

Mash-2
mammalian achaete-scute homologous protein-2

MASH POT
mashed potatoes

MASS
metastatic adenocarcinoma in the serosal surfaces
mitral valve (prolapse), aortic (anomalies), skeletal (changes), and skin (changes)

mass
massage (*See also* M, MSS, mss)
massive

massc
mass concentration (*See also* masc)

MAST
medical antishock trousers
Michigan Abuse Screening Test
Michigan Alcoholism Screening Test
military antishock trousers
motion artifact suppression technique
multiple antigen stimulation test
multithread allergosorbent test

mAST
mitochondrial aspartate aminotransferase

mast
mastectomy
mastoid

MAT
Manipulative Aptitude Test
manual arts therapist

maternal (*See also* mat.)
maternity (*See also* mat.)
mature (*See also* M, mat.)
mean absorption time
medication administration team
methionineadenosyltransferase
Metropolitan Achievement Test
microagglutination test
microscopic agglutination test
Miller-Abbott tube
Miller Analogies Test
motivation analysis test
multifocal atrial tachycardia
multiple agent therapy
Music Achievement Test (1-4)

MAT7
Metropolitan Achievement Test,
Seventh Edition

mat.
material
maternal (*See also* MAT)
maternity (*See also* MAT)
mature (*See also* M, MAT)

MATE
Marital Attitudes Evaluation
Maternal Attitudes Evaluation

MATHS
muscle (pain), allergy, tachycardia
and tiredness, headache syndrome

MATPP
Medical Audiologic Tinnitus Patient
Protocol

MATSA
Marek associated tumor-specific
antigen

MATV
Matucare virus

MAV
mechanical auxiliary ventricle
minimal apparent viscosity
minute alveolar volume
movement arm vector
multinucleated atypia of the vulva
myeloblastosis-associated virus

MAVA
multiple abstract variance analysis

MAVIS
mobile artery and vein imaging
system

MAVR
mitral and aortic valve replacement

max
maxilla
maxillary
maximal
maximum

MAX A
maximum assistance (assist)

MAXCONT
maximum contrast method

max EP
maximal esophageal pressure

MAxL
midaxillary line

MAYO
mayonnaise

MAYV
Mayaro virus

MB
buccal margin
Mallory body
mammillary body
mandible
margin, buccal
Marsh-Bendall (factor)
medical board
medulloblastoma
megabyte
mercury bougie
mesiobuccal
methyl bromide
methylene blue (*See also* MBl,
MEB, MeB)
microbiologic assay
microbubble
muscle balance
muscle-brain
myocardial band
myocardial bridging

6MB
six-meal bland (diet)

M/B
mother/baby

Mb
mandible body
myoglobin (*See also* MbCO, MbO$_2$)

MBA
Maxwell-Brancheau arthroereisis
methylbenzyl alcohol
methylbischloroethylamine (nitrogen
mustard)
methylbovine albumin

NOTES

M

MBAR
    myocardial β-adrenergic receptor
mbar
    millibar
MBAS
    methylene blue active substance
MBB
    modified barbital buffer
MBC
    bactericidal concentration
    male breast cancer
    maximum bladder capacity
    maximum breathing capacity
    mesiobuccal cusp
    metastatic breast cancer
    methylthymol blue complex
    microcrystalline bovine collagen
    minimal bacterial concentration
    minimal bactericidal concentration
    minimum bactericidal concentration
MB CK, MB-CK
    M and B isoenzyme (heart) of
    creatine kinase (*See also* CPK-
    MB)
    myocardial band enzymes of CPK
    (*See also* CPK-MB)
MBCL
    monocytoid B-cell lymphoma
MbCO
    carbon monoxide myoglobin
    myoglobin (*See also* Mb, MbO_2,
    MYO, MYOGLB)
MBCR
    mesiobuccal cusp ridge
MBCU
    metallic bead-chain
    cystourethrograph
MBD
    maximal bactericidal dilution
    maximum bactericidal dilution
    metabolic bone disease
    methylene blue dye
    minimal brain damage
    minimal brain dysfunction
    (syndrome)
MBDG
    mesiobuccal developmental groove
MBE
    may be elevated
    medium below elbow (cast)
MBEST
    modulus blipped echo-planar single-
    pulse technique
MBF
    meat base formula
    medullary blood flow
    muscle blood flow
    myocardial blood flow

MBFC
    medial brachial fascial compartment
MBFLB
    monaural bifrequency loudness
    balance
M-BFU-E
    mature burst-forming unit erythroid
MBG
    mean blood glucose
MBGS
    Morphine-Benzedrine Group Scale
MBGV
    Marburg virus
MBH
    maximal benefit from
    hospitalization
    medial basal hypothalamic region
    medial basal hypothalamus
MBH_2
    methylene blue, reduced (*See also*
    MBR)
MBHI
    Millon Behavioral Health Inventory
MBI
    Maslach Burnout Inventory
    methylene blue instillation
MBIP
    model-based image processing
MBK
    methyl butyl ketone
MBL
    mannan-binding lectin
    mannose-binding lectin
    medium brown loose (stool)
    menstrual blood loss
    minimal bactericidal level
MBl
    methylene blue (*See also* MB,
    MEB, MeB)
MBLA
    methylbenzyl linoleic acid
    mouse-specific bone marrow-derived
    lymphocyte antigen
MBM
    mineral basal medium
    mother's breast milk
MBNW
    multiple-breath nitrogen washout
MBO
    mesiobuccoocclusal
MbO_2
    myoglobin (*See also* Mb, MbCO,
    MYO, MYOGLB)
    oxymyoglobin
MBOT
    mucinous borderline ovarian tumors
MBP
    major basic protein

malignant brachial plexopathy
maltose-binding protein
mannan-binding protein
mannose-binding protein
mean arterial blood pressure
mean blood pressure
medullary bone pain
melitensis, bovine, porcine (antigen from *Brucella melitensis*, *B. bovis* and *B. suis*)
mesiobuccopulpal
modified Bagshawe protocol
myelin base protein
myelin basic protein

MBPA
malposition of the branch pulmonary artery

MBPS
multigated (cardiac) blood pool scanning

MBq
megabecquerel

MBR
major breakpoint region
mesiobuccal root
methylene blue, reduced (*See also* MBH$_2$)

MBRT
methylene blue reduction time

MBRVO
macular branch retinal vein occlusion

MBS
Martin-Bell syndrome
modified barium swallow
Multi Balance System

MBSA
methylated bovine serum albumin

MBSD
maple bark stripper disease

MBSP
Monitoring Basic Skills Progress

MBT
maternal blood type
mercaptobenzothiazole
mixed bacterial toxin
mucinous borderline tumor
multiple blunt trauma

MBTI
Myers-Briggs Type Indicator (psychologic test)

MBTS
modified Blalock-Taussig shunt

MBV
mitral balloon valvotomy

MBZ
mebendazole

M-C
Magovern-Cromie (prosthesis)
mineralocorticoid (*See also* MC)

MC
macroglobulinemia
male child
mass casualty
mast cell
maximal concentration
maximum control
medium-chain (triglyceride)
medullary carcinoma
medullary cavity
medullary cystic (disease)
megacoulomb
megacycle
melanoma cell
meningeal carcinomatosis
Merkel cell
mesangial cell
mesenchymal chondrosarcoma
mesenteric collateral
mesiocervical
mesocaval (shunt)
metacarpal
metatarsocuneiform
methyl cellulose
methylcholanthrene (*See also* MCA)
microcephaly
microciliary clearance
microcirculation
midcapillary
midcarpal
mineralocorticoid (*See also* M C)
minilaparotomy cholecystectomy
minimal change
Minkowski-Chauffard (syndrome)
mitotic cycle
mitral commissurotomy
mixed cellularity
mixed cryoglobulinemia
molluscum contagiosum
monkey cell
monocomponent highly purified pork insulin
mononuclear cell

M

NOTES

MC *(continued)*
    Moraxella catarrhalis
    mouth care
    mycelial phase (of fungi)
    myocarditis
MC-540
    merocyanine 540
M/C
    male, castrated (animal)
M&C
    morphine and cocaine
Mc
    mandible coronoid
mC
    millicoulomb
MCA
    major coronary artery
    medical care administration
    mesial contact area
    metacarpal amputation
    methylcholanthrene (*See also* MC)
    microcarcinoma
    micrometastases clonogenic assay
    middle cerebral aneurysm
    middle cerebral artery
    middle colic artery
    monocarboxylic acid
    monoclonal antibody (*See also* MA, MAB, MAb, MCAB, MoAb)
    motorcycle accident (*See also* MA)
    mucin-like carcinoma-associated antigen
    multichannel analyzer
    multiple congenital abnormalities
    multiple congenital anomalies
2-MCA
    2-methyl citric acid
MCAB, MC-Ab
    Minnesota Clerical Assessment Battery
    monoclonal antibody (*See also* MA, MAB, MAb, MCA, MoAb)
MCAD
    medium-chain acyl-coenzyme A dehydrogenase
MCAF
    monocyte chemoattractant and activity factor
    monocyte chemotactic and activating factor
MCA/MR
    multiple congenital anomalies/mental retardation (syndrome)
MCAO
    middle cerebral artery occlusion
MCAP
    middle cerebral artery pressure

MCAR
    melanocortin receptor type 4
    mixed cell agglutination reaction
MCAS
    middle cerebral artery syndrome
MCAT
    Medical College Admission Test
    middle cerebral artery thrombosis
    Minnesota Clerical Aptitude Test
    myocardial contrast appearance time
MCAV
    Macaua virus
MCB
    membranous cytoplasmic body
    midcycle bleeding
    middle chamber bubbling
    monochlorobenzidine
McB
    McBurney (point)
mCBF
    mean cerebral blood flow
MCBM
    muscle capillary basement membrane
MCBMT
    muscle capillary basement membrane thickening
MCBR
    minimal concentration of bilirubin
    minimum concentration of bilirubin
MCC
    marked cocontraction
    mean corpuscular (hemoglobin) concentration (*See also* MCHbC, MCHC)
    measure mucociliary clearance
    medial cell column
    metacarpocarpal (joints)
    metacerebral cell
    metastatic cord compression
    microcrystalline collagen
    midstream clean catch (urine)
    minimal complete-killing concentration
    minimum complete-killing concentration
    mucociliary clearance
    mucocutaneous candidiasis
    mutated in colon cancer
    mutated colorectal carcinoma
    Mycobacterium cell wall complex
McC
    McCarthy (panendoscope)
    McCoy (antibody)
MCCD
    minimal cumulative cardiotoxic dose

MCCN
mesangiocapillary glomerulonephritis
MCCS
Minnesota Cocaine Craving Scale
MCCU
mobile coronary care unit
MCD
magnetic circular dichroism
malformation of cortical
development
margin crease distance
mast cell degranulation
mean cell diameter
mean central dose
mean consecutive difference
mean corpuscular diameter
medullary collecting duct
medullary cystic disease
metabolic coronary dilation
metacarpal cortical density
metastatic Crohn disease
minimal cerebral dysfunction
minimal change disease
molecular coincidence detection
molybdenum cofactor deficiency
multicentric Castleman disease
multicystic disease
multicystic dysplasia
multiple carboxylase deficiency
muscle carnitine deficiency
MCDD
multiple complex developmental
disorder
MCDI
Minnesota Child Development
Inventory
MCDK
multicystic dysplasia kidney
multicystic dysplastic kidney
MCDP
mast cell degranulating peptide
MCDT
mast cell degranulation test
multiple choice discrimination test
MCDU
mercaptolactate-cysteine disulfiduria
MCE
major coronary event
medical care evaluation
minimal cytotoxic epitope
multicystic encephalopathy
multiple cartilaginous exostosis

myocardial contrast
echocardiography
MCES
multiple cholesterol emboli
syndrome
MCF
macrophage chemotactic factor
macrophage cytotoxicity factor
median cleft face
medium corpuscular fragility
microcomplement fixation
monocyte chemotactic factor
monocyte (leukotactic) factor
mononuclear cell factor
most comfortable frequency
multicentric foci
myocardial contractile force
MCFA
medium-chain fatty acid
miniature centrifugal fast analyzer
MCFP
mean circulating filling pressure
MCFSR
mean circumferential fiber-
shortening rate
MCG
magnetocardiogram
magnetocardiography
membrane coating granule
mesencephalic central gray
monoclonal gammopathy (*See also*
MG)
mcg
microgram (*See also* μg)
MCGC
metacerebral giant cell
MCGF
mast cell growth factor
mcg/kg/min
micrograms per kilogram per
minute
MCGN
mesangiocapillary glomerulonephritis
minimal-change glomerulonephritis
mixed cryoglobulinemia with
glomerulonephritis
MCH
maternal and child health
mean cell hemoglobin
mean corpuscular hemoglobin (*See
also* MCHb)
melanin-concentrating hormone

M

NOTES

MCH *(continued)*
    methacholine
    microfibrillar collagen hemostat
    mucous cell hyperplasia
    muscle contraction headache
MCHA
    microsome antibody
MCHb, MCHg
    mean corpuscular hemoglobin (*See also* MCH)
MCHbC
    mean cell hemoglobin concentration (*See also* MCHC)
    mean corpuscular hemoglobin concentration (*See also* MCHC, MCC)
    mean corpuscular hemoglobin count (*See also* MCHC)
MCHC
    maternal and child health care
    mean cell hemoglobin concentration (*See also* MCHbC)
    mean corpuscular hemoglobin concentration (*See also* MCHbC, MCC)
    mean corpuscular hemoglobin count (*See also* MCHbC)
MCHD
    mixed-cellularity Hodgkin disease
MCHS
    maternal and child health service
MCI
    mean cardiac index
    methicillin (*See also* METH)
    midcarpal instability
    mild cognitive impairment
MCi
    megacurie
mCi
    millicurie
MCID
    minimum clinically important difference(s)
mCid
    millicuries destroyed
mCi-hr
    millicurie-hour
MCINS
    minimal change idiopathic nephrotic syndrome
MCK
    multicystic kidney
MCKD
    multicystic kidney disease
MCL
    mantle cell lymphoma
    maximal comfort level
    maximal containment laboratory
    medial collateral ligament
    midclavicular line
    midcostal line
    minimal change lesion
    mixed culture, leukocyte
    modified chest lead
    most comfortable level
    most comfortable loudness
    mucocutaneous leishmaniasis
mcL
    microliter (1/1,000 of an mL) (*See also* μL)
MCLC
    medial collateral ligament complex
MCLL
    most comfortable listening level
    most comfortable loudness level
MCL-N
    midclavicular line to nipple
MCLNS, MCLS
    mucocutaneous lymph node syndrome
MCMI
    Millon Clinical Multiaxial Inventory (psychiatric battery)
MCMI-II
    Millon Clinical Multiaxial Inventory II
MCMI-III
    Millon Clinical Multiaxial Inventory III
MCN
    minimal-change nephropathy
    mixed cell nodular (lymphoma) (*See also* MC-N)
MC-N
    mixed cell nodular (lymphoma) (*See also* MCN)
MCNS
    minimal-change nephrotic syndrome
MCO
    managed care organization
    medical care organization
    mupirocin calcium ointment (Bactroban Nasal)
MCOV
    Marco virus
MCP
    maximal closure pressure
    mean carotid pressure
    medical control physician
    melanosis circumscripta precancerosa
    membrane cofactor protein
    metacarpal
    metacarpophalangeal (*See also* MP)
    metaclopramide
    methyl-accepting chemotaxis protein
    mitotic-control protein

monocyte chemoattractant protein
monocyte chemotactic protein
mucin clot-prevention (test)
mucopolysaccharidoses (plural)

MCP-1

monocyte chemoattractant protein-1
monocyte chemotactic peptide-1
monocyte chemotactic protein-1

MCPJ

metacarpophalangeal joint

MCPS

Missouri Children's Picture Series
(psychologic test)

Mcps

megacycles per second (*See also*
Mc/s)

MCPT

Monte Carlo photon transport

MCQ

multiple choice question

MCR

mesial cusp ridge
message competition ratio
metabolic clearance rate
midcarpal radial
minor cluster region
morphine controlled-release
mother-child relationship
mutation cluster region
myocardial revascularization
steroid metabolic clearance rate

MC=R

moderately constricted and equally
reactive (pupils)

MC2-R

melanocortin-2 receptor

MC3-R

melanocortin-3 receptor

MC4-R

melanocortin-4 receptor

MCRC

metastatic colorectal cancer

MCRE

Mother-Child Relationship
Evaluation

MCS

magnetic control suturing
malignant carcinoid syndrome
Marlow-Crowne Scale
massage of the carotid sinus
Mental Component Summary
mesocaval shunt

methylcholanthrene(-induced)
sarcoma
microculture and sensitivity
middle coronary sinus
Miles-Carpenter syndrome
moderate constant suction
multiple chemical sensitivity
multiple combined sclerosis
myocardial contractile state

Mc/s

megacycles per second (*See also*
Mcps)

MCSA

McCarthy Scales of Children's
Ability
minimal cross-sectional area
Moloney cell surface antigen

mCsA

maintenance cyclosporine
monotherapy

MCSDS

Marlowe-Crown Social Desirability
Scale

M-CSF

macrophage colony-stimulating
factor
monocyte colony-stimulating factor

MC-SR

moderately constricted and slightly
reactive (pupils)

MCSS

multiple chemical sensitivity
syndrome

MCT

manual cervical traction
mast cell containing tryptase but
not chymase
mean cell thickness
mean cell threshold
mean circulation time
mean colonic transit
mean corpuscular thickness
medium-chain triglyceride
medullary carcinoma of thyroid
medullary collecting tubule
microwave coagulation therapy
Minnesota Clerical Test
monocarboxylate/proton cotransporter
monocarboxylate transporter
monocrotaline
motor coordination test
mucinous cystic tumor

M

NOTES

MCT *(continued)*
mucociliary transport
multiple compressed tablet

MCTC
mast cell containing both tryptase and chymase
metrizamide computed tomographic cisternography
metrizamide computed tomography cisternography

MCTD
mixed connective-tissue disease

MCTF
mononuclear cell tissue factor

MCTT
mucociliary clearance time

MCU
malaria control unit
maximal care unit
micturating cystourethrography
midcarpal ulnar
motor cortex unit

mcU
microunit

MCUG
micturating urogram

MCV
mean cell volume
mean clinical value
mean corpuscular volume
melanoma whole-cell vaccine
molluscum contagiosum virus
motor conduction velocity

MCVr
reticulocyte mean corpuscular volume

MCVRI
minimal coronary vascular resistance index

MCYLS
marginal cost per year of life saved

MCZ
miconazole

MD
macula densa
macular degeneration
magnesium deficiency
main duct
maintenance dialysis
maintenance dose
major depression
malate dehydrogenase
malic dehydrogenase
malrotation of duodenum
mammary dysplasia
mandibular
manic depression

manic-depressive
Mantoux diameter
Marek disease
maternal deprivation
maximal dose
mean deviation
mean diastolic
measurable disease
Meckel diverticulum
medialis dorsalis (nucleus)
mediastinal disease
medical department
mediodorsal
medium dosage
Ménétrier disease
mental deficiency
mental depression
mentally deficient
mesiodistal
methyldichloroarsine
microtube dilution
Minamata disease
minimal dosage
mitral disease
mixed diet
moderate disability
moderately differentiated
monocular deprivation
movement disorder
multiple deficiency
multiple dose
muscular dystrophy
myeloproliferative disease
myocardial damage
myocardial disease
myotonic dystrophy

Md
mendelevium *(See also* Mv)

md
median *(See also* M, m)

MDA
malondialdehyde
manual dilatation of anus
methylenedioxyamphetamine
micrometastases detection assay
monodehydroascorbate
motor discriminative acuity
multivariant discriminant analysis
right mentoanterior (fetal position)
[L. *mento-dextra anterior*]

MDAC
multidose activated charcoal
multiple-dose activated charcoal
multiplying digital-to-analog converter

MDAD
mineral dust airway disease

MDA-LDL, MDALDL
   malondialdehyde conjugated low-density lipoprotein
   malondialdehyde modified low-density lipoprotein
MDAP
   Machover Draw-A-Person (Test)
MDB
   Mental Deterioration Battery
MDBK
   Madin-Darby bovine kidney (cell)
MDBP
   mean resting diastolic blood pressure
MDC
   macrophage-derived chemokine
   major diagnostic category
   medial dorsal cutaneous (nerve)
   minimal detectable concentration
   minimum detectable concentration
MDCA
   mean distal contraction amplitude
MDCK
   Madin-Darby canine kidney (cell)
MDCM
   mildly dilated congestive cardiomyopathy
MDCN
   medial dorsal cutaneous nerve
MDCV
   Mojui Dos Campos virus
MDD
   major depressive disorder
   manic-depressive disorder
   mean daily dose
   mesial developmental depression
MDDA
   Minnesota Differential Diagnosis of Aphasia
MDDC
   monocyte-derived dendritic cell
MDE
   major depressive episode
   mucinous ductal ectasia
MDEA
   N-ethyl-3,4-methylenedioxyamphetamine
MDEBP
   mean daily erect blood pressure
MDF
   mean dominant frequency
   myocardial depressant factor

MDG
   mean diastolic gradient
MDGF
   macrophage-derived growth factor
MDH
   malate dehydrogenase
   medullary dorsal horn
MDHR
   maximum determined heart rate
MDI
   manic-depressive illness
   mental development index
   metered-dose inhaler
   methylenedioxyindenes
   methylene diphenyl diisocyanate
   multidirectional instability
   multiple daily injection
   multiple dosage insulin
   Multiscore Depression Inventory
MDII
   multiple daily insulin injection
MDIS
   metered-dose inhaler-spacer (device)
MDIT
   mean disintegration time
MDK
   multicystic dysplastic kidney
MDL
   master drug list
MDLS
   Miller-Dieker lissencephaly syndrome
MDLVP
   mean diastolic left ventricular pressure
MDM
   middiastolic murmur
   minor determinant mix (penicillin)
MDMA
   3,4-methylelenedioxy-methamphetamine
   methylenedioxymethamphetamine
MDMQ
   Menstrual Distress Management Questionnaire (*See also* MDQ)
MDMS
   methylene dimethane sulfonate
mdn
   median
mDNA
   mitochondrial deoxyribonucleic acid

NOTES

MDNB
    mean daily nitrogen balance
    metadinitrobenzene
    methylene diphosphate

MDNCF
    monocyte-derived neutrophil
      chemotactic factor

MDNT
    midnight

MDO
    mentally disordered offender
    mesiodistocclusal

MDOT
    modified directly observed therapy
    modified double-opposing tab

MDOV
    Monte Dourado virus

MDP
    mandibular dysostosis and
      peromelia
    manic-depressive psychosis
    methylene diphosphate
    methylene diphosphonate
    muramyldipeptide
    muscular dystrophy, progressive
    right mentoposterior (fetal position)
      [L. *mento-dextra posterior*]

MDPD
    maximum dose permissible dose

MDPI
    maximal daily permissible intake

MDQ
    memory deviation quotient
    Menstrual Distress Questionnaire
      (*See also* MDMQ)
    minimal detectable quantity

MDR
    mammalian diving response
    median duration of response
    Medical Device Reporting
      (regulation)
    minimal daily requirement
    minimum daily requirement
    multidrug resistance (protein)
    multidrug-resistant
    multiple drug resistance
    multiple drug-resistant

MD=R
    moderately dilated and equally
      reactive (pupils)

MDR-1
    multidrug resistance gene

MD-50(r)
    diatrizoate sodium injection 50%

MDRE
    multiple-drug-resistant enterococci

MDREF
    multidrug resistant enteric fever

MDRH
    multidisciplinary rehabilitation
      hospital

MDRS
    Mattis Dementia Rating Scale

MDRSP
    multidrug-resistant *Streptococcus*
      pneumoniae

MDR-TB, MDRTB
    multidrug-resistant tuberculosis
    multiple-drug resistant tuberculosis

MDS
    maternal deprivation syndrome
    medical data screen
    medical data system
    membrane-spanning domain
    microdilution system
    microsurgical drill system
    milk drinker's syndrome
    minimum data set
    multidimensional scaling
    myelodysplastic syndrome
    myocardial depressant substance

MDSBP
    mean daily supine blood pressure

MDSO
    mentally disordered sex offender

MD-SR
    moderately dilated and slightly
      reactive (pupils)

MDSU
    medical day stay unit

MDT
    maggot debridement therapy
    mast (cell) degeneration test
    mean dissolution time
    median detection threshold
    motion detection threshold
    multidisciplinary team
    multidrug therapy
    right mentotransverse (fetal
      position) [L. *mento-dextra*
      transversa]

MDTA
    McDonald Deep Test of
      Articulation

MDTM
    multidisciplinary team meeting

MDTP
    multidisciplinary treatment plan

MDTR
    mean diameter-thickness ratio

MDU
    maintenance dialysis unit
    microvascular Doppler
      ultrasonography

MDUO

    myocardial disease of unknown origin

MDV

    Main Drain virus
    Marek disease virus
    mucosal disease virus
    multiple dose vial
    myocardial Doppler velocity

MDVP 4305

    Multi-Dimensional Voice Program 4305

MDY

    month, date, year

Mdyn

    megadyne

ME

    macular edema
    magnitude estimation
    male equivalent
    malic enzyme
    manic episode
    marginal excision
    maximal effort
    median eminence
    medical education
    medical events
    medical evidence
    meningoencephalitis
    mercaptoethanol
    mestranol
    metabolic and electrolyte (disorder)
    metabolic energy
    metabolism
    metabolizable energy
    metamyelocyte
    methionine enkephalin
    Methodist
    methyleugenol
    microembolization
    middle ear
    mouse embryo
    mouse epithelial (cell)
    muscle energy
    muscle examination
    myalgic encephalomyelitis

2ME, 2 ME, 2-ME

    2-mercaptoethanol

M/E, M:E

    metabolic/endocrine
    myeloid/erythrocyte
    myeloid to erythroid
    myeloid/erythroid (ratio)

ME$_{50}$

    50% maximal effect

Me

    megakaryocytic
    menton
    methyl (*See also* meth)

MEA

    measles virus vaccine
    mercaptoethylamine
    microwave endometrial ablation
    multiple endocrine abnormalities
    multiple endocrine adenomatosis
    multiple endocrine adenopathies

MEA-II

    multiple endocrine adenomatosis type II

MeAIB

    methylaminoisobutyric acid

MEAP

    Multiphasic Environmental Assessment Procedure

meas

    measurement

MEAT

    Minnesota Engineering Analogies Test

MEAV

    Meaban virus

MEB

    muscle-eye-brain (disease)

MeB

    methylene blue (*See also* MB, MBl)

MEBS

    muscle-eye-brain syndrome

MeBSA

    methylated bovine serum albumin

MEBV

    Mount Elgon bat virus

MEC

    mecillinam
    meconium
    median effective concentration
    middle ear canal
    middle ear cell
    minimum effective concentration
    mucoepidermoid carcinoma
    myoepithelial cell

M

NOTES

MECA
> Methodology for Epidemiology in Children and Adolescents
> Methods for Epidemiology of Child and Adolescent Mental Disorders

MECG
> maternal electrocardiogram
> mixed essential cryoglobulinemia

MeCP2
> methyl-CpG-binding protein 2

MECT
> maximal extrapolated clotting time

MECTA
> mobile electroconvulsive therapy apparatus

MED
> medial (*See also* med)
> median erythrocyte diameter
> medical (*See also* med)
> medication
> medicine (*See also* med)
> medium (*See also* med)
> medulloblastoma
> minimal effective diameter
> minimal effective dose
> minimal erythema dose
> minimum effective dose
> multiple epiphyseal dysplasia

med
> medial (*See also* MED)
> median
> medical (*See also* MED)
> medicine (*See also* MED)
> medium (*See also* MED)

MEDAC
> multiple endocrine deficiency, Addison disease, and candidiasis (syndrome)
> multiple endocrine deficiency-autoimmune candidiasis

MED-ART
> Medical Automated Records Technology

MedDRA
> Medical Dictionary for Regulatory Activities

MEDEX, Medex
> medication administration record
> military medical corpsmen [Fr. *médicin extension*]

MEDICS
> meat, eggs, dairy, invisible fat, condiments, snacks
> Medical Examination and Diagnostic Coding System

MED-IDDM
> multiple epiphyseal dysplasia-early onset diabetes mellitus syndrome

MEDLARS
> Medical Literature Analysis and Retrieval System

MEDLINE
> MEDLARS On-Line

med men
> medial meniscectomy
> medial meniscus

MED NEC
> medically necessary

MEDPAR
> Medical Provider Analysis and Review

MEdREP
> Medical Education Reinforcement and Enrichment Program

MEDS
> medications
> microsurgical extraction of ductal sperm

MedSurg
> medicine and surgery

Med Tech
> medical technology

MEE
> measured energy expenditure
> methylethyl ether
> middle ear effusion
> multilocus enzyme electrophoresis

M-EEG
> magnetoencephalogram

MEF
> maximal expiratory flow
> maximum expiratory flow
> middle ear fluid
> midexpiratory flow
> migration enhancement factor
> mouse embryo fibroblast

MEF$_{50}$
> maximum expiratory flow at 50% vital capacity
> mean maximal expiratory flow

MEFR
> maximal expiratory flow rate
> maximum expiratory flow rate

MEFSR
> maximal expiratory flow-static recoil (curve)

MEFV
> maximal expiratory flow volume
> maximum expiratory flow volume

MEFVC
> maximal expiratory flow volume curve

mechanical expiratory flow volume curve

MEG

magnetoencephalogram
magnetoencephalograph
magnetoencephalography
megakaryocyte
mercaptoethylguanidine
metabolic, endocrine, and gastrointestinal
multifocal eosinophilic granuloma

MEG-CSF

megakaryocyte colony-stimulating factor

MEGD

minimal euthyroid Graves disease

mEGF

mouse epidermal growth factor

MEGX

monoethylglycinexylidide

MeHg

methylmercury

MEI

medical economic index
metastatic efficiency index
middle ear implantable

MEIA

microparticle capture enzyme immunoassay
microparticle enzyme immunoassay
microparticulate enzyme immunoassay

MEK

MAP/ERK kinase
methylethylketone
methyl ethyl ketone

MEKC

micellar electrokinetic chromatography

MEKK

MEK kinase

MEKS

Mediterranean Kaposi sarcoma

MEL

melatonin
metabolic equivalent level
mouse erythroleukemia
murine erythroleukemia

mel

melanoma
melena

mel 1–3

Meleagris adenovirus 1–3

MELAN

melanin

MELAS

(mitochondrial) myopathy, encephalopathy, lactic acidosis, and stroke-like episodes syndrome
myopathy, encephalopathy, lactic acidosis, stroke-like episodes

MEL B

melarsoprol (Arsobal)

MELC

murine erythroleukemia cell

Mel-CAM

melanoma cell adhesion molecule

MELDOS

meliodosis

MELI

metenkephalin-like immunoreactivity

MELV

Melao virus

MEM

Eagle minimum essential medium
macrophage electrophoretic mobility
malignant epithelioid mesothelioma
memory
minimal essential solution
minimum essential medium
monocular estimate method

MEMA

methyl methacrylate (*See also* MMA)

memb

membrane

MEMPHIS

Memphis Educational Model Providing Handicapped Infant Services

MEMR

multiple exostoses-mental retardation (syndrome)

MEMS

medication monitoring event system

MEN

meningococcal (*Neisseria meningitidis*) (serogroups unspecified) vaccine
methylethylnitrosamine
multiple endocrine neoplasia
multiple endocrine neoplasms

M

NOTES

479

MEN 1, MEN1, MEN I
multiple endocrine neoplasia type 1
MEN 2, MEN-2, MEN2
multiple endocrine neoplasia type 2
MEN 3, MEN3, MEN-3, MEN III
multiple endocrine neoplasia type 3
men.
meningeal
meninges
meningitis
MEN 2A, MEN IIA
multiple endocrine neoplasia type 2A
MEN 2B, MEN-2b, MEN IIb
multiple endocrine neoplasia type 2B
MenCon
meningococcal conjugate
MEND
Medical Education for National Defense
minimum effective naproxen dose
MENS
microamperage electrical nerve stimulation
multiple endocrine neoplasia syndrome
menst
menstrual
menstruate
menstruating
MENT
7-alpha-methyl-19-nortestosterone
MEO
malignant external otitis
MeOH
methyl alcohol
MEOS
microsomal ethanol oxidizing system
MEP
maximal expiratory pressure
maximum expiratory pressure
mean effective pressure
meperidine (*See also* mep)
motor end plate
motor evoked potential
mucoid exopolysaccharide
multimodality evoked potential
mep
meperidine (*See also* MEP)
MEPC
miniature endplate current
MEPH
mephobarbital

MEPOP
mitochondrial encephalomyopathy with sensorimotor polyneuropathy, ophthalmoplegia, and paralysis
MEPP
miniature endplate potential
MePr
methylprednisolone
MEPS
means-end problem solving
mEq
milliequivalent
mEq/24 H
milliequivalents per 24 hours
mEq/L
milliequivalent per liter
MER
mean ejection rate
medical evidence of record
mersalyl (acid)
methanol extraction residue
methanol-extruded residue
molar esterification rate
motor-evoked response
multimodality-evoked response
MERAC
musculoskeletal evaluation, rehabilitation and conditioning
MERB
metenkephalin receptor binding
MERG
macular electroretinogram
MERRF
myoclonic epilepsy with ragged red fibers
myoclonus epilepsy with ragged red fibers
MERV
Mermet virus
MES
maintenance electrolyte solution
maximal electroshock seizure
mesial (*See also* M, m)
Metrazol-electroshock seizure
microembolic signal
morpholinoethanesulfonic acid
mucosal electrosensitivity
muscle in elongated state
myoelectric signal
Mes
mesencephalic
mesencephalon
MESA
microepididymal sperm aspiration
microsurgical epididymal sperm aspiration
mesc
mescaline

MESCH
    Multi-Environment Scheme
MESF
    molecule of equivalent soluble
        fluorochrome
MESGN
    mesangial glomerulonephritis
MeSH
    Medical Subject Heading (in
        MEDLARS)
MESI
    mangled extremity syndrome index
MESNA, mesna
    2-mercaptoethane sulfonate
    2-mercaptoethanesulfonic acid
    2-mercaptoethane sulphonate sodium
MESP
    maximal exercise systolic pressure
MesPGN
    mesangial proliferative
        glomerulonephritis
MESS
    Mangled Extremity Severity Score
mESS
    meridional end-systolic stress
    meridional ESS
MET
    medical emergency treatment
    metabolic (*See also* metab)
    metabolic equivalent (*See also*
        METS)
    metamyelocyte
    metastasis (*See also* M, met)
    metastatic (*See also* M, met)
    methionine
    metoprolol
    metronidazole
    midexpiratory time
    minimum elicitation threshold
    Minimum Essentials Test
    multistage exercise test
Met
    methionine (*See also* M)
met
    metallic (chest sounds)
    metastasis (*See also* M, MET)
    metastasize
    metastasizing
    metatarsal (*See also* MT)
META
    metamyelocyte

methacryloxyethyltrimellitic
    anhydride
methacryloxyethyl trimellitic
    anhydride
meta
    metacarpal
    metatarsal
metab
    metabolic (*See also* MET)
    metabolism
met-enkephalin
    methionine-enkephalin
METH
    methicillin (*See also* MCI)
Meth
    methamphetamine
    methedrine
meth
    methyl (*See also* Me)
Met-Hb, MetHb, metHb
    methemoglobin (*See also* HbMet,
        MHB, MHb, MHGB)
MeTHF
    methyltetrahydrofolic acid
methyl G, methyl GAG
    mitroguazone dihydrochloride
MetMb, metMb
    metmyoglobin
METS
    metabolic equivalents (multiples of
        resting oxygen consumption) (*See
        also* MET)
    metastases (*See also* mets)
mets
    metastases (*See also* METS)
METT
    maximal exercise tolerance test
metz
    Metzenbaum (scissors)
MEV
    maximal exercise ventilation
    murine erythroblastosis virus
MeV
    megaelectron volt
    million electron volts
MEWDS
    multiple evanescent white dot
        syndrome
MEX
    mexiletine
MF
    magnification factor

M

NOTES

MF *(continued)*
    Malassezia folliculitis
    Malassezia furfur
    masculinity/femininity
    mass fragmentography
    meat free
    medium frequency
    megafarad
    melamine-formaldehyde (resin)
    merthiolate formaldehyde (solution)
      (*See also* MFS)
    mesial facial
    methanol-formaldehyde
    methoxyflurane
    microfibrile
    microfilament
    microfilia
    microscopic factor
    midcavity forceps
    mitogenic factor
    mitotic figure
    mossy fiber
    mucosal fluid
    multifactorial
    multifactorial model
    multiplication factor
    mutation frequency
    mutton fat
    mycosis fungoides
    myelin figure
    myelofibrosis
    myocardial fibrosis
    myofibrillar

MF51
    polysorbate 80/sorbitan triolate
      emulsifier

M/F
    male to female (ratio)
    moment/force (ratio)

M&F
    male and female
    mother and father

Mf
    maxillofrontal
    microfilaria

mF
    millifarad

MFA
    malaise, fatigue, and anorexia
    methyl fluoracetate
    monofluoroacetate
    multifocal functional autonomy
    multifunctional acrylic
    multiple factor analysis
    Musculoskeletal Function
      Assessment

MFAT
    multifocal atrial tachycardia

MFB
    medial forebrain bundle
    metallic foreign body
    multiple-frequency bioimpedance

MFC
    mean frequency of compensation
    medial femoral condyle
    Micro-Flow compactor
    minimal fungicidal concentration

m-FC
    membrane focal coli (broth)

MFD
    mandibulofacial dysostosis
    Memory for Designs (test)
    midforceps delivery
    milk-free diet
    minimal fatal dose
    monorhythmic frontal delta (EEG)
    multiple fractions per day
      (radiotherapy)

MFEL
    medical free electron laser

MFEM
    maximal forced expiratory
      maneuver

MFF
    matching familiar figures (*See also*
      MFFT)
    metal fume fever

MFFT
    Matching Familiar Figures Test
      (*See also* MFF)

MFG
    magnetic field gradient
    manofluorography
    middle frontal gyrus
    milk fat globule
    modified heat-degraded gelatin

MFGM
    milk fat globule membrane

MFH
    malignant fibrohistiocytoma
    malignant fibrous histiocytoma
    membrane-free hemolysate

MFH-B
    malignant fibrous histiocytoma of
      bone

MFI
    malleable facial implant
    mean fluorescent intensity

MFID
    multielectrode flame ionization
      detector

M-FISH
    multispectral fluorescent in situ
      hybridization

MFM
  millipore filter method
  multifidus muscle
MFMN
  multifocal motor neuropathy
MFNS
  mometasone furoate nasal spray
MFO
  mixed function oxidase
MFP
  monofluorophosphate
  myofascial pain
MFPR
  multifetal pregnancy reduction
MFPS
  myofascial pain syndrome
MFPVC
  multifocal premature ventricular
    contraction
MFR
  mean flow rate
  midforceps rotation
  mucus flow rate
  myofascial release
MFRL
  maximal force at rest length
MFS
  medical fee schedule
  merthiolate formaldehyde solution
    (*See also* MF sol)
  mitral first sound
  monofixation syndrome
MF sol
  merthiolate formaldehyde solution
    (*See also* MFS)
MFSR
  maximum expiratory airflow-static
    lung elastic recoil pressure
MF/SS
  mycosis fungoides/Sézary syndrome
MFT
  medial femoral torsion
  multifocal atrial tachycardia
  muscle function test
MFU
  medical followup
MFVD
  midforceps vaginal delivery
MFVL
  maximal flow-volume envelope
  maximum flow-volume loop

MFVNS
  middle fossa vestibular nerve
    section
MFVPT
  Motor-Free Visual Perception Test
    (*See also* MVPT)
MFVR
  minimal forearm vascular resistance
MFW
  multiple fragment wounds
MG
  Marcus Gunn (pupil) (*See also*
    MGP)
  margin (*See also* mar., marg)
  medial gastrocnemius (muscle)
  membranous glomerulonephritis (*See
    also* MGN)
  membranous glomerulopathy
  menopausal gonadotropin
  mesiogingival
  methylglucoside
  methylguanidine
  Michaelis-Gutmann (body)
  minigastrin
  monoclonal gammopathy (*See also*
    MCG)
  monoglyceride
  mucigen granule
  mucous granule
  muscle group
  myasthenia gravis (*See also* MyG)
  myoglobin
Mg
  magnesium
mG
  milligauss
mg
  milligram
mg%
  milligrams percent
MGA
  malposition of great arteries
  medical gas analyzer
  melengestrol acetate
MGAB
  mucous gland adenoma of
    bronchus
MGB
  medial geniculate body
Mgb
  myoglobulin

M

NOTES

MGBG
>methylglyoxal-bis-guanylhydrazone
>methylglyoxal bisguanylhydrazone
>methylglyoxal *bis*-guanylhydrazone

MGC
>minimal glomerular change
>multinucleated giant cell

MgC
>magnocellular neuroendocrine cell

MGCE
>multifocal giant cell encephalitis

MgCO₃
>magnesium carbonate

MGCT
>malignant giant cell tumor
>malignant glandular cell tumor
>mixed germ cell tumor

MGD
>maximal glucose disposal
>meibomian gland dysfunction
>mixed gonadal dysgenesis

MGDF
>megakaryocyte growth and development factor

MGDI
>mammary-derived growth inhibitor

mg/dL
>milligram per deciliter

mg-el
>milligram-element

MGES
>multiple gated equilibrium scintigraphy

MGF
>macrophage growth factor
>mast cell growth factor
>maternal grandfather

MGG
>May-Grünwald-Giemsa (staining)
>molecular and general genetics
>mouse gamma globulin

MGGH
>methylglyoxal guanylhydrazone

MGGM
>maternal great grandmother

MGH
>microglandular hyperplasia
>monoglyceride hydrolase

mg/h, mg-hr
>milligram per hour

MGHL
>middle glenohumeral ligament

MGI
>macrophage and granulocyte inducer

MGIT
>*Mycobacteria* Growth Indicator tube

MGJ
>mucogingival junction

mg/kg
>milligram per kilogram (*See also* mpk)

mg/kg d
>milligram per kilogram per day

mg/kg hr
>milligram per kilogram per hour

MGL
>minor glomerular lesion

mg/L
>milligram per liter

MGM
>maternal grandmother

MGN
>medial geniculate nucleus
>membranous glomerulonephritis (*See also* MG)

MgO
>magnesium oxide

MG/OL
>molecular genetics/oncology laboratory

MGP
>Marcus Gunn pupil (*See also* MG)
>marginal granulocyte pool
>marginated granulocyte pool
>matrix Gla protein
>medical group practice
>membranous glomerulonephropathy
>methyl green pyronin (dye)
>mucinglycoprotein
>mucous glycoprotein

MGR
>modified gain ratio
>multiple gas rebreathing
>murmurs, gallops, or rubs

MGS
>malignant glandular schwannoma
>metric gravitational system

MGSA
>melanoma growth-stimulating activity
>melanoma growth stimulatory activity

MGSD
>mean gestational sac diameter

MgSO4, MgSO₄
>magnesium sulfate (Epsom salt)

MGT
>malignant glomus tumor
>management

mgtis
>meningitis

mgtt
>minidrop (60 minidrops = 1 mL)

MGUS
>monoclonal gammopathy of undetermined significance
>monoclonal gammopathy of unknown significance

MGW
>magnesium sulfate, glycerin, and water (enema)
>multiple gunshot wound

MGXT
>multistage graded exercise test

mGy
>milligray

M-H
>Mueller-Hinton (agar) (*See also* MHA)

MH
>macular hemorrhage
>macular hole
>maleic hydrazide
>malignant histiocytosis
>malignant hyperpyrexia
>malignant hypertension
>malignant hyperthermia
>mammotropic hormone
>mannoheptulose
>marital history
>medial hypothalamus
>medical history
>Medtronic-Hall (prosthesis)
>melanophore-stimulating hormone (*See also* MSH)
>menstrual history
>mental health
>mental hygiene
>mesothelial hyperplasia
>moist heat
>monosymptomatic hypochondriasis
>multiple handicapped
>murine hepatitis
>mutant hybrid
>myohyoid

M/H
>microcytic hypochromic (anemia)

Mh
>mandible head

mH
>millihenry

MHA
>May-Hegglin anomaly
>methemalbumin

>microangiopathic hemolytic anemia (*See also* MAHA)
>microhemagglutination assay
>middle hepatic artery
>mixed hemadsorption
>Mueller-Hinton agar (*See also* M-H)

MHAQ
>Modified Health Assessment Questionnaire

MHA-TP
>microhemagglutination assay for *Treponema pallidum*
>microhemagglutination-*Treponema pallidum*

MHA-TPA
>microhemagglutination assay-*Treponema pallidum* assay

MHB
>maximal hospital benefit
>mental health (insurance) benefit
>methemoglobin (*See also* HbMet, Met-Hb, MHb, MHGB)

MHb
>medial habenular
>methemoglobin (*See also* HbMet, Met-Hb, MHB, MHGB)
>myohemoglobin

MHBSS
>modified Hanks balanced salt solution

MHC
>major histocompatibility complex
>mental health care
>mental health center
>mental health clinic
>mental health counselor
>minor histocompatibility complex
>multiphasic health checkup
>myosin heavy chain

MHC-I
>major histocompatibility complex class I

MHC-II
>major histocompatibility complex class II

mhcp
>mean horizontal candle power

m/hct
>microhematocrit

MHCU
>mental health care unit

M

NOTES

MHD
maintenance hemodialysis
maximal human dose
mean hemolytic dose
mental health department
minimal hemolytic dilution
minimal hemolytic dose
minimum hemolytic dose

MHGB
methemoglobin (*See also* HbMet, Met-Hb, MHB, MHb)

MHH
mental health hold

MHI
malignant histiocytosis of intestine
Mental Health Index (information)
mild head injury

MHIP
mental health inpatient

MHLC
Multidimensional Health Locus of Control (test)

MHLS
metabolic heat load stimulator

MH/MR
mental health and mental retardation

MHN
massive hepatic necrosis
Mohs hardness number
morbus hemolyticus neonatorum

MHNTG
multiheteronodular toxic goiter

MHO
medical house officer
microsomal heme oxygenase

mho
reciprocal ohm
siemens unit (ohm spelled backward)

MHOCE
multiple hereditary osteochondral exostosis

MHP
hyperphenylalaninemia
maternal health program
1-mercuri-2-hydroxypropane
methoxyhydroxypropane
monosymptomatic hypochondriacal psychosis

MHPA
mild hyperphenylalaninemia
Minnesota-Hartford Personality Assay

MHPG
methoxyhydroxyphenylglycol
3-methoxy-4-hydroxyphenylglycol

MHR
major histocompatibility region
malignant hyperthermia resistance
maximal heart rate
methemoglobin reductase (*See also* MR, MR-E)

MHS
major histocompatibility system
malignant hypothermia susceptibility
multihospital system
multiple health screening

MHSA
microaggregated human serum albumin

MHST
multiphasic health screen test

MHT
meningohypophyseal trunk
mental health team
multiphasic health testing

MHTI
minor hypertensive infant

MHV
magnetic heart vector
Mahogany Hammock virus
middle hepatic vein
minimal height velocity
mouse hepatitis virus

MHVD
Marek herpesvirus disease

MHW
medial heel wedge
mental health worker

MHX
methohexital sodium

MHx
medical history

MhxR
medical history review

MHz
megahertz

MI
maturation index
meconium ileus
medical inspection
meiosis I
melanophore index
membrane intact
menstruation induction
mental illness
mental institution
mentally impaired
mercaptoimidazole
mesenteric ischemia
mesioincisal
metabolic index
metaproterenol inhaler
methyl indole

microsatellite instability
migration index
migration inhibition
mild irritant
mitotic index
mitral incompetence
mitral insufficiency
mononucleosis infectiosa
morphology index
motility index
myocardial infarct
myocardial infarction
myocardial ischemia
myoinositol

M&I
maternal and infant (care)

mi
mile

MIA
medically indigent adult
missing in action
multiinstitutional arrangement
multiple intracranial aneurysms

MIAA
microaggregated albumin (*See also* MAA)

MIAP
modified innervated antral pouch

MIBB
minimally invasive breast biopsy

MIBE
measles inclusion body encephalitis

MIBG, mIBG
metaiodobenzylguanidine
metaiodobenzyl-guanidine

MIBI
methoxyisobutyl isonitrile
methoxyisobutylisonitrile

MIBI-SPECT
methoxyisobutyl isonitrile single-photon emission computed tomography

MIBK
methylisobutyl ketone

MIC
maternal and infant care
mean intercriterion correlation
medical intensive care
methacholine inhalation challenge
microcytic erythrocyte
microscope
microscopic

minimal inhibitory concentration
minimal isorrheic concentration
minimum inhibitory concentration
mobile intensive care
model immune complex

MiC
minocycline

MICA
mentally ill chemical abuser
mirror-image complementary antibody

MICABG
minimally invasive coronary bypass grafting

MICG
macromolecular insoluble cold globulin

MICN
mobile intensive care nurse

MICR
methacholine inhalation challenge response

micro
microcyte
microcytic
microscopic

µA
microampere

µbar
microbar

microbiol
microbiological
microbiology

µC
microcoulomb

µCi
microcurie

µCi-hr
microcurie-hour

µ Eq
microequivalent

µg
microgram (*See also* mcg)

µγ
microgamma

µg/kg
microgram per kilogram

µg/L
microgram per liter

µGy
microgray

M

NOTES

μH
microhenry

μin
microinch

μkat
microkatal (micro-moles/sec)

μL
microliter (*See also* λ, mcL)

μM
micromolar

μm
micrometer
micromilli-

μm³
cubic micrometer

μmHg
micrometer of mercury

μμ
micromicro-
micromicron

μmm
micromillimeter (nanometer)

μmol, mcmol
micromole

μmol/L
micromolar

μΩ
microhm

μOsm
micro-osmolar

μR
microroentgen

μs
microsecond (*See also* μsec)

μU
microunit

μV
microvolt

μW
microwatt

MICS
minimally invasive cardiac surgery
Mother/Infant Communication
Screening

MICU
medical intensive care unit
mobile intensive care unit

MID
maximum inhibiting dilution
maximum inhibiting duration
maximum interincisal distance
mesioincisodistal
microvillus inclusion disease
midazolam
minimal infecting dose
minimal infective dose
minimal inhibitory dilution
minimal inhibitory dose
minimal irradiation dose
minimum infective dose
Modular Internal Distraction
(orthopedics)
multiinfarct dementia
multiple ion detection

mid
middle
midposition

mid/3
middle third (of long bone)

MIDA
mass isotopomer distribution
analysis

MIDAS
microphthalmia, dermal aplasia,
sclerocornea syndrome
Migraine Disability Assessment
Scale

MIDCAB
minimally invasive direct coronary
artery bypass

MIDCABG
minimally invasive direct coronary
artery bypass graft

MIDD
maternally inherited diabetes and
deafness

MID EPIS
midline episiotomy

MIDI
Microbial Identification System

Mid I
middle insomnia

midsag
midsagittal

MIE
maximim inspiratory effort
meconium ileus equivalent
medical improvement expected
methylisoeugenol

MIEI
medication-induced esophageal
injury

MIF
macrophage-inhibiting factor
maximum inspiratory flow
mean inspiratory flow
melanocyte-inhibiting factor
merthiolate, iodine, formaldehyde
(method)
merthiolate, iodine, formalin
(solution)
methylene-iodine-formalin
microimmunofluorescence (test)
midinspiratory flow
mifepristone (RU 486; Mifeprex)
migration-inhibiting factor

migration-inhibitory factor
mixed immunofluorescence
müllerian-inhibiting factor

MIFC

merthiolate, iodine, formaldehyde
concentration
minimally invasive follicular
carcinoma

MIFR

maximal inspiratory flow rate
midinspiratory flow rate

MIFT

merthiolate, iodine, formaldehyde
technique

MIF 50%VC

midinspiratory flow at 50% of
vital capacity

MIg

malaria immunoglobulin
measles immunoglobulin
membrane immunoglobulin

MIGB

metaiodobenzylguanidine

MIGET

multiple inert gas elimination
technique

MIGW

maximal increment in growth and
weight

MIH

medication-induced headache
melanotropin release-inhibiting
hormone
methylhydrazine
methylisopropylbenzamide
migraine with interparoxysmal
headache
minimal intermittent (dosage of)
heparin
monoiodohistidine
müllerian-inhibiting hormone
müllerian inhibitory hormone
myointimal hyperplasia

MIHR

magnetically influenced homeopathic
remedy

MII

McDowell Impairment Index
meiosis II

Mik

Mikulicz (disease, clamp)

MIKA

minor karyotype abnormality

MIKE

mass-analyzed ion kinetic energy

MIL

mesial incisal lingual (surface)
military
mother-in-law (*See also* M/L)

MILMD

Management Inventory on
Leadership, Motivation and
Decision-Making

MILP

mitogen-induced lymphocyte
proliferation

MILS

medication information leaflet for
seniors

MILTA

mucosal intact laser tonsillar
ablation

MIM

Mendelian Inheritance in Man

MIMCU

medical intermediate care unit

MIME

mean indices of meal excursions

MIMIC

multivane intensity modulation
compensator

MIMS

Medical Information Management
System
Medical Inventory Management
System

MIMV

Maferr Inventory of Masculine
Values

MIMyCA

maternally inherited myopathy and
cardiomyopathy

MIN

mammary intraepithelial neoplasia
medial interlaminar nucleus
melanocytic intraepidermal neoplasia
microsatellite instability
mineral (*See also* min)
minimal (*See also* min)
minimum (*See also* min, M)
minor (*See also* min)
minute (*See also* min, M, m)
multiple intestinal neoplasia

M

NOTES

min

mineral (*See also* MIN)
minimal (*See also* MIN)
minim (pharmacology)
minimum (*See also* MIN, M)
minor (*See also* MIN)
minute (*See also* MIN, M, m)

MINA

monoisonitrosoacetone

MIN A

minimal assistance (assist)

Mincep

Minnesota Comprehensive Epilepsy Program

MINE

medical improvement not expected

MINI

Mini International Neuropsychiatric Interview

MINIA

monkey intranuclear inclusion agent

mini-allo

allographic stem cell transplant

mini-FES

mini functional endoscopic sinus

minilap, mini-lap

minilaparotomy

mini-MUD

matched unrelated donor stem cell transplant

MINV

Minnal virus

MIO

minimal identifiable odor
monocular indirect ophthalmoscopy

MION

monocrystalline iron oxides

MIP

macrophage inflammatory protein
maximal inspiratory pressure
maximum inspiratory pressure
maximum-intensity pixel
maximum-intensity projection (radiology)
mean intrathoracic pressure
mean intravascular pressure
medical improvement possible
megameatus-intact prepuce
membrane integral protein
metacarpointerphalangeal
minimal inspiratory pressure
minimally invasive procedure

MIP-1

macrophage inflammatory protein-1

mip

macrophage infectivity potentiator

MIP-1 alpha, MIP-1-alpha

macrophage inflammatory protein alpha-1

MIP-1-beta

macrophage inflammatory protein-1-beta

MIPcor

coronal maximum-intensity projection
coronary maximum-intensity projection

MIPI

mean interpotential interval

MIPS

myocardial isotopic perfusion scan

MIQ

Minnesota Importance Questionnaire

MIR

multiple isomorphous replacement

MIRBI

Mini Inventory of Right Brain Injury

MIRD

medical internal radiation dose
medical internal radiation dosimetry

MIRF

macrophage immunogenic antigen-recruiting factor

MIRI

myocardial infarction recovery index

MIRP

myocardial infarction rehabilitation program

MIRS

Medical Improvement Review Standard

MIRU

myocardial infarction research unit

MIRV

Mirim virus

MIS

macrophage inflammatory protein
management information system
Medical Information Service
meiosis-inducing substance
melanoma in situ
microbial identification system
minimally invasive surgery
minimum incision surgery
mitral insufficiency
moderate intermittent suction
müllerian-inhibiting substance

Mis Astig

mixed astigmatism

misc

miscarriage
miscellaneous

M Isch
    myocardial ischemia
MISG
    modified immune serum globulin
MISH
    multiple in situ hybridization
MISHAP
    microcephalus, imperforate (anus),
    syndactyly, hamartoblastoma,
    abnormal (lung lobulation),
    polydactyly
MISO
    misonidazole
MISS
    minimally invasive spine surgery
    modified injury severity score
    (scale)
MISSGP
    mercury in Silastic strain gauge
    plethysmography
MIST
    Medical Information Service by
    Telephone
    minimally invasive surgical
    technique
MIT
    male impotence test
    marrow iron turnover
    mean input time
    meconium in trachea
    melodic intonation therapy
    metabolism inhibition test
    migration inhibition test
    miracidial immobilization test
    monoiodinated tyrosine
    monoiodotyrosine
    3-monoiodotyrosine
    Motor Impersistence Test
    multiple injection therapy (of
    insulin)
mit
    mitral
MITGCN
    malignant intratubular germ-cell
    neoplasia
MITI
    myocardial infarction triage and
    intervention
mit insuf
    mitral insufficiency
MITOX
    mitoxantrone

MIU
    million international units
mIU
    milli-International unit (one-
    thousandth of an International
    Unit)
MIV
    major injury vector
MIVA
    mivacurium
MIVAP
    minimally invasive video-assisted
    parathyroidectomy
MIVOD
    mesenteric inflammatory
    venoocclusive disease
MIVR
    minimally invasive valve repair
    minimally invasive valve
    replacement
MIW
    mental inquest warrant
MIX
    methylisobutylxanthine
mix.
    mixture (*See also* mixt)
mix. mon
    mixed monitor
mixt
    mixture (*See also* mix.)
MJ
    Machado-Joseph (disease)
    marijuana (*See also* POT)
    megajoule
mJ
    millijoule
MJA
    mechanical joint apparatus
MJAD
    Machado-Joseph Azorean disease
MJD
    Machado-Joseph disease
MJDQ
    Minnesota Job Description
    Questionnaire
MJL
    medial joint line
MJS
    medial joint space
MJT
    Mead Johnson tube
    Mowlem-Jackson technique

M

NOTES

MK
marked
menaquinone (vitamin K_2)
monkey kidney (*See also* MkK)
myokinase

M-K
McCarey-Kaufman (medium)

MK-6
menaquinone-6
vitamin K_2

MK-7
menaquinone-7

MK-639
indinavir

Mk
monkey

MKAB
may keep at bedside

MKAS
Meyer-Kendall Assessment Survey

mkat
millikatal

mkat/L
millikatal per liter

MKB
married, keeping baby
megakaryoblast

MKC
monkey kidney cell

MK-CSF
megakaryocyte colony-stimulating factor

mkg
meter-kilogram

MKHS
Menkes kinky hair syndrome

MKI
mitosis-karyorrhexis index
mitotic-karyorrhexis index

MkK
monkey kidney (*See also* MK)

MKM
microgram per kilogram per minute
myopic keratomileusis

MKP
monobasic potassium phosphate

MKS, mks
meter-kilogram-second

MKSAP
Medical Knowledge Self-Assessment Program

MKTC
monkey kidney tissue culture

MKV
killed measles vaccine

M-L
Martin-Lewis (medium)

ML
malignant lymph
malignant lymphoma
marked latency
maximal left
mediolateral
meningeal leukemia
mesiolingual
middle lobe
midline
molecular layer
monocytoid lymphocyte
motor latency
mucolipidosis
multiple lentiginosis
muscular layer
myeloid leukemia

ML2, ML-II
mucolipidosis type II

ML3, ML-III
mucolipidosis type III

ML4, ML-IV
mucolipidosis, type IV

M/L
mediolateral
monocyte/lymphocyte (ratio) (*See also* M:L)
mother-in-law (*See also* MIL)

M:L
maltase to lactase (ratio)
monocyte-lymphocyte ratio (*See also* M/L)

mL
millilambert
milliliter

ml
midline

MLA
left mentoanterior (fetal position) [L. *mento-laeva anterior*]
medical laboratory assay
medium long-acting
mesiolabial (*See also* MLa)
monocytic leukemia, acute
multilanguage aphasia

MLa
mesiolabial (*See also* MLA)

mLa
acute monocytic leukemia (*See also* AML, AMOL)

MLAB
Multilingual Aphasia Battery

MLAC
minimum local analgesic concentration

MLAI, MLaI
mesiolabioincisal

MLAP
    mean left atrial pressure
MLaP
    mesiolabiopulpal
MLB
    monaural loudness balance (test)
MLb
    macrolymphoblast
MLBP
    mechanical low back pain
MLBW
    moderately low birth weight
MLC
    chronic myelomonocytic leukemia
    Marginal Line Calculus (Index)
    mesiolingual cusp
    metastatic liver cancer
    minimal lethal concentration
    minimum lethal concentration
    mixed leukocyte concentration
    mixed leukocyte culture
    mixed ligand chelate
    mixed lymphocyte concentration
    mixed lymphocyte culture
    morphine-like compound
    multilamellar cytosome
    multileaf collimator
    multilevel care
    multilumen catheter
    myelomonocytic leukemia, chronic
    myosin light chain
MLCI
    marginal line calculus index
MLCK
    MLC kinase
    myosin light-chain kinase
MLCN
    multilocular cystic nephroma
MLCP
    myosin light-chain phosphatase
MLCR
    mesiolingual cusp ridge
    mixed lymphocyte culture reaction
MLCT
    metal-to-ligand charge transfer
ML-CVP
    multilumen central venous pressure
MLCW
    mixed lymphocyte culture, weak
MLD
    manual lymph drainage
    masking level difference

    median lethal dose (*See also* MLD_{50})
    melioidosis (*Pseudomonas pseudomallei*) vaccine
    metachromatic leukodystrophy
    microlumbar diskectomy
    microsurgical lumbar diskectomy
    minimal lesion disease
    minimal lethal dose (*See also* mld)
    minimum lethal dose
    minimum lumen diameter
MLD_{50}
    median lethal dose (*See also* MLD)
mld
    minimal lethal dose (*See also* MLD)
MLDG
    mesiolingual developmental groove
mL/dL
    milliliter per deciliter
MLE
    maximal likelihood estimation
MLEE
    multilocus enzyme electrophoresis
MLEpis
    mediolateral episiotomy
    midline episiotomy
MLF
    medial longitudinal fasciculus
    mesiolingual fossa
    morphine-like factor
MLG
    mesiolingual groove
    mitochondria lipid glucogen
MLGN
    minimal lesion glomerulonephritis
ML-H
    malignant lymphoma, histiocytic
MLH
    multiple lobar hemorrhage
MLI
    mesiolinguoincisal
    mixed lymphocyte interaction
    motilin-like immunoreactivity
mL/kg
    milliliter per kilogram
MLL
    malignant lymphoma, lymphoblastic (type)
    mixed lineage leukemia
mL/L
    milliliters per liter

M

NOTES

mL/min
milliliters per minute

MLN
manifest latent nystagmus
melanoma vaccine
membranous lupus nephropathy
mesenteric lymph node

MLNS
minimal lesions nephrotic syndrome
mucocutaneous lymph node
syndrome

MLO
mediolateral oblique
mesiolinguo-occlusal

MLP
left mentoposterior (fetal position)
[L. *mento-laeva posterior*] (*See
also* LMP)
mesiolinguopulpal
microsomal lipoprotein
midlevel provider
multiple lymphomatous polyposis

ML-PCR
mixed-linker PCR

MLPD
malignant lymphocytic proliferation
disease

ML-PDL
malignant lymphoma, poorly
differentiated lymphocytic

MLPP
maximum loose-packed position

MLQ
Multifactor Leadership Questionnaire

MLR
major liver resection
mean length of response
middle latency response
mixed leukocyte reaction
mixed leukocyte response
mixed lymphocyte reaction
mixed lymphocyte response
multiple logistic regression
myocardial laser revascularization

MLRA
multiple linear regression analysis

mlRNA
messenger-like RNA

MLS
macrolides, lincosamides, and
streptogramins
Maroteaux-Lamy syndrome
maximum likelihood score
mean life span
median life span
median longitudinal section
mediastinal B-cell lymphoma with
sclerosis

microphthalmia with linear skin
defects
middle lobe syndrome
mini lag screw system
mucolipidoses
multiple line scan
myelomonocytic leukemia, subacute

mL/sec
milliliters per second

MLSI
multiple line-scan imaging

MLST
multilocus sequence typing

MLT
mean latency time
median lethal time
melatonin

MLTC
mixed leukocyte-trophoblast culture

MLTI
mixed lymphocyte target interaction

MLU
mean length of utterance

MLUm
mean length of utterance in
morphemes

MLV
Moloney leukemogenic virus
monitored live voice
Mono Lake virus
mouse leukemia virus
multilaminar vesicle
murine leukemia virus

MLVDP
maximal left ventricular developed
pressure

MLWHF
Minnesota Living with Heart
Failure (questionnaire)

mlx
millilux

MM
macromolecule
major medical (insurance)
malignant melanoma
malignant mesothelioma
manubrium of malleus
Marshall-Marchetti (procedure for
urinary incontinence)
measuring-mounting
medial malleolus
megamitochondria
melanoma metastasis
member months
meningococcic meningitis
metastatic melanoma
methadone maintenance
micrometastases

middle molecule
milk and molasses (*See also* M&M)
minimal medium
mismatch
mist mask
modified Miller maneuver
morbidity and mortality (*See also* M&M)
motor meal
mucous membrane
Muller maneuver
multiple myeloma
muscle movement
muscles (*See also* mm)
muscularis mucosae
mycophenolate mofetil
myeloid metaplasia
myelomeningocele

M1 to M7
categories of acute nonlymphoblastic leukemia

M&M
milk and molasses (*See also* MM)
morbidity and mortality (*See also* MM)

Mm
mandible mentum

mM
millimolar
millimole (*See also* mmol)

mm
methylmalonyl
millimeter
mucous membrane
murmur
muscles (*See also* MM)

mm²
square millimeter

mm³
cubic millimeter (*See also* cmm, cu mm)

MMI
maternal meiosis I

MMII, MM2
maternal meiosis II

MMA
mastitis, metritis, agalactia (syndrome)
maxillomandibular advancement
medical materials account
methylmalonic acid

methylmalonic aciduria
methylmercuric acetate
methyl methacrylate (*See also* MEMA)
monocyte monolayer assay
monomethylarsonic acid

MMAA
mini-microaggregated albumin colloid

MMAD
mass median aerodynamic diameter

MMAT
Minnesota Mechanical Assembly Test

MMATP
methadone maintenance and aftercare treatment program

MMC
migrating motor complex
migrating myoelectric complex
minimal medullary concentration
mucosal mast cell
murine mesangial cell
myelomeningocele

mMCAI
malignant middle cerebral artery infarction

MMD
intramural microvessel density
malignant metastatic disease
mass median aerodynamic diameter
mass median diameter (of particles)
mean marrow dose
minimal morbidostatic dose
mucus membranes dry
myotonic muscular dystrophy (*See also* MyMD)

MMDA
5-methoxy-3,4-methylenedioxyamphetamine
methyoxymethylene dioxyamphetamine

MMDG
mesial marginal developmental groove

MME
malignant myoepithelioma
M-mode echocardiography
mouse mammary epithelium

MMECT
multimonitored electroconvulsive treatment

NOTES

M

MMECT *(continued)*
  multiple monitored electroconvulsive therapy

MMEF
  maximal midexpiratory flow (*See also* MMF)

MMEFR
  maximal midexpiratory flow rate (*See also* MMFR)

MMEP
  microcephaly, microphthalmia, ectrodactyly, prognathism syndrome

MMF
  magnetomotive force
  mandibulomaxillary fixation
  maxillomandibular fixation
  maximal midexpiratory flow (*See also* MMEF)
  mean maximal flow
  mycophenolate mofetil

MMFG
  mouse milk fat globule

MMFR
  maximal midexpiratory flow rate (*See also* MMEFR)
  maximal midflow rate
  maximum midexpiratory flow rate

MMFV
  maximal midexpiratory flow volume

MMG
  mean maternal glucose
  mechanomyography

MMH
  Marino, Muller-Hermelink
  monomethylhydrazine

mmHg
  millimeters of mercury

mmH$_2$O
  millimeters of water

MMI, MM1
  macrophage migration index
  macrophage migration inhibition
  maximal medical improvement
  medial medullary infarction
  methimazole
  methylmercaptoimidazole

mμ
  millimicron

MMIH
  megacystis, microcolon, intestinal hypoperistalsis

MMIHS
  megacystis-microcolon-intestinal hypoperistalsis syndrome

MMK
  Marshall-Marchetti-Krantz (cystourethropexy)

MML
  monomethyllysine
  myelomonocytic leukemia

mM/L
  millimoles per liter (*See also* mmol/L)

MMLV
  Moloney murine leukemia virus
  Montana myotis leukoencephalitis virus

MMM
  microsome-mediated mutagenesis
  mucous membranes moist
  myelofibrosis with myeloid metaplasia
  myeloid metaplasia with myelofibrosis
  myelosclerosis with myeloid metaplasia

mmm
  micromillimeter
  millimicron

MMMF
  man-made mineral fiber

MMMM
  megalocornea, macrocephaly, mental and motor retardation syndrome

mMMSE
  modified version of the mini mental status examination

MMMT
  malignant mixed mesodermal tumor
  malignant mixed müllerian tumor
  metastatic mixed müllerian tumor

MMN
  mismatch negativity
  morbus maculosus neonatorum
  multifocal motor neuropathy
  multiple mucosal neuroma

MMNC
  marrow mononuclear cell

MMO
  maxillomandibular osteotomy
  maximal mouth opening
  methane monooxygenase

MMOA
  maxillary mandibular odentectomy alveolectomy

M-mode
  motion mode
  time-motion mode

MMoL
  myelomonoblastic leukemia

mmol
  millimole (*See also* mM)

mmol/L
  millimole per liter

millimoles per liter (*See also* mM/L)

MMP

matrix metalloprotease

matrix metalloproteinase

multiple medical problems

MMP-2

matrix metalloproteinase-2

MMP-3

matrix metalloproteinase-3

MMP-7

matrix metalloproteinase-7

MMP-8

matrix metalloproteinase-8

MMP-9

matrix metalloproteinase-9

MMP-10

matrix metalloproteinase-10

MMP-12

matrix metalloproteinase-12

MMPC

metastatic malignant pheochromocytoma

MMPI

matrix metalloproteinase inhibitor

McGill-Melzack Pain Index

Minnesota Multiphasic Personality Inventory

MMPI-2

Minnesota Multiphasic Personality Inventory, Second Edition

MMPI-A

Minnesota Multiphasic Personality Inventory-Adolescent

MMPI-Adolescent

MMPI-D

Minnesota Multiphasic Personality Inventory Depression (Scale)

mmpp

millimeters partial pressure

MMPR

methylmercaptopurine riboside

6-MMPR

6-methylmercaptopurine riboside

mm-PTH

mid-molecule parathyroid hormone

MMR

mass miniature radiography

mass miniature roentgenography

maternal mortality rate

measles-mumps-rubella (vaccine)

megalocornea-mental retardation syndrome

meningitis or encephalitis, metabolic, Reye (syndrome)

mesial marginal ridge

midline malignant reticulosis

mild mental retardation

mismatch repair

mobile mass x-ray

mortality rate ratio

mutation mismatch repair

myocardial metabolic rate

MMRSA

mupirocin-resistant, methicillin-resistant *Staphylococcus aureus*

MMS

Maloney murine sarcoma

methyl methanesulfonate

mixed mesodermal sarcoma

Mohs micrographic surgery

MMSE

Mini Mental State Examination

mm/sec

millimeters per second

mm st

muscle strength

MMT

malignant mesenchymal tumor

manual muscle test

manual muscle testing

methadone maintenance treatment

microcephaly, mesobrachyphalangy, tracheoesophageal (fistula syndrome)

mixed müllerian tumor

mouse mammary tumor

MMTA

methylmetatyramine

MMTIC

Murphy-Meisgeier Type Indicator for Children

MMTP

methadone maintenance treatment program

MMTT

Multicenter Myocarditis Treatment Trial

MMTV

malignant mesothelioma of the tunica vaginalis

monomorphic ventricular tachycardia

mouse mammary tumor virus

M

NOTES

MMU
medical maintenance unit
mercaptomethyl uracil

mmu
millimass unit

MMUA
macromolecular uronate

mμc
millimicrocurie

mμg
millimicrogram

mμs
millimicrosecond

MMV
mandatory minute ventilation
mandatory minute volume

MMVF
manmade vitreous fiber

MMWR
Morbidity and Mortality Weekly
Report

MMY
Mental Measurements Yearbook

MN
blood group in MNS blood group
system
malignant nephrosclerosis
median nerve
meganewton
melanocytic nevus
melena neonatorum
membranous nephropathy
membranous neuropathy
mesenteric node
metanephrine
midnight (*See also* M/N, mn)
mononuclear
motor neuron
mucosal neurolysis
multinodular
myoneural

M/N
macrocytic/normochromic (anemia)
microcytic/normochromic (anemia)
midnight (*See also* MN, mn)

M&N
morning and night

Mn
manganese

mN
micronewton
millinormal

mn
midnight (*See also* MN, M/N)

MNA
maximal noise area

MNAP
mixed nerve action potential

MNB
monomicrobial nonneutrocytic
bacterascites
murine neuroblastoma

MNBCC
multiple nevoid-basal cell
carcinoma

MNC
monomicrobial necrotizing cellulitis
mononuclear cell
mononuclear leukocyte (*See also*
MNL)

MNCV
motor nerve conduction velocity

MND
minimal necrosing dose
minor neurologic dysfunction
modified neck dissection
motor neuron disease

MNE
monosymptomatic nocturnal enuresis

MNF
myelinated nerve fiber

MNG
multinodular goiter

mng
morning

MNGIE
mitochondrial neurogastrointestinal
encephalomyopathy
myoneuro-gastrointestinal
encephalopathy

MNHL
mixed large- and small-cell non-
Hodgkin lymphoma

MNJ
myoneural junction

MNL
maximal number of lamellae
mononuclear leukocyte (*See also*
MNC)

MNM
mononeuritis multiplex

MN/m²
meganewton per square meter

MNMCB
motor neuropathy with multifocal
conduction block

MNMK
maximal number of microbes killed

MNMS
myonephropathic metabolic
syndrome

MNNB
Monas-Nitz Neuropsychological
Battery

MNO
minocycline

MNOE
malignant necrotizing otitis externa
MNP
mononuclear phagocyte
MNPA
methoxynaphthyl propionic acid
MNPRT
mixed neutron and photon
radiotherapy
MNPV
multiple nucleopolyhedrovirus
MNR
marrow neutrophil reserve
MNS
blood group system consisting of
groups M, N, and MN
medial nuclear stratum
microamperage neural stimulation
a minor blood group
MNSER
mean normalized systolic ejection
rate
Mn-SOD
manganese superoxide dismutase
MnSSEP
median nerve somatosensory evoked
potential
MNTB
medial nucleus of trapezoid body
MNTI
melanotic neuroectodermal tumor of
infancy
Mn-TPPS$_4$
manganese tetrasodium-meso-tetra
MNTV
Minatitlan virus
MNU
methylnitrosourea
MNX
meniscectomy
MNZ
metronidazole
MO
manually operated
medial oblique (x-ray view)
medical officer
menhaden oil
mesioocclusal
mineral oil
minute output
mitral orifice
molecular orbital

monooxygenase
month (*See also* M, mo, mon)
months old (*See also* mo)
morbidly obese
mother (*See also* M, MOM, MTR)
myositis ossificans
sulfamethoxine
MO$_2$
myocardial oxygen consumption
Mo
mode
Moloney (strain)
molybdenum
monoclonal
^{99}Mo
molybdenum-99
mo
mode
month (*See also* M, MO, mon)
months old (*See also* MO)
MOA
mechanism of action
medical office assistant
metronidazole, omeprazole,
amoxicillin
monoamine oxidase
MoAb
monoclonal antibody (*See also* MA,
MAB, MAb, MCA, MCAB)
MOAHI
mixed obstructive apnea and
hypopnea index
MOB
medical office building
mob, mobil
mobility
mobilization
MOBV
Mobala virus
MOC
maximal oxygen consumption
medial olivocochlear
metronidazole, omeprazole, and
clarithromycin
mother of child
multiple ocular coloboma
MOCI
Maudsley Obsessional Compulsive
Inventory
MoCM
molybdenum-conditioned medium

M

NOTES

MOCS-III
    Minnesota Occupational
    Classification System
MOD
    maturity-onset diabetes (*See also*
        MODM)
    mean optical density
    mesial, occlusal, distal
    mesioocclusodistal
    mode of death
    moderate (*See also* mod)
    moment of death
    Multi-Operatory Dentalaser
    multiorgan dysfunction
    multiple organ dysfunction
mod
    moderate (*See also* MOD)
    moderation
    modification
    modulation
    module
MOD A
    moderate assistance (assist)
MODED
    microcephaly, oculodigital,
        esophageal, duodenal syndrome
modem
    modulator/demodulator
MODM
    maturity-onset diabetes mellitus
        (*See also* MOD)
MODS
    multiorgan dysfunction syndrome
    multiple organ dysfunction
        syndrome
MODY
    maturity-onset diabetes in the
        young
    maturity-onset diabetes of youth
MOE
    movement of extremities
MOF
    marine oxidation/fermentation
    mesial occlusal facial
    methoxyflurane
    multiorgan failure
    multiple organ failure
MOFS
    multiple-organ failure syndrome
MOG
    myelin-oligodendrocyte glycoprotein
MOI
    maximal oxygen intake
    mechanism of injury
    medical optimal imaging
    multiplicities of infection
MoICU
    mobile intensive care unit

MOIOD
    medial osseous interorbital distance
MOIVC
    membranous obstruction of the
        inferior vena cava
MOJAC
    mood, orientation, judgment, affect,
        content
MOJUV
    Moju virus
MOL
    molecular layer
mol
    mole
    molecular
    molecule
molc
    molar concentration
MOLDR
    mathematical optimization and
        logical dimensioning for
        radiotherapy
molfr
    mole fraction
mol/kg
    mole per kilogram
mol/L
    mole per liter
mol/m³
    mole per cubic meter
mol/s
    mole per second
mol wt
    molecular weight (*See also* MW,
        MWt)
MOM
    milk of magnesia
    mother (*See also* M, MO, MTR)
    mucoid otitis media
    multiples of median
M.O.M.
    mouse-on-mouse
MoM, mom
    multiples of the appropriate
        gestational median
MOMA
    methoxyhydroxymandelic acid
    methylhydroxymandelic acid
MOMO
    macrosomia, obesity, macrocephaly,
        ocular abnormality (syndrome)
MOMP
    major outer membrane protein
MOMS
    multiple organ malrotation
        syndrome
MoMSV
    Moloney murine sarcoma virus

MoMuLV
Moloney murine leukemia virus
(*See also* MML, MMLV)

MOMX
macroorchidism marker X

MON
maximum observation nursery
modifier of Min
Mongolian (gerbil)
monitor

mon
month (*See also* M, MO, mo)

MONO, mono
mononucleosis (*See also* mono)
Monospot (test)

mono, di
monochorionic, diamniotic (twins)

mono, mono
monochorionic, monoamniotic
(twins)

monos
monocytes

MOP
major organ profile
medical outpatient
medical outpatient program

5-MOP
5-methoxypsoralen

8-MOP
8-methoxypsoralen

MOPV
monovalent oral polio virus
vaccine

MOR
morphine (*See also* morph)

MORA
mandibular orthopedic repositioning
appliance

MORD
magnetic optical rotatory dispersion

MORFAN
mental (retardation), overgrowth,
remarkable face, and acanthosis
nigrans

morph
morphine (*See also* MOR)
morphological (*See also* morphol)
morphology (*See also* morphol)

morphol
morphological (*See also* morph)
morphology (*See also* morph)

mortal.
mortality

MORV
Moriche virus

MOS
medial orbital sulcus
medical optical spectroscopy
mirror optical system
missed ostium sequence
mitral opening snap
myelofibrosis osteosclerosis

mos
months

MOSD
multiple organ system dysfunction

MOSF
multiple organ system failure

MOSFET
metal oxide semiconductor field
effect transistor

mOsm, MOsm, mOsmol
milliosmole

mOsm/kg, mosm/kg
milliosmoles per kilogram

MOSP
myelin/oligodendrocyte-specific
protein

MOST
manual organ stimulation technique
Modern Occupational Skills Test

MOSV
Mossuril virus

MOT
mini object test
motility (examination)
mouse ovarian tumor

MOTS
mucosal oral therapeutic system

MOTSA
multiple overlapping thin-slab
acquisition

MOTT
mycobacteria other than
Mycobacterium tuberculosis
mycobacteria other than tuberculosis

MOU
medical oncology unit
memorandum of understanding

MOUS
multiple occurrence of unexplained
symptoms

M

NOTES

501

MOV
  minimum obstructive volume
  multiple oral vitamin
MOVC
  membranous obstruction (of
    inferior) vena cava
MOW
  Meals on Wheels
MOX
  moxalactam
MP
  machine preservation
  macrophage
  malignant pyoderma
  matrix protein
  mean pressure
  mechanical percussion
  mechanical percussor
  medial plantar
  membrane potential
  menstrual period
  mentoposterior (position)
  mentum posterior (fetal position)
  mesenteric panniculitis
  mesial pit
  mesiopulpal
  metacarpophalangeal (*See also* MCP)
  metatarsophalangeal (joint) (*See also*
    MTP, MTPJ)
  methylprednisolone (*See also* MPS)
  microfibrillar protein
  minimal pigment
  modulator protein
  moist pack
  monitor pattern
  monophasic
  monophosphate
  motor potential
  mouthpiece
  mouth pressure
  mucopolysaccharide (*See also* MPS)
  multiparous
  muscle potential
  mycoplasmal pneumonia
  myocardial perfusion
4MP4
  methylpyrazole
mp
  melting point
  millipond
MPA
  main pulmonary artery
  medial preoptic area
  medroxyprogesterone acetate
  metatarsus primus adductus
  methylprednisolone acetate
  microscopic polyangiitis
  microstomia prevention appliance

  minor physical anomaly
  mycophenolic acid
MPa
  megapascal
MPAA
  male pattern androgenetic alopecia
MPAC
  Memorial Pain Assessment Card
MPAP
  mean pulmonary artery pressure
  multipurpose access port
MPAPC
  mucus-producing adenopapillary
    carcinoma
MPAQ
  McGill Pain Assessment
    Questionnaire
MPAWP
  mean pulmonary artery wedge
    pressure
MPB
  male pattern baldness
  mephobarbital
  meprobamate
  modified piggyback
MPBFV
  mean pulmonary-blood-flow velocity
MPBNS
  modified Peyronie bladder neck
    suspension
MPC
  marine protein concentrate
  maximal permissible concentration
  maximum permissible concentration
  metallophthalocyanine
  micropapillary component
  minimal mycoplasmacidal
    concentration
  minimal protozoacidal concentration
  minimum mycoplasmacidal
    concentration
  Mooney Problem Checklist
  mucopurulent cervicitis
  myeloblast-promyelocyte
    compartment
MPCD
  minimal perceptible color difference
MPCh
  medial posterior choroidal
    (ophthalmology)
MPCN
  microscopically positive, culturally
    negative
MPCO
  micropolycystic ovary (syndrome)
MPCP
  mean pulmonary capillary pressure

M-PCR
multiplex polymerase chain reaction

MPCU
medical progressive care unit

MPCUR
maximal permissible concentration of unidentified radionuclides

MPCWP
mean pulmonary capillary wedge pressure

MPD
main pancreatic duct
main papillary duct
matched peripheral dose
maximal permissible dose
maximum permissible dose
mean population doubling
Measures of Psychosocial Development
membrane potential difference
minimal perceptible difference
minimal peripheral dose
minimal phototoxic dose
minimal popular dose
minimal port diameter
Minnesota Percepto-Diagnostic (Test) (*See also* MPDT)
multiplanar display
multiple personality disorder
myeloproliferative disease
myofascial pain-dysfunction

MPDS
mandibular pain dysfunction syndrome
myofascial pain dysfunction syndrome

MPDT
Minnesota Percepto-Diagnostic Test (*See also* MPD)

MPDW
mean percentage of desirable weight

MPE
malignant pleural effusion
maximal possible effect
maximal possible error
mean prediction error
multiphoton excitation

MPEAK
multipeak

MPEC
monopolar electrocoagulation
multipolar electrocoagulation

MPED
minimal phototoxic erythema dose

MPEG
methoxypolyethylene glycol

MPEH
methylphenylethylhydantoin

MPF
major proglucagon fragment
maturation-promoting factor
mean power frequency
methylparaben free
mitosis-promoting factor
myofascial pain syndrome

MPFBT
Minnesota Paper Form Board Test

MPFF
micronized purified flavonoid fracture

MPFL
medial patellofemoral ligament

MPFM
mini-Wright peak flow meter

MPG
magnetopneumography
malignant paraganglioma

MPGM
monophosphoglycerate mutase

MPGN
membranoproliferative glomerulonephritis (type I, II)
mesangiocapillary glomerulonephritis (type I, II)
mesangioproliferative glomerulonephritis

MPGR
multiplanar gradient recall
multiple planar gradient-recalled

MPH
male pseudohermaphroditism
mandibular plane to hyoid (*See also* MP-H)
massive pulmonary hemorrhage
methylphenidate
micronodular pneumocyte hyperplasia
midparental height
milk protein hydrolysate

M

NOTES

MP-H
>   mandibular plane to hyoid
>   (craniometric) (*See also* MPH)

mph
>   miles per hour

M phase
>   phase of mitosis in cell growth
>   cycle

MPHD
>   methoxyhydroxphenolglycerol
>   multiple pituitary hormone
>   deficiencies

MPHR
>   maximal predicted heart rate
>   maximum predicted heart rate

MPI
>   macrophage inflammatory protein
>   mannose phosphate isomerase
>   master patient index
>   Maudsley Personality Inventory
>   maximal permitted intake
>   maximal point of impulse
>   Multidimensional Pain Inventory
>   Multiphasic Personality Inventory
>   Multivariate Personality Inventory
>   myocardial perfusion imaging

MPIAS
>   multiparameter intraarterial sensor

MPIF-1
>   myeloid progenitor inhibitory
>   factor-1

M6P/IGF-2R
>   mannose-6-phosphate/IGF-2 receptor

MPI/MRI
>   myelofibrosis proliferation/regression
>   index

MPJ
>   metacarpophalangeal joint
>   metatarsophalangeal joint

mpk
>   milligram per kilogram (*See also*
>   mg/kg)

MPKV
>   Maprik virus

MPL
>   mesiopulpolabial (*See also* MPLA,
>   MPLa)
>   mesiopulpolingual (*See also* MPLA,
>   MPLa)

MP-L
>   midpapillary longitudinal

MPLA, MPLa
>   mesiopulpolabial (*See also* MPL)
>   mesiopulpolingual (*See also* MPL)

MPLC
>   medium pressure liquid
>   chromatography

MPL(r)
>   monophosphoryl lipid A

MPLV
>   myeloproliferative leukemia virus

MPM
>   malignant papillary mesothelioma
>   malignant pleural mesothelioma
>   medial pterygoid muscle
>   Mortality Probability Model
>   multiple primary malignancy
>   multiple primary melanoma
>   multipurpose meal
>   mycophenolate mofetil

MPMT
>   Murphy punch maneuver test

MPMV
>   Mason-Pfizer monkey virus

MPN
>   monthly progress note
>   most probable number
>   multiple primary neoplasms

MPNST
>   malignant peripheral nerve sheath
>   tumor

MPO
>   male pattern obesity
>   maximal power output
>   maximum power output
>   minimal perceptible odor
>   myeloperoxidase (bone marrow
>   stain)

MPOA
>   medial preoptic area

MPOS
>   myeloperoxidase system

MPP
>   massive periretinal proliferation
>   maximal perfusion pressure
>   maximal print position
>   maximum pressure picture
>   medial pterygoid plate
>   medical personnel pool
>   metacarpophalangeal profile
>   multiple presentation phenotype

MPPC
>   malignant primary
>   pheochromocytoma

mppcf
>   millions of particles per cubic foot
>   (of air)

MPPG
>   microphotoelectric plethysmography

MPPN
>   malignant persistent positional
>   nystagmus

MPPS
>   massive parallel processing system

MPPT
  methylprednisolone pulse therapy
MPPv
  main portal vein peak velocity
MPQ
  McGill Pain Questionnaire
  Multidimensional Personality
    Questionnaire
MPR
  mannose-6-phosphate receptor
  marrow production rate
  massive preretinal retraction
  maximal pulse rate
  myeloproliferative reaction
  myocardial perfusion reserve
MP-RAGE
  magnetization prepared-rapid
    gradient echo
MP-RAGE-WE
  magnetization-prepared rapid
    gradient echo-water excitation
MPRE
  minimal pure radium equivalent
MPRV
  Mapuera virus
MPR view
  multiplanar reformatting view
MPS
  Management Philosophies Scale (I-
    V)
  mean particle size
  methylprednisolone (*See also* MP)
  Michigan Picture Stories
  microbial profile system
  mononuclear phagocyte system
  Montreal platelet syndrome
  movement-produced stimulus
  mucopolysaccharide (*See also* MP)
  mucopolysaccharidoses (plural)
  mucopolysaccharidosis
  multiphasic screening
  myocardial perfusion scintigraphy
  myocardial protection system
  myofascial pain syndrome
MPS-I
  mucopolysaccharidosis I
MPS-IH
  mucopolysaccharidosis type I Hurler
MPS-IHS
  mucopolysaccharidosis type I
    Hurler-Scheie

MPS-IS
  mucopolysaccharidosis type I
    Scheie
MPS-II
  mucopolysaccharidosis type II
    Hunter
MPS-IIIA
  mucopolysaccharidosis type III
    Sanfilippo A
MPS-IIIB
  mucopolysaccharidosis type III
    Sanfilippo B
MPS-IIIC
  mucopolysaccharidosis type III
    Sanfilippo C
MPS-IV
  mucopolysaccharidosis type IV
    Morquio
MPS-VI
  mucopolysaccharidosis type VI
    Maroteaux-Lamy
MPS-VII
  mucopolysaccharidosis type VII Sly
mps
  meters per second
MPSC
  micropapillary serous carcinoma
MPSMT
  Merrill-Palmer Scale of Mental
    Tests
MPSRT
  matched pairs signed rank test
MPSS
  massively parallel signature
    sequencing
  methylprednisolone sodium succinate
  Mood and Physical Symptoms
    Scale
MPSV
  myeloproliferative sarcoma virus
MPT
  maximal predicted phonation time
  Michigan Picture Test
  multidisciplinary pain treatment
  multiple-parameter telemetry
  multiple-puncture test
  multipuncture test
MP-T
  midpapillary transverse

M

NOTES

MPTAH
> Mallory phosphotungstic acid hemotoxylin (stain)

MPTh
> mechanical pain threshold

MPTP
> methyl-phenyl-tetrahydropyridine
> N-methyl-4-phenyl-1,2,3,6-tetrahydropyridine

MPTR
> motor, pain, touch, reflex (deficit)

MPT-R
> Michigan Picture Test, Revised

MPTS
> minocycline periodontal therapeutic system

MPU
> maternal pediatric unit

MPV
> mean plasma volume
> mean platelet volume
> metatarsus primus varus
> mitral valve prolapse

mpz
> millipièze

MQ
> memory quotient
> menaquinone

MQC
> microbiologic quality control

MQOL-HIV
> multidimensional quality of life questionnaire for person with human immunodeficiency virus

MQOV
> Mosqueiro virus

MR
> Maddox rod
> magnetic resonance
> malar rash
> mandibular reflex
> manifest refraction
> mannose-resistant
> maximal right
> may repeat
> measles-rubella (vaccine)
> medial rectus (muscle)
> medial rotation
> median raphe
> medical record
> medical rehabilitation
> medication responder
> medium range
> megaroentgen
> menstrual regulation
> mentally retarded
> mental retardation
> mesencephalic raphe

> metabolic rate
> methemoglobin reductase (*See also* MHR, MR-E)
> methyl red
> milk ring
> mineralocorticoid receptor
> mitral reflux
> mitral regurgitation
> mixed respiratory
> moderate resistance
> modulation rate
> mortality rate
> mortality ratio
> motivation research
> multicentric reticulohistiocytosis
> multiplication rate
> multiplicity reactivation
> muscle receptor
> muscle relaxant
> myotactic reflex

MR2
> Microputor II

M&R
> measure and record

M$_r$, M_r
> molecular weight ratio
> relative molecular mass

Mr
> mandible ramus

mR
> milliroentgen

MRA
> magnetic resonance angiography
> magnetic resonance arteriography
> main renal artery
> marrow repopulation activity
> medical record administrator
> medical records administrator
> midright atrium
> multivariate regression analysis

MRAN
> medical resident admitting note

MRAP
> maximal resting anal pressure
> mean right atrial pressure

MRAr
> magnetic resonance arthrography

MRAS
> main renal artery stenosis

MRBC
> monkey red blood cell
> mouse red blood cell

MRBF
> mean renal blood flow

MRC
> magnetic resonance cholangiogram
> magnetic resonance cholangiography
> magnetic resonance colonography

maximal recycling capacity
medullary renal carcinoma
methylrosaniline chloride (gentian
violet, crystal violet)

MRCA
magnetic resonance coronary
angiography

MRCC
metastatic renal cell carcinoma

MRCNS
methicillin-resistant coagulase-
negative *Staphylococcus*

MRCP
magnetic resonance
cholangiopancreatography
mental retardation, cerebral palsy
movement-related cortical potential

MRCPs
movement-related cortical potentials

MRD
marginal reflex distance
margin reflex distance
matched related donor
mean reference diameter
medical records department
method of rapid determination
minimal reacting dose (*See also*
mrd)
Minimal Record of Disability
minimal renal disease
minimal residual disease

mrd
millirad
millirutherford
minimal reacting dose (*See also*
MRD)

MRDD
maximum recommended daily dose
mentally retarded and
developmentally disabled
Mental Retardation and
Development Disabilities

MRDM
malnutrition-related diabetes mellitus

MRE
magnetic resonance elastography
manual resistance exercise
maximal restrictive exercise
maximal risk estimate
most recent episode

MR-E
methemoglobin reductase (*See also*
MHR, MR)

MRELD
mixed receptive-expressive language
disorder

mrem
millirem
milliroentgen equivalent man

mrep
milliroentgen equivalent physical

MRF
magnetic resonance flowmetry
medical record file
melanocyte-releasing factor
melanocyte-stimulating factor
melanocyte-(stimulating hormone)-
releasing factor
mesencephalic reticular formation
midbrain reticular formation
mitral regurgitant flow
moderate renal failure
monoclonal rheumatoid factor
müllerian regression factor

mRF
monoclonal rheumatoid factor

MRFC
mouse rosette-forming cell

MRFT
modified rapid fermentation test

MRG
mean rejection grading
mean residual gap
median rhomboid glossitis
murmurs, rubs, and gallops

MRH
Maddox rod hyperphoria
melanocyte-releasing hormone
melanocyte(-stimulating hormone)-
releasing hormone
melanotropin-releasing hormone

MRHA
mannose-resistant hemagglutination

MRHD
maximal recommended human dose
maximum recommended human
dose

mrhm
milliroentgens per hour at one
meter

MRHT
modified rhyme hearing test

M

NOTES

MRI
machine-readable identifier
magnetic resonance imaging
medical records information
moderate renal insufficiency

MRIF
melanocyte release-inhibiting factor

MRIH
melanocyte release-inhibiting hormone

MRKHS
Mayer-Rokitansky-Küster-Hauser syndrome

MRL
medical research laboratory
minimal response level
moderate rubra lochia

MRLT
mesalamine-related lung toxicity

MRLVD
maximum residue limits of veterinary drugs

MRM
magnetic resonance mammography
modified radical mastectomy

MRN
magnetic resonance neurography
malignant renal neoplasm
medical record number
medical resident's note

mRNA
messenger ribonucleoprotein acid
messenger RNA

mRNP
messenger ribonucleoprotein

MRO
minimal recognizable odor
muscle receptor organ

MROU
medial rectus, both eyes

MRP
magnetic resonance pancreatography
mandibular reconstruction plate
maximal reimbursement point
maximum (anal) resting pressure
mean resting potential
medical reimbursement plan
multidrug resistance (associated) protein
multidrug resistance protein

MRPAH
mixed reverse passive antiglobulin hemagglutination

MRPN
medical resident progress note

MRR
marrow release rate

maximal relation rate
maximal relaxation rate

MRS
magnetic resonance spectroscopy
mania rating scale
median range score
medical receiving station
mental retardation syndrome
methicillin-resistant *Stapylococcus*

MRSA
methicillin-resistant *Staphylococcus aureus*

MRSD
mental retardation, skeletal dysplasia, abducens palsy (syndrome)

MRSE
methicillin-resistant *Staphylococcus epidermidis*

MRSI
magnetic resonance spectroscopic imaging

MRSS
methicillin-resistant *Staphylococcus* species

MRT
magnetic resonance tomography
major role therapy
malignant rhabdoid tumor
mean residence time
mean resistance time
median reaction time
median recognition threshold
median relapse time
Metropolitan Readiness Test
milk ring test
modified rhyme test
muscle response test

MRTA
magnetic resonance tomographic angiography

MRTK
malignant rhabdoid tumor of kidney

MRTS
malignant rhabdoid tumor of soft tissue

MRU
magnetic resonance urography
mass radiography unit
mean relational utterance
measure of resource use
medical resource utilization
minimal reproductive unit
molecular recognition unit

MRUS
maximal rate of urea synthesis

MRV
> magnetic resonance venography
> mammalian orthoreovirus
> minute respiratory volume
> Mitchell River virus
> mixed respiratory vaccine
> mononuclear Reed-variant (cell)

MRVP
> mean right ventricular pressure
> methyl red, Voges-Proskauer
> (medium)

MRX
> *Moraxella catarrhalis* vaccine

MR X 1, MRx1
> may repeat one time
> may repeat times one (once)

MRXA
> X-linked mental retardation-aphasia
> syndrome

MRXS1–6
> X-linked mental retardation
> syndrome 1–6

MRZ
> measles, rubella and zoster

MS
> main scale
> maladjustment score
> mannose-sensitive
> mass spectrometry
> mass spectrophotometer
> mean score
> mechanical stimulation
> Meckel syndrome
> medical services
> medical student
> medical supply
> medical surgical
> medical survey
> melanonychia striata
> menopausal syndrome
> mental status
> metabolic syndrome
> metaproterenolsulfate
> microscope slide
> milkshake
> minimal support
> mitral sound
> mitral stenosis
> mobile surgical (unit)
> modal sensitivity
> moderately susceptible
> molar solution
> mongolian spot
> morning stiffness
> morphine sulfate (*See also* ms,
> MSO4)
> motile sperm
> mucosubstance
> multilaminated structure
> multiple sclerosis
> muscle shortening
> muscle spasm
> muscle strength
> musculoskeletal (*See also* MSK)
> myasthenic syndrome
> myeloid sarcoma

3MS
> Modified Mini-Mental Status
> (examination)

MS-222
> tricaine methane sulfonate

M&S
> microculture and sensitivity

ms
> manuscript
> millisecond (*See also* msec, σ)
> morphine sulfate (*See also* MS,
> MSO4)
> murmurs
> musculoskeletal (*See also* MS,
> MSK)

m/s
> meters per second (*See also* m/sec)

m/s^2
> meters per second squared

MSA
> major serologic antigen
> male specific antigen
> mammary serum antigen
> mannitol salt agar
> Marriage Skills Analysis
> Medical Savings Accounts
> membrane stabilizing action
> membrane-stabilizing activity
> metropolitan statistical area
> microsomal autoantibodies
> mitotic spindle apparatus
> mouse serum albumin
> multichannel signed averager
> Multidimensional Scalogram
> Analysis
> multiple system atrophy
> multiplication-stimulating activity

NOTES

M

MSA (*continued*)
    muscle-specific actin (*See also* HHF-35)
    muscle sympathetic activity
    myositis-specific autoantibody

MSAA
    multiple sclerosis-associated agent

MSAD
    multiple scan average dose

MSAF
    meconium-stained amniotic fluid

MSAFP
    maternal serum alpha-fetoprotein

MSAO
    meal-stimulated acid output

MSAP
    mean systemic arterial pressure

MSAS
    Mandel Social Adjustment Scale
    Memorial Symptom Assessment Scale

MSAS-P
    Memorial Symptom Assessment Scale-Physical

MSAS-Psych
    Memorial Symptom Assessment Scale-Psychological

MSAS-SF
    Memorial Symptom Assessment Scale-short form

MSAT
    Minnesota Scholastic Aptitude Test

MSB
    mainstem bronchus
    martius scarlet blue
    mediastinal shed blood
    mid-small bowel
    most significant bit

MSBC
    maximal specific binding capacity

MSBLA
    mouse-specific B-lymphocyte antigen

MSBOS
    maximal surgical blood order schedule

MSBP
    mandibular staple bone plate
    Münchausen syndrome by proxy (*See also* MSP)

MSC
    major symptom complex
    midsystolic click
    MS Contin
    multiple sib case

MSCA
    McCarthy Scales of Children's Abilities

MSCC
    midstream clean-catch (urine culture)

MSCE
    monitored self-care evaluation

MSCLC
    mouse stem cell-like cell

MSCNS
    methicillin-susceptible coagulase-negative *Staphylococcus*

MSCP, mscp
    mean spherical candle power

MS-CRS
    morphine sulfate controlled-release suppository

MSCS
    Multidimensional Self Concept Scale

MSCs
    mesenchymal stem cells

MSCU
    medical special care unit

MSCWP
    musculoskeletal chest wall pain

MSD
    male sexual dysfunction
    mean sorted difference
    mean square deviation
    metabolic screening disorder
    microsurgical diskectomy
    midsagittal diameter
    midsleep disturbance
    mild sickle (cell) disease
    most significant digit
    multiple sulfatase deficiency

MSDBP
    mean sitting diastolic blood pressure

MSDI
    Martin Suicide Depression Inventory

MSDS
    material safety data sheet

MSE
    mean spherical equivalent
    medical support equipment
    mental status examination
    muscle-specific enolase

3MSE
    Modified Mini-Mental State Examination

mse
    mean square error

msec
    millisecond (*See also* ms, σ)

m/sec
    meter per second
    meters per second (*See also* m/s)

MSEL
> Mullen Scales of Early Learning
> myasthenic syndrome of Eaton-
> Lambert

MSER
> mean systolic ejection rate
> Mental Status Examination Record
> mental status examination report

MSES
> medical school environmental stress

MSET
> multistage exercise test

MSEV
> microsurgical epididymovasostomy

MSF
> macrophage slowing factor
> macrophage spreading factor
> meconium-stained fluid
> Mediterranean spotted fever
> megakaryocyte-stimulating factor
> migration-stimulating factor
> modified sham feeding

MSG
> massage
> methysergide
> monosodium glutamate

MSGV
> mouse salivary gland virus

MSH
> medical self-help
> melanocyte-stimulating hormone
> melanophore-stimulating hormone
> (See also MH)
> minimally symptomatic
> hypothyroidism

MSHA
> mannose-sensitive hemagglutination

MSH-IF
> melanocyte-stimulating hormone-
> inhibiting factor

MSHRF
> melanocyte-stimulating hormone-
> releasing factor

MSHSC
> multiple self-healing squamous
> carcinoma

MSI
> magnetic source imaging
> mass sociogenic illness
> medium-scale integration
> metered solution inhaler

> microsatellite instability
> microstructured implant
> multiple subcortical infarction
> musculoskeletal impairment

MSIS
> Multiple Severity of Illness System
> multistate information system

MSK
> medullary sponge kidney
> musculoskeletal (See also MS)

MSKP
> Medical Sciences Knowledge
> Profile

MSL
> mean sentence length
> midsternal line
> multiple symmetric lipomatosis

MSLA
> mouse-specific lymphocyte antigen
> multisample Luer adapter

MSLR
> mixed skin (cell) leukocyte
> reaction

MSLSS
> Multidimensional Student Life
> Satisfaction Scale

MSLT
> Multiple Sleep Latency Test

MSM
> magnetic starch microspheres
> men (who have) sex with men
> methsuximide (Celontin)
> methylsulfonylmethane
> midsystolic murmur
> mineral salts medium

MSN
> hereditary motor sensory neuropathy
> II-deafness-mental retardation
> medial septal nucleus
> mildly subnormal

MSNA
> muscle sympathetic nerve activity

MSO
> managed services organization
> medial superior olive
> mentally stable and oriented
> mental status, oriented
> most significant other

MSO4
> morphine sulfate (See also MS,
> ms)

NOTES

MSOF
    multiple system organ failure
    multisystem organ failure
MSP
    maximum squeeze pressure
    mouse serum protein
    Münchausen syndrome by proxy
      (*See also* MSBP)
MSPGN
    mesangial proliferative
      glomerulonephritis
MSPN
    medical student progress note
MSPQ
    Modified Somatic Perception
      Questionnaire
MSPS
    musculoskeletal pain syndrome
    myocardial stress perfusion
      scintigraphy
MSPSS
    Multidimensional Scale of
      Perceived Social Support
MSPU
    medical short procedure unit
MSPv
    midshunt peak velocity
MSQ
    Managerial Style Questionnaire
    mental status questionnaire
    meters squared (*See also* m^2)
    Minnesota Satisfaction Questionnaire
MSR
    mitral stenoregurgitation
    monosynaptic reflex
    muscle stretch reflex
MSRA
    maximal static response assay
MSRPP
    Multidimensional Scale for Rating
      Psychiatric Patients
MSRT
    Minnesota Spatial Relations Test
MSS
    Marital Satisfaction Scale
    massage (*See also* M, mass, mss)
    mean sac size
    mental status schedule
    metabolic support service
    microsatellite stable
    Minnesota Satisfaction Scale
    minor surgery suite
    monophasic synovial sarcoma
    motion sickness susceptibility
    mucus-stimulating substance
    multiple sclerosis susceptibility
    muscular subaortic stenosis

mss
    massage (*See also* M, mass, MSS)
MSSA
    methicillin-susceptible
      Staphylococcus aureus
MSSB
    MacArthur Story Stem Battery
MSS-CR
    mean sac size and crown-rump
      length
MSSG
    multiple sclerosis susceptibility gene
MSSST
    Meeting Street School Screening
      Test
MSSU
    midstream specimen of urine
MST
    maladies sexuellement transmissible
      (French-sexually transmitted
      disease)
    maximum stimulation test
    mean survival time
    mean swell time (botulism test)
    medial superior temporal
    median survival time
    mental stress test
    multiple subpial transection
    multisystemic therapy
MSTA
    mumps skin test antigen
MSTh
    mesothorium
MSTI
    multiple soft tissue injuries
MSU
    maple syrup urine
    medical studies unit
    memory for symbolic unit
    midstream specimen of urine
    midstream urine (specimen)
    monosodium urate
    myocardial substrate uptake
MSUA
    midstream urinalysis
MSUD
    maple syrup urine disease
MSUM
    monosodium urate monohydrate
MSV
    maximal sustained (level of)
      ventilation
    mean scale value
    Moloney sarcoma virus
    murine sarcoma virus
mSv
    millisievert (radiation unit)

MSVC
    maximal sustainable ventilatory capacity
    maximal sustained ventilatory capacity

MSVL
    maximal spatial vector to left

MSW
    multiple stab wounds

MSWYE
    modified sea water yeast extract (agar)

MSYN
    monophasic synovial sarcoma

MT
    antimetallothionein antibody
    empty
    macular target
    maggot therapy
    magnetization transfer
    maintenance therapy
    malaria therapy
    malignant teratoma
    mammary tumor
    Martin-Thayer (plate, medium)
    mastoid tip
    maximal therapy
    maximal toleration
    medial temporal
    medial thalamus
    medial thickening
    mediastinal tube
    medical treatment
    melatonin
    membrana tympani
    membrane thickness
    membrane type (types 1–6)
    mesangial thickening
    metallothionein
    metatarsal (*See also* met)
    metatarsophalangeal
    methyltyrosine
    microtome
    microtubule
    middle turbinate
    midtrachea
    minimal threshold
    Monroe tidal drainage (*See also* MTD)
    more than
    Muir-Torre (syndrome)
    multiple tics
    multitest (plate)
    muscle and tendon
    muscle test
    muscle testing
    muscle tone
    music therapy

M-T
    macroglobulin-trypsin

M/T
    masses (or) tenderness
    myringotomy (with) tubes

M&T
    myringotomy and tubes

mt
    tympanic membrane [L. *membrana tympani*]

3-MT
    3-methoxytyramine

MT6
    mercaptomerin

MTA
    malignant teratoma, anaplastic
    mammary tumor agent
    Management Transactions Audit
    medullary-type adenocarcinoma
    metatarsus adductus
    mineral trioxide aggregate
    multitargeted antifolate
    myoclonic twitch activity

MTAC
    mass transfer area coefficient

MTAD
    tympanic membrane of right ear [L. *membrana tympana auris dextrae*]

MTAI
    Minnesota Teacher Attitude Inventory

MT/AK
    music therapy/audiokinetics

MTAL
    medullary thick ascending limb

MTAS
    Maternal Trait Anxiety Score
    tympanic membrane of left ear [L. *membrana tympana auris sinistrae*]

MTAU
    tympanic membranes of both ears [L. *membranae tympani aures unitae*]

NOTES

MTB
methylthymol blue
Mycobacterium tuberculosis

MTBE
meningeal tick-borne encephalitis
methyl-*tert*-butyl ether (therapy)
methyl tertiary butyl ether

MTBF
mean time between (or before)
failures

mTBI
mild traumatic brain injury

MTBV
Marituba virus

MTC
magnetization transfer contrast
(radiology)
mass transfer coefficient
maximal tolerated concentration
medical test cabinet
medical training center
medullary thyroid cancer
medullary thyroid carcinoma
metatarsocuneiform
multilocular thymic cyst

MTC-DOX
doxorubicin adsorbed to magnetic
targeted carrier

MTCT
mother-to-child transmission

MTD
maximal tolerated dose
maximum tolerated dose
mean total dose
mean tubular diameter
metastatic trophoblastic disease
minimum toxic dose
Monroe tidal drainage (*See also*
MT)
multiple tic disorder
Mycobacterium tuberculosis direct
(test) (*See also* MTDT)

MTDDA
Minnesota Test for Differential
Diagnosis of Aphasia

MTDI
maximal tolerable daily intake

MT-DN
multitest, Dermatophytes, and
Nocardia (plate)

mtDNA
mitochondrial deoxyribonucleic acid

MTDT
modified tone decay test
Mycobacterium tuberculosis direct
test (*See also* MTD)

MTE
main timing event

medical toxic environment
multiple trace elements

MTE-4(r)
trace metal elements injection

MTET
modified treadmill exercise testing

MTF
maximal terminal flow
medical treatment facility
mesial triangular fossa
mithramycin
modulation transfer factor
modulation transfer function

MTG
middle temporal gyrus (gyri)
midthigh girth

MTg
mouse thyroglobulin

MTHF
methyl tetrahydrofolic acid

MTHFR
methylene tetrahydrofolate reductase
5,10-methylene-tetrahydrofolate
reductase

m-THPC
meso-tetra (hydroxyphenyl) chlorine
m-tetra (hydroxyphenyl) chlorine

MTI
magnetization transfer imaging
malignant teratoma, intermediate
minimal time interval

MTJ
midtarsal joint

MTL
Metropolitan Life Table (for
desirable weight)

MTLE
medial (mesial) temporal-lobe
epilepsy

MTLP
metabolic toxemia of late
pregnancy

MTM
mouth-to-mouth (resuscitation)
Thayer-Martin, modified (agar)

MT-M
multitest, mycology (plate)

MT-MMP
membrane-bound membrane-type
metalloproteinase

mtMRI
magnetization transfer magnetic
resonance imaging

MTMT
maximum tolerated medical therapy

MTMX
X-linked myotubular myopathy

MTOC
>   microtubule organizing center
>   mitotic organizing center

mTOR
>   mammalian target of rapamycin

MTP
>   master treatment plan
>   maximal tolerated pressure
>   medial tibial plateau
>   medical termination of pregnancy
>   metatarsophalangeal (joint) (*See also* MP, MTPJ)
>   methylprednisolone
>   microsomal triglyceride transfer protein
>   microtubule protein
>   multidisciplinary treatment plan
>   muramyl tripeptide

MTPI
>   metatarsophalangeal implant

MTPJ
>   metatarsophalangeal joint (*See also* MP, MTP)
>   MTP joint

MTPT
>   1-methyl-4-phenyl-1,2,3,6-tetrahydropyridine

MTQ
>   methaqualone

MTR
>   magnetization transfer ratio
>   mass, tenderness, rebound (abdominal examination)
>   Meinicke turbidity reaction
>   mental treatment rules
>   metronidazole
>   mother (*See also* M, MO, MOM)

MTR-0
>   no masses, tenderness, or rebound (abdominal examination)

M-tropic
>   macrophage tropic

MTRV
>   Matruh virus

MTS
>   medial tibial syndrome
>   mesial temporal sclerosis
>   mitochondrial targeting sequence
>   moderate tactile stimulus
>   Mohr-Tranebjaerg syndrome
>   multicellular tumor spheroid

MTSS
>   medial tibial stress syndrome
>   menstrual toxic shock syndrome

MTST
>   maximal treadmill stress test

MTT
>   malignant teratoma, trophoblastic
>   malignant triton tumor
>   malignant trophoblastic teratoma
>   mammillothalamic tract
>   maximal treadmill testing
>   meal tolerance test
>   mean pulmonary transit time
>   mean transit time
>   medial tibial torsion
>   methylthiotetrazole
>   monotetrazolium

MTU
>   malignant teratoma, undifferentiated
>   medical therapy unit
>   methylthiouracil

M-TURP
>   minimal transurethral resection of prostate

MTV
>   mammary tumor virus (of mice)
>   maximal toleration volume
>   maximum tolerable volume
>   metatarsus varus

MT-Y
>   multitest yeast (plate)

MTZ
>   mirtazapine (Remeron)
>   mitoxantrone

μ, mu
>   chemical potential
>   dynamic viscosity
>   electrophoretic mobility
>   heavy chain of immunoglobulin M
>   linear attenuation coefficient
>   magnetic moment (*See also* m)
>   mean (*See also* M, m)
>   mutation rate
>   mu (12th letter of Greek alphabet), lowercase
>   permeability
>   population mean (statistics)

MU
>   Mache unit
>   maternal uncle
>   megaunit
>   mescaline unit

M

NOTES

MU (*continued*)
    million units
    monitor unit
    Montevideo unit
    motor unit
    mouse unit (*See also* m.u.)
    Murphy unit

mU
    milliunit

m.u.
    mouse unit (*See also* MU)

MUA
    manipulation under anesthesia
    middle uterine artery
    multiple unit activity

MUAC
    middle upper arm circumference

MUAP
    (macro) motor unit action potential
    motor unit action potential

μ_β
    Bohr magneton

MUC
    maximal urinary concentration
    maximum urinary concentration
    mucosal ulcerative colitis

muc
    mucilage

MUCL
    medial ulnar collateral ligament

MUCP
    maximum urethral closure pressure

MUCV
    Mucambo virus

MUD
    matched unrelated donor
    minimal urticarial dose

MUDV
    Munguba virus

MUE
    medication use evaluation

μF
    microfarad

MUFA
    monounsaturated fatty acid

MUFR
    maximal urinary flow rate

MUGA
    multigated angiogram
    multiple gated acquisition

MUGEx
    multiple (blood pool scan during) exercise (*See also* MUGX)

MUGR
    multigated (blood pool image at) rest

MUGS
    monoclonal gammopathy of undetermined significance

MUGUS
    monoclonal gammopathy of unknown significance

MUGX
    multigated (blood pool image during) exercise (*See also* MUGEx)

mu-HCD
    mu-heavy-chain disease

μIU
    one-millionth International Unit

MULE
    microcomputer upper limb exerciser

mulibrey
    muscle, liver, brain, eye (disease)

mult
    multiple
    multiplication

multi-CSF
    multi-colony-stimulating factor

multip
    multiparous

MuLV, MuLv
    murine leukemia virus

μmg
    micromilligram (nanogram)

MUMPS
    Massachusetts General Hospital Utility Multi-Programming System

MuMTv
    murine mammary tumor virus

$\mu\mu Ci$
    micromicrocurie (picocurie)

$\mu\mu F$
    micromicrofarad (picofarad)

$\mu\mu g$
    micromicrogram (picogram)

MUNSH
    Memorial University of Newfoundland Scale of Happiness

MUNV
    Munguba virus

MUN(WI)
    Munich Wistar (rat)

μ_o
    permeability of vacuum

MUO
    myocardiopathy of unknown origin

$M\Omega$
    megohm

$m\Omega$
    milliohm

MUP
    major urinary protein
    maximal urethral pressure

4-methylumbelliferyl phosphate
motor unit potential
mouse urine protein

MUPAT
multiple-site perineal applicator
technique

MUPIT
Martinez universal interstitial
template

Mur
muramic acid

MURC, MURCS
measurable undesirable respiratory
contaminants

MURCS
müllerian, renal, cervicothoracic,
somite abnormalities

MURD
matched unrelated donor

MurNAc
N-acetylmuramate

MURV
Murutucu virus

mus 1–2
Mus adenovirus 1–2

musc
muscle
muscular
musculature

MUSE
medicated urethral system for
erection

μsec
microsecond (*See also* μs)

mus-lig
musculoligamentous

MUST
medical unit, self-contained and
transportable

MUSTPAC
medical ultrasound 3D portable,
with advanced communication

mut.
mutation

MUU
mouse uterine unit

mUW
modified University of Wisconsin
(solution)

MUWU
mouse uterine weight unit

MV
main venule
malignant (rabbit fibroma) virus
maternal venous
maximal ventilation
measles virus
mechanical ventilation
megavolt
microvilli
midventricular
minute ventilation
minute volume
mitral valve
mixed venous
multivesicular
multivessel

Mv
mendelevium (*See also* Md)

mV
millivolt

MVA
malignant ventricular arrhythmia
manual vacuum aspiration
mechanical ventricular assistance
mevalonic acid
microvascular angiopathy
microvillus atrophy
mitral valve area
modified vaccine (virus) Ankara
motor vehicle accident

MV·A
megavolt-ampere

mV·A
millivolt-ampere

MVB
manual ventilation bag
mixed venous blood
multivesicular body

MVC
maximal vital capacity
maximal voluntary contraction
maximum voluntary contraction
microvessel count
minute virus of canines
motor vehicle collision (crash)
myocardial vascular capacity

MVc
mitral valve closure

MV(c)ELISA
measles virus enzyme-linked
immunosorbent assay

M

NOTES

MVD
Marburg virus disease
microvascular decompression
microvessel density
mitral valve disease
mouse vas deferens
multivessel (coronary) disease
myocardial vasodilation

MVE
mitral valve echo
mitral valve (leaflet) excursion
Murray Valley encephalitis
Murray Valley encephalitis (virus)

MVG, MVgrad
mitral valve gradient

MVH
massive variceal hemorrhage
massive vitreous hemorrhage

MVI
motor vehicle injury
multiple vitamin injection
multivalvular involvement
multivitamin infusion

MVII
Minnesota Vocational Interest
Inventory

MVK
Massachusetts Vision Kit

MVL
mitral valve leaflet

MVLS
mandibular vestibulolingual
sulcoplasty
Mecham Verbal Language Scale
modified varicella-like syndrome

MVM
medullary venous malformation
microvillous membrane
minute virus of mice

MVMT
movement

MVN
medial ventromedial nucleus
medial vestibular nucleus

MVO
maximal venous outflow
maximum venous outflow
mean venous outflow
mitral valve opening
mitral valve orifice

MVO2, MVO$_2$
maximal venous oxygen
(consumption)
mixed venous oxygen saturation
(*See also* MVO$_2$S, SvO$_2$)
myocardial ventilation, oxygen
(rate)

oxygen content of mixed venous
blood

MVO$_2$
myocardial oxygen consumption

mVO$_2$
minimal venous oxygen
(consumption)

MVOA
mitral valve orifice area

MVO$_2$S
mixed venous oxygen saturation
(*See also* MVO2, SvO$_2$)

MVP
maximum vasal pressure
mean platelet volume
mean venous pressure
microvascular pressure
mitral valve prolapse

MVPS
mitral valve prolapse syndrome

MVPT
Mertens Visual Perception Test
Motor-Free Visual Perception Test
(*See also* MFVPT)

MVR
massive vitreous reaction
massive vitreous retraction
massive vitreous retractor (blade)
maximal ventilation rate
microvitreoretinal
minimal vascular resistance
mitral valve regurgitation
mitral valve replacement

MVRI
mixed vaccine, respiratory infection
mixed virus respiratory infection

MVS
Massachusetts XII Vitrectomy
System
mitral valve stenosis
motor, vascular, and sensory

MVSD
muscular ventricular septal defect

mV-sec
millivolt-second

MVT
maximal ventilation time
mesenteric vein thrombosis
monomorphic ventricular tachycardia
movement
multiform ventricular tachycardia
multivitamin

MV-T
mitral valve-transverse

MVTR
moisture vapor transmission rate

MVU
Montevideo units

MVV
>maximal ventilatory volume
>maximal voluntary ventilation
>maximum voluntary ventilation
>mixed vespid venom

MVV₁
>maximal ventilatory volume

M-W
>Mallory-Weiss syndrome
>men and women

MW
>mean weight
>megawatt
>microwave (*See also* mw)
>molecular weight (*See also* mol wt, MWt)
>Munich Wistar (rat)

mW
>milliwatt

mw
>microwave (*See also* MW)

MWAV
>Manawa virus

MWB
>minimal weight bearing

mWb
>milliweber

MWC
>Monod-Wyman-Changeux (model)

MWCB
>manufacturer's working cell bank

MWD
>maximum walking distance
>microwave diathermy
>molecular weight distribution

MWF
>metal working fluid

M-W-F
>Monday-Wednesday-Friday

MWI
>Medical Walk-In (Clinic)

MWLT
>Modified Word Learning Test

MWMT
>Monotic Word Memory Test

MwoA
>migraine without aura

MWP
>mean wedge pressure

MWPC
>multiwire proportional chamber

MWS
>Marden-Walker syndrome
>Mickety-Wilson syndrome
>Moersch-Woltman syndrome

MWT
>maintenance of wakefulness test
>Mallory-Weiss tear
>malpositioned wisdom teeth
>maximum walking time
>myocardial wall thickness

6-MWT
>6-minute walking test

MWt
>molecular weight (*See also* mol wt, MW)

MX
>matrix

MX2
>3'-deamino-3'-morpholino-13-deoxo-10-hydroxycarminomycin

Mx
>manifest refraction
>mastectomy
>maxillary
>maxwell
>MEDEX (physician assistant training program)
>movement
>multiple
>myringotomy (*See also* MYR)

M$_{xy}$
>transverse magnetization

My
>myopia
>myxedematous

my
>mayer (unit of heat capacity)

MyBP-C
>myosin-binding protein-C

Mycol
>mycologist
>mycology

MYD
>mydriatic

MyD
>myotonic (muscular) dystrophy

MYEL
>multiple myeloma

Myel
>myelocyte

M

NOTES

myel
  myelin
  myelinated
Myelo
  myelogram
  myelography
MyG
  myasthenia gravis (*See also* MG)
Myg
  myriagram
MYKV
  Mykines virus
MyL
  myrialiter
Mym
  myriameter
MyMD
  myotonic muscular dystrophy (*See also* MMD)
MYO
  myoglobin (*See also* Mb, MbCO, MbO$_2$, MYOGLB)
myo
  myocardial
  myocardium
MYOC
  myocilin
MyoD
  myogenic regulatory protein (family of genes)
MYOGLB
  myoglobin (*See also* Mb, MbCO, MbO$_2$, MYO)
myop
  myopia

MYR
  myringotomy (*See also* Mx)
MYS
  medium yellow soft (stools)
  myasthenia syndrome
MYST
  mediastinal yolk sac tumor
MYTGC
  Miller-Yoder Test of Grammatical Comprehension
MZ
  mantle zone
  marginal zone
  mezlocillin
  monozygotic (twin)
M$_z$
  longitudinal magnetization
m/z
  mass-to-charge ratio
MZA
  monozygotic (twins raised) apart
MZB
  mizoribine
MZBCL, MZBL
  marginal zone B-cell lymphoma
MZL
  mantle zone lymphoma
  marginal zone (cell) lymphoma
  marginal zone lymphocyte
  marginal zone lymphoma
MZT
  monozygotic (twins raised) together

N

antigenic determinant of erythrocytes
asparagine (*See also* Asn)
inherited blood factor in MNS blood group
loudness
nasal (*See also* n, NAS)
nasion
nausea
negative (*See also* neg)
Neisseria
neomycin (*See also* NE, neo, NM)
nerve (*See also* n)
Neumega
neural
neuraminidase
neurologist (*See also* neur, neuro, neurol)
neurology (*See also* neur, neuro, neurol)
neuropathy
neutron number
neutrophil
never
newton
nicotinamide
night
nipple
nitrogen (*See also* N2)
no
nodal
node
nodule
nonalcoholic
none
nonmalignant
Nonne (globulin test)
noon (*See also* M)
nor (*See also* n)
norepinephrine
normal (*See also* n, NL, nl, NOR, norm, NR)
normal concentration
normality (equivalent/liter)
north
not
notified
noun
NPH insulin
nucleoside (*See also* Nuc)
nucleus
number (*See also* n, NO, No, no.)
number of atoms

number density (number of moles of substance per unit of volume)
number of molecules
number of neutrons in an atomic nucleus
number of observations (in statistics) (*See also* n)
number in sample
numerical aptitude
numerical aptitude (General Aptitude Test Battery)
nu (13th letter of Greek alphabet), uppercase
population size
radiance
refractive index (*See also* n)
sample size (*See also* n)
spin density
unit of neutron dosage

0.02N

fiftieth normal (solution) (*See also* N/50)

0.1N

tenth-normal (solution) (*See also* N/10)

0.5N

half-normal (solution) (*See also* N/2)

2N

double-normal (solution)

2n

diploid chromosome number

N/2

half-normal (solution) (*See also* 0.5N)
seminormal

3n

triploid chromosome number

n-3

omega-3

4n

tetraploid

5'-N

5'-nucleotidase

N-9

nonoxynol-9

N/10

tenth-normal (solution) (*See also* 0.1N)

N-13

nitrogen-13

¹³N

ammonia-13
nitrogen-13

N

N/50
>fiftieth-normal (solution) (*See also* 0.02N)

n (*See also* N)
>amount of substance expressed in moles
>haploid chromosome number
>index of refraction
>nano- (prefix)
>nasal (*See also* N)
>nerve (*See also* N)
>neuter (*See also* neut)
>neutron
>neutron dosage (unit of)
>neutron number density
>night
>nor (*See also* N)
>normal (*See also* N, NL, nl, NOR, norm, NR)
>normal concentration
>number (*See also* N, NO, No, no.)
>number of density of molecule
>number of observations (*See also* N)
>principal quantum number
>refractive index (*See also* RI)
>rotational frequency
>sample size (*See also* N)

n̄
>mean value of n for a number of observations (in statistics)

n.
>born [L. *natus*]
>nostril [L. *naris*]

n_0
>Loschmidt's number

^{14}N
>nitrogen-14

^{15}N
>nitrogen-15

N2
>nitrogen (*See also* N)
>second nerve

N_2
>nitrogen

N 2.5
>phenylephrine HCl 2.5% ophthalmic solution (Neo-Synephrine)

N=1 trial
>number equal to one; single patient trial

NA
>Avogadro constant/number (*See also* L, Λ, NA)
>nalidixic acid
>nasopharyngeal angiofibroma
>Native American
>neuraminidase
>neurologic age
>neuropathic arthropathy
>neutralizing antibody
>neutrophil antibody
>new admission
>nicotinamide
>nicotinic acid
>nitric acid
>no abnormality
>nodular amyloidoma
>Nomina Anatomica
>nonadherent
>non-A (hepatitis)
>nonalcoholic
>nonamnionic
>nonmyelinated axon
>noradrenaline
>norethindrone acetate
>normal axis
>nosocomially acquired
>not admitted
>not antagonized
>not applicable (*See also* N/A)
>not attempted
>not available
>nuclear antibody
>nuclear antigen
>nucleic acid
>nucleus accumbens (septi)
>nucleus ambiguus
>numerical aperture
>numeric aperture
>nursing action

N&A
>normal and active

N/A
>no alternative
>not applicable (*See also* NA)

N.A.
>numerical aperture

Na
>natrium (sodium)
>sodium [L. *natrium*] (*See also* sod, Na+)

Na+
>sodium (*See also* sod, Na)

^{23}Na
>sodium-23

^{24}Na
>sodium-24

nA
>nanoampere

na
>nephrogenic adenoma

NAA
>*N*-acetylaspartate
>naphthalene acetic acid
>neutral amino acid

neutron activation analysis
neutrophil aggregation activity
nicotinic acid amide
no apparent abnormalities
nucleic acid amplification

NAAC
no apparent anesthetic complication

NAACP
neoplasia, allergy, Addison
(disease), collagen (vascular
disease), and parasites

NAA/Cr
N-acetylaspartate/creatine ratio

NAAG
N-acetylaspartylglutamate

NAAP
N-acetyl-4-amino-phenazone
National Arthritis Action Plan

NAAT
nucleic acid amplification
techniques (testing)

NAATPT
not available at the present time

NAB
nonweightbearing ambulation
not at bedside
novarsenobenzene

NABS
normoactive bowel sounds

NABX
needle aspiration biopsy

NAC
accessory nucleus (Monakow
nucleus)
N-acetyl-L-cysteine
nasal allergen challenge
neoadjuvant chemotherapy
nerve-approximating clamp
nipple-areola complex
no acute changes
nonadherent cell

NACD
no anatomical cause of death
not acidified

NAC-EDTA
N-acetyl-L-cysteine ethylenediaminetetraacetic acid

n-Ach
achievement need (in psychology)

NaCl
sodium chloride (salt)

NaClO
sodium hypochlorite

NaCMC
sodium carboxymethyl cellulose

NACS
Neurologic and Adaptive Capacity
Score

NACT
neoadjuvant chemotherapy

NAD
new antigenic determinant
nicotinamide adenine dinucleotidase
nicotinamide adenine dinucleotide
nicotinic acid dehydrogenase
no abnormal discovery
no abnormality demonstrable
no active disease
no acute disease
no acute distress
no apparent disease
no apparent distress
no appreciable disease
normal axis deviation
nothing abnormal detected
nothing abnormal discovered

NAD⁺
oxidized form of nicotinamide
adenine dinucleotide

NaD
sodium dialysate

NADA
New Animal Drug Application

NADG
nicotinamide adenine dinucleotide
glycohydrolase

NADH
nicotinamide adenine dinucleotide
(reduced form)

NaDodSO₄
sodium dodecyl sulfate (*See also*
SDS)

NADP⁺
nicotinamide adenine dinucleotide
phosphate positive
oxidized form of nicotinamide
adenine dinucleotide phosphate

NADPH, NADP
nicotinamide adenine dinucleotide
phosphate

NADSIC
no apparent disease seen in chest

NOTES

NAE
> net acid excretion

Na$_e$
> exchangeable body sodium (natrium)

NAF
> nafcillin (*See also* NF)
> Native American female
> net acid flux
> neutrophil activating factor
> neutrophil-activating factor
> normal adult female
> Notice of Adverse Findings (FDA post-audit letter)

NaFl
> sodium fluorescein

NAFLD
> nonalcoholic fatty liver disease

NAG
> N-acetyl-beta-glucosaminidase
> N-acetyl-β-glucosaminidase
> N-acetylglutamate
> narrow-angle glaucoma
> nonagglutinable
> nonagglutinating

NAGO
> neuraminidase and galactose oxidase

NAGS
> natural apophysial glides

NaHCO$_3$, NaHCO3
> sodium bicarbonate

NAI
> net acid input (urinary)
> neuraminidase inhibition (*See also* NI)
> no action indicated
> no acute inflammation
> nonaccidental injury
> nonadherence index
> Nuremberg Aging Inventory

NaI
> sodium iodide

NAIM
> nonvasculitic autoimmune inflammatory meningoencephalitis

NAION
> nonarteritic anterior ischemic optic neuropathy
> nonarteritic ischemic optic neuropathy

NAIR
> nonadrenergic inhibitory response

NAIT
> neonatal alloimmune thrombocytopenia

NaI(Tl)
> thallium-activated sodium iodide crystal (in gamma ray detectors)
> thallium-activated sodium iodide (sodium iodide crystal)

Na&K
> sodium and potassium (in urine)

Na$^+$-K$^+$
> sodium-potassium

NaK ATPase
> sodium- and potassium-activated adenosine triphosphatase

Na&KSP
> sodium and potassium spot (urine test)

NAL
> nasal angiocentric lymphoma
> nonadherent leukocyte

NALC
> *N*-acetyl-L-cysteine-sodium hydroxide (test)

NALD
> neonatal adrenoleukodystrophy

NALL
> null (cell line of) acute lymphocytic leukemia

NALP
> neuroadenolysis of pituitary

NALS
> neonatal adjuvant life support

NALT
> nasopharyngeal-associated lymphoid tissue

NAM
> nail-apparatus melanoma
> Native American male
> natural actomyosin
> normal adult male

NAME
> nevi, atrial myxoma, myxoid neurofibroma, and ephelides (syndrome)
> nevi, atrial myxomas, myxomas (of skin and mammary glands), and ephelides (syndrome)

NAMN
> nicotinic acid mononucleotide

NANB
> non-A, non-B (hepatitis) (hepatitis C)

NANBH
> non-A, non-B hepatitis

NANBNC, NANBNCH
> non-A, non-B, non-C hepatitis

NANBV
> non-A, non-B (hepatitis) virus

NANC
>nonadrenergic noncholinergic noncholinergic (neuron)

NAND
>not-and (result is false only if all arguments are true—otherwise, result is true)

NANIPER
>nonallergic noninfectious perennial rhinitis

N ant/post
>anterior and posterior "zones" (nerve cell groups—nuclei of hypothalamus)

NAP
>narrative, assessment, and plan
>nasion pogonion (angle of convexity in craniometrics)
>nerve action potential
>neutrophil-activating protein
>neutrophil alkaline phosphatase
>P-nitro-alpha-acetylamino-beta-hydroxypropiophenone
>nonacute profile
>nosocomial acquired pneumonia
>nucleic acid phosphatase

8NAP
>eighth nerve action potential

NaP
>sodium phosphate

NAPA
>N-acetyl procainamide

NAPD
>no active pulmonary disease

Na Pent
>sodium pentothal

NaPG
>sodium pregnanediol glucuronide

NAPH
>naphthyl

NAPI
>Neurodevelopmental Assessment (Procedure) for Preterm Infants

NAPQI
>N-acetyl-p-benzoquinoneimine

N$_{aqs}$
>number of planar acquisitions per phase-encoding step

NAR
>nasal airway resistance
>no action required
>no adverse reaction

nonambulatory restraint
nonanaphylactic reaction
not at risk

NARA
>Narcotics Addict Rehabilitation Act

NARC, narc
>narcotic (*See also* narco)
>narcotics (officer, slang) (*See also* narco, NO)

Narc
>nucleus arcuatus (nucleus infundibularis)

narco
>narcolepsy
>narcotic (*See also* NARC)
>narcotic addict (slang)
>narcotics (hospital, officer, treatment center—slang) (*See also* NARC, NO)

NARES
>nonallergic rhinitis with eosinophilia syndrome

NaRI
>noradrenaline reuptake inhibitor

NARP
>neurogenic muscle weakness, ataxia, and retinitis pigmentosa
>neuropathy, ataxia, retinitis pigmentosa

NARS
>neuropsychiatric acquired (immunodeficiency syndrome)
>rating scale

NART
>National Adult Reading Test (United Kingdom)

NAS
>nasal (*See also* N, n)
>Nasoule virus
>Neonatal Abstinence Score
>neonatal abstinence syndrome
>neonatal air leak syndrome
>neuroallergic syndrome
>no abnormality seen
>no added salt
>normalized alignment score

NAS-BA, NASBA
>nucleic acid sequence-based amplification
>nucleic acid sequence-based analysis

NOTES

NASDCA
    naphthol AS-D chloracetate
NASH
    nonalcoholic steatohepatitis
Na-Spt
    sodium spot (urine test)
NASS
    Neonatal Abstinence Scoring
      System
NaSSA
    noradrenergic and specific
      serotonergic antidepressant
NASTT
    nonspecific abnormality of ST
      segment and T wave
NAT
    N-acetyltransferase
    natal
    National Attention Test
    neonatal alloimmune
      thrombocytopenia
    no action taken
    no acute trauma
    nonaccidental trauma
    nonspecific abnormality of T wave
    Nonverbal Ability Test
    nucleic acid test (testing)
    Numerical Attention Test
nat
    national
    native
    natural
    nature
NATB
    Non-Reading Aptitude Test Battery
NATM
    sodium aurothiomalate
NATP
    neonatal alloimmune
      thrombocytopenic purpura
NAUC
    normalized area under the curve
NAVEL
    nerve, artery, vein, empty space,
      lymphatics
NAVV
    Navarro virus
NAW
    nasal antral window
NAWM
    normal-appearing white matter
NB
    nail bed
    needle biopsy
    Negri bodies
    nervus buccalis
    neuroblast
    neuroblastoma

    neurometric (test) battery
    newborn (*See also* nb)
    nitrogen balance
    nitrous oxide-barbiturate
    non-B (hepatitis)
    normoblast
    note well [L. *nota bene*] (*See also*
      n.b.)
    novobiocin
    nuclear bag (certain intrafusal
      muscle fiber nuclei of a
      neuromuscular spindle)
    nutrient broth
N/B
    neopterin to biopterin (ratio)
Nb
    niobium
n.b.
    note well [L. *nota bene*] (*See also*
      NB)
nb
    newborn (*See also* NB)
NBAS
    Neonatal Behavioral Assessment
      Scale
NBAS-K
    Neonatal Behavioral Assessment
      Scale with Kansas Supplements
NBC
    nasobiliary catheter
    nephroblastomatosis complex
    newborn center
    nonbacterial cystitis
    nonbattle casualty
    nonbed care
    nuclear, biologic, chemical
n-BCA
    n-butyl cyanoacrylate
NBCC
    nevoid basal cell carcinoma
NBCCS
    nevoid basal cell carcinoma
      syndrome
NBCIE
    nonbullous congenital ichthyosiform
      erythroderma
NBD
    nasobiliary drain
    necrotizing bowel disease
    neurogenic bladder dysfunction
    neurologic bladder dysfunction
    no brain damage
    nucleotide-binding domain
NBE
    northern bean extract
NBEI
    non–butanol-extractable iodine
      (syndrome)

NBF
not breastfed

NBH
new bag (bottle) hung

NBHH
newborn helpful hints

NBI
neutrophil bactericidal index
no bone injury
nonbattle injury
nosocomial bacterial infection

NBIC
newborn intensive care

NBICU
newborn intensive care unit (*See also* NB Int, NICU)

NBIL
neonatal bilirubin

NB Int
newborn intensive (care unit) (*See also* NBICU)

nBiPAP
nasal bilevel (biphasic) positive airway pressure

nbl
normoblast

NBL/OM
neuroblastoma and opsoclonus-myoclonus

NBM
no bowel movement
normal bone marrow
normal bowel movement
nothing by mouth (*See also* NPO)
nucleus basalis of Meynert

nbM
newborn mouse

nbMb
newborn mouse brain

NBME
normal bone marrow extract

NBN
narrow band noise
newborn nursery

NBNC CLD
HBsAg-negative, anti-HCV-negative chronic liver disease
non-B, non-C chronic liver disease

NBO
nonbed occupancy

NBP
needle biopsy of prostate

neoplastic brachial plexopathy
no bone pathology
nonbacterial prostatitis

NBQC
narrow-base quad cane

NBR
no blood return

NBRS
Nursery Neurobiological Risk Score

NBS
neonatal Bartter syndrome
Neri Barré syndrome
nevoid basal (cell carcinoma) syndrome
New Ballard Score
newborn screen (serum thyroxine and phenylketonuria)
Nijmegan breakage syndrome
no bacteria seen
normal blood serum
normal bowel sounds
normal brain stem
normal burro serum
nystagmus blockage syndrome

NBSCU
newborn special care unit

NBT
nitroblue tetrazolium (test)
normal breast tissue

NBTE
nonbacterial thrombotic endocarditis

NBTG
nitrobenzylthioguanosine

NBTNF
newborn, term, normal, female

NBTNM
newborn, term, normal, male

NBT-PABA
nitroblue tetrazolium-paraaminobenzoic acid

NBTV
nonbacterial thrombotic vegetation

NBUVB
narrowband UVB

NBV
Nelson Bay orthoreovirus

NBVV
nonbleeding visible vessel

NBW
normal birth weight

NC
nabothian cyst

N

NOTES

NC (*continued*)
    nasal cannula
    nasal clearance
    natural cytotoxicity
    neck complaint
    neonatal cholestasis
    nephrocalcin
    nerve conduction
    neural crest
    neurogenic claudication
    neurologic check
    neurologic control
    nevus comedonicus
    nitrocellulose
    nitrosocarbazole
    no casualty
    no change
    no charge
    no complaints
    noise criterion
    noncirrhotic
    noncontributory
    normal control
    normocephalic
    nose clamp
    nose clip
    nose cone
    not classified
    not completed
    not cultured
    nucleocapsid
    nursing coordination

N&C
    nerves and circulation

N:C
    nuclear-cytoplasmic (ratio) (*See also* N/C, NCR)

N/C
    neurocirculatory
    nuclear/cytoplasmic (ratio) (*See also* N:C, N&C, HCR)

nC
    nanocoulomb

n/c
    nuclear-to-cytoplasmic ratio

NCA
    neurocirculatory asthenia
    neutrophil chemotactic activity
    no congenital abnormalities
    nodulocystic acne
    noncontractile area
    nonspecific cross-reacting antigen
    normal coronary arteries
    nuclear cerebral angiogram

NCAH
    nonclassical adrenal hyperplasia

NCAM, N-CAM
    nerve-cell adhesion molecule
    neural cell-adhesive molecule

NcAMP
    nephrogenous cyclic adenosine monophosphate

N/CAN
    nasal cannula

NCAP
    nasal continuous airway pressure

NCAT, NC/AT
    normocephalic and atraumatic

NCB
    natural childbirth
    needle core biopsy
    no code blue

NCC
    neurocysticercosis
    no concentrated carbohydrates
    noncoronary cusp
    nucleus caudalis centralis
    nursing care card
    nursing care continuity

NC-CAH
    nonclassic congenital adrenal hyperplasia

NCCP
    noncardiac chest pain

NCCT
    noncontrast helical computed tomography

NCCU
    neurosurgical continuous care unit
    newborn convalescent care unit

NCD
    neck-capsule distance
    neurocirculatory dystonia
    nitrogen clearance delay
    no congenital deformities
    normal childhood diseases
    normal childhood disorders
    not considered disabling
    not considered disqualifying
    Nursing-Care Dependency (scale)

NCDV
    Nebraska calf diarrhea virus

NCE
    negative contrast echocardiography
    new chemical entity
    nonconvulsive epilepsy

NCF
    neutrophil chemotactic factor
    night care facility
    no cold fluids
    (polymorphonuclear) neutrophil chemotactic factor

NCF(C)
> neutrophil chemotactic factor (complement)

NCGL
> nucleus corporis geniculati lateralis

NCGN
> necrotizing crescentic glomerulonephritis

NCI
> naphthalene creosote and iodoform
> nuclear contour index
> nucleus colliculi inferioris
> nursing care integration

nCi
> nanocurie

NCIS
> nursing care information sheet

NCIT
> Nursing Care Intervention Tool

NCJ
> needle catheter jejunostomy

NCL
> neuronal ceroid lipofuscinosis
> nuclear cardiology laboratory

NCLD
> neonatal chronic lung disease

NCM
> nailfold capillary microscope
> nonclinical manager

N/cm²
> newton per square centimeter

NCMC
> natural cell-mediated cytotoxicity

NCNC
> normochromic, normocytic (anemia)
> normochromic normocytic (erythrocyte)

NCNCA
> normochromic normocytic anemia

NCO
> no complaints offered

NCP
> NeuroCybernetic prosthesis
> no caffeine or pepper
> nonclonogenic proliferating (cells)
> noncollagen protein
> noncontrast phase
> nursing care plan

NCPAP, n-CPAP
> nasal continuous positive airway pressure

NCPB
> neurolytic celiac plexus block

NCPE
> noncardiogenic pulmonary edema

NCPF
> noncirrhotic portal fibrosis

NcpPCu
> nonceruloplasmin plasma copper

NCPR
> no cardiopulmonary resuscitation

NCR
> neurologic/circulatory/range of motion
> neutrophil chemotactic response
> nuclear-cytoplasmic ratio (*See also* N/C, N:C)

nCR
> nodular complete response

NCRC
> nonchild-resistant container

NCRLM
> noncolorectal liver metastasis

NCS
> nasal congestion score
> nerve conduction study
> newborn calf serum
> no concentrated sweets
> noncircumferential stenosis
> noncontact supervision
> noncoronary sinus
> noncured sarcoidosis
> noncurrent serum
> Norian Craniofacial Repair System
> not clinically significant
> numb chin syndrome

NCSE
> nonconvulsive status epilepticus

NCT
> neoadjuvant chemotherapy
> nerve compression test
> nerve conduction test
> neural crest tumor
> neutron capture therapy
> noncontact tonometer
> noncontact tonometry
> number connection test

NCV
> nerve conduction velocity
> no commercial value
> noncholera *Vibrio*
> nuclear venogram

N

NOTES

NCVS
nerve conduction velocity study
ND
nasal deformity
nasoduodenal
nasolacrimal duct
natural death
neck dissection
neonatal death (*See also* NND)
neoplastic disease
nervous debility
neurologic development
neuropsychologic deficit
neurotic depression
neutral density
Newcastle disease
new drug
nifedipine (*See also* NIF)
no data
no date
no disease
nondetectable
nondetermined
nondiabetic
nondisabling
none detectable
normal delivery
normal deposition
normal development
normal dose
nose drops
not detected
not determined
not diagnosed
not done
nothing done
not nondetectable
nucleus of Darkschewitsch
nurse's diagnosis
nutritionally deprived
N&D
nodular and diffuse (lymphoma)
N/D
no defects
N$_D$, n$_D$
refractive index
Nd
neodymium
number of dissimilar (matches)
NDA
new device angioplasty
New Drug Application
no data available
no demonstrable antibodies
no detectable activity
no detectable antibody

NDC
nondifferentiated cell
nuclear dehydrogenating clostridia
NDD
no-dialysis days
NDE
near-death experience
nondiabetic extremity
NDEA
no deviation of electrical axis
NDEV
Ndelle virus
NDF
neutral density filter (test)
neutral detergent fiber
neutrophil diffraction factor
new differentiation factor
new dosage form
no disease found
NDFP
nodular and diffuse fibrous
    proliferation
NDGA
nordihydroguaiaretic acid
NDH
neurogenic dysplasia of hip
NDI
naphthalene diisocyanate
nephrogenic diabetes insipidus
NDIR
nondispersive infrared (analyzer)
NDIRS
nondispersive infrared spectrometer
NDK-K
nucleoside 5'-diphosphate kinase
NDM
neonatal diabetes mellitus
NDMA
nitrosodimethylamine
N dm/vm
nucleus dorsomedialis-ventromedialis
nDNA
native deoxyribonucleic acid
N/D NHL
nodular/diffuse non-Hodgkin
    lymphoma
Nd/NT
nondistended/nontender
NDOV
Nyando virus
NDP
net dietary protein
nucleoside diphosphate
NDP-K
nucleoside diphosphate kinase
NDR
neonatal death rate
neurotic depressive reaction

normal detrusor reflex
nucleus dorsalis raphe
NDS
 Neurologic Disability Score
 New Drug Submission
 normal dog serum
NDSA
 nondermatomal sensory abnormality
NDST
 neurodevelopmental screening test
NDT
 nasal duodenostomy tube
 neurodevelopmental techniques
 neurodevelopmental treatment
  (physical therapy)
 noise detection threshold
 nondestructive testing
NDUV
 Ndumu virus
NDV
 Newcastle disease virus
NDW
 number of different words
NDx
 nondiagnostic
Nd:YAG
 neodymium:YAG (laser)
 neodymium:yttrium-aluminum-garnet
  (surgical laser)
Nd:YLF
 neodymium: yttrium-lithium-fluoride
  (laser)
NE
 national emergency
 nausea and emesis
 necrotic enteritis
 neomycin (*See also* N, neo, NM)
 neonatal encephalopathy
 nephropathia epidemica
 nerve ending
 nerve excitability (test)
 neural excitation
 neuroendocrine
 neuroepithelium
 neurologic examination
 neutropenic enterocolitis
 neutrophil elastase
 never exposed
 no ectopia
 no effect
 no enlargement
 nonelastic

nonendogenous
norepinephrine (*See also* NOR-EPI)
norethindrone
not elevated
not enlarged
not equal
not evaluated
not examined
nutcracker esophagus
Ne
 neon
NEA
 neoplasm embryonic antigen
 no evidence of abnormality
NEAA
 nonessential amino acid
NEAC
 norethindrone acetate
NEAD
 nonepileptic attack disorder
NEAT
 nonexercise activity thermogenesis
 Norris Educational Achievement
  Test
NEB
 hand-held nebulizer
 neuroendocrine body
NEC
 necrotizing enterocolitis
 neuroendocrine cell
 Neurological Examination for
  Children
 no essential change
 noise equivalent counts
 nonesterified cholesterol
 not elsewhere classifiable
 not elsewhere classified
 not elsewhere coded
 not enough cells
nec
 necessary
NECT
 nonenhanced computed tomography
NED
 no evidence of disease
 no expiration date
 normal equivalent deviation
NED-SD
 no evidence of disease-stationary
  disease
NEEE
 Near East equine encephalomyelitis

NOTES

NEEG
neoelectroencephalography
normal electroencephalogram

NEEP
negative end-expiratory pressure

NEF
negative expiratory force
negative factor
nephritic factor (*See also* NF)

NEFA
nonesterified fatty acid

NEFG
normal external female genitalia

NEG
neglect
nonenzymatic glycation

neg
negative (*See also* N)

NEH
neutrophilic eccrine hidradenitis

NEJ
neuroeffector junction

NEM
N-ethylmaleimide
neurotrophic enhancing molecule
no evidence of malignancy
nonspecific esophageal motility
(disorder)

nem
nutritional milk unit [Ger.
Nährungs Einheit Milch]

nema
nematode (threadworm)

Nemb
Nembutal

NEMD
nonexudative macular degeneration
nonspecific esophageal motility
disorder
nonspecific esophageal motor
dysfunction

NENAR
noneosinophilic nonallergic rhinitis

NENT
nasal endotracheal tube

NEO
necrotizing external otitis
Neuroticism, Extroversion, and
Openness (test)

neo
neoarsphenamine
neomycin (*See also* N, NE, NM)
neonatal (*See also* neonat)
neovascularity

NEOH
neonatal/high (risk)

NEOM
neonatal/medium (risk)

neonat
neonatal (*See also* neo)

NEP
needle-exchange program
negative expiratory pressure
nephrology (*See also* NEPH)
neutral endopeptidase
no evidence of pathology
noise equivalent power

nep
nephrectomy

NEPD
no evidence of pulmonary disease

NEPH
nephrology (*See also* NEP)

neph
nephritis

NEPHGE
nonequilibrium pH (gradient) gel
electrophoresis

NEPHRO
nephrogram

NEP-I
neutral endopeptidase inhibition

NEPPK
nonepidermolytic palmoplantar
keratoderma

NEPV
Nepuyo virus

NER
no evidence of recurrence
nonionizing electromagnetic
radiation

NERD
no evidence of recurrent disease
nonerosive reflux disease

NERDS
nodules, eosinophilia, rheumatism,
dermatitis, and swelling

NERO
noninvasive evaluation of radiation
output

nerv, ner
nervous
nervousness

NES
nonepileptic seizure
nonstandard electrolyte solution
norepinephrine-selective
not elsewhere specified

NESP
novel erythropoiesis stimulating
protein

NESP55
neuroendocrine secretory protein 55

NET
choroidal or subretinal
neovascularization

nasoendotracheal tube (*See also* NETT)
nerve excitability test
netilmicin
neuroectodermal tumor
neuroendocrine tumor
norepinephrine transporter
norethisterone

net
Internet

NETA
norethindrone acetate (Aygestin)

NETEN, NET-EN
norethisterone enanthate

NETT
nasal endotracheal tube (*See also* NET)

NETZ
needle (diathermy) excision of the transformation zone

neu
neurilemma

NeuAc
N-acetylneuraminic acid

neur, neuro, neurol
neurologic
neurologist (*See also* N)
neurology (*See also* N)

neuropath
neuropathology (*See also* NP)

neurosurg
neurosurgeon (*See also* NSurg)
neurosurgery (*See also* NS, NSurg)

ncut
neuter (*See also* n)
neutral
neutralize
neutrophil

NEV
noninvasive extrathoracic ventilator

NEX
nose to ear to xiphoid
number of excitations (radiology)

NEY, NEYA
neomycin egg yolk (agar)

NF
nafcillin (*See also* NAF)
nasopharyngeal fibroma
National Formulary
necrotizing fasciitis
nephritic factor (*See also* NEF)
neurofibromatosis

neurofilament
neutral fraction
night frequency (of voiding)
Nissen fundoplication
noise factor
none found
nonfiltered
nonfluent
nonfront
nonfunction
nonwhite female
normal flow
not filtered
not found
nursed fair
nursing facility
nylon fiber

NF 1, NF1, NF-1
neurofibromatosis type 1

NF 2, NF2, NF-2
neurofibromatosis type 2

nF
nanofarad

NFA
Nerve Fiber Analyzer

NFA-I
normal fecal antigen

NFALO
Nerve Fiber Analyzer laser ophthalmoscope

NFAP
nursing facility-acquired pneumonia

NFAR
no further action required

NFAT
nuclear factor of activated T cell

NF-κB
nuclear factor-kappa B

NFB
nonfermentative gram-negative bacilli
nonfermenting bacteria

NFC
not favorably considered

NFCC
neighborhood family care center

NFCS
neonatal facial coding system

NFD
neurofibrillary degeneration
no family doctor

NOTES

N

NFDR
> neurofacial-digitorenal (syndrome)
> neurofaciodigitorenal

NFE
> nonferrous extract

NFFD
> not fit for duty

NFH
> nonfamilial hematuria

NFI
> nerve-function impairment
> no-fault insurance
> no further information

NF-KB, NF-kappa-B
> nuclear factor-κB
> nuclear factor kappa B

NFL
> nerve fiber layer

NFLD
> nerve-fiber-layer defect

NFLX
> norfloxacin (Noroxin)

NFM
> northern fowl mite

NF-NS, NFNS
> neurofibromatosis-Noonan syndrome

NFP
> natural family planning
> neurofilament protein
> neurofilament triplet polypeptide
> no family physician
> not for publication

NFPA
> nonfunctioning pituitary adenoma

NFS
> neural foraminal stenosis
> non-fire setter

NFT
> neurofibrillary tangle
> Nitrazine fern test
> no further treatment

NFTD
> normal full-term delivery

NFTE
> not found this examination

NFTSD
> normal full-term spontaneous
>   delivery

NFTT
> nonorganic failure to thrive

NFW
> nursed fairly well

N-G
> nasogastric (*See also* NG)

NG
> nasogastric (*See also* N-G)
> new growth
> nitroglycerin (*See also* nitro, NTG, NTZ)
> nodose ganglion
> no good
> no growth
> nongenetic
> nongroupable

ng
> nanogram

NGA
> nutrient gelatin agar

NGAV
> Ngaingan virus

NGB
> neurogenic bladder

NGC
> nucleus (reticularis) gigantocellularis

N-Ger
> neurologic geriatrics

NGF
> nerve growth factor

NG fdgs
> nasogastric feedings

NGFR
> nerve growth factor receptor
> neural growth factor receptor

NGGR
> nonglucogenic/glucogenic ratio

NGHD-SS
> non-growth hormone-deficient short
>   stature

NGI
> not guilty (by reason of) insanity
>   (*See also* NGRI)
> nuclear globulin inclusion
> Nurse's Global Impressions

n giv
> not given

NGJ
> nasogastro-jejunostomy

NGJT
> nasogastrojejunal tube

NGM
> norgestimate

ng/mL
> nanogram per mL
> nanograms per milliliter

NGOs
> nongovernmental organizations

NGR
> narrow gauze roll
> nasogastric replacement

NGRI
> not guilty by reason of insanity
>   (*See also* NGI)

NGS
> normal goat serum

NGSA
　　nerve growth stimulating activity
NGSF
　　nongenital skin fibroblast
　　nothing grown so far
NGT
　　nasogastric tube
　　normal glucose tolerance
NgTD
　　negative to date
NGU
　　nongonococcal urethritis
NGVB
　　nightguard vital bleaching
NH
　　natriuretic hormone
　　Naval Hospital
　　neonatal hemochromatosis
　　neonatal hepatitis
　　neurologically handicapped
　　nodular and histiocytic
　　nonhuman
　　nursing home
NH3, NH₃
　　ammonia
　　anhydrous ammonia
N(H)
　　hydrogen density
NHA
　　no histologic abnormalities
　　nonspecific hepatocellular
　　　abnormality
NHAIS
　　Naylor-Harwood Adult Intelligence
　　　Scale
NHBD, NHB
　　non-heart-beating donor
NHC
　　neighborhood health center
　　neonatal hypocalcemia
　　nonhistone chromatin
　　nonhistone chromosomal (protein)
　　nursing home care
NH4Cl
　　ammonium chloride
NHCP
　　nonhistone chromosomal protein
NHCU
　　nursing home care unit
NHD
　　normal hair distribution

NHDF
　　normal human diploid fibroblast
NHDL
　　non–high-density lipoprotein
NHE
　　Na^+/H^+ exchanger
　　sodium/hydrogen exchanger
NHEI
　　Na^+/H^+ exchange inhibitor
NHG
　　normal human globulin
NHGJ
　　normal human gastric juice
NHGU
　　net hepatic glucose uptake
NHH
　　neurohypophyseal hormone
NHI
　　National Health Insurance
　　Neisseria-Haemophilus Identification
NHIS
　　Naylor-Harwood Intelligence Scale
NHK
　　normal human kidney
NHL
　　nodular histiocytic lymphoma
　　non-Hodgkin lymphoma
nHL
　　normalized hearing level
NHLPP
　　hereditary neuropathy with liability
　　　for pressure palsy
NHM
　　no heroic measures
NHML
　　non-Hodgkin malignant lymphoma
NHO
　　notify house officer
NHP
　　nonhemoglobin protein
　　nonhistone protein
　　normal human (pooled) plasma
　　Nottingham Health Profile
　　nursing home placement
NHPA
　　no histopathologic abnormality
NHPP
　　normal human pooled plasma
NHR
　　net histocompatibility ratio
　　noise-to-harmonic ratio

NOTES

N

NHS
    Nance-Horan syndrome
    normal horse serum
    normal human serum
NHT
    neoadjuvant hormonal therapy
    nonpenetrating head trauma
    nursing home transfer
NHTR
    nonhemolytic transfusion reaction
nHuIFN-beta
    natural human interferon-beta
nHuIFN-gamma
    natural human interferon-gamma
NHW
    nonhealing wound
NHWM
    normal human white matter
NI
    neuraminidase inhibition (*See also*
        NAI)
    neurologic improvement
    neutralization index
    nitroxoline
    no improvement
    no information
    noise index
    none indicated
    not identified
    not isolated
    nucleus intercalatus
Ni
    nickel
NIA
    nephelometric inhibition assay
    neutrophil-inducing activity
    niacin
    no information available
NIAL
    not in active labor
NIB
    noninvolved bone
NIBP
    noninvasive blood pressure
NIBPM
    noninvasive blood pressure
        measurement
NIBS
    nearly ideal binary solvent
niBUT
    not invasive break-up time
NIC
    neurogenic intermittent claudication
    newborn intensive care
    Nomarsky interference contrast
    noninvasive carotid (study)
    Nursing Interventions Classification

Nic
    nicotinyl alcohol
NiCad
    nickel-cadmium
NICC
    neonatal intensive care center
    noninfectious chronic cystitis
NICE
    new, interesting, and challenging
        experiences
    noninvasive carotid examination
NICO
    neuralgia-inducing cavitational
        osteonecrosis
    noninvasive cardiac output
        (monitor)
NICS
    noninvasive carotid studies
NICTH
    non-islet cell tumor hypoglycemia
NICU
    neonatal intensive care unit
    neurologic intensive care unit
    neurosurgical intensive care unit
        (*See also* NSICU)
    newborn intensive care unit (*See
        also* NBICU)
    nonallergic contact urticaria
    nonimmunologic contact urticaria
NID
    no identifiable disease
    not in distress
NIDA five
    amphetamine/methamphetamine,
        opiates, and phencyclidine
NIDD
    non–insulin-dependent diabetes
NIDDM
    noninsulin-dependent diabetes
        mellitus
    non–insulin-dependent diabetes
        mellitus
NIDS
    nonionic detergent soluble
NIF
    negative inspiratory force (*See also*
        NiF)
    neutrophil-immobilizing factor
    nifedipine (*See also* N)
    nifuroquine
    nonintestinal fibroblast
    not in file
NiF
    negative inspiratory force (*See also*
        NIF)
nif genes
    nitrogen fixation (genes for)

NIFS
noninvasive flow study
nIg
nonimmunoglobulin
nig.
black [L. *niger*]
NIGS
NIH-CPSI
National Institutes of Health
Chronic Prostatitis Symptom
Index
NIHD
noise-induced hearing damage
NIHF
nonimmune hydrops fetalis
NIHL
noise-induced hearing loss
NIHSS
National Institutes of Health Stroke
Scale
NIID
neuronal intranuclear inclusion
disease
NIL
noise interference level
nothing in light
not in labor
nil.
nothing [L. *nihil*]
NIM2, NIM-2
Nerve Integrity Monitor 2
NIM-2
Nicolet Nerve Integrity Monitor
NIMA
noninherited maternal antigen
NIMAs
noninherited maternal antigens
NIMH-DIS
National Institute of Mental Health
Diagnostic Interview Schedule
NIMH-OC
National Institute of Mental
Health-Global Obsessive
Compulsive Scale
NIMV
noninvasive motion ventilation
NIN
nuclear excision repair instability
NI-NR
no infection-no rejection
NINU
neurointermediate nursing unit

NINVS
noninvasive neurovascular studies
NIOPCs
no intraoperative complications
NIP
catnip
negative inspiratory pressure
nipple
nitroiodophenyl
no infection present
no inflammation present
nonspecific (chronic) interstitial
pneumonitis
nonspecific interstitial pneumonia
nonspecific interstitial pneumonitis
NIPAs
noninherited paternal antigens
NIPB
noninvasive blood pressure
NIPD
nightly intermittent peritoneal
dialysis
NIPII
no improvement with pinhole
NIPPV
noninvasive positive pressure
ventilation
NIPS
Neonatal Infant Pain Scale
noninvasive programmed stimulation
noninvolved psoriatic skin
NIPTS
noise-induced permanent threshold
shift
NIQV
Nique virus
NIR
near infrared
near-infrared interactance
NIRA
nitrite reductase
NIRCA
nonisotopic RNase cleavage assay
NIRD
nonimmune renal disease
NIRP
near infrared photoplethysmography
NIRR
non–insulin-requiring remission

NOTES

N

NIRS
near-infrared spectroscopy (*See also* NIS)
normal inactivated rabbit serum

NIS
near-infrared spectroscopy (*See also* NIRS)
no inflammatory signs
nonimmune sheep (serum)
sodium-iodide symporter

NISD
neonatal iron-storage disease

NISH
nonisotopic in situ hybridization
nonradioactive in situ hybridization

NISM
(bed) nucleus of stria medullaris

NISs
New Injury Severity Score

NIST
(bed) nucleus of stria terminalis

NISV
nonionic surfactant vesicle

NIT
nasointestinal tube
neonatal isoimmune thrombocytopenia

NITD
neuroleptic-induced tardive dyskinesia
non–insulin-treated disease

nit. ox.
nitric oxide (*See also* NO)

Nitro
sodium nitroprusside

nitro
nitroglycerin (*See also* NG, NTG, NTZ)

NITTS
noise-induced temporary threshold shift

NIV
nodule-inducing virus
noninvasive ventilation

NIVA
noninvasive vascular assessment

NIVLS
noninvasive vascular laboratory studies

NIVS
noninvasive ventilatory support

NIZ
noninfarct zone

NJ
nasojejunal (tube)

NJLV
Naranjal virus

NK
natural killer (cell)
not known

N.K.
Nomenklatur Kommission

NKA
neurokinin A
no known allergies

nkat
nanokatal

NKB
neurokinin B
no known basis
not keeping baby

NKC
natural killer cell
nonketotic coma

NKCC2
sodium-potassium-2 chloride cotransporter

NKD
no known diseases

NKDA
no known drug allergies

NKE
needle-knife electrocautery

NKECN
nonkeratinizing epidermoid carcinoma

NKF
needle-knife fistulotomy

NKFA
no known food allergies

NKH
nonketotic hyperglycemia (*See also* NKHG)
nonketotic hyperglycinemia
nonketotic hyperosmolar
nonketotic hyperosmotic

NKHA
nonketotic hyperosmolar acidosis

NKHG
nonketotic hyperglycemia (*See also* NKH)
nonketotic hyperglycinemia

NKHHC
nonketotic hyperglycmic-hyperosmolar coma

NKHOC
nonketotic hyperosmolar coma

NKHS
nonketotic hyperosmolar syndrome
normal Krebs-Henseleit solution

NKMA
no known medication allergies

NKOV
Nkolbisson virus

NKP
  needle-knife papillotomy
NKPP
  needle-knife precut papillotomy
NKSF
  natural killer (cell)-stimulating
    factor
NKTS
  natural killer target structure
NL
  nasolacrimal
  neural lobe
  neutral lipid
  nodular lymphoma
  nonlatex
  normal (*See also* N, n, nl, NOR,
    norm, NR)
  normal libido
  normal limits
  normolipemic
  Nyhan-Lesch (syndrome)
nL
  nanoliter
nl
  normal limits
  normal (value) (*See also* n, NL,
    NOR, norm)
NLA
  neuroleptanalgesia
  neuroleptanesthesia
  normal lactase activity
NLAA
  naphthoxylactic acid
NLAL
  nodule-like alveolar lesion
NLB
  needle liver biopsy
NLC
  nasolabial crease
NL ClCl, NLC&C, NL C/Cl
  normal libido, coitus, and climax
NLD
  nasolacrimal duct
  necrobiosis lipoidica diabeticorum
  no local doctor
NLDL
  normal low-density lipoprotein
n-LDL
  native LDL
NLDO
  nasolacrimal duct obstruction

NLE
  neonatal lupus erythematosus
  nurse's late entry
Nle
  norleucine
NLEA
  Nutrition Labeling and Education
    Act of 1990
NLF
  nasolabial fold
  nelfinavir
  neonatal lung fibroblast
  nonlactose fermentation
NLFGNR
  nonlactose fermenting gram-negative
    rod
NLGCLS
  Noonan-like giant cell lesion
    syndrome
NLH
  nodular lymphoid hyperplasia
NLM
  noise level monitor
  no limitation of motion
NLMC
  nocturnal leg muscle cramp
NLN
  no longer needed
NLO
  nasolacrimal occlusion
NLOB
  needle-localized open biopsy
NLP
  natural language processing
  neurolinguistic program
  nodular liquefying panniculitis
  no light perception
  normal light perception
  normal luteal phase
NLPD
  nodular-lymphocytic, poorly
    differentiated
NLS
  neonatal lupus syndrome
  Neu-Laxova syndrome
  nonlinear least squares (method)
  normal lymphocyte supernatant
  nuclear localization signal
  nuclear localization signal (motif)
NLSD
  normal life span for dogs

NOTES

N

NLT

Names Learning Test
normal lymphocyte transfer (test)
not later than (*See also* nlt)
not less than (*See also* nlt)
nucleus lateralis tuberis

nlt

not later than (*See also* NLT)
not less than (*See also* NLT)

NLV

Norwalk-like virus

NLX

naloxone (*See also* Nx)

NM

neomycin (*See also* N, NE, neo)
neuromedical
neuromuscular
neuronal microdysgenesis
nevomelanocytic
nictitating membrane [L. *nictitare* to wink]
night and morning (*See also* N&M, n.m.)
nitrogen mustard (*See also* HN2)
nodular melanoma
nodular mixed (lymphocytic-histiocystic)
nonmalignant
nonmotile (bacteria)
nonwhite male
normetadrenaline
normetanephrine (*See also* NMN, normet)
not measurable
not measured
not mentioned
not motile
nuclear matrix
nuclear medicine
nuclear membrane
nurse manager

N/M

newton per meter

N&M

nerves and muscles
night and morning (*See also* NM, n.m.)

N/m²

newton per square meter

nM

nanomolar

n.m.

night and morning [L. *nocte et mane*] (*See also* N&M, n.m.)

nm

nanometer
nonmetallic
nux moschata (nutmeg)

NMA

neurogenic muscular atrophy

NMATWT

New Mexico Attitude Toward Work Test

NMB

neuromuscular blockade

NMBA

neuromuscular blocking agent
nitrosomethylbenzylamine

NMC

neuromuscular control
nodular, mixed cell (lymphoma)
no malignant cells
nucleus reticularis magnocellularis
nurse-managed center

NMCD

nephrophthisis-medullary cystic disease

NMCPT

New Mexico Career Planning Test

NMD

naturopathic doctor
neuromuscular disorder
neuromyodysplasia
neuronal migration disorders
normal muscle development

NMDA

N-methyl-D-aspartate

NME

necrolytic migratory erythema
new molecular entity

NMEP

neurogenic motor evoked potential

NMES

neuromuscular electrical stimulation
neuromuscular electrical stimulator

NMF

neuromuscular facilitation
nonmigrating fraction (of spermatozoa)

NMG

N-methyl-D-glucamide

NMGTD

nonmetastatic gestational trophoblastic disease

NMH

neurally mediated hypotension

NMHH

no medical health history

NMI

no manifest improvement
no mental illness
no middle initial
no more information
normal male infant

NMIS
    nuclear medicine information
      system
NMJ
    neuromuscular junction
NMJAPT
    New Mexico Job Application
      Procedures Test
NMKB
    not married, keeping baby
NMKOT
    New Mexico Knowledge of
      Occupations Test
NML
    nodular mixed lymphoma
NMM
    nevoid malignant melanoma
    nodular malignant melanoma
NMN
    neurotized melanocytic nevus
    nicotinamide mononucleotide
    N1-methylnicotinamide
    no middle name
    normetanephrine (*See also* NM,
      normet)
    Novy-McNeal-Nicolle (medium)
      (*See also* NNN)
NMN+
    nicotinamide mononucleotide
      (reduced form)
NMNKB
    not married, not keeping baby
NMO
    nitrogen mustard oxide
NMOH
    no medical ocular history
nmol
    nanomole
nmol/L
    millimicromolar
    nanomole per liter
NMOS
    N-type metal oxide semiconductor
NMP
    nail matrix phenolization
    neuromuscular pacification
    neutral metallopeptidase
    normal menstrual period
    nuclear matrix protein
    nucleoside 5'-monophosphate
NMP-22
    nuclear matrix protein

NMPCA
    nonmetric principal component
      analysis
NMR
    Neill-Mooser reaction
    neonatal mortality rate
    neonatal mortality risk
    nictitating membrane response
    nuclear magnetic resonance
    nuclear medicine
NMRI
    nuclear magnetic resonance imaging
NMRL
    normal-mode ruby laser
NMRS
    nuclear magnetic resonance
      spectroscopy
NMRT (R)
    Nuclear Medicine Radiologic
      Technologist (Registered)
NMS
    neonatal morphine solution
    neurally mediated syncope
    neuroleptic malignant syndrome
    neuromuscular spindle
    N-methylspiroperidol
    normal mouse serum
N·m/s
    newton meter per second
NMSC
    nonmelanoma skin cancer
NMSE
    normalized mean square root
NMSIDS
    near-miss sudden infant death
      syndrome
NMT
    nebulized mist treatment
    neuromuscular tension
    neuromuscular transmission
    no more than
    nuclear medicine technology
NMTB
    neuromuscular transmission blockade
NMTD
    nonmetastatic trophoblastic disease
NMTS
    neuromuscular tension state
NMTSS
    nonmenstrual toxic shock syndrome
NMU
    neuromuscular unit

N

NOTES

NMUT
nitrosomethylurethane
NMV
New Minto virus
NMVS
neurally mediated vasovagal syncope
N/N
negative/negative
nurse's notes (*See also* NN)
N-N
nurse-to-nurse (orders)
NN

narrative notes
Navajo neuropathy
neonatal
neural network
nevocellular nevus
normally nourished
normal nursery
nurse's notes (*See also* N/N)
N:N

azo group (chemical group with two nitrogen atoms)
n.n.

new name [L. *nomen novum*] (*See also* n. nov., nom. nov., nov. n.)
nn

nerves (*See also* Ns)
NNA

normochromic normocytic anemia
NNAS

neonatal narcotic abstinence syndrome
NNB

normal newborn
NNBC

node negative breast cancer
NND

neonatal death (*See also* ND)
New and Nonofficial Drugs
nonspecific nonerosive duodenitis
NNE

neonatal necrotizing enterocolitis
nonneuronal enolase
NNG

nonspecific nonerosive gastritis
NNI

noise and number index
NNL

no new laboratory (test orders)
NNM

neonatal mortality
NNN

nitrosonornicotine
normal neonatal nursery
normal newborn nursery

Novy, MacNeal, and Nicolle (medium) (*See also* NMN)
NNO

no new orders
n. nov.

new name [L. *nomen novum*] (*See also* n.n., nom. nov., nov. n.)
NNP

nerve net pulse
non-nociceptive pain
N:NPK

grams of nitrogen to non-protein kilocalories
NNR

New and Nonofficial Remedies
not necessary to return
NNRTI

nonnucleoside reverse transcriptase inhibitor
NNS

nasal nicotine spray
neonatal screen (hematocrit, total bilirubin, and total protein)
nicotine nasal spray
nonneoplastic syndrome
nonnutritive sucking
NNT

neonatally tolerant
nuclei nervi trigemini
number needed to treat
NNU

net nitrogen utilization
NNV

nasal nocturnal ventilation
NNWI

Neonatal Narcotic Withdrawal Index
NO

narcotics officer (*See also* NARC, narc, narco)
nasal oxygen
nitric acid
nitric oxide
nitroglycerin ointment
nitroso-
none obtained
nonobese
number (*See also* N, n, No, no.)
nursing office
N2O

nitrous oxide
NO₂

nitrogen dioxide
No

nobelium
no.

number [L. *numero*] (*See also* N, n, NO)

NOAEL
no observed adverse effect level
NOAR
Norfolk Arthritis Register
NOBT
nonoperative biopsy technique
NOC
N-nitroso compound
noc, noct
nocturia
nocturnal [L. *noctis* of the night]
NO-CCE
no clubbing, cyanosis, or edema
NOD
nodular (melanoma)
nondefinitive (pattern)
nonobese diabetic
notice of disagreement
notify of death
NOE
nasoorbitoethmoid
nuclear Overhauser effect
NOED
no observed effect dose
NOEL
no observed effect level (of toxin)
no ess abn
no essential abnormalities
NOF
nonossifying fibroma
N/OFQ
nociceptin/orphanin FQ
NOFT
nonorganic failure to thrive
NOGM
no gammopathy (detected)
NOH
neurogenic orthostatic hypotension
NOI
nature of illness
NOII
nonocclusive intestinal ischemia
NOK
next of kin
NOL
not on label
NOM
nonsuppurative otitis media
normal extraocular movements
nom. dub.
a doubtful name [L. *nomen dubium*]

NOMI
nonocclusive mesenteric infarction
nonocclusive mesenteric ischemia
NOMID
neonatal-onset multisystem
inflammatory disease
nom. nov.
new name [L. *nomen novum*] (*See also* n.n., n. nov., nov. n.)
nom. nud.
name without designation [L. *nomen nudum*]
NO/N2
nitric oxide/nitrogen
NOND
none detected
NONF
nonfasting
non-MALT
non–mucosa-associated lymphoid
tissue (lymphoma)
NONMEM
nonlinear mixed-effects model
(modeling)
non pal
not palpable
non-Q MI
non-Q-wave myocardial infarction
non reb
nonrebreathing (mask)
nonREM, non-REM
nonrapid eye movement (*See also* NREM)
NONS
nonspecific
NO-NSAIDs
nitric oxide-releasing NSAID
nonsegs
nonsegmented (neutrophils)
non-SSM
non-skin-sparing mastectomy
nonvis, nonviz
nonvisualized
N2O:O2
nitrous oxide to oxygen ratio
NOOB
not out of bed
N$_2$O/O$_2$/opioid
nitrous oxide-oxygen-opioid
(anesthetic technique)
NOP
national outpatient profile

NOTES

NOP (*continued*)
  not on patient
  not otherwise provided (for) (*See also* NP)

4NOQ
  4-nitroquinolin-1-oxide-induced tumor

NOR
  noradrenaline (*See also* Noradr)
  norethynodrel
  normal (*See also* N, n, NL, nl, norm, NR)
  nortriptyline
  nucleolar organizing region (cytogenetics)
  nucleolus-organizing region

Noradr
  noradrenaline (*See also* NOR)

NORC
  normal curve

NOR-EPI
  norepinephrine (*See also* NE)

norleu
  norleucine

norm
  normal (*See also* N, n, NL, nl, NOR, NR)

normet
  normetanephrine (*See also* NM, NMN)

NORV
  Northway virus

NOS
  neonatal opium solution (diluted deodorized tincture of opium)
  network operating system
  new-onset seizures
  nitrous oxide synthase
  no organisms seen
  not on staff
  not otherwise specified

NOS1
  nitric oxide synthase gene

nos
  numbers

NOSAC
  nonsteroidal antiinflammatory compound

NOSE
  normal ovarian surface epithelium

NOSI
  nitric oxide synthase inhibitors

NOSIE
  Nurses' Observation Scale for Inpatient Evaluation

NoSOS
  no surgery on site

NOT
  nocturnal oxygen therapy
  nucleus of optic tract

NOTT
  nocturnal oxygen therapy trial

NOU
  not on unit

Nov
  novobiocin

nov.
  new [L. *novum*]

NOV L
  human insulin zinc suspension (Novolin L)

NOV N
  human insulin isophane suspension (Novolin N)

nov. n.
  new name [L. *novum nomen*] (*See also* n.n., n. nov., nom. nov.)

NOV R
  human insulin regular (Novolin R)

nov. sp.
  new species [L. *novum species*]

NOW
  negotiable order of withdrawal

NP
  nasal prongs
  nasopharyngeal
  nasopharynx (*See also* NPhx)
  near point (ophthalmology)
  necrotizing pancreatitis
  neonatal-perinatal
  nephrographic phase
  nerve palsy
  neuritic plaque
  neuropathology (*See also* neuropath)
  neuropeptide
  neurophysin (*See also* Np)
  neuropsychiatrist
  neuropsychiatry
  neutrogenic precautions
  newly presented
  new patient
  Niemann-Pick (disease)
  nitrogen-phosphorus (detector in gas chromatography)
  nitrophenide
  nitrophenol
  nitroprusside
  nodular paragranuloma
  nonpalpable
  nonpathologic
  nonpaying
  nonphagocytic
  nonpracticing
  nonproducer (cell)
  no pain

no phone
no progression
normal plasma
normal pressure
nosocomial pneumonia
not (otherwise) provided (for) (*See also* NOP)
not palpable
not perceptible
not performed
not practiced
not pregnant
not present
nuclear pharmacist
nuclear pharmacy
nucleoplasmic (index)
nucleoprotein
nucleoside phosphorylase
nursed poorly
nursing practice
nursing procedure
proper name [L. *nomen proprium*] (*See also* n.p.)

N-P

need-persistence

Np

neper (unit for comparing magnitude of two powers, usually electrical or acoustic)
neptunium
neurophysin (*See also* NP)

n.p.

proper name [L. *nomen proprium*] (*See also* NP)

np

nucleotide pair

NPA

nasopharyngeal airway
nasopharyngeal aspirate
near point of accommodation
Niemann-Pick disease type A
no previous admission
nucleus of pretectal area

NPa

nail patella (syndrome)

NPAT

nonparoxysmal atrial tachycardia

Np-AVP

neurophysin associated with vasopressin

NPB

Nellcor Puritan Bennett (instrumentation)
Niemann-Pick (disease type) B
nodal premature beat
nonprotein bound

NPBC

node-positive breast cancer

NPBF

nonplacental blood flow

NPC

nasopharyngeal cancer
nasopharyngeal carcinoma (*See also* NPCa)
near point of convergence
negative peritoneal cytology
Niemann-Pick (disease type) C (sphingomyelin lipidosis)
nodal premature contractions
nonparenchymal (liver) cell
nonpatient contact
nonproductive cough
nonprotein calorie
no prenatal care (*See also* NPNC)
no previous complaint
nucleus of posterior commissure

NPCa

nasopharyngeal carcinoma (*See also* NPC)

NPCC

nonprotein carbohydrate calories

NPCIS

nasopharyngeal carcinoma in situ

NP-CPAP, NPCPAP

nasal prong continuous positive airway pressure

NPCR

normalized protein catabolic rate

NPD

narcissistic personality disorder
natriuretic plasma dialysate
negative pressure device
Niemann-Pick disease
Niemann-Pick (disease type) D
nitrogen-phosphorus detector
nonprescription drugs
no pathologic diagnosis

NPDL

nodular poorly differentiated lymphocytic (lymphoma)

NPDR

nonproliferative diabetic retinopathy

NOTES

NPE
neurogenic pulmonary edema
neuropsychologic examination
nonpulmonary route of elimination
no palpable enlargement
normal pelvic examination

NPEM
nocturnal penile erection monitoring

N periv
nuclei periventriculares

NPEV
nonpolio enterovirus

NPF
nasopharyngeal fiberscope
no predisposing factor

N-PFMSO4
nebulized preservative-free morphine
sulfate

NPFT
Neurotic Personality Factor Test

NPG
nonpregnant

NPGS
neopentyl glycol succinate

NPH
nephronophthisis
neutral protamine Hagedorn
(insulin)
no previous history
normal-pressure hydrocephalus
nucleus prepositus hypoglossi
nucleus pulposus herniation

NPH1
nephronophthisis type 1

NPhx
nasopharynx (See also NP)

NPI
Narcissistic Personality Inventory
neonatal perception inventory
Neuropsychiatric Inventory
no present illness
Nottingham Prognostic Index
nucleoplasmic index

NPIC
neurogenic peripheral intermittent
claudication

NPII
Neonatal Pulmonary Insufficiency
Index

NPIS
Numeric Pain Intensity Scale

NPJT
nonparoxysmal (atrioventricular)
junctional tachycardia

NPK
nonprotein kilocalories

NPL
insulin lispro protamine
(suspension)
nasopharyngolaryngoscopy
neoproteolipid
nodular poorly differentiated
lymphoma

NPLSM
neoplasm

NPM
nothing per mouth

NPN
nonprotein nitrogen

nPNA
normalized protein nitrogen
appearance

NPNC
no prenatal care (See also NPC)

NPNT
nonpalpable, nontender

NPO
nil per os
nothing by mouth [L. nil per os]
(See also NBM)
nucleus preopticus

n.p.o.
nothing by mouth (nil per os)

NPOC
nonpurgeable organic carbon

NPO/HS
nothing by mouth at bedtime [L.
nil per os hora somni]

NPOS
nitrite positive

NPOT
narrow pulmonary outflow tract

Np-OT
oxytocin-associated neurophysin

NPOW
not prisoner of war

NPP
nitrophenylphosphate
normally progressing pregnancy
normal pool plasma
normal postpartum

NPPB
normal perfusion pressure
breakthrough

NPPNG
non–penicillinase-producing Neisseria
gonorrheae

NP polio
nonparalytic poliomyelitis

NPPV
nasal positive pressure ventilation
noninvasive positive-pressure
ventilation

NPR
    nasopharyngeal reflux
    natriuretic peptide receptor
    net protein ratio
    normal pulse rate
    nothing per rectum
    nucleoside phosphoribosyl

NPRL
    normal pupillary reaction to light

NPRM
    notice of proposed rulemaking

NPS
    nasopharyngeal stenosis
    new patient set-up

Nps
    nitrophenylsulfenyl

NPSA
    nonphysician surgical assistant
    normal pilosebaceous apparatus

^{59}NP scintigraphy
    iodomethyl-norcholesterol-59
      scintigraphy

NPSD
    nonpotassium-sparing diuretics

NPSG
    nocturnal polysomnogram
    nocturnal polysomnography

NPSH
    nonprotein sulfhydryl (group)

NP-SLE, NPSLE
    neuropsychiatric syndrome of
      systemic lupus erythematosus
    neuropsychiatric systemic lupus
      erythematosus

NPT
    near patient test
    neoprecipitin test
    neopyrithiamin hydrochloride
    neuropsychological test
    nocturnal penile tumescence
    no prior tracings
    normal pressure and temperature

NPTS
    nocturnal painful tonic spasm

NPU
    net protein utilization

NPV
    negative predictive value
    negative pressure ventilation
    nothing per vagina
    nuclear polyhidrosis virus
    nucleus paraventricularis

NPY
    neuropeptide Y

NPZ
    neuropsychological test Z score

NQA
    nursing quality assurance

NQMI
    non–Q-wave myocardial infarction

NQR
    nuclear quadruple resonance

NR
    nephrogenic rest
    nerve root
    neural retina
    neutral red
    newly reformulated
    noise reduction
    none reported
    nonreactive
    nonrebreathing
    nonreimbursable
    nor
    no radiation
    no reaction
    no recurrence
    no refill
    no rehearsal
    no rejection
    no report
    no response
    no return
    normal (*See also* N, n, NL, nl,
      NOR, norm)
    normal range
    normal reaction
    normal record
    normotensive rat (*See also* NTR)
    not reached
    not reacting
    not readable
    not recorded
    not reported
    not resolved
    nuclear receptor
    nucleotide residue
    number
    nurse
    nutrition ratio
    Reynolds number (*See also* N_R)

N/R
    not remarkable

NOTES

N_R
  Reynolds number (*See also* NR)
n.r.
  do not repeat [L. *non repetatur*]
nr
  near
NRA
  nitrate reductase
  nucleus raphe alatus
  nucleus retroambigualis
NRAF
  nonrheumatic atrial fibrillation
Nramp
  natural resistance macrophage-
    associated protein
NRB
  nonrebreather (oxygen mask)
  nonrejoining (DNA strand) break
NRBA
  neutrophil respiratory burst activity
NRBC, NRbc
  normal red blood cell
  nucleated red blood cell (mass)
NRBS
  nonrebreathing system
NRC
  noise reduction coefficient
  normal retinal correspondence
  not routine care
NRCL
  nonrenal clearance
NRD
  nonrenal death
NRDS
  neonate respiratory distress
    syndrome
NREH
  normal renin essential hypertension
NREM, NREMS
  nonrapid eye movement (sleep)
    (*See also* nonREM, non-REM)
NRF
  normal renal function
NRFC
  non–rosette-forming cell
NRGC
  nucleus reticularis gigantocellularis
NRH
  nodular regenerative hyperplasia (of
    liver)
NRI
  nerve root involvement
  nerve root irritation
  neutral regular insulin
  nonrespiratory infection
  no recent illnesses
  norepinephrine reuptake inhibitor

NRIT
  Non-Reading Intelligence Test,
    Levels 1-3
NRIV
  Ngari virus
NRK
  normal rat kidney
NRL
  nucleus reticularis lateralis
N-RLX
  nonrelaxed
NRM
  nonrebreathing mask
  no regular medicines
  normal retinal movement
  normal rnage (of) motion (*See also*
    NROM)
  nucleus raphe magnus
  nucleus reticularis magnocellularis
NRN
  no return necessary
nRNA
  nuclear ribonucleic acid
nRNP
  nuclear ribonucleoprotein
NRO
  neurology
NROM
  normal range of motion (*See also*
    NRM)
NRP
  nonreassuring pattern
  nucleus reticularis parvocellularis
NRPAT
  net revenue, patient
NRPC
  nucleus reticularis pontis caudalis
NRPG
  nucleus reticularis
    paragigantocellularis
NRPR
  nonbreathing pressure relieving
NRR
  net reproduction rate
  Noise Reduction Rating
  note, record, report
NRS
  Neurobehavioral Rating Scale
  nonimmunized rabbit serum
  normal rabbit serum
  normal reference serum
  numerical rating scale
  numeric rating scale
nrsng
  nursing (*See also* NSG, nsg)
NRSTS
  nonrhabdomyosarcoma soft tissue
    sarcoma

NRT
> neuromuscular reeducation technique
> nicotine replacement therapy
> nitron radical trap

NRTI
> nucleoside (analog) reverse
>   transcriptase inhibitor
> nucleoside (analog) RT inhibitor
> nucleoside reverse transcriptase
>   inhibitor

NRTOT
> net revenue, total

NRV
> Neckar river virus
> nucleus reticularis ventralis

NS
> nasal steroid
> natural science
> needle shower
> nephrosclerosis
> nephrotic syndrome
> nerve sheath
> nervous system
> Netherton syndrome
> neurologic sign
> neurologic surgery
> neurologic survey
> neurosarcoidosis
> neurosecretory
> neurosurgery (*See also* neurosurg,
>   NSurg)
> neurosyphilis
> neurotic score
> nevus sebaceus
> nipple stimulation
> nodular sclerosis
> nodus sinuatrialis
> nonsmoker (*See also* NSM)
> nonsnorer
> nonspecific
> nonstimulation
> nonstructural (protein)
> nonstutterer
> nonsymptomatic
> Noonan syndrome
> normal saline (*See also* N/S)
> normal serum
> normal sodium (diet)
> normal study
> normospermic
> Norwegian scabies

> no sample
> no sequelae (*See also* ns)
> no-show
> no specimen (*See also* ns)
> not seen
> not significant (*See also* ns)
> not specified (*See also* NSP)
> not stated
> not sufficient
> not symptomatic
> nuclear sclerosis
> nursing services
> nutritive sucking
> nylon suture (*See also* ns)

N/S
> normal saline (*See also* NS)

Ns
> nasopinale
> nerves (*See also* nn)

ns
> nanosecond (*See also* nsec)
> no sequelae (*See also* NS)
> no specimen (*See also* NS)
> not significant (*See also* NS)
> nylon suture (*See also* NS)

NSA
> neck-shaft angle
> neuron-specific enolase
> nonspecific arrhythmia
> normal serum albumin
> no salt added
> no serious abnormality
> no significant abnormality
> no significant anomaly
> nutritional status assessment

NSAA
> nonsteroidal antiandrogen

NSAD
> no signs of acute disease

NSAE
> nonsupported arm exercise

NSAIA
> nonsteroidal antiinflammatory agent

NSAID
> nonsteroidal antiinflammatory drug

NSAP
> nonspecific abdominal pain

NSB
> nonspecific binding

NSBGP
> nonspecific bowel gas pattern

NOTES

N

NSBR
  Nottingham modification of Scarff-
  Bloom-Richardson grading
NSC
  neurosecretory cell
  non–service-connected (disability)
    (*See also* NSCD)
  nonspecific suppressor cell
  no significant change
NSCC
  non-small cell cancer
  non-small cell carcinoma
NSCD
  non–service-connected disability (*See
    also* NSC)
NSCFPT
  no significant change from
    previous tracing
NSCLC
  non-small cell lung cancer
  non-small cell lung carcinoma
NSCST
  nipple stimulation contraction stress
    test
NSD
  N-acetylneuraminic acid storage
    disease
  Nairobi sheep disease
  nasal septal deviation
  neonatal staphylococcal disease
  neurosensory deficit
  night sleep deprivation
  nitrogen-specific detector
  nominal single dose
  nominal standard dose
  normal single dose
  normal spontaneous delivery
  no significant defect
  no significant deficiency
  no significant deviation
  no significant difference
  no significant disease
NSDA
  nonsteroid-dependent asthmatic
NSDU
  neonatal stepdown unit
NSDV
  Nairobi sheep disease virus
NSE
  neuron-specific enolase
  nonspecific csterase
  normal saline enema
NS̄E
  nausea without emesis [Fr. *sans*]
nsec
  nanosecond (*See also* ns)
NSED
  nonsurgeon, emergency department

NSF
  nodular subepidermal fibrosis
  no significant findings
NSFTD
  normal spontaneous full-term
    delivery
NSG
  necrotizing sarcoid granulomatosis
  neurosecretory granule
  nursing (*See also* nrsng, nsg)
nsg
  nursing (*See also* nrsng, NSG)
NSGCT
  nonseminomatous germ cell tumor
NSGCTT, NSTGCT
  nonseminomatous germ cell
    testicular tumor
  nonseminomatous testicular germ
    cell tumor
NSGO
  nonspecific granulomatous orchitis
NSG STA
  nursing station
NSHD
  nodular sclerosing Hodgkin disease
NSHL
  nonsyndromic hearing loss
NSHPT
  neonatal severe hyperparathyroidism
NSI
  negative self-image
  neurosensory impairment
  nonsyncytium-inducing
  no sign of infection
  no sign of inflammation
NSICU
  neurosurgery intensive care unit
    (*See also* NICU)
NSIDS
  near-sudden infant death syndrome
NSILA
  nonsuppressible insulinlike activity
NSILP
  nonsuppressible insulin-like protein
NSIP
  nonspecific interstitial pneumonia
  nonspecific interstitial pneumonia-
    fibrosis
  nonspecific interstitial pneumonitis
NSJ
  nevus sebaceus of Jadassohn
NSL
  nonsalt loser
NSLF
  normal sheep lung fibroblast
NSM
  nerve sheath myxoma
  neurosecretory material

nonantigenic specific mediator
nonsmoker (*See also* NS)
nutrient sporulation medium
N·s/m²
newton-second per square meter
NSMMVT
nonsustained monomorphic
ventricular tachycardia
NSN
Neo-Synephrine
nephrotoxic serum nephritis
nicotine-stimulated neurophysin
number of similar negatives
NSND
nonsymptomatic, nondisabling
NSO
Neosporin ointment
nonnutritive sucking opportunity
nucleus supraopticus
NSol
nerve-to-soleus
NSOM
near field scanning optical
microscope
NSP
neck and shoulder pain
neuron-specific protein
neurotoxic shellfish poisoning
not specified (*See also* NS)
number of similar positives
NSP4
nonstructural protein 4
NSPE
no specimen (obtainable)
NSPs
nonstarch polysaccharides
NSPVT
nonsustained polymorphic ventricular
tachycardia
NSQ
Neuroticism Scale Questionnaire
not sufficient quantity
NSR
nasoseptal reconstruction
nasoseptal repair
nonspecific reaction
nonsystemic reaction
normal sinus rhythm
not seen regularly
nSRBC
normal sheep red blood cell

NSRP
nerve-sparing radical prostatectomy
NSRR
normal sinus rate and rhythm
NSRRL
neutral, sidebent right, rotated left
NSRT
nonsurgical septal reduction therapy
NSS
nasal symptom score
neurological signs stable
normal saline solution
normal size and shape
not statistically significant
nutritional support service
NSSC
normal size, shape, and consistency
NSSL
normal size, shape, and location
NSSP
normal size, shape, and position
NSSPAVAF
normal size, shape, and position,
anteverted and anteflexed (uterus)
NSST
nonspecific ST (wave segment
changes on electroencephalogram)
Northwestern Syntax Screening Test
NSSTT, NSST-TWCs
nonspecific ST and T (wave)
nonspecific ST-T wave changes
NST
neospinothalamic (tract)
nonshivering thermogenesis
nonstress test
nonstress test (fetal monitoring)
normal sphincter tone
no specific type
not sooner than
nutritional status type
nutritional support team
nutrition support team
NSTD
nonsexually transmitted disease
NSTI
necrotizing soft-tissue infection
NSTT
nonseminomatous testicular tumor
NSU
necrotizing sclerocorneal ulceration
neurosurgical unit
nonspecific urethritis

N

NOTES

NSurg
>neurosurgeon (*See also* neurosurg)
>neurosurgery (*See also* neurosurg, NS)

NSV
>nonspecific vaginitis

NSVD
>normal spontaneous vaginal delivery

NSVT
>nonsustained ventricular tachycardia

NSX
>neurosurgical examination

NSY
>nursery

N-T, N&T
>nose and throat

NT
>nasotracheal
>neotetrazolium
>neurofeedback training
>neurotensin
>neutralization technique
>neutralization test
>neutralizing (*See also* Nt)
>next time
>nicotine tartrate
>nontypable
>Nordic Track
>normal temperature
>normal tissue
>normotensive
>nortriptyline
>no test
>not tender
>not tested
>nourishment taken
>N-telopeptide
>nucleation time
>numbness and tingling
>nursing technician

NT-3
>neurotrophin-3

NT-4
>neurotrophin-4

NT-5
>neurotrophin-5

5'-NT
>5'-nucleotidase

N/T
>neck-to-thigh ratio

Nt
>amino terminal
>neutralizing (*See also* NT)

NTA
>natural thymocytotoxic autoantibody
>nitrilotriacetic acid
>Nurse Training Act

NTAB
>nephrotoxic antibody

N Tachy
>nodal tachycardia

NT-ANP
>N-terminal atrial natriuretic peptide

NTAV
>Ntaya virus

NTB
>necrotizing tracheobronchitis

N/TBC
>nontuberculous

NTBC therapy
>2-(2-nitro-4-trifluromethylbenzoyl)-3-cyclohexanedione

NTBR
>not to be resuscitated

NTC
>neurotrauma center

NTCC
>National Type Culture Collection

NTCS
>no tumor cells seen

NTD
>negative to date
>neural tube defect
>nitroblue tetrazolium dye
>noise tone difference

NTE
>neurotoxic esterase
>neutral thermal environment
>nontest ear
>not to exceed
>nuclear track emulsion

NTED
>neonatal toxic-shock-syndrome-like exanthematous disease

NTF
>nasogastric tube feeding
>normal throat flora

NTG
>nitroglycerin (*See also* NG, nitro, NTZ)
>nontoxic goiter
>nontreatment group
>normal-tension glaucoma
>normal triglyceridemia

NTGO
>nitroglycerin ointment

NTHH
>nontumorous hypergastrinemic hyperchlorhydria

NTHI
>native tissue harmonic imaging
>nontypeable *Haemophilus influenzae*

NTI
>narrow therapeutic index
>nasotracheal intubation

nonthyroid illness
nonthyroid index
no treatment indicated

NTL

nectar-thick liquid (diet consistency)
nortriptyline
no time limit

NTLE

neocortical temporal-lobe epilepsy

NTLI

neurotensin-like immunoreactivity

NTM

Neuman-Tytell medium
nocturnal tumescence monitor
nontuberculous mycobacteria (*See also* NTMB)

NTMB

nontuberculous mycobacteria (*See also* NTM)

NTMI

nontransmural myocardial infarction

NTMNG

nontoxic multinodular goiter

NTN

nephrotoxic nephritis
neurturin

NTND

not tender, not distended (abdomen)

NTNG

nontoxic nodular goiter

NTOM

nerve territory oriented macrodactyly

NTP

narcotic treatment program
nitropaste
nonthrombocytopenic preterm (infant)
normal temperature and pressure
nucleoside triphosphate
sodium nitroprusside

NTPD

nocturnal tidal peritoneal dialysis

NTPPH, NTPPPH

nucleoside triphosphate pyrophosphohydrolase

NTR

negative therapeutic reaction
normotensive rat (*See also* NR)
nutrition

NTRI

nucleoside reverse transcriptase inhibitor

NTRK1

neurotrophic tyrosine kinase receptor, type 1

NTS

nasotracheal suction
nephrotoxic serum
nicotine transdermal system
nonturning (against) self (psychology)
non-typhi *Salmonella*
nontyphoidal salmonellae
nucleus of the tractus solitarius
nucleus tractus solitarius

NTT

nasotracheal tube
nearly total thyroidectomy
nonthrombocytopenic term (infant)
nuchal translucency thickness

NTU

nephelometric turbidity units

NTV

nervous tissue vaccine

NTX

naltrexone

NTx

N-telopeptide

NTZ

nitazoxanide
nitroglycerin (*See also* NG, nitro, NTG)
normal transformation zone (colposcopy)

ν, nu

frequency
kinematic viscosity (*See also* υ)
neutrino
number of degrees of freedom
nu (13th letter of Greek alphabet), lowercase
stoichiometric number

NU

name unknown

Nu

nucleolus
nucleus

nU

nanounit

NOTES

nu
neurilemma
nude (mouse)

NUC
nuclear (*See also* nucl)
nuclear medicine
sodium urate crystal

Nuc
nucleoside (*See also* N)

nuc
nucleated

NU-CHIPS
Northwestern University Children's Perception of Speech Test

nucl
nuclear (*See also* NUC)

NUD
nonulcer dyspepsia

NUG
necrotizing ulcerating gingivitis
necrotizing ulcerative gingivitis

NUGV
Nugget virus

NUI
number user identification

nullip
nulliparous

num
numerator

NuMA
nuclear mitotic apparatus

numc
number concentration

NUN
nonurea nitrogen

NUP
necrotizing ulcerative periodontitis

NURB
Neville upper reservoir buffer

NURD
nonuniform rotational defect

NUV
near-ultraviolet
negative ulnar variance

NV
naked vision (*See also* Nv)
nausea and vomiting (*See also* N/V, N&V)
near vision
negative variation
neovascularization
neurovascular
new vessel
next visit
nodular vasculi
nonvegetarian
nonvenereal
nonveteran

normal value
normal volunteer
normovolemic
norverapamil
not vaccinated
not venereal
not verified
not volatile
trigeminal nerve

N/V, N&V
nausea and vomiting (*See also* NV)

Nv, Nv.
naked vision (*See also* NV)

nv
nonvolatile

NVA
near visual acuity
normal visual acuity

Nva
norvaline

NVAF
nonvalvular atrial fibrillation

NVB
neurovascular bundle

NVBG
nonvascularized bone graft

NVC
neurovascular checks
nonvalved conduit
normal vital capacity

NVCC
neurovascular cross compression

nvCJD
new variant Creutzfeldt-Jakob disease

NVD
nausea, vomiting, diarrhea
neck vein distention
neovascularization (of optic) disc
neurovesicle dysfunction
Newcastle virus disease
nonvalvular (heart) disease
normal vaginal delivery
no venereal disease
no venous distention

NVDC
nausea, vomiting, diarrhea, and constipation

NVE
native
native valve endocarditis
neovascularization elsewhere (on retina)
new vessels elsewhere

NVFS
nuclear ventricular function study

NVG
neovascular glaucoma

neoviridogrisein
nonventilated group

NVI

neovascularization of the iris

NVL

neurovascular laboratory

NVLD

nonverbal learning disability

NVM

neovascular membrane
nonvolatile matter

NVP

nausea and vomiting of pregnancy
near visual point
nevirapine

NVR

no radiographically visible
 recurrence

NVS

nasal vestibular stenosis
neurologic vital signs
neurovascular status
nonvaccine serotype
nutritionally variant streptococcus

NVSS

normal variant short stature

NW

naked weight
nasal wash
nonwithdrawn
not weighed

NWB

nonweightbearing
no weightbearing

NWBL

nonweightbearing, left

NWBR

nonweightbearing, right

NWC

number of words chosen

NWD

neuroleptic withdrawal
normal well developed

NWF

new working formulation

NWI

Neonatal Withdrawal Inventory
notch width index

NWm

nitrogen washout, multiple (breath)

NWR

normotensive Wistar rat

NWS

New World screwworm
 (*Cochliomyia hominivorax*
 [Coquerel])

NWs

nitrogen washout, single (breath)

NWSM

Nocardia water-soluble nitrogen

NWTS, NWTSG

National Wilms Tumor Study

NX, Nx

naloxone (*See also* NLX)
nephrectomy
regional lymph nodes cannot be
 addressed

Nx

next

N x m

newton by meter

NY

nystatin

NYC

New York City (medium)

NYD

not yet diagnosed
not yet discovered

NYHA

New York Heart Association
 (classification)

NYP

not yet published

nyst

nystagmus

NZ

enzyme
neutral zone
normal zone

NZB

New Zealand black (mouse)

NZGLM

New Zealand green-lipped mussel

NZO

New Zealand obese (mouse)

NZR

New Zealand red (rabbit)

NZW

New Zealand white (mouse)

N

NOTES

O

absence of sex chromosome
agglutinative reactions
blood type in ABO blood group
eye [L. *oculus*]
negative
nil
no
none
nonmotile microorganisms and their somatic antigens, antibodies, and
nonmotile organism
no special preparation necessary (for test)
obese (*See also* OB, ob)
objective (findings)
observation (*See also* OBS)
obstetrics (*See also* OB, OBS)
obvious
occipital (*See also* Occ, occip)
occiput (*See also* Occ, occip)
occlusal
often
old
open (*See also* o, opg)
opening (*See also* o, opg)
operator
operon (genetics)
opium
oprelvekin
oral (*See also* (O))
orally (*See also* (O))
orange (indicator color)
orbit
orderly (*See also* ord)
orotidine (*See also* Ord)
ortho
orthopedic (*See also* OR, Orth, ortho)
osteocyte
other
output
oxidative
oxygen (*See also* O2, O_2, OXY, oxy)
pint [L. *octarius*] (*See also* $\overline{O}$)
respirations (on anesthesia chart)
without (*See also* ō, S, s̄, WO, w/o, wo)
zero

1O2

singlet oxygen

O2

both eyes (*See also* O.U.)

oxygen (symbol for the diatomic gas) (*See also* OXY, oxy)

O2–

superoxide

O_2

oxygen

O_3

ozone

O-9

octyoxynol-9

^{15}O

oxygen-15

^{16}O

oxygen-16

^{17}O

oxygen-17

^{18}O

oxygen-18

Θ, omicron

omicron (15th letter of Greek alphabet), uppercase

$\overline{O}$

pint [L. *octarius*]

O-

blood type O negative

O+

blood type O positive

(O)

oral
orally

o

no
omicron (15th letter of Greek alphabet), lowercase
opening (*See also* opg)

ō

negative
none
without (*See also* S, s̄, WO, w/o, wo)

o-

ortho- (chemical symbol)

OA

object assembly (psychology)
obstructive apnea
occipital artery
occipitoanterior (fetal position)
occipitoatlantal
occiput anterior
occupational asthma
occupationally induced asthma
ocular albinism
old age
oleic acid
on admission

O

OA *(continued)*
    on arrival
    open adrenalectomy
    open appendectomy
    ophthalmic artery
    opiate analgesia
    opsonic activity
    optic atrophy
    oral airway *(See also* OAW)
    oral alimentation
    oral appliance
    orotic acid *(See also* Oro)
    orthophonic acid
    osteoarthritis *(See also* osteo)
    osteoid area
    ovalbumin *(See also* OVA, OV)
    ovarian ablation
    overall assessment
    oxalic acid
    oxolinic acid
    O. (subtest)

O-A
    Objective-Analytic (Anxiety Battery)

O&A
    observation and assessment
    odontectomy and alveoloplasty

O/A
    on or about

O₂a
    oxygen availability

OAA
    Old Age Assistance
    oxaloacetic acid (test)

OAAD
    ovarian ascorbic acid depletion
        (test)

OAAS, OAA/S
    Observer Assessment of Alertness
        and Sedation

OAB
    old age benefits
    overactive bladder

OABP
    organic anion-binding protein

OAC
    omeprazole, amoxicillin,
        clarithromycin
    oral anticoagulant
    overaction

OAD
    obstructive airway disease
    occlusive arterial disease
    organic anionic dye
    overall diameter
    overall diameter of contact lens
    overanxious disorder

OADC
    oleic acid, albumin, dextrose, and
        catalase (medium)

OADMT
    Oliphant Auditory Discrimination
        Memory Test

OADP-CDS
    Oregon Adolescent Depression
        Project-Conduct Disorder Screener

OAdV 1–6
    ovine adenovirus 1–6

OAE
    open access endoscopy
    otoacoustic emission (test)

OAF
    off-axis factor
    open air factor
    oral anal fistula
    osteoclast-activating factor

OAG
    open-angle glaucoma

OAH
    ovarian androgenic hyperfunction

OAI
    Ostomy Assessment Inventory

OAJ
    open apophyseal joint

OALF
    organic acid-labile fluoride

OALL
    ossification of anterior longitudinal
        ligament

OAM
    omeprazole, amoxicillin,
        metronidazole
    outer acrosomal membrane
    oxyacetate malonate

OAO
    ophthalmic artery occlusion

OAP
    Occupational Ability Pattern
    old age pension
    old age pensioner
    ophthalmic artery pressure
    osteoarthropathy
    oxygen at atmospheric pressure

OAPs
    Occupational Ability Patterns
        (psychologic test)

OAR
    off-axis ratio
    organs at risk
    orientation/alertness remediation
    other administrative reasons
    Ottawa Ankle Rules

OARSA
    oxacillin aminoglycoside-resistant
        Staphylococcus aureus

OAS
old age security
Older Adult Services
oral allergy syndrome
Oral Analogue Scale
orbital apex syndrome
organic anxiety syndrome
osmotically active substance
outpatient assessment service
overall survival
Overt Aggression Scale

OASIS
One Action Stent Introduction
System
osteotomy analysis simulation
software
Outcomes and Assessment
Information Set

OASO
overactive superior oblique

OASP
organic acid-soluble phosphorus

OASR
overactive superior rectus

OASS
Overt Agitation Severity Scale

OAST
Oliphant Auditory Synthesizing Test

OAT
ornithine aminotransferase

OATS
oligoasthenoteratozoospermia
syndrome
osteochondral autograft transfer
system

OAV
oculoauriculovertebral (dysplasia,
syndrome)

OAVS
oculoauriculovertebral spectrum

OAW
oral airway (See also OA)

OAWO
opening abductory wedge osteotomy

OB
obese (See also ob)
obesity
objective benefit
obliterative bronchiolitis
obstetrician
obstetrics (See also OBS)
occult bleeding

occult blood
olfactory bulb (See also OLB)
oligoclonal band
osteoblast
osteoblastoma

OB+
occult blood positive

O&B
opium and belladonna

ob
obese (See also OB)

OBA
office-based anesthesia
oral bile acid

OB-A
obstetrics-aborted

OBB
own bed bath

OBC
operable breast cancer

OBD
optimum biologic dose
organic brain disease
organic brain disorder

OB-Del
obstetrics-delivered

OBE
out-of-body experience

OBE-CALP
placebo capsule or tablet

OBF
organ blood flow

OB-GYN, OB/GYN
obstetrician-gynecologist
obstetrics and gynecology

obj
object
objective

OBK
obstructed kidney

obl
oblique

OBLA
onset of blood lactate accumulation

OB marg
obtuse marginal

OBN
occult blood-negative

OB-ND
obstetrics-not delivered

OBP
occult blood-positive

NOTES

O

559

OBP *(continued)*
    office blood pressure
    ova, blood, and parasites (stool exam)

OBS
    observation
    observed (*See also* obsd)
    obstetrical service
    obstetrics (*See also* OB)
    organic brain syndrome

obs
    obsolete

obsd
    observed (*See also* OBS)

obst
    obstipation
    obstructed
    obstruction

obstet
    obstetric

obt
    obtained

OBTM
    omeprazole, bismuth subcitrate, tetracycline, and metronidazole

OB-US
    obstetrical ultrasound

OBW
    open bed warmer

O-C, O&C
    onset and course (of disease)

OC
    obstetrical conjugate
    occlusocervical
    office call
    on call
    only child
    open cholecystectomy
    operative cholangiography
    optical chromatography
    optic chiasm (*See also* OX)
    oral care
    oral cavity
    oral contraceptive
    organ confined
    organ culture
    original claim
    Osteocalcin
    outer canthal (distance)
    ovarian cancer
    oxygen consumed

Oc
    ochre suppressor genetic mutation

OCA
    oculocutaneous albinism
    olivopontocerebellar atrophy (*See also* OPCA)
    open care area

    operant conditioning audiometry
    oral contraceptive agent

OCAD
    occlusive carotid artery disease

O₂ cap.
    oxygen capacity

OCB
    obsessive-compulsive behavior

OCBF
    outer cortical blood flow

OCBZ
    oxcarbazepine

OCC
    occlusal
    oculocerebrocutaneous
    old chart called
    oral cavity cancer

Occ
    occasional (*See also* occ, occas)
    occipital (*See also* occip)
    occiput (*See also* O, occip)
    occlusion (*See also* occl)
    occlusive

occ, occas
    occasional (*See also* Occ)
    occasionally
    occupation (*See also* occup)
    occurrence

OCCC
    open-chest cardiac compression
    ovarian clear cell carcinoma

occip
    occipital (*See also* O, Occ)
    occiput (*See also* Occ, O)

occip F
    occipitofrontal (*See also* OF)

occip-F HA
    occipitofrontal headache (*See also* OF-HA)

occl
    occlusion (*See also* Occ)

OCCM
    open-chest cardiac massage

OCCPR
    open-chest cardiopulmonary resuscitation

OccTh
    occupational therapy (*See also* Occup Rx, OT)

occup
    occupation (*See also* occ)
    occupational
    occupies
    occupying

Occup Rx
    occupational therapy (*See also* OccTh, OT)

OCD
> obsessive-compulsive disorder
> osteochondritis dissecans
> ovarian cholesterol depletion (test)

OCDS
> Obsessive-Compulsive Drinking Scale

OCE
> outpatient code editor

OCF
> osteopathy in the cranial field

OCG
> omnicardiogram
> oral cholecystogram
> oral cholecystography

OCH
> oral contraceptive hormone

Ochs
> Ochsner

OCI
> Obsessive-Compulsive Inventory
> Ophthalmic Confidence Index
> Organizational Culture Inventory

OCIF
> osteoclastogenesis inhibitory factor

OCL
> Occupational Check List (psychologic test)
> oral colonic lavage
> Orthopedic Casting Lab (splint)

OCLG
> osteoclast-like giant cell (*See also* OLGC)

OCM
> Odorant Confusion Matrix
> oral contraceptive medication

OCN
> obsessive-compulsive neurosis
> oculomotor nucleus (*See also* OMN)

OCNS
> Obsessive-Compulsive Neurosis Scale

O-CNV
> occult choroidal neovascularization

OCOR
> on-call to operating room

OCP
> octacalcium phosphate
> ocular cicatricial pemphigoid
> Onchocerciasis Control Program
> oral contraceptive pill

> ova, cysts, and parasites (stool exam)

OCPD
> obsessive-compulsive personality disorder

OCR
> ocular counterrolling
> ocular countertorsion reflex
> oculocardiac reflex
> oculocephalic reflux
> oculocerebrorenal (*See also* OCRL)
> off-center ratio
> optical character recognition

oCRF
> ovine corticotropin-releasing factor

OCRL
> oculocerebrorenal (*See also* OCR)

OCRS
> oculocerebrorenal syndrome

OCS
> Obsessive-Compulsive Scale
> Ondine curse syndrome
> open canalicular system (of platelets)
> oral cancer screening
> oral contraceptive steroid
> outpatient clinic substation
> oxycorticosteroid

11-OCS
> 11-oxycorticosteroid

OCT
> Object Classification Test
> octreotide
> optical coherence tomography
> optimal cutting temperature (medium)
> oral cavity tumors
> oral contraceptive therapy
> ornithine carbamoyltransferase
> osseous coagulum trap
> outer canthal distance
> oxytocin challenge test

O₂CT
> oxygen content

Oct-1
> octamer-binding

OCTD
> ornithine carbamoyltransferase deficiency

OCTR
> open carpal tunnel release

NOTES

OCTT
orocecal transit time
OCU
observation care unit
OCV
ordinary conversational voice
OCVM
occult cerebral vascular malformation
occult cerebrovascular malformation
occult vascular malformation
oculocerebrovasculometer
OCWO
oblique closing wedge osteotomy
OCX
oral cancer examination
OD
(drug) overdosage
(drug) overdose
occipital dysplasia
occupational dermatitis
occupational disease
oculus dexter (right eye)
Ollier disease
on duty
oocyte donation
open drop (anesthesia)
open duct
optical density
optic disk
optimal dose
oral-duodenal
organization development
originally derived
osteochondritis dissecans
outdoor
outer diameter
out-of-date
outside diameter
ovarian dysgerminoma
overdose
right eye (*See also* RE, O.D.)
O-D
obstacle-dominance
original-derived
O.D., o.d.
oculus dexter (right eye)
right eye [L. *oculus dexter*] (*See also* RE, OD)
od
daily
ODA
once-daily aminoglycoside
osmotic driving agent
right occipitoanterior (fetal position) [L. *occipitodextra anterior*]
ODAC
on-demand analgesia computer

ODAT
one day at a time
ODB
opiate-directed behavior
ODC
oral disease control
ornithine decarboxylase
orotidylate decarboxylase (deficiency)
outpatient diagnostic center
oxygen dissociation curve
ODCH
ordinary disease of childhood
ODD
oculodentodigital (dysplasia, syndrome)
once-daily dosing
oppositional defiant disorder
opposition defiance disorder
osteodental dysplasia
OD'd
(drug) overdosed
ODE
o–desmethylencainide
ODED
oculodigitoesophagoduodenal
ODF
osteoclast differentiation factor
ODM, ODm
occlusion dose monitor
ophthalmodynamometer
ophthalmodynamometry
opponens digiti minimi
ODN
oligodeoxynucleotide
optokinetic nystagmus
ODOD
oculodentoosseous dysplasia
Odont
odontology
odont
odontogenic
ODP
offspring of diabetic parents
right occipitoposterior (fetal position) [L. *occipitodextra posterior*]
OD/P
right eye patched
ODQ
on direct questioning
opponens digiti quinti (muscle)
Owestry Disability Questionnaire
ODRV
Odrenisrou virus
ODS
Operation Desert Storm
organized delivery system

ODSG
ophthalmic Doppler sonogram
ODSU
oncology day stay unit
one day surgery unit
ODT
oculodynamic test
orally disintegrating tablet
right occipitotransverse (fetal
position) [L. *occipitodextra
transversa*]
ODTS
organic dust toxic syndrome
ODU
optical density unit
OE
on examination (*See also* O/E)
orthopedic examination (*See also*
OX)
otitis externa
O-E
standard observed minus expected
O&E
observation and examination
O/E
on examination (*See also* OE)
(ratio of) observed to expected
Oe
oersted (centimeter-gram-second unit
of magnetic field strength)
OEC
outer ear canal
ovarian epithelial cancer
OEE
osmotic erythrocyte enrichment
outer enamel epithelium
OEF
oxygen extraction fraction
OEI
opioid escalation index
O2EI
oxygen extraction index
OEIS
omphalocele, exstrophy (of the
bladder), imperforate (anus), and
spinal (abnormalities)
OEM
occupational and environmental
medicine
open-end marriage
opposite ear masked

original equipment manufacturer
(computers)
OENT
oral endotracheal tube
OEP
oil of evening primrose (evening
primrose oil)
OER
osmotic erythrocyte (enrichment)
oxygen enhancement ratio
oxygen extraction rate
oxygen extraction ratio (*See also*
O_2ER)
O_2ER
oxygen extraction ratio (*See also*
OER)
OERP
odor event-related potential
OERR
entry system)
OES
Olympus endoscopy system
optical emission spectroscopy
oral esophageal stethoscope
oesoph
esophagus (oesophagus) (*See also*
E, ES, ESO, esoph)
OESP
orthopedic examination, special
OET
open epicutaneous test
oral endotracheal tube (*See also*
OETT)
oral esophageal tube
OETT
oral endotracheal tube (*See also*
OET)
OF
occipitofrontal (*See also* occip F)
optic fundi
orbitofrontal
osmotic fragility (test)
osteitis fibrosa
Ostrum-Furst (syndrome)
other (medical/surgical) facility
Ovenstone factor
oxidation-fermentation (medium)
(*See also* O-F, O/F)
O-F, O/F
oxidation-fermentation (medium)
(*See also* OF)

NOTES

O

OFA
oncofetal antigen
OFB
oval fat body
OFBM
oxidation-fermentation basal medium
OFC
occipitofrontal circumference
open food challenge
orbitofacial cleft
osteitis fibrosa cystica
ofc
office (*See also* off.)
OFCD
oculofaciocardiodental
OFCTAD
occipito-faciocervico-thoraco-
abdomino-digital (dysplasia)
OFD
object-film distance (radiology) (*See
also* ofd)
occipitofrontal diameter
oral-facial-digital (syndrome)
orofaciodigital (dysostosis,
syndrome)
ofd
object-film distance (radiology) (*See
also* OFD)
OFD syndrome
orofaciodigital syndrome
Off
official (*See also* off.)
off.
office (*See also* ofc)
official (*See also* Off)
OF-HA
occipitofrontal headache (*See also*
occip-F HA)
OFI
other febrile illness
OFLOX, OFLX
ofloxacin
OFM
open face mask
orofacial malformation
orofacial movement
OFNE
oxygenated fluorocarbon nutrient
emulsion
OFPF
optic fundi and peripheral fields
OFR
oxygen-free radicals
OF rad
occipitofrontal radiation
OFTT
organic failure to thrive

OG
obstetrics and gynecology (*See also*
OB-GYN, OB/GYN, O&G)
occlusogingival
oligodendrocyte
optic ganglion
oral gastric
orange green (stain)
orogastric
orogastric (feeding)
outcome goal (long-term goal)
O&G
obstetrics and gynecology (*See also*
OB/GYN, OG)
OGA
orogastric gonococcal aspirate
OGC
oculogyric crisis
OGCT
oral glucose challenge test
ovarian germ cell tumor
OGD
old granulomatous disease
OGF
opioid growth factor
ovarian growth factor
oxygen gain factor
OGH
ovine growth hormone
OGIMD
oculogastrointestinal muscular
dystrophy
OGM
outgrowth medium
OGS
oxygenic steroid
OGT
oral glucose tolerance
orogastric tube
OGTT
oral glucose tolerance test
oral glucose tolerance testing
OH
hydroxycorticosteroid (*See also*
HCS, OHCS)
hydroxyl group
hydroxyl radical
obstructive hypopnea
occipital horn
occupational health
occupational history
ocular history
on hand
open-heart (surgery)
oral hygiene
orthostatic hypotension
osteopathic hospital

out of hospital
outpatient hospital

17-OH
17-hydroxycorticosteroids

OHA
oral hypoglycemic agent

OHAHA
ophthalmoplegia-hypotonia-ataxia-
hypacusis-athetosis (syndrome)

24-OHase
vitamin D 24-hydroxylase

Ohase
hydroxylase

OHB$_{12}$
hydroxocobalamin (vitamin B$_{12}$)
(*See also* OH-Cbl)

O$_2$Hb
oxyhemoglobin

OHC
hydroxycholecalciferol (*See also*
OHD)
occupational health center
outer hair cell

OH-Cbl
hydroxocobalamin (*See also* OHB$_{12}$)

OHCS
hydroxycorticosteroid (*See also*
HCS, OH)

17-OHCS
17-hydroxycorticosteroid

OHD
hydroxycholecalciferol (*See also*
OHC)
hydroxy vitamin D
organic heart disease

25-OH-D3, 1,25(OH)2 D3, 25(OH)D3
1,25-dihydroxyvitamin D3
25-hydroxyvitamin D

OHDA
hydroxydopamine (*See also* HD,
HDA)
6-hydroxydopamine

OH-DOC
hydroxydeoxycorticosterone

OHF
old healed fracture
Omsk hemorrhagic fever
overhead frame

OHFA
hydroxy fatty acid

OHFT
overhead frame trapeze

OHFV
Omsk hemorrhagic fever virus

OHG
oral hypoglycemic

OHI
ocular hypertension indicator
Oral Hygiene Index
oral hygiene instructions

OH-IAA
hydroxyindoleacetic acid (*See also*
HIAA)

4-OHIPA
4-hydroxyifosfamide

OHI-S
Oral Hygiene Index-Simplified
Simplified Oral Hygiene Index

OHL
hydroxylysine
oral hairy leukoplakia

ohm-cm
ohm-centimeter

OHNS
otolaryngology, head, and neck
surgery (dept.)

OHP
hydroxyproline
obese hypertensive patient
orthogonal-hole test pattern
oxygen under high pressure

17-OHP
17-hydroxyprogesterone

OHRP
open-heart rehabilitation program

OHRR
open heart recovery room

OHS
obesity hypoventilation syndrome
occupational health and safety
occupational health service
ocular histoplasmosis syndrome
ocular hypoperfusion syndrome
open heart surgery
ovarian hyperstimulation syndrome
Overcontrolled Hostility Scale

OHSS
ovarian hyperstimulation syndrome

OHT
ocular hypertension
ocular hypertensive (glaucoma
suspect)
orthotopic heart transplant

O

NOTES

OHT *(continued)*
> orthotopic heart transplantation
> overhead trapeze

OHTN
> ocular hypertension

OHTx
> orthotopic heart transplantation

OHU
> hydroxyurea

1,25(OH)₂-VitD, 25OH-VitD
> 25-hydroxyvitamin D

OI
> objective improvement
> obturator internus
> occipitoiliacus
> oligoclonal immunoglobulin
> opportunistic illness
> opportunistic infection
> opsonic index
> orgasmic impairment
> Orientation Inventory (psychologic test)
> orthoiodohippurate (*See also* OIH)
> osteogenesis imperfecta (type I–IV)
> otitis interna
> ouabain insensitive
> oxygenation index
> oxygen income
> oxygen intake

O-I
> outer-to-inner

oi
> orbitale inferius

OIA
> optical immunoassay
> optimal immunoassay
> osmotically induced asthma

OIC
> osteogenesis imperfecta congenita

OID
> optimal immunomodulating dose
> organism identification (number)

OIE
> Occupational Interests Explorer

OIF
> observed intrinsic frequency
> oil immersion field (microscopy)

OIH
> iodine-123 orthoiodohippurate
> orthoiodohippurate (*See also* OI)
> ovulation-inducing hormone

OIHA
> orthoiodohippurate
> orthoiodohippuric acid

oint
> ointment

OIP
> organizing interstitial pneumonia

OIRDA
> occipital intermittent rhythmic delta activity

OIS
> Occupational Interests Surveyer
> ocular ischemic syndrome
> optical intrinsic signal (imaging)
> optimum information size
> Organ Injury Scaling

OIT
> Organic Integrity Test
> osteogenesis imperfecta tarda
> ovarian immature teratoma
> (Tien) organic integrity test (psychiatry)

OIU
> optical internal urethrotomy

OJ, oj
> orange juice (*See also* OrJ)
> orthoplast jacket

OK, ok
> all right
> approved
> correct

OKAN
> optokinetic after nystagmus

OKC
> odontogenic keratocyst

OKCE
> open kinetic chain exercises

OKHV
> Okhotskiy virus

OKN
> optokinetic nystagmus

OKOV
> Okola virus

OKQ
> Osteoporosis Knowledge Questionnaire

OKT
> ornithine-ketoacid transaminase
> Ortho-Kung T (cell)

OKT3
> ornithine-ketoacid transaminase
> orthoclone

OL
> open label (study)
> other location

O.L.
> left eye [L. *oculus laevus*] (*See also* LE, O.S.)

Ol, ol.
> oil [L. *oleum*]

ol
> orbitale laterale

OLA
> left occipitoanterior (fetal position) [L. *occipitolaeva anterior*]

OLB

olfactory bulb (*See also* OB)
open liver biopsy
open lung biopsy

OLBI

overlapping biphasic impulse

OLC

oligodendroglialike cell
ouabainlike compound

OLD

obstructive lung disease
occupational immunologic lung
disease
orthochromatic leukodystrophy

OLF

ouabainlike factor

OLGC

osteoclast-like giant cell (*See also*
OCLG)

OLH, oLH

ovine lactogenic hormone
ovine leuteinizing hormone

OLIB

osmiophilic lamellar inclusion body

OLIDS

open-loop insulin delivery system

OLIV

Olifantsvlei virus

OLM

ocular larva migrans
ophthalmic laser microendoscope

OLMAT

Otis-Lennon Mental Ability Test

OLNM

occult lymph node metastasis

OLP

abnormal lipoprotein
left occipitoposterior (fetal position)
[L. *occipitolaeva posterior*]

OLR

optic labyrinthine righting
otology, laryngology, and rhinology

ol res

oleoresin

OLS

ordinary least squares
ouabainlike substance

OLSID, OLSIDI

Oral Language Sentence Imitation
Diagnostic Inventory

OLSIST

Oral Language Sentence Imitation
Screening Test

OLT

left occipitotransverse (fetal
position) [L. *occipitolaeva
posterior*]
orthotopic liver transplantation (*See
also* Olt)
osteochondral lesion of the talus

Olt, OLTx

orthotopic liver transplant (*See also*
OLT)

OLTP

online transaction processing

OLULA

office laparoscopy under local
anesthesia

OLV

one-lung ventilation

OLZ

olanzapine

OM

obtuse marginal (coronary artery)
occipitomental
occupational medicine
ocular melanoma
oculomotor
oral motor
oral mucositis
organomegaly
Osborn-Mendel (rat)
osteomalacia
osteomyelitis (*See also* osteo)
osteopathic manipulation
osteopathic manipulative medicine
otitis media
outer membrane
ovulation method (birth control)

OM-1

first obtuse marginal artery

OM-2

second obtuse marginal artery

O2M

oxygen mask

OMA

obtuse marginal artery
older maternal age

OMAC

otitis media, acute, catarrhal (*See
also* OMCA)

NOTES

O

OMAS
>occupational maladjustment syndrome
>otitis media, acute, suppurating (*See also* OMSA)

OMB
>obtuse marginal branch

OMB$_1$
>first obtuse marginal branch

OMB$_2$
>second obtuse marginal branch

OMC
>omeprazole, metronidazole, clarithromycin
>open mitral commissurotomy
>short orientation-memory-concentration test

OMCA
>otitis media, catarrhal, acute (*See also* OMAC)

OMCC, OMCCH
>otitis media, catarrhal, chronic

OMChS
>otitis media, chronic, suppurating (*See also* OMSC)

OMD
>ocular muscle dystrophy
>oculomandibulodyscephaly
>organic mental disorder
>oromandibular dystonia

OME
>omeprazole
>otitis media with effusion

ω, omega
>angular frequency
>angular velocity
>carbon atom farthest from principal functioning group
>omega (24th and last letter of Greek alphabet), lowercase

Ω, omega
>ohm
>omega (24th and last letter of Greek alphabet), uppercase

OMENS
>orbital, mandibular, ear, neural, soft tissue
>orbit, mandible, ear, (cranial) nerves, soft tissue (syndrome)

OMF
>oculomandibulofacial (syndrome)

OMFAQ
>OARS Multidimensional Functional Assessment Questionnaire

OMFS
>oral and maxillofacial surgery

OMG
>ocular myasthenia gravis

OMI
>old myocardial infarction
>oocyte maturation inhibitor

OMJA
>oblique midtarsal joint axis

OML
>orbitomeatal line

OMM
>ophthalmomandibulomelic (dysplasia, syndrome)
>outer mitochondrial membrane

OMN
>oculomotor nerve
>oculomotor nucleus (*See also* OCN)

OMOV
>Omo virus

OMP
>oculomotor palsy (third nerve)
>olfactory marker protein
>orotidine 5'-monophosphate
>orotidylate
>orotidylic acid
>outer membrane protein

OMPA
>octamethyl pyrophosphoramide
>otitis media, purulent, acute

OMPC, OMPCh
>otitis media, purulent, chronic

OMR
>operative mortality rate

OMS
>not on my shift
>offshore medical school
>opsoclonus-myoclonus syndrome
>oral and maxillofacial surgery
>oral morphine sulfate
>organic mental syndrome
>organic mood syndrome
>otomandibular syndrome

OM&S
>osteopathic medicine and surgery

OMSA
>otitis media, suppurative, acute (*See also* OMAS)

OMSC, OMSCh
>otitis media, secretory, chronic
>otitis media, suppurative, chronic (*See also* OMChS)

OMT, OM/T
>oral mucosal transudate
>osteomanipulative therapy
>osteopathic manipulation treatment
>osteopathic manipulative technique
>osteopathic manipulative therapy
>osteopathic manipulative treatment

OMU
>ostiomeatal unit

OMVC
open mitral valve commissurotomy
OMVD
optimized microvessel density (analysis)
OMVI
operating motor vehicle while intoxicated
ON
occipitonuchal
onlay
ophthalmia neonatorum
optic nerve
optic neuritis
optic neuropathy
oronasal
Ortho-Novum
osteonecrosis
overnight
ONB
olfactory neuroblast
ONC
oncology (*See also* onco, oncol)
over-the-needle catheter
ONCG-A
oncogenic virus battery-acute
onco, oncol
oncology (*See also* ONC)
oncogene
gene
ONCORNA
oncogene ribonucleic acid
OncoScint CR/OV
OncoScint colorectal/ovarian carcinoma localization scintigraphy
OND
ondansetron
orbitonasal dislocation
other neurological disease
other neurologic disease
other neurologic disorder
ONDS
Oriental nocturnal death syndrome
ONDST
overnight high-dose dexamethasone suppression test
ONF
open Nissen fundoplication
ONH
optic nerve head
optic nerve hypoplasia

ONI
old nerve injury
ONL
olfactory nerve layer
ONM
ocular neuromyotonia
ONNV
O'nyong-nyong virus
ONP
operating nursing procedure
ONPG, ONP-GAL
omicron-nitrophenyl-beta-galactosidase
o-nitrophenyl-β-galactosidase
ON RR
overnight recovery room
ONSD
optic nerve sheath decompression
ONSF
optic nerve sheath fenestration
ONSM
optic nerve sheath meningioma
ONTG
oral nitroglycerin
ONTR
orders not to resuscitate
OO
oophorectomy
ophthalmic ointment
oral order
osteoid osteoma
other
out of
O-O
outer-to-outer
O&O
off and on
o/o
on account of
OOA
outer optic anlage
OOB
out of bed
out-of-body (experience)
OOBBRP
out of bed (with) bathroom privileges
OOBL
out of bilirubin light
OOC
onset of contractions
out of cast
out of control

O

NOTES

OOH&NS
>ophthalmology, otorhinolaryngology, and head and neck surgery

OOH-SCD
>out-of-hospital sudden cardiac death

OOI
>out of Isolette

OOL
>onset of labor

OOLR
>ophthalmology, otology, laryngology, and rhinology

OOM
>onset of menarche

OOP
>out on pass
>out of pelvis
>out of plaster (cast)

OOPS
>out of program status

OOR
>out of room

OORW
>out of radiant warmer

OOS
>out of sequence
>out of specification (deviation from standard)
>out of splint
>out of stock (*See also* OS)

OOT
>out of town

OOW
>out of wedlock (*See also* OW)

OP
>oblique presentation
>occipitoparietal
>occipitoposterior
>occiput posterior
>old patient (previously seen)
>olfactory peduncle
>open
>opening pressure
>operation (*See also* op)
>operative
>operative procedure
>ophthalmology
>opponens pollicis (muscle)
>organophosphorous
>original package
>oropharynx
>orthostatic proteinuria
>oscillatory potential
>osmotic pressure
>osteoporosis
>other (than) psychotic
>outpatient (*See also* O/P, OPT)
>overpressure
>overproof
>ovine prolactin

OP-1
>osteogenic protein-1

OP-3
>Orthopantomograph-3

OP-10
>Orthopantomograph-10

O/P
>outpatient (*See also* OP, OPT)

O&P
>ova and parasites (stool exam)

Op
>opisthocranion

op
>operation (*See also* OP)
>operational
>operator
>opposite
>work [L. *opus*]

OPA
>oral pharyngeal airway
>outpatient anesthesia

OPAC
>opacity (opacification)

OPAT
>outpatient parenteral antibiotic therapy

OPB
>outpatient basis

OPC
>oculopalatocerebral (syndrome)
>oligomeric proanthocyanidin
>operable pancreatic carcinoma
>oropharyngeal candidiasis
>outpatient care
>outpatient catheterization
>outpatient clinic
>oxypneumocardiogram

OPCA
>(neonatal) olivopontocerebellar atrophy
>olivopontocerebellar atrophy (*See also* OCA)
>(X-linked) olivopontocerebellar ataxia

OPCAB
>off-pump coronary artery bypass
>off-pump coronary artery bypass (grafting)

OPCD
>olivopontocerebellar degeneration

op. cit.
>in the work cited [L. *opere citato*]

OPCOS
>oligomenorrheic polycystic ovary syndrome

OPCP
orthocresolphthalein complex

OPCS-4
Classification of Surgical Operations and Procedures (4th revision)

OPD
obstetric prediabetes
obstructive pulmonary disease
optical path difference
optical penetration depth
oropharyngeal dysphagia
otopalatodigital (syndrome)
outpatient department
outpatient dispensary

OpDent
operative dentistry

OPDG
ocular plethysmodynamography

OPDUR
on-line prospective drug utilization review

OPE
oral peripheral examination
outpatient evaluation

OPERA
outpatient endometrial resection/ablation

OPG
ocular plethysmography
ocular pneumoplethysmography
oculoplethysmograph
oculoplethysmography
oculopneumoplethysmography (See also OPPG)
ophthalmoplethysmograph
ophthalmoplethysmography
osteoprotegerin
oxypolygelatin (plasma volume extender)

opg
opening (See also o)

OPG/CPA
oculoplethysmography/carotid phonoangiography

OPGF
osteoprotegerin factor

OPGL
osteoprotegerin ligand

OPGR
OptiMed glaucoma pressure regulator

OPH, Oph
obliterative pulmonary hypotension
ophthalmia
ophthalmologist (See also Ophth)
ophthalmology (See also Ophth)
ophthalmoscope (See also Ophth)
ophthalmoscopy (See also Ophth)

oph
ophthalmic
ophthalmologic

OphSeg
ophthalmic segment

Ophth
ophthalmologist (See also OPH, Oph)
ophthalmology (See also OPH, Oph)
ophthalmoscope (See also OPH, Oph)
ophthalmoscopy (See also OPH, Oph)

OPI
oculoparalytic illusion
Omnibus Personality Inventory

OPIM
other potentially infectious material

OPK
optokinetic

OPL
oral premalignant lesion
osmotic pressure (of proteins in) lymph
other party liability
outer plexiform layer
ovine placental lactogen

OPLL
ossification of posterior longitudinal ligament

OPM
occult primary malignancy
ophthalmoplegic migraine
opponens digiti minimi (muscle)

OPMD
oculopharyngeal muscular dystrophy

OpMNPV
Orgyia pseudotsugata MNPV

OPN
ophthalmic nurse
osteopontin

OPO
optical parametric oscillator
organ procurement organizations

O

NOTES

OPOC

oropharynx, oral cavity

OPP

ocular perfusion pressure
osmotic pressure of plasma
ovine pancreatic polypeptide
oxygen partial pressure

opp

opposing
opposite

OPPES

oil-associated pneumoparalytic
eosinophilic syndrome

OPPG

oculopneumoplethysmography (*See also* OPG)

OPPOS

opposition

OPPS

Outpatient Prospective Payment System

OPRDU

outpatient renal dialysis unit

op reg

operative region

oprg

operating

OPRT

orotate phosphoribosyl transferase

OPS

Objective Pain Scores
operations
Orpington prognostic scale
orthogonal polarization spectral
osteoporosis-pseudoglioma syndrome
osteoporosis-pseudolipoma syndrome
outpatient service
outpatient surgery
output signal processor

OPSA

ovarian papillary serous adenocarcinoma

OpScan

optical scanning

OPSI

overwhelming postsplenectomy infection

OPSU

outpatient surgical unit

O PSY

open psychiatry

OPT

Ohio pediatric tent
optimum
outpatient (*See also* OP, O/P)
outpatient treatment

Opt

optometrist

opt.

best [L. *optimus*]
optical
optician
optics
optimal
optimum
optional

OPT c̄ CA

Ohio pediatric tent with compressed air

OPT c̄ O₂

Ohio pediatric tent with oxygen

OPT-NSC

outpatient treatment, nonservice-connected

OPT-SC

outpatient treatment, service-connected

OPV

occult (trauma), postanoxia, ventriculoperitoneal
oral (attenuated) poliovirus vaccine
oral polio vaccine
oral poliovirus vaccine
outpatient visit

OPW, OPWL

opiate withdrawal

OQSMAT

Otis Quick Scoring Mental Abilities Test

O-R

oxidation-reduction (system)

OR

oblique ridge
odds ratio
oil retention (enema)
open reduction
operating room
operations research
optic radiation
oral rehydration
organ recovery
orienting reflex
orienting response
orthopedic (*See also* Orth, ortho)
orthopedic research
ovary reserve
overrefraction
own recognizance
oxidized-reduced

Or

outflow rate

ORA

occiput right anterior (fetal position)
opiate receptor agonist
opioid receptor agonist

ORAN
    orthopedic resident admit note
ORBC
    ox red blood cell
ORC
    order/results communication
    outpatient rehabilitation centers
    ox red cell
ORCH
    orchiectomy
orch
    orchitis
ORD
    optical rotary dispersion
    optical rotatory dispersion
    oral radiation death
Ord
    orotidine
ord
    orderly
    ordinate
OREF
    open reduction and external
        fixation
OR en
    oil-retention enema
ORF
    open reading frame
OR&F
    open reduction and fixation
org
    organ
    organic
    organism
ORIF
    open reduction and internal fixation
orig
    origin
    original
ORIV
    Oriboca virus
OrJ
    orange juice (*See also* OJ, oj)
ORL
    oblique retinacular ligament
    otorhinolaryngology
ORMF
    open reduction metallic fixation
ORN
    operating room nurse
    osteoradionecrosis

Orn
    ornithine
ORO
    oil red O
Oro
    orotate
    orotic acid (*See also* OA)
OROS
    oral osmotic
    ostomotic release oral system
OROV
    Oropouche virus
ORP
    occiput right posterior (fetal
        position)
    oxidation-reduction potential (*See
        also* E_h, eH, E_o+, $E°$)
ORPM
    orthorhythmic pacemaker
ORQ
    Occupational Roles Questionnaire
ORS
    olfactory reference syndrome
    oral rehydration salt
    oral rehydration solution
    oral surgeon
    oral surgery (*See also* OS)
    orthopedic surgeon (*See also* OS)
    orthopedic surgery (*See also* OS)
ORSA
    oxacillin-resistant *Staphylococcus
        aureus*
ORSIST
    Oral Language Sentence Imitation
        Screening Test
ORSP
    Optochin-resistant *Streptococcus
        pneumoniae*
O-R system
    oxidation-reduction system
ORT
    ocular radiation therapy
    oestrogen (estrogen)-replacement
        therapy
    oral rehydration therapy
    orthodromic reciprocating
        tachycardia
Orth, ortho
    orthopedic (*See also* OR)
    orthopedics
orthot
    orthotonus

NOTES

O

ORUV
Orungo virus
ORx
oriented
ORx4
oriented to time, place, person, and objects (watch, pen, book) (*See also* Ox4)
ORx1
oriented to time
ORx2
oriented to time and place (*See also* Ox2)
ORx3
oriented to time, place, and person (*See also* Ox3)
ORXV
Oriximina virus
OS
left eye
by mouth (*See also* m, (m), per os, PO, p.o.)
occipitosacral (fetal position)
occupational safety
oligospermic
Omenn syndrome
opening snap (heart sound)
open surgery
operating suite
ophthalmic solution
oral surgery (*See also* ORS)
orbitale superius
orthopedic surgeon (*See also* ORS)
orthopedic surgery (*See also* ORS)
osmium
osteogenic sarcoma
osteoid surface
osteosarcoma
osteosclerosis
ouabain sensitive
out of stock (*See also* OOS)
overall survival
oxidative stress
oxygen saturation (*See also* O_2 sat., SaO_2, SO_2)
O.S., o.s.
left eye [L. *oculus sinister*] (*See also* LE, O.L.)
oculus sinister (left eye)
Os
osmium
os
bone [L. pl. *ossa*]
mouth [L. pl. *ora*]
opening
OSA
obstructive sleep apnea

off-site anesthesia
osteosarcoma
OSA/H
obstructive sleep apnea/hypoventilation
OSA/HS
obstructive sleep apnea/hypopnea syndrome
OSAI
organism-specific antibody index
OSAP
Office Sterilization and Asepsis Procedures Research
OSAS
obstructive sleep apnea syndrome
O_2 sat.
oxygen saturation (*See also* OS, SaO_2, SO_2)
OSBCL
Ottawa School Behavior Checklist
OSBT
ovarian serous borderline tumor
osc
oscillate
OSCAR
On-line Survey Certification and Reporting
OSCC
oral squamous cell carcinoma
OSCE
objective structural clinical examination
OSCJ
original squamocolumnar junction
OSD
obstructive sleep disorder
ocular surface disease
Osgood-Schlatter disease
outside doctor
overseas duty
overside drainage
OSD-6
Obstructive Sleep Disorders-6 (test)
OSE
ovarian surface epithelium
OSESC
opening snap ejection systolic click
OSF
outer spiral fibers (of cochlea)
outlet strut fracture
overgrowth-stimulating factor
OSFI
organ system failure index
OSFT
outstretched fingertips
OSH
oral surgery handpiece
outside hospital

OSHA
Occupational Safety and Health Act

OSI
Occupational Stress Indicator
optical surface imaging
Orthopedic Systems Inc.

OSIQ
Offer Self-Image Questionnaire (for Adolescents)

OSL
Osgood-Schlatter lesion

OSM
osmolality
ovine submaxillary mucin
oxygen saturation meter

Osm
osmole

osM
osmolar

osm
osmosis
osmotic

OSMED
otospondylometaphyseal dysplasia

OSMF
oral submucous fibrosis

Osm/kg
osmole per kilogram (osmolality)

Osm/L, Osm/l
osmole per liter (osmolarity)

osmo
osmolality

OSM S
osmolality serum

OSM U
osmolality urine

OSN
off-service note

OSNP
one-step nested PCR

OSP
oncocytic schneiderian papilloma
output signal processor
outside pass

OS/P
left eye patched

Osp
outer surface protein

OspA
outer surface protein A

OSPL
output sound pressure level

OSS
Object Sorting Scales (psychologic test)
occupational stress syndrome
osseous
over-shoulder strap

OSSAV
Ossa virus

OS-SPT
osmolality urine spot (test)

OST
Object Sorting Test
optimal sampling theory

ost
osteotomy

Osteo
osteopathy

osteo
osteoarthritis (*See also* OA)
osteomyelitis (*See also* OM)
osteopathology

osteocart
osteocartilaginous

osteopath
osteopathologist (*See also* Osteo)

OSTI
Optimal Stent Implantation

OT
(Koch) old tuberculin
objective test
object test
oblique talus
occipitotransverse
occiput transverse
occlusion time
occupational therapy
ocular tension
Oestreicher-Turner (syndrome)
office treatment
old term
old terminology (anatomy)
old tuberculin
olfactory threshold
olfactory tubercle (*See also* OTU)
optic tract
oral transmucosal
orientation test
original tuberculin
orotracheal (tube)
orthopedic treatment

O

NOTES

OT *(continued)*
    otolaryngology (*See also* Ot, OTO, Oto, Otolar)
    otology (*See also* OTO, Oto, Otol)
    outer table
    outlier threshold
    oxytocin (*See also* OX, OXT, OXY, oxy)
O/T
    oral temperature
Ot
    otolaryngology (*See also* OT, OTO, Oto, Otolar)
OTA
    oligoteratoasthenozoospermia
    open to air
    Opinions toward Adolescents (psychologic test)
    ornithine transaminase
    orthotoluidine arsenite
OTAPS
    Ohio Tests of Articulation and Perception of Sounds
OTC
    ornithine transcarbamoylase
    ornithine transcarbamoylase (deficiency)
    oval target cell
    over-the-counter (nonprescription drug)
    oxytetracycline
OTc
    heartrate-corrected OT interval
OTC Rx
    over-the-counter prescription
OTD
    optimal therapeutic dose
    oral temperature device
    organ tolerance dose
    out the door
OTE
    (McMaster) Overall Treatment Evaluation
    optically transparent electrode
OTF
    oral transfer factor
OTFC
    oral transmucosal fentanyl citrate
OTH
    other
OTHS
    occupational therapy home service
OTI
    ovomucoid trypsin inhibitor
OTM
    orthotoluidine manganese (sulfate)
OTO, Oto
    one-time only

otolaryngology (*See also* OT, Ot, Otolar)
otology (*See also* OT, Otol)
Otol
    otologist
    otology (*See also* OT, OTO, Oto)
OtoLAM
    OtoScan laser-assisted myringotomy
Otolar
    otolaryngology (*See also* OT, Ot, OTO, Oto)
OTPT
    oral triphasic tablets (contraceptive)
OTR
    ocular tilt reaction
OT/RT
    occupational therapy/recreational therapy
OTS
    occipital temporal sulcus
    orotracheal suction
OTT, OT(T)
    orotracheal tube
    overall treatment time
OTU
    olfactory tubercle (*See also* OT)
    operational taxonomic unit
OTW
    off-the-wall
    over the wire
OU
    both eyes
    observation unit
O.U., o.u.
    both eyes (together) [L. *oculi unitas*]
    each eye [L. *oculi uterque*]
    oculus unitas (both eyes)
    oculus uterque (each eye)
OUAV
    Ouango virus
OUBIV
    Oubi virus
OUES
    oxygen uptake efficiency slope
OULQ
    outer upper left quadrant
OU/P
    both eyes patched
OURQ
    outer upper right quadrant
OUS
    obstetric ultrasound
    overuse syndrome
oUW
    original University of Wisconsin (solution)

OV
oculovestibular
office visit
Osler-Vaquez (disease)
osteoid volume
outflow volume
ovalbumin (*See also* OA, OVA)
overventilation
ovulating
ovulation
ovum
oyster virus

O₂V
oxygen ventilation equivalent

Oᵥ
outflow volume

Ov
ovary

ov
ovarian

OVA
chicken ovalbumin
ovalbumin (*See also* OA, OV)

OVAL
ovalocyte

OVAS
ocular vergance and accommodation sensor

OVC
ovarian carcinoma

OVD
occlusal vertical dimension

OvDF
ovarian dysfunction

OVDQ
Organizational Value Dimensions Questionnaire

OVEM
ovarian epithelial metasepithelial

OVET
ovarian epithelial tumor

OVF
Octopus visual field

OVIS
Ohio Vocational Interest Survey

OVIT
Oral Verbal Intelligence Test

OVLP
overlap myositis

OVLT
organum vasculosum laminae terminalis

organum vasculosum of lamina terminalis

OVS
obstructive voiding symptom

OVT
ovarian vein thrombosis

OVX
ovariectomized

OW
off work
once weekly
open wedge
open wedge (osteotomy)
open wound
ordinary warfare
outer wall
out of wedlock (*See also* OOW)
oval window
ova weight

O/W
oil in water (emulsion)
oil-water (ratio)

o/w
otherwise

OWA
organics-in-water (analyzer)

OWL
out of wedlock

OWNK
out of wedlock and not keeping (child)

OWR
ovarian wedge resection

OWRS
Osler-Weber-Rendu syndrome

OWS
overwear syndrome

OWT
zero work tolerance

OWVI
Ohio Work Values Inventory

OX
optic chiasm (*See also* OC)
orthopedic examination (*See also* OE)
oxacillin
oximeter
oxymel (honey, water, and vinegar)
oxytocin (*See also* OT, OXT, OXY, oxy)

NOTES

Ox

oxygen (*See also* O2, O$_2$, OXY, oxy)

Ox1

oriented to time

Ox2

oriented to time and place (*See also* ORx2)

Ox3

oriented to time, place, and person (*See also* ORx)

Ox4

oriented to time, place, person, and objects (watch, pen, book) (*See also* ORx4)

OXA

oxacillinase
oxaliplatin (Eloxatin)

OXC

oxcarbazepine

Oxi

oximeter
oximetry

OX40L

OX40 ligand

OXLAT

oxalate

Ox-LDL, oxLDL

oxidative modification of LDL
oxidized low-density lipoprotein

OXM

pulse oximeter

OXP

oxypressin

OXPHOS

oxidative phosphorylation

OXT

oxytocin (*See also* OT, OX, OXY, oxy)

OXY, oxy

oxygen (*See also* O2, O$_2$, Ox)
oxytocin (*See also* OT, OX, OXT)

Oxy-5

benzoyl peroxide

OXZ

oxazepam (Serax)

OYE

old yellow enzyme

OZ

optical zone

oz, oz.

ounce

oz ap

apothecary's ounce

oz t

ounce troy

after [L. *post*] (*See also* p)
by weight [L. *pondere*]
father [L. *pater*]
form perception (in General
 Aptitude Test Battery)
gas partial pressure (*See also* p,
 PP)
handful [L. *pugillus*]
near [L. *proximum*]
near point (of vision) [L. *punctum
 proximum*] (*See also* PP, pp)
page
pain
para (parity)
parent
parenteral
parietal (electrode placement in
 electroencephalography)
parity
parous
part (*See also* pt)
partial pressure (*See also* p, PP)
passive
paternal
paternally contributing
patient (*See also* PNT, PT, Pt, pt)
pelvis
penicillin (*See also* PCN, PEN,
 Pen, pen., PN, PNC)
per
percent
percentile
perceptual speed
percussion
perforation (*See also* perf)
peripheral
permeability
permeability constant
peta-
peyote
pharmacopoeia (British)
phenacetin
phenolphthalein
phon (unit of loudness)
phosphate (group)
phosphorus
physiology (*See also* PHY, PHYS)
pico-
pilocarpine
pin
pink (indicator color)
pint (*See also* p, PT, pt)
placebo (*See also* PBO, PL, PLBO,
 PCB, PLB)

plan
plasma
point
poise (unit of dynamic viscosity)
poison
poisoning
polarity
polarization
pole
polymyxin
pons
poor
popular response
population
porcelain
porcine
porphyrin
position (*See also* pos)
positive (*See also* POS, pos)
posterior (*See also* post, post.)
postpartum
power
precipitin
prednisone (*See also* PDN, PRED)
premolar
presbyopia (*See also* PR, Pr)
press
pressure (*See also* p, PR, press.)
primary
primipara (*See also* I-para, primip)
primitive (hemoglobin)
private (patient, room)
probability
probable error
product
progesterone
prolactin (*See also* P, PR, Pr,
 PRL, Prl)
proline (*See also* Pro)
properdin
propionate
protein (*See also* PR, Pr, PRO,
 prot)
Protestant
proximal
psoralen
psychiatry (*See also* PS, Psy,
 psychiat)
psychosis
pulmonary (*See also* P, PUL, pul,
 pulm)
pulse
pupil
P wave (in electrocardiography)
pyloroplasty

P

P *(continued)*
    radiant flux
    radiant power
    rho (17th letter of Greek
      alphabet), uppercase
    significance probability (value)
    sound power
    weight [L. *pondus*]

P1
    orthophosphate
    pilocarpine 1% ophthalmic solution

P_1
    first parental generation
    inorganic orthophosphate
    orthophosphate

P2
    pulmonic second heart sound

P_2
    pulmonic second (heart) sound

P-3
    Pain Patient Profile

P/3
    proximal third
    proximal third (of bone)

P_3
    luminous flux
    proximal third (of bone) (*See also*
      P/3)

P_4
    progesterone

P-32, ^{32}**P**
    phosphorus-32
    phosphorus-32
    radioisotope of phosphorus

^{33}**P**
    phosphorus-33

P-50
    oxygen half-saturation pressure of
      hemoglobin

/P
    partial lower denture

P/
    partial upper denture

p
    after (*See also* P)
    atomic orbital with angular
      momentum quantum number 1
    (freeze) preservation
    frequency of the more common
      allele of a pair
    momentum
    page
    papilla (optic)
    para
    partial (pressure) (*See also* P, PP)
    peripheral
    phosphate
    pico-

    pint (*See also* P, PT, pt)
    pond
    pressure (*See also* P, PR, press.)
    probability
    probable error
    proton
    pupil
    sample proportion (in statistics)
    short arm of chromosome
    sound pressure

p7
    cleaved polyprotein precursor
      molecule product
    HIV nucleocapsid protein

p9
    cleaved polyprotein precursor
      molecule product

p24
    cleaved polyprotein precursor
      molecule product

p55
    cleaved polyprotein precursor
      molecule

p̄
    after [L. *post*]
    mean pressure (gas)

p-
    para- (chemical prefix for two
      symmetrical substitutions in
      benzene ring)

PGTC
    partial seizures with or without
      generalized tonic-clonic seizures

PA
    alveolar partial pressure
    alveolar pressure
    panic attack
    pantothenic acid
    paralysis agitans
    paranoia
    parietal (cell) antibody
    partial pressure
    passive aggressive
    paternal aunt
    pathology
    pentanoic acid
    periarteritis
    peridural artery
    periodic acid
    periodontal abscess
    permeability area
    pernicious anemia
    peroxidatic activity
    phakic-aphakic
    phenol alcohol
    phenylacetate
    phosphatidic acid
    phosphoarginine

photo allergy
phthalic anhydride
physical assistance
Picture Arrangement (psychology)
pineapple (test for butyric acid in
  stomach)
pituitary-adrenal
plasma aldosterone
plasminogen activator
platelet adhesiveness
platelet aggregation
platelet associated
pleomorphic adenoma
polyacrylamide
polyarteritis (*See also* PAr)
polyarthritis
postaural
posteroanterior (position for x-ray)
prealbumin
predictive accuracy
pregnancy-associated
presents again
pressure augmentation
primary aldosteronism
primary amenorrhea
primary anemia
prior to admission
proactivator
proanthocyanidin
procainamide
professional association
proinsulin antibody
prolonged action
prophylactic antibiotic
propionic acid
prostate antigen
protective antigen
proteolytic activity
prothrombin activity
protrusio acetabuli
Pseudomonas aeruginosa
psychiatric aide
psychoanalysis (*See also* PYA)
psychoanalyst
psychogenic aspermia
psychosocial assessment
pulmonary angiography
pulmonary artery
pulmonary artery (banding)
pulmonary atresia
pulmonary autograft

pulpoaxial
puromycin aminonucleoside
pyrophosphate arthropathy
pyrrolizidine alkaloid
yearly [L. *per annum*]

P/A

percussion (and) auscultation (*See
  also* P&A)
position (and) alignment (*See also*
  P&A)

P&A, P & A

percussion and auscultation (*See
  also* P/A)
position and alignment (*See also*
  P/A)
present and active (reflex)
protection and advocacy

$P_2 = A_2$

pulmonic second heart sound equal
  to aortic second heart sound

$P_2 > A_2$

pulmonic second heart sound
  greater than aortic second heart
  sound

$P_2 < A_2$

pulmonic heart sound less than
  aortic second heart sound

Pa

arterial partial pressure
arterial pressure
pascal (unit of pressure
  measurement)
protactinium
pulmonary arterial (pressure)
pulmonary artery (line)

pA

picoampere

pA_2

affinity constant (binding drug to
  drug receptor)

PAA

partial agonist activity
periampullary adenoma
phenylacetic acid
physical abilities analysis
plasma angiotensinase activity
polyacrylamide
polyacrylic acid
polyamino acid
premarket approval application
pyridine acetic acid

NOTES

P(A-aDO₂)
> alveolar-arterial oxygen tension difference

PAAF
> pancreatitis-associated ascites fluid

p(A-a)O₂
> alveolar-arterial pressure difference

PAAP
> percutaneous alcohol ablation of the parathyroid gland

PAAS
> Pediatric Acute Admission Severity

PAAT
> Parent as a Teacher Inventory

pAAT
> plasma alpha 1-antitrypsin

PAB
> *para*-aminobenzoate
> p-aminobenzoic acid (*See also* PABA)
> *para*-aminobenzoate
> pharmacologic autonomic block
> polyacrylamide bead
> Positive Attention Behavior
> prealbumin
> premature atrial beat
> pulmonary artery banding
> purple agarbase (medium)

PAb
> protein antibody

PABA
> paraaminobenzoic acid (*See also* PAB)
> *para*-aminobenzoic acid (*See also* PAB)

PABD
> preoperative autologous blood donation

PABM
> peak adult bone mass

PABP
> pulmonary artery balloon pump

PAC
> pancreatic adenocarcinoma
> papular acrodermatitis of childhood
> *para*-aminoclonidine
> parent-adult-child (in transactional analysis)
> phenacemide
> phenacetin (acetophenetidin), aspirin, and caffeine
> Physical Assessment Center
> picture archiving communication (system)
> plasma aldosterone concentration
> preadmission certification
> premature atrial contraction
> premature auricular contraction
> Progress Assessment Chart (of Social and Personal Development)
> prophylactic anticonvulsant
> pulmonary artery catheter
> pulmonary artery catheterization

PACAP
> pituitary adenylate cyclase activating polypeptide

PACATH
> pulmonary artery catheter

PACC
> protein A (immobilized in) collodion charcoal

PACE
> performance and cost efficiency
> Personal Assessment for Continuing Education
> personalized aerobics for cardiovascular enhancement
> Professional and Administrative Career Examination
> promoting aphasics communicative effectiveness
> Psychosocial Assessment of Childhood Experiences
> pulmonary angiotensin I converting enzyme

PACG
> Prevocational Assessment and Curriculum Guide
> primary angle-closure glaucoma

PACI
> partial anterior cerebral infarct
> partial anterior circulation infarct

PACL
> Personality Adjective Check List

PACNS
> primary angiitis of the central nervous system
> primary angiitis of CNS

PaCO2, Pa_CO2, PaCO₂
> arterial carbon dioxide pressure (tension)
> arterial partial pressure of CO_2
> partial arterial gas tension of carbon dioxide
> partial pressure of arterial carbon dioxide
> partial pressure of carbon dioxide in arterial gas

PACONA
> periodic acid-concanavalin A

PACP
> pulmonary artery counterpulsation

PAC/PRA
> plasma aldosterone concentration/plasma renin activity

PACS

    partial anterior circulation syndrome
    picture archival communication
      system
    picture archiving and
      communication (system)

PACSRO

    picture archiving and
      communications systems in
      radiation oncology

PACT

    papillary carcinoma of thyroid
    precordial acceleration tracing
    Prescription Analyses and Cost
    prism and alternate cover test

PACU

    postanesthesia care unit

PACV

    Pacui virus

PAD

    pelvic adhesive disease
    per adjusted discharge
    percutaneous abscess drainage
    peripheral arterial disease
    pharmacologic atrial defibrillator
    phenacetin, aspirin, and
      desoxyephedrine
    phonologic-acquisition device
    photon absorption densitometry
    practical approach design
    pre-aid to the disabled
    preliminary anatomic diagnosis
    preoperative autologous donation
    primary affective disorder
    psychoaffective disorder
    public access defibrillation
    public access defibrillator
    pulmonary artery diastolic (*See also*
      PAd)
    pulmonary artery diastolic pressure
    pulsatile assist device

PAd

    pulmonary artery diastolic (*See also*
      PAD)

PADCAB

    perfusion-assisted direct coronary
      artery bypass

PADDS

    photon-activated drug delivery
      system

PADI

    posterior atlantodental interval

PADP

    pulmonary arterial diastolic pressure
    pulmonary artery diastolic pressure

PADP-PAWP

    pulmonary artery diastolic and
      wedge pressure

PADPRP

    poly (adenosine diphosphate-ribose)
      polymerase

PADS

    Post Anesthesia Discharge Scoring
      System

PAE

    paradoxical air embolism
    postanoxic encephalopathy
    postantibiotic effect
    progressive assistive exercise
    Pygeum africanum extract

PA&E

    present, active, equal

PAEC

    pig aortic endothelial cell

paed

    paediatrics (*See also* PD, PED,
      ped, Peds)

PAEDP

    pulmonary artery end-diastolic
      pressure

PAF

    paroxysmal atrial fibrillation (*See*
      also PAFIB)
    paroxysmal auricular fibrillation
    phosphodiesterase-activating factor
    platelet activating/aggregating factor
    platelet-activating factor
    platelet-aggregating factor (*See also*
      PAgF)
    platelet aggregation factor (*See also*
      PAgF)
    pollen adherence factor
    posterior auricular flap
    premenstrual assessment form
    pseudoamniotic fluid
    pulmonary arteriovenous fistula

PA&F

    percussion, auscultation, and
      fremitus

PAF-A

    platelet-activating factor of
      anaphylaxis

NOTES

P

PAF-AH
> platelet-activating factor acetylhydrolase

PAFD
> percutaneous abscess and fluid drainage
> pulmonary artery filling defect

PAFG
> picric acid formaldehyde-glutaraldehyde

PAFI
> platelet-aggregation factor inhibitor

PAFIB
> paroxysmal atrial fibrillation (*See also* PAF)

PAFP
> pre-Achilles fat pad

PAG
> periaqueductal gray (matter)
> phenylacetylglutamine
> pictorial anticipatory guidance
> pineal antigonadotropin
> polyacrylamide gel
> pregnancy alpha-2 glycoprotein
> pregnancy-associated globulin
> protein A-gold
> pulmonary angiography

pAg
> protein A-gold (technique)

PAGA
> premature appropriate for gestational age

PAGE
> perfluorocarbon-associated gas exchange
> polyacrylamide gel electrophoresis

PAGE-SS
> polyacrylamide gel electrophoresis with silver stain

PAgF
> platelet-aggregating factor (*See also* PAF)

PAGG
> penta-acetylglucopyranosyl guanine

PAGIF
> polyacrylamide gel isoelectric focusing

PAGMK
> primary African green monkey kidney

PAG/PVG
> periaqueductal-periventricular

PAH
> *p*-aminohippuric acid
> *para*-aminohippuric acid
> p-aminohippurate
> p-aminohippuric acid (*See also* PAHA)

> paraaminohippurate
> paraaminohippuric
> phenylalanine hydroxylase
> polycyclic aromatic hydrocarbon
> polynuclear aromatic hydrocarbon
> postatrophic hyperplasia
> prealbumin-associated hyperthyroxinemia
> predicted adult height
> pulmonary artery hypertension
> pulmonary artery hypotension

PAHA
> p-aminohippuric acid (*See also* PAH)

PAHV
> Pahayokee virus

PAHVC
> pulmonary alveolar hypoxic vasoconstriction

PAI
> Pain Appraisal Inventory
> Pair Attraction Inventory
> partial (incomplete) androgen insensitivity
> perforating artery infarct
> Personality Assessment Inventory
> plasminogen activator inhibitor
> platelet accumulation index

PAI-1
> plasminogen activator inhibitor type 1

PAI-2
> plasminogen activator inhibitor type 2

PAIC
> procedures, alternatives, indications and complications

PAIDS
> pediatric acquired immunodeficiency syndrome

PAIg
> platelet-associated immunoglobulin

PAIgG
> platelet-associated immunoglobulin G

PAIR
> percutaneous aspiration, instillation of hypertonic saline, respiration
> Personal Assessment of Intimacy in Relationships
> puncture, aspiration, injection, reaspiration

PAIS
> partial androgen insensitivity syndrome
> Psychosocial Adjustment to Illness Scale
> punctate area of increased signal

PAIVMs
> passive accessory intervertebral movements

PAIVS
> pulmonary atresia with intact ventricular septum

PAJ
> paralysis agitans juvenilis

PAJB
> primary antecubital jump bypass

PAK
> pancreas after kidney
> pancreas after kidney transplant
> pancreas and kidney
> percutaneous access kit

PAL
> pathology laboratory
> peptidyl-alpha-hydroxyglycine alpha-amidating lyase
> phenylalanine ammonia lyase
> posterior axillary line
> posteroanterior and lateral
> powered air loss
> product of activated lymphocyte
> Profile of Adaptation to Life
> pyogenic abscess of liver

pal.
> palate

PALA
> N-phosphoacetate-L aspartate
> *N*-phosphonoacetyl-*l*-aspartic acid

PA&Lat
> posteroanterior and lateral

Pa Line
> pulmonary artery line

PALM
> premature accelerated lung maturation

PALN
> paraaortic lymph node

PALP
> placental alkaline phosphatase

palp
> palpable
> palpate
> palpation
> palpitation

PALS
> Paired Associate Learning Subtest
> pediatric advanced life support
> pediatric life support

> periarterial lymphatic sheath
> periarteriolar lymphocyte sheath
> prison-acquired lymphoproliferative syndrome

PA-LS-ID
> pernicious anemia-like syndrome and immunoglobulin deficiency

PALST
> Picture Articulation and Language Screening Test

PALT
> Paired Associate Learning Task

PALV
> Palyam virus

Palv
> alveolar pressure

PAM
> (crystalline) penicillin (G in 2%) aluminum monostearate
> pancreatic acinar mass
> pancreatic acinar metaplasia
> partial allosteric modulators
> penicillin aluminum monostearate
> peptidylglycine alpha-amidating monooxygenase
> periodic acid-silver methenamine
> phenylalanine mustard
> postauricular myogenic
> potential acuity meter
> pralidoxime
> primary acquired melanosis
> primary amebic meningoencephalitis (*See also* PAME)
> pulmonary alveolar macrophage
> pulmonary alveolar microlithiasis
> pulmonary artery mean pressure
> pyridine aldoxime methiodide

2-PAM
> 2-pralidoxime

PAMBA
> paraaminomethylbenzoic acid

PAMC
> pterygoarthromyodysplasia, congenital

PAMD
> primary adrenocortical micronodular dysplasia

PAME
> primary amebic meningoencephalitis (*See also* PAM)

NOTES

P

585

PAMP
proadrenomedullin N-20 terminal peptide
pulmonary artery mean pressure

PAN
panoral x-ray examination
periarteritis nodosa (*See also* PN)
periodic alternating nystagmus
peroxyacetyl nitrate
polyacrylonitrile
polyacrylonitryl
polyarteritis nodosa (*See also* PN)
positional alcohol nystagmus
posterior ampullary nerve
primary afferent nociceptor neuron
puromycin aminonucleoside (*See also* PANS)
puromycin aminonucleoside nephropathy
puromycin aminonucleoside nephrosis

pan.
pancreas
pancreatectomy
pancreatic

p-ANC
perinuclear antineutrophil cytoplasmic

P-ANCA, p-ANCA, pANCA
perinuclear antineutrophil cytoplasmic antibody

PANCH
pituitary adenoma-adenohypophyseal neuronal choristoma

PAND
primary adrenocortical nodular dysplasia

PANDAS
pediatric autoimmune neuropsychiatric disorders associated with streptococcus infections

PANDO
primary acquired nasolacrimal duct obstruction

PANESS
physical and neurologic examination for soft signs

PANP
pelvic autonomic nerve preservation

PANS
puromycin aminonucleoside (*See also* PAN)

PANSS
Positive and Negative Stroke Scale
Positive and Negative Syndrome Scale

PANTA
polymyxin B, amphotericin B, nalidixic acid, trimethoprim, azlocillin

PAO
peak acid output
peripheral airway obstruction
peripheral arterial occlusion
plasma amine oxidase
polyamine oxidase

PAO$_2$
alveolar oxygen partial pressure
arterial oxygen pressure (tension)
partial pressure alveolar oxygen
partial pressure arterial oxygen

P$_{ao}$
airway opening pressure

PAo
pulmonary artery occlusion (pressure)

Pao
ascending aortic pressure

PAO$_2$–PaO$_2$
alveolar-arterial difference in partial pressure of oxygen

PAOD
peripheral arterial occlusive disease
peripheral arteriosclerotic occlusive disease
popliteal artery occlusive disease

PAOG
primary open-angle glaucoma

PAOGRP
peak acid output after gastrin-releasing peptide

PAOI
peak acid output insulin-induced

PAOP
pulmonary artery occluded pressure
pulmonary artery occlusion pressure

PAOPg
peak acid output after pentagastrin stimulation

PAOx
phenylacetone oxime

PAP
pancreatitis-associated protein
Papanicolaou (smear, test) (*See also* Pap)
papaverine
para-aminophenol
passive-aggressive personality
Patient Assessment Program
peak airway pressure
peroxidase antibody to peroxidase
peroxidase-antiperoxidase (technique, complex)
3'-phosphoadenosine 5'-phosphate

placental acid phosphatase
placental alkaline phosphatase
positive airway pressure
preoperative antimicrobial
  prophylaxis
primary atypical pneumonia
prostatic acid phosphatase
pulmonary alveolar proteinosis
pulmonary artery pressure (*See also*
  PA)
purified alternate pathway

Pap

Papanicolaou (smear, test) (*See also*
  PAP)
papillary

pap

papilloma

pap.

papilla

PAPA

preschool-age psychiatric assessment
pyogenic sterile arthritis, pyoderma
  gangrenosum, and acne

PAPase

phosphatidate phosphohydrolase
phosphatidic acid phosphohydrolase

PAPF

platelet adhesiveness plasma factor

PAPI

PAP immunoperoxidase

pap in. canthus

papilloma, inner canthus

PAPm

mean pulmonary artery pressure

papova

papilloma-polyoma-vacuolating agent
  (virus)
papilloma virus, polyoma virus,
  vacuolative virus

PAPP

p-aminopropiophenone
Pappenheimer bodies
pregnancy-associated plasma protein

PAPP-A, PAPPA

pregnancy-associated plasma protein
  A

PAPPC

pregnancy-associated plasma protein
  C

PAPS

adenosine 3'-phosphate 5'-
  phosphosulfate

3'-phosphoadenosine 5'-
  phosphosulfate
primary antiphospholipid (antibody)
  syndrome
primary antiphospholipid syndrome

PA/PS

pulmonary atresia/pulmonary
  stenosis

PAPUFA

physiologically active
  polyunsaturated fatty acid

PAPV

partial anomalous pulmonary veins
peak hyperemic average velocity
positive airway pressure ventilation

Pa-Pv

pulmonary arterial pressure-
  pulmonary venous pressure

PAPVC

partial anomalous pulmonary
  venous connection

PAPVD

partial anomalous pulmonary
  venous drainage

PAPVR

partial anomalous pulmonary
  venous return

PAPW

posterior aspect (of the) pharyngeal
  wall

PAQ

Personal Attributes Questionnaire
Position Analysis Questionnaire (job
  analysis)

PAQLQ

Pediatric Asthma Quality of Life
  Questionnaire

PAR

paraffin
parainfluenza (paramyxovirus)
  vaccine
parallel (*See also* par.)
passive avoidance reaction
perennial allergic rhinitis
pharyngeal acid reflux
photosynthetically active radiation
physiologic aging rate
plain abdominal radiography
plasma appearance rate
platelet aggregate ratio
positive attention received
possible allergic reaction

NOTES

P

PAR *(continued)*
  postanesthesia recovery (room) *(See also* PARR, PARU)
  posterior apical radius
  probable allergic rhinitis
  problem-analysis report
  Proficiency Assessment Report
  protease-activated receptor
  proximal alveolar region
  pulmonary arteriolar resistance
  pulse amplitude ratio

PAr
  polyarteritis *(See also* PA)

Par
  paranoid

par.
  paraffin
  parallel *(See also* PAR)
  paralysis

para
  number of pregnancies producing viable offspring
  paraparesis
  paraplegic
  parathyroid *(See also* PT, PTH)
  parathyroidectomy
  parous (having borne one or more children)
  woman who has given birth

para 0
  nullipara (no child borne)

para 1, I-para
  primipara (first pregnancy) *(See also* P, primip)
  unipara (having borne one child)

para 2, II-para
  bipara (having borne two children)
  secundipara (second pregnancy)

para 3, III-para
  tertipara (third pregnancy)
  tripara (having borne three children)

para 4
  quadripara (having borne four children)

para C, para c
  paracervical

Paraflu
  Parainfluenza

para L
  paralumbar

parapsych
  parapsychology

PARAS
  postauricular and retroauricular scalping

parasit
  parasite

parasitic
parasitology

parasym
  parasympathetic (division of antonomic nervous system) *(See also* PS)

para T
  parathoracic

PARC
  perennial allergic rhinoconjunctivitis

PARD
  platelet aggregation as a risk of diabetes

parent.
  parenteral
  parenterally

PARH
  plasminogen activator-releasing hormone

PARK
  photoastigmatic refractive keratectomy

PAROM
  passive assistance range of motion

parox
  paroxysm
  paroxysmal

PARP
  poly(ADP-ribose)polymerase (autoantibody)

PAR-Q
  Physical Activity Readiness Questionnaire

PARR
  postanesthesia recovery room *(See also* PAR, PARU)

PARS
  Personal Adjustment and Role Skills (Scale)
  Personal and Role Skills
  postanesthesia recovery score

PaRS
  pararectal space

part.
  of a part [L. *partis*]
  partly [L. *partim*]
  parturition

PARU *(See also* PAR, PARR)
  postanesthetic recovery unit

PARV
  Paraná virus

PAS
  p-aminosalicylic acid *(See also* PASA)
  para-aminosalicylate *(See also* PASA)
  paraaminosalicylic acid *(See also* PASA)

Parent Attitude Scale
patient appointments and scheduling
periodic acid-Schiff (stain)
peripheral access system
peripheral anterior synechia
persistent atrial standstill
personality assessment system
phosphatase acid serum
photoacoustic spectroscopy
pneumatic antiembolic stocking
postanesthesia score
posterior airway space
preadmission screening
pregnancy advisory service
premature atrial stimulus
premature auricular systole
progressive accumulated stress
pseudoachievement syndrome
pulmonary arterial stenosis
pulmonary artery stenosis
pulmonary artery systolic

Pa·s

pascal-second (*See also* Pa x s)

PASA

p-aminosalicylic acid (*See also* PAS)
para-aminosalicylic acid (*See also* PAS)
primary acquired sideroblastic anemia
proximal articular set angle

PAS-AB

periodic acid Schiff-Alcian blue (stain)

PASAT

Paced Auditory Serial Addition Test

PaSat

saturation of oxygen in arterial blood

PAS-C

para-aminosalicylic acid crystallized (with ascorbic acid)

PASCC

pseudovascular adenoid squamous cell carcinoma

PASCCL

pseudovascular adenoid squamous cell carcinoma of the lung

PASD

after diastase digestion

PA/S/D

pulmonary artery systolic/diastolic

PASE

Pacemaker Selection in the Elderly

P'ase

alkaline phosphatase (*See also* AKP, ALK-P, alk phos, alk p'tase, ALP, AlPase, AP, KA)

PASES

Performance Assessment of Syntax Elicited and Spontaneous (test)

Pas Ex

passive exercise

PASG

pneumatic antishock garment

PASH

periodic acid-Schiff hematoxylin (stain)
pseudoangiomatous stromal hyperplasia

PASI

psoriasis area sensitivity index
psoriasis area and severity index

PASK

peripheral anterior stent keratopathy

PASM

periodic acid-silver methenamine (stain)

PASP

pulmonary artery systolic pressure

PASS

Pain Anxiety Symptoms Scale
Parent Awareness Skills Survey
Perception of Ability Scale for Students

pass.

here and there [L. *passim*]
passive

PASSA

proximal articular set angle

PAST

periodic acid-Schiff technique

PASVR

pulmonary anomalous superior venous return

PAT

Pain Apperception Test
paroxysmal atrial tachycardia
passive alloimmune thrombocytopenia
patella (*See also* pat.)
patient

NOTES

P

PAT *(continued)*
    percentage of acceleration time
    percutaneous aspiration
      thromboembolectomy
    peripheral arterial tone
    Photo Articulation Test
      (psychology)
    Physical Ability Test
    picric acid turbidity
    platelet aggregation test
    polyamineacetyltransferase
    preadmission (screening and)
      assessment team
    preadmission testing
    Predictive Ability Test (psychology)
    pregnancy at term
    preventive allergy treatment
    prism adaptation test
    prophylactic antibiotic treatment
    psychoacoustic test
    psychoacoustic testing
    pulmonary artery trunk

pat.
    patella (*See also* PAT)
    patent
    paternal origin

PATAV
    Pata virus

PATE
    prolonged acute tissue expansion
    psychodynamic and therapeutic
      education
    pulmonary artery thromboembolism
    pulmonary artery
      thromboendarterectomy

PATH (*See also* path.)
    pathologic
    pathology (*See also* path.)
    pituitary adrenotropic hormone

path.
    pathogen
    pathogenesis
    pathogenic
    pathologic (*See also* PATH)
    pathologist
    pathology (*See also* PATH)

path. fx
    pathologic fracture

PATI
    Penetrating Abdominal Trauma
      Index

PATLC
    Progressive Achievement Tests of
      Listening Comprehension

pat. med.
    patent medicine

PATP
    preadmission testing program

PATS
    payment at time of service

PA-T-SP
    periodic acid-thiocarbohydrazide-
      silver proteinate (stain)

pat. T
    patellar tenderness

PAT/TM
    patient's time

PATV
    Patois virus

PAU
    penetrating aortic ulcer
    penetrating atherosclerotic ulcer

PAV
    partial atrioventricular
    Pavulon (pancuronium bromide)
    percutaneous aortic valvuloplasty
    poikiloderma atrophicans vasculare
    posterior arch vein
    proportional assist ventilation
    proportional assist ventilator

Pa Va Ex
    passive vascular (or venoarterial)
      exercise (a negative pressure)

PAVe
    L-phenylalanine mustard, vinblastine

PA-VF
    pulmonary arteriovenous fistula

PAVM
    pulmonary arteriovenous
      malformation

PAVN
    paraventricular nucleus

PAVNRT
    paroxysmal atrioventricular nodal
      reciprocal tachycardia

PAVSD
    pulmonary atresia with ventricular
      septal defect

PAW
    peak airway pressure
    peripheral airway
    pulmonary artery wedge

Paw
    mean airway pressure

Pawo
    pressure at airway opening

PAWP
    pulmonary artery wedge pressure

PAX
    periapical x-ray

PAX3
    paired box homeotic 3 (gene)

PAX8
    paired box homeotic 8 (gene)

Pa x s
    pascal per second (*See also* Pa·s)

PB
    barometric pressure
    British Pharmacopeia
        [*Pharmacopoeia Britannica*] (*See
        also* BP)
    pancreaticobiliary
    paraffin bath
    Paul-Bunnell (antibody, test) (*See
        also* PBT)
    pentobarbital
    perineal body
    periodic breathing
    peripheral blood
    peroneus brevis
    phenobarbital
    phenylbutyrate
    phonetically balanced (word lists)
    piggyback
    pinch biopsy
    pinealoblastoma
    piperonyl butoxide
    polymyxin B
    posterior baffle
    powder bed
    powder board
    power building
    premature beat
    Presbyterian
    pressure balanced
    pressure breathing
    protein binding
    protein bound
    pudendal block
    punch biopsy
    pyridostigmine bromide (Mestinon)
PB%
    phonetically balanced percentage (of
        word lists)
P&B
    pain and burning
    phenobarbital and belladonna
P_B
    barometric pressure
Pb
    lead [L. *plumbum*] (*See also*
        plumb.)
    phenobarbital
    presbyopia
    probenecid
PBA
    percutaneous bladder aspiration
    percutaneous breathing assister

    polyclonal B-cell activity
    pressure breathing assister
    prolactin-binding assay
    prune belly anomaly
    pulpobuccoaxial
P_BA
    brachial arterial pressure
PBAL
    protected bronchoalveolar lavage
P-BAP
    Behavioral Assessment of Pain
        Questionnaire
PBB
    polybromated biphenyl
    polybrominated biphenyl
Pb-B
    lead level in blood
PBC
    perfusion balloon catheter
    periodic breathing cycle
    peripheral blood cell
    plasma bilirubin concentration
    point of basal convergence
    prebed care
    pregnancy and birth complication
    primary biliary cirrhosis
    progestin-binding complement
    protected brush catheter
PBCL
    parafollicular B-cell lymphoma
PBD
    percutaneous biliary drainage
    postburn day
    proliferating bile ductules
    proliferative breast disease
PBE
    partial breech extraction
    power building exercise
PBF
    percent body fat
    peripheral blood flow
    phosphate-buffered formalin
    placental blood flow
    pulmonary blood flow (*See also*
        Qp)
PB-Fe
    protein-bound iron
PBFS
    penile blood flow study
PBG
    Penassay broth plus glucose
    porphobilinogen

NOTES

P

PBG-D
porphobilinogen deaminase
PBGM
Penassay broth plus glucose plus menadione
PBG-S
porphobilinogen synthase
PBH
pulling-boat hands
PBHA
porous block hydroxyapatite
PBI
parental bonding instrument
partial bony impaction
penile-brachial index
phenformin
protein-bound iodine
PbI
lead intoxication
PBK
Phonetically Balanced Kindergarten
phosphorylase *b* kinase
pseudophakic bullous keratopathy
PBL
peripheral blood leukocyte
peripheral blood lymphocyte
primary bone lymphoma
primary brain lymphoma
PBLC
premature birth live child
PBLI
premature birth live infant
PBLT
peripheral blood lymphocyte transformation
PBM
peripheral basement membrane
peripheral blood monocyte
peripheral blood mononuclear (cell) (*See also* PBMC)
PBMC
peripheral blood mononuclear cell (*See also* PBM)
PBMNC
peripheral blood mononuclear cell
PBMTx
porcine bone marrow transplantation
PBMV
pulmonary blood mixing volume
PBN
paralytic brachial neuritis
peripheral benign neoplasm
polymyxin B sulfate, bacitracin, and neomycin
PBNA
partial body neutron activation
PB:ND
problem: nursing diagnosis

PBNS
percutaneous bladder neck stabilization
percutaneous bladder neck suspension
PBO
penicillin in beeswax and oil
placebo (*See also* P, PL, PLBO, PCB, PLB)
PbO
lead monoxide
PBP
peak blood pressure
penicillin-binding protein
percutaneous balloon pericardiotomy
phantom breast pain
porphyrin biosynthetic pathway
progressive bulbar palsy
prostate-binding protein
protein-bound polysaccharide
pseudobulbar palsy
purified *Brucella* protein
PBPC
peripheral blood progenitor cell
PBPCT
peripheral blood progenitor cell transplant
PBPI
penile-brachial pressure index
penile-brachial pulse index
PBQ
phenylbenzoquinone
Preschool Behavior Questionnaire
PBR
peripheral-type benzodiazepine receptor
PBRT
phonetically balanced rhyme test
PBRVO
peripheral branch retinal vein occlusion
PBS
Pediatric Behavior Scale
peripheral-blood smear
peroneus brevis split
phenobarbital sodium
phosphate-buffered saline
phosphate-buffered sodium
polybrominated salicylanilide
prune belly syndrome
pulmonary branch stenosis
PBSC
penicillin, bacitracin, streptomycin, caprylate
peripheral blood stem cell
PBSCR
peripheral blood stem cell reserve

PBSCT
>peripheral blood stem cell transplantation

PBSP
>prognostically bad signs during pregnancy

PBT
>Paul Bunnell test (*See also* PB)
>phenacetin breath test
>primary brain tumor
>profile-based therapy

PBT4, PBT$_4$
>protein-bound thyroxine

PBTE
>percutaneous transhepatic liver biopsy with tract embolization

PbtO2
>brain tissue partial pressure of oxygen

PBV
>percutaneous balloon valvuloplasty
>predicted blood volume
>pulmonary balloon valvuloplasty
>pulmonary blood volume

PbV
>*Penicillium brevicompactum* virus

PBVI
>pulmonary blood volume index

PBW
>posterior bite wing

PB word
>phonetically balanced word

PBZ
>phenoxybenzamine
>phenylbutazone
>Pyribenzamine (tripelennamine)

PC
>avoirdupois weight [L. *pondus civile*]
>packed cells
>palmitoyl carnitine
>pancreatic cancer
>paper chromatography
>parent cell
>parent to child
>particulate component
>partition coefficient
>pathologic consultation
>peak clipping
>pelvic cramp
>penicillin
>pentose cycle

peritoneal cell
pharmacology
pheochromocytoma (*See also* PCC, pheo)
phosphate cycle
phosphatidylcholine (lecithin)
phosphocreatine
phosphorylcholine
photocoagulation
photoconductive
phrase construction
picryl chloride
picture completion
pill counter
piriform cortex
placebo-controlled (study)
plasma cell
plasma concentration
plasma cortisol
plasma cytoma
platelet concentrate
platelet count
Pneumocystis carinii
pneumotaxic center
politically correct
polycentric
polyposis coli
poor condition
popliteal cyst
portacaval (shunt)
portal cirrhosis
postcoital
posterior cervical
posterior chamber
posterior circulation
posterior circumflex artery
posterior column
posterior commissure
posterior cortex
precordial
premature contractions
prepiriform cortex
present complaint
pressure control
primary cleavage
primary closure
principal cell
printed circuit
procollagen
producing cell
productive cough
professional corporation

NOTES

PC *(continued)*
proliferative capacity
proprotein convertase
prostatic carcinoma
provisional cortex
proximal colon
pseudocyst
Psychodevelopment Checklist
pubococcygeus (muscle) (*See also* PCG)
pulmonary capillary
pulmonic closure
pulp canal
Purkinje cell
pyloric canal
pyruvate carboxylase

P-C
phlogistic corticoid

PC1
prohormone convertase 1

PC2
prohormone convertase 2

PC3
prohormone convertase 3

P&C
prism and (alternative) cover test (crossover test, screen and cover test in ophthalmology)
prism and cover test

p.c.
after a meal [L. *post cibum*]
post cibum (after meals)

pc
parsec
percent

pc1
platelet count pretransfusion

pc2
platelet count posttransfusion

PCA
pancreatic carcinoma
para-chloramphetamine
parenteral-controlled analgesia
parietal cell antibody
passive cutaneous anaphylaxis
patient care aide
patient care assistant
patient-controlled analgesia
patient-controlled analgesic
patient-controlled anesthesia
penicillamine
perchloric acid
percutaneous carotid arteriogram
percutaneous coronary angioplasty
personal care attendant
phenylcarboxylic acid
photocontact allergic
plasma catecholamine concentration
porous coated anatomic (prosthesis)
portacaval anastomosis
postcardiac arrest
postciliary artery
postconceptional age
posterior cerebral artery
posterior communicating aneurysm
posterior communicating artery
posterior cricoarytenoid
precoronary care area
principal components analysis
procainamide
procoagulant activity
prostate cancer
prostatic carcinoma
protected catheter aspirate
pyrrolidone carboxylic acid

PcA
prostatic adenocarcinoma

pCa
prostate cancer

PCAR
presumed circle area ratio

PCAS
Psychotherapy Competence Assessment Schedule

PCASSO
patient-centered access to secure systems online

PCAV
Pacora virus

PCAVC
persistent complete atrioventricular canal

PCB
pancuronium bromide
pancuronium (Pavulon)
paracervical block
placebo (*See also* P, PBO, PL, PLBO, PLB)
polychlorinated biphenyl
polychlorobiphenyl
portacaval bypass
postcoital bleeding
prepared childbirth
protected catheter brushing
proximal communicating branch
Pseudomonas cepacia bacteremia

PcB, Pcb
near point of convergence to intercentral baseline [L. *punctum convergens basalis*]

PCBH
personal care boarding home

PCBM
particulate cancellous bone and marrow

PCBMN
palmar cutaneous branch of the median nerve

PC-BMP
phosphorylcholine-binding myeloma protein

PCBS
percutaneous cardiopulmonary bypass support

PCBUN
palmar cutaneous branch of the ulnar nerve

PCC
Pasteur Culture Collection
patient care coordinator
percutaneous cecostomy
percutaneous cervical cordotomy
peripheral cholangiocarcinoma
personal care clinic
petrous carotid canal
pheochromocytoma (*See also* pheo, PC)
phosphate carrier compound
plasma catecholamine concentration
pneumatosis cystoides coli
postcoital contraception
posterior central curve
precipitated calcium carbonate
precoronary care
premature chromosome condensation
primary care clinic
progressive cardiac care
propagating clustered contraction
prothrombin complex concentration

PCc
periscopic concave

PCCC
pediatric critical care center

PCCI
penetrating craniocerebral injuries

PCCL
percutaneous cholecystolithotomy

PCCM
primary care case management

PCCP
percutaneous cord cyst puncture

PCC-R
Percentage of Consonants Correct-Revised

PCCS
parent-child communication schedule

PCCU
post-coronary care unit

PCD
pacer-cardioverter defibrillator
papillary collecting duct
paroxysmal cerebral dysrhythmia
peritoneal dialysis catheter
phosphate-citrate-dextrose
plasma cell dyscrasia
pneumatic compression device
polycystic disease
posterior corneal deposit
postmortem cesarean delivery
postparacentesis circulatory dysfunction
primary ciliary dyskinesia
programmable cardioverter-defibrillator
programmed cell death
prolonged contractile duration
pulmonary clearance delay

PCDAI
Paediatric Crohn Disease Activity Index (British)
Pediatric Crohn Disease Activity Index

PCDC
plasma clot diffusion chamber

PCDF
polychlorinated dibenzofuran

PCDUS
plasma cell dyscrasia of unknown significance

PCE
physical capacity evaluation
potentially compensable event
pseudocholinesterase (*See also* PCHE)
pseudophakic corneal edema
pulmocutaneous exchange
Smith physical capacities evaluation

PCEA
patient-controlled epidural analgesia (*See also* PEA)

pCEA
polyclonal carcinoembryonic antigen

PCEC
purified chick embryo cell (culture)

P-cell
Purkinje cell

PCF
partial conjunctival flap

NOTES

P

PCF *(continued)*
>peak cough flow
>peripheral circulatory failure
>pharyngoconjunctival fever
>posterior cranial fossa
>prothrombin conversion factor

pcf
>pound per cubic foot

PCFIA
>particle concentration fluorescence immunoassay

PCFT
>platelet complement fixation test

Pc-fV
>*Penicillium cyaneo-fulvum* virus

PCG
>paracervical ganglion
>phonocardiogram
>Planning Career Goals (psychologic test)
>plasma cell granuloma
>pneumocardiogram
>primate chorionic gonadotropin
>pubococcygeus (muscle) (*See also* PC)

PCGG
>percutaneous coagulation of gasserian ganglion

PCGLV
>poorly contractile globular left ventricle

PCH
>paroxysmal cold hemoglobinuria
>periocular capillary hemangioma
>personal care home
>polycyclic hydrocarbon
>pulmonary capillary hemangiomatosis
>pulp chamber

PCHE
>pseudocholinesterase (*See also* PCE)

PCHI
>permanent childhood hearing impairment

PCHL
>permanent childhood hearing loss

PC&HS
>after meals and at bedtime

PCI
>percutaneous coronary intervention
>pneumatosis cystoides intestinalis
>posterior curve intermediate (cornea)
>Premarital Communication Inventory
>prophylactic brain irradiation
>prophylactic cranial irradiation
>prothrombin consumption index

PCi, pCi
>picocurie

PCINA
>patient-controlled intranasal analgesia

PCIOL, PC-IOL
>posterior chamber intraocular lens

PCIRF
>radiologic contrast-induced renal failure

PCIRV, PC-IRV
>pressure control inverse ratio ventilation
>pressure-controlled inverse ratio ventilation

PCIS
>Patient Care Information System
>postcardiac injury syndrome

PCK
>polycystic kidney

PCKD
>polycystic kidney disease

PCL
>pacing cycle length
>persistent corpus luteum
>plasma cell leukemia
>posterior chamber lens
>posterior collagenous layer
>posterior cruciate ligament
>proximal collateral ligament

PCLBCL
>primary cutaneous large B-cell lymphoma

PCLC
>Paneth cell-like change

PCLD
>polycystic liver disease (*See also* PLD)

PCLI
>plasma cell labeling index
>posterior chamber lens implant

P closure
>plastic closure

PCLR
>paid claims loss ratio

PCM
>paracoccidioidomycosis
>pericellular matrix
>primary cutaneous melanoma
>protein-calorie malnutrition
>protein carboxymethylase
>pubococcygeal muscle
>pulse code modulation

PCMB, p-CMB
>p-chloromercuribenzoate

PCMBSA
>*para*-chloromercuribenzine sulfonic acid

PCMC
Primary Children's Medical Center

PCMF
perceptual cognitive motor function

PC-MRI
phase-contrast magnetic resonance imaging

PCMT
pacemaker circus-movement tachycardia

PCMX
parachlorometaxylenol
para–chloro-*m*-xylenol
p-chloro-meta-xylenol

PCN
penicillin (*See also* P, PEN, Pen, pen., PN, PNC)
percutaneous nephrolithotomy
percutaneous nephrostomy
pregnenolone carbonitril
primary care network
primary care nursing

PCNA
proliferating cell nuclear antigen

PCNA-LI
PCNA-labeling index

PCNB
pentachloronitrobenzene

PCNHL
primary cerebral non-Hodgkin lymphoma

PCNL
percutaneous nephrolithotomy (*See also* PNL)
percutaneous nephrolithotripsy
percutaneous nephrostolithotomy

PCNS
primary central nervous system

PCNs
posterior cervical nodes

PCNSL
primary central nervous system lymphoma

PCNT
percutaneous nephrostomy tube

PCNV
postchemotherapy nausea and vomiting

PCO
patient complains of
polycystic ovary

posterior capsular opacification
posterior capsule opacification
predicted cardiac output
procyanidol oligomer
procytoxid

PCO$_2$, PCO2, P$_{CO2}$, Pco2
carbon dioxide pressure
carbon dioxide pressure
carbon monoxide pressure or tension
partial pressure of carbon dioxide
pressure of carbon dioxide
pressure of CO$_2$

PCoA
posterior communicating artery (*See also* PCom)

PCOD
polycystic ovarian disease
polycystic ovary disease

PCOE
prescriber (physician) computer order entry

PCom
posterior communicating artery (*See also* PCoA)

PComA
posterior communicating artery

PCOS
polycystic ovarian syndrome
polycystic ovary syndrome (*See also* POS)

PCP
parachlorophenate
patient care plan
pentachlorophenol
peripheral coronary pressure
persistent cough and phlegm
phencyclidine
phencyclidine hydrochloride
pneumocystic pneumonia
Pneumocystis carinii pneumonia
postoperative constrictive pericarditis
primary care person
primary care physician
primary care provider
prochlorperazine
procollagen peptide
pulmonary capillary pressure
pulse cytophotometry

PCPA
para-chlorophenylalanine

NOTES

P

PCPB
>percutaneous cardiopulmonary
>bypass
>procarboxypeptidase B

PCPL
>pulmonary capillary protein leakage

pcpn
>precipitation (*See also* pcpt, precip)

PCPS
>percutaneous cardiopulmonary
>support
>peroral cholangiopancreatoscopy
>phosphatidylcholine-
>phosphatidylserine

pcpt
>perception
>precipitate
>precipitation (*See also* pcpn, precip)

PCQ
>Pain Coping Questionnaire

PCR
>pathologically confirmed complete
>remission
>patient care report
>patient contact record
>percutaneous coronary
>revascularization
>phosphocreatine
>plasma clearance rate
>polymerase chain reaction
>probable causal relationship
>progressive condylar resorption
>protein catabolic rate
>reverse transcription polymerase
>chain reaction

PCr
>phosphocreatine

PCRA
>percutaneous coronary rotational
>atherectomy
>pure red-cell aplasia

PCRC
>primary colorectal cancer

PCR-ISH
>polymerase chain reaction in situ
>hybridization

PCR/PSA
>polymerase chain reaction analysis
>of prostate-specific antigen

PCR-RFLP
>polymerase chain reaction-restriction
>fragment length polymorphism

PCR-SSCP
>polymerase chain reaction–single-
>strand conformation polymorphism

PCS
>palliative care service
>patient care system
>patient-controlled sedation
>patterns of care study
>pelvic congestion syndrome
>peroral cholangioscopy
>personal care service
>pharmacogenic confusional
>syndrome
>Physical Component Summary
>portable cervical spine
>portacaval shunt
>postcardiac surgery
>postcardiotomy syndrome
>postcholecystectomy syndrome
>postconcussion syndrome
>precordial stethoscope
>primary cancer site
>primary cesarean section
>Priority Counseling Survey
>proportional counter spectrometry
>proximal coronary
>proximal coronary sinus
>pseudotumor cerebri syndrome
>pulp canal sealer

P c/s
>primary cesarean section

pcs
>preconscious

PCSD
>prone cranial support device

PCSM
>percutaneous stone manipulation

PCT
>patient care technician
>Physiognomic Cue Test
>(psychology)
>plasma clotting time
>plasmacrit test (for syphilis)
>plasmacytoma
>platelet hematocrit
>polychlorinated triphenyl
>porcine calcitonin
>porphyria cutanea tarda
>portacaval transportation
>portacaval transposition
>positron computed tomography
>postcoital test
>posterior chest tube
>primary chemotherapy
>procalcitonin
>progestin challenge test
>prothrombin consumption time
>proximal convoluted tubule
>pulmonary care team

pct
>percent

PCTA
>percutaneous coronary transluminal
>angioplasty

PC/TC
power cut/tungsten carbide

PCTCL
percutaneous transhepatic cholecystolithotomy

PCU

pain control unit
palliative care unit
patient care unit
primary care unit
progressive care unit
protective care unit
protein-calorie undernutrition
pulmonary care unit

p cut
percutaneous

PCV

packed cell volume
parietal cell vagotomy
polycythemia vera (*See also* PV)
postcapillary venule
pressure-controlled ventilation
pressure control ventilation

PCV7
pneumococcal 7-valent conjugate vaccine

PcV
Penicillium chrysogenum virus

PCVC
percutaneous central venous catheter

PCVD
pulmonary collagen vascular disease

PCV-M
polycythemia vera (with myeloid) metaplasia

PCW

pulmonary capillary wedge (pressure) (*See also* PCWP)
purified cell walls

PCWP
pulmonary capillary wedge pressure (*See also* PCW)

PCX
paracervical

PCx
periscopic convex

PCXR
portable chest radiograph
portable chest x-ray

PCZ
prochlorperazine

PD

(inter)pupillary distance
Paget disease
pancreas divisum
pancreatic duct
pancreaticoduodenectomy
pancreatoduodenectomy
panic disorder
papilla diameter
paralyzing dose
Parkinson disease
parkinsonian dementia
paroxysmal discharge
pars distalis (pituitary)
patent ductus
patient day
patient demonstration
pediatric dose
pediatrics (*See also* paed, PED, ped, Peds)
percutaneous diskectomy
percutaneous drain
peritoneal dialysis
personality disorder
pharmacodynamics
phenyldichlorarsine
phenyldichloroarsine
phosphate dehydrogenase
photosensitivity dermatitis
Pick disease
plasma defect
pocket depth (dental)
poorly differentiated
Porak-Durante (syndrome)
porphobilinogen deaminase
posterior division
postnasal drainage
postural drainage
potential difference
present disease
pressor dose
pressure dressing
primary dendrite
prism diopter (*See also* p.d.)
probing depth
problem drinker
process diagnostic
progression (of) disease
prostatodynia
protein degradation
protein deprived
protein diet

NOTES

P

PD *(continued)*
> provocation dose
> psychopathic deviate
> psychotic dementia
> psychotic depression
> pulmonary disease (*See also* PUD, PuD)
> pulpodistal
> pulse duration
> pupillary distance
> pure dysarthria
> pyloric dilator

2PD
> two-point discrimination

P/D, p/d
> packs per day (cigarettes) (*See also* PPD)

P(D+)
> probability of having disease

P(D−)
> probability of not having disease

Pd
> palladium

pd
> papilla diameter
> period

p.d.
> by the day [L. *per diem*]
> prism diopter (*See also* PD)

PD$_{50}$
> median paralyzing dose

PDA
> parenteral drug abuser
> patent ductus arteriosus
> patient distress alarm
> pediatric allergy
> personal digital assistant
> plantar digital artery
> polymorphic delta activity
> poorly differentiated adenocarcinoma
> posterior descending (coronary) artery
> predialyzed human albumin
> property damage accident
> pulmonary disease anemia

PDAB
> *para*-dimethylaminobenzaldehyde

PDAF
> platelet-derived angiogenesis factor

PDAI
> Perianal Crohn Disease Activity Index

PDAP
> peritoneal dialysis-associated peritonitis

PDB
> Paget disease of bone

> *para*-dichlorobenzene (*See also* PDCB)
> phosphorus-dissolving bacteria
> preperitoneal distention balloon
> preventive dental (health) behavior

PDC
> pancreatic duct cell carcinoma
> parkinsonism-dementia complex
> patient denies complaints
> pediatric cardiology
> pentadecylcatechol
> peritoneal dialysis catheter
> physical dependence capacity
> plasma digoxin concentration
> plasma disappearance curve
> poorly differentiated carcinoma
> postdecapitation convulsion
> preliminary diagnostic clinic
> private diagnostic clinic
> property damage collision (crash)
> pyrindinol carbamate
> pyruvate dehydrogenase complex

PD&C
> postural drainage and clapping

PdC
> pediatric cardiology

PDCA
> Plan-Do-Check-Act (process improvement)

PDCB
> *para*-dichlorobenzene (*See also* PDB)

PDCD
> primary degenerative cerebral disease

PD-CSE
> pulsed Doppler cross-sectional echocardiography

PDD
> percentage depth dose
> pervasive developmental disorder
> premenstrual dysphoric disorder
> primary degenerative dementia
> pyridoxine-deficient diet

PDDAT
> primary degenerative dementia of Alzheimer type

PDDB
> phenododecinium bromide

PDD-NOS
> pervasive developmental disorder not otherwise specified

PDE
> paroxysmal dyspnea on exertion
> peritoneal dialysis effluent
> personality disorder examination
> phosphodiesterase
> phosphodiesterase (inhibitor)

progressive dialysis encephalopathy
pulsed Doppler echocardiography

PDE5, PDE 5
cyclic guanosine monophosphate-
specific phosphodiesterase 5
phosphodiesterase 5
phosphodiesterase type 5

PdE
pediatric endocrinology

PD-ECGF
platelet-derived endothelial cell
growth factor

PDEGF
platelet-derived epidermal growth
factor

PDE-1
phosphodiesterase inhibitor

PDE3I
phosphodiesterase III inhibition

PDE5I
phosphodiesterase type 5 inhibitor

PDET
poorly differentiated embryonal cell
tumor

PDF
peritoneal dialysis fluid
Portable Document Format
probability density function

PDFC
premature dead female child

PDG
parkinsonism dementia (complex of)
Guam
phosphate-dependent glutaminase
phosphogluconate dehydrogenase

PDGA
pteroyldiglutamic acid

PDGF
platelet-derived growth factor

PDGF-A
platelet-derived growth factor A

PDGS
partial form of DiGeorge syndrome

PDGXT
predischarge graded exercise test

PDH
past dental history
phosphate dehydrogenase
progressive disseminated
histoplasmosis
pyruvate dehydrogenase

PDHC
pyruvate dehydrogenase complex
(deficiency)

PdHO
pediatric hematology-oncology

PDHRF
platelet-derived histamine-releasing
factor

PDI
Pain Disability Index
Periodontal Disease Index
phasic detrusor instability
phosphodiesterase inhibitor
plan-do integration
power Doppler imaging
protein disulfide isomerase
psychiatric diagnostic interview
Psychomotor Development Index

Pdi
transdiaphragmatic pressure

PDIE
phosphodiesterase

PDIg
platelet-directed immunglobulin

PDIGC
patient dismissed in good condition

P-diol
pregnanediol

Pdisniff
maximal sniff-induced
transdiaphragmatic pressure

PDK
3-phosphoinositide-dependent protein
kinase

PDL
periodontal ligament
polycystic disease of liver
poorly differentiated lymphocyte
population doubling level
postures of daily living
primary dysfunctional labor
progressively diffused
leukoencephalopathy
pulsed-dye laser
pulsed-dye laser (therapy)

Pdl
pudendal

pdl
poundal (force of acceleration)

PDLC
poorly differentiated lung cancer

NOTES

P

601

PDLD
poorly differentiated lymphocytic-diffuse

PDLL
poorly differentiated lymphocytic lymphoma

PDLN
poorly differentiated (lymphocytic) lymphoma-nodular

PDLP
predigested liquid protein

PDLS
physical daily living skills

PDM
polydimethylsiloxane
polymyositis and dermatomyositis
predentin matrix

PDMC
premature dead male child

PDMEA
phosphoryldimethylethanolamine

PDMS
Patient Data Management Systems
Peabody Developmental Motor Scale
pharmacokinetic drug-monitoring service
polydimethylsiloxane

PDN
Paget disease of the nipple
prednisone (*See also* P, PRED)
private day nurse
private duty nurse
prosthetic disk nucleus

PdNEO
pediatric neonatology

PdNEP
pediatric nephrology

PDP
pancreatic duct pressure
papular dermatitis of pregnancy
passive-dependent personality
pattern disruption point
peak diastolic pressure
piperidinopyrimidine
platelet-depleted plasma
positive distending pressure
primer-dependent deoxynucleic acid polymerase
product development protocol

PD&P
postural drainage and percussion

PDPD
prolonged-dwell peritoneal dialysis

PDPH
postdural puncture headache

PDPI
primer-dependent deoxynucleic acid polymerase index

PDPV
postural drainage, percussion and vibration

PDQ
parental development questionnaire
Personality Diagnostic Questionnaire
Physician Data Query
Premenstrual Distress Questionnaire
Prescreening Development Questionnaire
pretty damn quick (slang)
protocol data query

PDQ-R
Personality Diagnostic Questionnaire-Revised

PDR
pandevelopmental retardation
patients' dining room
pediatric radiology
peripheral diabetic retinopathy
Physician's Desk Reference
pleiotropic drug resistance
postdelivery room
primary drug resistance
proliferative diabetic retinopathy
prospective drug review
pulsed dose rate

PdR
pediatric radiology

pdr
powder (*See also* powd, pwd)

PDRB
Permanent Disability Rating Board

PDRc̄VH
proliferative diabetic retinopathy with vitreous hemorrhage

PDRP
proliferative diabetic retinopathy

PDS
pain-dysfunction syndrome
pancreatic duct sphincter
paroxysmal depolarization shift
paroxysmal depolarizing shift
patient data system
pediatric surgery (*See also* PdS, PS)
Pendred syndrome
peritoneal dialysis system
pigment dispersion syndrome
polydioxanone
polydioxanone suture
predialyzed (human) serum
primary dependence study
Progressive Deterioration Scale

PdS

 pediatric surgery (*See also* PDS, PS)

 psychiatric deviate, subtle

PDT

 percutaneous dilational tracheostomy

 percutaneous dilational tracheotomy

 phenyldimethyltriazine

 photodynamic therapy

 population doubling time

 postdisaster trauma

PDTA

 propanoldiaminotetraacetic acid

PDTC

 pyrrolidine dithiocarbamate

PDU

 pulsed Doppler ultrasonography

PDUF

 pulsed Doppler ultrasonic flowmeter

PDUFA

 Prescription Drug User Fee Act (1992)

PDUR

 Predischarge Utilization Review

PDV

 peak diastolic velocity

PDW

 platelet distribution width

PDWHF

 platelet-derived wound healing factor

PDx

 principal diagnosis

pDXA

 peripheral dual-energy x-ray absorptiometry

PE

 dipalmitoyl phosphatidylethanolamine

 expiratory pressure (*See also* P_E)

 pancreatic extract

 paper electrophoresis

 parallel elastic (component of muscle)

 partial epilepsy

 pedal edema

 Pel-Ebstein (disease)

 pelvic examination

 penile erection

 percutaneous endoscopic

 pericardial effusion

 peritoneal exudate

 phakoemulsification

 pharyngoesophageal

 phenylephrine

 phosphatidylethanolamine

 photographic effect

 phycoerythrin

 physical education (*See also* PED, P Ed, Phys Ed)

 physical evaluation

 physical examination (*See also* PEx, PX, Px)

 physical exercise

 physiologic ecology

 pigmented epithelium

 plasma exchange

 plating efficiency

 pleiotrophic functional defect

 pleural effusion

 point of entry

 polyethylene

 polynuclear eosinophil

 portal embolization

 potential energy

 powdered extract

 preeclampsia

 preexcitation

 present examination

 pressure equalization

 prior to exposure

 probable error

 probe excision

 protein excretion

 Pseudomonas exotoxin

 pulmonary edema

 pulmonary embolism

 pulmonary embolus

 pulmonary emphysema

 pyramidal eminence

 pyroelectric

 pyrogenic exotoxin

P-E

 portal (venous and) enteric (drainage technique)

PE2

 secondary plating efficiency

PE-3

 phosphatidylinositol

PE24

 Preemie Enfamil 24

P_E

 expiratory pressure (*See also* PE)

Pe

 Peclet number

NOTES

P

Pe *(continued)*
    perylene
    pregnenolone
    pressure on expiration

pe
    pericardium channel (acupuncture)

PEA
    patient-controlled epidural analgesia
      (*See also* PCEA)
    pelvic examination under anesthesia
    phenylethyl alcohol (agar)
    phenylethylamine
    polysaccharide egg antigen
    preemptive analgesia
    pulseless electrical activity

PE↓A
    pelvic examination under anesthesia
      (*See also* PEA)

PEACH
    Preschool Evaluation and
    Assessment for Children with
    Handicaps

PEAO
    phenylethylamine oxidase

PEAP
    positive end-airway pressure

PEAQ
    Personal Experience and Attitude
    Questionnaire

PEARL
    physiologic endometrial
    ablation/resection loop

PEBB
    percutaneous excisional breast
    biopsy

PEBD
    partial external biliary diversion

PEBG
    phenethylbiguanide

PEC
    parallel elastic component
    patient evaluation center
    pectoralis
    peduncle of cerebrum
    peritoneal exudate cell
    perivascular epithelioid cell
    politico-economic-conservatism
    protein-induced eosinophilic colitis
    pulmonary ejection click
    pyrogenic exotoxin C

PECAM-1
    platelet endothelial cell adhesion
    molecule-1

PECCE
    planned extracapsular cataract
    extraction

PECHO, Pecho
    prostatic echogram

PECHR
    peripheral exudative choroidal
    hemorrhagic retinopathy

PECO$_2$
    mixed expired carbon dioxide
    tension

PECT
    positron emission computed
    tomography

PED
    paroxysmal exertion-induced
    dyskinesia
    pediatric emergency department
    pediatrics (*See also* paed, PD, ped,
    Peds)
    peduncle (cerebral)
    percutaneous external drainage
    pharyngoesophageal diverticulum
    pigment epithelial detachment
    pollution and environmental
    degradation
    postentry day
    postexertional dyspnea
    prenatally exposed to drugs

P Ed
    physical education (*See also* PE,
    Phys Ed)

ped
    pedestrian
    pediatrics (*See also* paed, PD,
    PED, Peds)

PEDD
    proton-electron dipole-dipole

ped ed
    pedal edema

PEDG
    phenylethyldiguanide

PEDI
    Pediatric Evaluation of Disability
    Inventory

PEDI-DEG
    pediatric deglycerolized red blood
    cells

PED/MV
    pedestrian hit by motor vehicle

PeDS
    Pediatric Drug Surveillance

Peds
    pediatrics (*See also* paed, PD,
    PED, ped)

PEE
    parallel elastic element
    punctate epithelial erosion

PEEP
    peak end-expiratory pressure
    positive end-expiratory pressure

PEEP/CPAP

positive end-expiratory pressure/continuous positive airway pressure

PEEPi

intrinsic positive end-expiratory pressure

PEER

Pediatric Examination of Educational Readiness
pronation-eversion-external rotation

PEET

Pediatric Extended Examination at Three

PEEX

Pediatric Early Elemental Examination

PEF

peak expiratory flow (rate) (*See also* PEFR)
pharyngoepiglottic fold
Psychiatric Evaluation Form
pulmonary edema fluid

%PEF

percent predicted peak expiratory flow

PEFR

peak expiratory flow rate (*See also* PEF)
peak flowmeter

PEFSR

partial expiratory flow-static recoil (curve)

PEFT

peak expiratory flow time

PEFV

partial expiratory flow volume

PEG

Patient Evaluation Grid
pegylated
percutaneous endoluminal gastrostomy
percutaneous endoscopic gastrostomy
pericyte edema generation
pneumoencephalogram
pneumonencephalography
polyethylene glycol

PEG-ADA

pegademase bovine
polyethylene glycol-adenosine deaminase

polyethylene glycol-modified adenosine deaminase

PEG-ELS

polyethylene glycol electrolyte lavage solution

PEGG

Parent Education and Guidance Group

PEG-IL-2

polyethylene glycol-modified interleukin-2

PEG-J

percutaneous endoscopic gastrojejunostomy

PEG-JET

percutaneous endoscopic gastrostomy and jejunal extension tube
percutaneous endoscopic gastrostomy with jejunal extension tube

PEG-L-ASP, PEG-*l*-ASP

polyethylene glycol-conjugated *l*-asparaginase

PEG-LES

polyethylene glycol electrolyte lavage solution

PEG-SOD

polyethylene glycol-conjugated superoxide dismutase (pegorgotein)

PEH

palmoplantar eccrine hidradenitis
postexercise hypotension

PEHO

progressive encephalopathy, edema, hypsarrhythmia, optic atrophy

PEI

percutaneous ethanol injection
phosphate excretion index
phosphorus excretion index
physical efficiency index
polyethylenimine
postexercise index

PEIT

percutaneous ethanol injection therapy

PEITC

phenethyl isothiocyanate

PEJ

percutaneous endoscopic jejunostomy

PEK

punctate epithelial keratopathy

NOTES

P

PEL
>peritoneal exudate lymphocyte
>permissible exposure limit
>primary effusion lymphoma

Pel
>elastic recoil pressure of lung
>lung elastic recoil pressure

PELA
>peripheral excimer laser angioplasty

PELCA
>percutaneous excimer laser coronary angioplasty

PELD
>percutaneous endoscopic lumbar diskectomy

PELISA
>paper enzyme-linked immunosorbent assay

PELs
>permissible exposure limits

PELV
>pelvimetry

Pel-V
>elastic pressure-volume

PEM
>pediatric emergency medicine
>peritoneal exudate macrophage
>polymorphic epithelial mucin
>precordial electrocardiographic mapping
>prescription event monitoring
>primary enrichment medium
>probable error of measurement
>protein-energy malnutrition
>pulmonary endothelial membrane

PEMA
>phenylethylmalonamide

P$_{Emax}$
>maximal expiratory mouth pressure

PEMF
>pulsating electromagnetic field
>pulsed electromagnetic field

PEMS
>physical, emotional, mental, and safety
>pulsed electromagnetic stimulator

PEN
>palisaded encapsulated neuroma
>pancreatic endocrine neoplasm
>parenteral and enteral nutrition
>Pharmacy Equivalent Name

Pen, pen.
>penicillin (*See also* P, PCN, PEN, PN, PNC)

pen.
>penetrating

PENG
>photoelectronystagmography

PENL
>primary extranodal lymphoma

PENS
>percutaneous electrical nerve stimulation
>percutaneous epidural nerve stimulator
>percutaneous epidural neurostimulator

Pent
>pentothal

PEO
>progressive external ophthalmoparesis
>progressive external ophthalmoplegia

PEP
>patient education program
>peptidase
>performance evaluation procedure
>pharmacologic erection program
>phosphoenolpyruvate
>polyestradiol phosphate
>positive expiratory pressure
>postencephalitic parkinsonism
>postexposure prevention/postexposure prophylaxis
>postexposure prophylaxis
>preejection period
>progestogen-dependent endometrial protein
>protein electrophoresis
>Psychiatric Evaluation Profile
>Psychoeducational Profile
>Psycho-Epistemological Profile

Pep
>peptidase

PEPA
>peptidase A
>protected environment (units and) prophylactic antibiotics

PEPAP
>analog of meperidine

PEPC
>peptidase C

PEPc
>corrected preejection period

PEPCK, PEPK
>phosphoenolpyruvate carboxykinase

PEPD
>peptidase D

PEPI
>preejection period index

PEP/LVET
>preejection period/left ventricular ejection time

PEPP
>payment error prevention program
>positive expiratory pressure plateau

PEPR
> precision encoder and pattern recognizer

PEPS
> peptidase S
> peroral electronic pancreatoscope

PER
> peak ejection rate
> pediatric emergency room
> period
> periodic evaluation record
> pertussis (whooping cough) vaccine, antigens not otherwise unspecified
> protein efficiency ratio
> pudendal evoked response

P-ER
> pronation-external rotation

per
> perineal
> periodic
> periodicity
> person
> through, by [L. per]

PERa
> pertussis, acellular antigen(s), vaccine

PERC
> perceptual
> percutaneous
> potential erythropoietin-responsive cell

percus, PERCUSS
> percussion

PERD
> photoelectric registration device

PERF
> peak expiratory flow rate

perf
> perfect
> perforation (See also P)

PERG
> pattern-evoked electroretinogram

PERI
> peritoneal fluid

peri
> perineal

periap
> periapical

Peri Care
> perineum care

perim
> perimeter

Perio
> periodontics

peri-pads, Per pad
> perineal pads

PERK
> prospective evaluation of radial keratotomy

PERL
> pupils equal accommodation, reactive to light
> pupils equal and reactive to light
> pupils equal and react to light

PERLA, PEARLA
> pupils equal, reactive to light and accommodation
> pupils equal and react to light and accommodation

PERM
> progressive encephalomyelitis with rigidity and myoclonus

perm
> permanent
> permutation

per os
> by mouth (See also m, (m), OS, PO, p.o.)

perp
> perpendicular

PerQ SANS
> Percutaneous Stoller Afferent Nerve Stimulation System

PERR
> pattern evoked retinal response

PERRL
> pupils equal, round, and reactive to light

PERRLA
> pupils equal, round, reactive to light and accommodation

PERR-LADC
> pupils equal, round, reactive to light and accommodation directly and consensually

PERS
> patient evaluation rating scale
> personal emergency response system

pers
> personal

PERT
> product-enhanced reverse transcriptase

NOTES

P

607

PERT (continued)
program evaluation and review technique

PERV
Perinet virus
porcine endogenous retrovirus

PERw
pertussis, whole-cell antigens, vaccine

PES
pacing esophageal stethoscope
papillary fibroelastoma
photoelectron spectroscopy
plastic endosurgical system
Pleasant Events Schedule
polyethersulfone
postextrasystolic
preepiglottic space
preexcitation syndrome
primary empty sella (syndrome)
programmed electrical stimulation
pseudoexfoliation syndrome (*See also* PXS)
psychiatric emergency service

P.E.S.
Plastic Endosurgical System

PESA
percutaneous epididymal sperm aspiration

PESDA
perfluorocarbon-exposed sonicated dextrose albumin

Pesend
end-expiratory esophageal pressure

PESP
postextrasystolic potentiation

pe SPL
peak equivalent sound pressure level

PESQ
Personal Experience Screening Questionnaire

PESS
powered endoscopic sinus surgery

Pess
pessary

Pessniff
maximal sniff-induced esophageal pressure

PESST
Patterned Elicitation Syntax Screening Test

PEST
point estimation by sequential testing

PET
paraffin-embedded tissue
parent effectiveness training
peak ejection time
pear-shaped extension tube
peritoneal equilibration test
polyethylene terephthalate
polyethylene tube
poor exercise tolerance
positron emission tomography
postexposure treatment
predominantly epithelial thymoma
preeclamptic toxemia
pressure equalization tube
pressure equalizing tube
problem elicitation technique
Professional Employment Test
progressive exercise test
psychiatric emergency team
pulmonary endodermal tumor

PETA
pentaerythritol triacrylate

PET balloon
positron emission tomography balloon

PETCO$_2$
extrapolated end-tidal carbon dioxide tension
partial pressure of end-tidal CO_2

PET-FDG
positron emission tomography with 2-[F-18]-fluoro-2-deoxy-D-glucose
positron emission tomography with [^{18}F]-labeled fluorodeoxyglucose

PETH
pink-eyed, tan-hooded (rat)

PETINIA
particle-enhanced turbidimetric inhibition immunoassay

PETN
pentaerythritol tetranitrate

petr
petroleum

PETT
pendular eye-tracking test
phenethylthiazolethiourea
positron emission transaxial tomography
positron emission transverse tomography

PEU
plasma equivalent unit
polyether urethane

PEV
pulmonary extravascular (fluid) volume

PeV
peripheral vein (*See also* PV)

peV
peak electron volt

PEVN
periventricular nucleus
PEWV
pulmonary extravascular water volume
PEX
phosphate-regulating gene with homologies to endopeptidases found at the HYP locus on the X chromosome
PEx
physical examination (*See also* PE, PX, Px)
PEX#3
plasma exchange number three
PEXG
pseudoexfoliative glaucoma
PF
parafascicular (nucleus)
parallel fiber
parotid fluid
pars flaccida
partially follicular
patellofemoral (joint)
peak flow
pemphigus foliaceus
pericardial fluid
perifolliculitis
peripheral field
peritoneal fluid
permeability factor
personality factor
phenol formaldehyde
physicians' forum
picture-frustration (study, test) (*See also* P-F)
plantar flexion
plasma factor
plasma fibronectin
platelet factor
pleural fluid
power factor
precursor fluid
preservative free
proflavin
prostatic fluid
protection factor
pterygoid fossa
pulmonary factor
pulmonary fibrosis
pulmonary function
Purkinje fiber

purpura fulminans
push fluids
P-F
picture-frustration (study, test) (*See also* PF)
PF1
parainfluenza virus type 1
platelet factor 1
PF2
parainfluenza virus type 2
platelet factor 2
PF3
parainfluenza virus type 3
platelet factor 3
PF4
parainfluenza virus type 4
platelet factor 4
16 PF, 16PF
16 Personality Factor Questionnaire
The Sixteen Personality Factors test
P/F
pass/fail (system)
pF
picofarad
PF$_{1-4}$
platelet factors 1 through 4
PFA
foscarnet
phosphonoformic acid
platelet function analysis
profunda femoris artery
proximal reference axis
psychological first aid
pure free acid
PFAGH
penalty, frustration, anxiety, guilt, hostility
PFAPA
periodic fever, aphthous stomatitis, pharyngitis, cervical adenitis
PFAPE
perfluoroalkylpolyether
PFAS
performic acid-Schiff (reaction)
performic acid-Schiff (stain)
PFB
potential for breakdown
properdin factor B
pseudofolliculitis barbae
PFC
pancreatic fluid collection

NOTES

P

PFC *(continued)*
    patient-focused care
    pelvic flexion contracture
    perfluorocarbon
    perfluorochemical
    pericardial fluid culture
    permanent flexure contracture
    persistent fetal circulation
    plaque-forming cell
    Press-Fit component
    prolonged febrile convulsions
    purified fibrillar collagen

pFc
    noncovalently bonded dimer of C-terminal immunoglobulin of Fc fragment

PFCPH
    persistent fetal circulation with pulmonary hypertension

PFD
    pancreatic functioning diagnostant
    patellofemoral dysfunction
    perfluorodecaline
    polyostotic fibrous dysplasia
    polyurethane foam dressing
    primary flash distillate

PFE
    pelvic floor exercise

PFEAAC
    posterior fossa extra-axial arachnoid cyst

PFeeds
    after feedings

PfEMP-1
    Plasmodium falciparum erythrocyte membrane protein-1

PFF
    perifollicular fibroma
    polymer fume fever

PFFD
    proximal femoral focal deficiency
    proximal femur focal deficiency
    proximal focal femoral deficiency

PFG
    peak-flow gauge

PFGC
    pseudofollicular growth center

PFGE
    pulsed-field gel electrophoresis
    pulsed-field gradient gel electrophoresis

PfHRP-2
    Plasmodium falciparum histidine-rich protein 2

PFHx
    positive family history

PFI
    progression-free interval

PFIB
    perfluoroisobutylene

PFIC
    progressive familial intrahepatic cholestasia
    progressive familial intrahepatic cholestasis

PFJ
    patellofemoral joint

PFJS
    patellofemoral joint syndrome

PFK
    periodically fluctuating protein kinase
    phosphofructoaldolase
    phosphofructokinase

PFKL
    phosphofructokinase, liver (type)

PFKM
    phosphofructokinase, muscle (type)

PFKP
    phosphofructokinase, platelet (type)

PFL
    profibrinolysin

PFM
    peak flow meter
    porcelain fused to metal
    primary fibromyalgia

PFME
    pelvic floor muscle exercise

PFN
    partially functional neutrophil

PFNA
    percutaneous fine-needle aspiration

PFNAB
    percutaneous fine-needle aspiration biopsy

PFNEI
    percutaneous fine-needle ethanol injection

PFNP
    peripheral facial nerve palsy

PFO
    patent foramen ovale
    plantar fasciitis orthosis

PFOB
    perfluorooctyl bromide

PFOE
    peripheral fractional oxygen extraction

PFP
    patellofemoral pain
    pentafluoropropionic anhydride
    pentafluoropropionyl
    platelet-free plasma
    preceding foreperiod
    progression free probability
    purified fusion protein

PFPC
> Pall-filtered packed cells

PFPS
> patellofemoral pain syndrome

PFQ
> personality factor questionnaire

PFR
> parotid flow rate
> peak filling rate
> peak flow rate
> pericardial friction rub

PFRC
> plasma-free red cell
> predicted functional residual
> capacity

PFROM
> pain-free range of motion

PFS
> patellar femoral syndrome
> pelvic floor electrical stimulation
> penile flow study
> picture frustration study
> prefilled syringe
> preservative-free solution (system)
> pressure-flow study
> primary fibromyalgia syndrome
> progression-free survival
> protein-free supernatant
> pulmonary function score

PFSDQ
> Pulmonary Functional Status and
> Dyspnea Questionnaire

PFST
> positional feedback stimulation
> trainer

PFT
> pancreatic function test
> parafascicular thalamotomy
> placentofetal transfusion
> posterior fossa tumor
> postoperative flexor tendon
> pulmonary function test

PFT$_4$
> proportion free thyroxine

PFTBE
> progressive form of tick-borne
> encephalitis

PFTC
> primary fallopian tube carcinoma

PFU
> plaque-forming unit
> pock-forming unit

PFUO
> prolonged fever of unknown origin

PFV
> physiologic full value
> portal-vein blood flow velocity

PFW
> peak flow whistle
> pHisoHex face wash

PFWB
> Pall-filtered whole blood
> Psychological General Well-Being
> (index)

PFWT
> pain-free walking time

PG
> paged in hospital
> parapsoriasis guttata
> paregoric
> parotid gland
> partial gastrectomy
> pentagastrin
> pepsinogen
> peptidoglycan
> percutaneous gastrostomy
> performance goal (short-term goal)
> pergolide
> *Pharmacopoeia Germanica* (*See also*
> PhG)
> phosphate glutamate
> phosphatidylglycerol
> phosphatidyl glycine
> phosphogluconate
> phosphoglycerate
> pigment granule
> pituitary gonadotropin
> placental grade (biophysical profile)
> plasma gastrin
> plasmaglucose
> plasma triglyceride
> polygalacturonate
> postgraduate
> postgraft
> postprandial glucose
> pregnanediol glucuronide
> pregnant
> propylene glycol
> prostaglandin
> proteoglycan
> pyoderma gangrenosum

PG1
> pepsinogen 1

NOTES

P

P_G
  plasma glucose
Pg
  gastric pressure
  nasopharyngeal electrode placement
    in electroencephalography
  pogonion
  pregnancy
  pregnant
  pregnenolone
pg
  page
  picogram
PGA
  pancreaticogastrostomy anastomosis
  phosphoglyceric acid
  polyglandular autoimmune
    (syndrome) (*See also* PGAS)
  polyglycolic acid
  prostaglandin A
  pteroylglutamic acid
PGAC
  phenylglycine acid chloride
PGA-I
  polyglandular autoimmune syndrome
    type I
PGA-II
  polyglandular autoimmune syndrome
    type II
PGA-PLA
  polyglycolic acid-polylactic acid
PGAS
  persisting galactorrhea-amenorrhea
    syndrome
  polyglandular autoimmune syndrome
    (*See also* PGA)
Pgasniff
  maximal sniff-induced gastric
    pressure
PGAV
  Pongola virus
PGB
  prostaglandin B
PGC
  percentage of goblet cells
  pontine gaze center
  primordial germ cell
  prostaglandin C
PGCMS
  Philadelphia Geriatric Center
    Morale Scale
PGD
  phosphogluconate dehydrogenase
  phosphoglyceraldehyde
    dehydrogenase
  preimplantation genetic diagnosis
  prostaglandin D
  pure gonadal dysgenesis

PGD2, PGD_2
  prostaglandin D2
  prostaglandin D_2
PGDH
  phosphogluconate dehydrogenase
PGDR
  plasma glucose disappearance rate
PGE
  percutaneous gastroenterostomy
  platelet granule extract
  posterior gastroenterostomy
  primary generalized epilepsy
  prostaglandin E
  proximal gastric exclusion
PGE2, PGE_2
  prostaglandin E2
  prostaglandin E_2
PGE1, PGE_1
  prostaglandin E1
  prostaglandin E_1
PGEM
  prostaglandin E metabolite
PGF
  paternal grandfather (*See also* pgf)
  placental growth factor
  primary graft failure
  prostaglandin F
PGF_{2alpha}, PGF_{2a}, PGF2-alpha
  prostaglandin F_{2alpha}
  prostaglandin F_{2a}
  prostaglandin F2-alpha
PGF_2
  prostaglandin F2
pgf
  paternal grandfather (*See also* PGF)
PGG
  polyclonal gamma globulin
  prostaglandin G
PGG_2
  prostaglandin G_2
PGGF
  paternal great-grandfather
PGGM
  paternal great-grandmother
PGG-Q
  porphobilinogen—quantitative
PGH
  pituitary growth hormone
  placental growth hormone
  plasma growth hormone
  porcine growth hormone
  prostaglandin H
PGH2, PGH_2
  prostaglandin H2
  prostaglandin H_2
PGHS
  prostaglandin H synthase

PGI
peripheral glycerol injection
phosphoglucose isomerase
potassium, glucose, and insulin
prostaglandin I

PGI2, PGI$_2$
prostacyclin
prostaglandin I (*See also* PGI)
prostaglandin I2
prostaglandin I$_2$

PGJ
prostaglandin J

PGK
phosphoglycerate kinase
phosphoglycerokinase

PGL
persistent generalized
lymphadenopathy
phosphoglycolipid
primary gastric lymphoma
primary gastric non-Hodgkin
lymphoma

PGlyM
phosphoglyceromutase

PGM
paternal grandmother
phosphoglucomutase

PGMA
polyglycerol methacrylate

PGN
proliferative glomerulonephritis

PGO
pontogeniculooccipital (spike)

PGP
postgamma proteinuria
prepaid group practice
protein gene product

Pgp, P-gp
P-glycoprotein

Pg-Ppl
gastric-intrapleural pressure

PGR
pelvic girdle relaxation
percutaneous glycerol rhizolysis
progesterone receptor (*See also*
PgR)
psychogalvanic reflex
psychogalvanic response

PgR
progesterone receptor (*See also*
PGR, PR)
progestin receptor

P-graph
penile plethysmograph

1,3-P$_2$Gri
1,3-diphosphoglycerate

2,3-P$_2$Gri
2,3-diphosphoglycerate

P-GRN
progranulocyte

PGS
Persian Gulf syndrome
persistent gross splenomegaly
Pettigrew syndrome
pineal gonadal syndrome
plant growth substance
posterior glottic stenosis
postsurgical gastroparesis syndrome
prolapse gastropathy syndrome
prostaglandin synthetase
proteoglycan subunit

PGSE
pulsed-gradient spin echo

PGSI
prostaglandin synthetase inhibitor

PGSR
psychogalvanic skin resistance
psychogalvanic skin response

PGSRA
psychogalvanic skin response
audiometry

PGT
play group therapy

PGTP
primary glaucoma triple procedure

PGTR
plasma glucose tolerance rate

PGTT
prednisolone glucose tolerance test

PG-TXL
poly (L-glutamic acid)-paclitaxel

PGU
peripheral glucose uptake
postgonococcal urethritis

PGUT
phosphogalactose uridyl transferase

PGV
proximal gastric vagotomy

PGVS
postganglionic vagal stimulation

PGW
person gametocyte week

NOTES

P

PGWB
Psychological General Well-Being Scale

PGWBI
Psychological General Well Being Index

PGX
prostaglandin X

PGY
postgraduate year

PGYE
peptone, glucose, and yeast extract (medium)

PH
parathyroid hormone (*See also* PTH)
parenchymal hematoma
parenchymal hemorrhage
partial hepatectomy
passive hemagglutination
past history (*See also* Px)
peliosis hepatitis
perianal herpes
persistent hepatitis
personal history
pharmacopeia (*See also* Ph, PHAR, pharm)
phenethicillin
phenylalanine hydroxylase
pinhole
polycythemia hypertonica
poor health
porphyria hepatica
posterior hypothalamus
post history
previous history
primary hyperparathyroidism
prolylhydroxylase
prostatic hypertrophy
pseudohermaphroditism
pubic hair
public health
pulmonary hypertension
pulp horn
punctate hemorrhage

PH-1
primary hyperoxaluria type 1

Ph
pharmacopeia
phenanthrene
phenyl (*See also* Φ)
Philadelphia
phosphate

Ph1, Ph^1
Philadelphia chromosome

Ph+, PH-positive
Philadelphia chromosome-positive

pH
hydrogen ion concentration

pH$_{im}$
intramucosal pH

pH$_i$
isoelectric point (*See also* IEP, IP, i.p., PI, pI, pIs)

ph
phase
phial
phote (unit of surface illumination)

PHA
passive hemagglutination
peripheral hyperalimentation
photometer
phytohemagglutinin
phytohemagglutinin activation
phytohemagglutinin antigen
polyhydroxy acid
posterior hypothalamic area
postoperative holding area
pseudohypoaldosteronism
pulse-height analyzer

pH$_A$, pHa
arterial blood hydrogen tension
arterial pH

PHACE
posterior (fossa malformation), (large facial) hemangiomas, (coarctation of) aorta, cardiac (defects), arterial (abnormalities), eye (abnormalities)

PHACES
posterior (fossa malformation), (large facial) hemangiomas, (coarctation of) aorta, cardiac (defects), arterial (abnormalities), eye (abnormalities), sternal clefting (or supraumbilical raphe)

PHACO
phacoemulsification

PHACO OD
phacoemulsification of the right eye

PHACO OS
phacoemulsification of the left eye

PHA I
pseudohypoaldosteronism type I

PHA II
pseudohypoaldosteronism type II

PHAL
peripheral hyperalimentation
phytohemagglutinin-stimulated lymphocyte

phal
phalanges (plural)
phalanx

PHAlb
polymerized human albumin
PHA-m
phytohemagglutinin-mucopolysaccharide (fraction)
PHA-P, PHA-p
phytohemagglutinin-P
phytohemagglutinin-protein (fraction)
PHAR, phar
pharmaceutical
pharmacist
pharmacopeia (*See also* pharm)
pharmacy (*See also* PHARM)
pharynx
PHARM, pharm
pharmacopeia (*See also* PHAR, phar)
pharmacy (*See also* PHARM)
PHAT
pleomorphic hyalinizing angiectatic tumor
PHB
preventive health behavior
PHb
pyridoxylated hemoglobin
PHBB
propylhydroxybenzyl benzimidazole
PHBD
predominant hyperparathyroid bone disease
PHC
permissive hypercapnia
personal health cost
posthospital care
premolar hypodontia, hyperhidrosis, and canities prematura (Böök syndrome)
primary health care
primary hepatic carcinoma
primary hepatocellular carcinoma
proliferative helper cell
PHCA
profound hypothermic circulatory arrest
profoundly hypothermic circulatory arrest
PHCC
primary hepatocellular carcinoma
Ph-CML
Philadelphia chromosome-negative chronic myelogenous leukemia

Ph^{1+}-CML
Philadelphia chromosome-positive chronic myelogenous leukemia
PHCO$_3$
plasma bicarbonate
PHD
paroxysmal hypnogenic dyskinesia
pathological habit disorder
personal heart device
photoelectron diffraction
potentially harmful drug
pulmonary heart disease
PHDD
personal history of depressive disorders
PHDPE
porous high-density polyethylene
PHE
periodic health examination
postheparin esterase
proliferative hemorrhagic enteropathy
Phe
phenylalanine (*See also* F)
PhEEM
photoemission electron microscopy
PHEMA
polyhydroxyethylmethacrylate
phen
phenformin
PHEN-FEN, phen-fen
phentermine and fenfluramine
pheo
pheochromocytoma (*See also* PCC, PC)
PHEP
progressive home exercise program
PHF
paired helical filaments
personal hygiene facility
PHFG
primary human fetal glia
PHG
portal hypertensive gastropathy
pulmonary hyalinizing granuloma
PhG
Pharmacopoeia Germanica (*See also* PG)
phgly
phenylglycine

NOTES

P

PHH
paraesophageal hiatus hernia
posthemorrhagic hydrocephalus
PHHI
persistent hyperinsulinemic
hypoglycemia of infancy
φ, phi
ability continuum
magnetic flux
osmotic coefficient
phi coefficient (statistics)
phi (21st letter of Greek alphabet),
lowercase (*See also* Φ)
quantum yield
Φ, phi
phenyl (*See also* Ph)
phi (21st letter of Greek alphabet),
uppercase (*See also* φ)
PHI
passive hemagglutination inhibition
peptide histidine isoleucine
phosphohexose isomerase
physiologic hyaluronidase inhibitor
pontine hyperintensity
prehospital index
PH-I
primary hyperoxaluria type I
PhI
Pharmacopoeia Internationalis
pHi
intracellular hydrogen ion
concentration
PHIM
posthypoxic intention myoclonus
PHIQ
Philadelphia Head Injury
Questionnaire
PHIS
post-head injury syndrome
PHIV
portal hypertensive intestinal
vasculopathy
PHK
platelet phosphohexokinase
postmortem human kidney
PHKC
postmortem human kidney cell
PHLA
postheparin lipolytic activity
PHM
peptide histidine methionine
peptidylglycine alpha-hydroxylating
monooxygenase
posterior hyaloid membrane
Preventive Health Model
psyllium hydrophilic mucilloid
PHM-27
peptide hystidyl-methionine-27

PhM
pharyngeal musculature
PHMB
polyhexamethylene biguanine
(Baquacil, a pool cleaner)
PHN
paroxysmal noctural hemoglobinuria
postherpetic neuralgia
public health nursing
Puritan heated nebulizer
Ph-negative
Philadelphia chromosome-negative
PHNI
pinhole no improvement
PHO
periarticular heterotopic ossification
public health official
PH$_2$O
partial pressure of water vapor
PHOB
phobic anxiety
phorbol ester TPA
phorbol ester 12-O-
tetradecanoylphorbol-13-acetate
phos
phosphatase
phosphate
PHP
panhypopituitarism
partial hospitalization program
passive hyperpolarizing potential
persistent hyperphenylalaninemia
pooled human plasma
postheparin phospholipase
postheparin plasma
prehospital program
prepaid health plan
primary hyperparathyroidism
pseudohypoparathyroidism (*See also*
PHPT)
pyridoxylated hemoglobin-
polyoxyethylene
PH-positive (*var. of* Ph+)
PHPP, *p*-HPPO
p-hydroxyphenyl pyruvate oxidase
PHPPA
parahydroxyphenylpyruvic acid
PHPT
pseudohypoparathyroidism (*See also*
PHP)
pHPT
primary hyperparathyroidism
PHPV
persistent hyperplasia of primary
vitreous
persistent hyperplastic primary
vitreous

PHR
    peak heart rate
    photoreactivity
PHS
    partial hospitalization program
    patient-heated serum
    phenylalanine hydroxylase stimulator
    pooled human serum
    posthypnotic suggestion
    pseudoprogeria/Hallermann-Streiff
PHSC
    pluripotent hemopoietic stem cell
PHSL
    primary hepatosplenic lymphoma
PHSQ
    Psychosocial History Screening
      Questionnaire
PHST
    Psychosocial History Screening Test
pH-stat
    apparatus for maintaining pH of
      solution
PHT
    peroxide hemolysis test
    phentolamine
    phenytoin
    portal hypertension
    primary hyperthyroidism
    pulmonary hypertension
PHTN
    portal hypertension
    pulmonary hypertension
PHV
    peak height velocity
    persistent hypertrophic vitreous
    Prospect Hill virus
PHVD
    posthemorrhagic ventricular
      dilatation
    posthemorrhagic ventricular dilation
PHVE
    partial hepatic vascular exclusion
PHVM
    posthemorrhagic ventriculomegaly
PHx
    past history
Phx
    pharynx
PHY, phy
    pharyngitis
    physical

    physiology (*See also* P, PHYS)
    phytohemagglutinin
PhyO
    physician's orders
PHYS
    physiology (*See also* P, PHY)
PhyS
    physiologic saline (solution)
phys dis
    physical disability
Phys Ed
    physical education (*See also* PE,
      PED, P Ed)
physio
    physiologic
    physiotherapy
Physiol
    physiology
Phys Med
    physical medicine
Phys Ther
    physical therapy (*See also* PT)
π, pi
    pi (16th letter of Greek alphabet)
    ratio of circumference to diameter
      (3.1415926536)
PI
    international protocol
    isoelectric point (*See also* IEP, IP,
      i.p., pH_i, pI, pIs)
    pacing impulse
    package insert
    pallidal index
    pancreatic insufficiency
    paradoxical intention
    parainfluenza (virus)
    pars intermedia
    paternity index
    patient's interest
    Pearl Index
    percutaneous injury
    performance improvement
    performance index
    performance intensity
    perinatal injury
    Periodontal Index
    peripheral iridectomy
    permanent incidence
    permeability index
    persistent illness
    personal injury
    Personality Index

NOTES

P

PI *(continued)*

personality inventory
phagocytic index
phosphate ion
phosphatidylinositol (*See also* PtdIns)
physically impaired
pineal body
plaque index
pneumatosis intestinalis
poison ivy
polyphosphoinositide
ponderal index
pontine infarct
posteroinferior
postictal immobility
postincident
postinfection
postinjury
postinoculation
preinduction (examination)
premature infant
prematurity index
preparatory interval
present illness
pressure on inspiration
primary immunodeficiency
primary infarction
primary infection
principal investigator
proactive inhibition
proactive interference
programmed instruction
proinsulin
prolactin inhibitor
proliferative index
propidium iodine
protamine insulin
protease inhibitor
proximal intestine
pulmonary incompetence
pulmonary infarction
pulmonic insufficiency
pulsatility index

P of I

proof of illness

PI-3

parainfluenza 3 virus

PI3

phosophoinositol-3

P$_i$

inorganic orthophosphate

Pi

inorganic phosphate
inorganic phosphorus
parental generation
pressure in inspiration
protease inhibitor

pI

isoelectric point (*See also* IEP, IP, i.p., pH$_i$, PI, pIs)
platelet count increment

pi

platelet count increment (*See also* pI)

pi *(var. of π)*

PIA

peripheral interface adapter
personal injury accident
phenylisopropyladenosine
photoelectronic intravenous angiography
plasma insulin activity
porcine intestinal adenomatosis
preinfarction angina
purinergic agonist

PIAP

placental alkaline phosphatase (*See also* PLAP)

PIAPACS

psychological information, acquisition, processing, and control system

PIAT

Peabody Individual Achievement Test

PIAV

Picola virus

PIAVA

polydactyly, imperforate anus, vertebral anomalies (syndrome)

PIB

partial ileal bypass
periinfarction block
professional information brochure
psi-interactive biomolecule

PIBC

percutaneous intraaortic balloon counterpulsation

PIBD

paucity of interlobular bile ducts

PIBF

progesterone-induced blocking factor

PIBIDS

photosensitivity, ichthyosis, brittle hair, impaired intelligence, decreased fertility, and short stature

PIC

penicillin-inhibitor combinations
peripherally inserted catheter
personal injury collision (crash)
Personality Inventory for Children
plasmin-inhibitor complex
polysaccharide-iron complex
posterior intermediate curve

postinflammatory corticoid
postintercourse

PICA

Pictorial Instrument for Children and Adolescents
Porch Index of Communicative Abilities
posterior inferior cerebellar artery
posterior inferior communicating artery
posteroinferior cerebellar artery

PICAC

Porch Index of Communicative Abilities in Children

PICC

percutaneously inserted central line catheter
peripherally inserted central catheter

PICD

periinfarction conduction defect
primary irritant contact dermatitis

PICH

primary intracerebral hemorrhage

PICHI

pulse-inversion contrast harmonic imaging

PiCO$_2$

partial pressure of intramuscular carbon dioxide

PICP

carboxyterminal propeptide of type 1 procollagen

PICS

Parent Interview for Child Syndrome
Patterns of Individual Change Scale

PICSES

pancreatic islet cell-specific enhancer sequence

PICSI

Picture Identification for Children-Standardized Index

PICSO

pressure-controlled intermittent coronary sinus occlusion

PICSYMS

picture symbols

PICT

pancreatic islet cell transplantation

PICU

pediatric intensive care unit

psychiatric intensive care unit
pulmonary intensive care unit

PICV

Pichinde virus

PICVC

peripherally inserted central venous catheter

PID

pain intensity difference (score)
pelvic inflammatory disease
photoionization detector
plasma iron disappearance
position indicating device
primary immune deficiency
prolapsed intervertebral disk
proportional-integral-derivative
protruded intervertebral disk

PIDDST

pediatric infectious disease developmental screening test

PIDRA

portable insulin dosage-regulating apparatus

PIDS

primary immunodeficiency syndrome (*See also* PIS)

PIDT

plasma iron disappearance time

PIE

postinfectious encephalomyelitis
preimplantation embryo
prosthetic infectious endocarditis
pulmonary infiltrate with eosinophilia
pulmonary infiltration with eosinophilia
pulmonary interstitial edema
pulmonary interstitial emphysema

PIEE

pulsed irrigation for enhanced evacuation

PIEF

isoelectric focusing in polyacrylamide

PIES

Picture Interest Exploration Survey

PIEx

posteroinferior external

PIF

peak inspiratory flow
pigment inspiratory factor
point of identical flow

NOTES

P

619

PIF *(continued)*
    premorbid inferiority feeling
    proinsulin-free
    prolactin-inhibiting factor
    proliferation-inhibiting factor
    proliferation inhibitory factor
    prostatic interstitial fluid

PIFG
    poor intrauterine fetal growth

PIFR
    peak inspiratory flow rate

PIFT
    platelet immunofluorescence test

PIG
    pertussis immune globulin
    phosphate-independent glutaminase

PIGI
    pregnancy-induced glucose
      intolerance

pigm
    pigment
    pigmented

PIGN
    postinfectious glomerulonephritis

PIGPA
    pyruvate, inosine, glucose
      phosphate, and adenine

pIgR
    polyimmunoglobulin receptor

PIH
    pregnancy-induced hypertension
    preventricular intraventricular
      hemorrhage
    prolactin-inhibiting hormone
    prolactin inhibitory hormone
    pseudointimal hyperplasia

PIHH
    postinfluenza-like hyposmia and
      hypogeusia

PII
    plasma inorganic iodine
    primary irritation index

PIIID
    peripheral indwelling intermediate
      infusion device

PIIn
    posteroinferior internal

PIIP
    portable insulin infusion pump

PIIS
    posterior inferior iliac spine

PI3-K
    phosphatidylinositol 3′-kinase

PI3′K
    phosphoinositide 3′kinase

PIL
    patient information leaflet
    primary intestinal lymphangiectasia
    purpose in life

PILBD
    paucity of interlobular bile duct

PILO
    pilocarpine

PIM
    penicillamine-induced myasthenia
    pulse-inversion mode (ultrasound)

P$_{Imax}$
    maximal inspiratory mouth pressure

PIMIA
    potentiometric ionophore mediated
      immunoassay

PIMS
    programmable implantable
      medication system

PIN
    personal identification number
    posterior interosseous nerve
    prostatic intraepithelial neoplasia

PIN-1
    prostatic intraepithelial neoplasia,
      mild dysplasia or low grade

PIN-2
    prostatic intraepithelial neoplasia,
      moderate dysplasia or high grade

PIN-3
    prostatic intraepithelial neoplasia,
      severe dysplasia or high grade

PIND
    progressive intellectual and
      neurological deterioration

PINN
    proposed international nonproprietary
      name

PINS
    person in need of supervision

PINV
    postimperative negative variation

PIO
    pemoline
    progesterone in oil

PIO$_2$
    inspired oxygen tension
    intraalveolar oxygen tension
    partial pressure of inspiratory
      oxygen

P$_{IO_2}$
    partial pressure of inspiratory
      oxygen

PION
    posterior interosseous nerve
    posterior ischemic optic neuropathy

PIP
    paraffin immunoperoxidase
    paralytic infantile paralysis
    peak inflation pressure

peak inspiratory pressure
personal injury protection
piperacillin
plasma cell interstitial pneumonitis
positive inspiratory pressure
postictal psychosis
postinflammatory polyposis
postinfusion phlebitis
postinspiratory pressure
pressure inversion point
prolactin inducible protein
proximal interphalangeal (joint) (*See also* PIPJ)
psychosis, intermittent hyponatremia, polydipsia (syndrome)
Psychotic Inpatient Profile
pulmonary immaturity of prematurity
pulmonary insufficiency of the premature

PIP$_2$, PI4P, PI4,5P2
phosphatidylinositol 4,5-bisphosphate

PIPA
platelet ^{125}I-labeled (staphylococcal) protein A

PI-PB
performance versus intensity function for phonetically balanced words

PIP/DIP
proximal interphalangeal/distal interphalangeal (joints)

PIPE
persistent interstitial pulmonary emphysema

PIPES
piperazine diethanesulfonic acid

PIPIDA
paraisopropyliminodiacetic acid (scan)

PIPIS
Rhode Island Pupil Identification Scale

PIPJ
proximal interphalangeal joint (*See also* PIP)

PIPP
Premature Infant Pain Profile

PIP/TZ
piperacillin-tazobactam (Zosyn)

PIQ
Performance Intelligence Quotient

PIR
piriform
postinhibition rebound
pressure increment rate

P-IRI
plasma immunoreactive insulin

PIRS
plasma immunoreactive secretion

PIRYV
Piry virus

PIS
pregnancy interruption service
primary immunodeficiency syndrome (*See also* PIDS)
Provisional International Standard
pulmonary intimal sarcoma

pIs
isoelectric point (*See also* IEP, IP, i.p., pH$_i$, PI, pI)

PISA
phase-invariant signature algorithm
proximal isovelocity surface area

PISCES
percutaneously inserted spinal cord electrical stimulation

PIT
pacing-induced tachycardia
peak isometric torque
perceived illness threat
Picture Identification Test
pin-in-tube
Pitocin (oxytocin)
Pitressin (vasopressin)
plasma iron turnover
pulsed inotrope therapy

Pit
patellar inhibition test

Pit-1
pituitary-specific transcription factor-1

pit.
pituitary

PITC
phenylisothiocyanate

PITP
pseudoidiopathic thrombocytopenic purpura

PITR
plasma iron turnover rate

PITS
parent-infant traumatic stress

NOTES

P

PIU
    polymerase-inducing unit
PI-urea
    phosphate ion-urea
PIV
    parainfluenza virus
    peripheral intravenous
    polydactyly, imperforate anus,
      vertebral anomalies (syndrome)
PIV-3
    parainfluenza virus type 3
PIVD
    protruded intervertebral disk
PIVH
    peripheral intravenous
      hyperalimentation
    periventricular-intraventricular
      hemorrhage
PIVKA-II
    prothrombin induced by vitamin K
      absence or antagonist-II
PIVM
    passive intervertebral motion
PIWT
    partially impacted wisdom teeth
PIXE, PIXIE
    particle-induced x-ray emission
    proton-induced x-ray emission
pixel
    picture element
PIXV
    Pixuna virus
PJ
    pancreatic juice
    patellar jerk
    Peutz-Jeghers (syndrome)
    porcelain jacket (crown)
PJA
    pancreaticojejunostomy anastomosis
PJB
    premature junctional beat
PJC
    premature junctional contraction
PJI
    prosthetic joint infection
PJP
    pancreatic juice protein
PJRT
    permanent junctional reciprocating
      tachycardia
PJS
    peritoneojugular shunt
    Peutz-Jeghers syndrome
PJT
    paroxysmal junctional tachycardia
PJVT
    paroxysmal junctional ventricular
      tachycardia

PK
    pack (cigarette)
    penetrating keratoplasty (*See also*
      PKP)
    pericardial knock
    pharmacokinetic
    pig kidney
    Prausnitz-Küstner (antibodies,
      reaction) (*See also* PKT)
    protein kinase
    psychokinesis
    psychokinetic
    pyruvate kinase
P_K
    plasma potassium
pK
    ionization constant of acid
pK′, pK-
    apparent value of pK
    negative logarithm of dissociation
      constant of acid
pK_a
    negative logarithm of acid
      ionization constant
pk
    peck
PKA
    prekallikrein activator
    prokininogenase
    protein kinase A
pKa
    measure of acid strength
PKAR
    protein kinase activation ratio
PKase
    protein kinase
pkat
    picokatal
PKB
    prone knee bend
    protein kinase B
PKC
    protein kinase C
PKD
    paroxysmal kinesigenic dyskinesia
    polycystic kidney disease
    proliferative kidney disease
    proteinase K digestion
PKDL
    post-kala azar dermal leishmaniasis
PKF
    phagocytosis and killing function
PKG
    protein kinase G
PKI
    potato kallikrein inhibitor

PKK

    plasma prekallikrein
    prekallikrein

PKN

    parkinsonism

PKND

    paroxysmal nonkinesigenic
      dyskinesia

PKP

    penetrating keratoplasty (*See also*
      PK)

PKPG

    penetrating keratoplasty and
      glaucoma

PKR

    phased knee rehabilitation
    phosphorylation by the cellular
      double-stranded RNA-activated
      kinase

PKRS

    Phelps Kindergarten Readiness
      Scale

PKS

    pulmonary Kaposi sarcoma

PKSAP

    Psychiatric Knowledge and Skills
      Self-Assessment Program

PKT

    Prausnitz-Küstner test (*See also* PK)

PKU

    phenylketonuria

PKV

    killed poliomyelitis vaccine

pkV

    peak kilovoltage

pkyrs

    pack-year of smoking (2 packs a
      day for 20 years would be 40
      pack-years)

PL

    palmaris longus
    pancreatic lipase
    perception of light
    phospholipase
    phospholipid (*See also* PPL)
    photoluminescence
    place
    placebo (*See also* P, PBO, PLBO,
      PCB, PLB)
    placental lactogen
    plantar
    plasma lemma

    plastic surgery
    platelet (*See also* PLT, Plt)
    platelet antigen
    platelet lactogen
    plural
    polymer of lactic (acid)
    posterior lip (of acetabulum)
    preferential looking
    preleukemia platelet (*See also* PLT,
      Plt)
    premature labor
    problem list
    proboscis lateralis
    procaine and lactic acid
    psychosocial-labile
    pulpolingual
    pulpolinguoaxial
    Purkinje layer
    transpulmonary pressure

PL/1

    programming language 1 (one)

P$_L$

    pulmonary venous pressure (*See
      also* PVP)
    transpulmonary pressure

Pl

    plasma
    Poiseuille (law, space)

pL

    picoliter

pl

    place
    pleural
    plural

PLA

    peripheral laser angioplasty
    peroxidase-labeled antibodies (test)
    phospholipase A
    Plasma-Lyte A
    platelet antigen
    polylactic acid
    posterolateral (coronary) artery
    potentially lethal arrhythmia
    Product License Application
    pulpolabial
    pulpolinguoaxial

PLA2, PLA$_2$

    phospholipase A2
    phospholipase A$_2$

PLa

    pulpolabial

NOTES

P

Pla
> left atrial pressure

PLAD
> proximal left anterior descending (artery)

PL-ADOS
> prelinguistic autism diagnostic observation

plague
> bubonic plague

PLAI
> Preschool Language Assessment Instrument

Plan B
> levonorgestrel (a progestogen emergency contraceptive)

PLAP
> placental alkaline phosphatase (*See also* PIAP)
> polyclonal antiplacental alkaline phosphatase

plat
> platelet

PLAT C
> platelet concentration

PLAT P
> platelet pheresis

PLAV
> Playas virus

PLAX
> parasternal long axis

PLB
> parietal lobe battery
> percutaneous liver biopsy
> phospholamban
> phospholipase B
> placebo (*See also* P, PBO, PL, PLBO, PCB)
> porous layer bead
> posterolateral branch
> primary lymphoma of bone
> primary non-Hodgkin lymphoma of bone

PLBO
> placebo (*See also* P, PBO, PL, PCB, PLB)

PLC
> peripheral lymphocyte count
> personal locus of control
> phospholipase C
> pityriasis lichenoides chronica
> pleomorphic lobular carcinoma
> primary liver cell
> proinsulin-like component
> protein-lipid complex
> pseudolymphocytic choriomeningitis

PLCC
> primary liver cell cancer

PLCL
> polyclonal gammopathy identified

PL-CLP
> platelet clump

PLCO
> postoperative low cardiac output

PLD
> partial lower denture
> percutaneous laser diskectomy
> peripheral light detection
> phospholipase D
> platelet defect
> polycystic liver disease (*See also* PCLD)
> posterior latissimus dorsi (muscle)
> postlaser day
> potentially lethal damage
> pregnancy, labor, and delivery

PLDD
> percutaneous laser disk decompression
> poorly differentiated lymphoma, diffuse

PLDH
> plasma lactic dehydrogenase

PLDR
> potentially lethal damage repair

PLE
> panlobular emphysema
> paraneoplastic limbic encephalopathy
> pleura
> polymorphous light eruption (*See also* PMLE)
> protein-losing enteropathy
> pseudolupus erythematosus (syndrome)

PLED
> periodic lateralizing epileptiform discharge

PLES
> parallel line equal spacing

PLET
> polymyxin, lysozyme, EDTA, and thallous acetate (in heart infusion agar)

PLEU
> pleural (fluid)

PLEVA
> pityriasis lichenoides et varioliformis acuta

PLF
> perilymphatic fistula
> prior level of function

PLFC
> premature living female child

PLFD
> perilunate fracture-dislocation

PLFS
   perilymphatic fistula syndrome
PLG
   photoablative laser goniotomy
   plague (*Yersinia pestis*) (la Peste)
      vaccine
   plasminogen
PLGA
   polymorphous low-grade
      adenocarcinoma
P-LGV
   psittacosis lymphogranuloma
      venereum
PLH
   paroxysmal localized hyperhidrosis
   placental lactogenic hormone
   pulmonary lymphoid hyperplasia
PLHB
   percutaneous left heart bypass
PLIC
   posterior limb of the internal
      capsule
PLIF
   posterior lumbar interbody fusion
   posterolateral interbody fusion
PLISSIT
   permission, limited information,
      specific suggestions, and intensive
      therapy
PLL
   peripheral light loss
   poly-L-lysine
   posterior longitudinal ligament
   pressure length loop
   prolymphocytic leukemia
PLLA
   poly-L-lactic acid
PLM
   percentage of labeled mitoses
   periodic leg movement
   periodic limb movement
   plasma level monitoring
   Plasma-Lyte M
   polarized light microscopy
   precise lesion measuring
   product-line manager
PLMC
   premature living male child
PLMD
   periodic limb movement disorder

PLMS
   periodic limb movements during
      sleep
PLMT
   plasmacytoid lymphocyte
PLMV
   posterior leaf mitral valve
PLN
   pelvic lymph node
   peripheral lymph node
   popliteal lymph node
   posterior lip nerve
PLND
   pelvic lymph node dissection
PLNR
   perilobar nephrogenic rest
PLO
   pluronic lecithin organogels
   polycystic lipomembranous
      osteodysplasia
PLOF
   previous level of functioning
PLOP
   partial laryngopharyngectomy
PLOSA
   physiologic low stress angioplasty
PLP
   paraformaldehyde-lysine-periodate
   parathyroid hormonelike protein
   partial laryngopharyngectomy
   phantom limb pain
   plasma leukopheresis
   polystyrene latex particle
   proteolipid protein
   protolipid protein
   pyridoxal phosphate
   pyridoxal 5'-phosphate
PLPD
   pseudoperiodic lateralized
      paroxysmal discharge
PLPH
   postlumbar puncture headache
PLR
   persistent reactivity to light
   pronation-lateral rotation (fracture)
   pupillary light reflex
PLS
   plastic leafspring
   plastic surgery
   point locator stimulator
   preleukemic syndrome
   Preschool Language Scale

NOTES

P

PLS *(continued)*
>primary lateral sclerosis
>prostaglandin-like substance

PLs
>premalignant lesions

pls
>please

PLSA
>posterolateral spinal artery

PLSI
>Psoriasis Life Stress Inventory

PLSO
>posterior leafspring orthosis

PLST
>progressively lowered stress
>threshold

PLSURG
>plastic surgery

PLSV
>Palestina virus

PLT
>pancreatic lymphocytic infiltration
>peroneus longus tendinopathy
>platelet *(See also* PL, Plt)
>primed lymphocyte test
>primed lymphocyte typing
>psittacosis, lymphogranuloma
>venereum, trachoma

Plt
>platelet *(See also* PL, PLT)

PLT EST
>platelet estimate

PLTF
>plaintiff

PLT-G
>giant platelet

PLTSS
>Pediatric Liver Transplant-Specific
>Scale

PLUG
>plug the lung until it grows

plumb.
>lead [L. *plumbum*] *(See also* Pb)

PLUT
>Plutchnik (geriatric rating scale)

PLV
>panleukopenia virus
>partial liquid ventilation
>phenylalanine, lysine, and
>vasopressin
>poliomyelitis live vaccine
>posterior left ventricular

plx
>plexus

PLYM
>prolymphocyte

PLYO
>plyometric

PLZF
>promyelocytic leukemia zinc finger

PM
>after death [L. *post mortem*]
>afternoon [L. *post meridiem*] *(See
>also* p.m.)
>evening
>pacemaker
>pagetoid melanocytosis
>papillae mammae
>papillary muscle
>papular mucinosis
>paromycin
>partially muscular
>partial meniscectomy
>particulate matter
>pectoralis major
>perinatal mortality
>periodontal membrane
>peritoneal macrophage
>petit mal (epilepsy)
>photomultiplier
>physical medicine
>plasma membrane
>platelet membrane
>platelet microsome
>pneumomediastinum
>poliomyelitis
>polymorphonuclear
>polymyositis
>poor metabolizer
>porokeratosis of Mibelli
>posterior mitral
>postmenopausal
>postmortem *(See also* post, post.)
>premamillary nucleus
>premarketing (approval)
>premolar
>presents mainly
>presystolic murmur
>pretibial myxedema
>preventive medicine *(See also* PRM,
>PrM, PVMed)
>primary motivation
>prostatic massage
>protein methylesterase
>psammomatous meningioma
>pterygoid muscle
>puberal macromastia
>pulmonary macrophage
>pulpomesial

PM10
>particulate matter less than 10
>micrometers diameter

P/M
>parent-metabolite (ratio)

Pm
>promethium

pM

picomolar

p.m.

afternoon [L. *post meridiem*] (*See also* PM)

pm

picometer

PMII

paternal meiosis II

PMA

papillary, marginal, attached (gingiva)
para-methoxyamphetamine
phenylmercuric acetate
phorbolmyristate acetate
phorbol myristate acetate
phosphomolybdic acid
positive mental attitude
premenstrual asthma
premenstrual exacerbation of asthma
primary mental abilities
Prinzmetal angina
progressive muscular atrophy
psychomotor agitation
pyridylmercuric acetate

PMAA

Premarket Approval Application (medical devices)

PMAC

phenylmercuric acetate

PMAT

Primary Mental Abilities Test

PMB

papillomacular bundle
para-hydroxymercuribenzoate
polychrome methylene blue (stain)
polymorphonuclear basophil
polymyxin B
postmenopausal bleeding

PMBC

percutaneous mitral balloon commissurotomy

PMBV

percutaneous mitral balloon valvotomy
percutaneous mitral balloon valvuloplasty

PMC

percutaneous mitral commissurotomy
peripheral multifocal chorioretinitis
phenylmercuric chloride
pleural mesothelial cell

pontine micturition center
premature mitral closure
premotor cortex
pseudomembranous colitis

PMCP

para-monochlorophenol
perinatal mortality counseling program

PMCT

perinatal mortality counseling team

PMD

papillary muscle dysfunction
Pelizaeus-Merzbacher disease
perceptual motor development
piecemeal degranulation
posterior mandibular depth
primary myocardial disease
primidone (Mysoline)
private medical doctor
programmed multiple development
progressive muscular dystrophy

PMDD

premenstrual dysphoric disorder

pMDI

pressurized metered-dose inhaler

PM-DM, PM/DM

polymyositis-dermatomyositis

PMDS

persistent müllerian duct syndrome
premenstrual dysphoric syndrome
primary myelodysplastic syndrome

PME

pelvic muscle exercise
phosphomonoester
polymorphonuclear eosinophil
postmenopausal estrogen
progressive myoclonus epilepsy

PMEA

adefovir
phosohonylmethoxycthyladenine
9-2-phosphonylmethoxyethyl-adenine

PMEALS

after meals

PMEC

pseudomembranous enterocolitis

PMEOAT

Photo-Mask-and Etch-on-a-Tube

PMF, pmf

progressive massive fibrosis
proton motive force
pterygomaxillary fossa
pupils mid-position, fixed

NOTES

P

PMFAC
    prednisone, methotrexate, FAC
PMFBW
    paramedian frontal bone window
PMGCT
    primary mediastinal germ-cell tumor
PMH
    past medical history (*See also*
        PMHx)
    posteromedial hypothalamus
    programmed medical history
    pure motor hemiparesis
PMHR
    predicted maximal heart rate
PMHx
    past medical history (*See also*
        PMH)
PMI
    Pain Management Index
    past medical illness
    paternal meiosis I
    patient medical instruction
    patient medication instruction
    perioperative myocardial infarction
    petition of mental illness
    phosphomannose isomerase
    plea of mental incompetence
    point of maximal impulse
    point of maximal intensity
    point of maximum impulse
    posterior myocardial infarction
    postmyocardial infarction
    present medical illness
    previous medical illness
PMID
    painful minor intervertebral
        dysfunction
    PubMed Unique Identifier (National
        Library of Medicine)
PMIS
    postmyocardial infarction syndrome
PMJ
    progressive multifocal leuko-J
        encephalopathy
PMK
    pacemaker
    primary monkey kidney
PML
    posterior mitral leaflet
    premature labor
    progressive multifocal
        leukodystrophy
    progressive multifocal
        leukoencephalopathy
    prolapsing mitral leaflet
    promyelocytic leukemia
    pulmonary microlithiasis

pML
    posterior mitral valve leaflet
PMLCL
    primary mediastinal large-cell
        lymphoma
PMLE
    polymorphous light eruption (*See
        also* PLE)
PMLS
    primary mediastinal large cell
        lymphoma with sclerosis
PMM
    perilacunar mineral matrix
    protoplast maintenance medium
PMMA
    polymethylmethacrylate
    polymethyl methacrylate
PMME
    primary malignant melanoma of
        the esophagus
PMMF
    pectoralis major myocutaneous flap
PMN
    polymodal nociceptors
    polymorphonuclear
    polymorphonuclear (leukocyte) (*See
        also* POLY, poly)
    polymorphonuclear neutrophil (*See
        also* M_7)
    Premarket Notification (medical
        devices)
PMN-3
    plasma polymorphonuclear elastase
PMNC
    percentage of multinucleated cells
    peripheral blood mononuclear cell
PMNG
    polymorphonuclear granulocyte
PMNR
    periadenitis mucosa necrotica
        recurrens
PMNS
    postmalarial neurological syndrome
PMO
    postmenopausal osteoporosis
pmol
    picomole
PMP
    pain management program
    past menstrual period
    patient management problem
    patient medication profile
    peripheral myelin protein
    persistent mentoposterior (fetal
        position)
    previous menstrual period
    psychotropic medication plan

PMPA
r-9-2-phosphonylmethoxpropyl adenine
tenofovir

PMP22 gene
peripheral myelin protein 22 gene

PMPM
per member per month

PMPO
postmenopausal palpable ovary

PMPS
postmastectomy pain syndrome

PMPY
per member per year

PMQ
phytylmenaquinone (vitamin K1)

PMR
pacemaker rhythm
papillary muscle rupture
percutaneous myocardial revascularization
percutaneous revascularization
percutaneous transmyocardial laser revascularization
perinatal morbidity rate
perinatal mortality rate
periodic medical review
physical medicine and rehabilitation
polymorphic reticulosis
polymyalgia rheumatica
posteromedial release
premedication regimen
prior medical record
progressive muscle relaxation
proportional morbidity ratio
proportional mortality ratio
proportionate morbidity ratio
proton magnetic resonance
psychomotor retardation

PM&R
physical medicine and rehabilitation

³¹P MRI
phosphorus magnetic resonance imaging

PMRP
portable monitor of respiratory parameters

P-MRS
phosphorus magnetic resonance spectroscopy
phosphorus nuclear magnetic resonance spectroscopy

PMRS
physical medicine and rehabilitation service

³¹P-MRS
phosphorus-31 magnetic resonance spectroscopy

PMRV
Paramushir virus

PMS
patient management system
performance measurement system
perimenstrual syndrome
peripheral muscle strength
phenazine methosulfate
poor miserable soul
postmarketing surveillance
postmenopausal syndrome
postmenstrual stress
postmitochondrial supernatant
pregnant mare serum
premenstrual symptoms
premenstrual syndrome
pulse, motor, and sensory
pureed, mechanical, soft (diet)

PMSC
pluripotent myeloid stem cell

PM-Scl
polymyositis-scleroderma

PMSF
phenylmethyl sulfonyl fluoride

PMSG
pregnant mare serum gonadotropin

PMT
pacemaker-mediated tachycardia
percutaneous mechanical thrombectomy
photoelectric multiplier tube
photomultiplier tube
point of maximum tenderness
Porteus maze test
postmenstrual tension
premenstrual tension
pseudosarcomatous myofibroblastic tumor

PMTS
premenstrual tension syndrome

PMTT
pulmonary mean transit time

PMV
paralyzed and mechanically ventilated
percutaneous mitral valvuloplasty

NOTES

P

PMV *(continued)*
  prolapsed mitral valve
  prolapse of mitral valve
PMV 1–9
  avian paramyxovirus virus 1–9
PmvCO$_2$
  partial pressure of mesenteric
    venous carbon dioxide
PMVL, pMVL
  posterior mitral valve leaflet
PMVP
  pulmonary microvascular
    permeability to protein
PMW
  pacemaker wire
PMZ
  pentamethylenetetrazol
  postmenopausal zest
PN
  nightmare [L. *pavor nocturnus*]
  papillary necrosis
  parenteral nutrition
  penicillin (*See also* P, PCN, PEN,
    Pen, pen., pen., PNC)
  perceived noise
  percussion note
  percutaneous nephrostogram
  percutaneous nucleotomy
  periarteritis nodosa (*See also* PAN)
  peripheral nerve
  peripheral neuropathy (*See also*
    PNP)
  peripheral node
  phrenic nerve
  plaque neutralization
  pneumonia (*See also* pneu, PNM)
  polyarteritis nodosa (*See also* PAN)
  polynephritis
  polyneuritis
  pontine nucleus
  poorly nourished
  positional nystagmus
  posterior nares
  postnasal
  postnatal
  predicted normal
  premie nipple
  primary nurse
  progress note
  pronucleus
  propoxyphene napsylate
  psychiatry-neurology
  psychoneurologist
  psychoneurology
  psychoneurotic
  pulmonary disease
  pyelonephritis

  pyridine nucleotide
  pyrrolinitrin
P&N
  psychiatry and neurology
P/N
  positive to negative (ratio)
PN$_2$, P$_{N2}$, P$_{n2}$
  nitrogen partial pressure
  partial pressure of nitrogen
PNA
  Paris Nomina Anatomica
  peanut agglutinin
  pentose nucleic acid
  peptide nucleic acid
  polynitroxyl albumin
P$_{Na}$
  plasma sodium
PNAB
  percutaneous needle aspiration
    biopsy
PNAC
  parenteral nutrition-associated
    cholestatic
PNAH
  polynuclear aromatic hydrocarbon
PNAS
  prudent no-salt-added (diet)
PNAvQ
  positive-negative ambivalent quotient
PNB
  percutaneous needle biopsy
  polymyxin, neomycin, bacitracin
  popliteal nerve block
  premature newborn
  premature nodal beat
  prostatic needle biopsy
PNBT
  para-nitroblue tetrozolium
PNC
  paranasal cancer
  penicillin (*See also* P, PCN, PEN,
    Pen, pen., PN)
  peripheral nerve conduction
  peripheral nucleated cell
  pneumotaxic center
  postnecrotic cirrhosis
  premature nodal contraction
  prenatal care
  prenatal course
  purine nucleotide cycle
PNCA
  proliferating nuclear cell antigen
PNCS
  primary neuroendocrine carcinoma
    of skin
PnCV
  nonvalent pneumococcal conjugate
    vaccine

PND

paroxysmal nocturnal dyspnea
partial neck dissection
pelvic node dissection
postnasal drainage
postnasal drip
postnatal depression
postneonatal death
pregnancy, not delivered
purulent nasal drainage

pnd.

pound (*See also* lb.)

PNdB

perceived noise level

PND-Rh

postnasal drip due to rhinitis

PNDS

postnasal drainage syndrome
postnasal drip syndrome

PND-Si

postnasal drip due to sinusitis

PNE

peripheral nerve evaluation
peripheral neuroepithelioma
plasma norepinephrine
pneumoencephalography
primary nocturnal enuresis
pseudomembranous necrotizing
enterocolitis

PNEC

pulmonary neuroendocrine cell

PNEE

pulmonary neuroepithelial endocrine

PNET

peripheral neuroectodermal tumor
primary neuroectodermal tumor
primitive neuroectodermal tumor

PNET-MB

primitive neuroectodermal tumor-
medulloblastoma

pneu

pneumonia (*See also* PN, PNM)

PNEUMO

pneumothorax

PNF

prenatal fluoride
primary nonfunction
proprioceptive neuromuscular
facilitation
proprioceptive neuromuscular
fasciculation (reaction)

PNG

penicillin G
pneumogram

PNH

paroxysmal nocturnal
hemoglobinuria
polynitroxyl-hemoglobin

PNI

perineural invasion
peripheral nerve injury
postnatal infection
prognostic nutritional index
pseudoneointimal
psychoneuroimmunology

PNID

Peer Nomination Inventory for
Depression

PNIF

peak nasal inspiratory flow

PNK

polynucleotide kinase

PNKD

paroxysmal nonkinesigenic
dyskinesia

PNL

percutaneous nephrolithotomy (*See
also* PCNL)
percutaneous nephrostolithotomy
peripheral nerve lesion
polymorphonuclear neutrophilic
leukocyte

PNLA

percutaneous needle lung aspiration

PNM

perinatal mortality
peripheral dysostosis, nail
hypoplasia, mental retardation
peripheral nerve myelin
pneumonia (*See also* PN, pneu)
postneonatal mortality (syndrome)

PNMG

persistent neonatal myasthenia
gravis

PNMR

perinatal mortality rate

PNMT

phenylethanolamine N-
methyltransferase
phenylethylamine N-methyl
transferase

PNN

probabilistic neural network

NOTES

P

P-NP

para-nitrophenol (See also PNP)

PNP

paraneoplastic pemphigus
para-nitrophenol (See also P-NP)
peak negative pressure
peripheral neuropathy (See also PN)
platelet neutralization procedure
polyneuropathy
progressive nuclear palsy
psychogenic nocturnal polydipsia

PNPase

purine nucleoside phosphorylase

PNPB

positive-negative pressure breathing

PNPG

p-nitrophenylglycerol
para-nitrophenyl-β-galactoside

pNPP, *p*NPP

para-nitrophenylphosphate

PNPR

positive-negative pressure respiration

PNPS

para-nitrophenylsulfate

PNR

physician's nutritional
recommendation

PNRB

partial non-rebreather (oxygen
mask)

PNRS

premature nursery

PNS

paraneoplastic syndrome
parasympathetic nervous system
partial nonprogressive stroke
peripheral nervous stimulator
peripheral nervous system
posterior nasal spine

PNSH

perimesencephalic nonaneurysmal
subarachnoid hemorrhage

PNSP

penicillin-nonsusceptible
Streptococcus pneumoniae
posterior nasal spine to soft palate

PNSS

Pediatric Nutrition Surveillance
System

PNST

peripheral nerve sheath tumor

PNT

paroxysmal nodal tachycardia
partial nodular transformation
percutaneous nephrostomy tube
percutaneous neuromodulatory
therapy

pnthx

pneumothorax

PNTML

pudendal-nerve terminal motor
latency

PNU

pneumococcal (Streptococcus
pneumoniae) vaccine, not
otherwise specified
protein nitrogen unit

PNUcn

pneumococcal (Streptococcus
pneumoniae) conjugate vaccine

PNUps

pneumococcal (Streptococcus
pneumoniae) polysaccharide

PNV

postoperative nausea and vomiting
prenatal vitamin

pnx

pneumonectomy
pneumothorax (See also PT, PTX,
Px)

PNZ

posterior necrotic zone

PO

by mouth [L. per os] (See also
p.o., m, (m), OS, per os)
parapineal organ
parietal operculum
parietooccipital
perceptual organization
period of onset
perioperative
periosteum
per os
phone order
physician only
posterior
postoperative (See also P-O, POP,
POp, postop, post-op)
postoperatively (See also postop)
predominating organism

P-O

postoperative (See also PO, POP,
POp, postop, post-op)

PO4

phosphate

P/O

oxidative phosphorylation ratio
protein to osmolar (ratio)

P&O

parasites and ova
prosthesis and orthosis
prosthetic and orthotic

PO$_2$, P$_{O2}$, P$_{o2}$

partial pressure of oxygen
pressure of oxygen

Po
    polonium
    porion
    position response
    progesterone

p.o.
    by mouth, orally [L. *per os*] (*See also* PO, m, (m), OS, per os, PO)

POA
    pancreatic oncofetal antigen
    phalangeal osteoarthritis
    point of application
    power of attorney
    preoptic area (of the hypothalamus)
    primary optic atrophy

POAD
    peripheral occlusive arterial disease

POADS
    postaxial acrofacial dysostosis syndrome

POAG
    primary open-angle glaucoma

POAH
    posterior occipitoatlantal hypermobility

POA-HA
    preoptic anterior hypothalamic area

POB
    penicillin, oil, and beeswax
    phenoxybenzamine
    place of birth

POBC
    primary operable breast cancer

POBE
    Profile of Out-of-Body Experiences

POC
    particulate organic carbon
    plans of care
    point of care
    polyolefin copolymer
    position of comfort
    postoperative care
    presurgical orthopedic correction
    products of conception

Po/C
    ocular pressure

POCI
    posterior circulation infarct

POCS
    posterior circulation syndrome

POCT
    point-of-care testing

POCY
    postoperative chronologic year

POD
    pacing on demand
    peroxidase
    place of death
    podiatry
    polycystic ovary disease
    postoperative day
    postovulatory day

POD 1
    postoperative day one

PODCO
    power-oriented depth controlled osteotomy cutter

PODQ
    Perceptual Organization Deviation Quotient

PODVT
    postoperative deep venous thrombosis

PODx
    preoperative diagnosis

POE
    patient-oriented evidence
    pediatric orthopedic examination
    port of entry
    position of ease
    postoperative endophthalmitis
    postoperative exercise
    prone on elbows
    proof of eligibility
    provider order entry

POEMS
    polyneuropathy, organomegaly, endocrinopathy, monoclonal component, skin changes
    polyneuropathy, organomegaly, endocrinopathy, monoclonal gammopathy, and skin changes (syndrome)
    polyneuropathy, organomegaly, endocrinopathy, M protein, and skin changes (syndrome)

POET
    pulse oximeter/end tidal (carbon dioxide)
    pulse oximeter/end tidal (CO_2)

POET2
    point of entry, traction and twist

NOTES

P

POEx
postoperative exercise

POF
physician's order form
position of function
premature ovarian failure
primary ovarian failure
pyruvate oxidation factor

POG
Penthrane, oxygen, and gas (nitrous oxide)
polymyositis ossificans generalisata
products of gestation

Pog
pogonion

POH
past ocular history
perillyl alcohol
personal oral hygiene
postoperative hemorrhage

pOH
hydroxide ion concentration in a concentration/solution
hydroxyl concentration

POHA
preoperative holding area

POHI
physically or otherwise health-impaired

POHS
presumed ocular histoplasmosis syndrome

POI
Personal Orientation Inventory
postoperative instructions

POIB
place outpatient in inpatient bed

POIK, poik
poikilocyte
poikilocytosis

point-EXACCT
point mutation detection using exonuclease amplification couple capture technique

pois
poison
poisoned
poisoning

POL
physician's office laboratory
poliovirus vaccine, not otherwise specified
posterior oblique ligament
premature onset of labor

pol
polish
polishing

polio
poliomyelitis

POLIP
polyneuropathy, ophthalmoplegia, leukoencephalopathy, and intestinal pseudoobstruction

poll.
pollicis

POLS
postoperative length of stay

POLY
polychromic erythrocytes
polymorphonuclear (leukocyte) (*See also* PMN, poly)

poly
polydipsia
polymorphonuclear (leukocyte) (*See also* PMN, PML, POLY)
polymorphonuclear neutrophilic granulocyte (leukocyte)
polyphagia
polyuria

poly-A, poly(A)
polyadenylic (acid)

poly-C, poly(C)
polycytidylic (acid)

POLY-CHR
polychromatophilia

poly-G, poly(G)
polyguanylic (acid)

poly-HEMA
poly-(2-hydroxyethyl methacrylate)

poly-I, poly(I)
polyinosinic (acid)

poly-LC, poly-L:C
copolymer of polyinosinic and polycytidylic acids
synthetic RNA polymer

% POLYS
percent of polymorphonuclear leukocytes

poly-T, poly(T)
polythymidylic (acid)

polytef
polytetrafluoroethylene

poly-U, poly(U)
polyuridylic (acid)

POM
pain on motion
peripheral osteoma of mandible
polyoximethylene
prescription-only medicine
pulse oximetry monitoring
purulent otitis media

POMA
Performance-Oriented Mobility Assessment

POMC
proopiomelanocortin
propiomelanocortin
POMES
prospective outcomes monitoring evaluation system
POMP
phase-offset multiplanar
phase-ordered multiplanar
principal outer material protein
POMR
problem-oriented medical record (*See also* POR)
POMS
Profile of Mood States
POMS-FI
Fatigue-Inertia Subscale of the Profile of Mood States
PON
paraxonase
particulate organic nitrogen
postoperative note
PONI
postoperative narcotic infusion
PONS
Profile of Nonverbal Sensitivity
PONV
postoperative nausea and vomiting
POO
prostatic outlet obstruction
POOH
postoperative open heart (surgery)
POOR
poor clot
POP
diphosphate group
pain on palpation
paroxypropione
PCL-oriented placement
persistent occipitoposterior (fetal position)
pituitary opioid peptide
plasma oncotic pressure
plasma osmotic pressure
plaster of Paris (*See also* PP)
polymyositis ossificans progressiva
popliteal (*See also* Pop., poplit)
posterior oropharynx
postoperative (*See also* PO, P-O, POp, postop, post-op)
progestin-only pill

POp
postoperative (*See also* PO, P-O, POP, postop, post-op)
Pop.
popliteal (*See also* POP, poplit)
population
POPC
Pediatric Overall Performance Category (scale)
poplit
popliteal (*See also* POP, Pop.)
POPP
psoriatic onychopachydermoperiostitis
POP-Q
Pelvic Organ Prolapse-Quantified system
POPS
peroral pancreatoscopy
POPs
persistent organic pollutants
POR
physician of record
postocclusive oscillatory response
problem-oriented (medical) record (*See also* POMR)
PORD
posterior reduction device
PORH
postocclusive reactive hyperemia
postoperative reactive hyperemia
PORN
progressive outer retinal necrosis
PORP
partial ossicular reconstruction prosthesis
partial ossicular replacement prosthesis
porph
porphyrin
PORR
postoperative recovery room
PORT
Patient Outcomes Research Team
Perception of Relationships Test
perioperative respiratory therapy
postoperative radiation therapy
postoperative radiotherapy
postoperative respiratory therapy
port
portable
POS
paraosteal osteosarcoma

NOTES

P

POS (*continued*)
    physician's order sheet
    point of service
    polycystic ovary syndrome (*See also* PCOS)
    positive (*See also* P, pos)
    psychoorganic syndrome

pos
    position (*See also* P)
    positive (*See also* P, POS)

POSC
    problem-oriented system (of) charting

POSIT
    Problem-Oriented Screening Instrument for Teenagers

POSM
    patient-operated selector mechanism
    plasma osmolality

pos pr
    positive pressure

POSS
    percutaneous on-surface stimulation
    proximal over-shoulder strap

poss
    possible

POST
    peritoneal oocyte and sperm transfer
    peritoneal oocyte sperm transfer
    Police Officer Selection Test

post, post.
    posterior (*See also* P)
    postmortem (*See also* PM)

PostC
    posterior chamber

POST-CABG
    post coronary artery bypass graft

PostCap
    posterior capsule

postgangl
    postganglionic

Post-M
    urine specimen after prostate massage

postop, post-op
    postoperative (*See also* PO, P-O, POP, POp)
    postoperatively (*See also* PO)

post prand.
    after dinner [L. *post prandium*]

POSTS
    positive occipital sharp transients of sleep

post sag D
    posterior sagittal diameter

post tib
    posterial tibial

PostVD
    posterior vitreous detachment

POSYC
    Pain Observation Scale for Young Children

POT
    marijuana (*See also* MJ)
    peak occupancy time
    periostitis ossificans toxica
    plans of treatment
    postoperative treatment
    purulent otitis media

pot.
    a drink [L. *potus*]
    potash
    potassium (*See also* K, kal, potass)
    potential (*See also* poten)
    potion

PotAGT
    potential abnormality of glucose tolerance

potass
    potassium (*See also* K, kal, pot.)

poten
    potential (*See also* pot.)

POTF
    preocular tear film

POTS
    postural orthostatic tachycardia syndrome

POU
    placenta, ovary, uterus

POV
    privately owned vehicle

PoV
    portal vein

POVT
    pelvic ovarian vein thrombosis
    puerperal ovarian vein thrombophlebitis
    puerperal ovarian vein thrombosis

POW
    Powassan (encephalitis)
    prisoner of war

powd
    powder (*See also* pdr, pwd)

POWSBP
    pulse oximetry waveform systolic blood pressure

POWV
    Powassan virus

POX
    pulse oximeter (reading)

POZ
    posterior optical zone

P-P
    probability-probability (plots)

PP

diphosphate group
near point of accommodation [L. *punctum proximum*] (*See also* P, pp)
pacesetter potential (*See also* PCP)
pancreatic polypeptide
paradoxical pulse
parietal pleura
partial pressure (*See also* P, p)
partial upper and lower dentures
pathology point
pedal pulse
pellagra preventive
pentose pathway
perfusion pressure
periodontal pockets
peripheral pulse
peritoneal pseudomyxoma
permanent partial
per protocol
persisting proteinuria
Peyer patch
phosphorylase phosphatase
pink puffer (sign of emphysema)
pinpoint
pinprick
placental protein
plane polarization
planned parenthood
plasma pepsinogen
plasmapheresis
plasma protein
plaster of Paris (*See also* POP)
polypeptide
polystyrene agglutination plate
poor person
population planning
porcine pancreatic
posterior papillary
posterior pituitary
postpartum (*See also* pp)
postprandial (*See also* pp, PPD)
precocious pubarche
preferred provider
presenting part
private patient
private practice
prophylactics
prothrombin-proconvertin
protoporphyria
protoporphyrin

proximal phalanx
pseudomyxoma peritonei
pterygoid process
pulse pressure
pulsus paradoxus
punctum proximum (of convergence) (*See also* p.p.)
purulent pericarditis
push pills
pyrophosphate (*See also* PYP, Pyro, PPi)

P&P

pins and plaster
policy and procedure
prothrombin and proconvertin (test)

PP₁

free pyrophosphate

p.p.

punctum proximum (*See also* PP)

pp

after meals [L. *post prandial*] (*See also* p̄p̄, post prand.)
near point of accommodation [L. *punctum proximum*] (*See also* P, PP)
polyphosphate
postpartum (*See also* PP)
postpill (amenorrhea)
postprandial (*See also* PP, PPD)
private patient

p̄p̄

after meals [L. *post prandial*] (*See also* pp, post prand.)

pIIIp

procollagen-III peptide

PPIX

protoporphyrin IX
protoporphyrin nine

PIIIP

aminoterminal type three procollagen propeptide
procollagen type III aminoterminal peptide

PP5

placental protein 5

PPA

palpation, percussion, and auscultation (*See also* PP&A, pp&a)
pelvic phased-array coil
pepsin A
phenylpropanolamine

NOTES

P

PPA *(continued)*
 phenylpyruvic acid
 Pittsburgh pneumonia agent
 plasmid pattern analysis
 polyphosphoric acid
 postpartum amenorrhea
 postpill amenorrhea
 propanolamine
 pulmonary artery pressure (*See also*
  PAP)
 pure pulmonary atresia
 pyrophosphate arthritis-pseudogout
PP&A, pp&a
 palpation, percussion, and
  auscultation (*See also* PPA)
Ppa
 pulmonary artery
PPACK
 D-Phe-L-Pro-L-Arg-chloromethyl
  ketone
 D-phenylalanyl-L-prolyl-L-arginine-
  chloromethyl ketone
PPAF
 progressive perivenular alcoholic
  fibrosis
PPAR
 peroxisomal proliferator receptor
 peroxisome proliferator-activated
  receptor
PPARg, PPAR-gamma
 peroxisome-proliferator-activated
  receptor gamma
PPAS
 peripheral pulmonary artery stenosis
 postpolio atrophy syndrome
Ppaw
 pulmonary artery wedge pressure
PPB, ppb
 parts per billion
 platelet-poor blood
 pleuropulmonary blastoma
 positive pressure breathing
 prostate puncture biopsy
PPBE
 postpartum breast engorgement
 proteose-peptone beef extract
PPBS
 postprandial blood sugar
PPBV
 Phnom Penh bat virus
PPC
 pentose phosphate cycle
 peripheral posterior curve
 Personal Problems Checklist
 Personal Problems Checklist for
  Adolescents
 plasma prothrombin conversion
 plaster of Paris cast

 pneumopericardium
 pooled platelet concentrate
 positive peritoneal cytology
 posterior peripheral curve
 primary peritoneal carcinoma
 progressive patient care
 prostatic pressure coefficient
 proximal palmar crease
PPCA
 percent of the periphery that has
  ciliary activity
 plasma prothrombin conversion
  accelerator
 proserum prothrombin conversion
  accelerator
PPCD
 polymorphous posterior corneal
  dystrophy
 posterior polymorphous corneal
  dystrophy
PPCF
 peripartum cardiac failure
 plasma prothrombin conversion
  factor
PPCH
 piperazinylmethyl cyclohexanone
PPCM
 postpartum cardiomyopathy
PPCP
 Parent Perception of Child Profile
PPD
 packs per day (cigarettes) (*See also*
  P/D)
 paraphenylenediamine
 percussion and postural drainage
  (*See also* P and PD, P&PD)
 permanent partial disability
 phenyldiphenyloxadiazole
 photodynamic diagnosis
 posterior polymorphous dystrophy
 postpartum day
 postprandial (*See also* PP, pp)
 primary peritoneal drainage
 primary physical dependence
 progressive perceptive deafness
 purified protein derivative (of
  tuberculin)
 purified protein derivative (test)
 (Siebert) purified protein derivative
  (of tuberculin)
 (5 tuberculin unit strength) purified
  protein derivative
P and PD, P&PD
 percussion and postural drainage
  (*See also* PPD)
ppd
 prepared (*See also* Ppt)

PPDA
paraphenylenediamine
PPD-B
purified protein derivative–Battey
pp'-DDE
pp'-dichlorodiphenyldichloroetene
PPDR
preproliferative diabetic retinopathy
PPD-S
purified protein derivative–standard
PPDS
phonologic programming deficit syndrome
PPE
palmoplantar erythrodysesthesia
partial plasma exchange
permeability pulmonary edema
personal protective equipment
polyphosphoric ester
porcine pancreatic elastase
postpartum endometritis
professional performance evaluation
programmed physical examination
pruritic papular eruption
Ppeak
peak airway pressure
PPEM
potentially pathogenic environmental mycobacterial
PPES
palmar-plantar erythrodysesthesia syndrome
pedal pulses equal and strong
PPF
pellagra preventive factor
percutaneous plantar fasciotomy
phagocytosis promoting factor
plasma protein fraction
p-p factor
pellagra-preventing factor (niacin)
PPG
pediatric pneumogram
phalloplethysmography
photoplethysmography (*See also* ppg)
polypropylene glycol
polyurethane-polyvinyl graphite
postprandial glucose
pretragal parotid gland
pylorus-preserving gastrectomy

ppg
photoplethysmography (*See also* PPG)
picopicogram
PPGA
postpill galactorrhea/amenorrhea
PPG-AFO
polypropylene glycol-ankle-foot orthosis
PPGF
polypeptide growth factor
PPGI
psychophysiologic gastrointestinal (reaction)
PPGP
prepaid group practice
PPG-TLSO
polypropylene glycol-thoracolumbosacral orthosis
PPH
past pertinent history
persistent postdrainage hypotony
persistent pulmonary hypertension
postpartum hemorrhage
primary postpartum hemorrhage
primary pulmonary hypertension
protocollagen proline hydroxylase
pphm
parts per hundred million
PPHN
persistent pulmonary hypertension of newborn
PPHP
pseudoPHP
pseudopseudohypoparathyroidism
PPHT
primary plexogenic hypertension
ppht
parts per hundred thousand
PPHTN
portopulmonary hypertension
PPHx
previous psychiatric history
PPI
partial permanent impairment
patient package insert
permanent pacemaker insertion
Plan-Position-Indication
preceding preparatory interval
prepulse inhibition
present pain intensity
proton pump inhibitor

NOTES

P

PPI *(continued)*
purified porcine insulin
purified pork insulin

PPi, PP$_i$
inorganic pyrophosphate (*See also* IPP)
pyrophosphate (*See also* PYP, PP)

PPID
peak pain intensity difference (score)

PPIE
prolonged postictal encephalopathy

PPIM
postperinatal infant mortality

PPIVMs
passive physiological intervertebral movements

PPJ
pure pancreatic juice

PPK
palmoplantar keratoderma
palmoplantar keratosis
partial penetrating keratoplasty
population pharmacokinetics

PPL
pars plana lensectomy
penicilloylpolylysine
penicilloyl-polylysine
phospholipid (*See also* PL)
postprandial lipemia
primary pulmonary non-Hodgkin lymphoma
protein polysaccharide

Ppl
intrapleural pressure
pleural pressure

PPLF
postperfusion low flow

PPLO
pleuropneumonia-like organism

PPLOV
painless progressive loss of vision

PPM
parts per million (*See also* ppm)
permanent pacemaker
persistent pupillary membrane
phosphopentomutase
physician practice management
pigmented pupillary membrane
posterior papillary muscle

ppm
parts per million (*See also* PPM)
pulses per minute

PPMA
postpoliomyelitis muscular atrophy
progressive postmyelitis muscular atrophy

PPMD
posterior polymorphic dystrophy (of cornea)

PPMM
postpolycythemia myeloid metaplasia

PPMS
primary-progressive multiple sclerosis
psychophysiologic musculoskeletal (reaction)
Purdue Perceptual-Motor Survey

PPN
partial parenteral nutrition
pedunculopontine nucleus
peripheral parenteral nutrition

PPNA
peak phrenic nerve activity

PPNAD
pigmented nodular adrenocortical disease
primary pigmented nodular adrenocortical disease

PPNET
peripheral primitive neuroectodermal tumor

PPNG
penicillinase-producing gonococci
penicillinase-producing *Neisseria gonorrhoeae*

PPO
diphenyloxazole
2,5-diphenyloxazole
passive prehension orthosis
peak pepsin output
platelet peroxidase
preferred provider organization
prepatient periods to oocyst

PPOB
postpartum obstetrics

PPO-HSA
penicillin-penicilloyl human serum albumin

PPoma
pancreatic polypeptide-secreting tumor

PPP
Pain Perception Profile
palatopharyngoplasty
palmoplantar pustulosis
passage, power, and passenger (progress of labor)
patient prepped and positioned
pearly penile papules
pedal pulse present
pentose phosphate pathway
peripheral pulse palpable
Pickford Projectives Picture
plasma protamine precipitating

platelet-poor plasma
point-to-point protocol
polyglactin 910-polydioxanon
polyphoretic phosphate
poor platelet plasma
porcine pancreatic polypeptide
postnatal penicillin prophylaxis
postpartum psychosis
posttraumatic persistent
  pneumothorax
preferred practice patterns
proportional pulse pressure (SBP
  minus DBP)/SBP
protamine paracoagulation
  phenomenon
purified placental protein
pustulosis palmaris et plantaris

PP&P

posterior pole and periphery

PPPBL

peripheral pulses palpable both legs

PPPD

pylorus-preserving
  pancreatoduodenectomy

PPPE

prolonged postpeel erythema

PPPG

postprandial plasma glucose

PPPH

purified placental protein, human

PPPI

primary private practice insurance

PPPM

Parents' Postoperative Pain Measure
per patient per month

PPPMA

progressive postpolio muscle
  atrophy

PPPPP

pain, pallor, pulse loss, paresthesia,
  and paralysis

PPPPPP

pain, pallor, paraesthesia,
  pulselessness, paralysis, prostration

PPQ

Postoperative Pain Questionnaire

PPR

patient-physician relationship
patient progress record
photopalpebral reflex
physiologic pattern release
pitch period perturbation

poor partial response
Price precipitation reaction

PPr

paraprosthetic
periodontal prophylactics

PPRE

peroxisome proliferator response
  element

PPRF

paramedian pontine reticular
  formation
pontine paramedian reticular
  formation
pontine parareticular formation
postpartum renal failure

PPRibp, PPRP

5-phospho-α-d-ribosyl 1-
  pyrophosphate (*See also* PRPP)
phosphoribosyl pyrophosphate

PPROM

preterm premature rupture of
  membranes
prolonged premature rupture of
  membranes

PPRST

Printing Performance School
  Readiness Test

PPRWP

poor precordial R-wave progression

PPS

Pap plus speculoscopy
parapharyngeal space
patellofemoral pain syndrome
pepsin
pepsin A
peripheral pulmonary stenosis
personal portable stimulator
Personal Preference Scale
phosphoribosylpyrophosphate
  synthetase
point-prevalent survey
polyvalent pneumococcal
  polysaccharide
postpartum sterilization
postperfusion syndrome
postpericardiotomy syndrome
postphlebitic syndrome
postpoliomyelitis syndrome
postpolio syndrome
postpump syndrome
Prausnitz-Küstner sclerosis
presurgical psychological screening

NOTES

P

PPS (*continued*)
 primary acquired preleukemic
 syndrome
 prospective payment system
 prospective pricing system
 protein plasma substitute
 pulse per second
 sodium pentosan polysulfate

PPSB
 prothrombin, proconvertin, Stuart
 factor, antihemophilic B factor

PPSEQ
 Postpartum Self-Evaluation
 Questionnaire

PPSH
 pseudovaginal perineoscrotal
 hypospadias

PPSS
 peripheral protein sparing solution

PPT
 parietal pleural tissue
 partial prothrombin time
 peak-to-peak threshold
 person, place, and time
 Physical Performance Test
 plant protease test
 posterior pelvic tilt
 postpartum thyroiditis
 potassium phosphotungstate
 pressure pain threshold
 pulmonary platelet trapping

Ppt
 parts per trillion
 precipitate (*See also* ppt)
 prepared

ppt
 precipitate (*See also* Ppt)
 precipitation (*See also* pptn)

pPTCA
 primary percutaneous transluminal
 coronary angioplasty

PPTD
 postpartum thyroid disease

pptd
 precipitated

PPTL
 postpartum tubal ligation
 pressure pain tolerance level

pptn
 precipitation (*See also* ppt)

PPTT
 postpartum painless thyroiditis (with
 transient) thyrotoxicosis
 prepubertal testicular tumor

PPU
 perforated peptic ulcer

PPV
 pars plana vitrectomy

patent processus vaginalis
 pneumococcal polysaccharide
 vaccine
 porcine parvovirus
 positive predictive value
 positive-pressure ventilation
 Precarious Point virus
 progressive pneumonia virus

Ppv
 pulmonary vein

PPVT
 Peabody Picture Vocabulary Test

PPVT-R
 Peabody Picture Vocabulary Test-
 Revised

PPW
 plantar puncture wound
 pylorus-preserving Whipple
 modification

Ppw
 pulmonary wedge pressure (*See also*
 PWP)

PPY
 packs per year (cigarettes)

PPZ
 perphenazine

PPZSO
 perphenazine sulfoxide

PQ
 paraquat
 permeability quotient
 plastoquinone
 pronator quadratus
 pyrimethamine-quinine

PQ-9
 plastoquinone-9

pQCT
 computer tomographic methods of
 peripheral skeleton
 peripheral quantitative computed
 tomography

PQD
 protocol data query

PQNS
 protein, quantity not sufficient

PQOCN
 Psychiatric Questionnaire Obsessive-
 Compulsive Neurosis

PQOL
 perceived quality of life

PQRST
 palliation, quality, radiation,
 severity, time
 position, quality, radiation, severity,
 time

PR
 far point (of accommodation) [L.
 punctum remotum]

pack removal
palindromic rheumatism
Panama red (variety of marijuana)
parallax (and) refraction
pars recta
partial reinforcement
partial remission
partial response
patient relations
peer review
pelvic rock
percentile rank
peripheral resistance
per rectum
phenol red
photoreaction
photoreactivation
physical rehabilitation
physician reviewer
pityriasis rosea
polymyalgia rheumatica
posterior root
postural reflex
potency ratio
potential relation
preference record
pregnancy (*See also* preg, pregn)
pregnancy rate
premature (*See also* Pr, prem)
presbyopia (*See also* P, Pr)
pressoreceptor
pressure (*See also* P, press.)
prevention
Preyer reflex
proctology
production rate
professional relations
profile
progesterone receptor (*See also* PgR)
progressive relaxation
progressive resistance
progressive resistive exercise (*See also* PRE)
prolactin (*See also* P, Pr, PRL, Prl)
prolonged remission
prone
propicillin
propranolol
prosthion
protease

protein (*See also* P, Pr, PRO, prot)
Protestant
psychotherapy responder
public relations
Puerto Rican
pulmonary regurgitation
pulmonary rehabilitation
pulmonic regurgitation
pulse rate
pulse repetition
pyramidal response

P=R
pupils equal in size and reaction

PR-2
Bennett pressure ventilator

PR3
proteinase 3

P–R
time between P wave and beginning of QRS complex in electrocardiography

P/R
productivity to respiration (ratio)

P&R
pelvic and rectal (examination)
pulse and respiration

P.r.
punctum remotum (*See also* p.r.)

Pr
pair
praseodymium
premature (*See also* PR, prem)
presbyopia (*See also* P, PR)
primary
prism
proctologist
production rate (of steroid hormones)
prolactin (*See also* P, PR, PRL, Prl)
propyl
protein (*See also* P, PR, PRO, prot)

p.r.
far point of accommodation [L. *punctum remotum*]
per rectum
punctum remotum (*See also* P.r.)
by way of rectum [L. *per rectum*]

PRA
panel of reactive antibodies
percent reactive antibody

NOTES

P

643

PRA *(continued)*
    percent reactive antibody/panel reactive antibody
    phonation, respiration, articulation-resonance
    phosphoribosylamine
    plasma renin activity
    plasmin renin activity
    progesterone receptor assay
    proximal reference axis
prac, pract
    practice
    practitioner
PRAFO
    pressure-relief ankle-foot orthosis
    pressure-relief ankle-foot orthotic
PrA-HPA
    protein A hemolytic plaque assay
PRAMS
    Pregnancy Risk Monitoring System
prand.
    dinner [L. *prandium*]
PRAS
    Patient Rated Anxiety Scale
    prereduced anaerobically sterilized (medium)
    pseudo-renal-artery syndrome
PRAT
    platelet radioactive antiglobulin test
pRB
    retinoblastoma protein
pRb
    Rb protein expression
PRBC
    packed red blood cells (*See also* PRC)
PRBV
    placental residual blood volume
PRC
    packed red (blood) cells (*See also* PRBC)
    peer review committee
    phase response curve
    plasma renin concentration
    polymerase chain reaction
PRCA
    pure red (blood) cell agenesis
    pure red (blood) cell aplasia
PrCa
    prostate cancer
PRCC
    papillary renal cell carcinoma
PRD
    partial reaction of degeneration
    phosphate restricted diet
    polycystic renal disease
    postradiation dysplasia

PRDS
    Pitt-Rogers-Danks syndrome
PRDX
    postradiation dysplasia
PRE
    Parkland Rapid Exam
    partial-reinforcement effect
    passive resistance exercise
    photoreacting enzyme
    physical reconditioning exercise
    Picture Reasoning Test
    pigmented retina epithelial (cell)
    progressive resistance exercise (*See also* PR)
    progressive-resistive exercise
    proton relaxation enhancement
pre
    preliminary
pre-AIDS
    pre-acquired immune deficiency syndrome
PREB
    Pupil Record of Education Behavior
preChx
    preoperative chemotherapy
precip
    precipitate
    precipitated
    precipitation (*See also* pcpn)
PRED, Pred
    prednisone (*See also* P, PDN)
pred
    predicted
PREE
    partial reinforcement extinction effect
preemie, premie
    premature
Pref-1
    preadipocyte factor-1
prefd
    preferred
PREG
    Pregestimil (infant formula)
    pregnelone
preg, pregn
    pregnancy (*See also* PR)
    pregnant (*See also* PR)
prelim
    preliminary
PREM
    Prematurity Risk Evaluation Measure
Pre-M
    urine specimen before prostate massage

prem
> premature (*See also* PR, Pr)
> prematurity

PR enzyme
> phosphorylase-rupturing enzyme
> photoreactivating enzyme

preop, pre-op
> preoperative
> preoperatively

prep
> preparation
> prepare (for surgery)
> preposition

prepd, prepped
> prepared (for surgery)

PRERLA
> pupils round, equal, react to light and accommodation

preRx
> preoperative radiotherapy

preserv
> preservation
> preserve

PRESS
> point-resolved spectroscopy
> Pre-Reading Expectancy Screening Scale

press.
> pressure (*See also* P, p, PR)

PREV
> Pretoria virus

prev
> prevent
> prevention
> preventive
> previous

PrevAGT
> previous abnormality of glucose tolerance

PREZ
> posterior root entry zone

PRF
> partial reinforcement
> patient report form
> peak repetition frequency
> peptide regulatory factor
> percutaneous radiofrequency rhizolysis
> Personality Research Form
> plasma-resistant fiber oxygenator
> pontine reticular formation
> progressive renal failure
> prolactin-releasing factor
> pulse repetition frequency
> pyrogen-releasing factor

pRF
> polyclonal rheumatoid factor

PRFA
> plasma-recognition-factor activity

PRFD
> percutaneous radio-frequency denervation

PRFM
> premature rupture of fetal membranes (*See also* PROM)
> prolonged rupture of fetal membranes (*See also* PROM)

PRFN
> percutaneous radiofrequency

PRFNB
> percutaneous radio-frequency facet nerve block

PRFR
> pressure-retaining flow-relieving

PRG
> phleborheogram
> phleborheography
> purge

PRGI
> percutaneous retrogasserian glycerol injection

PRH
> past relevant history
> postocclusive reactive hyperemia
> preretinal hemorrhage
> prolactin-releasing hormone

PRHBF
> peak reactive hyperemia blood flow

PrHPT
> primary hyperparathyroidism

PRI
> Pain Rating Index
> Partner Relationship Inventory
> Patient Review Instrument
> Personal Relationship Inventory
> phosphate reabsorption index
> phosphoribose isomerase
> plexus rectales inferiores (venous plexus) (*See also* VvRI)
> Prescriptive Reading Inventory

PRIAS
> Packard radioimmunoassay system

NOTES

P

PRICE
> protection, restricted activity, ice, compression, elevation

PRICES
> protection, rest, ice, compression, elevation, support (first aid)

PRIH
> prolactin release-inhibiting hormone

prim
> primary

PRIME
> preinversion multiecho

PRIME-MD
> Primary Care Evaluation of Mental Disorders

primip, PRIMP
> primipara (*See also* I-para, P)

PRIND
> prolonged reversible ischemic neurologic deficit

PRINS
> primed in situ labeling

PR interval
> onset of ventricular depolarization

PRISM
> Pediatric Risk of Mortality (Score)

PRIST
> paper radioimmunosorbent technique
> paper radioimmunosorbent test

priv
> private

PRK
> photorefractive keratectomy
> photorefractive keratoplasty
> primary rabbit kidney

PRL, Prl
> preferred retinal locus
> prolactin (*See also* P, PR, Pr)

PRLA
> pupils react to light and accommodation (*See also* PERRLA)

PRM
> partial rebreathing mask
> phosphoribomutase
> photoreceptor membrane
> prematurely ruptured membrane
> preventive medicine (*See also* PM, PrM, PVMed)
> Primary Reference Material
> primidone

PrM
> preventive medicine (*See also* PM, PRM, PVMed)

PRM-SDX, PRM-SOX
> pyrimethamine sulfadoxine

PRN, p.r.n.
> as needed [L. *pro re nata*]

PRNF
> primary nonfunction

PRO
> projection
> prolapse
> pronation (*See also* pron)
> protein (*See also* P, PR, Pr, prot)

PRO2000
> sulfonated polymer

Pro
> proline (*See also* P)

proANF
> proatrial natriuretic factor

prob
> probability
> probable
> problem

proc
> procedure
> proceeding
> process

proct, PROCTO, procto
> procotoscopic
> proctology
> proctoscopy

prod.
> product
> production

PROEF
> postoperative regimen for oral early feeding

Pro El
> protein electrophoresis

PROG
> progesterone
> prognathism
> program
> progressive

prog, progn
> prognosis (*See also* Prx, Px)

progr
> progress

prolong.
> prolongation
> prolonged

PROM
> passive range of motion
> prelabor rupture of the membranes
> premature rupture of (fetal) membranes (*See also* PRFM)
> programmable read-only memory
> prolonged rupture of (fetal) membranes (*See also* PRFM)

ProMACE-CytaBOM
> methotrexate

PROMIN
> programmable multiple ion monitor

PROMM
    proximal myotonic myopathy
Promy, PROMYEO
    promyelocyte
pron
    pronation (*See also* PRO)
    pronator (*See also* PRO)
PROP
    propranolol
PROP-1
    prophet of Pit-1 (gene)
proph, prop., prophy
    prophylactic
    prophylaxis
PROPLA
    prophospholipase A
pros, prostat
    prostate
    prostatic
PROSO
    protamine sulfate
PROST
    pronuclear stage transfer
    pronucleate stage embryo transfer
    pronucleate stage tubal transfer
PROSTALAC
    prosthetic antibiotic-loaded acrylic
    cement
prosth, PROS
    prosthesis
    prosthetic
prot
    protein (*See also* P, PR, Pr, PRO)
protime, pro time, pro-time
    prothrombin time (*See also* PT)
PROTO
    protoporphyrin
PROT REL
    protrusive relationship
prov
    provisional (diagnosis)
PROVIMI
    proteins, vitamins, and minerals
prox
    proximal
PRP
    panretinal photocoagulation
    patient recovery plan
    penicillinase-resistant penicillin
    penicillin-resistant pneumococci
    physiologic rest position
    pityriasis rubra pilaris

platelet-rich plasma
polymer of ribose phosphate
polyribophosphate
polyribosyl ribitol phosphate
polyribosylribitol phosphate
poor progression of R wave in
    precordial leads
postreplication repair
postural rest position
premenopausal hormone receptor
    positive
pressure rate product
problem reporting program
progressive rubella panencephalitis
proliferative retinopathy
    photocoagulation
Psychotic Reaction Profile
pulse repetition frequency
PrP
    prion protein
PrP^{Sc}
    prion protein scrapie isoform
PrP^c
    prion protein normal isoform
PRP-D
    polyribosylribitol phosphate-
    diphtheria toxoid conjugate
PRPP
    5-phospho-alpha-d-ribosyl
        pyrophosphate (*See also* PPRibp)
    5-phospho-α-d-ribosyl pyrophosphate
        (*See also* PPRibp)
    phosphoribosylpyrophosphate
PrP^{Sc}-reactive plaque
    prion protein scrapie isoform-
    reactive plaque
PRP-T
    polysaccharide tetanus conjugate
    vaccine
PRQ
    Personal Resource Questionnaire
PRR
    proton relaxation rate
    pulmonary reimplantation response
PRRE
    pupils round, regular, and equal
        (*See also* PERRL)
PRRERLA
    pupils round, regular, equal; react
    to light and accommodation (*See
    also* PEARLA, PERRLA)

NOTES

P

PR-RSV
Prague Rous sarcoma virus
PRS
parent's rating scale
Personality Rating Scale
photon-radiosurgical therapy
plasma renin substrate
positive rolandic spike
Prieto syndrome
prolonged respiratory support
pupil rating scale
PRSA
plasma renin substrate activity
PRSL
potential renal solute load
PRSM
peripheral smear
PRSP
penicillinase-resistant synthetic
penicillin
penicillin-resistant *Streptococcus
pneumoniae*
PRSs
positive rolandic spikes
PRSV
Prague strain Rous sarcoma virus
PRT
Pantomime Recognition Test
Penicillium roqueforti toxin
percutaneous rotational
thrombectomy
pharmaceutical research and testing
phosphoribosyltransferase (*See also*
PRTase)
phosphoribosyl transferase
photoradiation therapy
photostress recovery time
physiologic reflux test
Picture Reasoning Test
postoperative respiratory treatment
progressive relaxation training
protamine response test
psychotic trigger reaction
PRt
prospective randomized trial
PRTase
phosphoribosyltransferase (*See also*
PRT)
PRTCA
percutaneous rotational transluminal
coronary angioplasty
PRTH
pituitary resistance to thyroid
hormone
pituitary RTH
selective pituitary resistance to
thyroid hormone

PRTH-C
prothrombin (time) control (*See also*
PT-C)
PRTS
Partington syndrome
PRU
percent reduction in urea
peripheral resistance unit
PRUJ
proximal radioulnar joint
PRV
Paroo River virus
polycythemia rubra vera
pseudorabies virus
PRVA
peripheral vein renin activity
PRVC
pressure-regulated volume control
PRVEP
pattern reversal visual evoked
potential
PRVR
peak-to-resting-velocity ratio
PrVS
prevesicle space
PRW
past relevant work
polymerized ragweed
PRWP
poor R-wave progression
(electrocardiogram)
Prx
prognosis (*See also* prog, progn,
Px)
PRZ
prazepam
PRZF
pyrazofurin
PS
chloropicrin
pacemaker syndrome
paired stimulation
Palmaz-Schatz (stent) (*See also*
PSS)
pancreas sufficient
pancreozymin secretin
paradoxical sleep
paralaryngeal space
paranoid schizophrenia
paraseptal
parasternal
parasympathetic (division of
autonomic nervous system) (*See
also* parasym)
partial shoulder
pathologic stage
patient's serum

pediatric surgery (*See also* PDS, PdS)
performance status
performing scale (IQ)
periodic syndrome
peripheral smear
permeability surface
phosphate saline (buffer)
phosphatidylserine
photosynthesis
phrenic (nerve) stimulation
physical status
phytosterol
pigeon serum
plastic surgery (*See also* PSurg)
point of symmetry
polysaccharide
polystyrene
polysulfone (filter)
population sample
Porter-Silber (*See also* PSC)
postcardiotomy shock
posterior synechiae
posterior synechiotomy
postmaturity syndrome
pregnancy serum
prescription
pressure sore
pressure support
prestimulus
primary stem
principal sulcus
prognostic score
programmed symbols
prostatic secretion
protamine sulfate
protective services
protein synthesis
Proteus syndrome
psychiatric (*See also* psychiat)
pulmonary sequestration
pulmonary stenosis
pulmonic stenosis
pulse sequence
pyloric stenosis
pyrimethamine; sulfadoxine

PS I
healthy patient with localized pathological process

PS II
a patient with mild to moderate systemic disease

PS III
a patient with severe systemic disease limiting activity but not incapacitating

PS IV
a patient with incapacitating systemic disease

P-S
pancreozymin-secretin
pyramid surface

P/S
polisher-stimulator
polyunsaturated-to-saturated fatty acids ratio

P&S
pain and suffering
paracentesis and suction
permanent and stationary
pharmacy and supply

Ps
prescription
pseudocyst

ps
per second
picosecond (*See also* psec)

PSA
pathologic spontaneous activity
picryl sulfonic acid
Pisum sativum agglutinin
polyethylene sulfonic acid
polysubstance abuse
power spectral analysis
procedural sedation and analgesia
product selection allowed
progressive spinal ataxia
prolonged sleep apnea
proportion of survivors affected
prostate-specific antigen
public service announcement

PsA
psoriatic arthritis

Psa
systemic blood pressure (*See also* SBP)

PSA-ACT
prostate-specific antigen bound to alpha-1 antichymotrypsin

PSAD
prostate-specific antigen density
PSA density

NOTES

P

PSAD *(continued)*
> psychoactive substance abuse and dependence

PSADT
> prostate-specific antigen doubling time

PSAG
> *Pseudomonas aeruginosa*

PSAGN
> poststreptococcal acute glomerulonephritis

PSAN
> psychoanalyst

PSAn
> psychoanalysis
> psychoanalytic

PSAP
> peak systolic aortic pressure
> prostate-specific acid phosphatase

PSA-TZ
> prostate-specific antigen transition zone

PSAV
> prostate-specific antigen velocity
> PSA velocity

PSAX
> parasternal short axis

PSB
> patellar stabilizing brace
> protected specimen brush
> protected specimen brushing

PSBO
> partial small bowel obstruction

PSC
> partial subligamentous calcification
> patient services coordination
> Pediatric Symptom Checklist
> percutaneous suprapubic cystostomy
> physiologic squamocolumnar
> pigmented spindle cell
> pluripotential stem cell
> Porter-Silber chromogen (*See also* PS)
> posterior semicircular canal
> posterior subcapsular cataract (*See also* PSCC)
> primary sclerosing cholangitis
> pronation spring control
> propagated sensation along the channel
> pubosacrococcygeal (diameter)
> pulse-synchronized contractions

PSCA
> proximal subcontact area

PSCC
> posterior subcapsular cataract (*See also* PSC)

P450SCC
> P450 side chain cleavage

PSC Cat
> posterior subcapsular cataract

PSCE
> presurgical coagulation evaluation

PSCH
> peripheral stem cell harvest

PsChE
> pseudocholinesterase

PSCI
> Primary Self-Concept Inventory

Psci
> pressure at slow component intercept

PSCM
> pokeweed activated spleen conditioned medium

PSCN
> plexiform spindle cell nevus

P/score
> pressure score

PSCP
> papillary serous carcinoma of the peritoneum
> posterior subcapsular cataractous plaque
> posterior subcapsular precipitates

PSCT
> peripheral stem cell transplant

PSCU
> pediatric special care unit

PSD
> particle size distribution
> pediatric spectrum of disease
> peptone-starch-dextrose
> percutaneous stricture dilatation
> periodic synchronous discharge
> phosphate supplemental diet
> photon-stimulated desorption
> pilonidal sinus disease
> pituitary stalk distortion
> pneumosinus dilatans
> posterior sagittal diameter
> poststenotic dilation
> poststroke depression
> postsynaptic density
> power spectral density
> psychosomatic disease

PSDES
> primary symptomatic diffuse esophageal spasm

PSDI
> Positive Symptom Distress Index

PSDK
> poststatic dyskinesia

PSDS
> palmar surface desensitization

PSE
    paradoxical systolic expansion
    partial splenic embolization
    penicillin-sensitive enzyme
    Pidgin Sign English
    point of subjective equality
    portal-systemic encephalopathy
    portosystemic encephalopathy
    postshunt encephalopathy
    preparticipation sports examination
    Present State Examination
    pseudoephedrine
    purified spleen extract

PSEC
    poststress ethanol (alcohol)
        consumption

psec
    picosecond (*See also* ps)

PSEK
    progressive symmetric
        erythrokeratodermia

pseudoPHP
    pseudopseudohypoparathyroidism

pseudo POHS
    pseudopresumed ocular
        histoplasmosis syndrome

PSF
    peak scatter factor
    point spread function
    posterior spinal fusion
    posterior spine fusion
    prostacyclin-stimulating factor
    pseudosarcomatous fasciitis

psf
    pound per square foot

PSFMT
    pseudosarcomatous fibromyxoid
        tumor

PSFR
    pancreatic secretory flow rate
    peak secretory flow rate

PSG
    peak systolic gradient
    phosphate, saline, glucose
    polysomnogram
    polysomnograph
    polysomnography
    portosystemic gradient
    presystolic gallop

PSGN
    poststreptococcal glomerulonephritis

PSH
    past surgical history
    postspinal (anesthetic) headache

P&SH
    personal and social history

PSH II
    Physicians' Health Study II

PsHD
    pseudoheart disease

PSHx
    past surgical history

ψ, psi
    psi (23rd letter of Greek alphabet),
        lowercase
    wave function

Ψ
    pseudouridine (*See also* Q)
    psi (23rd letter of Greek alphabet),
        uppercase
    psychology

PSI
    Parental Stress Index
    Parenting Stress Index
    Pediatric Speech Intelligibility Test
    pelvic support index
    personal security index
    Personal Style Inventory
    physiologic stability index
    Pneumonia Severity Index
    portal shunt index
    posterior sagittal index
    posterior superior iliac (spine) (*See
        also* PSIS)
    postponing sexual involvement
    pound per square inch
    Predictive Salvage Index
    problem solving information
    prostaglandin synthetic inhibitor
    Psychological Screening Inventory
    psychosomatic inventory
    punctate subepithelial infiltrate

psi, p.s.i.
    pounds per square inch

psia
    pounds per square inch absolute

PSIC
    pediatric surgical intensive care

pSIDS
    partially unexplained sudden infant
        death syndrome

NOTES

P

PSIF

reverse fast imaging with steady-state free precession

PSIFT

platelet suspension immunofluorescence test

psig

pounds per square inch gauge

PSIL

percentage signal intensity loss
preferred frequency speech interference level

PSIS

posterior sacroiliac spine
posterior superior iliac spine (*See also* PSI)

PSK

polysaccharide Kreha

p70S6k

protein 70-kDa S6 ribosomal subunit kinase

PSL

parasternal line
percent stroke length
potassium, sodium chloride, and sodium lactate (solution)

PSLL

pancreatoscopic laser lithotripsy

PSLT

Picture Story Language Test

PSM

polysomnogram
presystolic murmur
propagated sensation along the meridian
prostate-specific membrane

PSMA

personal self-maintenance activities
progressive spinal muscular atrophy
prostate-specific membrane antigen
proximal spinal muscular atrophy

PSMed

psychosomatic medicine (*See also* PsychosMed)

PSMF

protein-sparing modified fast

PSM-R

Optimism-Pessimism Scale, revised

PSMS

Physical Self Maintenance Scale

PSN

pontosubicular neuron necrosis

PSNP

progressive supranuclear palsy

PSNS

parasympathetic nervous system

PSO

pelvic stabilization orthosis

physician supplemental order
physostigmine salicylate ophthalmic
Polysporin ointment
proximal subungual onychomycosis

pSO2

arterial oxygen saturation

PsoE

erythrodermic psoriasis

Psol

partly soluble

PSOR

psoralen

P/sore

pressure sore

PSP

pacesetter potential (*See also* PP)
pancreatic spasmolytic peptide
pancreatic stone protein
paralytic shellfish poisoning
parathyroid secretory protein
periodic short pulse
persephin
Personnel Security Preview
phenolsulfonphthalein (phenol red)
photostimulable phosphor dental radiography
pigeon serum protein
positive spike pattern
post space preparation
postsynaptic potential
primary spontaneous pneumothorax
professional simulated patient
progressive supranuclear palsy
pseudopregnancy

psp

posterior subcapsular plaque

PSPDV

posterior superior pancreaticoduodenal vein

PSPF

prostacyclin synthesis-stimulating plasma factor

PSPUMP

prostatic stromal proliferation of uncertain malignant potential

PSQ

Parent Symptom Questionnaire
patient satisfaction questionnaire
Personal Strain Questionnaire

PSR

(extrahepatic) portal-systemic resistance
pain sensitivity range
percutaneous stereotactic radiofrequency (rhizotomy)
point-spread function
problem status report
proliferative sickle retinopathy

Psychiatric Status Rating (scale)
pulmonary stretch receptor

PSRA

poststreptococcal reactive arthritis
pressure sore risk assessment

PSRBOW

premature spontaneous rupture of
bag of waters

PSReA

poststreptococcal reactive arthritis

PSRI

Professional Sexual Role Inventory

PSROM

preterm spontaneous rupture of
membranes

PSRS

Process Skills Rating Scale

PSRT

photostress recovery test

PSS

painful shoulder syndrome
Palmaz-Schatz stent (*See also* PS)
pediatric surgical service
Peritonitis Severity Score
physiologic saline solution
physiologic salt solution
porcine stress syndrome
portosystemic shunting
primary Sjögren syndrome
progressive systemic scleroderma
progressive systemic sclerosis
psoriasis severity scale
psychiatric services section
Psychiatric Status Schedule
pure sensory stroke
pure sensory syndrome
quantitative sacroiliac scintigraphy

PSSE

partial saturation spin echo

PSS-HN

performance status scale for head
and neck cancer

PSS:NICU

Parental Stressor Scale: Neonatal
Intensive Care Unit

PSSP

penicillin-sensitive *Streptococcus
pneumoniae*

PST

pancreatic suppression test
paroxysmal supraventricular
tachycardia

Pascal-Suttle Test (psychiatry)
penicillin, streptomycin, tetracycline
perceptual span time
peristimulus time
phenolsulfotransferase
phonemic segmentation test
platelet survival time
positive symptom total
poststenotic
poststimulus time
posttransfusion hepatitis
postural stimulation test
postural stress test
prefrontal sonic treatment
promontory stimulation test
protein-sparing therapy
proximal straight tubule

PSTH

poststimulus time histogram
poststimulus time histograph

PSTI

pancreatic secretory trypsin inhibitor

PSTO

Purdue Student-Teacher
Opinionnaire

PSTP

pentasodium triphosphate

PSTT

placental site trophoblastic tumor

PSTV

potato spindle tuber viroid

PSU

pediatric sedation unit
photosynthetic unit
postsurgical unit
primary sampling unit
pseudomonas (*P. aeruginosa*)
vaccine

PSUD

psychoactive substance use disorder

PSUR

periodic safety update reporting

PSurg, P-Surg

plastic surgery (*See also* PS)

PSV

peak systolic velocity
positive support ventilator
pressure supported ventilation
pressure support ventilation
primary systemic vasculitides
primary systemic vasculitis

NOTES

P

PSV *(continued)*
    psychological, social, and vocational (adjustment factors)
    Punta Salinas virus
PS V
    physical status patient classifications. Emergency operations are designated by E after the classification.)
PSVER
    pattern-shift visual-evoked response
PsV-F
    Penicillium stoloniferum F virus
PsV-S
    Penicillium stoloniferum S virus
PSVT
    paroxysmal supraventricular tachycardia
PSW
    past sleepwalker
    primary surgical ward
    psychiatric social worker
PSWC
    periodic sharp wave complex
PSWF
    positive sharp wave fibrillations (electromyograph)
PSWL
    peroral shock wave lithotripsy
PSX
    pseudoexfoliation
PSY, Psy
    presexual youth
    psychiatry (*See also* P, PS, psychiat)
    psychology (*See also* psych, psychol)
psych
    pscyhiatry (*See also* psychol)
    psychologic (*See also* psychol)
    psychology (*See also* psychol, PSY)
psychiat
    psychiatric (*See also* P, PS, Psy)
    psychiatry (*See also* P, PS, Psy)
psychoan
    psychoanalysis
    psychoanalytical
psychol
    psychologic
    psychology (*See also* PSY, psych)
psychopath.
    psychopathic
    psychopathologic
    psychopathology
PsychosMed
    psychosomatic medicine (*See also* PSMed)

psychother
    psychotherapeutic
    psychotherapy
psy-path
    psychopathic (*See also* psychopath.)
PSZ
    pseudoseizure
ps-ZES
    pseudo-Zollinger-Ellison syndrome
PT
    parathormone (*See also* PTH)
    parathyroid (*See also* para, PTH)
    paroxysmal tachycardia
    patient (*See also* P, PNT, Pt, pt)
    pericardial tamponade
    permanent and total
    pertussis toxin
    pertussis toxoid
    pharmacy and therapeutics
    phenytoin
    phonation time
    phosphotransferase
    photophobia
    phototoxicity
    physical therapist
    physical therapy (*See also* Phys Ther)
    physical training
    physiotherapy
    pine tar
    pint (*See also* P, p, pt)
    plasma thromboplastin
    pluridirectional tomography
    pneumothorax (*See also* pnx, PTX, Px)
    polyvalent tolerance
    posterior tibial
    posterior tibial (artery pulse)
    posttransplantation
    preterm
    primary thrombocythemia
    pronator teres
    propylthiouracil
    prothrombin time (*See also* protime)
    protriptyline
    proximal tubule
    pulmonary thrombosis
    pulmonary toilet
    pulmonary trunk
    pulmonary tuberculosis (*See also* PTB)
    pure tone (audiometry)
    pyramidal tract
    temporal plane
P1/2T
    pressure one-half time

P/T
- pain and tenderness
- piperacillin/tazobactam (Zosyn)

P&T
- paracentesis and tubing (of ears)
- peak and trough
- permanent and total
- pharmacy and therapeutics

P$_T$
- total pressure

Pt
- patient (*See also* P, PNT, PT, pt)
- platinum
- psychasthenia

pt
- part (*See also* P)
- patient (*See also* P, PNT, PT, Pt)
- pint (*See also* P, p, PT)
- point

PTA
- pancreas transplant alone
- pancreas transplantation alone
- pancreatic transplantation alone
- parathyroid adenoma
- patellar tendon autograft
- percutaneous transluminal angioplasty (*See also* PTAB)
- peritonsillar abscess
- persistent trigeminal artery
- persistent truncus arteriosus
- phosphotungstic acid
- physical therapy assistant
- plasma thromboplastin antecedent
- platelet thromboplastin antecedent
- posttraumatic amnesia
- pretreatment anxiety
- primitive trigeminal artery
- prior to admission
- prior to arrival
- prothrombin activity
- pure tone acuity
- pure tone average (*See also* PT(A))

PT(A)
- pure tone average (*See also* PTA)

PTAB
- popliteal-tibial artery bypass
- pterygoalar bar

PTAF
- policy target adjustment factor

P-TAG
- target-attaching globulin precursor

PTAH
- phosphotungstic acid-hematoxylin (stain)

PTAP
- purified (diphtheria) toxoid (precipitated by) aluminum phosphate

PTARF
- posttraumatic acute renal failure

PTAS
- percutaneous transluminal angioplasty with stent placement
- percutaneous transluminal angioscopy

PTB
- patellar tendon-bearing (cast prosthesis)
- phosphotyrosine-binding domain
- pretibial bearing
- pretibial buttress
- prior to birth
- pulmonary tuberculosis (*See also* PT)

PTBA
- percutaneous transluminal balloon angioplasty (*See also* PTA)

PTBD
- percutaneous transhepatic biliary drainage
- percutaneous transluminal balloon dilatation

PTBD-EF
- percutaneous transhepatic biliary drainage-enteric feeding

PTBE
- pyretic tick-borne encephalitis

PTBNA
- protected transbronchial needle aspirate

PTBO
- patellar tendon-bearing orthosis

PTBP
- *para*-tertiary butylphenol

PTBS
- patellar tendon-bearing suspension
- posttraumatic brain syndrome

PTB-SC-SP
- patellar tendon-bearing–supracondylar-suprapatellar (prosthesis)

NOTES

P

655

PT-C

prothrombin time control (*See also* PRTH-C)

PTC

papillary thyroid carcinoma
patient to call
percutaneous transhepatic cholangiogram
percutaneous transhepatic cholangiography
peritubular capillary
phase transfer catalyst
phenylthiocarbamide
phenylthiocarbamoyl
pheochromocytoma, thyroid carcinoma (syndrome)
plasma thromboplastin component
post-tetanic count
premature tricuspid closure
primary thymic carcinoma
prior to conception
prothrombin complex
pseudotumor cerebri
pulmonary tissue concentration

PTCA

percutaneous transhepatic cholangiogram (*See also* PTHC)
percutaneous transhepatic cholangiography (*See also* PTHC)
percutaneous transluminal coronary angioplasty
percutaneous transluminal coronary arteriography

PTCC

percutaneous transhepatic cholecystoscopy

PtcCO$_2$

transcutaneous carbon dioxide tension

PTCD

percutaneous transhepatic cholangio-drainage

PTCDLF

pregnancy, term, complicated delivered, living female

PTCDLM

pregnancy, term, complicated delivered, living male

PTCL

peripheral T-cell lymphoma
postthymic T-cell lymphoma

PTCP

pseudothrombocytopenia

PTCR

percutaneous transluminal coronary recanalization
percutaneous transluminal coronary revascularization

PTCRA

percutaneous transluminal coronary rotational ablation
percutaneous transluminal coronary rotational atherectomy

PTCS

percutaneous transhepatic cholangioscopy
Primary Test of Cognitive Skills

PTCSL

percutaneous transhepatic cholangioscopic lithotomy

PT-CT

prothrombin time control

PTD

para-toluenediamine
percutaneous thrombolytic device
percutaneous transhepatic drainage
percutaneous transluminal dilatation
percutaneous transpedicular diskectomy
period to discharge
permanent total disability
persistent trophoblastic disease
personality trait disorder
pharmacy to dose
photodynamic therapy
prevention and treatment of depression
prior to delivery
prior to discharge
psychotropic drug

Ptd

phosphatidyl

PtdCho

phosphatidylcholine

PtdEth, PtdEtn

phosphatidylethanolamine

PtdIns

phosphatidylinositol (*See also* PI)

PtdIns(4,5)P$_2$

phosphatidylinositol 4,5-bisphosphate

PTDM

posttransplant diabetes mellitus

PTDP

permanent transvenous demand pacemaker

PtdSer

phosphatidylserine

PTE

parathyroid extract
peritumoral edema
posttraumatic endophthalmitis
posttraumatic epilepsy
pretibial edema
proximal tibial epiphysis
pulmonary thromboembolectomy

pulmonary thromboembolism
pulmonary thromboendarterectomy

PTED

pulmonary thromboembolic disease

PTEF

peak tidal expiratory flow
time to peak tidal expiratory flow

PteGlu

pteroylglutamic (acid)

PTEN

pentaerythritol tetranitrate
phosphatase and tensin homologue
deleted on chromosome

PTER

percutaneous transluminal
endomyocardial revascularization

PTE-4(r)

trace metal elements injection

pter

end of short arm of chromosome

PTF

patient transfer form
patient treatment file
pentoxifylline
plasma thromboplastin factor
posterior talofibular
post-tetanic facilitation

PTFA

prothrombin time fixing agent

PTFE

polytetrafluorethylene
polytetrafluoroethylene

PTFL

posterior talofibular ligament

PTFS

posttraumatic fibromyalgia syndrome

PTG

parathyroid gland
photoplethysmogram

PTGA

pteroyltriglutamic acid

PTGBD

percutaneous transhepatic gallbladder
drainage

PTGC

progressive transformation of
germinal center

PTGDS

patellar tendon graft donor site

PTH

parathormone (*See also* PT)

parathyroid (*See also* para, PT)
parathyroid hormone (*See also* PH)
phenylthiohydantoin
plasma parathyroid hormone
plasma thromboplastin (component)
posttransfusion hepatitis
prior to hospitalization

PTh

primary thrombocythemia

Pth

chest wall elastic recoil pressure

PTHBD

percutaneous transhepatic biliary
drain(age)

PTHC

percutaneous transhepatic
cholangiogram (*See also* PTCA)
percutaneous transhepatic
cholangiography (*See also* PTCA)

PThHR

pituitary thyroid hormone resistance

PTH-LP

parathyroid hormonelike polypeptide

PTHR

pituitary thyroid hormone resistance

PTHRP, PTH-rP, PTHrP

parathyroid hormone-related peptide
parathyroid hormone-related protein
PTH-related protein

PTHS

parathyroid hormone secretion
parathyroid hormone secretion (rate)
posttraumatic hyperirritability
syndrome

PTHV

Pathum Thani virus

PTI

pancreatic trypsin inhibitor
persistent tolerant infection
Personnel Tests for Industry
Pictorial Test of Intelligence
pressure time index
pressure-time integral

PTIF

peak tidal inspiratory flow

PTJV

percutaneous transtracheal jet
ventilation

PTK

phototherapeutic keratectomy
protein tyrosine kinase

NOTES

P

PTL
> perinatal telencephalic leukoencephalopathy
> peripheral T-cell lymphoma
> pharyngeotracheal lumen
> pharyngotracheal lumen (airway)
> posterior tricuspid leaflet
> posterior tricuspid (valve) leaflet
> preterm labor
> protriptyline
> pudding-thick liquid (diet consistency)
> (sodium thiopental) Pentothal

PTLC
> precipitation thin-layer chromatography

PTLD, PTLPD, PT-LPD
> posttransplantation lymphoproliferative disease
> posttransplantation lymphoproliferative disorder
> posttransplant lymphoproliferative disease
> posttransplant lymphoproliferative disorder

PTM
> patient monitored
> posterior trabecular meshwork
> posttransfusion mononucleosis
> posttraumatic meningitis
> pressure time per minute
> preterm milk
> pretibial myxedema

Ptm
> pterygomaxillary (fissure)
> transmural pressure (airway, blood vessel)

PTMA
> phenyltrimethylammonium

PTMC
> percutaneous transvenous mitral commissurotomy

PTMDF
> pupils, tension, media, disc, and fundus

PTMR
> percutaneous (transluminal) myocardial revascularization
> percutaneous transmyocardial revascularization

PTN
> pain transmission neuron
> posterior tibial nerve

PT-NANB
> posttransfusion non-A, non-B (hepatitis)

PT-NANBH
> parenterally transmitted non-A non-B hepatitis

PTNB
> percutaneous transthoracic needle biopsy
> preterm newborn

pTNM
> pathological tumor, nodes, metastases (pathological staging of cancer)

PTN/MK
> pleiotrophin/midkine growth enhancer

PTO
> Klemperer tuberculin [Ger. *Perlsucht Tuberculin Original*]
> part-time occlusion (eye patch)
> percutaneous transhepatic obliteration
> personal time off
> please turn (the patient) over
> proximal tubal obstruction
> Purdue Teacher Opinionnaire

P to P
> point to point

PTP
> percutaneous transhepatic portography
> Physical Tolerance Profile
> posterior tibial pulse
> posttetanic potentiation
> posttransfusion purpura
> pressure time product
> prior to program
> prothrombin-proconvertin
> proximal tubular pressure
> pseudothrombophlebitis

Ptp
> transpulmonary pressure

PTPI
> posttraumatic pulmonary insufficiency

PTPM
> posttraumatic progressive myelopathy

PTPN
> peripheral (vein) total parenteral nutrition

PTPS
> postthrombophlebitis syndrome

PT-PTT
> prothrombin time and partial thromboplastin time

PTQ
> Parent-Teacher Questionnaire
> Purdue Teacher Questionnaire

PTR

paratesticular rhabdomyosarcoma
patella tendon reflex
patient to return
patient termination record
peripheral total resistance
pressure transmission ratio
prothrombin time ratio
psychotic trigger reaction
tuberculin *Mycobacterium tuberculosis bovis* [Ger. *Perlsucht Tuberculin Rest*]

PTr

porcine trypsin

PTRA

percutaneous transluminal renal angioplasty
percutaneous transluminal rotational atherectomy

PTRIA

polystyrene-tube radioimmunoassay

PTRTH

peripheral tissue resistance to thyroid hormone

Ptrx

pelvic traction

PTS

painful tonic seizure
para-toluenesulfonic (acid)
patellar tendon socket
patellar tendon stabilization
patellar tendon suspension
patella tendon socket
Pediatric Trauma Scale
Pediatric Trauma Score
permanent threshold shift
phosphotransferase system
postthrombotic syndrome
posttraumatic syndrome
prior to surgery

6-PTS

6-pyruvoyltetrahydropterin synthase

pts

patients

PTSD

posttraumatic stress disorder

PTSMA

percutaneous transluminal septal myocardial ablation

PTSS

posttraumatic signs or symptoms

PTT

partial thromboplastin time
particle transport time
patellar tendon transfer
platelet transfusion therapy
posterior tibial tendinitis
posterior tibial tendon
posterior tibial transfer
protein truncation testing
pulmonary transit time
pulse transmission time
pure tone threshold

PTT-CT

partial thromboplastin time control

PTTD

posterior tibial tendon dysfunction

PTTG

pituitary tumor transforming gene

PTTH

prothoracotropic hormone

PTTW

patient tolerated traction well

PTU

pain treatment unit
pregnancy, term, uncomplicated

PTUCA

percutaneous transluminal ultrasonic coronary angioplasty

PTUDLF

pregnancy, term, uncomplicated delivered, living female

PTUDLM

pregnancy, term, uncomplicated delivered, living male

P-TUMT

periurethral transurethral microwave thermotherapy

PTV

percutaneous transtracheal jet ventilation
planning target volume
posterior terminal vein
posterior tibial vein
Punta Toro virus

PTVV

Ponteves virus

PTWTKG

patient's weight in kilograms

PTX

pancreas transplant
parathyroidectomy (*See also* PTx)
pelvic traction

NOTES

P

PTX *(continued)*
> pentoxifylline
> phototherapy
> phototoxic reaction
> picrotoxinin
> pneumothorax (*See also* pnx, PT, Px)

PTx
> parathyroidectomy (*See also* PTX)
> pelvic traction

PTXA
> parathyroidectomy and autotransplantation

PTZ
> pentamethylenetetrazole
> pentylenetetrazol
> phenothiazine

PU
> passed urine
> paternal uncle
> pelvic-ureteric
> pelviureteral
> pepsin unit
> peptic ulcer
> polyurethane
> posterior urethra
> precursor uptake
> pregnancy urine
> prostatic urethra
> by way of urethra [L. *per urethra*]

Pu
> plutonium

PUA
> pelvic (examination) under anesthesia

PUB
> pubic

pub, publ
> public

PUBS
> percutaneous umbilical blood sampling
> purple urine bag syndrome

PUC
> pediatric urine collector

PUCV
> Puchong virus

PUD
> partial upper denture
> peptic ulcer disease
> percutaneous ureteral dilatation
> pulmonary disease (*See also* PD, PuD)

PuD
> pulmonary disease (*See also* PD, PUD)

PUE
> pyrexia of unknown etiology

PUF
> polyurethane film
> polyurethane foam
> pure ultrafiltration

PUFA
> polyunsaturated fatty acid

PUFFA
> polyunsaturated free fatty acid

PUH
> pregnancy urine hormone

PUI
> posterior urethral injury

PUK
> peripheral ulcerative keratitis

PUL, pul
> percutaneous ultrasonic lithotripsy
> pubourethral ligament
> pulmonary (*See also* P, pulm)

pulm
> gruel [L. *pulmentum*]
> pulmonary (*See also* P, PUL, pul)
> pulmonic

PULP
> pulpotomy

Pulse A
> pulse apical

PULSE OX, pulsox
> pulse oximetry

Pulse R
> pulse radial

PULSES
> (general) physical, upper extremities, lower extremities, sensory, excretory, social support (physical profile)

PUN
> plasma urea nitrogen

PUND
> pregnancy, uterine, not delivered
> pregnancy uterine, undelivered

PUNL
> percutaneous ultrasonic nephrolithotripsy

PUO
> pyrexia of undetermined origin
> pyrexia of unknown origin

PUP
> percutaneous ultrasonic pyelolithotomy

PU-PC
> polyunsaturated phosphatidylcholine

PU/PL
> partial upper and lower dentures

PUPP
> pruritic urticarial papules and plaques

PUPPP
   pruritic urticarial papules and
     plaques of pregnancy
PUR
   polyurethane
Pur
   purine
   purple
purg
   purgative
PURV
   Purus virus
PUS
   percutaneous ureteral stent
   preoperative ultrasound
PUSH
   Pressure Ulcer Scale for Healing
PUT
   provocative use test
   putamen
   putrescine
PUU
   Puumala hantavirus
PUUV
   Puumala virus
PUV
   positive ulnar variance
   posterior urethral valve (type I–IV)
PUVA
   photochemotherapy with oral
     methoxypsoralen therapy followed
     by UVA
   psoralen plus ultraviolet light of A
     wavelength
   pulsed ultraviolet actinotherapy
PUVD
   pulsed ultrasonic (blood) velocity
     detector
PUVT
   paraumbilical vein tumor
PUW
   pick-up walker
PV
   pancreatic vein
   papillomavirus
   paraventricular
   Parvovirus
   pemphigus vulgaris
   peripheral vascular
   peripheral vein (See also PeV)
   peripheral vessel
   per vagina

   phonation volume
   photovoltaic
   pinocytotic vesicle
   pityriasis versicolor
   plasma viscosity
   plasma volume
   pneumococcus vaccine
   polio vaccine
   polycythemia vera (See also PCV)
   polyoma virus
   polyvinyl
   popliteal vein
   portal vein
   postvasectomy
   postvoiding
   predictive value
   prenatal vitamins
   pressure-volume
   projectile vomiting
   pulmonary vein
   pulmonic valve
   pure vegetarian
   by way of vagina [L. per
     vaginam]
P-V
   Paton-Valentine (leukocidin)
   pressure-volume (curve)
P/V
   pressure-to-volume (ratio)
P&V
   peak and valley
   percuss and vibrate
   pyloroplasty and vagotomy
Pv
   venous pressure (See also VP)
PVA
   partial villous atrophy
   Personal Values Abstract
   polyvinyl alcohol (fixative)
   polyvinyl alcohol foam
   Prinzmetal variant angina
   ventricular pseudoaneurysm
PVAB
   postventricular atrial blanking
PVAc
   polyvinyl acetate
PVAD
   prolonged venous access devices
PVAM
   potential visual acuity meter
PVAR
   pulmonary vein atrial reversal

NOTES

P

661

PVARP
postventricular atrial refractory
period

PVAS
postvasectomy (specimen)

PVB
paravertebral block
pigmented villonodular bundle
porcelain veneer bridge
premature ventricular beat

PVBS
possible vertebrobasilar system

PVC
persistent vaginal cornification
polyethylene vacuum cup
polyvinyl chloride
porcelain veneer crown
postvoiding cystogram
predicted vital capacity
premature ventricular contraction
primary visual cortex
pulmonary venous capillary
pulmonary venous congestion

PVCI
portal vein congestive index

PVCM
paradoxical vocal cord motion

Pvco2, Pv$_{CO2}$
partial pressure of carbon dioxide
in mixed venous blood
partial pressure (tension) of carbon
dioxide, vein

PVD
patient very disturbed
percussion, vibration, and drainage
peripheral vascular disease
peripheral vestibular deficit
portal vein dilation
posterior vitreal detachment
posterior vitreous detachment
postural vertical dimension
postvagotomy diarrhea
premature ventricular depolarization
pulmonary valve dysplasia
pulmonary vascular disease

PVDF
polyvinylidene difluoride

PVE
perivenous encephalomyelitis
periventricular echogenicity
premature ventricular extrasystole
prosthetic valve endocarditis

PVEL
periventricular echolucency

PVEP
pattern visual evoked potential

PVER
pattern visual evoked response

P vera
polycythemia vera

PVF
peripheral visual field
portal venous flow
primary ventricular fibrillation
pulmonary venous flow

PVFD
paradoxical vocal fold dysfunction

PVFS
postviral fatigue syndrome

PVG
periventricular gray matter
pulmonary valve gradient

PVGM
perifoveolar vitreoglial membrane

PVH
periventricular hemorrhage
periventricular hyperintensity
persistent viral hepatitis
pulmonary vascular hypertension

PVH-B
persistent viral hepatitis, type B

PVH-NANB
persistent viral hepatitis, non-A,
non-B

PVI
pelvic venous incompetence
peripheral vascular insufficiency
periventricular inhibitor
Personal Values Inventory
portal vein infusion
protracted venous infusion

PVK
penicillin V potassium

P-VL
Panton-Valentine leukocidin

PVL
peripheral vascular laboratory
perivalvular leakage
periventricular leukomalacia
periventricular radiolucency
plasma viral load
proliferative verrucous leukoplakia

PVM
parallel virtual machine
paravertebral muscle
pneumonia virus of mice
proteins, vitamins, and minerals

PVMed
preventive medicine (*See also* PM,
PRM, PrM)

PVMS
paravertebral muscle spasm

PVMT
Primary Visual Motor Test

PVN
paraventricular nucleus

peripheral venous nutrition
predictive value of a negative
(test)

PVNPS

post-Vietnam psychiatric syndrome

PVNS

pigmented villonodular synovitis
pigmented villonodular
tenovagosynovitis

PVO

peripheral vascular occlusion
portal vein obstruction
portal vein occlusion
pulmonary vascular obstruction
pulmonary venous obstruction
pulmonary venous occlusion

PVo

pulmonary valve opening

PvO2, Pvo2

partial pressure (tension) of
oxygen, vein
partial venous gas tension of
oxygen

Pv$_{O2}$

partial oxygen pressure in mixed
venous blood

PVOD

peripheral vascular occlusive
disease
pulmonary vascular obstructive
disease
pulmonary venoocclusive disease

PVP

penicillin V potassium
peripheral vein plasma
peripheral venous pressure
polyvidone
polyvinylpyrrolidone (povidone)
portal venous phase
portal venous pressure
posteroventral pallidotomy
predictive value of a positive (test)
pulmonary venous pressure (*See
also* P$_L$)

PVPG

paravertebral paraganglioma

PVP-I

polyvinylpyrrolidone
(povidone)–iodine

PVR

paraventricular nuclear stratum
peripheral vascular resistance

perspective volume rendering
postvoiding residual
postvoid residual
proliferative vitreoretinopathy
prosthetic valve regurgitation
pulmonary vascular resistance
pulmonary venous redistribution
pulse value recording
pulse volume recorder
pulse volume recording

pVR

perspective volume rendering

PVRI

peripheral vascular resistance index
pulmonary vascular resistance index

PVS

Beery Picture Vocabulary Screening
paravesical space
percussion, vibration, and suction
peripheral vascular surgery
peripheral vascular system
peritoneovenous shunt
persistent vegetative state
persistent viral syndrome
pigmented villonodular synovitis
poliovirus sensitivity
polyvinyl sponge
portal venous sampling
premature ventricular systole
programmed ventricular stimulation
prosthetic valve stenosis
pulmonary vein stenosis
pulmonic valve stenosis

PVST

prevertebral soft tissue

PVT

paraventricular thalamic nucleus
paroxysmal ventricular tachycardia
Peabody Vocabulary Test
physical volume test
portal vein thrombosis
pressure, volume, temperature
previous trouble
primary ventricular tachycardia
private (patient) (*See also* pvt)
proximal vein thrombosis

pvt

private (patient) (*See also* PVT)

PVTT

portal vein tumor thrombus
tumor thrombus in the portal vein

NOTES

P

PVV

persistent varicose veins
portal venous velocity

PVW

posterior vaginal wall

PW

pacing wire
patient waiting
peristaltic wave
plantar wart
posterior wall
posterior wall (of heart)
psychological warfare
pulmonary wedge (pressure)
pulsed wave
pulse width
puncture wound

P&W

pressures and waves

Pw

progesterone withdrawal

PWA

people with acquired
immunodeficiency syndrome
person with AIDS

P wave

part of the electrocardio-graphic
cycle representing atrial
depolarization

PWB

partial weightbearing
Positive Well-being (scale)
psychologic wellbeing
Puno-Winter-Byrd (spine fixation
system)

PWBC

peripheral white blood cell

PWBL

partial weight bearing, left

PWBR

partial weight bearing, right

PWBRT

prophylactic whole brain radiation
therapy

PWC

peak work capacity
physical work capacity

PWCA

personal watercraft accident

PWD

patients with diabetes
person(s) with a disability
precipitated withdrawal diarrhea
pulsed-wave Doppler

pwd

powder (*See also* pdr, powd)

PWE

people with epilepsy
posterior wall excursion

PWI

pediatric walk-in clinic
perfusion-weighted (magnetic
resonance) imaging
posterior wall infarct

PWLV

posterior wall of left ventricle

PWM

pokeweed mitogen

PWMI

posterior wall myocardial infarction

PWO

persistent withdrawal occlusion

PWP

pulmonary wedge pressure (*See also*
Ppw)

PWS

port-wine stain
pulse-wave speed

PWT

posterior wall thickness

pwt

pennyweight

PWTD

pulsed-wave tissue Doppler

PWTd

posterior wall thickness at end-
diastole

PWV

peak weight velocity
Polistes wasp venom
posterior wall velocity
pulse wave velocity

PX

pancreatectomized
peroxidase
physical examination (*See also* PE,
PEx, Px)

Px

past history (*See also* PH)
physical examination (*See also* PE,
PEx, PX)
pneumothorax (*See also* pnx, PT,
PTX)
prognosis (*See also* prog, progn,
Prx)
prophylaxis

PXA

pleomorphic xanthoastrocytoma

PXAT

paroxysmal atrial tachycardia

PXE

pseudoxanthoma elasticum

PXF

pseudoexfoliation

PXM
projection x-ray microscopy
PXS
dental prophylaxis (cleaning)
pseudoexfoliation syndrome (*See also* PES)
PXT
piroxantrone
PY, P/Y
pack-year (cigarettes)
person-year
Py
phosphopyridoxal
polyoma (virus)
pyrene
pyridine
PYA
psychoanalysis (*See also* PA)
PYC
proteose-yeast castione (medium)
PyC
pyogenic culture
PYD
pyridinium
pyridinoline
PYE
peptone-yeast extract
person-years of exposure
PYG
peptone-yeast(extract)-glucose (broth)
PYGM
peptone-yeast-glucose-maltose (broth)
PYHx
packs per year history
PYLL
potential years of life lost
PYM
psychosomatic
PYP
pyrophosphate (*See also* PP, Pyro)
PYP(r)
technetium Tc 99m pyrophosphate kit
PYR
person-year rad
pyrrolidonyl arylamidase
PyR
L-pyrrolidonyl-beta-naphthylamide
Pyr
pyridine

pyrimidine
pyroglutamic acid
pyruvate
Pyro
pyrophosphate (*See also* PP, PYP)
pyro-Glu-His-Pro-amide
pyroglutamyl-histidyl-prolineamide
PyrP
pyridoxal phosphate
PYS
pyriform sinus
PYY
peptide YY
PZ
pancreozymin
peripheral zone
prazosin
pregnancy zone
proliferative zone
Pz
parietal midline (zero) electrode placement in electroencephalography
pz
pieze (unit of pressure)
PZA
pyrazinamide
pyrazoloacridine (a drug class of sidatine/hyponotics)
PzB
parenzyme, buccal
PZ-CCK
pancreozymin-cholecystokinin
PZD
partial zona dissection
partial zona drilling
partial zonal dissection
piperazinedione
PZE
piezoelectric
Pzf
zero-flow pressure
PZI
protamine zinc insulin
PZM
pressure zone microphone
PZP
pregnancy zone protein

NOTES

P

Q

cardiac output (*See also* CO)
clerical perception
clerical perception (General
  Aptitude Test Battery)
coenzyme Q. (ubiquinone) (*See also*
  CoQ)
coulomb (*See also* C, coul)
each, every [L. *quaque*] (*See also*
  q)
electrocardiographic wave
1,4-glucan branching enzyme
glutamine (*See also* Gln)
perfusion (flow)
pseudouridine
Quaalude
quadriceps
quantitative (*See also* qt, quant)
quantitative test
quantity (of heat)
quart (*See also* q, qt)
quarter (*See also* q, qr)
quartile
quaternary
question (*See also* quest.)
quinacrine (fluorescent method)
quinidine
quinone
quotient
radiant energy
reaction energy
reactive power
volume of blood flow

Q-6, Q$_6$, -Q$_6$

ubiquinone-6
ubiquinone-Q$_6$

Q$_9$

ubichromenol-9

Q$_{10}$, -Q$_{10}$

temperature coefficient
ubiquinone-50

Q°, q°

every hour

Q̇

blood flow (*See also* B, Q$_B$)

Q1°

every hour around the clock

Q2°

every two hours around the clock

q

each, every [L. *quaque*] (*See also*
  Q)
electric charge
four [L. *quattuor*]

frequency of rarer allele of a gene
  pair
long arm of chromosome
quantity (*See also* Q, qt, qty,
  quant)
quart (*See also* Q, qt)
quarter (*See also* Q, qr)
quintal
quodque
volume (*See also* V, vol)

q.

each
every

QA

quality assessment
quality assurance
quinaldic acid
quisqualic acid

QAC

before every meal
quaternary ammonium compound

QAFT

quantitative autonomic functioning
  testing

QALE

quality-adjusted life expectancy

QALY

quality-adjusted life-years

QAM

quality assurance monitor

q.a.m.

every morning [L. *quaque ante
  meridiem*]

Q angle

Quatrefages angle (parietal angle)

Q-angle

quadriceps angle

QAP

quality assurance program
quinine, Atabrine (quinacrine
  hydrochloride), and pamaquine

QAR

quality assurance reagent
quantitative autoradiographic

QA/RM

quality assurance/risk management

QAS

quality-adjusted survival
quality assurance standards

QAT

quality assurance technical
  (material)

QAUR

quality assurance and utilization
  review

QB

Quantitative (Electrophysiological) Battery

whole blood (*See also* B, WB, W Bld)

Q$_B$

blood flow (*See also* BF, Q̇)

total body clearance (*See also* TBC)

QBC

quality buffy coat

quantitative buffy coat

QBCA

quantitative buffy-coat analysis

QBV

whole blood volume

QC

quad cane

quality control

quick catheter

quinine and colchicine

Qc

pulmonary capillary blood flow (perfusion)

QCA

quantitative coronary angiography

quantitative coronary arteriography

QCD

quantum chromodynamics

QCL

quadrigeminal cistern lipoma

Q$_{CO2}$

microliters of carbon dioxide given off per mg of dry weight of tissue per hour

Q compound

Chinese cucumber

QC-PCR

quantitative competitive PCR

quantitative competitive polymerase chain reaction

Q$_{CSF}$

rate of bulk flow of cerebrospinal fluid from cerebrospinal space by arachnoid villi uptake

QCT

quantified computed tomography

quantitative computed tomography

QCU

qualitative coronary ultrasound

QD

dialysate flow

every day [L. *quaque die*] (*See also* q.d.)

q.d.

every day [L. *quaque die*]

QDAM, q.d.a.m.

once daily in the morning

QDE

quantum detection efficiency

QDPM, q.d.p.m.

once daily in the evening

QDR

quantitative digital radiography

QDS

qigong deviation syndrome

QE

quinidine effect

QED

every even day

quantum electrodynamics

quick and early diagnosis

q.e.d.

that which is to be demonstrated [L. *quod erat demonstrandum*]

QEE

quadriceps extension exercise

QEEG

quantitative electroencephalogram

quantitative electroencephalography

QET

Quality Extinction Test

QEW

quick early warning

QF

quadratus femoris

quality factor (relative biologic effectiveness)

quick freeze

Qf

rate of fluid filtration

Q fever

Queensland (Australian) fever (*See also* QF)

Q fract

quick fraction

QFV

Q fever (*Coxiella burnetii*) vaccine

QGS

quantitative gated SPECT

Q-H$_2$

ubiquinol (*See also* H$_2$Q)

q.h.

every hour [L. *quaque hora*]

q.2h.

every two hours [L. *quaque secunda hora*]

q.3h.

every three hours [L. *quaque tertia hora*]

q.4h.

every four hours [L. *quaque quarta hora*]

QHS

at bedtime [L. *hora somni hour of sleep*]

Q

quantitative hepatobiliary scintigraphy

q.h.s.

each bedtime, every night [L. *quaque hora somni* every hour of sleep] (*See also* HS, h.s., QHS)
every night

QI

quality improvement

QIAD

Quantitative Inventory of Alcohol Disorders

QID

four times daily [L. *quater in die*] (*See also* q.i.d.)
Quantum inflation device

q.i.d.

four times daily [L. *quater in die*] (*See also* QID)
quater in die (four times a day)

QIE

quantitative immunoelectrophoresis

QIg

quantitative immunoglobulin

QJ

quadriceps jerk

QKD **interval**

Korotkoff sounds interval

QL

quality of life

QLF

quantitative light induced fluorescence

QLI

Quality of Life Index

QLQ

Quality of Life Questionnaire

QLQ-C30

Quality of Life Questionnaire-C30

QLS

Quality of Life Scale
quasielastic laser light-scattering spectroscope

qlty

quality

QM

quantization matrix
Quénu-Muret (sign)
quinacrine mustard

QMB

qualified Medicare beneficiary

QMI

Q-wave myocardial infarction

QMM

qigong meridian massage

QMT

quantitative muscle testing

QMV

quadricusp mitral valve

QMWS

quasimorphine withdrawal syndrome

QNA

quadriceps neutral angle

QNB

quinuclidinyl benzilate

QNS, q.n.s., qns

quantity not sufficient

QO_2, Q_{O2}

oxygen consumption
oxygen quotient
oxygen utilization

QOC

Quality of Contact

q.o.d.

every other day [L. *quaque altera die*]

QOL

quality of life

QOLI

Quality of Life Interview
Quality of Life Inventory

QOLIE-31

quality of life in epilepsy

QOM

quality of motion
quality of movement

QP

quadrant pain
quanti-Pirquet (reaction)

Qp

pulmonary blood flow (*See also* PBF)

QPC

quadrigeminal plate cistern
quality of patient care

Qpc

pulmonary capillary blood flow

QPCR, Q-PCR

quantitative polymerase chain reaction

QPD

quadrature phase detector

NOTES

QPEEG
quantitative pharmacoelectroencephalography

QPM, q.p.m.
each evening [L. *quaque post meridiem*]

QPOS
Quality Point of Service

QP/QS, Qp/Qs
flow ratio
left-to-right shunt ratio (electrocardiography)
pulmonary-to-systemic flow ratio
ratio of pulmonary to systemic circulation

QPT
quick prothrombin time

QPVT
Quick Picture Vocabulary Test

Q$_s$/Q$_t$
intrapulmonary shunt fraction

QQH, q.q.h.
every four hours [L. *quaque quarta hora*] (*See also* q.4h.)
United Kingdom abbreviation for every four hours

QR
quadriradial
quality review
Quick Recovery (Defibrillator)
quieting reflex
quieting response
quiet room
quinaldine red

Q.R.
quantity is correct [L. *quantum rectum*] (*See also* QR)

qr
quadriradial
quarter (*See also* Q, q)

QRB
Quality Review Bulletin

Q-RB
electrocardiographic time-wave interval

QRC
qualitative radiocardiography

QRE
quality-related event

QRN
quasiresonant nucleus

QRNG
quinolone-resistant *Neisseria gonorrhoeae*

QRS
electrocardiographic wave (complex or interval)

QRS-ST
electrocardiographic junction between QRS complex and ST segment

QRS-T
electrocardiographic angle between QRS and T vectors

QRZ
wheal reaction time [Ger. *Quaddel Reaktion Zeit*]

QS
every shift
Q-switched
quadriceps set
quadrilateral socket
quantitation standard
quantity sufficient
quiet sleep

QS2
total electromechanical systole

Qs
systemic blood flow

QSAC
quadrant sparing acetabular component

QSAR
quantitative structure-activity relationship

Q-SART
Quantitative Sudomotor Axon Reflex Test

QSART
quantitative sudomotor axon reflex test

QSC
quasistatic compliance

QS$_2$I
shortened electrochemical systole

Q sign
Quant sign

Qsp
physiologic shunt flow

QSPV
quasistatic pressure volume

Qs/Qt
intrapulmonary shunt fraction
intrapulmonary shunt ratio
right-to-left shunt ratio

Qsrel
relative shunt flow

QSRL
Q-switched ruby laser

QSS
quantitative sacroiliac scintigraphy

QST
Quantitative Sensory Testing

Q-S test
Queckenstedt-Stookey test

QSYAG
> Q-switched neodymium:YAG laser

Q-T
> electrocardiographic interval from the beginning of QRS complex to end of the T wave
> Quick Test (psychology, pregnancy, prothrombin)

QT$_c$ (*var. of* QTc)

Qt
> quiet (*See also* qt)

qt
> quantitative (*See also* Q, quant)
> quantity (*See also* Q, q, qty, quant)
> quart (*See also* Q, qt)
> quiet (*See also* Qt)

QTB
> quadriceps tendon bearing

QTC
> quantitative tip culture

QTc, QT$_c$
> QT corrected for heart rate

QTd
> QT dispersion

qter
> end of long arm of chromosome

QTL
> quantitative trait locus

Q-TWIST, Q-TWiST
> quality-adjusted time without symptoms (of disease) and toxicity
> quality-adjusted time without symptoms or toxicity

qty
> quantity (*See also* Q, q, qt, quant)

QU
> quiet

quad
> quadrant
> quadriceps
> quadrilateral
> quadriplegia
> quadriplegic

quad ex
> quadriceps exercise

quadrupl.
> four times as much [L. *quadruplicato*]

qual
> qualitative
> quality

qual anal
> qualitative analysis

QUALY
> quality adjusted life-year

QUALYS
> quality-adjusted life-year saved

quant
> quantitative (*See also* Q, qt)
> quantity (*See also* Q, q, qt, qty)

quar
> quarantine

QUART
> quadrantectomy, axillary dissection, radiation therapy

quart.
> fourth [L. *quartus*]
> quarterly

quasi-CW
> quasi-continuous wave

quats
> quaternary ammonium compounds

quer
> querulous

QUEST
> Quality of Upper Extremities Test
> Quality, Utilization, Effectiveness, Statistically Tabulated

quest.
> question (*See also* Q)
> questionable

QuICCC
> Questionnaire for Identifying Children with Chronic Conditions

QUICHA
> quantitative inhalation challenge apparatus

QUICKI
> quantitative insulin sensitivity check index

quint.
> fifth [L. *quintus*]

quotid.
> daily [L. *quotidie*]

QUS
> quantitative (bone) ultrasound
> quantitative ultrasound

q.v.
> which see (literature citation) [L. *quod vide*]

NOTES

QW
　　every week
　　quality of working (life) (*See also* QWL)

QWB
　　Quality of Well-Being (scale)

QWB-SA
　　Quality of Well-Being Scale Self-Administered

QWE
　　every weekend

q. 4 wk.
　　every four weeks

q. wk
　　once a week

QWL
　　quality of working life (*See also* QW)

QWMS
　　quantitative wall motion score

QYBV
　　Qalyub virus

QYD
　　Qi (and) Yin deficiency

QYS
　　Qingyangshen

R

arginine (*See also* Arg)
Behnken unit (of roentgen-ray exposure)
Broadbent registration point
drug-resistant plasmid
electrocardiographic wave in QRS complex
far point [L. *remotum*] (*See also* r)
gas constant (8.315 joules)
metabolic respiratory quotient
organic radical
race
racemic
rad
radial
radioactive (*See also* RA)
radiology
radius (*See also* r, Ra, rad)
ramus
range
Rankine (scale)
rare
rate
ratio
rationale
raw
reacting
reaction
reading
Réaumur (scale)
recessive
rectal
rectified average
rectum (*See also* rect)
red (indicator color)
reference (*See also* ref)
regimen
registered (trademark) (*See also* Reg)
regression coefficient
regular (*See also* reg)
regular insulin
regulator (gene)
rejection (factor)
relapse
relation
relaxation
release (factor)
remission
remote point of convergence
repressor
resazurin
resident
residuum
resistance
resistance determinant (plasmid)
resistance (electrical) (*See also* RES)
resistance unit (in cardiovascular system) (*See also* RU)
resistant
respiration (*See also* resp)
respiratory exchange ratio (*See also* R_E, RER)
response (*See also* resp)
rest (cell cycle)
resting
restricted
reticulocyte (*See also* RET, RETIC)
retinoscopy
reverse (banding) (*See also* REV)
review (*See also* REV)
rhythm
rib
ribose (*See also* r, Rib)
right (*See also* (R), RT, Rt, rt)
Rinne (hearing test)
roentgen (*See also* r, ROE, roent)
root
rough (bacterial colony)
routine
rub
side chain in amino acid formula
stimulus [G. *Reiz*] (*See also* S, ST)
take [L. *recipe*] (*See also* Rx)
total response (*See also* TR)

R1
longitudinal relaxivity

R2
transverse relaxivity

RI, R1
type I regulatory dimer

RII, R2
type II regulatory dimer

R#1
good risk (for anesthesia)

R#2
fairly good risk (for anesthesia)

R#3
poor risk (for anesthesia)

R#4
very poor risk (for anesthesia)

°R
(degree) Rankine
(degree) Réaumur

+R
Rinne test positive

(R)

rectal
right (*See also* R, RT)

R$_i$

inhibitory receptor

R$_{rs}$

respiratory system resistance

R$_s$

stimulatory receptor

-R

Rinne (hearing) test negative

(r)

registered trademark

r

angle of refraction
correlation coefficient
product moment
racemic
radius (*See also* R, Ra, rad)
recombinant
reproductive potential
ribose (*See also* R, Rib)
ring chromosome 1–22
roentgen (*See also* R, ROE, roent)
round
sample correlation coefficient

r.

far point [L. *remotum*] (*See also* R)

r^2

coefficient of determination

RA

radioactive (*See also* R)
radiographic absorptiometry
radionuclide angiography (*See also* RNA)
ragocyte (rheumatic arthritis cell)
ragweed antigen
rales
Raynaud (phenomenon)
reading age
readmission
reciprocal asymmetrical
refractory anemia
refractory ascites
regional anesthesia
remittance advice
renal artery
renin activity
renin-angiotensin
repeat action (drugs)
residual air
retinoic acid
rheumatoid agglutinin (*See also* Rh agglut)
rheumatoid arthritis
rhinocerebral aspergillosis
rifampicin

right angle
right arm
right atrial (pressure)
right atrium
right auricle
Rokitansky-Aschoff (sinus)
room air
rotational atherectomy

5α-RA

5-alpha-reductase activity

R$_A$

airway resistance (*See also* AR, RAW, R$_{AW}$, R (AW))

Ra

radial (*See also* rad)
radium
radius (*See also* R, r, rad)
Rayleigh number

^{226}Ra

radium-226

rA

riboadenylate

RAA

renin-angiotensin-aldosterone (system)
right aortic arch
right atrial abnormality
right atrial appendage

RAAA

ruptured abdominal aortic aneurysm

RAAGG

rheumatoid arthritis agglutinin

RAAPI

resting ankle-arm pressure index

RAAS

renin-angiotensin-aldosterone system

rAAT

recombinant alpha-1 antitrypsin
recombinant alpha$_1$ antitrypsin

RAB

rabies vaccine, not otherwise specified
remote afterload brachytherapy
remote afterloading brachytherapy
rice, applesauce, and banana (diet)

Rab

rabbit

RABA

rabbit antibladder antibody
radioantigen-binding assay

RABCa

rabbit antibladder cancer

RABDEV

rabies vaccine, duck embryo culture

RABFRhl-2

rabies vaccine, diploid fetal-rhesus-lung-2 cell line

RABG
room air blood gas
RABHDCV
rabies vaccine, human diploid cell culture
RAbody
right atrium body
RABP
retinoic acid-binding protein
RABPCEC
rabies vaccine, purified chick embryo cell culture
RAC
radial artery catheter
ranitidine bismuth citrate, amoxicillin, clarithromycin
right antecubital
right atrial contraction
RAC3
receptor-associated coactivator 3
rac
racemate
racemic
RACAT
rapid acquisition computed axial tomography
RACCO
right anterior caudocranial oblique
RACT
recalcified (whole-blood) activated clotting time
RAD
ionizing radiation unit
radiation absorbed dose (*See also* rad)
radical (*See also* rad)
radiology (*See also* Rad, Radiol)
reactive airways disease
regional alveolar damage
right anterior descending
right atrial diameter
right axis deviation
roentgen administered dose
Rad
radiologist (*See also* Radiol)
radiology (*See also* RAD, Radiol)
radiotherapist
radiotherapy (*See also* RADIO, RT, Rx)
rad
radial (*See also* Ra)
radian

radiation-absorbed dose (*See also* RAD)
radical (*See also* RAD)
radiculitis
radius (*See also* R, r, Ra)
roentgen absorbed dose
root [L. *radix*]
RADA
right acromiodorsoanterior (fetal position)
RADCA
right anterior descending coronary artery
rad imp
radium implant
RADIO
radiotherapy (*See also* Rad, Rad Ther, RT, Rx)
Radiol
radiologist (*See also* Rad)
radiology (*See also* RAD, Rad)
RADISH
rheumatoid arthritis, diffuse idiopathic skeletal hyperostosis
RAD ISO VENO BILAT
radioactive isotopic venogram, bilateral
RADIUS
routine antenatal diagnostic imaging with ultrasound
RADIV
Radi virus
RadLV
radiation leukemia virus
RADP
right acromiodorsoposterior (fetal position)
RADS
ionizing radiation units
rapid assay delivery systems
reactive airways disease syndrome
reactive airways dysfunction syndrome
retrospective assessment of drug safety
Reynolds Adolescent Depression Scale
rad/s
radian per second
RADT
rapid antigen-detection test

NOTES

Rad Ther
> radiotherapy (*See also* Rad, RADIO, RT, Rx)

RADTS
> rabbit antidog-thymus serum

Rad Ul
> radius-ulna

RADWASTE
> radioactive waste

RAE
> right atrial enlargement

RaE
> rabbit erythrocyte

RAEB
> refractory anemia, erythroblastic
> refractory anemia with excess blasts

RAEB-T
> refractory anemia with excess of blasts in transformation

RAEBT, RAEB-t
> refractory anemia with excess blasts in transition

RAEM
> refractory anemia with excess myeloblasts

RAF
> rapid atrial fibrillation
> rheumatoid arthritis factor

Ra-F
> radium-F

RAFF
> rectus abdominis free flap

RAFT
> Rehabilitative Addicted Family Treatment

RAG
> ragweed
> room air gas

Ragg
> rheumatoid agglutinator

RAH
> radioactive Hippuran (test)
> regressing atypical histiocytosis
> right anterior hemiblock (*See also* RAHB)
> right atrial hypertrophy

RAHB
> right anterior hemiblock (*See also* RAH)

rAHF
> antihemophilic factor (recombinant)

RAHO
> rabbit antibody to human ovary

RAHTG
> rabbit antihuman-thymocyte globulin

RAI
> radioactive iodine (*See also* [131]I)

Resident Assessment Instrument
resting ankle index
right atrial involvement

RAID
> radioimmunodetection (*See also* RID)
> radiolabeled antibody imaging

RAIR
> rectoanal inhibitory reflex

RAIS
> reflection-absorption infrared spectroscopy

RAIT
> radioimmunotherapy

RAIU
> radioactive iodine uptake (*See also* RIU)
> radioiodine uptake
> (thyroidal) radioactive iodine uptake (test)

RAL
> resorcylic acid lactone

RALPH
> renal-anal-lung-polydactyly-hamartoblastoma (syndrome)

RALT
> Riley Articulation and Language Test
> routine admission laboratory test

RAM
> radar absorbent material
> radioactive material
> random-access memory
> rapid alternating movements
> rectus abdominis muscle
> rectus abdominis musculocutaneous (flap)
> rectus abdominis myocutaneous (flap)
> reduced-acquisition matrix
> research aviation medicine
> right anterior measurement

RAMBA
> retinoic acid metabolism blocking agent

RAMCF
> rectus abdominis myocutaneous flap

RAMI
> Risk-Adjusted Mortality Index

RAMP
> radioactive antigen microprecipitin
> Rate Modulated Pacing
> right atrial mean pressure

RAMT
> rabbit antimouse-thymocyte

RAN
> resident's admission notes

R2AN
> second year resident's admission notes

RANA
> rheumatoid arthritis nuclear antigen

RAND
> random (sample, specimen)

RANK
> receptor activator of NF-κB
> receptor activator of nuclear factor-kappa B

RANKL
> RANK-ligand
> receptor activator of nuclear factor kappa B ligand

RANS
> retinal arterial narrowing and straightening

RANT
> right anterior

RANTES
> regulated on activation, normal T-cell expressed and secreted
> regulated upon activation, normal T-cell expressed and secreted

RAO
> right anterior oblique
> right anterior occipital

RaONC
> radiation oncology

RAP
> receptor-associated protein
> recurrent abdominal pain
> regression-associated protein
> Relative Aspects of Potential
> relative average perturbation
> remote access perfusion
> renal artery pressure
> resident assessment protocol
> rheumatoid arthritis precipitin
> right abdominal pain
> right atrial pressure

RAPA
> radial artery pseudoaneurysm
> rapamycin

RAPC
> resistance activated protein C

RAPD
> random amplified polymorphic DNA
> rapid amplification of polymorphic DNA
> relative afferent pupillary defect

RAPE
> right atrial pressure elevation

RAPM
> refractory anemia with partial myeloblastosis

RAPO
> rabbit antibody to pig ovary

RAPS
> recurrent abdominal pain syndrome

RAQ
> right anterior quadrant

RAR
> rat insulin receptor
> retinoic acid receptor
> right arm reclining
> right arm recumbent
> *trans*-retinoic acid

RARE
> rapid acquisition with relaxation enhancement
> rapid acquisition with resolution enhancement

RARLS
> rabbit antirat-lymphocyte serum

RARS
> refractory anemia with ring sideroblasts
> retinoic acid receptor

RARs
> retinoic acid receptors

RARTS
> rabbit antirat-thymocyte serum

RAS
> reality-adaptive supportive
> recurrent aphthous stomatitis
> reflex-activating stimulus
> renal artery stenosis
> renin-angiotensin system
> reticular activating system
> rheumatoid arthritis serum (factor)
> right arm, sitting
> Rokitansky-Aschoff sinus
> rotational atherectomy system

RASE
> rapid-acquisition spin echo

RASP
> radial artery systolic pressure
> Rapidly Alternating Speech Perception (Test)

R

NOTES

RASS
  rheumatoid arthritis and Sjögren syndrome
RAST
  radioallergosorbent assay test
  radioallergosorbent test
RASV
  recovered avian sarcoma virus
RAT
  rat aortic tissue
  Remote Associates Test
  repeat action tablet
  rheumatoid arthritis (factor) test
  right anterior thigh
  rotating aspiration thromboembolectomy
RATA
  radioimmunologic assay antithyroid antibody
RATC
  Robert Apperception Test for Children
RA test
  test for rheumatoid factor
RATG
  rabbit antithymocyte globulin
RATHAS
  rat thymus antiserum
RATS
  rabbit antithymocyte serum
RATx
  radiation therapy
RAU
  radioactive uptake
  recurrent aphthous ulcer
RAUC
  raw area under curve
RAV
  Rous-associated virus
RAVLT
  Rey Auditory Verbal Learning Test
RAW, R (AW), R_{AW}
  airway resistance (*See also* AR, R_A)
  resistance airway
R_{AW}
  regional gas exchange
RAZ
  razoxane
RAZV
  Razdan virus
RB
  rating board
  rebreathing
  relieved by
  Renaut body
  respiratory bronchiole
  respiratory bronchiolitis

  respiratory burst
  reticulate body
  retinoblastoma
  retrobulbar
  right breast
  right bundle
  right buttock
  round body
R&B
  right and below
Rb
  retinoblastoma gene
  retinoblastoma protein
  rubidium
RBA
  relative binding affinity
  rescue breathing apparatus
  right basilar artery
  right brachial artery
  risks, benefits, and alternatives (discussion with patient)
  rose bengal antigen
RBAF
  rheumatoid biologically active factor
RBAP
  repetitive bursts of action potential
RBAS
  rostral basilar artery syndrome
RBB
  right breast biopsy
  right bundle branch
RBBB
  right bundle branch block
RBBsB
  right bundle branch system block
RBBX
  right breast biopsy examination
RBC
  ranitidine bismuth citrate
  red blood cell
  red blood (cell) count (*See also* RCC)
  red blood corpuscle
RBC-ADA
  red blood cell adenosine deaminase
RBCD
  right border cardiac dullness
RBC FO
  red blood cell fallout
RBC frag
  red blood cell fragility
RBCM
  red blood cell mass
RBC/P
  red blood cell to plasma (ratio)
RBC s/f
  red blood cell spun filtration

RBCV
> red blood cell volume (*See also* VRBC)

RBD
> REM (rapid eye movement sleep) behavior disorder
> right border of dullness (percussion of heart)
> right brain damage

RBE
> radiobiologic equivalent
> relative biologic effectiveness

RBF
> regional blood flow
> renal blood flow
> riboflavin

RBG
> random blood glucose
> retinol-binding globulin

RB-ILD, RBILD
> respiratory bronchiolitis-associated interstitial lung disease

Rb Imp
> rubber base impression

RBL
> radiographic baseline
> rat basophilic leukemia
> Reid baseline
> rubber band ligation
> rubber band ligator

RBM
> Raji (cell)-binding material
> regional bone mass
> resorbable blast media
> ribonucleic acid-binding motif
> RNA-binding motif

RBME
> regenerating bone marrow extract

RBMT
> Rivermead Behavioral Memory Test

RBN
> retrobulbar neuritis

RBON
> retrobulbar optic neuritis

RBOW
> rupture of bag of waters

RBP
> resting blood pressure
> retinol-binding protein
> riboflavin-binding protein

Rb-82 PET
> rubidium-82 positron emission tomography

RBPS
> Rasor blood pumping system

RBR
> radiation bowel reaction

RBRVS
> resource-based relative value scale

RBS
> Randall-Baker Soucek
> random blood sugar
> rapid body shaper
> rutherford backscattering

RbSA
> rabbit serum albumin (*See also* RSA)

RBSI
> radiographic bone strength index

RBSP
> ramus, body, symphysis, palate

RBT
> rational behavior therapy

RBU
> Raji (cell)-binding unit

RBUV
> Rochambeau virus

RBV
> right brachial vein
> Rio Bravo virus

RB-V
> right bundle ventricular

RBVO
> right brachial vein occlusion

RBW
> relative body weight

RBZ
> rubidazone (zorubicin)

RC
> race
> radiocarpal
> reaction center
> receptor-chemoeffector (complex) (*See also* RCC)
> recrystallized
> red cell
> red (cell) cast (*See also* RCC)
> red corpuscle
> referred care
> reflection coefficient
> regenerated cellulose
> rehabilitation counseling

NOTES

RC *(continued)*
    report called
    resistance and capacitance
    respiration cease
    respiratory care
    respiratory center
    response, conditioned *(See also* Rc)
    response criteria
    rest cure
    retention catheter *(See also* ret cath)
    retrograde cystogram
    retruded contact (position)
    rib cage
    right coronary
    right (ear), cold (stimulus)
    Roman Catholic
    root canal
    rotator cuff
    routine cholecystectomy

R & C
    reasonable and customary

R/C
    reclining chair

Rc
    receptor
    response, conditioned *(See also* RC)

RCA
    radiographic contrast agent
    radionuclide cerebral angiogram
    Raji cell assay
    reactive cutaneous
      angioendotheliomatosis
    red (blood) cell adherence
    red (blood) cell agglutination
    relative chemotactic activity
    renal cell carcinoma
    retained cortical activity
    right carotid artery
    right coronary angiography
    right coronary artery
    root cause analysis
    rotational coronary atherectomy

rCABG
    reoperative coronary artery bypass
      graft

RCB
    rotator cuff buttress

RCBF
    renal cortical blood flow

rCBF
    regional cerebral blood flow

RCBV
    regional cerebral blood volume

RCC
    radiographic coronary calcification
    radiologic control center
    rape crisis center
    ratio of cost to charges

    receptor-chemoeffector complex *(See
      also* RC)
    red (blood) cell cast *(See also* RC)
    red (blood) cell concentrate
    red (blood) cell count *(See also
      RBC)*
    renal cell carcinoma
    right common carotid
    right coronary cusp
    Roman Catholic Church

Rcc
    radiochemical

RCCA
    right common carotid artery

RCC-CC
    clear cell renal cell carcinoma

RCCT
    randomized controlled clinical trial
    results of clinical controlled trial

RCD
    relative (area of) cardiac dullness

RCDA
    recurrent chronic dissecting
      aneurysm

RCDP
    rhizomelic chondrodysplasia punctata

RCDR
    relative corrected death rate

RCDS
    Revised Children's Depression
      Scale
    Reynolds Child Depression Scale

RCE
    reasonable compensation equivalent
    renal cholesterol embolization
    right carotid endarterectomy

RCF
    red (blood) cell filter ability
    red (blood) cell folate
    Reiter complement fixation
    relative centrifugal field
    relative centrifugal force
    ristocetin cofactor *(See also* RCoF)
    Ross carbohydrate free

RCFA
    right common femoral angioplasty
    right common femoral artery

RCFE
    residential care facility for the
      elderly

RCFR
    relative coronary flow reserve

RCFS
    reticulocyte cell-free system

RCG
    radioelectrocardiography *(See also*
      RECG)

R

RCH
rectocolic hemorrhage
residential care home
RCHF
right-sided congestive heart failure
RCI
rate change induced
respiratory control index
RCIA
red (blood) cell immune adherence
RCIP
rape crisis intervention program
RCIT, RCITR
red (blood) cell iron turnover
red (blood) cell iron turnover rate
RCL
radial collateral ligament
range of comfortable loudness
recurrent corneal lesion
renal clearance
RCLAAR
red (blood) cell-linked antigen-
antiglobulin reaction
RCM
radiocontrast material
radiographic contrast media
radiographic contrast medium
red (blood) cell mass
reinforced clostridial medium
replacement culture medium
restricted cardiomyopathy
restrictive cardiomyopathy
retinal capillary microaneurysm
rheumatoid cervical myelopathy
right costal margin
Roux conditioned medium
RCMAS
Revised Children's Manifest
Anxiety Scale
RCMI
red cell morphology index
rCMRO$_2$
regional cerebral metabolic rate for
oxygen
RCN
right caudate nucleus
RCoF
ristocetin cofactor (*See also* RCF)
RCP
random chemistry profile
respiratory care plan
retrocorneal pigmentation

retrograde cerebral perfusion
riboflavin carrier protein
rcp
reciprocal (translocation)
RCPH
red cell peroxide hemolysis
RCPM, RCPMT
Raven Colored Progressive Matrices
Test (*See also* CPM)
rCPP
regional cerebral perfusion pressure
RCQG
right caudal quarter ganglion
RCR
relative consumption rate
replication-competent retrovirus
(assay)
respiratory control ratio
rotator cuff repair
RCRC
recurrent colorectal cancer
RCRS
Rehabilitation Client Rating Scale
RCS
rabbit (aorta)-contracting substance
Reality Check Survey
red (blood) cell suspension
red color sign
repeat cesarean section (*See also*
R/CS)
reticulum cell sarcoma (*See also*
RSA)
right coronary sinus
R/CS
repeat cesarean section (*See also*
RCS)
RCSP
resting calcaneal stance position
RCT
randomized clinical trial
randomized controlled trial
rectal carcinoid tumor
red colloidal test
retrograde conduction time
root canal therapy
Rorschach content test
RC TNTC
red cells too numerous to count
RCU
recurrent calcium urolithiasis
respiratory care unit

NOTES

RCV
> red cell volume
> right colic vein

RCVA
> right cerebrovascular accident

RCVR
> renal cortical vascular resistance

RCX
> ramus circumflexus

RD
> radial deviation
> rate difference
> Raynaud disease
> reaction of degeneration
> reaction of denervation
> reflex decay
> Reiter disease
> renal disease
> Rénon-Delille (syndrome)
> resistance determinant
> respiratory disease
> respiratory distress
> restricted duty
> reticular dysgenesis
> retinal detachment
> Reye disease
> rhabdomyosarcoma (*See also* RMS)
> rheumatoid disease
> right deltoid
> right dorsoanterior
> Riley-Day (syndrome)
> Rolland-Desbuquois (syndrome)
> rubber dam
> ruptured disk

R&D
> research and development

Rd
> reading
> rutherford (unit of radioactivity)

RDA
> recommended daily allowance
> recommended dietary allowance
> representational difference analysis
> right dorsoanterior (fetal position)
> right ductus arteriosus
> rubidium dihydrogenarsenate

RdA
> reading age

RDB
> randomized double-blind (trial)
> research and development board

RDC
> research diagnostic criteria

RDD
> renal dose dopamine
> Rosai-Dorfman disease

RDDA
> recommended daily dietary allowance

RDDP
> ribonucleic acid-dependent deoxynucleic acid polymerase (*See also* RDPase)

RDE
> receptor-destroying enzyme
> remote data entry

RDEA
> right deviation of electrical axis

RDEB
> recessive dystrophic epidermolysis bullosa

RDES
> remote data entry system

RDF
> rapid dissolution formula
> rotary door flap

RDFC
> recurring digital fibroma of childhood

RDFS
> ratio of decayed and filled surfaces

RDFT
> ratio of decayed and filled teeth

RDG
> retrograde duodenogastroscopy
> right dorsogluteal

RDHBF
> regional distribution of hepatic blood flow

RDI
> recommended daily intake
> recommended dietary intake
> relative dose intensity
> respiratory distress index
> respiratory disturbance index
> Retirement Descriptive Index
> rupture-delivery interval

RDIH
> right direct inguinal hernia

RDLBBB
> rate-dependent left bundle branch block

RDLS
> Reynell Development Language Scales (psychologic test)

RDM
> readmission (*See also* Rdm)
> right deltoid muscle
> rod disk membrane

Rdm
> readmission (*See also* RDM)

RDMs
> reactive drug metabolites

rDNA

    recombinant deoxyribonucleic acid
    recombinant DNA
    ribosomal deoxyribonucleic acid
    ribosomal DNA

RDOD

    retinal detachment, oculus dexter
      (right eye)

RDOS

    retinal detachment, oculus sinister
      (left eye)

RDP

    radiopharmaceutical drug product
    random-donor platelet
    right dorsoposterior (fetal position)

RDPA

    right descending pulmonary artery

RDPase

    ribonucleic acid-dependent
      deoxyribonucleic acid polymerase
      (*See also* RDDP)

RDPE

    reticular degeneration of pigment
      epithelium

RDQ

    respiratory disease questionnaire

RdQ

    reading quotient (*See also* RG)

RDR

    rate-drop response

RDRC

    radioactive drug research committee

RDRV

    Rhesus diploid (cell strain) rabies
      vaccine

RDS

    research diagnostic (criteria)
    respiratory distress syndrome (of
      newborn)
    reticuloendothelial depressing
      substance

rDsg

    recombinant desmoglein

RDT

    regular (hemo)dialysis treatment
    retinal damage threshold
    routine dialysis therapy

RDTD

    referral, diagnosis, treatment, and
      discharge

RDU

    recreational drug use

RDVT

    recurrent deep vein thrombosis

RDW

    red (blood cell) diameter width
    red (blood cell) distribution width
      (index)
    reticulocyte distribution width

RE

    concerning (*See also* re)
    racemic epinephrine
    radiodermatitis emulsion
    radium emanation
    Rasmussen's encephalitis
    readmission
    rectal examination
    reflux esophagitis
    regional enteritis
    regular education
    renal and electrolyte
    renal excretion
    resting energy
    reticuloendothelial
    retinol equivalent
    right ear
    right eye (*See also* OD, O.D.)
    ring enhancement
    rostral end
    rowing ergometer

R&E

    research and education
    rest and exercise
    round and equal

R↑E

    right upper extremity

RE√

    recheck

R_E

    respiratory exchange ratio (*See also*
      R, RER)

R_e

    Reynolds number

Re

    rhenium

^{186}Re

    rhenium-186

^{188}Re

    rhenium-188

re

    concerning (*See also* RE)
    regarding

REA

    radiation emergency area

NOTES

REA *(continued)*
  radioenzymatic assay
  renal anastomosis
  restriction endonuclease analysis
  restriction enzyme analysis
  right ear advantage
ReA
  reactive arthritis
READ
  restriction endonuclease analysis
readm
  readmission
REAL
  Revised European-American
    (Classification of) Lymphoid
    Neoplasms
  Revised European-American
    Lymphoma (classification)
REALM
  Rapid Estimation of Adult Literacy
    in Medicine
REAS
  reasonably expected as safe
REAT
  radiologic emergency assistance
    team
REB
  roentgen-equivalent biologic
  rubber-reinforced bandage
R-EBD-HS
  recessive epidermolysis bullosa
    dystrophica–Hallopeau-Siemens
    (syndrome)
REC
  radioelectrocomplexing
  rearend collision
  receptor
  recommend
  record (*See also* rec)
  recovery
  recreation (*See also* rec)
  recur
  right external carotid
rec
  reactive
  recent
  recombinant chromosome
  recommendation
  record (*See also* REC)
  recreation (*See also* REC)
  recurrence (*See also* recur, recur)
  recurrent (*See also* recur, recur)
RECA
  right external carotid artery
recd, rec'd
  received
RE CEL
  reticulum cell

RECG
  radioelectrocardiography (*See also*
    RCG)
recip
  recipient
  reciprocal
recom
  smallest unit of DNA capable of
    recombination
recond
  reconditioned
  reconditioning
reconstr
  reconstruction
RecOS
  reconstruction occlusal surface
recryst
  recrystallization
rect
  rectal (*See also* R)
  rectification
  rectified
  rectum (*See also* R)
  rectus (muscle)
recur
  recurrence (*See also* rec)
  recurrent (*See also* rec)
RED
  radiation experience data
  rapid erythrocyte degeneration
  rectal evacuatory disorder
Re-D
  reevaluation deadline
red.
  reduce
  reducing
  reduction (*See also* redn)
redn
  reduction (*See also* red.)
redox
  oxidation-reduction
RED SUBS
  reducing substances
REE
  rapid extinction effect
  rare earth element
  resting energy expenditure
re-ed
  reeducation
REEDS
  retention (of tears), ectrodactyly,
    ectodermal dysplasia, and strange
    (hair, skin, and teeth syndrome)
REEG
  radioelectroencephalography
R-EEG
  resting electroencephalogram

R

REEL
>Receptive-Expressive Emergent Language (Scale)

REEL-2
>Receptive-Expressive Emergent Language (Scale), Second Edition

ReEND
>reproductive endocrinology

REEP
>right end-expiratory pressure
>role exchange/education-practice

REF
>ejection fraction at rest
>referred
>refused
>renal erythropoietic factor

ref
>reference (*See also* R)
>reflex (*See also* Refl)

Ref Doc
>referring doctor

REFI
>regional ejection fraction image
>regional ejection fraction imaging

ref ind
>refractive index (*See also* RI)

Refl
>reflect
>reflection
>reflex (*See also* ref)

Ref Phys
>referring physician

REFRAD
>released from active duty

REG
>radiation exposure guide
>radioencephalogram
>radioencephalography
>regression analysis
>rheoencephalography

Reg
>registered (*See also* R)

reg
>regarding
>region
>regular (*See also* R)
>regulation

Reg block
>regional block anesthesia

regen
>regenerate
>regeneration

reg rhy
>regular rhythm

reg R&R
>regular rate and rhythm (*See also* RRR)

reg. umb.
>umbilical region [L. *regio umbilici*]

regurg
>regurgitation

REH
>renin essential hypertension

REHAB, rehab
>rehabilitated
>rehabilitation

REL
>rate of energy loss
>recommended exposure level
>relative
>religion
>resting expiratory level

rel
>related
>relation
>relative

RELE
>resistive exercises, lower extremities

REM
>radiation-equivalent-man
>rapid eye movements
>rapid eye movement (sleep)
>recent event memory
>remarried
>remission
>reticular erythematous mucinosis
>return electrode monitor
>roentgen-equivalent-man (*See also* rem)

rem
>radiation equivalent in man
>removal
>roentgen-equivalent-man (*See also* REM)

REMA
>repetitive excess mixed anhydride (method)

REMAB
>radiation-equivalent-manikin absorption

REMCAL
>radiation-equivalent-manikin calibration

NOTES

REMP
roentgen-equivalent-man period

REMS
rapid eye movement sleep (*See also* REM)

REN, ren
renal (*See also* RN)

ren
ren mai channel (acupuncture)

REO
Receptive-Expressive Observation (Scale)
respiratory enteric orphan (virus)

REON
renal epithelioid oxyphilic neoplasm

REP
rapid electrophoresis
reactive eosinophilic pleuritis
repair
repeat (*See also* rept, rep)
report (*See also* rep, rept)
resistive exercise products
rest-exercise program
retrograde pyelogram (*See also* RP)
Rochester Epidemiology Project
roentgen equivalent-physical (*See also* rep)
(surgical) repair

rep
repeat (*See also* REP, rept)
replication
report (*See also* REP, rept)
roentgen equivalent-physical (*See also* REP)

rep.
let it be repeated [L. *repetatur*]

rep B&S
repetitive bending and stooping

REPC
reticuloendothelial phagocytic capacity

REP CK
rapid electrophoresis creatine kinase

REPL
recurrent early pregnancy loss

r-EPO
recombinant human erythropoietin

repol
repolarization

REP-PCR, Rep-PCR
repetitive extragenic palindromic polymerase chain reaction
repetitive polymerase chain reaction

reprep
re-preparation

REPS
reactive extensor postural synergy
repetitions

rept
repeat (*See also* REP, rep)
report (*See also* REP, rep)

Re-PUVA
combination retinoid and PUVA therapy

req
requested
required

REQF
wrong test requested-floor error

RER
peak respiratory ratio
renal excretion rate
respiratory exchange ratio (*See also* R, R_E)
rough endoplasmic reticulum

RER+
replication error positive

RER-
replication error negative

RES
(electrical) resistance (*See also* R)
radionuclide esophageal scintigraphy
recurrent erosion syndrome
resection
resident
reticuloendothelial system

res
research
reserve
residence
resident
residue

RESC, resc
resuscitation (*See also* resus)

ReSCU
Respiratory Special Care Unit

resist. ex.
resistive exercise

resp
respective
respectively
respiration (*See also* R)
respiratory (*See also* R)
response (*See also* R)
responsible

RESP-A
respiratory battery, acute

REST
Raynaud (phenomenon), esophageal (motor dysfunction), sclerodactyly, and telangiectasia (syndrome)
regressive electric shock therapy
regressive electroshock treatment
restoration
Restricted Environment Stimulation Therapy

restriction of environmental stimulation therapy
reticulospinal tract

resus

resuscitation (*See also* RESC, resc)

RESV

Restan virus

RET

rational-emotive therapy
rearranged during transfection
retention
reticulocyte (*See also* R, RETIC)
retina
retired (*See also* ret)
return
right esotropia

Ret

retarded

ret

rad equivalent therapeutic
retired (*See also* RET)

RETA

rete testis aspiration

RETC

rat embryo tissue culture

ret cath

retention catheter (*See also* RC)

ret detach

retinal detachment

RE-TEM

rectal-expander-assisted transanal endoscopic microsurgery

RETHINK

recognize, empathize, think, hear, integrate, notice, keep

RETIC, retic

reticulocyte (*See also* R, RET)

retro pyelo

retrograde pyelogram (*See also* REP, RP)

RETRX

retraction

RETUL

reticulum cell

Re-Tx

retransplantation

REU

rectal endoscopic ultrasonography

reu

radiation effect unit

REUE

resistive exercises to upper extremities

REUS

rectal endoscopic ultrasonography

REV, rev

reticuloendotheliosis virus
reversal
reverse (*See also* R)
review (*See also* R)
revolution (*See also* rev)
room's eye view

REVL

to be reviewed by laboratory (pathologist)

rev/min

revolution per minute

Rev of Sys

review of systems

re-x

reexamination

REZ

root exit zone

RF

radial fiber (of cochlea)
rapid filling
rate of flow (chromatography) (*See also* R_F)
receptive field (of visual cortex)
recognition factor
reduction fixation
reflecting (platelet)
regurgitant fraction
Reitland-Franklin (unit)
relative flow
relative fluorescence
release factor
releasing factor
renal failure
replicative form
resistance factor
resorcinol formaldehyde
respiratory failure
respiratory frequency
restricted fluids
retardation factor
reticular formation
retroflexed
retroperitoneal fibromatosis
rheumatic fever
rheumatoid factor
riboflavin

NOTES

RF *(continued)*
>   right foot
>   risk factor
>   root (canal) filling
>   rosette formation

R&F
>   radiographic and fluoroscopic

R$_F$
>   rate of flow (*See also* RF)

Rf
>   rutherfordium

rFVIII FS
>   antihemophilic factor (recombinant),
>   formulated with sucrose
>   (Kogenate)

RFA
>   radiofluorescent antibody
>   radiofrequency ablation
>   right femoral artery
>   right forearm
>   right frontoanterior (fetal position)

RFB
>   radial flow chromatography
>   residual functional capacity
>   retained foreign body
>   rheumatoid factor binding

RFb
>   respiratory feedback

RFC
>   radiofrequency coil
>   radiofrequency current
>   reduced folate carrier
>   retrograde femoral catheter
>   right frontal craniotomy
>   rosette-forming cell

RFCA
>   radiofrequency catheter ablation

RFD
>   residue-free diet

RFDT
>   Reach in Four Directions Test

RFE
>   relative fluorescence efficiency
>   return flow enema

RFFF
>   radial forearm free flap

RFFIT
>   rapid fluorescent focus inhibition
>   test

RFg
>   visual fields by Goldmann-type
>   perimeter

RFI
>   recurrence-free interval
>   renal failure index

RFIPC
>   Rating Form of IBD (inflammatory
>   bowel disease) Patient Concerns

RFL
>   radionuclide functional
>   lymphoscintigraphy
>   recurrent fetal loss
>   right frontolateral (fetal position)

RFLA
>   rheumatoid factorlike activity

RFLC
>   resistant Friend leukemia cell

RFLF
>   retained fetal lung fluid

RFLP
>   restriction fragment length
>   polymorphism (*See also* RLP)

RFLS
>   rheumatoid factorlike substance

RFM, rfm
>   rifampin

RFOL
>   results to follow

RFP
>   rapid filling period
>   renal function panel
>   request for payment
>   request for proposal
>   ret-fused protein
>   right frontoposterior (fetal position)

RF-PMR
>   radiofrequency percutaneous
>   myocardial revascularization

RFR
>   rapid filling rate
>   refraction

RFS
>   rapid frozen section
>   refeeding syndrome
>   relapse-free survival
>   renal function study

rFSH
>   recombinant follicle-stimulating
>   hormone

RFT
>   right fibrous trigone
>   right frontotransverse (fetal
>   position)
>   rod-and-frame test
>   routine fever therapy

RFTA
>   radiofrequency thermal ablation

RFTB
>   riboflavin tetrabutyrate

RFTC
>   radiofrequency thermocoagulation

RFTSW
>   right foot switch

RFTVR
>   radiofrequency tissue volume
>   reduction

RFUT
    radioactive fibrinogen uptake
RFV
    reason for visit
    right femoral vein
    Royal Farm virus
rFVIIa
    recombinant factor VIIA
RFVII
    Reading-Free Vocational Interest
      Inventory
RFW
    rapid filling wave
RFXAP
    RFX-associated protein
RG
    regurgitated (infant feeding)
    retrograde
    right gluteal
R/G
    red/green
Rg
    Rodgers antibody
RGA
    right gastroepiploic artery
RGAS
    retained gastric antrum syndrome
RGBMT
    renal glomerular basement
      membrane thickness
RGC
    radio-gas chromatography
    remnant gastric cancer
    respiratory glycoconjugate
    retinal ganglion cell
    right giant cell
RGD
    range-gated Doppler
RGE
    relative gas expansion
    respiratory gas equation
RGEA
    right gastroepiploic artery
RGEPS
    Rucker-Gable Educational
      Programming Scale
RGH
    rat growth hormone
    recurrent gross hematuria
RGM
    recurrent glioblastoma multiforme

    right gluteus maximus
    right gluteus medius
rGM-CSF
    recombinant (human) granulocyte-
      macrophage colony-stimulating
      factor (*See also* rhGM-CSF)
RGMT
    reciprocal geometric mean titer
RGO
    reciprocating gait orthosis
    reciprocation gait orthosis
RGP
    retrograde pyelogram
    rigid gas-permeable (contact lens)
    rural general practitioner
RGR
    relative growth rate
RGT
    reversed gastric tube
RGV
    Rio Grande virus
RH
    radial hemolysis
    radiant heat
    radiologic health
    reactive hyperemia
    recurrent herpes
    reduced haloperidol
    regional heparinization
    regulatory hormone
    relative humidity
    releasing hormone
    rest home
    retinal hemorrhage
    rheumatoid
    Richner-Hanhart (syndrome)
    right hand
    right hemisphere
    right hyperphoria
    room humidifier
Rh
    Rhesus (blood factor)
    rhinion (craniometric point)
    rhodium
Rh+, Rh pos
    Rhesus positive
Rh−, Rh neg
    Rhesus negative
rh
    rheuma (*See also* rheum)
    rheumatic (*See also* rheum)
    rhonchi

NOTES

r/h
> roentgen per hour

RHA
> right hepatic artery

Rha.
> l-rhamnose

rHA
> recombinant human albumin

R-HAB
> Rincoe human action bionic

Rh agglut
> rheumatoid agglutinins (*See also* RA)

RHAMM
> receptor for hyaluronan-mediated motility

rhAPC
> recombinant human activated protein C

RHB
> raise head of bed
> right heart border
> right heart bypass

rHBcAg
> recombinant HBcAg

RHBF
> reactive hyperemia blood flow

rhBMP-2, rHuBMP-2
> recombinant human bone morphogenetic protein

RH/BSO
> radical hysterectomy and bilateral salpingo-oophorectomy

RHBV
> right heart blood volume

RHC
> resin hemoperfusion column
> respiration has ceased
> right heart catheterization
> right hemicolectomy
> right hypochondrium
> routine health care

RhC
> rhesus antigen C

RhCE
> rhesus gene CE

RHCT
> renal helical computed tomography

RHD
> radial head dislocation
> radiant heat device
> radiologic health data
> relative hepatic dullness
> renal hypertensive disease
> rheumatic heart disease (*See also* rheu ht dis)
> right-hand dominant

> right hemisphere (brain) damage
> round heart disease

RhD
> rhesus D antigen
> rhesus gene D
> Rhesus (hemolytic) disease

rh-DNase
> dornase alfa (Pulmozyme)

RHE
> respiratory heat exchange
> retinohepatoendocrinologic (syndrome)

RhE
> rhesus E antigen

RHEED
> reflection high-energy electron diffraction

rheo
> rheostat

rh-EPO
> recombinant human erythropoietin

rheu ht dis
> rheumatic heart disease (*See also* RHD)

rheum
> rheuma (*See also* rh)
> rheumatic (*See also* rh)

RHF
> rheumatic fever vaccine
> right heart failure

RHG
> radial hemolysis in gel
> relative hemoglobin
> right hand grip

rhG-CSF
> recombinant human granulocyte colony-stimulating factor

rhGH
> recombinant human growth hormone

rhGH(m)
> mammalian-cell-derived recombinant human growth hormone (Serostim)

rhGM-CSF
> recombinant human granulocyte-macrophage colony-stimulating factor (*See also* rGM-CSF)

RHH
> right homonymous hemianopia

Rhi
> rhinology (*See also* Rhin)

RhIG, RhIg
> Rhesus immune globulin

rhIGF
> recombinant human insulinlike growth factor

R

rhIGF-1
> recombinant human insulin-like growth factor-1

RhIGIV
> Rh immune globulin intravenous

rhIL, rHuIL
> recombinant human interleukin

rhIL-2, rHuIL-2
> recombinant human interleukin-2

rhIL-3, rHuIL-3
> recombinant human interleukin-3

rhIL-10, rhuIL-10
> recombinant human IL-10

rhIL-11
> recombinant human interleukin-11

Rhin
> rhinologist
> rhinology (*See also* Rhi)

rhin
> rhinitis

rhino
> rhinoplasty

RHINOS
> fiberoptic rhinoscopy

r-hirudin
> recombinant hirudin

RHL
> recurrent herpes labialis
> right hemisphere lesion
> right hepatic lobe

RHLB
> Right Hemisphere Language Battery

RHLN
> right hilar lymph node

RHM
> routine health management

Rhm
> roentgen per hour at one meter

rhMCAF
> human macrophage-monocyte chemotactic and activating factor

rHM-CSF
> recombinant human macrophage colony-stimulating factor

rHm EPO, rHuEPO
> recombinant human erythropoietin

RhMK, RhMk, RhMkK
> Rhesus monkey kidney (*See also* RMK)

RHMV
> right heart mixing volume

RHN
> Rockwell hardness number

Rh$_{null}$
> Rhesus factor null (all Rh factors are lacking)

ρ, rho
> electrical resistivity
> electric charge density
> mass density
> population correlation coefficient
> reactivity
> rho
> rho (17th letter of Greek alphabet), lowercase

RHO
> right heeloff

RHOCS
> right-handed orthogonal coordinate system

Rho(D)
> immune globulin to an Rh-negative woman

RhoGAM
> RhO (D) immune globulin

rhom
> rhomboid (muscle)

RHP
> resting head pressure
> right hemiparesis
> right hemiplegia

RHPA
> reverse hemolytic plaque assay

rhPDGF, rHuPDGF
> recombinant human platelet-derived growth factor

RHR
> resting heart rate

R/hr
> roentgens per hour

RHS
> radial head subluxation
> Ramsay Hunt syndrome
> reciprocal hindlimb-scratching (syndrome)
> right hand side
> right heel strike
> rough hard sphere

rhSOD
> recombinant human superoxide dismutase

NOTES

RHT
    renal homotransplantation
    right hypertropia
r-hT-FPI
    recombinant human tissue factor
      pathway inhibitor
rhTSH
    recombinant human thyroid-
      stimulating hormone
    recombinant human TSH
RHU
    rheumatology
rhuMAb HER2
    recombinant anti-p185HER2
      monoclonal antibody
RHV
    right hepatic vein
    rotating hemostatic valve
rhVEGF
    recombinant human vascular
      endothelial growth factor
RHW
    radiant heat warmer
RI
    input resistor
    radiation intensity
    radioimmunology
    radioisotope
    ramus intermedius (coronary artery)
    recession index
    recombinant inbred (strain)
    reference interval
    refractive index (*See also* ref ind,
      n)
    regenerative index
    regional ileitis
    regular insulin
    relapse incidence
    relative intensity
    release inhibition
    remission induced
    remission induction
    renal insufficiency
    replicative intermediate
    resistance index
    resistive index
    respiratory illness
    respiratory index
    reticulocyte index
    retroactive inhibition
    retroactive interference
    rhythmic initiation
    ribosome
    right iliac (crest)
    Rohrer index
    rooming in
    rosette inhibition

R/I
    rule in
RIA
    radioimmunoassay
    relaxation-induced anxiety
    reversible ischemic attack
    right iliac artery
RIA-DA
    radioimmunoassay double antibody
      (test)
RIAST
    Reitan Indiana Aphasic Screening
      Test
RIAT
    radioimmune antiglobulin test
Rib
    ribose (*See also* R, r)
RIBA
    radioimmunoblot assay
    recombinant immunoblot assay
    recombinant immunosorbent assay
RIBLS
    Riley Inventory of Basic Learning
      Skills
RIBS
    rutherford ion backscattering
RIC
    renomedullary interstitial cell
    right iliac crest
    right internal capsule
    right internal carotid
RICA
    reverse immune cytoadhesion
    right internal carotid artery
RICE
    rest, ice, compresses, elevation
    rest, ice, compression, elevation
RICM
    right intercostal margin
RICS
    right intercostal space
RICU
    respiratory intensive care unit
RID
    radioimmunodetection (*See also*
      RAID)
    radioimmunodiffusion
    remission-inducing drug
    remove intoxicated driver
    right (ventricular) internal diameter
    ruptured intervertebral disk
RIDCSF
    radial immunodiffusion cerebrospinal
      fluid
RIE, RIEP
    radiation induced emesis
    relative inspiratory effort
    rocket immunoelectrophoresis

RIF
>   radiation-induced fibrosis
>   release-inhibiting factor
>   resistance-inducing factor
>   rifampin
>   right iliac fossa
>   right index finger
>   rigid internal fixation
>   rosette inhibitory factor

RIFA
>   radioiodinated fatty acid

RIFC
>   rat intrinsic factor concentrate

rIFN-A, rIFN-α, rIFN-a, rIFN-alpha
>   recombinant interferon alpha

rIFN-gamma
>   recombinant interferon gamma

RIG
>   rabies immune globulin
>   rabies immunoglobulin

RIGH
>   rabies immune globulin, human

RIGS
>   radioimmunoguided surgery

RIH
>   right inguinal hernia

RIHD
>   radiation-induced heart disease

RIHSA
>   radioactive iodinated human serum
>   albumin

RIIE
>   respiratory isolation implementation
>   efficiency

RIIS
>   respiratory isolation implementation
>   sensitivity

RIJ
>   right internal jugular (vein or
>   catheter)

RILD
>   radiation-induced liver disease

RILT
>   rabbit ileal loop test

RIM
>   radioisotope medicine
>   rapid identification method
>   recurrent induced malaria
>   relative-intensity measure

RIMA
>   reversible inhibitor of monoamine
>   oxidase-type A

>   right internal mammary anastomosis
>   right internal mammary artery

RIM-*Neisseria*
>   rapid identification method-*Neisseria*

RIMS
>   resonance ionization mass
>   spectrometry

RIN
>   radiation-induced neoplasm
>   rat insulinoma

RINB
>   Reitan-Indiana Neuropsychological
>   Battery

RIND
>   resolving ischemic neurologic
>   deficit
>   reversible ischemic neurologic
>   deficit
>   reversible ischemic neurologic
>   disability

RINN
>   recommended international
>   nonproprietary name

R_{int} R_{int}
>   intrinsic flow resistance

RINV
>   radiation-induced nausea and
>   vomiting

RIO
>   right inferior oblique (muscle)

RIOJ
>   recurrent intrahepatic obstructive
>   jaundice

R-IOL
>   remove intraocular lens

RIP
>   radioimmunoprecipitation (test)
>   rapid infusion pump
>   receptor interacting protein
>   reflex-inhibiting pattern
>   respiratory inductance
>   plethysmograph
>   respiratory inductance
>   plethysmography
>   respiratory inductive
>   plethysmography
>   respiratory inversion point
>   rhythmic inhibitory pattern

RIPA
>   radioimmunoprecipitation assay
>   ristocetin-induced platelet
>   agglutination

NOTES

RIPIS
Rhode Island Pupil Identification Scale

RIR
right iliac region
right inferior rectus

RIRB
radioiodinated rose bengal (dye)

RIS
radiographic imaging system
radioimmunoglobulin scintigraphy
rapid immunofluorescence staining
resonance ionization spectroscopy
respiratory index score
responding to internal stimuli

RIs
Rehabilitation Indicators

RISA
radioactive iodinated serum albumin
radioimmunosorbent assay
radioiodinated serum albumin
Responsibility and Independence Scale for Adolescents

RISB
Rotter Incomplete Sentences Blank

RISE
rifampin-isoniazid-streptomycin-ethambutol

RISHN
radiation-induced sarcoma of the head and neck

RIST
radioimmunosorbent test

RIT
radioimmunoglobulin therapy
radioimmunotherapy
radioiodinated triolein
ritonavir
Rorschach Inkblot Test (*See also* Ror)
rosette inhibition titer

RITA
right internal thoracic artery

RITC
rhodamine isothiocyanate
rhodamine isothiocyanate conjugated

RIU
radioactive iodine uptake (*See also* RAIU)
radioiodine uptake

RIV
ramus interventricularis
right innominate vein

RIVC
radionuclide (imaging of) inferior vena cava
right inferior vena cava

RIVD
ruptured intervertebral disk

RIVS
ruptured interventricular septum

RIX
radiation-induced xerostomia

RJ
radial jerk (reflex)
right jugular

RJA
regurgitant jet area

RJI
radionuclide joint imaging

RJS
reduced joint survey

RK
rabbit kidney
radial keratotomy
right kidney

RKG
radio(electro)cardiogram

RKH
Rokitansky-Kuster-Hauser (syndrome)

RKID
right kidney (urine sample)

RKS
renal kidney stone
retrograde kidney study

RKV
rabbit kidney vacuolating (virus)

RKW
renal kalium (potassium) wasting

RKY
roentgen kymography

R L, R-L, R→L, R/L
right-to-left (shunt)

RL
coarse rales
radiation laboratory
reduction level
resistive load
reticular lamina
right lateral (*See also* R LAT, R Lat, RT LAT, rt lat)
right leg
right lower
right lung
Ringer lactate (solution) (*See also* RLS)
rotation left

R or L
right or left

RL$_3$
numerous coarse rales

R$_L$
pulmonary resistance (*See also* R$_L$R$_P$)

Rl
medium rales
Rl$_2$
moderate number of medium rales
rl
fine rales
rl$_1$
few fine rales
RLA
radiographic lung area
right lower arm
R LAT, R Lat
right lateral (*See also* RL)
RLB
right lateral bending
RLBCD
right lower border of cardiac
dullness
RLC
rectus and longus capitis (muscle)
residual lung capacity
rhodopsin-lipid complex
RLD
related living donor
resistive load detection
right lateral decubitus (position)
ruptured lumbar disk
RLDP
right lateral decubital position
RLDS
Reynell Language Developmental
Scale
RLE
recent life event
recent life events
right lower extremity
RLF
retained lung fluid
retrolental fibroplasia
right lateral femoral
RLFP
Remaining Lifetime Fracture
Probability
RLG
right lateral gaze
RLGS
restriction landmark genomic
scanning
RLH
reactive lymphoid hyperplasia
recurrent lobar hemorrhage

RLI
Reasons for Living Inventory
RLL
right liver lobe
right lower lid
right lower limb
right lower lobe
RLMD
rat liver mitochondria (and
submitochondrial particles derived
by) digitonin (treatment)
RLN
recurrent laryngeal nerve
regional lymph node
RLNC
regional lymph node cell
RLND
regional lymph node dissection
retroperitoneal lymph node
dissection
RLO
residual lymphocyte output
Right-Left Orientation Test
RLP
radiation leukemia protection
rectal linitis plastica
remnant-like lipoprotein particle
remnant lipoprotein
restriction fragment length
polymorphism (*See also* RFLP)
ribosome-like particle
RLQ
right lower quadrant
RLQD
right lower quadrant defect
RLR
right lateral rectus (muscle)
R$_L$R$_P$
pulmonary resistance
RLRTD
recurrent lower respiratory tract
disease
RLS
person who stammers having
difficulty enunciating R, L, and
S
rat lung strip
Reaction Level Scale
restless legs syndrome
right-to-left shunt

R

NOTES

RLS *(continued)*
Ringer lactate solution (*See also* RL)
Roussy-Levy syndrome

RLSB
right lower scapular border
right lower sternal border

rl-sh
right-left shunt

RLT
reactive lymphoid tissue
red light therapy
reduced liver transplant
right lateral thigh

RLTCS
repeat low transverse cesarean section

RLUs
relative light units

RLV
Rauscher leukemia virus

RLWD
routine laboratory work done

RLX
right lower extremity

RM
radical mastectomy
random migration
range of movement
red marrow
reference material
regional myocardial
rehabilitation medicine
repetition maximum
resistive movement
respiratory metabolism
respiratory movement
rhabdomyosarcoma
Riehl melanosis
right median
risk management
risk model
room
Rosenthal-Melkersson (syndrome)
Rothmann-Makai (syndrome)
ruptured membranes

1-RM
one-repetition maximum

R&M
routine and microscopic

Rm
relative mobility
remission

rm
room

RMA
relative medullary area (of kidney)

right mentoanterior (fetal position)
Rivermead motor assessment

RMB
right main-stem bronchus

RMBF
regional myocardial blood flow

RMBPC
Revised Memory and Behavior Problems Checklist

RMC
right middle cerebral (artery)

RMCA, R-MCA
right main coronary artery
right middle cerebral artery

RMCAT
right middle cerebral artery thrombosis

RMCL
right midclavicular line

RMCP
rat mast cell protease

RMCT
rat mast cell technique

RMD
rapid movement disorder
ratio of midsagittal diameter
retromanubrial dullness
right manubrial dullness
rippling muscle disease

RME
rapid maxillary expansion
resting metabolic expenditure
right mediolateral episiotomy (*See also* RMLE)

RMEE
right middle ear exploration

rMET
recombinant methioninase

R meter
roentgen meter

RMF
right middle finger

RMI
Reading Miscue Inventory
Rivermead Mobility Index

RMIC
renomedullary interstitial cell

RMK
Rhesus monkey kidney (*See also* RhMK, RhMk, RhMkK)

RMK #1
remark number 1

RML
radiation myeloid leukemia
right mediolateral
right mentolateral (fetal position)
right middle lobe (of lung)

R

RMLB
   right middle lobe bronchus
RMLE
   right mediolateral episiotomy (*See also* RME)
RMLS
   right middle lobe syndrome
RMLV
   Rauscher murine leukemia virus (*See also* RMuLV)
RMM
   rapid micromedia method
RMP
   rapidly miscible pool
   rapid manual processing
   resting membrane potential
   rifampin
   right mentoposterior (fetal position)
RMQ
   Roland-Morris Questionnaire
RMR
   resting metabolic rate
   right medial rectus (muscle)
   root mean square residue
rMRGlu
   glucose metabolism
RMRM
   right modified radical mastectomy
RMS
   rectal morphine sulfate (suppository)
   red-man syndrome
   rehabilitation medicine service
   repetitive motion syndrome
   respiratory muscle strength
   rhabdomyosarcoma (*See also* RD)
   rheumatic mitral stenosis
   rigid-man syndrome
   Rocky Mountain spotted fever vaccine
   root-mean-square (*See also* rms)
   Ruvalcaba-Myhre-Smith
rms
   root-mean-square (*See also* RMS)
RMSB
   right middle sternal border
RMSD
   root-mean-square deviation
RMSE
   root-mean-square error
RMSF
   Rocky Mountain spotted fever

RMSS
   Ruvalcaba-Myhre-Smith syndrome
RMT
   ranitidine bismuth citrate, metronidazole, tetracycline
   relative medullary thickness
   retromolar trigone
   right mentotransverse (fetal position)
RMTD
   rhythmical midtemporal discharge
RMUl
   relief medication unit index
rMu IL-6
   murine interleukin-6
RMuLV
   Rauscher murine leukemia virus (*See also* RMLV)
RMV
   respiratory minute volume
RN
   radionucleotide (scanning)
   radionuclide
   red nucleus
   reflex nephropathy
   renal (disease) (*See also* REN, ren)
   reticular nucleus
   right nostril (naris)
R/N
   renew
Rn
   radon
²²²Rn
   radon-222
RNA
   radionuclide angiogram
   radionuclide angiography (*See also* RA)
   ribonucleic acid
   rough, noncapsulated, avirulent (bacterial culture)
RNAA
   radiochemical neutron activation analysis
RNA-PCR
   ribonucleic acid-polymerase chain reaction
RNASe, RNase
   ribonuclease
RNase D
   ribonuclease D

NOTES

RNase H
 ribonuclease H
RNase P
 ribonuclease P
RND
 radical neck dissection
 reactive neurotic depression
RNEF
 resting (radio)nuclide ejection
  fraction
RNF
 regular nursing floor
RNFL
 retinal nerve fiber layer
RNG
 radionuclide angiography
RNI
 reactive nitrogen intermediates
 recommended nutrient intake
RNICU
 regional neonatal intensive care
  unit
RNL
 renal laboratory profile
RNP
 restorative nursing program
 ribonucleoprotein
RNR
 ribonucleotide reductase
RNS
 reference normal serum
 repetitive nerve stimulation
 replacement normal saline (0.9%
  sodium chloride)
RNSC
 radionuclide superior cavography
RNST
 reactive nonstress test
RNT
 radioassayable neurotensin
Rnt
 roentgenology (*See also* roent)
RNTC
 rat nephroma tissue culture
RNUD
 recurrent nonulcer dyspepsia
RNV
 radionuclide venography
 radionuclide ventriculogram
 radionuclide ventriculography (*See
  also* RNVG)
rNV
 recombinant (capsid protein of)
  Norwalk virus
RNVG
 radionuclide ventriculography (*See
  also* RNV)

RO
 reality orientation
 reality oriented
 relative odds
 report of
 reverse osmosis
 Ritter-Oleson (technique)
 routine order
 rule out (*See also* R/O)
 Russian Orthodox
R/O
 rule out (*See also* RO)
R$_0$
 resting radium
ROA
 radiologic osteoarthritis
 regurgitant orifice area
 reversal of antagonist
 right occipitoanterior (fetal position)
 right occipitoanterior position
ROAC
 repeated oral (doses of) activated
  charcoal
ROAD
 reversible obstructive airways
  disease
ROAF
 reversed ophthalmic artery flow
ROAM
 roaming optical access multiscope
ROAT
 repeat open-application testing
ROATS
 rabbit ovarian antitumor serum
rob.
 robertsonian (translocation)
ROC
 receiver operating characteristic
 record of contact
 relative operating characteristic
 resident on call
 residual organic carbon
roc
 reciprocal ohm centimeter
ROC curve
 receiver operating characteristic
  curve
ROCF, ROCFT
 Rey-Estreich Complex Figure Test
 Rey-Osterrieth complex figure
Roch-Ochs
 Rochester-Ochsner
ROCV
 Rocio virus
ROD
 rapid opioid detoxification

RODA
  rapid opiate detoxification under anesthesia

RODAC
  replicate organism detection and counting

RODAC-TM
  replicate organism direct agar contact

RODEO
  rotating delivery of excitation off resonance

ROE
  report of event
  return on equity
  right otitis externa
  roentgen (*See also* R, r, roent)

roent
  roentgen (*See also* R, r, ROE)
  roentgenologist
  roentgenology (*See also* Rnt)

ROF
  review of outside films

ROG
  rogletimide

ROH
  rat ovarian hyperemia
  rat ovarian hyperemia (test)
  rubbing alcohol

ROI
  reactive oxygen intermediate
  region of interest
  release of information

ROIDS
  hemorrhoids

ROIH
  right oblique inguinal hernia

ROJM
  range of joint motion

ROL
  right occipitolateral (fetal position)

ROLC
  roentgenographically occult lung cancer
  roentgenologically occult lung cancer

ROLS
  Reinverting Operating Lens System

ROM
  range of motion
  range of movement
  read-only memory

rifampicin 600 mg, ofloxacin 400 mg, and minocycline 100 mg
right otitis media
rupture of membranes

Rom, Romb
  Romberg (sign)

rom
  reciprocal ohm meter

ROM C P
  range of motion complete and pain-free

ROMI
  rule out myocardial infarct
  rule out myocardial infarction

romied
  ruled out for myocardial infarction

ROMSA
  right otitis media, suppurative, acute

ROMSC
  right otitis media, suppurative, chronic

ROM WNL
  range of motion within normal limits

RON
  radiation optic neuropathy

ROOF
  retroorbicularis oculi fat

ROP
  regional organ procurement
  retinopathy of prematurity
  right occipitoposterior (fetal position)

ROPE
  respiratory ordered phase encoding

ROR
  the French acronym for measles-mumps-rubella vaccine
  retinoic acid-related orphan receptor

Ror
  Rorschach (Inkblot Test) (*See also* RIT)

RoRx
  radiation therapy

ROS
  reactive oxygen species
  review of systems (*See also* Rev of Sys)
  rod outer segment

RoS
  rostral sulcus

NOTES

ROSA
    rank-order stability analysis
ROSC
    restoration of spontaneous
        circulation
    return of spontaneous circulation
ROSNI
    round spermatid nuclei injection
rOspA
    recombinant outer surface protein
        A
ROSS
    review of signs and symptoms
    review of subjective symptoms
    review other subjective symptoms
ROT
    real oxygen transport
    remedial occupational therapy
    right occipitotransverse (fetal
        position)
    rotating (*See also* Rot, rot.)
    rotator
    rule of thumb
Rot, rot.
    rotating (*See also* Rot, rot.)
    rotation (*See also* ROT)
rot. ny
    rotatory nystagmus
ROU
    recurrent oral ulcer
ROUL
    rouleaux (rouleau)
rout.
    routine
ROW
    rat ovarian weight
    Rendu-Osler-Weber (syndrome)
    rest of (the) week
ROWPVT
    Receptive One-Word Picture
        Vocabulary Test
RP
    radial pulse
    radical prostatectomy
    radiographic planimetry
    radiopharmaceutical
    rapid processing (of film)
    Raynaud phenomenon
    reaction product
    reactive protein
    readiness potential
    rectal prolapse
    reduced profile
    reentrant pathway
    refractory period
    regulatory protein
    relapsing polychondritis
    relative potency

    respiratory (rate):pulse (rate) (index)
    responsible party
    resting position
    resting potential
    resting pressure
    restorative proctocolectomy
    rest pain
    retinitis pigmentosa
    retinitis proliferans (*See also* R Pr)
    retrograde pyelogram (*See also*
        REP)
    retroperitoneal
    reverse phase
    rheumatoid polyarthritis
    ribose phosphate
    root plane
R$_p$, Rp
    pulmonary resistance
RPA
    radial photon absorptiometry
    recurrent pleomorphic adenoma
    restenosis postangioplasty
    resultant physiologic acceleration
    reverse passive anaphylaxis
    ribonuclease protection assay
    right pulmonary artery
r-PA
    recombinant plasminogen activator
RPAB
    Rivermead Perceptual Assessment
        Battery
RPAW
    right pulmonary artery withdrawal
RPBD
    rating of perceived breathing
        difficulty
rPBF
    regional pulmonary blood flow
RPC
    reactive perforating collagenosis
    recurrent pyogenic cholangiogram
    recurrent pyogenic cholangiohepatitis
    relapsing polychondritis
    relative proliferative capacity
    restorative proctocolectomy
    retained products of conception
    root planing and curettage
RPCF, RPCFT
    Reiter protein complement-fixation
        (test)
RPCGN
    rapidly progressive crescenting
        glomerulonephritis
RPCV
    retropubic cytourethropexy
RPD
    removable partial denture

R-PDQ
Revised Denver Prescreening Development Questionnaire

RPDSI
Riley Preschool Developmental Screening Inventory

RPE
rated perceived exertion
rate of perceived exertion
rating of perceived exertion
recurrent pulmonary emboli
retinal pigment epithelial (cell)
retinal pigment epithelium

RPED
retina pigment epithelium detachment

r-PEG
recombinant polyethylene glycol

RPEP
rabies postexposure prophylaxis
right pre-ejection period

RPF
relaxed pelvic floor
renal plasma flow
retroperitoneal fibrosis

rPF4
recombinant platelet factor-4

RPFᵃ
arterial renal plasma flow

RPFS
Rosenzweig Picture-Frustration Study

RPFᵛ
venous renal plasma flow

RPG
radiation protection guide
retrograde percutaneous gastrostomy
retrograde pyelogram
rheoplethysmography

RPGG
retroplacental gamma globulin

RPGN
rapidly progressive glomerulonephritis
rapidly progressive (necrotizing) glomerulonephritis

RPGR
retinitis pigmentosa GTPase regulator gene

RPH
retroperitoneal hemorrhage

RPHA
reversed passive hemagglutination
reversed passive hemagglutination reaction

RPHAMCFA
reversed passive hemagglutination by miniature centrifugal fast analysis

RP-HPLC
reversed phase high-performance liquid chromatography

RPI
Racial Perceptions Inventory
resting pressure index
reticulocyte production index
reticulocytic production index

RPICA
right posterior internal carotid artery

RPICC
regional perinatal intensive care center

RPICCE
round pupil intracapsular cataract extraction

RPIPP
reversed phase ion-pair partition

RPL, RPLAD
retroperitoneal lymphadenectomy

RPLA
reversed passive latex particle agglutination

R-plasmid
resistance plasmid

RPLC
reversed-phase liquid chromatography

RPLD
repair of potentially lethal damage
retroperitoneal lymph node dissection (*See also* RPLND)

RPLND
retroperitoneal lymph node dissection (*See also* RPLD)
retroperitoneal pelvic lymph node dissection

RPLS
reversible posterior leukoencephalopathy
reversible posterior leukoencephalopathy syndrome

R

NOTES

RPM, rpm
radical pair mechanism
rapid processing mode
Raven Progressive Matrices
real-time position management
revolutions per minute
rotations per minute

RPMD
rheumatic pain modulation disorder

RPMPR
radical posteromedial and plantar release

RPN
renal papillary necrosis
resident's progress note

R2PN
second year resident's progress notes

RPND
retroperitoneal (lymph) node dissection

RPO
reflectance pulse oximetry
right posterior oblique (radiologic view)

RPP
(heart)rate-(systolic blood) pressure product
radical perineal prostatectomy
rate-pressure product
retropubic prostatectomy

RPPC
regional pediatric pulmonary center

RPPI
role perception picture inventory

RPPR
red (blood cell) precursor production rate

RPPS
retropatellar pain syndrome

RPR
rapid plasma reagent (test)
rapid plasma reagin
Reiter protein reagin

R Pr
retinitis proliferans (*See also* RP)

RPRCF
rapid plasma reagin complement fixation

RPRCT
rapid plasma reagin card test

RPR-CT
rapid plasma reagin circle card test

RPS, rps
renal pressor substance
reverse pivot shift
revolutions per second

RPT
rapid pull-through
rapid pull-through (technique)
refractory period of transmission

rpt
report

RPTA
renal percutaneous transluminal angioplasty

rptd
ruptured

RPTK
receptor protein tyrosine kinase

RPU
retropubic urethropexy

RPV
right portal vein
right pulmonary vein

RPVP
right posterior ventricular pre-excitation

Rpx
Rathke pouch homeobox transcription factor

RQ
reading quotient (*See also* RdQ)
recovery quotient
respiratory quotient

RQLQ
Respiratory Quality of Life Questionnaire
rhinoconjunctivitis-specific quality of life questionnaire

RQS
repeated quick stretch

RQS-E
repeated quick stretch from elongation

RQS-SEC
repeated quick stretch superimposed upon an existing contraction

RR
radial rate
radiation reaction
radiation response
rapid radiometric
rate ratio
reading retarded
recovery room
red reflex
regular rate
regular respiration
relative response
relative risk
renin release
respiratory rate
respiratory reserve
response rate

retinal reflex
rheumatoid rosette
right rotation
risk ratio
Riva-Rocci (sphygmomanometer)
  (*See also* RRS)
road rash
roentgenographic pelvimetry
rotation right
ruthenium red

R/R
rales/rhonchi

R&R
rate and rhythm
recent and remote
recession and resection
recession-resection
recess-resect
rest and recuperation

RRA
radioreceptor activity
radioreceptor assay
right radial artery
right renal artery

RRAM
rapid rhythmic alternating
  movements
relative response attributable to the
  maneuver

RRB
rigid rockerbottom

RRC
relative risk cohort
residency review committee
risk reduction component
routine respiratory care

RRCT no (m)
regular rate, clear tones, no
  murmurs

RRD
rhegmatogenous retinal detachment

RRE
radiation-related eosinophilia
regressive resistive exercise
Rev response element
round, regular, and equal (pupils)
  (*See also* RR&E)

RR&E
round, regular, and equal (pupils)
  (*See also* RRE)

RRED(r)
Rapid Rare Event Detection

RREF
resting radionuclide ejection fraction

RREID
rapid rabies enzyme
  immunodiagnosis

RRF
ragged red fiber
residual renal function
right rectus femoris

RRFC
renal reserve filtration capacity

RR-IIPO
rapid recompression-high pressure
  oxygen

RRI
recurrent respiratory infection
reflex relaxation index
relative response index
renal resistive index

RR-IOL
remove and replace intraocular lens

RRM
reduced renal mass
right radial mastectomy

RRMS
relapsing-remitting multiple sclerosis

rRNA
ribosomal ribonucleic acid
ribosomal RNA

RRND
right radical neck dissection

RROM
resistive range of motion

R rot
right rotation

RRP
radical retropubic prostatectomy
recurrent respiratory papilloma
recurrent respiratory papillomatosis
relative refractory period

RRpm
respiratory rate per minute

RRQG
right rostral quarter ganglion

RRR
recovery room routine
regular rate and rhythm
relative risk reduction
renin-release rate
renin-release ratio
risk rescue rating

NOTES

RRRN
round, regular, react normally (pupils)

RRS
retrorectal space
Riva-Rocci sphygmomanometer (*See also* RR)

Rrs
respiratory resistance

RRT
randomized response technique
relative retention time
resazurin reduction time

RRTM
retroperitoneal residual tumor mass

RRU
rapid reintegration unit
respiratory resistance unit

RRV
Rhesus rotavirus
right renal vein
Ross River virus

RRVN
retrolabyrinthine/retrosigmoidal vestibular neurectomy
retrolabyrinthine/retrosigmoid vestibular neurectomy

RRVO
repair relaxed vaginal outlet

RRVS
recovery room vital signs

RRV-TV
rhesus rotavirus-tetravalent vaccine

RRW
rales, rhonchi or wheezes

RS
random sample
rapid smoking
rating schedule
Raynaud syndrome
reactive site
reading of standard
recipient's serum
rectal sinus
rectal swab
rectosigmoid
recurrent seizures
Reed-Sternberg (cell) (*See also* R-S)
rehydrating solution
reinforcing stimulus
relative survival
remnant stomach
renal specialist
Repression-Sensitization (Scale)
reproductive success
reschedule
resolved sarcoidosis
resorcinol-sulfur

respiratory symptom
respiratory syncytial (virus)
respiratory system
response to stimulus (ratio)
restart
reticulated siderocyte (*See also* R-S)
Reye syndrome
rhythm strip
right sacrum
right septum
right side
right stellate (ganglion)
right subclavian
Ringer solution
ring sideroblast
Ritchie sedimentation
Roberts syndrome
rumination syndrome

RS-61443
mycophenolate mofetil

R-S
Reed-Sternberg (cell) (*See also* RS)
reticulated siderocyte (*See also* RS)
rough-smooth (variation)

R/S
reschedule
rest stress
rupture spontaneous

R&S
restraint and seclusion

R/s
roentgen per second

Rs
respond
response
(total) systemic resistance

r$_s$
rank correlation coefficient

R/S I
resuscitation status one (full resuscitative effort)

R/S II
resuscitation status two (no code, therapeutic measures only)

R/S III
resuscitation status three (no code, comfort measures only)

RSA
rabbit serum albumin (*See also* RbSA)
rat serum albumin
recurrent spontaneous abortion
regular spiking activity
relative specific activity
relative standard accuracy
respiratory sinus arrhythmia
reticulum (cell) sarcoma (*See also* RCS)

right sacroanterior (fetal position)
right sacrum anterior
right subclavian artery
roentgen stereophotogrammetric
   analysis

Rsa
   (total) systemic arterial resistance
RSAPE
   remitting seronegative arthritis with
      pitting edema
RSB
   reticulocyte standard buffer
   right sternal border
RSBI
   Rapid Shallow Breathing Index
RSBT
   rhythmic sensory bombardment
      therapy
RSC
   radioscaphocapitate
   rat spleen cell
   rectosigmoid neocolpopoiesis
   rested state contraction
   reversible sickle cell
   right side colon (cancer)
   right subclavian (artery) (vein)
RScA
   right scapuloanterior (fetal position)
RSCCD
   Rating Scale of Communication in
      Cognitive Decline
rsCD4
   recombinant soluble CD4
RSCL
   Rotterdam Symptom Check List
RSCN
   reactive spindle cell nodule
RScP
   right scapuloposterior (fetal
      position)
RSCS
   respiratory system compliance score
RSCT
   Rach Sentence Completion Test
   Rotter Sentence Completion Test
rscu-PA
   recombinant, single-chain, urokinase-
      type plasminogen activator
RSCVP
   right subclavian central venous
RSD
   rad surface dose

reflex sympathetic dystrophy
relative sagittal depth
relative standard deviation
RSDP
   random single donor platelet
RSE
   rat synaptic ending
   reactive subdural effusion
   refractory status epilepticus
   reverse sutured eye
   right sternal edge
RSEP
   right somatosensory evoked
      potential
RSES
   Rosenberg Self-Esteem Scale
RSF
   raw soybean flour
RSG
   Reitan Strength of Grip
RSH
   rectus sheath hematoma
   reduced sulfhydryl group
RSI
   rapid-sequence induction
   rapid sequence intubation
   repetitive strain injury
   repetitive stress injury
R-SICU
   respiratory-surgical intensive care
      unit
RSIVP
   rapid-sequence intravenous
      pyelography
RSL
   renal solute load
   right sacrolateral (fetal position)
R SL brace
   right short leg brace
RSLD
   repair of sublethal damage
RSLR
   reverse straight leg raise
RSLT
   reduced-size liver transplant
   reduced-size liver transplantation
RSLTx
   right single lung transplant
RSM
   remote study monitoring
   risk-screening model

NOTES

r-Sm
> reversal speed of bronchoconstriction in response to methacholine

RSMR
> relative standardized mortality ratio

RSN
> right substantia nigra

RSNI
> round spermatid nuclear injection

RSO
> right salpingo-oophorectomy
> right superior oblique (muscle)

rSO2, rSO$_2$
> regional oxygen saturation

RSOP
> right superior oblique palsy

RSP
> rapid straight pacing
> rat serum protein
> recirculating single pass
> removable silicone plug
> rhinoseptoplasty
> right sacroposterior (fetal position)

RS3PE
> remitting seronegative symmetric synovitis with pitting edema

RSPK
> recurrent spontaneous psychokinesis

RSPM
> Raven Standard Progressive Matrices

RSR
> rectosphincteric reflex
> regular sinus rhythm
> relative survival rate
> response-stimulus ratio
> right superior rectus (muscle)

rSR′
> RSR prime

RSRI
> renal:systemic renin index

RSS
> rat stomach strip
> rearfoot stability system
> rectosigmoidoscope
> reduced space symbologies
> repetitive stress syndrome
> representative sample sectioned
> rotatory subluxation of scaphoid

RSs
> relative supersaturation

RSSE
> Russian spring-summer encephalitis (See also RSS)

RSSEV
> Russian spring-summer encephalitis virus

RSSR
> relatively slow sinus rate

RST
> radiosensitivity test
> rapid simple tests
> rapid surfactant test
> reagin screen test
> right sacrotransverse (fetal position)
> rubrospinal tract

RSTL
> relaxed skin tension line

RSTS
> retropharyngeal soft tissue space

RSTs
> Rodney Smith tubes

RSV
> regurgitant stroke volume
> respiratory syncytial virus
> right subclavian vein

RSVA
> ruptured sinus of Valsalva aneurysm

RSVB
> respiratory syncytial virus bronchiolitis

RSVC
> right superior vena cava

RSV-IG, RSVIG
> respiratory syncytial virus immunoglobulin

RSV-IGIV, RSV-IVIG
> respiratory syncytial virus immune globulin intravenous
> respiratory syncytial virus intravenous immunoglobulin
> Rous sarcoma virus immune globulin intravenous
> Rous sarcoma virus immunoglobulin intravenous

RSVP
> rejuvenation with sparing of vascular perforators

RSW
> right-sided weakness

RT
> rabbit trachea
> radiation therapy (See also RXT, XRT)
> radiologic technology
> radiotelemetry
> radiotherapy (See also Rad, RADIO, Rad Ther, Rx)
> radium therapy
> random transfusion
> raphe transection
> rational therapy
> reaction time
> reading task

reading test
reading time
receptor transforming
reciprocating tachycardia
recovery time
recreational therapy
rectal temperature (*See also* R/T)
red tetrazolium
reduction time
relaxation time
renal transplant
repetition time
Reporter's Test
reptilase time
resistance training
resistance transfer
respiratory technology
respiratory therapy
rest tremor
retransformation
reverse transcriptase
right (*See also* R, (R), Rt, rt)
right thigh
right triceps
room temperature (*See also* rt)
running total

rT$_3$

reverse T$_3$

RT$_3$

resin triiodothyronine
(serum) resin triiodothyronine
(uptake) (*See also* RT$_3$U)

RT$_4$

resin thyroxin

R/T

rectal temperature (*See also* RT)
related to (*See also* R/t)

R$_T$

total pulmonary resistance

Rt

right (*See also* R, (R), RT, Rt)

R/t

related to (*See also* R/T)

rT

ribothymidine
reverse triiodothyronine

rt

right (*See also* (R), RT, Rt, rt)
room temperature (*See also* RT)

RTA

renal tubular acidosis

renal tubular antigen
road traffic accident

RTAH

right anterior hemiblock

RTAS

radiology telephone access system

RTAT

right anterior thigh

RTAV

Resistencia virus

RTAVI

Risk-Taking, Attitude, Values
Inventory

RTB

return to baseline

RTC

(a)round the clock
randomized trial, controlled
Readiness to Change (questionnaire)
renal tubular cell
research and training center
residential treatment center
return to clinic

RTCA

ribavirin

RTD

renal tubular dysgenesis
repetitive trauma disorder
residual thermal damage
resubmission turnaround document
routine test dilution

RTD-1

rhesus theta defensin 1

rtd

retarded
retired

RTE

rabbit thymus extract
renal tubular epithelial

RTER

return to emergency room

RTF

replication and transfer
resistance transfer factor
respiratory tract fluid
return to flow

RTFNA

real-time fine-needle aspiration

RTH

resistance to thyroid hormone

RtH

right-handed

NOTES

RTI

respiratory tract infection
reverse transcriptase inhibitor

Rti

resistance to movement of lung
tissue
tissue resistance

RTK

receptor tyrosine kinase
rhabdoid tumor of the kidney

RTKP

radiothermokeratoplasty

RTL

reactive to light (pupils)

rtl

rectal

RT LAT, rt lat

right lateral (*See also* RL, RT LAT,
rt lat)

RTLF

respiratory tract lining fluid

RTLX

real-time, low-intensity x-ray

RTM

reciprocal tension membrane
routine medical care

R_{tmf}

total matrix formation rate

rTMP

ribothymidylic acid (*See also* TMP)

RTN

renal tubular necrosis
routine

rtn

return

rTNFα

recombinant tumor necrosis factor
alpha

rTNM

retreatment (staging of cancer)

RTO

return to office
right toe off

RTOG

radiation therapy oncology group

Rtot

total airway resistance

RTP

radiation therapy planning
radiation treatment planning
renal transplant patient
return to play
reverse transcriptase-producing
(agent)

RTPA, rt PA, rtPA, rt-PA

recombinant tissue-type plasminogen
activator

RT-PCR

reverse transcriptase polymerase
chain reaction
reverse transcription polymerase
chain reaction

RTPE

reverse transcriptase primer
extension

RTPS

radiation therapy planning system

RTR

red (blood cell) turnover rate
renal transplant recipient
retention time ratio
return to room

RTRR

return to recovery room

RTS

real-time scan
relative tumor size
return to sender
Revised Trauma Score
right toe strike

rTSAB

rodent thyroid-stimulating antibody

rt scap bord

right scapular border

RTSW

Repeated Test of Sustained
Wakefulness

r_{tt}

obtained coefficient
reliability coefficient

RTU

ready to use
real-time ultrasonography (*See also*
RTUS)
relative time unit

RT₃U

resin triiodothyronine uptake (*See
also* RT₃)

rTU

ribosomal ribonucleic acid
transcription unit

RTUS

real-time ultrasonography (*See also*
RTU)

RTV

ritonavir
room temperature vulcanization
room temperature vulcanized
room temperature vulcanizing

RTW

return to work (*See also* R/W)

RTWD

return to work determination

RTx

radiation therapy

RU

radioactive uptake
radioulnar
rat unit
reading of unknown
recall urticaria
rectourethral
recurrent ulcer
residual urine
resin uptake
resistance unit (*See also* R)
retrograde urogram
retroverted uterus
right uninjured
right uninvolved
right upper
rodent ulcer
roentgen unit
routine urinalysis

RU-1

human embryonic lung fibroblast

RU 486

mifepristone

Ru

ruthenium

⁸²Ru

rubidium-82

RUA

routine urine analysis

RuBP

ribulose bisphophate

RUDS

reactive upper airways dysfunction
syndrome

RUE

right upper extremity

RUG

resource utilization group
retrograde urethrogram
retrograde urethrography

r-UK

recombinant urokinase

RUL

right upper (eye)lid
right upper lateral
right upper limb
right upper lobe
right upper lung

RUM

right upper medial

RUMI

Rowden uterine manipulator-injector

RUO

right ureteral orifice

RUOQ

right upper outer quadrant

RUP

rat urine protein
right upper pole

rupt

ruptured

RUQ

right upper quadrant

RUR

resin uptake ratio

RURTI

recurrent upper respiratory tract
infection

RUS

radioulnar synostosis
real-time ultrasonography
recurrent ulcerative stomatitis

RUSB

right upper sternal border

RUSS

recurrent ulcerative scarifying
stomatitis

RUT

rapid urease test

RUV

residual urine volume

RUX

right upper extremity

RV

random variable
rat virus
Rauscher virus
rectal vault
rectovaginal
reference value
reinforcement value
renal venous
reovirus
reserve volume
residual volume
respiratory volume
retinal vasculitis
retrovaginal
retroversion
return visit
rheumatoid vasculitis
rhinovirus
right ventricle
right ventricular

R

NOTES

RV *(continued)*
    rubella vaccine
    rubella virus
    Russell viper (time) *(See also* RVT, RVVT)

R_V
    radius of view

Rv
    rotavirus

RVA
    rabies vaccine adsorbed
    recombinant virus assay
    reentrant ventricular arrhythmia
    right ventricular activation
    right ventricular apex
    right ventricular apical
    right vertebral artery

RVAD
    right ventricular assist device

RVAW
    right ventricle anterior wall

RVB
    red venous blood

RVBF
    reversed vertebral blood flow

RVC
    radioactivity of vegetative cells
    respond to verbal command

RVCB
    right ventricular copulsation balloon

RVD
    reference vessel diameter
    relative vertebral density
    relative volume decrease
    right ventricular dimension
    right vertebral density

RVDO
    right ventricular diastolic overload

RVDP
    right ventricular diastolic pressure

RVDT
    retinal venous dilation and tortuosity

RVDV
    right ventricular diastolic volume

RVE
    right ventricular enlargement

RVECP
    right ventricular endocardial potential

RVEDD
    right ventricular end-diastolic diameter

RVEDP
    right ventricular end-diastolic pressure

RVEDV
    right ventricular end-diastolic volume

RVEDVI
    right ventricular end-diastolic volume index

RVEF
    right ventricular ejection fraction
    right ventricular end-flow

RVERP
    right ventricular refractory period

RVESV
    right ventricular end-systolic volume

RVESVI
    right ventricular end-systolic volume index

RVET
    right ventricular ejection time

RVF
    renal vascular failure
    Rift Valley fever
    right ventricular failure
    right ventricular function
    right visual field

RVFP
    right ventricular filling pressure

RVFV
    Rift Valley fever virus

RVG
    radionuclide ventriculogram
    radionuclide ventriculography
    radiovisiography
    relative value guide
    right ventrogluteal
    right visceral ganglion

RVH
    renal vascular hypertension
    renovascular hypertension
    right ventricular hypertrophy

RVHD
    rheumatic valvular heart disease

RVI
    relative value index
    right ventricle infarction

RVID
    right ventricular internal diameter
    right ventricular internal dimension

RVIDd
    right ventricle internal dimension diastole

RVIDP
    right ventricular initial diastolic pressure

RVIT
    right ventricular inflow tract (view)

RVL
    right vastus lateralis

RVLG
right ventrolateral gluteal
RVLM
rostral ventrolateral medulla
RVM
right ventricular mass
RVN
radionuclide ventriculogram
retrolabyrinthine vestibular
neurectomy
RVO
relaxed vaginal outlet
retinal vein occlusion
right ventricular outflow
right ventricular overactivity
RVol
regurgitant volume
RVOT
right ventricular outflow tract
RVP
red veterinary petrolatum
renovascular pressure
resting venous pressure
right ventricular pressure
RVPFR
right ventricular peak filling rate
RVPRA
renal vein plasma renin activity
RVR
rapid ventricular response
reduced vascular response
reduced vestibular response
relative vascular resistance
renal vascular resistance
renal vein renin
repetitive ventricular response
resistance to venous return
RVRA
renal vein renin activity
renal vein renin assay
renal venous renin assay
RV/RA
renal vein/renal activity (ratio)
RVRC
renal vein renin concentration
RV/RF
retroverted/retroflexed
RVRI
renal vascular resistance index
RVS
rabies vaccine, adsorbed
recognizable viral syndrome

relative value scale
relative value schedule
relative value study
reported visual sensation
retrovaginal space
Rokeach Value Survey (psychologic
test)
RVSO
right ventricle stroke output
RVSP
right ventricular systolic pressure
RVSW
right ventricular stroke work
RVSWI
right ventricular stroke work index
RVT
renal vein thrombosis
Russell viper (venom) time (*See
also* RV, RVVT)
RVTE
recurring venous thromboembolism
RV/TLC
residual volume to total lung
capacity (ratio)
residual volume/total lung capacity
(ratio)
RVU
relative value unit
RVV
rubella vaccine-like virus
Russell's viper venom
RVVT
Russell's viper venom time (*See
also* RV, RVT)
RVWD
right ventricular wall device
RW
radiologic warfare
ragweed
respiratory work
right (ear), warm (stimulus)
round window
R-W
Rideal-Walker (coefficient)
R/W
return to work (*See also* RTW)
RWAGE
ragweed antigen E
RWBT
rapid whole blood test
RWECochG
round window electrocochleography

NOTES

RWG
　rye whole-grain
RWIS
　restraint and water immersion
　　stress
RWJF
　Robert Wood Johnson Foundation
RWM
　regional wall motion
RWMA
　regional wall motion abnormality
RWP
　ragweed pollen
　R-wave progression
　　(electrocardiography)
RWS
　ragweed sensitivity
RWT
　relative wall thickness
　Roche, Wainer, and Thissen
　　method of height prediction
　R-wave threshold
　　(electrocardiography)
RX
　rapid exchange
Rx
　drug
　medication
　pharmacy
　prescribe
　prescription

prescription drug
radiotherapy (*See also* Rad, RADIO,
　Rad Ther, RT)
take [L. *recipe*] (*See also* R)
r(X)
　right X (chromosome)
Rxd
　treatment (prescribed)
Rx'd US
　treated with ultrasound, diathermy,
　　and traction
RXLI
　recessive X-linked ichthyosis
RXN
　reaction
Rx Phys
　treating physician
RXR
　9-*cis* retinoic acid
　9-cis retinoic acid receptor
　retinoid X receptor
RXT
　radiation therapy (*See also* RT)
　right exotropia
R-Y
　Roux-en-Y (anastomosis)
RZ
　reserve zone
RZR
　retinoid Z receptor

S

apparent power
area (*See also* A, a)
entropy (in thermodynamics)
exposure time (radiology)
foreskin
half [L. *semis*] (*See also* HF, hf, sem., semi, ss)
label [L. *signa* mark, write on] (*See also* s, sig)
left [L. *sinister*] (*See also* s)
mean dose per unit cumulated activity
midpoint of sella turcica (point)
relative storage capacity
response to white space
sacral
saline (*See also* SA, Sa, SAL, sal)
same
saturated
saturation (of hemoglobin)
schizophrenia
screen-containing cassette
second (*See also* s, sec)
section (*See also* s, SEC, sec, sect)
sedimentation coefficient
sella (turcica)
semilente (insulin)
senile
senility
sensation (*See also* s)
sensitivity (*See also* sen, sens)
sensory
septum
sequential (analysis)
series (*See also* s, ser)
serine (*See also* Ser)
serum
sick
siderocyte
siemens
sign (*See also* /S/, /s/, s)
signature (prescription) (*See also* /S/)
signed (*See also* /S/, s)
silicate
single (marital status)
singular
sinus
sister
small (*See also* Sm, sm)
smooth (bacterial colony)
soft
soil
solid

soluble
solute (*See also* SOL, solu)
son
sone (unit of loudness)
south
space (*See also* sp)
spasm
spatial aptitude (in General Aptitude Test Battery)
specific activity (*See also* SA)
spherical (lens) (*See also* Sph, sph)
spleen
sponge
sporadic
standard normal deviation
stem (cell)
stimulus (*See also* R, ST)
storage
streptomycin (*See also* SM, STM)
subject
subjective (findings)
substrate
suction
suicide
sulcus
sulfur
sum (of arithmetic series)
supervision
supravergence
surface
surgery (*See also* SURG, surg)
susceptible
suture
Svedberg (unit of sedimentation coefficient)
swine
Swiss (mouse)
symmetrical
sympathetic
synthesis (phase in cell cycle)
systole
without (*See also* ō, s̄, WO, w/o, wo)
write, let it be written [L. *signa*]

S1, S2, S3, S4

first through fourth heart sounds
suicide risk classification

S_1–S_4

first to fourth heart sounds

S1–S5

first to fifth sacral nerves
first to fifth sacral vertebrae

S7

summation gallop

S'
shoulder

/S/, /s/
sign (*See also* S, /s/, s)
signature (prescription) (*See also* S)
signed (*See also* S, s)

s
atomic orbital with angular
momentum quantum number zero
distance
label [L. *signa*] (*See also* S, sig)
left [L. *sinister*] (*See also* S)
length of path
sample standard deviation
sample variance (*See also* s²)
satellite (chromosome)
scruple
second (*See also* S)
section (*See also* S, SEC, sec,
sect)
sedimentation coefficient
selection coefficient
sensation (*See also* S)
series (*See also* S, ser)
sign (*See also* S, /S/, /s/)
signed (*See also* S)
steady state (*See also* ss)
suckling

7's
serial sevens test

s̄
conductivity (*See also* cond)
cross-section
millisecond (*See also* msec, ms, σ)
population standard deviation
reflection coefficient
standard deviation (*See also* SD)
Stefan-Boltzmann constant
stress
surface tension (*See also* ST)
type of molecular bond
wave number
wavenumber
without (*See also* ō, S, WO, w/o,
wo)
without spectacles

s²
sample variance (*See also* s)

³⁵S
sulfur-35

SA
according to art [L. *secundum
artem*]
sacroanterior
salicylamide
salicylic acid
saline (*See also* S, Sa, SAL, sal)
salt added

salvage angioplasty
sarcoma (*See also* sarc)
second antibody
secondary amenorrhea
secondary anemia
secondary arrest
self-agglutinating
self-analysis
semen analysis
sensitizing antibody
sensory awareness
septal apical
serratus anterior
serum albumin (*See also* SAB)
serum aldolase
short acting
sialic acid
sialoadenectomy
siblings (raised) apart
simian adenovirus
sinoatrial (node) (*See also* S-A,
SN, SAN)
sinus arrest
sinus arrhythmia
skeletal age
sleep apnea
slightly active
slow acetylator
social acquiescence
social age
soluble in alkaline (medium)
Spanish American
spatial average
specific activity (*See also* S)
spectrum analysis
sperm abnormality
sperm agglutinin
spiking activity
spinal anesthesia
splenic artery
standard accuracy
stimulus artifact
Stokes-Adams (attack, syndrome)
(*See also* SAA)
subarachnoid
substance abuse
suicide alert
suicide attempt
surface antigen
surface area
sustained action
sympathetic activity
systemic artery
systemic aspergillosis

S-A
sinoatrial (node) (*See also* SA, SN,
SAN)

S/A

same as
sugar and acetone (*See also* S&A)

S&A

sickness and accident (insurance)
sugar and acetone (*See also* S/A)

Sa

most anterior point of anterior
contour of the sella turcica
(point)
saline (*See also* S, SA, SAL, sal)
samarium

SAA

same as above
serum amyloid (type) A
severe aplastic anemia
splenic artery aneurysm
Stokes-Adams attack (*See also* SA)
synthetic amino acids

SAAG

serum ascites-albumin gradient

SAANDs

selective apoptotic antineoplastic
drugs

SAARD

slow-acting antirheumatic drug

SAAST

Self-Administered Alcoholism
Screening test

SAB

serum albumin (*See also* SA)
short-acting block
significant asymptomatic bacteriuria
sinoatrial block
Spanish American black
spontaneous abortion
streptavidin-biotin
streptavidin-biotin peroxidase
complex
subarachnoid bleed
subarachnoid block

SABOV

Sabo virus

SABP

spontaneous acute bacterial
peritonitis

SABR

screening auditory brainstem
response

SABV

Saboya virus

SAC

saccharin
screening and acute care
seasonal allergic conjunctivitis
segmental antigen challenge
serial autocorrelation
serum aminoglycoside concentration
short arm cast
sideline assessment of concussion
space available for the cord
splenic adherent cell
stable access cannula

SACA

Service Assessment for Children
and Adolescents

SACC.

short arm cylinder cast

sacc

cogwheel respiration [Fr. *saccades*
to jerk]

SACD

subacute combined degeneration
(*See also* SCD)

SACE

serum angiotensin-converting
enzyme (activity)

SACH

small animal care hospital
soft ankle, cushioned heel
(orthopaedic appliance)

SACHT

serum antichymotrypsin

sac-il

sacroiliac (*See also* SI)

SACL

Sales Attitude Check List

SACQ

Student Adaptation to College
Questionnaire

SACS

secondary anticoagulation system

SACSF

subarachnoid cerebrospinal fluid

SACT

sinoatrial conduction time

SAD

Scale of Anxiety and Depression
seasonal affective disorder
Self-Assessment Depression (Scale)
separation anxiety disorder
serial-agitated dilution
severe autoimmune disease

S

NOTES

SAD *(continued)*
  sinoaortic denervation
  small airway dysfunction
  social anxiety disorder
  social avoidance and distress
  source-to-axis distance
  specific antibody deficiency
  subacromial decompression
  subacute dialysis
  sugar and acetone determination
  sugar, acetone, diacetic acid (test)
  superior axis deviation
  suppressor-activating determinant

SADBE
  squaric acid dibutylester

SADD
  Standardized Assessment of
    Depressive Disorders

SADIA
  small-angle double-incidence
    angiogram

SADL
  simulated activities of daily living

SADQ
  Self-Administered Dependency
    Questionnaire

SADR
  suspected adverse drug reaction

SADS
  Schedule for Affective Disorders
    and Schizophrenia
  seasonal affective disorder
    syndrome
  Shipman Anxiety Depression Scale

SADS-C
  Schedule for Affective Disorders
    and Schizophrenia-Change

SADS-L
  Schedule for Affective Disorders
    and Schizophrenia-Lifetime
    (Version)

SADT
  Stetson Auditory Discrimination
    Test

SAE
  serious adverse event
  short above-elbow (cast)
  specific action exercise
  subcortical atherosclerotic
    encephalopathy
  supported arm exercise

SAEB
  sinoatrial entrance block

SAECG, SaECG, SAEG, SAEKG
  signal-averaged electrocardiogram
  signal-averaged electrocardiography
  signal-averaging electrocardiogram

SAEP
  Salmonella abortus equi pyrogen

SAESU
  substance abuse evaluation screen
    unit

SAF
  Self-Analysis Form
  self-articulating femoral (hip
    prosthesis)
  serum accelerator factor
  simultaneous auditory feedback
  Spanish American female

SAFA
  soluble antigen fluorescent antibody
    (test)

SAFE
  sexual assault forensic evidence
  simulated aircraft fire and
    emergency
  solid ankle flexible endoskeletal
  stationary ankle flexible
    endoskeleton
  stationary attachment flexible
    endoskeletal

SAFHS
  sonic-accelerated fracture-healing
    system

SAFK
  single-axis friction knee (prosthesis)

SAFTEE
  Systematic Assessment for
    Treatment of Emergent Events

SAFV
  Saint-Floris virus

SAG
  sodium antimony gluconate
  Swiss(-type) agammaglobulinemia

sag
  sagittal

SAGB
  Swedish Adjustable Gastric Band

Sag D
  sagittal diameter

SAGE
  serial analysis of gene expression

SAGES-P
  Screening Assessment for Gifted
    Elementary Students, Primary

SAGM
  sodium chloride, adenine, glucose,
    mannitol

SAGV
  Sagiyama virus

SAH
  S-adenosylhomocysteine (*See also*
    AdoHcy)
  S-adenosyl-L-homocysteine (*See also*
    AdoHcy)

subarachnoid hemorrhage

systemic arterial hypertension

SAHEM

self-applied health enhancement method

SAHIOES

Staphylococcus aureus hyperimmunoglobulinemia E syndrome

SAHS

sleep apnea-hypersomnolence syndrome

sleep apnea-hypopnea syndrome

SAHS-UAO

sleep apnea hypersomnolence syndrome associated with upper airway obstruction

SAI

Schedule for Assessment of Insight

Schema Assessment instrument

Self-Analysis Inventory

Sexual Arousability Inventory

Social Adequacy Index

sodium amytal interview

Student Adjustment Inventory

surface asymmetry index

systemic active immunotherapy

SAICAR

succinoaminoimidazole carboxamide (ribonucleotide)

succinyl aminoimidazole carboxamide ribotide

SAIDS

simian acquired immunodeficiency syndrome

SAKV

Sakhalin virus

SAL

salbutamol

salicylate (*See also* sal)

salicylic and lactic acid paint

saline (*See also* S, SA, Sa, sal)

Salmonella

self-aligning knee (prosthesis)

sensorineural acuity level

sensory acuity level

specified antilymphocytic

sterility assurance level

suction-assisted lipectomy

suction-assisted lipoplasty

SAL 12

sequential analysis of twelve chemistry constituents

sal

salicylate

salicylic

saline (*See also* S, SA, Sa, SAL)

saliva

salt

SALF

subacute liver failure

SALK

single-axis locking knee (prosthesis)

SALT

skin-associated lymphoid tissue

SALT-P

Slosson Articulation Language Test with Phonology

SALV

Salehabad virus

SAM

metaproterenol

S-adenosyl-L-methionine

salicylamide

scanning acoustic microscope

self-administered medication

sex arousal mechanism

short arc motion

sleep apnea monitor

smart anesthesia multigas

Spanish American male

spinal analysis machine

structural aluminum malleable

subcutaneous augmentation material

sulfated acid mucopolysaccharide

surface-active material

surface adherent monocyte

synthetic, adhesive, moisture (vapor permeable)

systemic anterior motion

systolic anterior motion (of mitral valve)

SAMBA

simultaneous areolar mastopexy and breast augmentation

SAMe, SAM-e

S-adenosylmethionine

SAMF

single antibody millipore filtration

SAMI

socially acceptable monitoring instrument

S

NOTES

717

sAMP
adenylosuccinic acid

SAMS
Study Attitudes and Methods Survey

S-AMY
serum amylase

SAN
side-arm nebulizer
sinoatrial node (*See also* SA, S-A, SN)
sinuatrial node
slept all night
solitary autonomous nodule

SANA
sinoatrial node artery

sanat
sanatorium

SANC
short arm navicular cast

SANDO
sensory ataxic neuropathy with dysarthria and ophthalmoplegia

SANDR
sinoatrial nodal reentry

sang.
sanguineous

sanit
sanitarium
sanitary
sanitation

SANS
Scale for the Assessment of Negative Symptoms
schedule for negative symptoms
Stoller afferent nerve stimulation
sympathetic autonomic nervous system

SANV
Sango virus

SAO
small airway obstruction
Southeast Asian ovalocytosis
splanchnic artery occlusion

SaO$_2$, S$_{Ao2}$
arterial oxygen saturation
oxygen saturation (*See also* OS, O$_2$ sat., SO$_2$)

SAP
saline-assisted polypectomy
sensory action potential
serum acid phosphatase
serum alkaline phosphatase
serum amyloid P (component)
severe acute pancreatitis
situs ambiguus with polysplenia
sporadic adenomatous polyps
stable angina pectoris

Staphylococcus aureus protease
systemic arterial pressure
systolic arterial pressure

SAP1
sphingolipid activator protein-1

SAP-1
stress-activated protein 1

sap.
saponification
saponify

SAPA
spatial average-pulse average

SAPD
self-administration of psychoactive drug
self-administration of psychotropic drug
signal-averaged P-wave duration

SAPH
saphenous

SAPHO
synovitis, acne, pustulosis, hyperostosis, osteomyelitis (syndrome)

SAPMS
short arm posterior-molded splint

sapon
saponification

SAPP
sodium acid pyrophosphate

SAPS
Scale for the Assessment of Positive Symptoms
short arm plaster splint
Simplified Acute Physiology Score
single-action pumping system

SAPS II
Simplified Acute Physiology Score version II

SAQ
saquinavir
School Atmosphere Questionnaire
Seattle angina questionnaire
Sexual Adjustment Questionnaire
short-arc quadriceps (test)
Substance Abuse Questionnaire

SAQC
statistical analysis and quality control

SAQLI
Sleep Apnea Quality of Life Index

SAR
scaffold-associated regions
scatter-air ratio
seasonal allergic rhinitis
sexual attitude reassessment
sexual attitude restructuring

specific absorption rate
structure-activity relationship
Sar
sarcosine
sulfarsphenamine
SARA
sexually acquired reactive arthritis
system for anesthetic and
respiratory administration
SARAN
senior admitting resident's
admission note
SARC
seasonal allergic rhinoconjunctivitis
sarc
sarcoma (*See also* SA)
SarCNU
sarcosinamide chloroethyl
nitrosourea
SARM
selective androgen-receptor
modulator
SARME
surgically assisted rapid maxillary
expansion
SARPE
surgically assisted rapid palatal
expansion
S Arrh
sinus arrhythmia
SART
Sexual Assault Response Team
sinoatrial recovery time
standard acid reflux test
SARV
Santa Rosa virus
SAS
saline, agent, and saline
scalenus anticus syndrome
School Assessment Survey
School Attitude Survey
see assessment sheet
self-rating anxiety scale
short arm splint
shoulder arm system
simultaneous analog stimulation
Situational Attitude Scale
Sklar Aphasia Scale
sleep apnea syndrome
small animal surgery
small aorta syndrome
Social Adaptation Status

Social Adjustment Scale
sodium amylosulfate
space-adaptation syndrome
Specific Activity Scale
statistical analysis system
statistical applications software
sterile aqueous solution
sterile aqueous suspension
subaortic stenosis
subarachnoid space
subaxial subluxation
sulfasalazine
supravalvular aortic stenosis (*See
also* SVAS)
surface-active substance
synthetic absorbable suture
SASH
saline, agent, saline, and heparin
SASI
Separation Anxiety Symptom
Inventory
SASMAS
skin-adipose superficial
musculoaponeurotic system
SASP
salazosulfapyridine
salicylazosulfapyridine
SASPP
septum pellucidum absent with
porencephalia syndrome
syndrome of absence of septum
pellucidum with poerencephaly
SASRS
Social Adjustment Self-Report Scale
SASS
Social Adaptation Self-Evaluation
Scale
SASSAD
six-area, six-sign atopic dermatitis
SASSI
Substance Abuse Subtle Screening
Inventory
SAT
satellite
saturated (*See also* sat., sat'd, std)
saturation (*See also* sat.)
Scholastic Aptitude Test
School Ability Test
School Attitude Test
self-administered therapy
Senior Apperception Technique
Senior Apperception Test

S

NOTES

SAT *(continued)*
    serum antitrypsin
    Shapes Analysis Test
    single-agent (chemo)therapy
    slide agglutination test
    specific antithymocytic
    speech awareness threshold
    spermatogenic activity test
    spinal attunement technique
    spontaneous activity test
    spontaneous autoimmune thyroiditis
    Stanford Achievement Test
    structural atypia
    subacute thrombosis
    subacute thyroiditis
    symptomless autoimmune thyroiditis
    systematized assertive therapy
    systemic assertive therapy
    terbutaline

sat.
    satisfactory
    saturated (*See also* SAT, sat'd, std)
    saturation (*See also* SAT)

SATA
    Scholastic Abilities Test for Adults
    spatial average-temporal average

SATB
    Special Aptitude Test Battery

SATC
    substance abuse treatment clinic

sat. cond
    satisfactory condition

sat'd
    saturated (*See also* std)

SATL
    surgical Achilles tendon lengthening

SATM
    sodium aurothiomalate

satn
    saturation

SATP
    spatial average temporal peak
    substance abuse treatment program

SATS
    refers to oxygen saturation levels

sat. sol., sat. soln.
    saturated solution

SATU
    substance abuse treatment unit

SATV
    Sathuperi virus

SAU
    statistical analysis unit

SAV
    San Angelo virus
    sequential atrioventricular (pacing)
    streptavidin
    supraannular valve

SA/V
    surface area to volume ratio

SAVD
    spontaneous assisted vaginal delivery

SAVED
    saphenous vein graft de novo

SAWV
    sawgrass virus

SAX
    short axis

SAZ
    sulfasalazine

SB
    safety belt
    sandbag
    scleral buckle
    seat belt
    Sengstaken-Blakemore (tube)
    septal basal
    serum bilirubin
    shortness of breath
    sick bay (military)
    sick boy
    side bend
    sideroblast
    Silvestroni-Bianco (syndrome)
    single blind
    single breath
    sinus bradycardia
    slide board
    small bowel
    sodium balance
    Southern blot
    soybean
    spina bifida
    sponge bath
    spontaneous blastogenesis
    spontaneously breathing
    stand by (*See also* ST BY)
    Stanford-Binet (Intelligence Scale) (*See also* SBIS)
    stereotyped behavior
    sternal border
    stillbirth
    stillborn (*See also* Stb, stillb)
    stone basketing
    suction biopsy
    surface binding (protein)

+SB
    wearing seat belt

S/B
    seen by
    side bending

SB-
    not wearing seat belt

Sb

antimony [L. *stibium*]
strabismus (*See also* strab)

sb

stilb (unit of luminous intensity)

SBA

serum bactericidal activity
serum bile acid
soybean agglutinin
spina bifida aperta
standby angioplasty
standby assistance
Summary Basis of Approval

SBAC

small bowel adenocarcinoma

SBAI

Social Behavior Assessment
Inventory

SBB

simultaneous binaural bithermal
small bowel biopsy
stereotactic breast biopsy
stimulation-bound behavior
Sudan Black B

SBBO

small bowel bacterial overgrowth

SBC

sensory binocular cooperation
serum bactericidal concentration
single base cane
standard bicarbonate
strict bed confinement
sunburn cell
superficial bladder cancer

S-BD

seizure-brain damage

SBD

straight bag drainage
suggested brain dysfunction
Supervisory Behavior Description

SbDH

sorbitol dehydrogenase

SBDX

scanning-beam digital x-ray

SBE

breast self-examination
saturated base excess
self-breast examination
short below-elbow (cast)
shortness of breath on exertion
small bowel enteroscopy
subacute bacterial endocarditis

SBEP

somatosensory brainstem evoked
potential

S/β

sickle cell beta

SBF

serologic-blocking factor
serum blocking factor
specific blocking factor
splanchnic blood flow
splenic blood flow
systemic blood flow

SBFE

Stanford-Binet Fourth Edition

SBFT

small bowel followthrough (*See also*
SMBFT)

SBG

selenite brilliant green
standby guard

SBGM

self blood-glucose monitoring

SBH

sea-blue histiocyte
sequencing by hybridization

SBHC

school-based health center

SBI

silent brain infarction
silicone (gel-containing) breast
implant
soybean trypsin inhibitor
systemic bacterial infection

SBIS

Stanford-Binet Intelligence Scale
(*See also* SB)

SBJ

skin, bones, joints

SBK

spinnbarkeit

SBL

serum bactericidal level
soybean lecithin
sponge blood loss

sBLA

supplemental Biologics License
Application

SBLLA

sarcoma, breast and brain tumors,
leukemia, laryngeal and lung
cancer adenoma

S

NOTES

SB-LM
Stanford-Binet Intelligence Test-Form LM

SBM
selective broth medium
subbasement membrane
subepithelial basement membrane

SBMPL
simultaneous binaural midplace localization

SBN₂, SB_{N2}, SBNT
single-breath nitrogen (test)

SBNW
single-breath nitrogen washout

SBO
small bowel obstruction
specified bovine offals
spina bifida occulta

SBOD
scleral buckle, right eye (oculus dexter)

SBOE
surgical blood order equation

SBOH
State Board of Health

SBOM
soybean oil meal

SBOS
scleral buckle, left eye (oculus sinister)

SBP
school breakfast program
scleral buckling procedure
serotonin-binding protein
small bowel phytobezoar
spontaneous bacterial peritonitis
spontaneous biliary perforation
steroid-binding plasma (protein)
sulfobromophthalein
systemic blood pressure (*See also* Psa)
systolic blood pressure (*See also* SYS BP)

SBPC
sulfobenzyl penicillin

SBPN
simultaneous bilateral percutaneous nephrolithotomy

SBQ
Smoking Behavior Questionnaire

SBQC
small-based quad cane

SBR
sluggish blood return
spleen-to-body (weight) ratio
stillbirth rate
strict bedrest
styrene-butadiene rubber

SBRN
sensory branch of radial nerve

SBS
serum blood sugar
shaken baby syndrome
short bowel syndrome
sick building syndrome
side to back to side
side by side
sinobronchial syndrome
small bowel series
social breakdown syndrome
staff burnout scale
straight back syndrome

SBSE
supine bicycle stress echocardiography

SBSM
self-blood sugar monitoring

SBSP
simultaneous bilateral spontaneous pneumothorax

SBSRT
Spreen-Benton Sentence Repetition Test

SBSS
Seligmann buffered salt solution

SBT
sequenced-based typing
serous borderline tumor
serum bactericidal test
serum bactericidal titer
serum bacteriologic titer
single-breath test
skin bleeding time
special baby Travesol
sulbactam

SBTB
sinus breakthrough beat

SBTI
soybean trypsin inhibitor (*See also* STI)

SBTPE
State Boards Test Pool Examination

SBTT
small bowel transit time

SBTx
small bowel transplantation

SBV
single binocular vision

SBW
seat belts worn

SBX
symphysis, buttocks, and xiphoid

SC
sacrococcygeal
schedule change

schizophrenia
Schüller-Christian (disease)
Schwann cell
Sciana (blood group)
sciatic (nerve)
science
scruple (*See also* scr)
secondary cleavage
secretory coil
secretory component
self-care
self-control
semicircular
semiclosed
semilunar-valve closure
serum complement
serum creatinine (*See also* SCr)
service connected
sex chromatin
Sezary cell
shallow compartment
short circuit
sick call
sickle cell
sieving coefficient
silicone coated
single chemical
skin conduction
slow component
small (blood pressure) cuff
Smeloff-Cutter
Snellen chart
sodium citrate
soluble complex
special care
specific characteristic
spinal cord
spleen cell (*See also* SPC)
sport cord
squamous carcinoma
statistical control
stellate cell
stem cell
stepped care
sternoclavicular
stimulus, conditioned
stratum corneum
stroke count
subcellular
subclavian
subclavian catheter
subcoastal (view)

subcorneal
subcortical
subcutaneous (*See also* sc, SQ, subcu, subcut, subq)
subtotal colectomy
succinylcholine (*See also* SCH)
sugar coated
sulfur colloid
sulfur containing
superior colliculus
superior constrictor (muscles of pharynx)
superior cornu
supplementary canal
supportive care
suppressor cell
supracondylar (suspension)
surface colony
surgical cone
surveillance cultures
systemic candidiasis
systolic click

S&C

sclera and conjunctiva (singular)
sclerae and conjunctivae (plural)
singly and consensually

99mTc-SC

technetium-99m sulfur colloid

Sc

scandium
scapula
science (*See also* Sci)
scientific (*See also* Sci)

47Sc

scandium-47

sc

scant
sclera
subcutaneous (*See also* subcu, subq, SQ, SC)
subcutaneously

s̄c

without correction (without glasses) [L. *sine correctione*] (*See also* s̄ gl)

SCA

School and College Ability (tests)
selfcare agency
severe congenital anomaly
sickle cell anemia
single-chain antigen-binding (protein)

NOTES

S

SCA *(continued)*
single-channel analyzer
sperm-coating antigen
spinocerebellar ataxia
spleen colony assay
steroidal-cell antibody
subclavian artery
subcutaneous abdominal (block)
superior cerebellar artery
suppressor cell activity

SCa, S$_{Ca}$
serum calcium

ScA
scapuloanterior

SCAA
sporadic cerebral amyloid
angiopathy

SCAb
autoantibody to stratum corneum

SCABG
single coronary artery bypass graft

SCAD
short-chain acyl-CoA dehydrogenase
deficiency
short-chain acyl coenzyme A
dehydrogenase
spontaneous coronary artery
dissection

sCAD
spontaneous cervical artery
dissection (*See also* SCAD)

SCAG
single coronary artery graft

SCAL
Self-Concept as a Learner

SCALE
Scaled Curriculum Achievement
Levels Test
Scales of Creativity and Learning
Environment

SCAMI
Self-Concept and Motivation
Inventory

SCAN
Screening (Test for Identifying)
Central Auditory Disorder
suspected child abuse (and) neglect
suspected child abuse or neglect
systolic coronary artery narrowing

SCAP
scapulae (plural)
scapular
scapula (singular)
stem cell apheresis

SCARED
Screen for Child Anxiety-Related
Emotional Disorders

SCARF
skeletal (abnormalities), cutis (laxa),
craniostenosis, (psychomotor)
retardation, facial (abnormalities)

SCARMD
severe childhood autosomal
recessive muscular dystrophy

SCAS
Self Care Assessment Schedule
semicontinuous activated sludge

SCAT
School and College Ability Test
sheep cell agglutination test
sheep cell agglutination titer
short-contact treatment
sickle cell anemia test

SCATBI
Scales of Cognitive Ability for
Traumatic Brain Injury

SCAV
Sunday Canyon virus

SCB
sedative cabinet bath
stratum corneum basic
strictly confined to bed

SCBA
self-contained breathing apparatus

SCBC
small cell bronchogenic carcinoma

SCBE
single-contrast barium enema

SCBF
spinal cord blood flow

SCBG
symmetrical calcification of basal
(cerebral) ganglia

SCBH
systemic cutaneous basophil
hypersensitivity

SCBP
stratum corneum basic protein

SCBU
special care baby unit

ScBU
screening bacteriuria

SCC
sequential combination
chemotherapy
services for crippled children
short calcaneocuboid
short circuit current
short course chemotherapy
sickle cell crisis
side-chain cleavage
small cell cancer
small cell carcinoma
small cleaved cell
spinal cord compression

squamous carcinoma of cervix
squamous cell cancer
squamous cell carcinoma (*See also* SCCA, SqCCA, sq cell ca)

SCCA

semiclosed circle absorber (system)
squamous cell carcinoma (*See also* SCC, SqCCA, sq cell ca)
squamous cell carcinoma antigen

SCCB

small cell cancer of the bladder
small cell carcinoma of bronchus

SCCD

Schnyder crystalline corneal dystrophy
subacute cortical cerebellar degeneration

SCCE

squamous cell carcinoma of the esophagus

SCCH

sternocostoclavicular hyperostosis

SCCHN

squamous cell carcinoma of head and neck

SCCHO

sternocostoclavicular hyperostosis

SCCI

subcutaneous continuous infusion

S-CCK-Pz

secretin, cholecystokinin, pancreozymin

SCCL

small cell carcinoma of lung

SCCM

Sertoli cell culture medium

SCCMS

slow-channel congenital myasthenic syndrome

SCD

sequential compression device
service-connected disability
sickle cell disease
spinal cord disease
spinocerebellar degeneration
subacute combined degeneration (*See also* SACD)
subacute combined degeneration (of spinal cord)
sudden cardiac death
sudden coronary death

sulfur-carbon drug
systemic carnitine deficiency

sCD4

soluble recombinant human CD4

ScDA

right scapuloanterior (fetal position) [L. *scapulodextra anterior*]

S-C disease

sickle cell-hemoglobin C disease

SCDM

soybean-casein digest medium

ScDP

right scapuloposterior (fetal position) [L. *scapulodextra posterior*]

SCE

saturated calomel electrode
secretory carcinoma of the endometrium
sister chromatid exchange
soft cooked egg
specialized columnar epithelium
split hand-cleft lip/palate and ectodermal dysplasia
subcutaneous emphysema

SCEMIA

self-contained enzymatic membrane immunoassay

SCEP

sandwich counterelectrophoresis
somatosensory cortical evoked potential

SCER

sister chromatid exchange rate

SCF

somatic cell-derived growth factor
special care formula
stem cell factor
supercritical fluid

SCFA

short-chain fatty acid

SCFE

slipped capital femoral epiphysis

SCFGT

Southern California Figure Ground Test

SCFI

specific clotting factor and inhibitor

scFv

single-chain variable fragment

NOTES

SCG
  seismocardiography
  serum chemistry graft
  serum chemogram
  sodium cromoglycate
  superior cervical ganglion

SCGYEM
  serum, casein, glucose, yeast
    extract medium

SCH
  Schirmer (test)
  schistosomiasis (*Schistosoma* sp.)
    vaccine
  sole community hospital
  succinylcholine (*See also* SC)
  suprachiasmatic
  suprachoroidal hemorrhage

SCh
  succinylcholine chloride

SCHAD
  short-chain hydroxyacyl-coenzyme A
    dehydrogenase

SChE
  serum cholinesterase

sched
  schedule

SCHISTO, SCHIZ
  schizocyte

schiz
  schizophrenia

SCHL
  subcapsular hematoma of liver

SCHLP
  supracricoid
    hemilaryngopharyngectomy

SCHNC
  squamous cell head and neck
    cancer

SCI
  Science Citation Index
  Sertoli cell index
  short crus of incus
  silent cerebral infarct
  silent cerebral infarction
  specific COX-2 inhibitor
  spinal cord injury
  structured clinical interview
  subcoma insulin

Sci
  science (*See also* Sc)
  scientific (*See also* Sc)

SCIA
  superficial circumflex iliac artery

SCIBTA
  stem cell indicated by
    transplantation assay

SCID
  severe combined immune deficiency
    (*See also* SCIDS)
  severe combined immunodeficiency
    (disorder)
  Structured Clinical Interview for
    DSM

SCIDA
  severe combined immunodeficiency
    disease, Athabascan

SCID-CV
  Structured Clinical Interview (for
    DSM-IV Axis I Disorders):
    Clinician Version

SCID-D
  Structured Clinical Interview (for
    DSM-IV) Dissociative Disorders

SCID-II
  Structured Clinical Interview (for
    DSM-IV) Axis II Personality
    Disorders

SCID-IV
  Structured Clinical Interview for
    DSM-IV Dissociative Disorders

SCID mice
  severe combined immunodeficient
    mice

SCID-P
  Structured Clinical Interview (for
    DSM-IV) Patient Version

SCID-PD
  Structured Clinical Interview (for
    DSM-IV) Psychotic Disorders

SCIDS
  severe combined immunodeficiency
    syndrome (*See also* SCID)

SCIG
  subcutaneous immunoglobulin

SCII
  Strong-Campbell Interest Inventory

SCIP
  Screening and Crisis Intervention
    Program

SCIPP
  sacrococcygeal to inferior pubic
    point

SCIS
  surface carcinoma in situ

SCIU
  spinal cord injury unit

SCIV
  subclavian intravenous
  subcutaneous intravenous

SCIWORA, SCIWOA
  spinal cord injury without
    radiographic abnormality
  spinal cord injury without
    radiological abnormality

SCJ
> squamocolumnar junction
> sternoclavicular joint

SCK
> serum creatine kinase

sc-kit
> soluble c-kit

SCL
> scaphocapitolunate arthrodesis
> scleroderma (*See also* SD)
> serum copper level
> sinus cycle length
> skin conductance level
> soft contact lens
> spinocervicolemniscal
> symptom checklist
> syndrome checklist

SCL-90
> Symptoms Checklist 90 (items)

Scl, scl
> sclerosis
> sclerotic

ScLA
> left scapuloposterior (fetal position)
> [L. *scapulolaeva anterior*]

SCLAX
> subcostal long axis

SCLBCL
> secondary cutaneous large B-cell
> lymphoma

SCLC
> small-cell lung cancer
> small-cell lung carcinoma

SCLD
> sickle cell chronic lung disease
> sickle cell lung disease

SCLE
> subacute cutaneous lupus
> erythematosus
> subcutaneous lupus erythematosis

SCLND
> selective complete lymph node
> dissection

ScLP
> left scapuloposterior (fetal position)
> [L. *scapulolaeva posterior*]

SCL-90R, SCL-90-R
> Symptoms Checklist 90 Revised

SCLS
> systemic capillary leak syndrome

SCLs
> synthetic combinatorial libraries

SCM
> scalene muscle
> Schwann cell membrane
> sensation, circulation, motion
> soluble cytotoxic medium
> spleen-cell conditioned medium
> split-cord malformation
> spondylotic caudal myelopathy
> steatocystoma multiplex
> sternocleidomastoid
> streptococcal cell membrane
> structure of the cytoplasmic matrix
> supraclavicular muscle
> surface-connecting membrane
> synovial chondromatosis

ScM
> scalene muscle

SCMC
> sodium carboxymethylcellulose
> sperm-cervical mucus contact
> spontaneous cell-mediated
> cytotoxicity

SCMD
> senile choroidal macular
> degeneration

SCMI
> single central maxillary incisor

SCML
> small cell malignant lymphoma

SCMV
> serogroup C meningococcal vaccine

SCN
> serum thiocyanate
> severe chronic neutropenia
> severe congenital neutropenia
> sodium thiocyanate
> special care nursery
> suprachiasmatic nucleus

SC$_{Na}$
> sieving coefficient for sodium

SCNB
> stereotactically guided core needle
> biopsy
> stereotactic core-needle biopsy

SCNC
> small cell neuroendocrine carcinoma

SCNS
> subcutaneous nerve stimulation

SCO
> Sertoli-cell-only (tumor)
> somatic crossing-over
> subcommissural organ

S

NOTES

SCOB
Schedule-Controlled Operant Behavior

SCOOP
Spofford-Christopher oxygen optimizing program

SCOP, scop
scopolamine
Structural Classification of Proteins

SCOPE
arthroscopy
Surveillance and Control of Pathogens of Epidemiologic Importance
systematic, complete, objective, practical, empirical

scope
perform endoscopy

SCOR
skin conductance orienting response

SCORAD
Severity Scoring of Atopic Dermatitis

SCORE
Simple Calculated Osteoporosis Risk Estimation

SCOT
succinyl CoA:3-ketoacid CoA transferase

SCP
secondary care provider
single-celled protein
sodium cellulose phosphate
soluble cytoplasmic protein
squamous cell papilloma
standardized care plan
submucous cleft palate
superior cerebellar peduncle
supracristal plane

SCP-2
sterol carrier protein-2

ScP
scapuloposterior

scp
spherical candle power

SCPF
stem cell proliferation factor

SCPK, S-CPK
serum creatine phosphokinase

SCPL-CHEP
supracricoid partial laryngectomy with cricohyoidoepiglottopexy

SCPN
serum carboxypeptidase N

SCPNT
Southern California Postrotary Nystagmus Test

SCPP
spinal cord perfusion pressure

SCPUFA
short-chain polyunsaturated fatty acid

SCR
silicon-controlled rectifier
skin conductance response
special care room
spondylotic caudal radiculopathy
stem cell rescue

SCr
serum creatinine (*See also* SC)

sCR
soluble complement receptor

sCR1
soluble complement receptor type 1

scr
scruple (*See also* SC)

sCRAG
serum cryptococcal antigen

SCRAM
speech-controlled respirometer for ambulatory measurement

SCRAP
Simple-Complex Reaction-Time Apparatus

SCREEN
Screening Children for Related Early Educational Needs

script
prescription

SC-RNV
subcutaneous radionuclide venography

SC/RP
scaling and root planing

SCRS
Short Clinical Rating Scale

SCS
Self-Control Scale
silicon-controlled switch
Social Climate Scale
spinal canal stenosis
spinal cord stimulation
splatter control shield
stem cell support
subacute confusional state
suspected catheter sepsis
synovial chondrosarcoma
systolic click syndrome

SCSAX
subcostal short axis

SCSIT
Southern California Sensory Integration Tests

SCSP, SC-SP
supracondylar-suprapatellar

SCSVT
> Southern California Space Visualization Test

SCT
> allogeneic stem-cell transplantation
> salmon calcitonin
> Sentence Completion Test
> Sertoli-cell tumor
> sex chromatin test
> Sexual Compatibility Test
> sickle cell trait
> solid cystic tumor
> sperm cytotoxic
> spinal computed tomography
> spinocervicothalamic
> spiral computed tomography
> squamous cell carcinoma of the thyroid
> staphylococcal clumping test
> Star Cancellation Test
> star-cancellation test
> stem cell transplant
> stem cell transplantation
> sugar-coated tablet

SCTA
> spiral computed tomography arteriography
> spiral CT angiography

SCTAT
> sex cord tumors with annular tubules

SCTP
> solid and cystic tumor of the pancreas

SCTX
> static cervical traction

SCU
> selfcare unit
> special care unit

SCUBA
> self-contained underwater breathing apparatus

SCUCP
> small cell undifferentiated carcinoma of the prostate

SCUD
> septicemic cutaneous ulcerative disease

SCUF
> slow continuous ultrafiltration

SCUM
> secondary carcinoma of the upper mediastinum

SCUNC
> small cell undifferentiated neuroendocrine carcinoma

SCUT
> schizophrenia, chronic undifferentiated type

SCV
> sensory conduction velocity
> Sixgun City virus
> slow-component velocity
> smooth, capsulated, virulent (bacteria)
> squamous cell carcinoma (of) vulva
> subclavian vein
> subcutaneous vaginal (block)

SCV-CPR
> simultaneous compression ventilation-cardiopulmonary resuscitation
> simultaneous compression-ventilation CPR

SCY
> scytonemin

S-D
> sickle cell (hemoglobin) D (disease)
> strength-duration (curve)
> suicide-depression

SD
> sagittal depth (of cornea)
> Sandhoff disease
> scleroderma (*See also* SCL)
> seborrheic dermatitis
> secretion droplet
> senile dementia
> sensory deficit
> septal defect
> serologically defined
> serologically detectable
> serologically determined
> serum defect
> severe deficit
> severe disability
> severely disabled
> shallow distance (aquatic therapy)
> shoulder disarticulation
> shoulder dislocation
> Shy-Drager (disease, syndrome)
> single dose

NOTES

S

SD *(continued)*
skin destruction
skin dose
sleep deprived
social desirability
socialized delinquency
socialized dementia
solvent-detergent
somadendritic
somatic dysfunction
spasmodic dysphonia
speech discrimination
spontaneous delivery
sporadic depression
Sprague-Dawley (rat)
spreading depression
stable disease
standard deviation
standard diet
statistical documentation
Stensen duct
stepdown (unit) *(See also* SDU)
sterile dressing
Still disease
stimulus drive *(See also* Sd)
stone disintegration
straight drainage
streptodornase
streptozocin and doxorubicin
succinate dehydrogenase *(See also* SDG)
sudden death
suicide-depression
sulfadiazine
superoxide dismutase
surgical drain
systolic discharge

S/D
sharp/dull
systolic/diastolic (ratio)

S&D
seen and discussed
stomach and duodenum

S^d
stimulus, discriminative

Sd
stimulus drive *(See also* SD)

SDA
right sacroanterior (fetal position) [L. *sacrodextra anterior*]
Sabouraud dextrose agar
salt-dependent agglutinin
same day admission
serotonin/dopamine antagonist
sialodacryoadenitis (virus)
specific dynamic action
steroid-dependent asthmatic
strand displacement amplification

succinic dehydrogenase activity
superficial distal axillary (node)

SDAP
single donor apheresis platelet

SDAT
senile dementia, Alzheimer type

SDAVF
spinal dural arteriovenous fistula

SDB
Sabouraud dextrose broth
self-destructive behavior
sleep-disordered breathing

SDBP
seated diastolic blood pressure
standing diastolic blood pressure
supine diastolic blood pressure

SDC
salivary duct carcinoma
sensitivity depth compensation (ramp)
serum digoxin concentration
serum drug concentration
size/date consistency
sleep disorders center
sodium deoxycholate
subacute combined degeneration
subclavian hemodialysis catheter
succinyldicholine
sulfodeoxycholate

SD&C
suction, dilation, and curettage

SDCL
symptom distress check list

SDD
selective digestive decontamination
selective digestive (tract) decontamination
specific developmental disorder
sporadic depressive disease
sterile dry dressing
subantimicrobial dose doxycycline

SDDT
selective decontamination of the digestive tract

SDE
specific dynamic effect
subdural empyema

SDEEG
stereotactic depth electroencephalogram

SDES
symptomatic diffuse esophageal spasm

SDF
sexual dysfunction
slow death factor
stream dilution factor

stress distribution factor
stromal-cell-derived factor
SDF-1
stromal cell-derived factor-1
SDFP
single-donor frozen plasma
SDG
short distance group
succinate dehydrogenase (*See also* SD)
sucrose density gradient
SDGC
sucrose density gradient centrifugation
SDGU
sucrose density gradient ultracentrifugation
SDH
serine dehydrase
sorbitol dehydrogenase
spinal detrusor hyperreflexia
spinal dorsal horn
subdural hematoma
subdural hemorrhage
subjacent dorsal horn
succinate dehydrogenase (activity)
systolic-diastolic hypertension
SDHD
sudden death heart disease
SDI
Self-Description Inventory
size/date inconsistency (fetus)
standard deviation interval
State Disability Insurance
Surtees Difficulties Index
SDIHD
sudden death ischemic heart disease
SDII
sudden death in infancy
SDKT
simultaneous double kidney transplantation
SDL
self-directed learning
serum digoxin level
serum drug level
speech discrimination loss
SDLE
sex difference in life expectancy
somatic dysfunction lower extremity

SDLRS
self-directed-learning readiness scale
sdly
sidelying
SDM
sensory detection method
single, divorced, married
soft drusen maculopathy
standard deviation of mean
sulfadimidine
S/D/M
systolic, diastolic, mean (blood pressure)
SDMT
Symbol Digit Modalities Test
SDN
sexually dimorphic nucleus
SD/N
signal-difference to noise ratio
SDNA
single-strand deoxyribonucleic acid
SDNN
standard deviation of normal-to-normal beats
SDNV
Serra do Navio virus
SDO
sudden-dosage onset
surgical diagnostic oncology
SDP
right sacroposterior (fetal position) [L. *sacrodextra posterior*]
single-donor platelets
stomach, duodenum, and pancreas
SDPC
Suicide-Depression Proneness Checklist
SDPH
sodium diphenylhydantoin
SDQII
Self-Description Questionnaire II
SDR
selective dorsal rhizotomy
short-duration response
spontaneously diabetic rat
surgical dressing room
SDRI
small, deep, recent infarct
small, deep, recent infarction
SDRT
Stanford Diagnostic Reading Test

S

NOTES

SDS

same day surgery
school dental service
Self-Directed Search
Self-Rating Depression Scale
sensory deprivation syndrome
sexual differentiation scale
simple descriptive scale
single dose suppression
sodium dodecyl sulfate (*See also* NaDodSO$_4$)
somatropin deficiency syndrome
specific diagnosis service
speech discrimination score
standard deviation score
stent delivery system
Student Disability Survey
sudden death syndrome
sulfadiazine silver
sustained depolarizing shift
Symptom Distress Scale
syringe-driven system

Sds, sds

sounds

SD-SK

streptodornase-streptokinase

SDSO

same day surgery overnight

SDS-PAGE

sodium dodecyl sulfate-polyacrylamide gel electrophoresis

SDT

right sacrotransverse (fetal position) [L. *sacrodextra transversa*]
sensory decision theory
single-donor transfusion
speech detectability threshold
speech detection threshold

SDU

short double upright
Standard Deviation Unit
stepdown unit

SDUE

somatic dysfunction upper extremity

SDW

separated, divorced, widowed

SDYS

Simpson dysmorphia syndrome

SE

saline enema
sanitary engineering
Seeing Eye
self-examination
self-explanatory
sheep erythrocyte
side effect
Signed English
smoke exposure
smoke extract
soft exudate
solid extract
sphenoethmoidal
spherical equivalent
spin-echo
spongiform encephalopathy
squamous epithelium
staff escort
standard error
starch equivalent
Starr-Edwards (prosthesis)
status epilepticus
sterol ester
subendocardial
subendothelial
supernormal excitability
supportive-expressive
surgical excision
sustained engraftment

S&E

safety and efficiency

S/E

suicidal and eloper

Se

selenium

^{75}Se

selenium-75

SEA

seronegativity, enthesopathy, arthropathy
sheep erythrocyte agglutination
shock-elicited aggression
side-entry access
soluble egg antigen
Southeast Asia
spinal epidural abscess
spondylitis, enthesitis, arthritis
spontaneous electrical activity
staphylococcal enterotoxin A
subdural electrode array
Survey of Employee Access
synaptic electronic activation

SEAR

Southeast Asia refugee

SEAT

sheep erythrocyte agglutination test

SEB

Scale for Emotional Blunting
staphylococcal enterotoxin B
surrogate end-point biomarker

SEBA

staphylococcal enterotoxin B antiserum

seb derm

seborrheic dermatitis

SEBI

stereotactic external-beam irradiation

seb ker
  seborrheic keratosis (*See also* SK)
SEBL
  self-emptying blind loop
SEC
  according to [L. *secundum*]
  school handicap condition
  secondary (*See also* sec)
  secretin
  secretion
  section (*See also* S, s, sec, sect)
  series elastic component (of
    muscles)
  sertoliform endometrioid carcinoma
  Singapore epidemic conjunctivitis
  sinusoidal endothelial cell
  size exclusion chromatography
  soft elastic capsule
  spontaneous echo contrast
  squamous epithelial cell
  steric exclusion chromatography
  strong exchange capacity (resin)
  superficial esophageal carcinoma
Sec
  Seconal
sec
  second (*See also* S, s)
  secondary (*See also* SEC)
  secretary
  section (*See also* S, s, SEC, scct)
SECG
  scalp electrocardiogram
  stress electrocardiography
SECL
  seclusion
SECPR
  standard external cardiopulmonary
    resuscitation
SE-CPT
  single-electrode current perception
    threshold
SECSY
  spin-echo correlated spectroscopy
sect
  section (*See also* S, s, SEC, sec)
SECTL
  single enhancing CT lesion
SED
  sedimentation (rate) (*See also* SED,
    sed rt)
  semielemental diet
  serious emotional disturbance

skin erythema dose
socially and emotionally disturbed
spondyloepiphyseal dysplasia
standard error of difference
staphylococcal enterotoxin D
strain energy density
suberythemal dose
sed.
  sedate
  sedative
  sedimentation (rate) (*See also* SED,
    sed rt)
  stool [L. *sedes*]
SEDC
  spondyloepiphyseal dysplasia
    congenita
SEDD
  Szondi Experimental Diagnostics of
    Drives
SED-NET
  severely emotional disturbed -
    network
sed rate, sed rt
  sedimentation rate (*See also* SED,
    sed rt)
SEE
  scopolamine-Eukodal-Ephetonin
  series elastic element
  standard error of estimate
  Surgical Eye Expeditions
SEE$_1$
  Seeing Essential English
SEE$_2$
  Signing Exact English
SEEG
  stereotactic electroencephalogram
SEEP
  small end-expiratory pressure
SEER
  Surveillance, Epidemiology, and
    End Results (network, program)
SEF
  somatically evoked field
  spectral edge frequency
  staphylococcal enterotoxin F
SEG
  segment
  soft elastic gelatin (capsule)
  sonoencephalogram
seg
  segmented neutrophil

NOTES

SEGA
    subependymal giant cell
    astrocytoma
SEG-CES
    segmental cement extraction system
sEGF
    salivary epidermal growth factor
segm
    segment
    segmented
SEH
    School Handicap Condition Scale
    severe emotional handicap
    spinal epidural hematoma
    spinal epidural hemorrhage
    subdural effusion with
        hydrocephalus
    subependymal hemorrhage
SeHCAT
    selenium-labeled homocholic acid
        conjugated with taurine
SEI
    Self-Esteem Index
    Self-Esteem Inventory
    subendocardial infarct
    subepithelial (corneal) infiltrate
    Suretee Events Index
SELCA
    smooth excimer laser coronary
        angioplasty
SELD
    slow expressive language
        development
SELDI
    surface enhanced laser
        desorption/ionization
SELF
    Self-Evaluation of Life Function
        scale
SELFVD
    sterile elective low forceps vaginal
        delivery
SELI
    specific expressive language
        impairment
SELU
    seromuscular enterocystoplasty lined
        with urothelium
SELV
    Seletar virus
SEM
    scanning electron micrograph
    scanning electron microscope
    scanning electron microscopy
    secondary enrichment medium
    semen (*See also* sem)
    serum methylguanidine
    skin, eye, mucocutaneous

slow eye movement
smoke exposure machine
standard error of mean
systolic ejection murmur
(verbal) sample evaluation method
sem
    semen (*See also* SEM)
    seminal
sem.
    half [L. *semis*] (*See also* HF, hf,
        S, semi, ss)
SEMD
    spondyloepimetaphyseal dysplasia
SEMDJL
    spondyloepimetaphyseal dysplasia
        (with) joint laxity
SEMG, sEMG
    surface electromyography
SEMI
    subendocardial myocardial infarction
    subendocardial myocardial injury
semi
    half [L. *semis*] (*See also* HF, hf,
        S, sem., ss)
semid
    half a dram
SEMS
    self-expanding metallic stent
    self-expanding microporous stent
sen
    sensitive
    sensitivity (*See also* S, sens)
SENA
    sympathetic efferent nerve activity
sens
    sensation
    sensitivity (*See also* S, sen)
    sensorium
    sensory
SEOC
    serous epithelial ovarian carcinoma
SEOV
    Seoul virus
SEP
    multiple sclerosis [F. *sclerose en
        plaques*]
    sclerose en plaques
    sclerosing encapsulating peritonitis
    sensory evoked potential
    separate
    separation of ghosts
    serum electrophoresis
    somatosensory evoked potential
        (*See also* SSEP, S-SEP)
    sperm entry point
    spinal evoked potential
    Stroke Education Program
    surface epithelium

syringe exchange program
systolic ejection period
SEPA
superficial external pudendal artery
separ
separately
separation
SEPS
subfascial endoscopic perforator
surgery
sept
septum
sept.
seven [L. *septem*]
SEPV
Sepik virus
SEQ
side-effects questionnaire
simultaneous equation
seq
sequel
sequelae (plural)
sequela (singular)
sequence
sequestrum
seq dev ex
sequential developmental exercises
SER
scanning equalization radiography
sebum excretion rate
sensory evoked response
sertraline (Zoloft)
service (*See also* serv)
side effects records
signal enhancement ratio
smooth endoplasmic reticulum (*See also* sER)
somatosensory evoked response
supination-external rotation
supination external rotation (type of fracture)
suppressive E-receptor
systolic ejection rate
Ser
serine (*See also* S)
sER
smooth endoplasmic reticulum (*See also* SER)
ser
serial
series (*See also* S, s)

SERCA
sarcoplasmic-endoplasmic reticulum calcium ATPase
SERI
Spondee Error Index
serial 7's
a mental status examination (starting with a 100, count backward by 7s)
serial sevens test
ser ind
serum index
SER-IV
supination-external rotation IV (fracture)
SERLINE
Serials on Line
SERM
selective estrogen receptor modulator
selective estrogen response modifier
SERO
serologic typing
sero, serol
serologic
serology
SERPACWA
skin exposure reduction paste against chemical warfare agents
SERPIN
serine protease inhibitor
ser sect
serial sections
SERT
serotonin reuptake transporter
sustained ethanol release tube
serv
service (*See also* SER)
SERVHEL
service and health (records)
SES
seroepidemiological study
socioeconomic status
spatial emotional stimuli
standard electrolyte solution
subendothelial space
sess
sessile
SEST
supine empty stress test

NOTES

SET
shredding embolectomy thrombectomy
signal extraction technology
skin endpoint titration
social environmental therapy
support, empathy, and truth
systolic ejection time

SETTLE
spindle-cell epithelial tumor with thymus-like differentiation

SEV
sevoflurane (Ultane)

sev
sever
several
severe
severed

SEW
slice excitation wave

SEWHO
shoulder, elbow, wrist, hand orthosis

SEXAF
surface extended x-ray absorption fine (structure)

SeXO
serum xanthine oxidase

SF
Sabin-Feldman (dye test)
safety factor
salt free
saturated fat
scarlet fever
seizure frequency
seminal fluid
serosal fluid
serum factor
serum ferritin
serum fibrinogen
sham feeding
shell fragment
shrapnel fragment
shunt flow
sickle (cell hemoglobin) F
simian foam-virus
skin fibroblast
skin fluorescence
skull fracture
slow function
slow (initial) function
snack food
sodiumazide, fecal (medium)
soft feces
sound field
spinal fluid (*See also* sp fl)
spontaneous fibrillation
spontaneous fission (radioactive isotopes)
spontaneous fluctuation
spontaneous fracture
stable factor
starch-free
sterile female
stimulating factor
stress formula
sucrose-free
sugar-free
sulfation factor (of blood serum)
superior facet
suppressor factor
suprasternal fossa
survival fraction
Svedberg flotation (unit)
symptom free
synovial fluid (*See also* syn fl)

SF-1
steroidogenic factor-1

SF-6, SF$_6$
sulfahexafluoride
sulfur hexafluoride

SF-36
36-item short form health survey
Short Form-36 General Health Survey

S&F
soft and flat

SF%
shortening fraction percentage

S$_f$, Sf
flotation constant
negative sedimentation Svedberg unit
Svedberg flotation (unit)

SFA
saturated fatty acid
seminal fluid analysis
seminal fluid assay
serum folic acid
stimulated fibrinolytic activity
subclavian flap aortoplasty
superficial femoral angioplasty
superficial femoral artery

sFas
soluble Fas

sFasL
soluble FasL

SFB
saphenofemoral bypass
single frequency bioimpedance
surgical foreign body

SFBL
self-filling blind loop

SFC
serum fungicidal

soluble fibrin-fibrinogen complex
spinal fluid count
subaracyhnoid fluid collection

SFD

sheep factor delta
short foot drape
skin-film distance
small for dates (gestational age)
source film distance
soy-free diet
spectral frequency distribution

SFE

supercritical fluid extraction

SFEMG

single fiber electromyography

SFF

speaking fundamental frequency

SFFA

serum-free fatty acid

SFFF

sedimentation field flow
  fractionation

SFFV

(Friend) spleen focus virus

SFG

spotted fever group

SFH

schizophrenia family history
serum-free hemoglobin
stroma-free hemoglobin

SFHb

pyridoxalated stroma-free
  hemoglobin
stroma-free hemoglobin
  pyridoxalated

SFI

sciatic function index
Sexual Functioning Index
sexual function score
Social Function Index

SFIQ

Sexual Function Inventory
  Questionnaire

SFL

synovial fluid lymphocyte

SFLE

Stress From Life Experience

SFM

scanning force microscopy
soluble fibrin monomer

SFMC

soluble fibrin monomer complex

SFMS

Smith-Fineman-Myers syndrome

SFNV

sandfly fever Naples virus

SFO

subfornical organ

SFo

speaking phonation

SFP

screen filtration pressure
simulated fluorescence process
simultaneous foveal perception
spinal fluid pressure
stopped flow pressure
synostotic frontal plagiocephaly

SFPT

standard fixation preference test

SFR

screen-filtration resistance
stenotic flow reserve
stroke with full recovery

SFS

serial focus seizures
serum fungistatic
skin and fascia stapler
split function study
superficial fascial system

SFSV

sandfly fever Sicilian virus

SFT

sensory feedback therapy
serum-free thyroxin
skinfold thickness
solitary fibrous tumor

SFTAA

Short Form Test of Academic
  Aptitude

SFTR

sagittal, frontal, transverse, rotation

SFUP

surgical followup

SFV

simian foamy viruses
superficial femoral vein

SFW

sexual function of women
shell fragment wound
shrapnel fragment wound
slow filling wave

SFWB

social/family well-being

S

NOTES

SFWD
symptom-free walking distance
SG
Sachs-Georgi (test)
salivary gland
scrotography
sebaceous gland
secretory granule
serous granule
serum globulin
serum glucose
side glide
sign
skin graft
soluble gelatin
specific gravity (*See also* SPG, SpG, sp gr, sp. gr.)
stent graft
stratum granulosum
substantia gelatinosa
supplemental groove
Swan-Ganz (catheter) (*See also* SGC)
S/G
swallow/gag
SGA
small for gestational age
subjective global assessment (dietary history and physical examination)
substantial gainful activity (employment)
S-GAP
superior gluteal artery perforator
SGAR
spectral gradient acoustic reflectometry
SGAT
salivary gland anlage tumor
SGAV
Salanga virus
SGAW, SG$_{AW}$
specific airway conductance
SGB
Simpson-Golabi-Behmel (syndrome) (*See also* SGBS)
Swiss gym ball
SGBI
silicone gel-filled breast implant
SGBS
Simpson-Golabi-Behmel syndrome (*See also* SGB)
SGC
salivary gland carcinoma
spermicide-germicide compound
Swan-Ganz catheter (*See also* SG)
sweat gland carcinoma

SG-C
serum gentamicin concentration
SGc
specific conductance
SGCNB
stereotactic guided core-needle biopsy
SgCV
saguaro cactus virus
SGD
straight gravity drainage
SGE
secondary generalized epilepsy
significant glandular enlargement
SGF
sarcoma growth factor
silica gel filtered
simulated gastric fluid
skeletal growth factor
SGFR
single-nephron glomerular filtration rate (*See also* SNGFR)
SGGT
serum gamma-glutamyltransferase
SGH
sebaceous gland hyperplasia
subgaleal hematoma
SGIB
severe gastrointestinal bleeding
SGL
salivary gland lymphocyte
s̄ gl
without correction/without glasses (*See also* SC)
SGLPG
sulfate-3-glucuronyllactosaminyl paragloboside
SGLT
sodium glucose cotransporter
SGLT1
sodium glucose co-transporter-1
SGM
serum glucose monitoring
SGMI
silicone gel-filled mammary implant
SGO
surgery, gynecology, and obstetrics
SGOT
serum glutamic-oxaloacetic transaminase
serum glutamic-oxaloacetic transferase
SGP
serine glycerophosphatide
sialoglycoprotein
soluble glycoprotein
stress-generated potential

SGP-2
  sulfated glycoprotein-2
SGPA
  supragenicular popliteal artery
SGPG
  sulfate-3-glucuronyl paragloboside
SGPT
  serum glutamic pyruvic
    transaminase
  serum glutamic-pyruvic transaminase
SGR
  Sachs-Georgi reaction
  Shwartzman generalized reaction
  submandibular gland renin
SGRQ
  St. Georges Respiratory
    Questionnaire
SGRQ-A
  St. Georges Respiratory
    Questionnaire translated into
    American English
SGS
  Schinzel-Giedion syndrome
  second generation sulfonylurea
  short gut syndrome
  silicone gel sheeting
  stroke guidance system
  subglottic stenosis
sGS
  surgical Gleason score
S-Gt
  Sachs-Georgi test (*See also* SG)
SGTCS
  secondarily generalized tonic-clonic
    seizure
SGTT
  standard glucose tolerance test
SGV
  salivary gland virus
  selective gastric vagotomy
  small granular vesicle
SH
  Salter-Harris (fracture)
  Schönlein-Henoch (purpura) (*See
    also* SHP)
  serum hepatitis
  service hours
  sex hormone
  sexual harassment
  sham (operation)
  shared haplotypes
  Sherman (rat)

  short
  short hydrophobic
  shoulder (*See also* sh, SHLD)
  shower
  sick (in) hospital
  sinus histiocytosis
  sitting height
  social history
  somatotropic hormone (*See also*
    STH)
  spontaneously hypertensive (rat)
  state hospital
  sulfhydryl
  suprachoroidal hemorrhage
  surgical history
  symptomatic hypoglycemia
  systemic hyperthermia
S/H
  sample and hold
  suicidal/homicidal (ideation)
S&H
  speech and hearing
SH2
  Src-homology 2
sh
  sheep
  short
  shoulder (*See also* SH, SHLD)
SHA
  soluble HLA antigen
  staphylococcal hemagglutinating
    antibody
  super-heated aerosol
SHAA
  serum hepatitis-associated antigen
SHAA-Ab
  serum hepatitis-associated antigen
    antibody
SHAART
  salvage highly active antiretroviral
    therapy
SHAFT
  sad, hostile, anxious, frustrated,
    tenacious (patient)
SHAL
  standard hyperalimentation
SHARP
  School Health Additional Referral
    Program
SHAS
  Supplement to HIV/AIDS
    Surveillance

S

NOTES

SHAS *(continued)*
supravalvular hypertrophic aortic stenosis

SHAV
Shamonda virus
superior hemiazygos vein

SHB
sequential hemibody (irradiation)
subacute hepatitis with bridging
sulfhemoglobin (*See also* HbS, SHb, SULFHB)

S Hb
sickle hemoglobin (screen)

SHb, S-Hb
sulfhemoglobin (*See also* HbS, SHB, SULFHB)

SHBD
serum hydroxybutyrate dehydrogenase
serum hydroxybutyric dehydrogenase

SHBG
sex hormone-binding globulin
steroid hormone-binding globulin

sHBO2T
systemic hyperbaric oxygen therapy

SHC
sclerosing hepatic carcinoma
subsequent hospital care

SHCO
sulfated hydrogenated caster oil

SHCU
state hospital children's unit

SHD
structural heart disease

SHDI
supraoptical hypophysial diabetes insipidus

SHE
spinal epidural hemorrhage
subclinical hepatic encephalopathy
Syrian hamster embryo

SHEENT
skin, head, eyes, ears, nose, and throat

SHF
simian hemorrhagic fever

shf
super high frequency

SHG
shigellosis (*Shigella* sp.) vaccine
sonohysterography
synthetic human gastrin

SHGT
somatic cell human gene therapy

SHH
syndrome of hyporeninemic hypoaldosteronism

SHHP
semihorizontal heart position

SHI
second harmonic imaging
severe head injury
standard heparin infusion

Shig
Shigella

SHIP
Sgarlato hammertoe implant

SHL
sensorineural hearing loss (*See also* SNHL)
sudden hearing loss
supraglottic horizontal laryngectomy

sHLA
soluble human leukocyte antigen

SHLD
shoulder (*See also* SH, sh)

SHM
simple harmonic motion

SHMF
Similac Human Milk Fortifier

SHML
sinus histiocytosis with massive lymphadenopathy

SHMT
serine hydroxymethyltransferase

SHN
spontaneous hemorrhagic necrosis
subacute hepatic necrosis

SHO
secondary hypertrophic osteoarthropathy

SHORT, S-H-O-R-T
short (stature), hyperextensibility (of joints or) hernia (or both), ocular (depression), Rieger (anomaly), teething (delayed)

SHOV
Shokwe virus

SHOX
short stature homeobox (gene)

SHP
Schönlein-Henoch purpura (*See also* SH)
secondary hyperparathyroidism
secondary hypertension, pulmonary
state health plan
summer-type hypersensitivity pneumonitis
surgical hypoparathyroidism

SHPL
sacral horizontal plane line

sHPT
secondary hyperparathyroidism

SHQ
self-healing style of qigong

SHR
    scapulohumeral rhythm
    sinusoidal heart rate
    spontaneously hypertensive rat
ShR
    shading response
SHRC
    shortened, held, resisted, contracted
SHS
    Sayre head sling
    sheep hemolysate supernatant
    Shipley-Hartford Scale
    shoulder-hand syndrome
    student health service
    super high speed
    Sutherland-Haan syndrome
SHSP
    spontaneously hypertensive stroke-
      prone (rat)
SHSS
    Stanford Hypnotic Susceptibility
      Scale
SHT
    simple hypocalcemic tetany
    STYCAR Hearing Test
    subcutaneous histamine test
    symptomatic hemorrhage
SHUR
    System for Hospital Uniform
      Reporting
SHUV
    Shuni virus
SHV
    simian herpes virus
    sulfhydryl variant
SHVC
    suprahepatic inferior vena cava
SHx
    social history
SI
    fusin 29
    International System of Units [Fr.
      Système International d'Unites]
    sacroiliac (*See also* sac-il)
    Salience Inventory
    saline infusion
    saline injection
    saturation index
    self-inflicted
    sensitive index
    sensory integration
    serious illness

    serum insulin
    serum iron
    service index
    severity index
    sex inventory
    sexual intercourse
    signal intensity
    Singh Index
    single injection
    sinus irregularity
    small intestine
    social introversion
    soluble insulin
    special intervention
    spirochetosis icterohaemorrhagica
    stimulation index
    stress incontinence
    strict isolation
    stroke index
    structure of intellect
    sucrase-isomaltase
    suicidal ideation
    sulfated insulin
    suppression index
    syncytium-inducing
    syncytium-inhibiting
    Systematic Inquiry
    systolic index
S/I
    sucrose-to-isomaltase (ratio)
    superior/inferior
S&I
    suction and irrigation
Si
    most anterior point on lower
      contour of sella turcica (point)
    silicon
    (venous) sinus
si
    small intestine channel
      (acupuncture)
SIA
    serum inhibitory activity
    small intestinal atresia
    stimulation-induced analgesia
    stress-induced analgesia
    stress-induced anesthesia
    subacute infectious arthritis
    synalbumin-insulin antagonism
    syncytia induction assay
Sia
    sialic acids

S

NOTES

SIAD
> syndrome of inappropriate antidiuresis

SIADH
> syndrome of inappropriate antidiuretic hormone (secretion)
> syndrome of inappropriate (excretion) of antidiuretic hormone

SIAT
> supervised intermittent ambulatory treatment

SIB
> self-inflating bulb
> self-injurious behavior

sib, sibs
> sibling

SIBC
> serum iron-binding capacity
> synchronous ipsilateral breast cancer

SIBD
> silent ischemic brain damage

SIBDQ
> Short Inflammatory Bowel Disease Questionnaire

SIBIS
> self-injurious-behavior inhibiting system

SIBO
> small intestine bacterial overgrowth

SIC
> dry [L. siccus]
> selective intrapartum chemoprophylaxis
> self-intermittent catheterization
> serum inhibitory concentration
> serum insulin concentration
> squamous intraepithelial cell
> Standard Industrial Classification

SiC
> silicon carbide

sICAM
> soluble intracellular adhesion molecule

SICD
> Sequenced Inventory of Communication Development
> serum isocitrate dehydrogenase
> sudden infant crib death

SICH
> spontaneous intracerebral hemorrhage

SICSVA
> sequential impaction cascade sieve volumetric air (sampler)

SICT
> selective intracoronary thrombolysis

SICU
> spinal intensive care unit
> surgical intensive care unit

SID
> selective intestinal decontamination
> source image distance
> source-to-image (receptor) distance
> sucrase-isomaltase deficiency
> sudden inexplicable death
> sudden infant death
> suggested indication of diagnosis
> systemic inflammatory disease

s.i.d.
> once a day [L. semel in die]

SIDA
> French and Spanish abbreviation for AIDS

SIDAM
> structured interview for diagnosis of Alzheimer dementia

SIDAM-A
> infarct dementia, and dementias of other etiology according to ICD-10 and DSM-III-R

SIDD
> syndrome of isolated diastolic dysfunction

SIDER
> siderocyte

SIDFF
> superimposed dorsiflexion of foot

SIDS
> sudden infant death syndrome
> sulfoiduronate sulfatase deficiency

SIE
> stroke in evolution

SIEA
> superficial inferior epigastric artery

SIEP
> serum immunoelectrophoresis

SIER
> sonication-induced epitope retrieval

SIESTA
> snooze-induced excitation of sympathetic triggered activity

SIF
> sacral insufficiency fracture
> serum inhibitory factor
> simulated intestinal fluid
> small, intensely fluorescent (ganglia)
> somatotropin release-inhibiting factor (See also SRIF)

Sif
> segment inferior

SIFE
> serum immunofixation electrophoresis

SIFT

    selected ion flow tube

    transvaginal intrafallopian sperm transfer

SIFTER

    Screening Instrument for Targeting Educational Risk

SIG

    sigmoidoscope

    special interest group

SIg, sIg

    serum immunoglobulin

Sig

    signature (*See also* /S/, /s/)

    signed

sig

    sigmoidoscopy

    signal

    significant

sig.

    label, write [L. *signa*] (*See also* S, s)

    let it be written, labeled [L. *signetur*]

SIgA

    surface immunoglobulin A

sIgA

    secretory IgA

SIGI

    System for Interactive Guidance Information

Siglish

    Signed English

Σ, sigma

    foaminess

    sigma (18th letter of Greek alphabet), uppercase

    sum

    summation of all quantities following the symbol

    syphilis

σ, sigma

    millisecond (*See also* msec, ms, s̄)

    sigma (18th letter of Greek alphabet), lowercase

Signal 99

    patient in cardiac or respiratory distress

SIGSS

    selective imaging and graphics for stereotactic surgery

SIH

    somatotropin release-inhibiting hormone

    spontaneous intracranial hypotension

    stimulation-induced hypalgesia

    stress-induced hyperthermia

SIHC

    surgically implanted hemodialysis catheter

SIHE

    spontaneous intramural hematoma of the esophagus

SI-I

    shunt index via the inferior mesenteric vein

SIJ, SI jt

    sacroiliac joint

SIJS

    sacroiliac joint syndrome

SIL

    seriously ill list

    sister-in-law

    speech interference level

    squamous intraepithelial lesion

SIL/ASCUS

    squamous intraepithelial lesion/atypical squamous cell of undetermined significance

SILD

    Sequenced Inventory of Language Development

SILFVD

    sterile indicated low forceps vaginal delivery

SILL

    subischial leg length

SILS

    Shipley Institute of Living Scale

SILV

    Silverwater virus

    simultaneous independent lung ventilation

SIM

    selected ion monitoring

    Similac

    small intestine mesentery

    specialized intestinal metaplasia

    sucrose-isomaltose

    sulfide, indole, motility (medium)

sim 1–27

    simian adenovirus 1–27

NOTES

S

SIMA
single internal mammary artery

Sim c̄ Fe
Similac with iron

SIMCU
surgical intermediate care unit

simkin
simulation kinetics (analysis)

simp.
simple [L. *simplex*]

SIMS
secondary ion mass spectroscopy

simul
simultaneously

SIMV
Simbu virus
spontaneous intermittent mandatory
ventilation
synchronized intermittent mandatory
ventilation

SIN
salpingitis isthmica nodosa

sin.
without [L. *sine*]

SINES
short interspersed elements

sing.
singular

SINV
Sindbis virus

SIO
sacroiliac orthosis

SiO₂
silica

SIP
saturation inversion projection
segment inertial properties
Sickness Impact Profile
slow inhibitory potential
stroke in progression
surface inductive plethysmography
sympathetically independent pain

SIPI
Short Imaginal Processes Inventory

SIPS
sympathetically independent pain
syndrome

SIPT
Sensory Integration and Praxis
Tests

sIPTH
serum immunoreactive parathyroid
hormone

SIQ
sick in quarters (military)

SIR
single isomorphous replacement

specific immune release
standardized incidence ratio

SIREF
specific immune-response-enhancing
factor

SIRF
severely impaired renal function

SIRS
soluble immune response suppressor
Structured Interview of Reported
Symptoms
systemic inflammatory response
syndrome

SIS
saline infusion sonography
saline infusion sonohysterography
Second International Standard
sisomicin
sister
Skin Intensity Score
small intestinal submucosa
social information system
spontaneous interictal spike
sterile injectable solution
sterile injectable suspension
Stress Impact Scale
Stroke Impact Scale
Surgical Infection Stratification
(system)

SI-S
shunt index (via) superior
(mesenteric vein)

SISA
stenting in small arteries

SISI
short increment sensitivity index
small increment sensitivity index

SISPA
sequence-independent single primer
amplification

SISS
serum inhibitor of streptolysin S
severe invasion streptococcal
syndrome

SIT
serum-inhibiting titer
serum inhibitory titer
silicon-intensified target
Simultaneous Interview Technique
Slosson Intelligence Test
specific immunotherapy (allergy)
specific injection immunotherapy
sperm immobilization test
stress inoculation training
supraspinatus, infraspinatus, teres
(muscle insertions)
surgical intensive therapy

SITA
> standard infertility treatment algorithm
> Swedish interactive thresholding algorithm

SIT BAL
> sitting balance

SIT-F
> Sperm Immobilization Test-Fjabrant

SIT-I
> Sperm Immobilization Test-Isojima

SIT TOL
> sitting tolerance

SITx
> small-intestine transplantation

SIV
> simian immunodeficiency virus
> Sprague-Dawley-Ivanovas (rat)
> Survey of Interpersonal Values

SIVP
> slow intravenous push

SIW
> self-inflicted wound

SIWIP
> self-induced water intoxication (and) psychosis

sj
> sanjiao channel (acupuncture)

SJA
> subtalar joint axis

SJAV
> Sandjimba virus

SJC
> swollen joint count

SJF
> subtalar joint function

SJK
> Scheuermann juvenile kyphosis

SjO₂, SjVO₂
> jugular venous oxygen saturation

SJR
> Shinowara-Jones-Reinhart (unit)

S-JRA
> systemic juvenile rheumatoid arthritis

SJV
> San Juan virus

SK
> seborrheic keratosis (*See also* seb ker)
> senile keratosis
> skin (*See also* Sk, SKI)

> solar keratosis
> spontaneous killer (cell)
> streptokinase (*See also* STK)
> striae keratopathy
> swine kidney

Sk
> skin (*See also* SK, SKI)

sk
> skeletal (*See also* skel)
> skimmed

SKA, SKAO
> supracondylar knee-ankle orthosis (*See also* SKA)
> supracondylar knee-ankle (orthosis) (*See also* SKAO)

SKAB
> skeletal antibody

SKAT
> Sex Knowledge and Attitude Test

SKC
> single knee to chest

skel
> skeletal (*See also* sk)
> skeleton

SKI
> Skill Indicators
> skin (*See also* SK, Sk)

SKL
> serum-killing level

SKOLD
> Screening Kit of Language Development

SKPT
> simultaneous kidney-pancreas transplantation

SKSD, SK-SD
> streptokinase-streptodornase

SKT
> simple knee test

sk tr
> skeletal traction

SKU
> stock keeping unit (related to product identification)

SKY
> spectral karyotype
> spectral karyotyping

SL
> salt loser
> sarcolemma
> satellite-like
> scapholunate

NOTES

SL *(continued)*
Schwalbe line
sclerosing leukoencephalopathy
secondary leukemia
sensation level (of hearing)
sensory latency
sentinel lymphadenectomy
serious list
short leg (cast) (*See also* SLC)
Sibley-Lehninger (unit)
side-lying
signal level
slight
slit lamp
small leukocyte
small lymphocyte
soda lime
sodium lactate
solidified liquid
sound level
spinal length
standard laparoscopy
stereolithography
streptolysin
sublingual (ly)

S/L, S:L
sucrase-to-lactase (ratio)

Sl
slight
Steel (mouse)

sl
slice
slight
slow
slyke (unit of buffer value)
sublingual

SLA
left sacroanterior (fetal position)
[L. *sacrolaeva anterior*]
sex and love addictions
single-cell liquid cytotoxic assay
slide latex agglutination
soluble liver antigen
superficial linear array
surfactant-like activity
(The) Satisfaction with Life Areas
(test)

SLAC
scaphoid-lunate advanced collapse
scapholunate advanced collapse
scapholunate arthritic collapse

SLAM
scanning laser acoustic microscope
signaling lymphocytic activation
molecule
simultaneous latram and
mastectomy
Systemic Lupus Activity Measure

SLAP
serum leucine aminopeptidase
superior labrum anterior and
posterior (lesion)

SLAS
salt-losing adrenogenital syndrome

SLB
short leg brace
surgical lung biopsy

SLC
short leg cast (*See also* SL)
Sociopolitical Locus of Control
sodium-lithium countertransport
sodium-lithium countertransporter
synovial lining cell

SLC-90
Symptom Checklist 90

SLCC
short leg cylinder cast
sulfated lithocholic conjugate

SLCG
sulfolithocholylglycine

SLCT
Sertoli-Leydig cell tumor

SLD
second-line drug
serum lactate dehydrogenase
Spatz-Lindenberg disease
specific language disorder
stealth liposomal doxorubicin

SLDH
serum lactate dehydrogenase

SLE
slit-lamp examination (*See also* S/L)
St. Louis encephalitis
systemic lupus erythematosus

SLEA
sheep erythrocyte antibody
sheep erythrocyte antigen

SLED
slow low-efficiency dialysis
sustained low-efficiency dialysis

SLEDAI
SLE Disease Activity Index
Systemic Lupus Erythematosus
Disease Activity Index

SLEM
slow lateral eye movement

SLEP
short latent-evoked potential

SLEV
St. Louis encephalitis virus
(serology)

SLEX
slit-lamp examination
(ophthalmology, biomicroscopy)
(*See also* SLEX)

SLFIA
    substrate-labeled fluorescent
      immunoassay
    substrate-linked fluorescent
      immunoassay

SLFVD
    sterile low forceps vaginal delivery

SLGXT
    symptom-limited graded exercise
      test

SLHR
    sex-linked hypophosphatemic rickets

SLI
    secretin-like immunoreactivity
    selective lymphoid irradiation
    somatostatin-like immunoreactivity
      (*See also* SLIR)
    specific language impairment
    speech and language impaired
    splenic localization index
    subdermal levonorgestrel implant

SLIP
    Singer-Loomis Inventory of
      Personality

SLIR
    somatostatin-like immunoreactivity
      (*See also* SLI)

SLIT
    sublingual immunotherapy

SLJD
    Sinding-Larsen-Johansson disease

SLJM
    syndrome of limited joint mobility

SLK, SLKC
    superior limbic keratoconjunctivitis

SLL
    second-look laparotomy
    serum lidocaine level
    small lymphocytic lymphoma

SLM
    sound level meter

SLMC
    spontaneous lymphocyte-mediated
      cytotoxicity

SLMFD, SLMFVD
    sterile low midforceps (vaginal)
      delivery

SLMMS
    slightly more marked since

SLMN
    sarcoma-like mural nodule

SLMP
    since last menstrual period

SLN
    sentinel lymph node
    sublentiform nucleus
    superior laryngeal nerve

SLND
    sentinel lymph node detection

SLNM
    sentinel lymph node mapping

SLNTG
    sublingual nitroglycerin

SLNWBC
    short leg nonweightbearing cast

SLNWC
    short leg nonwalking cast

SLO
    scanning laser ophthalmoscope
    second-look operation
    shark liver oil
    Smith-Lemli-Opitz (syndrome)
    streptolysin O

SLOtest
    streptolysin O test

SLP
    left sacroposterior (fetal position)
      [L. *sacrolaeva posterior*]
    segmental limb (systolic) pressure
    sex-limited protein
    short luteal phase
    single-limb progression
    speech-language pathologist
    subluxation of patella

SLPI
    secretory leukocyte protease
      inhibitor
    secretory leukoprotease inhibitor
    secretory leukoproteinase inhibitor

SLPMS
    short leg posterior-molded splint

SLPP
    serum lipophosphoprotein

SLR
    Shwartzman local reaction
    single lens reflex
    straight-leg raise
    straight-leg raising
    Streptococcus lactis R

SLRT
    straight-leg raising tenderness
    straight-leg raising test

S

NOTES

SLS
scleroderma-like syndrome
second-look sonography
segment long-spacing (collagen)
short leg splint
shrinking lungs syndrome
single limb support
Spectranetics laser sheath
stagnate loop syndrome

SLSQ
Speech and Language Screening
Questionnaire

SLT
left sacrotransverse (fetal position)
[L. *sacrolaeva transversa*]
scanning laser tomography
secondary lymphatic tissue
selective laser trabeculoplasty
Shiga-like toxin
single-lung transplant
split-liver transplantation
STYCAR Language Test
swing light test

SLT-1
Shiga-like toxin I

SLTA
standard language test for aphasia

SLTEC
Shigella-like toxin-producing
Escherichia coli

SlTr
silent treatment

sl.tr.
slight trace

SLUD
salivation, lacrimation, urination,
and defecation

SLUDGE
salivation, lacrimation, urination,
defecation, gastrointestinal distress
and emesis

SLV
since last visit

SLVL
splenic lymphoma with villous
lymphocyte

SLWB
severely low birth weight

SLWC
short leg walking cast

SLZ
serum lysozyme

SM
sadomasochism
self-monitoring
self-mutilation
semimembranous
service mark

Sexual Myths (Scale)
Shigella mutant
simple mastectomy
skim milk
small
smoker
smooth muscle
somatomedin
sonomicrometry
space medicine
sphingomyelin
splenic macrophage
splenomegaly
sports medicine
Stairmaster
stapedius muscle
staphylococcus medium
streptomycin (*See also* S, STM)
submandibular
submucosal
submucous
substituted metabolite
substitute for morphine
suckling mouse (*See also* sM)
sucrose medium
suction method
sulfamerazine
superior mesenteric
supramamillary (nucleus)
sustained medication
symptoms (*See also* Sx, S_x)
synaptic membrane
synovial membrane
systolic mean (pressure)
systolic motion
systolic murmur

SM1
primary sensorimotor cortex

S&M, S/M
sadism/masochism
sadomasochism

Sm
samarium
small (*See also* S, sm)
Smith (antigen)
speed of bronchoconstriction in
response to methacholine
symptom (*See also* sx, sym, symp,
sympt)

153Sm
samarium 153

sM
suckling mouse (*See also* SM)

sm
small (*See also* S)

SM-A
somatomedin A

SMA
> schedule of maximal allowance
> sequential multichannel autoanalyzer
> sequential multiple analysis
> sequential multiple analyzer
> serial multiple analysis
> serum muramidase activity
> shape memory alloy
> simultaneous multichannel autoanalyzer
> simultaneous multiple analyzer
> small muscle atrophy
> smooth muscle actin
> smooth muscle antibody
> smooth muscle autoantibody
> spinal muscular atrophy
> spontaneous motor activity
> standard method agar
> superior mesenteric artery
> supplemental motor area
> supplementary motor area

SMA-6
> Sequential Multiple Analysis—six different blood tests

SMA 6/60
> Sequential Multiple Analysis—six different blood tests in sixty minutes

SMA-12
> Sequential Multiple Analysis—twelve different blood tests (biochemical profile)

SMA 12/60
> Sequential Multiple Analysis—twelve different blood tests in sixty minutes

SMA-20
> Sequential Multiple Analysis—twenty chemical constituents of blood

SMA-60
> Sequential Multiple Analysis—sixty chemical constituents of blood

SMABF
> superior mesenteric artery blood flow

SMABV
> superior mesenteric artery blood velocity

SMAC
> Sequential Multiple Analyzer Computer

SMAD
> Sma- and Mad-related protein

SMAE
> superior mesenteric artery embolus

SMAF
> smooth muscle activating factor
> specific macrophage-arming factor
> superior mesenteric artery (blood) flow

SMAL
> serum methyl alcohol level

SMALL
> same-day microsurgical arthroscopic lateral-approach laser-assisted

sm an
> small animal

SMAO
> superior mesenteric artery occlusion

SMAP
> systemic mean arterial pressure

SMAR
> self-medication administration record

SMART
> simultaneous multiple-angle reconstruction technique
> sperm microaspiration retrieval technique
> surgical myomectomy as reproductive therapy

SMAS
> submucosal aponeurotic system (flap)
> superficial musculoaponeurotic system
> superior mesenteric artery syndrome

SMASH
> self-massage acupressure for self-healing

SMAST
> Short Michigan Alcoholism Screening Test

SMAT
> School Motivation Analysis Test

SMB
> selected mucosal biopsy
> simulated moving bed (chromatography)
> standard mineral base

sMB
> suckling mouse brain

S

NOTES

SMBFT
small bowel followthrough (*See also* SBFT)

SMBG
self-monitored blood glucose

SMBP
serum myelin basic protein

SM-C, Sm-C
somatomedin C

SMC
sensorimotor cortex
skeletal myxoid chondrosarcoma
smooth muscle cell
somatomedin C
special monthly compensation
special mouth care
succinylmonocholine
supernumerary marker chromosome

SMCA
smooth muscle contracting agent
sorbitol MacConkey agar

SMCD
senile macular chorioretinal degeneration
systemic mast cell disease

SM-C/IGF
somatomedin C/insulin-like growth factor

SMD
senile macular degeneration
stereotypic movement disorder
sternocleidomastoid diameter
submanubrial dullness

SMDA
Safe Medical Device Act
starch methylenedianiline

SMDS
secondary myelodysplastic syndrome

SME
severe myoclonic epilepsy
significant medial event

SMECE
sclerosing mucoepidermoid carcinoma with eosinophilia

SMEDI
stillbirth, mummification, embryonic death, infertility (syndrome)

SMEI
severe myoclonic epilepsy in infancy

SMEM
supplemented (Eagle) minimal essential medium

SMEPP
subminiature end-plate potential

SMFA
Short Musculoskeletal Function Assessment
sodium monofluoroacetate

sm-FeSV
McDonough feline sarcoma virus

SMFP
state medical facilities plan

SMFVD
sterile midforceps vaginal delivery

SMG
submandibular gland
supramarginal gyrus

SMH
state mental hospital
strongyloidiasis with massive hyperinfection

SMI
Self-Motivation Inventory
sensory motor integration
severely mentally impaired
silent myocardial infarction
small volume infusion
stress myocardial image
Style of Mind Inventory
suggested minimum increment
supplementary medical insurance
sustained maximal inspiration

SMIDS
suppertime mixed insulin and daytime sulfonylureas

SmIg
surface membrane immunoglobulin

SMILE
safety, monitoring, intervention, length of stay, and evaluation
subperiosteal minimally invasive laser endoscopic (facelift)
sustained maximal inspiratory lung exercise

SMIT
standard mycological identification technique

SML
single major locus

SMM
scintimammography

SMMD
specimen mass measurement device

SMMI
Senoussi Multiphasic Marital Inventory

SMMVT
sustained monomorphic ventricular tachycardia

SMN
second malignant neoplasm
surgical microscope navigation

SMNB
submaximal neuromuscular block
SMN telomeric gene
survival motor neuron telomeric
gene
SMO
Sarns membrane oxygenator
serum monoamine oxidase
site management organization(s)
slip made out
supramalleolar orthosis
SMo
stainless steel and molybdenum
SMON
subacute myelooptic neuropathy
SMP
self-management program
simultaneous macular perception
skeletal muscle protein
slowest moving protease
slow-moving protease
special monthly pension
standard medical practice
standard medical procedure
submitochondrial particle
sympathetic maintained plan
SMPN
sensorimotor polyneuropathy
SMPS
sympathetically mediated pain
syndrome
SMR
scatter-maximum ratio
senior medical resident
sensorimotor rhythm
severe mental retardation
sexual maturity rating
skeletal muscle relaxant
somnolent metabolic rate
standardized metabolic rate
standardized mortality ratio
standard morbidity ratio
standard mortality ratio
stroke with minimal residuum
submucous resection
SMRD
stress-related mucosal damage
SMRR
submucous resection and
rhinoplasty

SMRT
silencing mediator of retinoic acid
and thyroid hormone receptor
SMS
scalded mouth syndrome
senior medical student
Smith-Magenis syndrome
somatostatin (*See also* SOM, SS,
SST)
stiff-man syndrome
supplemental minimal sodium
SMSA
standard metropolitan statistical area
SMT
Sertoli-cell mesenchyme tumor
smooth muscle tumors
Snider Match Test
spinal manipulative therapy
spindle microtubule
spontaneous mammary tumor
stereotactic mesencephalic
tractotomy
SMV
Sena Madureira virus
slow-moving vehicle
small volume
spiral vein of modiolus
submental vertex (view)
submentovertical
superior mesenteric vein
SMVR
supraannular mitral valve
replacement
SMVT
sustained monomorphic ventricular
tachycardia
SMX
sulfamethoxazole
SMX-TMP, SMX/TMP, SMZ/TMP
sulfamethoxazole and trimethoprim
SMZ
sulfamethazine
SMZL
splenic marginal zone lymphoma
SN
school of nursing
sciatic notch
sclerema neonatorum
scrub nurse
SeniorNet
sensorineural
sensory neuron

S

NOTES

SN *(continued)*
> seronegative
> serum neutralization
> serum-neutralizing
> single nephron
> sinoatrial node (*See also* SA, S-A, SAN)
> sinuatrial node (*See also* SA)
> sinus node
> spinal needle
> spontaneous nystagmus
> staff nurse
> standard nomenclature
> streptonigrin
> subnormal
> substantia nigra
> superior nasal
> supernatant
> supernormal
> suprasternal notch (*See also* SSN)

S-N
> sella to nasion (cephalometrics)

S/N
> sample to negative (control ratio)
> signal-to-noise ratio
> speech-to-noise (ratio)

SN$_B$, S-N-B
> sella-nasion-supramentale angle
> sella-nasion-supramentale (point B, in cephalometrics)

SN$_A$, S-N-A
> sella-nasion-subspinale (point A, in cephalometrics)

Sn
> subnasale
> tin [L. *stannum*]

^{113}Sn
> tin-113

SNA
> sinonasal adenocarcinoma
> specimen not available
> superior nasal artery
> sympathetic nerve activity
> systems network architecture

SNa
> serum sodium (concentration)

SNAC
> scaphoid nonunion advanced collapse

SNagg
> serum normal agglutinator

SNAGS
> sustained natural apophysial glides

SNAI
> Standard Nomenclature of Athletic Injuries

SNAP
> scheduled nursing activities program

> Score for Neonatal Acute Physiology
> sensory nerve action potential

SNAP-PE
> Score for Neonatal Acute Physiology-Perinatal Extension

SNARE
> soluble *N*-ethylmaleimide-sensitive factor attachment protein receptor

SNaRI
> serotonin noradrenergic reuptake inhibitor

SNAT
> suspected nonaccidental trauma

SNB
> scalene node biopsy
> sella-nasion-supramentale angle
> sentinel (lymph) node biopsy
> sentinel node biopsy
> Silverman needle biopsy

SNBR
> sentinel node-to-background ratio

SNC
> skilled nursing care
> small noncleaved cell (lymphoma)
> spontaneous neonatal chylothorax

SNc, Snc
> substantia nigra pars compacta

SNCC
> small noncleaved cell

SNCCL
> small noncleaved cell lymphoma

SNCL
> sinus node cycle length

SNC, n-B/B
> small noncleaved cell, non-Burkitt lymphoma

SNCV
> sensory nerve conduction velocity

SND
> selective neck dissection
> single needle device
> sinus node dysfunction
> striatonigral degeneration

SNDA
> Supplemental New Drug Application

SNDO
> Standard Nomenclature of Diseases and Operations

SNE
> sinus node electrogram
> spatial non-emotional (stimuli)
> subacute necrotizing encephalomyelopathy

SNEF
> skilled nursing extended (care) facility

SNEP
  student nurse extern program
SNES
  supracapsular nerve entrapment syndrome
SnET2
  tin ethyl
SNF
  sinus node formation
  skilled nursing facility
SnF2
  stannous fluoride
SNFH
  schizophrenia non-family history
SNF/MR
  skilled nursing facility for the mentally retarded
SNGBF
  single-nephron glomerular blood flow
SNGFR
  single-nephron glomerular filtration rate (*See also* SGFR)
SNGP
  supranuclear gaze palsy
SNGPF
  single-nephron glomerular plasma flow
SNHHD
  simplified nocturnal home hemodialysis
SNHL
  sensorineural hearing loss (*See also* SIIL)
SNIP
  silver nitrate immunoperoxidase
  strict no information in paper
SNIPPV
  synchronized nasal intermittent positive-pressure ventilation
SNJ
  nevus sebaceous of Jadassohn
SNM
  sentinel (lymph) node mapping
  sulfanilamide
SnMP, SnMp
  Sn(tin)-mesoporphyrin
  tin mesoporphyrin
SNMT
  systematic nutritional muscle testing
SN-N
  sternal notch to nipple

SnO₂
  tin oxide
SNOBOL
  String-Oriented Symbolic Language
SNODO
  Standard Nomenclature of Diseases and Operations
SNOMED
  Standardized Nomenclature of Medicine
  Systemized Nomenclature of Medicine
SNOMED CT(r)
  Systematized Nomenclature of Medicine Clinical Terms
SNOMED RT(r)
  Systematized Nomenclature of Medicine Reference Terminology
SNOOP
  Systematic Nursing Observation of Psychopathology
SNOP
  Systematized Nomenclature of Pathology
SNOs
  S-nitrosothiols
SNOT-16
  Sinonasal Outcome Test-16
SNP
  simple neonatal procedure
  single nucleotide polymorphism
  sinus node potential
  sodium nitroprusside
SNP-LP
  single nucleotide polymorphisms - linkage disequilibrium
SnPP
  tin protoporphyrin
SNPs
  single nucleotide polymorphisms
SNPV
  single nucleopolyhedrovirus
SNQ
  superior nasal quadrant
SNR
  substantia nigra zona reticulata
  supernumerary rib
Snr
  substantia nigra pars reticulata
SNRB
  selective nerve root block

NOTES

SNRI
> serotonin-norepinephrine reuptake inhibitor

snRNA
> small nuclear ribonucleic acid

SNRP, snRNP
> small nuclear ribonucleoprotein

SNRPN
> small nuclear ribonucleoprotein-associated polypeptide

SNRT
> sinus node recovery time (*See also* SRT)

SNRTd
> sinus node recovery time, direct (measuring)

SNS
> sacral nerve stimulation
> sterile normal saline
> surgical navigation system
> sympathetic nervous system

SNSA
> seronegative spondyloarthropathy

SNT
> sinuses, nose, throat
> suppan nail technique

SNUC
> sinonasal undifferentiated carcinoma

SNV
> Sin Nombre virus
> skilled nursing visit
> small-volume nebulizer
> spleen necrosis virus
> superior nasal vein
> systemic necrotizing vasculitis

SO
> salpingo-oophorectomy (*See also* S-O)
> second opinion
> sex offender
> shoulder orthosis
> significant other
> slow oxidative
> special observation
> sphenooccipital (synchondrosis)
> sphincter of Oddi
> spinal orthosis
> standing orders
> suboccipital
> suggestive of
> superior oblique
> supraoptic
> supraorbital
> sutures out
> sympathetic ophthalmia

SO$_2$
> oxygen saturation (*See also* OS, O$_2$ sat., SaO$_2$)

SO3
> sulfite

SO4, SO$_4$
> sulfate

S-O
> salpingo-oophorectomy (*See also* SO)
> sulfur dioxide

^{82}So
> strontium-82

SOA
> serum opsonic activity
> shortness of air
> spinal opioid analgesia
> supraorbital artery
> swelling of ankles

SOAA, SOAMA
> signed out against (medical) advice (*See also* SOAMA)

SOAE
> spontaneous otoacoustic emission

SOAM
> stitches out in morning
> sutures out in morning

SOA-MCA
> superficial occipital artery to middle cerebral artery

SOAP
> subjective (data), objective (data), assessment, and plan (problem-oriented record)

SOAPIE
> subjective (data), objective (data), assessment, plan, implementation, and evaluation (problem-oriented record)

SOAPS
> suction, oxygen, apparatus, pharmaceuticals, saline (anesthesia equipment)

SOB
> see order blank
> see order book
> shortness of breath
> side of bed
> suboccipitobregmatic

SOBOE
> shortness of breath on exertion

SOC
> see old chart
> sequential oral contraceptive
> socialization
> standard of care
> start of care
> state of consciousness (*See also* SoC)
> surgical overhead canopy

syphilitic steochondritis
system organ class

S&OC

signed and on chart

SoC

state of consciousness (*See also* SOC)

soc

social
society

SOCD

separation of circle-diamond

SOCS-3

suppressor of cytokine signaling 3

SocSec

Social Security

S-OCT

serum ornithine carbamoyltransferase

SOD

sinovenous occlusive disease
sphincter of Oddi dysfunction
spike occurrence density
superoxide dismutase
surgical officer of the day

sod

sodium (*See also* Na+, Na)

SODAS

spheroidal oral drug absorption system

sod bicarb

sodium bicarbonate

SODD

silencer of death domain (gene)

SOE

source of embolism

SOF

superior orbital fissure

SOFA

sepsis-related organ failure assessment
sequential organ failure assessment
stromal osteoclast-forming activity

SOFAS

Social and Occupational Functioning Assessment

SOFS

spontaneous osteoporotic fracture of sacrum
superior orbital fissure syndrome

SOFT

Sorting of Figures Test

SOG

suggestive of good
supraorbital groove

SOH

sexually oriented hallucination
sympathetic orthostatic hypotension

SOHN

supraoptic hypothalamic nucleus

SOHS

severe ovarian hyperstimulation syndrome

SoHx

social history

SOI

slipped on ice
Student Opinion Inventory
surgical orthotopic implantation (implant)
syrup of ipecac

SOKV

Sokuluk virus

SOL

solute (*See also* S, solu)
solution
space-occupying lesion

sol.

soluble
solution

SOLER

squarely (face person), open (posture), lean (toward person), eye (contact), relaxed

SOL I

special observations level one (there are also SOL II and SOL III)

soln.

solution (*See also* SOL, sol.)

SOLST

Stephens Oral Language Screening Test

solu

solute (*See also* S, SOL)

SOLV

Soldado virus

solv

dissolve [L. *solve*]
solvent

SOM

secretory otitis media
sensitivity of method
serous otitis media

NOTES

S

SOM *(continued)*
somatization
somatostatin (*See also* SMS, SS)
somatotropin
somnolent
sphincter of Oddi manometry
sulformethoxine
supraorbital margin

SOMA
subjective, objective, management, and analytic
System of Multicultural Assessment

somat
somatic

SOMI
sternal occipital mandibular immobilization
sternooccipital-mandibular immobilization (brace, orthosis)
sternooccipital-mandibular immobilizer

SOMPA
System of Multicultural Pluralistic Assessment

SOMT
Spatial Orientation Memory Test

SON
supraoptic nucleus (of the hypothalamus)

SONK
spontaneous osteonecrosis of knee

sono
sonogram
sonography

SONP
soft organs not palpable
solid organs not palpable

SOOF
suborbicularis oculi fat

SOOL
spontaneous onset of labor

SOP
sphincter of Oddi pressure
standard operating procedure

SOPA
Survey of Pain Attitudes
syndrome of primary aldosteronism

SOPCA
sporadic olivopontocerebellar ataxia

SOPM
stitches out in afternoon

SOPP
splanchnic occluded portal pressure

SOQ
Suicide Opinion Questionnaire

SOR
sign own release
stimulus-organism response

SOr
supraorbitale (craniometric)

sorb
sorbitol

SOREMP
sleep-onset rapid eye movement period

SORT-R
Slosson Oral Reading Test-Revised

SORV
Sororoca virus

SOS
save our ship (universal call for emergency)
self-obtained smear
silicone-only suspension
son of sevenless
speed of sound
stimulation of senses
Student Orientations Survey
suicidal observation status
supplemental oxygen system
Surgitek One-Step

SOSOB
sit on side of bed

SOT
sacrooccipital technique
Sensory Organization Test
solid organ transplant
something other than
squamous odontogenic tumor
stream of thought
superficial ocular trauma
systemic oxygen transport

SOTO
step out, turn out

SOTT
synthetic medium old tuberculin trichloroacetic acid (precipitated)

SP
sacral promontory
sacroposterior
sacrum posterior
sacrum to pubis
salivary progesterone
scale of psychosis
schizotypal personality
secretory piece
semiprivate
senile plaque
septal pore
septum pellucidum
sequential pulse
serine proteinase
seropositive
serum protein
shoulder press
shunt pressure

S

shunt procedure
silent period
skin potential
sleep deprivation
small protein
sodium perborate
soft palate
solid phase
spastic dysphonia
spastic paraplegia
spatial peak
speech
speech pathology
spike potential
spine
spiramycin
spirometry
spleen
spontaneous pneumothorax
spouse
standard of performance
standard practice
standard procedure
stand and pivot (*See also* S/P)
staphylococcal protease
status post (*See also* S/P)
steady potential
stool preservative
Streptococcus pneumoniae
subdural peritoneal
subliminal perception
substance
substance P
subtilopeptidase
sulfapyridine
summating potential
suprapatellar
suprapatellar pouch
suprapubic puncture
surfactant protein
symphysis pubis
synthase phosphatase
systolic pressure (*See also* S/P)

S/P

stand and pivot (*See also* SP)
status post (*See also* SP)

S&P

sharp and pink

Sp

most posterior point on posterior
contour of sella turcica
sacropubic

speech
spine (*See also* sp, spin)
summation potential

sP

senile parkinsonism

sp

space (*See also* S)
spec
specific (*See also* spec)
spinal
spine (*See also* Sp, spin)
spleen channel (acupuncture)

sp.

spirit, alcohol [L. *spiritus*] (*See also* spir.)

SP 1

suicide precautions number 1

SP1

stimulatory protein 1

SP 2

suicide precautions number 2

SP-A

surfactant protein-A

SPA

salt-poor albumin
schizophrenia with premorbid asociality
schizophrenia with premorbid association
serum prothrombin activity
sheep pulmonary adenomatosis
single-photon absorptiometry
speech pathology and audiology
sperm penetration assay
sphenopalatine artery
spinal progressive amyotrophy
spondyloarthropathy
spontaneous platelet aggregation
staphylococcal protein A (*See also* SpA)
stimulation-produced analgesia
subperiosteal abscess
suprapatellar amputation
suprapubic aspiration

SpA

spondyloarthropathy
staphylococcal protein A (*See also* SPA)

SPAC

satisfactory postanesthesia course
sectionally processed antibody coated

NOTES

SPACE
single potential analysis cavernous electrical activity

SPAD
selective antipolysaccharide antibody deficiency
stenosing peripheral arterial disease
subcutaneous peritoneal administration device

SPAG
small-particle aerosol generator

SPAI
steroid protein activity index

SPAM
scanning photoacoustic microscopy

SPAMM
spatial modulation of magnetization

span.
spansule

SPAQ
Seasonal Pattern Assessment Questionnaire

SPAR
sensitivity prediction by acoustic reflex

SPARS
spatially resolved spectroscopy

SPAT
side platelet aggregation test
slow paroxysmal atrial tachycardia

SPB
solitary plasmacytoma of bone

SP-B
surfactant protein-B

SPBE
saw palmetto berry extract

SPBI
serum protein-bound iodine

S-PBIgG
serum-platelet bindable immunoglobulin G

SPBT
suprapubic bladder tap

SPC
salicylamide, phenacetin, caffeine
saturated phosphatidylcholine
scaphopisocapitate
sclerosing pancreatocholangitis
serum phenylalanine concentration
sickle-shaped particle cell
simultaneous prism cover test
single palmar crease
single photoelectron counting
single proton counting
small pyramidal cell
spike-processed contraction
spleen cell (*See also* SC)
standard platelet count
statistical process control
Summary of Product Characteristics
suprapatellar cuff
suprapubic catheter
synthesizing protein complex

SP-C
surfactant protein-C

sPC
sequential postremission chemotherapy

SPCA
serum prothrombin conversion accelerator (factor VII)

sp cd
spinal cord

SPC system
single-photon counting system

SPCT
simultaneous prism and cover test

SPD
salmon-poisoning disease
schizotypal personality disorder
silicon photodiode
sociopathic personality disorder
sociopathic personality disturbance
specific paroxysmal discharge
spectral power distribution
spermidine
standard peak dilution
subcorneal pustular dermatosis
supply, processing, and distribution (department)
suprapubic drainage
synpolydactyly

S-2PD
static two-point discrimination

Spd
spermidine

SPDC
striopallidodentate calcinosis

SPDP
N-succinimidylproprionate

SPDT
single-pole, double-throw (switch)

SPE
saw palmetto extract
Sensory Perceptual Examination
septic pulmonary edema
serum protein electrolytes
serum protein electrophoresis
serum protein electrophoretogram
solid-phase extraction
soy phytoestrogen extract
streptococcal pyrogenic exotoxin
subjective paranormal experience
sucrose polyester
superficial punctate erosion

SPEA
streptococcal exotoxin-A
SPEAK
spectral peak
SPEB
streptococcal pyrogenic exotoxin B
SPEC
streptococcal pyrogenic exotoxin C
spec
special
specialist
specialty
specific (*See also* sp)
specimen
Spec Ed
special education
SPECS
System to Plan Early Childhood
Services
SPECT
single-photon emission computed
tomography
technetium-99m sestamibi single-
photon emission computed
tomography
SPEEP
spontaneous positive end expiratory
pressure
SPEG
serum protein electrophoretogram
SPELT-P
Structure Photographic Expressive
Language Test-II
SPEM
smooth pursuit eye movement
SPEP
serum protein electrophoresis
SPET
single-photon emission tomography
SPF
semipermeable film
skin protection factor
specific pathogen free
spectrophotofluorometer
split products of fibrin
standard perfusion fluid
streptococcal proliferative factor
Stuart-Prower factor
sun protection factor
sun protective factor
suntan photoprotection factor

SPFIA
solid phase fluorescence
immunoassay
sp fl
spinal fluid (*See also* SF)
SPFT
Sixteen Personality Factors Test
SPG
scrotopenogram
serine phosphoglyceride
specific gravity (*See also* SG, SpG,
sp gr, sp. gr.)
sphenopalatine ganglion
sucrose-phosphate-glutamic acid
symmetrical peripheral gangrene
SpG
specific gravity (*See also* SG, SPG,
sp gr, sp. gr.)
spg
sponge
SP-GCT
soft parts giant cell tumor
SPGR
spoiled gradient recalled
sp gr, sp. gr.
specific gravity (*See also* SG, SPG,
SpG)
SPH
secondary pulmonary hemosiderosis
severely and profoundly
handicapped
sighs per hour
spherocyte
sphingomyelin (*See also* Sph)
SPh
simple phobia
Sph
sphenoidale
spherical
spherical (lens) (*See also* S, sph)
spherocytosis
sphingomyelin (*See also* SPH)
sph
sphere
spherical (lens) (*See also* S, Sph,
sph)
spheroid
SPHE, SPHER
spherocyte
sp ht
specific heat

NOTES

SPI

selective protein index
Self-Perception Inventory
sensor position indicator
serum precipitable iodine
Shipley Personal Inventory
somatotyping ponderal index
speech processor interface
Standards for Pediatric
    Immunization
structured pain interview
subclinical papillomavirus infection
surgical peripheral iridectomy
symptom problem index

SPIA

solid-phase immunoabsorbent assay
solid-phase immunoassay

SPIB

Social and Prevocational
    Information Battery

SPICU

surgical pulmonary intensive care
    unit

SPID

summed pain intensity difference

SPIF

solid-phase immunoassay
    fluorescence
spontaneous peak inspiratory force

SPIFE

serum protein and immunofixation
    electrophoresis (system)

SPIH

superimposed pregnancy-induced
    hypertension

S-PIN

Steinmann pin

spin

spinal
spine

SPIO

superparamagnetic iron oxide
    (imaging agent)

spir

spiral

spir.

spirit, alcohol [L. *spiritus*] (*See
    also* sp.)

spiss.

dried [L. *spissus*]
inspissated, thickened by
    evaporation [L. *spissatus*]

SPK

serum pyruvate kinase
simultaneous pancreas-kidney
    (transplant)
single parent keeping (baby)

spinnbarkeit
superficial punctate keratitis

spkr

speaker

SPL

Staphylococcal Phage Lysate

SPL

short plantar ligament
skin potential level
sound pressure level
spontaneous lesion
staphylococcal phage lysate
superior parietal lobule

SPLATT

split anterior tibial tendon (transfer)
    (*See also* SPLATTT)

SPLATTT

split anterior tibial tendon transfer
    (*See also* SPLATT)

SPLV

serum parvo virus-like virus

Splx

splenectomy

SPM

scanning probe microscopy
second primary malignancy
self-phase modulation
shocks per minute
significance probability mapping
spectinomycin
spermine
subhuman primate model
suspended particulate matter
syllables per minute
synaptic plasma membrane

SpM

spiriformis medialis (nucleus)

spm

suppression and mutation

SPMA

spinal progressive muscular atrophy

SPMB

strong partial maternal behavior

SPME

solid-phase microextraction

SPMI

status post myocardial infarction

SPMR

standardized proportionate mortality

SPMSQ

Short Portable Mental Status
    Questionnaire

SPN

pneumolysin
solitary pulmonary nodule
supplementary parenteral nutrition
support parenteral nutrition
sympathetic preganglionic neuron

sp. n.
new species [L. *species novum*]
SPNK
single parent not keeping (baby)
SPO
sphincter-preserving operation
status postoperative
SpO₂
arterial oxyhemoglobin saturation
oxygen saturation as measured
using pulse oximetry
SPOA
subperiosteal orbital abscess
SPOCS
Surgical Planning and Orientation
Computer System
SpoCS
space of the cavernous sinus
SPOD
spouse's perception of disease
spon, spont
spontaneous
SPONASTRIME
spondylar changes, nasal anomaly,
striated metaphyses
SponVe
spontaneous ventilation
SPOOL
simultaneous peripheral operation
on-line
SPOP
sequential paired opposed plaque
SPORO
sporatrichosis
Sport Px
sport physical
SPOT
salpingitis after previous tubal
occlusion
salpingitis in previously occluded
tubes
sonographic planning of oncology
treatment
SPOV
Spondweni virus
SPP
Sexuality Preference Profile
single presentation phenotype
skin perfusion pressure
stannous pyrophosphate
super packed platelets
suprapubic prostatectomy

Spp, spp.
species (plural)
SPPS
single-photon planar scintigraphy
solid phase peptide synthesis
stable plasma protein solution
SPPT
superprecipitation (response)
SP-PVC
superior mesenteric-portal vein
confluence
SPQ
Sales Personality Questionnaire
SPR
scanned projection radiography
scan projection radiography
selective posterior rhizotomy
serial probe recognition
simultaneous pancreatic-renal
skin potential reflex
solid phase radioimmunoassay (*See
also* SPRIA)
solid phase receptacle
superior peroneal retinaculum
surface plasmon resonance
SPRAS
Sheehan Patient Rated Anxiety
Scale
SPRIA
solid phase radioimmunoassay (*See
also* SPR)
SPROM
spontaneous premature rupture of
membranes
SPRT
sequential probability ratio test
SPS
shoulder pain and stiffness
simple partial seizure
single patient system
slow-progressive schizophrenia
sodium polyanetholesulfonate
sodium polyethylene sulfonate
sound production sample
special Pap smear
status post surgery
stimulated protein synthesis
sulfite polymyxin sulfadiazine
(agar)
Symonds Picture-Story (Test) (*See
also* SPST)
systemic progressive sclerosis

NOTES

S

SpS
sphenoid sinus
spSHR
stroke-prone spontaneous hypertensive
SPSI
School Problem Screening Inventory
SPSS
spontaneous portal-systemic shunt
Statistical Package for Social Sciences
SPST
single-pole, single-throw (switch)
Symonds Picture-Story Test (*See also* SPS)
SPT
second primary tumor
septic pelvic thrombophlebitis
skin prick test
slow pullthrough
sound production tasks
spectinomycin
spinal tap
Spondee Picture Test
standing pivotal transfer
station pull-through
Supervisory Practices Test
suprapubic tenderness
Symbolic Play Test
SPTA
spatial peak temporal average
Sp tap
spinal tap
SPTB
spontaneous preterm birth
SPTI
systolic pressure time index
SPTL
subcutaneous panniculitis-like T-cell lymphoma
SPTP
spatial peak temporal peak
SPTS
subjective posttraumatic syndrome
SP TUBE
suprapubic tube
SPTURP
status post transurethral resection of prostate
SPTx
static pelvic traction
SPU
short procedure unit
SPUT
sputum
SPV
San Perlita virus

selective proximal vagotomy
Shope papillomavirus
slow-phase velocity
stentless porcine valve
sulfophosphovanillin
SPVR
systemic peripheral vascular resistance
SPX
smallpox vaccine (not otherwise specified)
SPXv
smallpox vaccine (vaccinia virus)
SPZ
secretin pancreozymin
sulfinpyrazone
SQ
social quotient
squalene
square
status quo
subcutaneous (*See also* SC, sc, subcu, subcut, subq)
survey question
symptom questionnaire
sq
square (*See also* SQ)
SQC
semiquantitative culture
squamous cell carcin
SqCCA, sq cell ca
squamous cell carcinoma (*See also* SCC, SCCA)
sq cm
square centimeter
SQE
subcutaneous emphysema
sq m
square meter
sq mm
square millimeter
SQMP
subcutaneous morphine pump
SQ3R
survey, question, read, review, recite
SQUID
superconducting quantum interference device
SQUIDS
superconducting quantum interference device susceptometer
SQV
saquinavir
SR
sarcoplasmic reticulum
saturation recovery
scanning radiometer

schizophrenic reaction
screen
secretion rate
sedimentation rate
see report
seizure resistant
self-recording
senior
sensitivity response
sensitization response (cell)
sentence repetition
seroreversion
service record
sex ratio
short hair (guinea pig)
side rails
sigma reaction
silicone rubber
sinus rhythm
skin resistance
slew rate
slow release
smooth-rough (bacterial colony)
social recreation
soluble repository
specific release
specific resistance
specific response
speech reception
stabilizing reversal
stage of resistance
stimulation ratio
stimulus response
stress relaxation
stretch reflex
sulfonamide-resistant
superior rectus
supply room
sustained release
suture removal
systemic reaction
systemic resistance
systems research
systems review

S-R

smooth-rough (bacterial colony)
(*See also* SR)
stimulus-response

3SR

self-sustained sequence replication
self-sustaining sequence replication

S&R

seclusion and restraints

S/R

schizophrenic reaction
strong/regular (pulse)

SR$_{AW}$

specific airway resistance

Sr

strontium

^{85}Sr

strontium-85

^{87m}Sr

strontium-87m

^{89}Sr

strontium-89

^{90}Sr

strontium-90

sr

steradian (unit of three-dimensional measure)

SRA

segmented renal artery
sewing ring area
spleen repopulating activity
steroid resistant asthma

SRAM

static random access memory

SRAN

surgical resident admission note

SR/AP

schizophrenic reaction, acute, paranoid

SR/AU

schizophrenic reaction, acute undifferentiated

SRAV

Saraca virus

SRBC

sheep red blood cell (*See also* SRC)
sickle red blood cell

SRBOW

spontaneous rupture of bag of waters

SRC

scleroderma renal crisis
sedimented red cell
sheep red cell (*See also* SRBC)
Student Reactions to College

SRCA

specific red cell adherence

NOTES

763

SRCBC
> serum reserve cholesterol binding capacity

SRCC
> sarcomatoid renal cell carcinoma

SRCP
> superficial renal cortical perfusion

SR/CP
> schizophrenic reaction, chronic, paranoid

SRCT
> small round-cell tumor

SR/CU
> schizophrenic reaction, chronic, undifferentiated

SRD
> service-related disability
> sodium-restricted diet
> specific reading disability

SRDS
> Self-Rating Depression Scale

SRDT
> single radial diffusion test

SRE
> Schedule of Recent Experiences
> skeletal related event

SREBP
> sterol regulatory element binding protein

SREDA
> subclinical rhythmic epileptiform discharge of adult

S-REM
> simulated real ear measurement

SREV
> Saumarez Reef virus

SRF
> semirigid fiberglass cast
> severe renal failure
> skin-reactive factor
> slow-reacting factor
> somatotropin-releasing factor
> split renal function
> subretinal fluid

SRF-A, SRFOA
> slow-reacting factor of anaphylaxis (*See also* SRFOA)

SRFC
> sheep (red cell) rosette-forming cell

SRFS
> split renal function study

SRGVHD
> steroid resistant graft-versus-host disease

SRH
> signs of recent hemorrhage
> single radial hemolysis

> somatotropin-releasing hormone
> spontaneously responding hyperthyroidism
> stigmata of recent hemorrhage

SRI
> serotonin reuptake inhibitor
> severe renal insufficiency
> surface regularity index

SRICU
> surgical respiratory intensive care unit

SRID
> single radial immunodiffusion

SRIF
> somatotropin release-inhibiting factor (*See also* SIF)

SRIH
> somatotropin release-inhibiting hormone

SRIV
> Sripur virus

SRK
> Sanders-Retzlaff-Kraff formula

SRL
> short radiolunate

SRM
> standardized response mean
> Standard Reference Material
> subretinal membrane
> superior rectus muscle

SRMD
> stress-related mucosal damage

SRMS
> sustained-release morphine sulfate

SRMs
> specified risk materials

SRN
> subretinal neovascularization (*See also* SRNV)
> superficial radial nerve

SRNA, sRNA, sRNA
> soluble ribonucleic acid
> soluble RNA

SR-NaF
> sustained-release sodium fluoride

SR/NE
> sinus rhythm, no ectopy

SRNG
> sustained-release nitroglycerin

SRNP
> soluble ribonuclear protein

SRNS
> steroid-responsive nephrotic syndrome

SRNV
> subretinal neovascularization (*See also* SRN)

SRNVM

    senile retinal neovascular membrane
    subretinal neovascular membrane

SRO

    sagittal ramus osteotomy
    single room occupancy
    sustained-release oral

SROA

    sports-related osteoarthritis

SROCPI

    Self-Rating Obsessive-Compulsive
    Personality Inventory

SROM

    spinal range of motion
    spontaneous rupture of membranes

SRP

    scaling and root planing (dental)
    septorhinoplasty
    short rib-polydactyly (syndrome)
    (*See also* SRPS)
    signal recognition particle
    signal recognition protein
    simple response paradigm
    single reference point
    stapes replacement prosthesis

SR-PLLA

    self-reinforced poly-L-lactide
    self-reinforcing polylevolactic acid

SRPS

    short rib-polydactyly syndrome (*See
    also* SRP)

SRR

    slow rotation room
    specific reading retarded
    stabilized relative response
    standardized rate ratio
    surgical recovery room
    systematic rational restructuring

SRRS

    Social Readjustment Rating Scale

SR-RSV

    Schmidt-Ruppin (strain) Rous
    sarcoma virus

SRS

    schizophrenic residual state
    sex reassignment surgery
    skeletal repair system
    slow-reacting substance
    Snyder-Robinson syndrome
    somatostatin receptor scintigraphy
    stereotactic radiosurgery

    suicide risk screen
    Symptom Rating Scale

s̄RS

    without redness or swelling

SRSA, SRS-A

    slow-reacting substance of
    anaphylaxis

SRSH

    self-reported self-harm

SRSV

    small round structured virus

SRT

    Seashore Rhythm Test
    sedimentation rate test
    segmented ring tripolar
    sick role tendency
    simple reaction time
    sinus (node) recovery time (*See
    also* SNRT)
    sleep-related tumescence
    smoke removal tube
    Social Relations Test
    speech reception test
    speech reception threshold
    speech recognition threshold
    spontaneously resolving
    thyrotoxicosis
    surfactant replacement therapy
    sustained release theophylline
    Symptom Rating Test

SRU

    side rails up
    solitary rectal ulcer
    structural repeating unit

SRUS

    solitary rectal ulcer syndrome

SRV

    Schmidt-Ruppin virus
    Shark River virus
    small round virus
    superior radicular vein

SRVG

    silicone elastomer ring vertical
    gastroplasty

SRVGB

    Silastic ring vertical-banded gastric
    bypass

SRVT

    sustained reentrant ventricular
    tachyarrhythmia

SRW

    short ragweed (test)

S

NOTES

SRY

sex-determining region (Y chromosome)

SS

sacrosciatic
saline soak
saline solution
saliva sample
saliva substitute
Salmonella-Shigella (agar) (*See also* SSA)
salt substitute
saturated solution (*See also* sat. soln.)
schizophrenia spectrum
Schizophrenia Subscale
schizophrenic spectrum
scleral spur
seizure sensitive
septic shock
serotonin syndrome
serum sickness
Sézary syndrome
short stature
siblings
sickle cell (anemia) (*See also* SSA)
side-to-side
signs and symptoms
single stranded (*See also* ss)
sliding scale
slip sent
slow-wave sleep
soapsuds (*See also* ss)
Social Security
social services
somatostatin (*See also* SMS, SOM)
sorbitan sesquioleate
sparingly soluble
special service
sport sheath
stable sarcoidosis
staccato syndrome
standard score
statistically significant
steady state (*See also* s, ss)
sterile solution
steroid sensitivity
steroid sulfurylation
Stickler syndrome
subaortic stenosis
subscapularis
subsegmental
subsequent sibling
substernal
suction socket
sulfasalazine
sum (of) squares
supersaturated

support (and) stimulation
susceptible
suture system
symmetrical strength
synovial sarcoma
syringosubarachnoid shunting
systemic sclerosis

S&S

shower and shampoo
signs and symptoms
sling and swathe
soft and smooth (prostate)
support and stimulation
swish and spit
swish and swallow

Ss

serum soluble (antigen)
subjects

ss

half [L. *semis*] (*See also* HF, hf, S, sem., semi)
single stranded (*See also* SS)
soapsuds (*See also* SS)
steady state (*See also* SS, s)
subspinale

SSA

sagittal split advancement
salicylsalicylic acid
Salmonella-Shigella agar (*See also* SS)
sickle cell anemia
Sjögren syndrome (antigen) A
skin-sensitizing antibody
skin sympathetic activity
special somatic afferent
sperm-specific antigen
sperm-specific antiserum
streptococcal superantigen
subsegmental airway
subsegmental atelectasis
sulfosalicylic acid

SSAER

steady-state auditory evoked response

SSAV

simian sarcoma-associated virus

SSB

short small bowel
short spike burst
stereospecific binding

SSBE

short-segment Barrett esophagus

SSBG

sex steroid-binding globulin

SSBR

see separate bacteriology report

SSC

saline sodium citrate

sign symptom complex
single-stripe colitis
sodium chloride-sodium citrate
  solution
somatosensory cortex
stainless steel crown
standard saline citrate
Stein Sentence Completion (test)
superior semicircular canal
suprascapular nerve compression
syngeneic spleen cell

SSc

systemic sclerosis

SSCA

sensitized sheep cell agglutination
single shoulder contrast
  arthrography
spontaneous suppressor cell activity

SSCCS

slow spinal cord compression
  syndrome

SSCD

superior semicircular canal
  deficiency

SSCF

sleep stage change frequency

SSCIF

squamous cell carcinoma inhibitory
  factor

SSCM

split spinal cord malformation

SSCP

single-strand conformation
  polymorphism
single-stranded conformational
  polymorphism
substernal chest pain

SSCr

stainless steel crown

SSCS

segmental spinal correction system

SSCT

Sacks Sentence Completion Test

SSCVD

sterile spontaneous controlled
  vaginal delivery

SSD

serosanguineous drainage
shaded-surface display (imaging)
shock(-induced) suppression of
  drinking

sickle cell disease
silver sulfadiazine
single saturating dose
Social Security Disability
source-skin distance
source-surface distance
source-to-skin distance
speech-sound discrimination
succinate semialdehyde
  dehydrogenase
sudden sniffing death
sum of square deviations
syndrome of sudden death

SSDBS

symptom schedule for the
  diagnosis of borderline
  schizophrenia

SSDI

Social Security Disability Insurance

SS-DNA, ssDNA

single-stranded deoxyribonucleic
  acid
single-stranded DNA

SSDP

sequence-specific DNA primer

SSE

saline solution enema
skin self-examination
soapsuds enema
steady-state exercise
systemic side effects

SSEA

stage-specific embryonic antigen

SSEEG

scalp-sphenoidal
  electroencephalography

SSEH

spontaneous spinal epidural
  hematoma

S-SEP, SSEP

short-latency somatosensory-evoked
  potential
somatosensory-evoked potential (*See
  also* SEP, SSEP)

SSER

somatosensory evoked response
  (*See also* SER)

SSF

soluble suppressor factor
subscapular skinfold (thickness)
supplementary sensory feedback

S

NOTES

SSFI
social stress and functionality inventory

SSFP
steady-state free precession
steady-state free progression

SSFSE
single shot fast spin echo

SSG
sublabial salivary gland

SSH
spinal subdural hemorrhage

SSHA
Survey of Study Habits and Attitudes

SSHb
homozygous for sickle cell hemoglobin

SSHL
severe sensorineural hearing loss

SSHR
steady state heart rate

SSHV
snowshoe hare virus

SSI
segmental sequential irradiation
segmental spinal instrumentation
semistructured psychiatric interview
shoulder subluxation inhibitor
sliding scale insulin
small-scale integration
stuttering severity instrument
subshock insulin
superior sector iridectomy
Supplemental Security Income
surgical site infection
symptom severity index
synthetic sentence identification
System Sign Inventory

SSIAM
Structured and Scaled Interview to Assess Maladjustment

SSIDS
sibling of sudden infant death syndrome (victim)

SSII
Safran Student's Interest Inventory

SSIS
side-to-side isoperistaltic strictureplasty

SSIT
subscapularis, supraspinatus, infraspinatus, and teres minor (muscles)

SSKI
saturated potassium iodide solution
saturated solution of potassium iodide
supersaturated potassium iodide

SSL
skin surface lipid
subtotal supraglottic laryngectomy
synthetic sentence list

S-sleep
synchronized sleep

SSM
scaphoid shift maneuver
skin-sparing mastectomy
skin surface microscopy
subsynaptic membrane
superficial spreading melanoma

S-SMase
secretory sphingomyelinase

SSN
severely subnormal
Social Security number
subacute sensory neuropathy
suprasternal notch (*See also* SN)

SSNS
steroid-sensitive idiopathic nephrotic syndrome
steroid-sensitive nephrotic syndrome

SSO
sagittal split osteotomy
Spanish-speaking only
special sense organs

SSOP
sequence-specific oligonucleotide probe (hybridization)
Standard System of Psychiatry

SSP
Sanarelli-Shwartzman phenomenon
sequence-specific primer
simultaneously stapled pneumonectomy
slice sensitivity profile
small spherical particle
stereotactic surface projection
subacute sclerosing panencephalitis (*See also* SSPE)
subclavian steal syndrome
supersensitivity perception

Ssp, ssp
subspecies (*See also* subsp)

SSPCS
side-to-side portacaval shunt

SSPD
schizoid-schizotypal personality disorder

SSPE
subacute sclerosing panencephalitis (*See also* SSP)

SSPG
steady-state plasma glucose

SSPI
steady-state plasma insulin
SSPL
saturation sound pressure level
SSPP
subsynaptic plate perforation
SSPS
side-to-side portacaval shunt
SS-PSE
Schizophrenic Subscale of Present State Examination
SSPT
Speech-Sound Perception Test
SSPU
surgical short procedure unit
SSQ
sequential scalar quantization
Social Support Questionnaire
SS-QOL
stroke-specific quality of life
SSR
somatosensory response
somatostatin receptor
steady-state rest
steroid-resistant rejection
substernal retraction
surgical supply room
sympathetic skin response
SSRFC
surrounding subretinal fluid cuff
SSRI
selective serotonin reuptake inhibitor
SSRO
sagittal split ramus osteotomy
SSRS
Social Skills Rating System
SSS
scalded skin syndrome
School Situation Survey
secondary Sjögren syndrome
sensation-seeking scale
sick sinus syndrome
Simple Scoring System
small sharp spike
soluble specific substance
specific soluble substance
Stanford Sleepiness Scale
sterile saline soak
strong soap solution
structured sensory stimulation

superior sagittal sinus
systemic sicca syndrome
SSS-58
58-point Scandinavian Stroke Scale
SSSB
sagittal split setback
SSSC
Social Support Scale for Children (test)
SSSS
staphylococcal scalded skin syndrome
ssSSc
systemic sclerosis sine scleroderma
SSST
superior sagittal sinus thrombosis
SSSV
superior sagittal sinus velocity
SST
sagittal sinus thrombosis
sclerosing stromal tumor
simple shoulder test
Slingerland Screening Tests
social skills training
sodium sulfite titration
somatosensory thalamus
somatostatin
SSTE
skin-soft tissue envelope
SSTN
Sandostatin
SSU
self-service unit
sterile supply unit
SSV
sheep seminal vesicle
simian sarcoma virus
SSVC
systemic venous collateral
SSVD
sterile, spontaneous vaginal delivery
SSW
short-stay ward
Staggered Spondaic Word Test
SSX
sulfisoxazole
S/SX
signs/symptoms
SSZ
sulfasalazine
ST
electrocardiographic wave segment

NOTES

ST *(continued)*
esotropia
(heat-)stable (entero)toxin
sacrotransverse
sacrum transverse
scala tympani
scapulothoracic
sclerotherapy
sedimentation time
semitendinosus
septal thickness
serum transferrin
shock therapy
siblings (raised) together
similarly tested
sinus tachycardia
sinus tympani
skin temperature
skin test
skin thickness
slight trace
slow twitch
soft tissue treatment
speech therapist
sphincter tone
split thickness
standardized test
standard test
starting time
stent thrombosis
sternothyroid
stimulus *(See also* R, S)
stomach *(See also* st, stom)
store *(See also* STO)
straight
stress test
stretcher
striatum *(See also* Str)
sublingual tablet
subtalar
subtotal
sulfathiozole
surface tension *(See also* σ)
surgical therapy
surrogate tolerogenesis
survival time
systolic time

S-T
sickle cell thalassemia

ST37
hexylresorcinol

St.
Saint
stomion

st
stage (of disease)
stere (measure of capacity)
stokes (unit of kinematic viscosity)

stomach *(See also* ST, stom)
stomion (median point of oral slit when lips are closed)
stone (measure of weight)
straight
stroke
subtype

STA
second trimester abortion
serum thrombotic accelerator
serum tobramycin assay
standard tube agglutination test
superficial temporal artery
superior temporal artery

Sta
staphylion
station

stab
stabilization
stabkernige (band neutrophil)
stab neutrophil

STABS
Suinn Test Anxiety Behavior Scale

STACL
Screening Test for Auditory Comprehension of Language

STAE
subsegmental transcatheter arterial embolization

St AE
standard above-elbow (cast)

S-TAG
slow-binding target-attaching globulin

STAG
split thickness autogenous graft
striped tag myocardial tagging system

STAI
Spielberger State-Trait Anxiety Inventory
State-Trait Anxiety Inventory

STAIC
State-Trait Anxiety Inventory for Children

STAI-I
State Trait Anxiety Index-I

STALD
Sheffield Screening Test for Acquired Language Disorders

STA-MCA
superficial temporal artery-middle cerebral artery

StanPsych
standard psychiatric (nomenclature)

STA-PCA
superficial temporal artery-posterior cerebral artery

STA-peg
> Smith subtalar joint arthroereisis peg

staph
> staphylococcus

STAPP
> short-term anxiety-provoking psychotherapy

STAR
> Scandinavian total ankle replacement
> Simultaneous Technique for Acuity and Readiness Testing
> specialized tissue aspirating resectoscope
> staged abdominal repair
> steroidogenic acute regulatory

StAR
> steroid acute regulatory protein
> steroid acute respiratory protein
> steroidogenic acute regulatory protein

STARRT
> selective tubal assessment to refine reproductive therapy

STARS
> Short-Term Auditory Retrieval and Storage (Test)

START, StaRT
> stereotactic-assisted radiation therapy

STAS
> State-Trait Anger Scale
> Support Team Assessment Schedule

STA-SCA
> superficial temporal artery-superior cerebellar artery

STAT
> at once [L. *statim*] (*See also* stat.)
> Suprathreshold Adaptation Test

Stat
> signal transducer and activator of transcription

Stat4
> signal transducer and activator of transcription-4

Stat5
> signal transducer and activator of transcription-5

stat
> radiation emanation unit (German)

stat.
> at once [L. *statim*] (*See also* STAT)
> statim

statA
> statampere (*See also* A-esu)

statC
> statcoulomb

STAXI
> State-Trait Anger Expression Inventory

STB, Stb
> stillborn (*See also* SB, stillb)

STBAL
> standing balance

ST BY
> stand by (*See also* SB)

STC
> sarcomatoid thymic carcinoma
> serum theophylline concentration
> sexually transmitted condition
> slow transit constipation
> soft tissue calcification
> stimulate to cry
> stroke treatment center
> subtotal colectomy
> sugar-tong cast

sTCC
> superficial transitional cell carcinoma

STCL
> Standardized Test of Computer Literacy

STD
> sexually transmitted disease
> skin test done
> skin test dose
> skin-to-tumor distance
> sodium tetradecyl (sulfate)
> source-tray distance
> standard density (reference)
> standard test dose
> ST segment depression

std
> saturated (*See also* SAT, sat., sat'd)
> standardized

STDH
> skin test for delayed-type hypersensitivity

STDS
> stone-tissue detection system

S

NOTES

STDT
standard tone-decay test
STD TF
standard tube feeding
STE
subperiosteal tissue expander
STEAM
stimulated echo acquisition mode
STEC
Shiga toxin-producing *Escherichia coli*
Stx 2-producing *Escherichia coli* (strain)
STEL
short-term exposure limit
STEM
scanning transmission electron microscope
sten
stenosed
stenosis
STEP
Sequential Tests of Educational Study
S.T.E.P.
Short Transitional Edge Protection
STEP-III
Sequential Tests of Educational Progress, Series III
STEPS
Screening Test for Educational Prerequisite Skills
sequential treatment employing pharmacologic support
system for thalidomide education and prescription safety
stereo
stereogram
stereophonic
STET
single photon emission tomography
submaximal treadmill exercise test
STETH
stethoscope
STF
serum thymus factor
slow twitch fiber
small third-trimester fetus
specialized treatment facility
special tube feeding
standard tube feeding
sudden transient freezing
superficial temporal fascia
sTf-R, sTfR
soluble transferrin receptor
STG
short-term goal

split-thickness graft
superior temporal gyrus
STGC
syncytiotrophoblastic giant cell
STH
soft tissue hemorrhage
somatotroph hormone
somatotropic hormone (*See also* SH)
subtotal hysterectomy
supplemental thyroid hormone
STh, S-Thal
sickle cell thalassemia
STHB
said to have been
ST/HR
ST segment/heart rate (slope)
STI
scientific and technical information
serum trypsin inhibitor
sexually transmitted infection
short-term immunotherapy
soft tissue injury
soybean trypsin inhibitor (*See also* SBTI)
systolic time interval
STIC
serum trypsin inhibition capacity
solid-state transducer intracompartment
STIF
spinopelvic transiliac fixation
stillb
stillborn (*See also* SB, Stb)
stim, stimn
stimulation
STING
subureteric Teflon injection
STIP
(basophilic) stippling
STIR
short inversion (imaging) recovery
short tau inversion recovery
short T1 inversion recovery
STJ
scapulothoracic joint
subtalar joint
STK
streptokinase (*See also* SK)
STK11
serine threonine kinase gene 11
STL
serum theophylline level
status thymicolymphaticus
swelling, tenderness, limited (motion)
STLE
St. Louis encephalitis

STLI
subtotal lymphoid irradiation

STLOM
swelling, tenderness, limitation of motion

STLS
subacute thyroiditis-like syndrome

STLV
simian T-cell lymphotropic virus
simian T-lymphotropic virus

STM
scanning tunneling microscope
scanning tunneling microscopy
short-term memory
streptomycin (*See also* SM)

StMPM
syncytiotrophoblast microvillar plasma membrane

STMV
Santarem virus

STN
subthalamic nucleus
supratrochlear nucleus

STn
sialyl-Tn

sTNF-RI
soluble tumor necrosis factor-a receptor type I

STNI
subtotal nodal irradiation

STNP
subtalar joint neutral position

STNR
symmetric tonic neck reflex

STNS
sham transcutaneous nerve stimulation

STNV
satellite tobacco necrosis virus

STO
store (*See also* ST)
surgical treatment objective

stom
stomach (*See also* ST, st)

STOP
selective tubal occlusion procedure
surgical termination of pregnancy

STORCH
syphilis, toxoplasmosis, other agents, rubella, cytomegalovirus, herpes simplex (virus)

STP
scientifically treated petroleum
serenity, tranquility, peace (user's term for dimethoxymethylamphetamine)
Sibling Training Program
sodium thiopental
standard temperature and pressure
standard temperature and pulse

S-TPA
serum tissue polypeptide antigen

STPD
standard temperature and pressure, dry

STPI
State-Trait Personality Inventory

STPP
sodium tripolyphosphate

STPS
specific thalamic projection system

STQ
superior temporal quadrant

STR
short tandem repeat
skin test reactivity
soft-tissue rheumatism
special treatment room
stone tissue recognition (system)
subtotal resection

Str
striatum (*See also* ST)

strab
strabismus (*See also* Sb)

StrAbs
striated muscle

STRAN
surgical resident's admission note

Strep
streptomycin

strep
streptococcus

strep TSS
streptococcal toxic shock syndrome

STRESS
subject's treatment-emergent symptom scale

STRP
short tandem repeat polymorphism
simple tandem repeat polymorphism

STRR
Slosson Test of Reading Readiness

NOTES

STRT
  simultaneous thermoradiotherapy
  skin temperature recovery time
struct
  sructural
  structure
STRV
  Stratford virus
STS
  serologic test for syphilis
  serology test for syphilis
  sexual tubal sterilization
  short-term storage
  silicone thermoplastic splinting
  sodium tetradecylsulfate
  sodium thiosulfate
  soft tissue sarcoma
  soft tissue swelling
  standard test for syphilis
  steroid sulfatase
  steroid sulfate
  subtrapezial space
  sugar-tong splint
STSE
  split-thickness skin excision
STSG
  split-thickness skin graft
STSS
  staphylococcal toxic shock
    syndrome
  streptococcal toxic shock syndrome
STSs
  sequence-tagged sites
STT
  scaphoid, trapezium, trapezoid
  scaphotrapeziotrapezoid (joint)
  scaphotrapezoid-trapezial
  sensitization test
  serial thrombin time
  skin temperature test
  soft tissue tumor
  spinothalamic tract
  standard triple therapy
  superficial tibiotalar
STTOL
  standing tolerance
STU
  shock trauma unit
  skin test unit
STUMP
  stromal tumor of unknown
    malignant potential
STV
  short-term variability
  soft tissue view
  superior temporal vein

STVA
  subtotal villous atrophy (*See also*
    SVA)
STVS
  short-term visual storage
STX
  saxitoxin
  stricture
  structure
Stx
  Shiga toxin
STYCAR
  Sheridan Tests for Young Children
    and Retardates
STZ
  streptozocin (*See also* SZ, Sz,
    SZN)
  streptozyme
SU
  salicyluric (acid)
  sensation unit
  sensory urgency
  solar urticaria
  Somogyi unit
  sorbent unit
  spectrophotometric unit
  stroke unit
  strontium unit
  subunit
  sulfonamide (*See also* Su)
  sulfonylurea
  supine
SU5416
  semoxinal
S/U
  shoulder/umbilicus
S&U
  supine and upright
Su
  sulfonamide (*See also* SU)
SUA
  serum uric acid
  single umbilical artery
  single unit activity
SUB
  Skene, urethral and Bartholin
    (glands)
subac
  subacute
subconj
  subconjunctival
subcu, subcut, subq
  subcutaneous (*See also* SC, sc, SQ,
    subq)
subl, subling
  sublingual
submand
  submandibular

SubN
    subthalamic nucleus
subsp
    subspecies (*See also* Ssp, ssp)
substd
    substandard
SUCC
    succinylcholine
Succ
    succinate
    succinic
SUD
    skin unit dose
    substance use disorder
    sudden unexpected death
    sudden unexplained death
SUDI
    sudden unexpected death in infants
    sudden unexplained death in
     infants
SUDS
    single-unit delivery system
    Single Use Diagnostic System
    Subjective Units of Distress Scale
    sudden unexplained death syndrome
SUE
    single-use electrode
SUF
    sequential ultrafiltration
SUFE
    slipped upper femoral epiphysis
suff
    sufficient
SUHT
    subject's height (in inches)
SUI
    stress urinary incontinence
    suicide
SUID
    sudden unexpected infant death
    sudden unexplained infant death
SUKA
    subungual keratoacanthoma
sulf
    sulfate
sulfa
    sulfonamide
SULFHB
    sulfhemoglobin (*See also* HbS,
     SHB, SHb)
SULF-PRIM
    sulfamethoxazole (and) trimethoprim

sum.
    summation
SUMD
    Scale for the Assessment of
     Unawareness of Mental Disorder
SUN
    serum urea nitrogen
    Standard Units and Nomenclature
SUNCT
    short duration, unilateral, neuralgic,
     conjunctival injection and tearing
SUND
    sudden unexplained death
SUO
    syncope of unknown origin
SUP
    stress ulcer prophylaxis
    superficial (*See also* sup)
    superior (*See also* sup)
    supination (*See also* supin)
    supinator (muscle) (*See also* sup)
    symptomatic uterine prolapse
sup
    superficial (*See also* SUP)
    superior (*See also* SUP)
    supervision
    supervisor
    supinator (muscle) (*See also* SUP)
SupHypArt
    superior hypophyseal artery
supin
    supination (*See also* SUP)
supp, suppos
    support
    suppository
suppl
    supplement
    supplementary
SUR
    sulfonylurea receptor
    suramin
SURF
    Service Utilization and Risk
     Factors
SURG, surg
    surgeon
    surgery (*See also* S)
    surgical
SURS
    solitary ulcer of rectum syndrome
SUS
    solitary ulcer syndrome

S

NOTES

SUS (*continued*)
  strained urinary sediment
  suppressor sensitive
susp
  suspended
  suspension
SUTI
  sperm-ubiquitin tag immunoassay
  symptomatic urinary tract infection
SUUD
  sudden unexpected, unexplained
    death
SUV
  standardized uptake value
  standard uptake value
SUVAG
  system universal verbotonol
    audition Guberina
SUX
  succinylcholine
  suction
SUZI
  subzonal injection
  subzonal insemination
  subzonal insertion
SV
  saphenous vein
  sarcoma virus
  satellite virus
  selective vagotomy
  semilunar valve
  seminal vesicle
  Sendai virus
  severe
  sigmoid volvulus
  simian virus
  single ventricle
  sinus venosus
  snake venom
  splenic vein
  spoken voice
  spontaneous ventilation
  stroke volume
  Study of Values
  subclavian vein
  subventricular
  supravital
S/V
  surface/volume (ratio)
SV40
  simian vacuolating virus 40
  simian virus 40
Sv
  sievert (unit)
sv
  single vibration
sv.
  serovar

SVA
  selective vagotomy with antrectomy
  selective visceral angiography
  sequential ventriculoatrial (pacing)
  spatial voltage (at maximal)
    anterior (force)
  special visceral afferent
  subtotal villous atrophy (*See also*
    STVA)
SVAS
  supravalvular aortic stenosis (*See
    also* SAS)
SVB
  saphenous vein bypass
SVBG
  saphenous vein bypass graft
SVC
  segmental venous capacitance
  selective vascular clamping
  slow vital capacity
  subclavian vein catheterization
  subclavian vein compression
  superior vena cava
  suprahepatic vena cava
  supraventricular crest
SV-CAH
  simple virilizing congenital adrenal
    hyperplasia
SVCCS
  superior vena cava compression
    syndrome
SVCG
  spatial vectorcardiogram
SVCO
  superior vena cava obstruction
SVC-PA
  superior vena cava-pulmonary artery
    (shunt)
SVCPMS
  segmental vertebral
    cellulotenoperiosteomyalgic
    syndrome
SVCR
  segmented venous capacitance ratio
SVC-RPA
  superior vena cava-right pulmonary
    artery (shunt)
SVCS
  superior vena cava syndrome
SVCT
  spiral x-ray computed tomography
SVD
  single-vessel disease
  singular value decomposition
  small vessel disease
  spontaneous vaginal delivery
  spontaneous vertex delivery

structural valve deterioration
swine vesicular disease

SVDV
swine vesicular disease virus

SVE
slow volume encephalography
soluble viral extract
special visceral efferent
sterile vaginal examination
Streptococcus viridans endocarditis
subcortical vascular encephalopathy
supraventricular ectopy

SVG
saphenous vein graft
scatter and veiling glare
seminal vesiculography

SVI
seminal vesicle invasion
small-vessel infarction
stroke volume index
systolic velocity integral (Doppler)

SVIB
Strong Vocational Interest Blank

S VISC
serum viscosity

SVL
severe visual loss
superficial vastus lateralis

SVM
seminal vesicle microsome
spatial voltage at maximal
(posterior force)
syncytiovascular membrane

SVN
small-volume nebulizer

SVO
splenic vein obstruction

SvO₂, S$_{VO2}$
mixed venous oxygen saturation
(*See also* MVO2, MVO₂S)
systemic vascular resistance index
venous oxygen saturation

SVOM
sequential volitional oral movement

SVP
selective vagotomy with
pyloroplasty
small volume parenteral (infusion)
spatial voltage (at maximal)
posterior (force)
spontaneous venous pulsation
spontaneous venous pulse

standing venous pressure
static volume pressure
superficial vascular plexus

SVPB
supraventricular premature beat

SVPC
supraventricular premature
contraction

SVR
sequential vascular response
supraventricular rhythm
systemic vascular resistance

SVRI
systemic vascular resistance index

SVS
slit ventricle syndrome

SVSe
supravaginal septum

SVT
sinoventricular tachyarrhythmia
sinus-vein thrombosis
STYCAR Vision Test
subclavian vein thrombosis
supraventricular tachyarrhythmia
supraventricular tachycardia

SVV
Sal Vieja virus

SVVD
spontaneous vertex vaginal delivery

SW
seriously wounded
short wave
slow wave
social worker
spherule wall
spike wave
spiral wound
stab wound
sterile water
stroke work
Swiss Webster (mouse)

S&W
soap and water

Sw
swine

sw
switch

SWA
seriously wounded in action

SWAMI
Speech with Alternating Masking
Index

S

NOTES

SWAMP
swine-associated mucoprotein
SWAP
short wavelength automated perimetry
SWBS
Spiritual Well-Being Scale
SWC
submaximal working capacity
SW-CAH
salt-wasting congenital adrenal hyperplasia
SWD
shortwave diathermy
SWE
slow-wave encephalography
SWFI
sterile water for injection (*See also* SWI)
SWG
standard wire gauge
SWGD
sterile water gastric drip
SWI
skin and wound isolation
sterile water for injection (*See also* SWFI)
stroke-work index
surgical wound infection
SWIM
sperm-washing insemination method
SWIORA
spinal cord injury without radiologic abnormality
SWL
shock wave lithotripsy
SWM
segmental wall motion
SWMA
segmental wall motion abnormality
SWMF
Semmes-Weinstein monofilament
SWO
superficial white onychomycosis
SWORD
Surveillance of Work-related and Occupational Respiratory Disease
SWP
small whirlpool
SWR
serum Wassermann reaction
surface wrinkling retinopathy
SWS
slow-wave sleep
spike-wave stupor
Sturge-Weber syndrome (*See also* SW)
Stüve-Wiedemann syndrome

SWT
shock-wave therapy
sine-wave threshold
Speech Weber Test
stab wound of throat
SWU
septic workup
SX
sulfamethoxypyridazine
Sx, S$_x$, sx
signs
surgery
symptom
SXA
single-energy x-ray absorptiometer
SXPL
strictureplasty
SXR
skull x-ray
SXT
sulfamethoxazole/trimethoprim (*See also* SMX/TMP, SULF-PRIM, TMP-SMX)
SY
syphilis (*See also* syph)
syphilitic (*See also* syph)
SYA
subacute yellow atrophy
SYC
small, yellow, constipated (stool)
sym
symmetrical
symptom (*See also* sx)
symb
symbol
symbolic
symp, sympt
symptom (*See also* Sm, sym)
sympath
sympathetic
symph
symphysis
SYN
synaptophysin
syn, synd
syndrome
synonym
synovial
sync
synchronous
syndet
synthetic detergent
syn fl
synovial fluid (*See also* SF)
synth
synthetic

syph

syphilis (*See also* SY)
syphilitic (*See also* SY)

SYR

Syrian (hamster)

syr

syringe

SYS

stretching-yawning syndrome
synovial sarcoma

sys

system (*See also* syst)
systemic (*See also* syst)

SYS BP

systolic blood pressure (*See also* SBP)

syst

system (*See also* sys)
systemic (*See also* sys)
systole
systolic

SZ

schizophrenic
seizure (*See also* Sz)
Skevas-Zerfus (disease)
streptozocin (*See also* STZ, Sz, SZN)
suction
sulfamethizole

Sz

schizophrenia
seizure (*See also* SZ)
skin impedance
streptozocin (*See also* STZ, SZ, SZN)

SZD

streptozocin diabetes

SZN

streptozocin (*See also* STZ, SZ, Sz)

S

NOTES

T⁻

temperature

T

absolute temperature (Kelvin)
electrocardiographic wave
   corresponding to repolarization of
   ventricles
inverted T. wave
life (time) (*See also* t)
obtained under test conditions
period (time)
ribothymidine (*See also* Thd)
tablespoonful (*See also* tbs)
tanycyte (ependymal cell)
tau (19th letter of Greek alphabet),
   uppercase
T bandage
T bar
telomere (banding of chromosomes)
temperature (*See also* temp)
temporal (electrode placement in
   electroencephalography)
temporary (*See also* temp)
tender
tension (intraocular) (*See also* TEM)
tera-
terminal (banding of chromosomes)
tertiary (*See also* t, ter, tert)
tesla (unit of measure)
testicle
testosterone
tetra
tetracycline (*See also* TC, Tc,
   TCN, TCNE, TE, TET)
T fiber
theophylline
thoracic (*See also* Th, thor)
thoracoabdominal (stapler)
thorax (*See also* Th, thor)
threatened (animal)
threonine (*See also* Thr)
thrombus (*See also* throm, thromb)
thymidine (*See also* TdR)
thymine (*See also* Thy)
thymus (cell) (*See also* thy.)
thymus-derived (lymphocyte)
thyroid
tidal (gas)
time
timolol
tincture (*See also* TR, Tr, tr)
tocopherol
tone
tonometer (reading)
topical (*See also* top.)

torque
total
toxicity (*See also* tox)
trace (*See also* TR, Tr, tr)
tracheotomy (set)
training (group)
transition (point) (*See also* TP)
transmittance
transverse (*See also* trans)
tray
triangulation
triggered
tritium (*See also* t)
tuberculin
tuberculum
tuberosity
tumor (antigen)
turnkey (system)
type

T+

increased intraocular tension
increased tension (pressure)

T 1/2

terminal half-life

T-

decreased tension (pressure)

T1–T12

first to twelfth thoracic nerves
first to twelfth thoracic vertebrae
   (*See also* D1–D12)

T2

spin-spin or transverse relaxation
   time (MRI scan)

T3

transurethral thermo-ablation therapy
   (Targis)
Tylenol with codeine (30 mg)

T-1824

Evans blue (dye)

²⁰¹T1

thallium-201

Tα₁

thymosin alpha₁

T₁

monoiodotyronine
tricuspid first heart sound

T_mg

maximal tubular reabsorption of
   glucose

t

duration
life (time) (*See also* T)
student test variable
teaspoonful
temperature (Celsius, Fahrenheit)

t *(continued)*
    temporal
    terminal
    tertiary *(See also* T, ter, tert)
    test (of significance)
    time
    ton (metric)
    tonne
    transformer
    translocation
    tritium *(See also* T)

t.
    three (times) [L. *ter*]

T1
    first twitch height
    spin-lattice or longitudinal
      relaxation time (MRI scan)

T12
    terminal half-life

T½
    (mitral) pressure half-time (Doppler)
    terminal half-life (of isotopes)

t½
    reaction half-time
    time taken for half of initial
      concentration of deoxyribonucleic
      acid to renature

2,4,5–T
    2,4,5-trichlorophenoxyacetic acid

T₂
    diiodothyronine
    second stage of decreased
      intraocular tension
    tricuspid second heart sound

T28
    Trapezoidal-28

T₃
    3,5,3'-triiodo-I-thyronine
    triiodothyronine *(See also* TIT,
      TITh, TRIT)
    3,5,3'-triiodothyronine *(See also*
      TITh)

T4
    CD4 (helper-inducer cells)
    thyroxine

T₄
    levothyroxine
    tetraiodothyronine (thyroxine)
    thyroxine

T-7
    free thyroxine factor

T>MIC
    time above minimum inhibitory
      concentration

TA
    alkaline tuberculin
    tactile afferent

Takayasu arteritis
T-amplifier
technical assistance
teichoic acid
temperature, axillary *(See also*
  T(A))
temporal arteritis
temporal average
tendon of Achilles
tension by applanation
tension, arterial
terminal antrum
terminal arteriole
Terminologia Anatomica
test age
thermophilic *Actinomyces*
thoracoabdominal
thymocytotoxic autoantibody
thyroarytenoid
thyroglobulin autoprecipitation
thyroglobulin autoprecipitin
thyroid antibody
thyroid autoantibody
tibialis anterior
titratable acid
total alkaloids
toxic adenoma
toxin-antitoxin *(See also* TAT)
tracheal aspirate
traffic accident *(See also* T/A)
transactional analysis
transaldolase
transantral
transplantation antigen
trapped air
treatment assignment
triamcinolone acetonide *(See also*
  TAA)
tricholomic acid
tricuspid anuloplasty
tricuspid atresia
trophoblast antigen
true anomaly
truncus arteriosus
tryptamine
tryptophan-acid (reaction)
tryptose agar
tube agglutination
tuberculin, alkaline
tumorantigen
tumor associated

TA-4
    tumor-antigen 4

T of A
    transposition of aorta

T + A
    ticlopidine plus aspirin

T/A
>time and amount
>traffic accident (*See also* TA, TAT)

T&A
>tonsillectomy and adenoidectomy
>tonsils and adenoids

T(A)
>temperature, axillary (*See also* TA)

Ta
>tantalum

¹⁷⁸Ta
>tantalum-178

¹⁸²Ta
>tantalum-182

TAA
>premature top codon
>thoracic aortic aneurysm
>total ankle arthroplasty
>transcoronary alcohol ablation
>transverse aortic arch
>triamcinolone acetonide (*See also* TA)
>tumor-associated antigen

TAAA
>thoracoabdominal aortic aneurysm

TAAF
>thromblastic activity of amniotic fluid

TA-AIDS
>transfusion-associated AIDS

TAB
>tablet (*See also* tab.)
>temporal artery biopsy
>therapeutic abortion (*See also* TAb)
>total atrial blanking
>triple antibiotic
>tumescent absorbent bandage
>typhoid, paratyphoid A, and paratyphoid B (vaccine)

TAb
>therapeutic abortion (*See also* TAB)

tab.
>tablet (*See also* TAB)

TABC
>total aerobic bacteria count
>typhoid, paratyphoid A, paratyphoid B, and paratyphoid C (vaccine)

TABTD
>typhoid, paratyphoid A, paratyphoid B, tetanus toxoid, and diphtheria toxoid (vaccine)

TAC
>tacrolimus
>terminal antrum contraction
>tetracaine, Adrenalin, and cocaine
>time-activity curve
>total abdominal colectomy
>total aganglionosis coli
>total allergen content
>transient aplastic crisis
>transiently amplifying cell
>triamcinolone acetonide cream
>triamcinolone cream

TACC
>thoracic aortic cross-clamping

TACE
>teichoic acid crude extract
>transarterial catheter embolization
>transarterial chemoembolization
>transcatheter arterial chemoembolization
>trianisylchloroethylene

tach, tachy
>tachycardia

TACI
>total anterior circulation infarct

TACK
>Translating and Congruent Mobile-Bearing Knee (test)

TACL
>Tests for Auditory Comprehension of Language

TACL-R
>Tests for Auditory Comprehension of Language-Revised

TACS
>total anterior circulation syndrome

TACurea
>timed average concentration, urea

TAD
>Test of Auditory Discrimination
>thiazolidinedione
>thoracic asphyxiant dystrophy
>thrombin activation device
>total administered dose
>*trans*-activation domain
>transient acantholytic dermatosis
>transverse abdominal diameter
>tricyclic antidepressant drug

TADAC
>therapeutic abortion, dilation, aspiration, and curettage

NOTES

TAE
> right atrial enlargement
> total abdominal evisceration
> transcatheter arterial embolization

TAER
> transient auditory-evoked response

TAES
> transcutaneous acupoint electrical
> stimulation

TAF
> tissue angiogenesis factor
> toxoid-antitoxin floccule
> toxoid-antitoxoid floccule
> tracheobronchial aspirate fluid
> transactivation factor
> trypsin-aldehyde-fuchsin
> tuberculin, albumose-free [Ger.
> *Tuberculin Albumose frei*]
> tumor angiogenesis factor
> tumor angiogenic factor

TAG
> target-attaching globulin
> thymine, adenine, and guanine
> tissue anchor guide
> triacylglycerol
> tumor-associated glycoprotein

TAG-72
> tumor-associated glycoprotein-72

TAGH
> triiodothyronine, amino acids,
> glucagon, and heparin

TAGV
> Taggert virus

TA-GVHD
> transfusion-associated graft-versus-
> host disease

TAH
> total abdominal hysterectomy
> total artificial heart

TAHBSO
> total abdominal hysterectomy and
> bilateral salpingo-oophorectomy

TAHV
> Tahyna virus

TAI
> thoracoabdominal irradiation
> tissue antagonist of interferon

TAIV
> Tai virus

TAL
> Achilles tendon lengthening
> tendo Achillis lengthening
> thick ascending limb
> thymic alymphopla
> thymic alymphoplasia
> total arm length
> total autogenous latissimus

> triamcinolone lotion
> tumor-associated lymphocyte

TALC
> transairway laryngeal control

talc
> talcum

t. ALCON
> Alcon tonometry

TALH
> thick ascending limb of Henle
> (loop)

TALL, T-ALL
> T-cell acute lymphoblastic leukemia

TALP
> total alkaline phosphatase
> tumor-assisted lymphoid proliferation

TALPS
> Transactional Analysis Life Position
> Survey

TALT
> testicular adrenal-like tissue

TALTFR
> tendo Achillis lengthening and toe
> flexor release

TAM
> Technology Assessment Methods
> Project
> teenage mother
> thermoacidurans agar modified
> total active motion
> toxoid-antitoxoid mixture
> transient abnormal myelopoiesis
> transtelephonic ambulatory
> monitoring (system)
> tricuspid annular motion
> tumor-associated macrophage

TAMBA
> talar axis–first metatarsal base
> angle

TAME
> tosylarginine methyl ester

TAMe
> toxoid-antitoxoid mixture esterase

TAMIS
> Telemetric Automated Microbial
> Identification System

TAML, t-AML
> therapy-related acute myelogenous
> leukemia
> therapy-related acute myeloid
> leukemia

TAMMAS
> temporary articulating
> methylmethacrylate antibiotic
> spacer

TAMV
> Tamiami virus

TAN

total adenine nucleotide
total ammonia nitrogen
Treatment Authorization Number
tropical ataxic neuropathy

tan.

tandem translocation
tangent

TANI

total axial (lymph) node irradiation

TANV

Tanga virus

TAO

thromboangiitis obliterans
thyroid-associated ophthalmopathy
triacetyloleandomycin
triamcinolone ointment
troleandomycin
turning against object

TAP

tension by applanation
Thornton anterior positioner
tone and positioning
tonometry by applanation (*See also*
AT, T APPL)
Trainer's Assessment of Proficiency
transabdominal preperitoneal
(laparoscopic hernia repair)
transesophageal atrial pacing (*See
also* TEAP)
transport-associated protein
transvaginal amniotic puncture
trypsin activation peptide
trypsinogen-activating peptide
tumor-activated prodrug

TAPC

total anomalous pulmonary
circulation

TAP-D

Test of Articulation Performance-
Diagnostic

TAPET

tumor amplified protein expression
therapy

TAPP

transabdominal preperitoneal
polypropylene (meshplasty)

T APPL

applanation tonometry (*See also*
AT, TAP)

TAPS

training and placement service
trial assessment procedure scale

TAP-S

Test of Articulation Performance-
Screen

TAPVC

total anomalous pulmonary venous
connection

TAPVD

total anomalous pulmonary venous
drainage

TAPVR

total anomalous pulmonary venous
return

TAQW

transient abnormal Q wave

TAR

thrombocytopenia & absent radius
tissue-air ratio
total abortion rate
total ankle replacement
total anorectal reconstruction
transactivator
treatment administration record
treatment authorization request

TARA

total articular replacement
arthroplasty
total articular resurfacing
arthroplasty
tumor-associated rejection antigen

TARC

thymus and activation-regulated
chemokine

TARP

total atrial refractory period

TART

tenderness, asymmetry, restricted
(motion), and tissue (texture
changes)
tissue (texture changes), asymmetry,
restriction (of motion,) tenderness
tumorectomy, axillary (dissection),
radiotherapy

TARTI

total apexcardiographic relaxation
time index

TAS

test for ascendance-submission
Test of Attitude Toward School
tetanus antitoxic serum

NOTES

T

TAS *(continued)*
thoracoabdominal syndrome
Toronto Alexithymia Scale
turning against self
typical absence seizure

TASA
tumor-associated surface antigen

TASB
Teacher Assessment of Social
Behavior

T'ase, Tase
tryptophan synthetase

TASH
transcoronary ablation of septal
hypertrophy

T-ASI
Teen Addiction Severity Index

TASI
transperitoneal anterior subcostal
incision

TASS
thyroiditis, Addison disease, Sjögren
syndrome, sarcoidosis (syndrome)

TAS/TVS
transabdominal/transvaginal
ultrasound

TAT
tandem autotransplants
tandem transplant
Tell a Tale (psychiatry)
tetanus antitoxin
thematic apperception test
thematic aptitude test
thrombin-antithrombin
thrombin-antithrombin III
thromboplastin activation test
till all taken
total abdominal fat
total adipose tissue
total antitryptic activity
toxin-antitoxin *(See also* TA)
transactivator of transcription
transaxial tomogram
transplant-associated
thrombocytopenia
transverse axial tomography
tray agglutination test
treponemal antibody test
triple advancement transposition
tumor activity test
turnaround time
tyrosine aminotransferase

TATA
tumor-associated transplantation
antigen

TATBA
triamcinolone acetomide *tert*-butyl
acetate

TATD
tyrosine aminotransferase deficiency

TATE
tumor-associated tissue eosinophilia

TATR
tyrosine aminotransferase regulator

TATST
tetanus antitoxin skin test

TATV
Tataguine virus

τ, tau
life (of radioisotope)
relaxation time
shear stress
spectral transmittance
tau (19th letter of Greek alphabet),
lowercase
transmission coefficient

TAUC
target area under the curve
time-averaged urea concentration

TAV
transcutaneous aortovelography
transvenous aortovelography
trapped air volume

TAWF
Test of Adolescent/Adult Word
Finding

TAX
cefotaxime *(See also* CTX)

TB
Tapes for the Blind
terminal bronchiole
terrible burning
thought broadcasting
thromboxane B
thymol blue
toluidine blue
toothbrush
total base
total bilirubin *(See also* TBIL, T
Bili, TOT BILI)
total body
total bound
tracheal bronchial (region)
tracheobronchitis
trapezoid body
tub bath
tubercle bacillus *(See also* TBA)
tuberculin
tuberculosis
tumor bearing

T-B
Thomas-Binetti (test)

T$_b$
buildup time
temperature, body

Tb
    terbium

Tb$_4$
    thymosin b$_4$
    thymosin beta$_4$

tb
    biologic half-life

TBA
    to be absorbed
    to be added
    to be administered
    to be admitted
    to be announced
    to be arranged
    to be assessed
    to be evaluated
    tertiary butyl acetate
    testosterone-binding affinity
    thiobarbituric acid
    thyroxine-binding albumin
    total bile acid
    total body (surface) area
    traditional birth attendant
    trypsin-binding activity
    tubercle bacillus (*See also* TB, Tb)
    tumor-bearing animal

TBAB
    thyroid-blocking antibody
    tryptose/blood/agar base

TBAGA
    term birth appropriate for
      gestational age

T-bar
    tracheotomy bar (a device used in
      respiratory therapy)

TBARS
    thiobarbituric acid-reactive substance

TBB
    transbronchial biopsy

TBBC
    total (vitamin) B$_{12}$ binding capacity

TBBM
    total body bone mineral

TBBMD
    total body bone mineral density

TBC
    to be canceled
    thyroxine-binding coagulin
    total-blood cholesterol
    total body calcium
    total body clearance (*See also* Q$_B$)
    total body counting

    traumatic bone cyst
    tubercidin
    tuberculous

TBD
    to be determined
    total body density
    Toxicology Data Base

TBE
    tick-borne encephalitis
    tuberculin bacillary emulsion

TBEV
    tick-borne encephalitis virus

TBF
    total body fat
    tracheal blood flow

TBFB
    tracheobronchial foreign body

TBFV
    tidal breathing flow-volume

TBFVL
    tidal breathing flow-volume loop

TBG
    testosterone-binding globulin
    thyroid-binding globulin
    thyroxine-binding globulin
    tracheobronchogram
    tris-buffered Grey (solution)

TBGE
    thyroxine-binding globulin, estimated

TBGI
    thyroid-binding globulin index
    thyroxine-binding globulin index

TBGP
    total blood granulocyte pool

TBH
    total body hematocrit

TBHT
    total body hyperthermia

TBI
    thrombotic brain infarction
    thyroid-binding index
    thyroxine-binding index
    tooth-brushing instruction
    total body irradiation (*See also*
      TBX)
    tracheobronchial injury
    traumatic brain injury
    tumor burden index

TBIAb
    thyroid-stimulating hormone-binding
      inhibitor antibody

T

NOTES

787

TBII
thyroid-binding inhibitory
immunoglobulin
thyrotropin-binding inhibitory
immunoglobulin
TSH-binding inhibitory
immunoglobulin

TBIL, T Bili
total bilirubin (assay)

TBK
total body kalium (potassium)
total body potassium (kalium)

TBLB
transbronchial lung biopsy

TBLC
term birth, living child

TBLF
term birth, living female

TBLI
term birth, living infant

TBLM
term birth, living male

TBLR
transconjunctival blepharoplasty laser
resurfacing

TBM
thin basement membrane
thyroxine-binding meningitis
total body mass
tracheobronchomalacia
tuberculous meningitis
tubular basement membrane

TBMD
thin basement membrane disease

TBMg
total-body magnesium

TBN
bacillus emulsion
total body nitrogen

TBNA
total body neutron activation
total body sodium
transbronchial needle aspiration
treated but not admitted

TBNAA
total body neutron activation
analysis

t-BOC, tBoc
t-butoxycarbonyl

TBOCS
Tale-Brown Obsessive-Compulsive
Scale

TBP
testosterone-binding protein
thiobisdichlorophenol (bithionol)
thyroxine-binding protein
toe blood pressure
total body phosphorus

total body photograph
total body protein
total bypass
tributyl phosphate
tuberculous peritonitis

TBPA
thyroid-binding prealbumin
thyronine-binding prealbumin
thyroxine-binding prealbumin

TBPT
total body protein turnover

TBR
total bed rest
tumor-bearing rabbit

TB-RD
tuberculosis-respiratory disease

TBRS
Timed Behavioral Rating Sheet

TBS
tablespoon
The Bethesda System
total body scan
total body solids
total body solute
total body surface
total burn size
total-serum bilirubin
tracheobronchial submucosa
tracheobronchoscopy
Transition Behavior Scale
tribromsalan (tribromosalicylanilide)
triethanolamine-buffered saline
tris-buffered saline

tbs, tbsp
tablespoon (*See also* TBS)

TBSA
total body surface area
total burn surface area

TBT, TbT
tolbutamide test
tracheal bronchial toilet
tracheobronchial toilet
tracheobronchial tree
transbronchoscopic balloon tipped
transcervical balloon tuboplasty

TBTNR
Toronto Biculture Test of
Nonverbal Reasoning

TBTT
tuberculin tine test

TBTV
Timboteua virus

TBUT
tear break-up test
tear breakup time

TBV
total blood volume

trabecular bone volume
transluminal balloon valvuloplasty
TBV$_p$
total blood volume predicted (from
body surface)
TBW
total body washout
total body water (*See also* TBWA)
total body weight
TBWA
total body water (*See also* TBW)
TBX
thromboxane (*See also* Thx, TX)
total body irradiation (*See also*
TBI)
TBZ
tetrabenazine
thiabendazole
TC
to contain
talocalcaneal
tandem colonoscopy
target cell
taurocholate
taurocholic (acid)
team conference
telephone call (*See also* T/C)
temperature compensation
teratocarcinoma
terminal cancer
tertiary cleavage
testicular cancer
tetracycline (*See also* T, Tc, TCN,
TCNE, TE, TET)
to (the) chest
therapeutic community
therapeutic concentrate
thermal conductivity (detector) (*See
also* λ, TCD)
thermocouple
thoracic cage
thoracic circumference
throat culture (*See also* TH-CULT)
thyrocalcitonin (*See also* TCA,
TCT)
tissue culture
tolonium chloride
tonsillar coblation
total calcium
total capacity
total cholesterol
total colectomy

total colonoscopy
total correction
tracheal collar
transcobalamin
transcutaneous (*See also* tc)
transhepatic cholangiography (*See
also* THC)
transplant center
transverse colon
trauma center
treatment completed
true conjugate
tuberculosis, contagious
tubocurarine
tumor cell
tungsten carbide
type (and) crossmatch (*See also*
T&C, T&M)
typical carcinoid
TC I
transcobalamin I
TC II
transcobalamin II
3TC
2',3'-dideoxy-3'thiacytidine
lamivudine (Epivir)
lamivudine triphosphate
TC7
Interceed
T:C
tumor:cerebellum (ratio)
T&C
test and crossmatch
turn and cough
type and crossmatch (*See also* TC,
T&M)
T/C
to consider
telephone call (*See also* TC)
TC$_{50}$
median toxic concentration
T$_c$
generation time of cell cycle
Tc
core temperature
cytotoxic T-cell
T (cell) cytotoxic
technetium
temporal complex
tetracycline (*See also* T, TC, TCN,
TCNE, TE, TET)
transcobalamin

NOTES

789

⁹⁹Tc
technetium-99

⁹⁹ᵐTc
⁹⁹ᵐtechnetium
technetium-99m

tc
transcutaneous (*See also* TC)
translational control

TC-III
total condylar III

T₄(C)
serum thyroxine measured by
column chromatography

TCA
talocalcaneal angle
tentorium cerebelli attachment
terminal cancer
terminal carcinoma
tetracyclic antidepressant
thyrocalcitonin (*See also* TC, TCT)
tissue concentrations of antibiotic(s)
tissue culture assay
total cholic acid
total circulating albumin
total circulatory arrest
total colonic aganglionosis
transcondylar axis
transluminal coronary angioplasty
tricalcium aluminate
tricarboxylic acid
trichloroacetate
trichloroacetic acid
tricuspid atresia
tricyclic amine
tricyclic antidepressant (*See also*
TCAD)
tricyclic antipsychotic
trihydrocoprostanic acid
tumor chemosensitivity assay
tumor clonogenic assays

TCABG, TCAG
triple coronary artery bypass graft

TCAD
transplant coronary artery disease
tricyclic antidepressant (*See also*
TCA)
tricyclic antidepressant drug

TCAR
tiazofurin

TCAT
Toglia Category Assessment Test
transmission computer-assisted
tomography

TCB
to call back
tetrachlorobiphenyl
total cardiopulmonary bypass

total counts bound
transcatheter biopsy
transconjunctival blepharoplasty
tumor cell burden

TcB
transcutaneous bilirubin

TCBF
total cerebral blood flow

Tc bond
technetium bond

TCBS
thiosulfate-citrate-bile salts-sucrose
(agar)

TCC
thromboplastic cell component
toroidal coil chromatography
total contact casting
transcatheter closure
transitional cell carcinoma
trichlocarban
trichlorocarbanilide

TCCA
transitional cell cancer-associated
(virus)
transitional cell cancer (of the
bladder) (*See also* TCCB)

TCCB
transitional cell carcinoma of
bladder (*See also* TCCA)

⁹⁹ᵐTc Ceretec
technetium-99m Ceretec

TCCL
T-cell chronic lymphocytic
(leukemia)

TC/CL
ticarcillin-clavulanate

TC CO₂
transcutaneous carbon dioxide
(monitor)

TCCS
transcranial color-coded (duplex)
sonography
transcranial color-coded (real-time)
sonography

TCD
thermal conductivity detector (*See
also* λ, TC)
tissue culture dose
transcerebellar diameter
transcranial Doppler (sonography,
ultrasound)
transcystic duct
transverse cardiac diameter

TCD₅₀
median tissue culture dose
tissue culture infectious dose (*See
also* TCID₅₀)

TC&DB
turn, cough, deep breath (*See also* CT&DB)

TCDC
taurochenodeoxycholate

TCD/CBDE
transcystic duct/common bile duct exploration

TCDD
2,3,7,8-tetrachlorodibenzo-*p*-dioxin
tetrachlorodibenzo-p-dioxin (dioxin)

TcDISIDA
technetium diisopropyliminodiacetic acid (scan)

Tc-99 DISIDA
technetium-99m DISIDA

99mTc-DMSA
technetium-99m dimercaptosuccinic acid

99mTc-DPTA, 99mTc DPTA, 99mTc DTPA
technetium-99m diethylenetriamine pentaacetic acid

TCE
T-cell enriched
tetrachlorodiphenyl ethane
total colon examination
transcatheter embolotherapy
trichloroethanol
trichloroethylene

T cell
small lymphocyte (*See also* T)

TCES
transcutaneous cranial electrical stimulation

TCESOM
trichloroethylene-extracted soybean-oil meal

TCET
transcerebral electrotherapy

TCF
tissue-coding factor (*See also* TSF)
total conjunctival flap
total coronary flow

TCFO
Therapy Carrot finger contracture orthosis

TCFU
tumor colony-forming unit

TCG
time compensation gain

TCGF
T-cell growth factor
thymus cell growth factor

99mTc glucoheptanoate
technetium-99m glucoheptanoate

99mTc-GSA
technetium-99m galactosyl-human serum albumin

TCH
tanned cell hemagglutination
thiophen-2-carboxylic acid hydrazide
total circulating hemoglobin
turn, cough, and hyperventilate

TChE
total cholinesterase

TcHIDA
technetium hepatoiminodiacetic acid (scan)

99mTc-HMPAO
99mTc-hexamethylpropyleneamine oxime

TCHR
traditional Chinese herbal remedy

TCHT
traditional Chinese herbal therapy

TCI
to come in (to hospital)
target-controlled infusion
total cerebral ischemia
Totman Change Index
transient cerebral ischemia
tricuspid insufficiency

TCi
teracurie

TCID
tissue culture infective dose
tissue culture inoculated dose

TCID$_{50}$
median tissue culture infective dose
tissue culture infectious dose (*See also* TCD$_{50}$)

TcIDA
technetium iminodiacetic acid

TCIE
transient cerebral ischemic episode

TCIFTT
transcervical intrafallopian tube transfer

TCIPA
tumor-cell-induced platelet aggregation

NOTES

T

TCIS
total corrected incremental score
transitional carcinoma in situ

TCL
thermochemiluminescence
thyroid T-cell line
tibial collateral ligament
total capacity of lung
transverse carpal ligament
triazine chlorguanide

T-CLL
T-cell chronic lymphatic leukemia

TCM
thick cutaneous melanoma
tissue culture medium
traditional Chinese medicine
transcutaneous monitor

Tc-99m
technetium-99m

TCMA
transcortical motor aphasia

^{99m}Tc-MAA
technetium-99m macroaggregated
albumin

^{99m}Tc MDP uptake
technetium-99m MDP uptake

tc-MER
motor-evoked response to
transcranial (stimulation)

TCMH
tumor-direct cell-mediated
hypersensitivity

TCMM
traditional Chinese materia medica

^{99m}Tc MMAA
technetium-99m mini-
microaggregated albumin

Tc-99m MIBI
technetium-99m
methoxyisobutylisonitrile

TCMP
thematic content modification
program

TCMS
transcranial cortical magnetic
stimulation
transcranial magnetic stimulation

Tc-99m-TcO4
technetium-99m pertechnetate

TCMV
Tacaiuma virus

TCMZ
trichloromethiazide

TCN
talocalcaneonavicular (joint)
terminal capillary network
tetracycline (*See also* T, TC, Tc,
TCNE, TE, TET)
triciribine phosphate (tricyclic
nucleoside)

TCNB
Tru-Cut needle biopsy

TCNE
tetracycline (*See also* T, TC, Tc,
TCN, TE, TET)

TcNM
tumor with lymph node metastases

TCN-P
triciribine phosphate

TCNS
transcutaneous nerve stimulator (*See
also* TNS)

TCNU
tauromustine

TCO
total contact orthosis

TcO^{4-}, TcO4–
free pertechnetate
pertechnetate

TCOM
transcutaneous oxygen monitor (*See
also* TOM)

T Con
temporary conservatorship

TCP
teacher-child-parent
therapeutic class profile
therapeutic continuous penicillin
thrombocytopenia
total cavopulmonary connection
total circulating protein
transcutaneous pacing
tranylcypromine
tricalcium phosphate
trichlorophenol
tricresyl phosphate
tropical calcific pancreatitis
tumor control probability

TCP-III
total condylar prosthesis III

TCPA
tetrachlorophthalic anhydride

TCPC
total cavopulmonary connection

TCPCO$_2$, tcPCO$_2$
transcutaneous carbon dioxide
pressure

TCPE
trichlorophenoxyethanol

^{99m}Tc phosphate
technetium-99m phosphate

TCPO$_2$, tcPO$_2$
transcutaneous oxygen pressure
(measurement)
transcutaneous (partial) pressure of
oxygen

TCPS

total cavopulmonary shunt

⁹⁹ᵐTc pyrophosphate

technetium-99m pyrophosphate

TCR

T-cell antigen receptor

T-cell reactivity

T-cell receptor

T-cell rosette

thalamocortical relay

total cytoplasmic ribosome

TCRBCL

T-cell-rich B-cell lymphoma

TCRE

transcervical resection of the
endometrium

tcRNA

translational control ribonucleic acid

TCRP

total cellular receptor pool

TCRV

Tacaribe virus

total red cell volume

TCR Vb

T cell antigen receptor Vb

TCS

T-cell supernatant

tethered-cord syndrome

tonic-clonic seizure

total cellular score

total coronary score

transcranial stimulation

Treacher Collins syndrome

Tricomponent Coaxial System

Tcs

T-cell-mediating contact sensitivity

TCSA

tetrachlorosalicylanilide

⁹⁹ᵐTc-SC

technetium-99m sulfur colloid

TCSM

Test of Cognitive Style in
Mathematics

TCSW

thinking creatively with sounds and
words

TCT

taurine cotransporter

thoracic computed tomography

thrombin clotting time

thymic carcinoid tumor

thyrocalcitonin (*See also* TC, TCA)

tincture

tracheal cytotoxin

transcatheter therapy

triple combination tablet (abacavir,
lamivudine, and zidovudine)

Trunk Control Test

TCU

Test of Concept Utilization

transitional care unit

tcu-PA

two-chain urokinase plasminogen
activator

TCV

tall cell variant

thoracic cage volume

three concept view

TCVA

thromboembolic cerebral vascular
accident

TD

to deliver

tardive dyskinesia (*See also* TDK)

T-cell dependent

temperature differential

temporary disability

teratoma differentiated

terminal device

test dose

tetanus-diphtheria (toxoid) (*See also*
Td)

tetrodotoxin

therapeutic dietitian

therapy discontinued

thermal dilution

thermodilution

thoracic duct

three (times per) day

threshold of detectability

threshold of discomfort

threshold dose

thymus-dependent

thyroid dysgenesis

tidal volume (*See also* TV, VT,
V_T)

timed disintegration

tocopherol deficient

tolerance dose

tone decay

torsion dystonia

total disability

total dose

totally disabled

NOTES

TD (*continued*)
>   toxic dose
>   tracheal diameter
>   tracking dye
>   transdermal
>   transverse diameter (*See also* trans D)
>   traveler's diarrhea
>   treatment discontinued
>   trichodiscoma
>   tuberoinfundibular dopaminergic
>   typhoid dysentery

TD$_{50}$
>   median toxic dose

T$_4$(D)
>   serum thyroxine measured by displacement analysis

T$_D$
>   time required to double number of cells in given population

T$_d$
>   diffusion time

Td
>   tetanus-diphtheria (toxoid; adult type)

tD
>   tetanus and diphtheria

TDA
>   testis-determining antigen
>   therapeutic drug assay
>   thyrotropin-displacing activity
>   tryptophan deaminase agar
>   TSH-displacing antibody

TDAC
>   tumor-derived activated cell

TDC
>   taurodeoxycholic (acid)
>   thermal dilution catheter
>   total dietary calories

TDCO
>   thermodilution cardiac output

TDD
>   telecommunication device (for the) deaf
>   telephone device for the deaf
>   tetradecadiene
>   thoracic duct drainage
>   total daily dose
>   total digitalizing dose
>   transpulmonary thermal-dye dilution

TDDA
>   tetradecadiene acetate

TDE
>   tetrachlorodiphenylethane
>   thiamine deficiency encephalopathy
>   time-delayed exponential
>   total daily energy (requirement)
>   total digestible energy
>   triethylene (glycol) diglycidyl ether

TDEC
>   test declined (no longer offered)

TDEE
>   total daily energy expenditure

TDF
>   testis-determining factor
>   Thinking Disturbance Factor
>   thoracic duct fistula
>   thoracic duct flow
>   time-dose fractionation (factor)
>   tissue-damaging factor (*See also* TF)
>   total-dietary fiber
>   tumor dose fractionation

TDH
>   thermostable direct hemolysin
>   threonine dehydrogenase
>   total decreased histamine
>   toxic dose, high

TDI
>   temperature difference integrator
>   therapeutic donor insemination
>   three-dimensional interlocking (hip)
>   tissue Doppler imaging
>   tolerable daily intake
>   toluene diisocyanate
>   total-dose infusion

TDK
>   tardive dyskinesia (*See also* TD)

TDL
>   temporal difference limen
>   thoracic duct lymphocyte
>   thymus-dependent lymphocyte
>   toxic dose, low

TDLN
>   tumor-draining lymph node

TDLNC
>   tumor-draining lymph node cell

TDLU
>   terminal ductal lobular unit
>   terminal duct lobular unit

TDM
>   tartaric dimalonate
>   therapeutic drug monitoring
>   thermodeltameter
>   trehalose dimycolate

T1DM
>   type 1 diabetes mellitus

T2DM
>   type 2 diabetes mellitus

TDMAC
>   tridodecylmethyl ammonium chloride
>   tridodecylmethylammonium chloride graft coating material

TDMS
>   Trex digital mammography system

tropical diarrhea-malabsorption
syndrome

TDMV

Tindholmur virus

TDN

total digestible nutrients
transdermal nitroglycerin (*See also*
TDNTG)

tDNA

transfer deoxyribonucleic acid

TDNTG

transdermal nitroglycerin (*See also*
TDN)

TDNWB

touchdown nonweightbearing

TDO

trichodentoosseous (syndrome)

TDP

tenderness to digital palpation
therapist-driven protocol
thermal death point
thiamine diphosphate
thoracic duct pressure
thymidine diphosphate
torsade de pointes (*See also* TdP)

TdP

torsade de pointes (*See also* TDP)

TdPVT

torsade de pointes ventricular
tachycardia

TDPWB

touchdown partial weightbearing

TdR

thymidine (*See also* T)

TDS

temperature, depth, and salinity

TDSP

time domain signal processor

TDT

tentative discharge tomorrow
terminal deoxynucleotidyl transferase
(*See also* TdT)
thermal death time
tone decay test
transmission disequilibrium test
Trieger Dot Test
tumor doubling time

TdT

terminal deoxynucleotide transferase
terminal deoxynucleotidyl transferase
(*See also* TDT)

TDU

time domain ultrasound

TDW

target dry weight

TDWB

touchdown weightbearing

TDx(r)

fluorescence polarization
immunoassay

TDYV

Tamdy virus

TDZ

thymus-dependent zone (of lymph
node)

TE

echo delay time
echo time
tennis elbow
terminal extension
test ear
tetanus (*See also* Te, tet)
tetracycline (*See also* T, TC, Tc,
TCN, TCNE, TET)
threshold energy
thromboembolic
thromboembolic event
thromboembolism
thymus epithelium
thyrotoxic exophthalmos
time estimation
tissue equivalent
tonsillectomy
tooth extracted
total estrogen (excretion)
Toxoplasma encephalitis
trace element
tracheoesophageal
transepithelial elimination
(terminated)
transesophgeal echocardiography
treadmill exercise
trial (and) error (*See also* T&E)
trichoepithelioma

T&E

testing and evaluation
training and experience
trial and error (*See also* TE)

T/E

testosterone to epitestosterone ratio

T$_E$

duration of expiration
expiratory time

NOTES

795

TE$_{mic}$
  tonsillectomy with operating microscope

Te
  tellurium
  tetanic (contraction)
  tetanus (*See also* TE, tet)

tE
  total expiratory time

te
  effective half-life (*See also* teff)

TEA
  temporal external artery
  tetraethylammonium
  thermal energy analyzer
  thromboendarterectomy
  total elbow arthroplasty
  transient emboligenic aortoarteritis
  transluminal extraction atherectomy
  transversely excited atmospheric (pressure)
  triethanolamine

TEAB
  tetraethylammonium bromide

TEAC
  tetraethylammonium chloride

TEACCH
  treatment and education of autistic and related communications handicapped children

TEAE
  triethylaminoethyl

TEAP
  transesophageal atrial pacing (*See also* TAP)

TEB
  thoracic electrical bioimpedance
  tris-ethylenediaminetetraacetate borate

TEBG, TeBG
  testosterone-estradiol-binding globulin

TeBIDA
  technetium 99m trimethyl 1-bromo-imono diacetic acid

T4/ebp-1
  thyroid-specific enhancer binding protein-1

TEBS
  transurethral electrical bladder stimulation

TEC
  thromboembolic complication
  Total Environment Control
  total eosinophil count
  total exchange capacity
  toxic *Escherichia coli*
  transient erythroblastopenia of childhood
  transluminal endarterectomy catheter
  transluminal extraction catheter
  transluminal extraction-endarterectomy catheter
  transpapillary endoscopic cholecystotomy
  triethyl citrate

T&EC
  trauma and emergency center

TECA
  technetium albumin (study)
  titrated extract of *Centella asiatica*

TECAB
  totally endoscopic coronary artery bypass

tech
  technical
  technique

TECV
  traumatic epiphyseal coxa vara

TED
  Tasks of Emotional Development
  threshold erythema dose
  thromboembolic disease (hose, stockings)
  thyroid eye disease
  tracheoesophageal dysraphism
  tris-ethylenediaminetetraacetate dithiothreitol

TEDD
  total end-diastolic diameter

TEDP
  tetraethyl dithionopyrophosphate

TEE
  thermal effect of exercise
  thermic effect of exercise
  total energy expended
  total energy expenditure
  transesophageal echocardiogram
  transesophageal echocardiograph
  transesophageal echocardiography
  transnasal endoscopic ethmoidectomy
  tyrosine ethyl ester

TEE-DSE
  transesophageal echocardiography-dobutamine stress echocardiography

TEEM
  tanned erythrocyte electrophoretic mobility
  Test for Examining Expressive Morphology

TEEP
  tetraethylpyrophosphate
  transesophageal echocardiography with pacing

TEF
  thermal effect of food

thermic effect of feeding
thermic effect of food
thyrotroph embryonic factor
tracheoesophageal fistula
trunk extension-flexion (unit)

TEF$_{25}$

tidal expiratory flow at 25% of tidal volume

TEF$_{75}$

tidal expiratory flow at 75% of tidal volume

TEF$_{50}$

tidal expiratory flow at 50% of tidal volume

teff

effective half-life (*See also* te)

TEF$_{25}$/PTEF

ratio of tidal expiratory flow at 25% of tidal volume and peak tidal expiratory flow

TEFS

transmural electrical field stimulation

TEF$_{50}$/TIF$_{50}$

ratio of tidal expiratory and inspiratory flow at 50% of tidal volume

TEG

thromboelastogram
thromboelastograph
thromboelastographic (monitor device)
thromboelastography

TEGDMA

tetraethylene glycol dimethacrylate

TEH

theophylline, ephedrine, and hydroxyzine

TEHV

Tehran virus

TEI

total episode of illness
transesophageal imaging

TEIB

triethyleneiminobenzoquinone

TEK

total exchangeable potassium

TEL

telemetry (*See also* tele)
telephone
Test of Economic Literacy
tetraethyl lead

TELD

Test of Early Language Development

TELD-2

Test of Early Language Development, Second Edition

tele

telemetry (*See also* TEL)

t½elim

elimination half-life

TEM

terminal extensor mechanism
therapeutic electromembrane
transanal endoscopic microsurgery
transmission electron microscope
transmission electron microscopy
transtelephonic exercise monitor
transverse electromagnetic
transverse electromagnetic mode
triethylenemelamine

TEMAC

tetramethyl ammonium chloride

TEMAS

Tell-Me-A-Story

TEMI

transient episodes of myocardial ischemia

temp

temperature (*See also* T)
temple
temporal
temporary (*See also* T)

TEN

tension (intraocular pressure) (*See also* T)
titanium elastic nailing
total enteral nutrition
total epidermal necrolysis
total excretory nitrogen
toxic epidermal necrolysis
toxic epidermal necrosis

TENa

total exchangeable sodium

tenac

tenaculum

TENS

transcutaneous electrical nerve stimulation
transcutaneous electrical nerve stimulator

TENV

Tensaw virus

NOTES

T

797

TENVAD
Test of Nonverbal Auditory Discrimination

TEOAE
transient evoked otoacoustic emission

TEP
thromboendophlebectomy
total endoprosthesis
total extraperitoneal (laparoscopic hernia repair)
totally extraperitoneal
tracheoesophageal prosthesis
tracheoesophageal puncture
transesophageal puncture
trigeminal evoked potential
tubal ectopic pregnancy

TeP
tender point

TEPA
thermic effect of physical activity
triethylenethiophosphoramide (*See also* TESPA)

TEPG
triethylphosphine gold

TEPP
tetraethylpyrophosphate
tetraethyl pyrophosphate

TEQ
toxic equivalents

TEQU
test equivocal (possible low titer)

TER
terlipressin
therapeutic external radiation
thermal enhancement ratio
total elbow replacement
total endoplasmic reticulum
total energy requirement
transcapillary escape rate
transurethral electroresection

ter
terminal or end (*See also* term., TRML, trml)
ternary
tertiary (*See also* T, t, tert)
threefold
three times

terb
terbutaline

TERC
Test of Early Reading Comprehension

TERIS
TERM
temporary endodontic restorative material

term.
full term (infant)
terminal (*See also* ter, TRML, trml)

TERT
total end-range time

tert
tertiary (*See also* T, t, ter)

TERV
Termeil virus

TES
Teacher Evaluation Scale
Team Effectiveness Survey
tetradecyl sulfate, ethanol, and saline
therapeutic electrical stimulation
therapeutic error signal
thoracic endometriosis syndrome
thymic epithelial supernatant
toxic epidemic syndrome
transcutaneous electrical stimulation
transcutaneous electric stimulation
transmural electrical stimulation
treatment of emergent symptom
tridimensional evaluation scale

TESA
testicular sperm aspiration

TESD
total end-systolic diameter

TESE
testicular sperm extraction

TESI
thoracic epidural steroid injection

TESPA
triethylenethiophosphoramide (thiotepa)

TESS
Treatment Emergent Symptom Scale

TEST
tubal embryo stage transfer

testos
testosterone

TET
tetanus (*See also* TE, Te, tet)
tetracycline (*See also* T, TC, Tc, TCN, TCNE, TE)
tetralogy (of Fallot) (*See also* TF, TOF)
tetroxiprim
total exchangeable thyroxine
transcranial electrostimulation therapy
treadmill exercise test
triethyltryptamine
tubal embryo transfer

tet
tetanus (*See also* TE, Te, TET)

TETA
test-estrin timed action
triethylenetetramine
TETCYC
tetracycline (*See also* T, TC, Tc,
TCN, TCNE, TE, TET)
TETD
tetraethylthiuram disulfide
(disulfiram)
TETE
too early to evaluate
TETEV
Tete virus
TETRAC
tetraiodothyroacetic acid
tE/tTOT
ratio of expiration time and total
time of breathing cycle
tet tox
tetanus toxoid (*See also* TT)
TEU
token economy unit
TEV
talipes equinovarus
TEVAP
transurethral electrovaporization of
the prostate
TEVP
transesophageal ventricular pacing
TEWL
transepidermal water loss (*See also*
TWL)
TEZ
transthoracic electric impedance
respirogram
TF
to follow
tactile fremitus
tail flick (reflex)
temperature factor
testicular feminization
tetralogy of Fallot (*See also* TET,
TOF)
Thomsen-Friedenreich
thymol flocculation
thymus (tolerance) factor
thymus (transfer) factor
tissue-damaging factor (*See also*
TDF)
tissue factor
total flow
transfer factor

transferrin (*See also* Tf, TFN)
transformation frequency
transfrontal
transvestic fetishism
tube feeding
tuberculin filtrate
tubular fluid
tuning fork
TF5
thymosin fraction 5
T$_f$
temperature, freezing
Tf
transferrin (*See also* TF, TFN)
TFA
thigh-foot angle
tibiofemoral angle
topical fluoride application
total fatty acids
trans fatty acids (*See also* tFA)
transverse fascicular area
trifluoroacetic acid
tFA
trans fatty acid (*See also* TFA)
TFAA
trifluoroacetic anhydride
TFAV
Thiafora virus
TFB
trifascicular block
TFB-PS
tibial fracture brace proximal
support
TFC
thoracic fluid content
threaded fusion cage
time to following commands
triangular fibrocartilage
TFCC
transjugular fibrocartilage complex
triangular fibrocartilage complex
triangular fibrocartilaginous complex
TFCQ
Toronto Functional Capacity
Questionnaire
TFD
target-film distance
thin film dressing
transdermal fentanyl device
TFd
transfer factor, dialyzable

NOTES

T

799

TFE
polytetrafluoroethylene (Teflon)
TFEV
timed forced expiratory volume
TFF
tangential flow filtration
trefoil factor family
tube-fed food
Tf–Fe
transferrin-bound iron
TFI
tubular-fertility index
tumor of the follicular
infundibulum
TFL
tensor fasciae latae
transnasal fiberoptic laryngoplasty
TFM
testicular feminization mutation
total fat mass
total fluid movement
transmission electron microscopy
transverse friction massage
trifluoromethylnitrophenol
Tfm
testicular feminization (syndrome)
(*See also* TFS)
TFN
total fecal nitrogen
totally functional neutrophil
transferrin (*See also* TF, Tf)
TFNE
transient focal neurologic event
TFO
triplex-forming oligonucleotide
TFP
temporalis fascia proper
treponemal false positive
trifluoperazine (*See also* TFZ)
trifunctional protein deficiency
TF/P
tubule fluid to plasma (ratio)
TFPI
tissue factor pathway inhibitor
(TF/P) In
tubule fluid to plasma insulin
(ratio)
TFR
total fertility rate
total flow resistance
TfR
transferrin receptor
TFRT
Tactile Finger Recognition Test
Tactile Form Recognition Test

TFS
testicular feminization syndrome
(*See also* Tfm)
tube-fed saline
T1FS
T1-weighted fat-suppressed (image)
TFT
Thought Field Therapy
thrombus formation time
thumb-finding test
thyroid function test
tight filum terminale
transfer factor test
trifluorothymidine
TF/UF
tubular fluid:ultrafiltrate (ratio)
TFV
Telok Forest virus
TFVL
tidal flow-volume loop
TFZ
trifluoperazine (*See also* TFP)
TG
tendon graft
testosterone glucuronide
tetraglycine
theophylline-guaifenesin
thioglucose
thioglycolate (broth) (*See also*
THIO)
thyroglobulin (*See also* thg)
total gastrectomy
toxic goiter
Toxoplasma gondii
transglutaminase
transmissible gastroenteritis (*See also*
TGE)
treated group
triacylglycerol
trigeminal (neuralgia)
triglyceride (*See also* TRIG, trig)
tumor growth
type genus (*See also* tg)
T_g
glass transition temperature
Tg
generation time (*See also* GT)
thyroglobulin
tG_1
time required to complete G_1
phase of cell cycle
tG_2
time required to complete G_2
phase of cell cycle
tg
type genus (*See also* TG)
TGA
taurocholate gelatin agar

third-generation antidepressant
thyroglobulin antibody (*See also* TgAb)
total glycoalkaloids
transient global amnesia
transposition of the great arteries
tumor glycoprotein assay

TgAb
thyroglobulin antibody (*See also* TGA)

TGAR
total graft area rejected

TGB
thyroid-binding globulin

Tgb
thyroglobulin

TGBI
thyroid growth-blocking immunoglobulin

TGC
tailgut cyst
time-gain compensation
time-gain compensator
time-gain control
time-varied gain control (*See also* TVGC)

TGCT
testicular germ cell tumor(s)

TGD
thermal green dye
thyroglossal duct
tumor growth delay

TGDC
thyroglossal duct cyst

TGE
theoretical growth evaluation
transgastrostomic enteroscopy
transmissible gastroenteritis (virus) (*See also* TG)
tryptone glucose extract

TGEF
transabdominal thin-gauge embryofetoscopy

TG ELISA
tissue transglutaminase ELISA

TGF
T-cell growth factor
therapeutic gain factor
transforming growth factor
trypanosome growth factor
tubuloglomerular feedback
tumor growth factor

TGFα, TGF-A, TGF-alpha
transforming growth factor α
transforming growth factor alpha

TGFβ, TGF-beta
transforming growth factor β
transforming growth factor beta

TGF-β1
transforming growth factor beta-1

TGF-1
transforming growth factor-1

TGF-β2, TGF-beta-2
transforming growth factor β2
transforming growth factor beta-2

TGF-β3, TGF-beta-3
transforming growth factor β3
transforming growth factor beta-3

TGFA
triglyceride fatty acid

TGG
turkey gamma globulin

TGGE
temperature-gradient gel electrophoresis

TGHA
thyroglobulin antibody

TGI
thyroid growth immunoglobulin
tracheal gas insufflation

TGL
triglyceride
triglyceride lipase

TGOR
transverse groove of oblique ridge

TGP
tobacco glycoprotein

TGR
tenderness, guarding, rigidity (abdominal exam)

T group, T-group
training group

TGS
tincture of green soap
triglycine sulfate

TGT
thromboplastin generation test
thromboplastin generation time
tolbutamide-glucagon test
transdermal glyceryl trinitrate

TGTL
total glottic transverse laryngectomy

TGV
thoracic gas volume

NOTES

T

TGV *(continued)*
transposition of great vessels
trapped gas volume

TGXT
thallium-graded exercise test

TGY, TGYA
tryptone glucose yeast (agar) (*See also* TGYA)

TGZ
troglitazone (Rezulin)

TH
tetrahydrocortisol
T helper (cell)
theophylline
thrill
thyrohyoid
thyroid hormone
thyrotropic hormone (*See also* TTH)
topical hypothermia
torcular herophili
total hydroperoxide
total hysterectomy
tube holder
tyrosine hydroxylase

TH2 (*var. of* Th2)

T&H
type and hold

Th
T-helper cell (*See also* TH)
thenar
thoracic (*See also* T, thor)
thorax (*See also* T, thor)
thorium
throat
thyroid

Th1, TH1
T-helper (cell) type 1

Th2, TH2
T-helper (cell) type 2

Th3, TH3
T-helper (cell) type 3

THA
tetrahydroacridine
tetrahydroaminoacridine
total hip arthroplasty
total hydroxyapatite
transient hemispheric attack
Treponema hemagglutination

ThA
thoracic aorta

THAA
thyroid hormone autoantibodies
tubular hypoplasia aortic arch

THAL, Thal
thalassemia

THAM
Tris(hydroxymethyl)-aminomethane (*See also* TRIS)
tromethamine

THAM-E
tromethamine E

THAN
transient hyperammonemia of newborn

THARIES
total hip articular replacement by internal eccentric shells

THb
total hemoglobin

THBI
thyroid hormone binding index

THbO$_2$, THb O$_2$
total oxyhemoglobin

THBR
thyroid hormone-binding ratio

THC
tetrahydrocannabinol (*See also* δ-9-THC)
tetrahydrocortisol
thigh circumference
thiocarbanidin
transhepatic cholangiogram
transhepatic cholangiography (*See also* TC)
transplantable hepatocellular carcinoma

δ-9-THC
delta-9-tetrahydrocannabinol (*See also* THC)

THCA
trihydroxycoprostanoic acid

THCCRC
tetrahydrocannabinol cross-reacting cannabinoids

THCT
triple-phase helical computer tomography

TH-CULT
throat culture (*See also* TC)

tHcy
total homocysteine (level)

THC:YAG
thulium-holmium-chromium:YAG (laser)

THD
thioridazine
transverse heart diameter

Thd
ribothymidine (*See also* T)

THDA
tuberohypophyseal dopaminergic neuron

THDOC
> tetrahydrodeoxycorticosterone

THE
> tetrahydrocortisol
> tetrahydrocortisone E
> tonic hind (limb) extension
> total-head excursion
> transhepatic embolization
> transhiatal esophagectomy
> tropical hypereosinophilia

theor
> theoretical
> theory

ther
> therapeutic (*See also* therap)
> therapy (*See also* therap)
> thermometer (*See also* therm)

therap
> therapeutic (*See also* ther)
> therapy (*See also* ther)

ther ex
> therapeutic exercise

therm
> thermometer (*See also* ther)

θ, theta
> angular coordinate variable
> customary temperature
> latent trait (statistics)
> temperature interval
> theta (eighth letter of Greek
> alphabet), lowercase

Θ, theta
> thermodynamic temperature
> theta (eighth letter of Greek
> alphabet), uppercase

THF
> humoral thymic factor
> tetrahydrocortisone F
> tetrahydrofluorenone
> tetrahydrofolate
> tetrahydrofolic
> tetrahydrofuran
> thymic humoral factor

THFA
> tetrahydrofolic acid
> tetrahydrofurfuryl alcohol

thg
> thyroglobulin (*See also* TG)

THH
> targetoid hemosiderotic hemangioma
> telangiectasia hereditaria
> haemorrhagica

THI
> therapeutic husband-insemination
> transient hypogammaglobulinemia of
> infancy
> trihydroxyindole

THIO
> thioglycolate (*See also* TG)

thio-T, thio-TEPA
> thiotriethylene phosphoramide

THIP
> tetrahydroisoxazolopyridinol

THIQ
> tetrahydraisoquinolon

THIV
> Thimiri virus

THKAFO
> trunk-hip-knee-ankle-foot orthosis

THL
> transvaginal hydrolaparoscopy
> true histiocytic lymphoma

THLAA
> tubular hypoplasia left aortic arch

THM
> Tamm-Horsfall mucoprotein
> total heme mass

TH₂O
> titrated water

THOR
> thoracentesis (fluid)

thor
> thoracic (*See also* T, Th)
> thorax (*See also* T, Th)

THORP
> titanium hollow osseointegrating
> reconstruction plate
> titanium hollow-screw
> osseointegrating reconstruction
> plate

thou.
> thousand

THOV
> Thogoto virus

THP
> take home pack
> Tamm-Horsfall protein
> tetrahydropapaveroline
> tissue hydrostatic pressure
> total hip prosthesis
> total hip replacement
> total hydroxyproline
> transhepatic portography
> trihexyphenidyl

NOTES

THPA
  tetrahydropteric acid
THPC
  tetrabis (hydroxymethyl)
    phosphonium chloride
tHPT
  tertiary hyperparathyroidism
THPV
  transhepatic portal vein
THQ
  tetroquinone
THR
  target heart rate
  thrombin receptor
  total hip replacement
  training heart rate
  transhepatic resistance
Thr
  threonine (*See also* T)
thr
  thyroid
  thyroidectomy
THR-CT
  thrombin control
THRF
  thyrotropic hormone-releasing factor
THRL
  total hip replacement, left
throm, thromb
  thrombosis
  thrombus (*See also* T)
THRR
  total hip replacement, right
THS
  tetrahydro-compound S
  tetrahydrodeoxycortisol
THSC
  totipotent hematopoietic stem cell
THSP
  titanium hollow screw plate
    (system)
THTV
  therapeutic home trial visit
THU
  tetrahydrouridine
THUG
  thyroid uptake gradient
THV
  therapeutic home visit
THVO
  terminal hepatic vein obliteration
Thx
  thromboxane (*See also* TBX, TX)
Thy
  thymine (*See also* T)
thy.
  thymectomy
  thymus (*See also* T)

THz
  terahertz
TI
  inversion time
  temporal integration
  terminal ileum
  thalassemia intermedia
  thallium
  therapeutic index
  thoracic index
  thought insertion
  threshold of intelligibility
  thymic irradiation
  thymus independent
  thyroxine iodine
  time information
  time interval
  tonic immobility
  total iron
  transischial
  translational inhibition
  transverse (diameter between) ischia
  transverse inlet
  tricuspid incompetence
  tricuspid insufficiency
  trunk index
  tubulointerstitial
  tumor inducing
  tumor induction
TI-201
  thallium chloride
T_I
  duration of inspiration
  inspiratory time
Ti
  titanium
TIA
  T-cell-restricted intracellular antigen
  Test Anxiety Inventory
  transient ischemic attack
  tumor-induced angiogenesis
TIAH
  total implantation of artificial heart
TIA-IR
  transient ischemic attack,
    incomplete recovery
TIB
  This I Believe (test)
  tumor immunology bank
Tib, tib
  tibia
TIBC
  total iron-binding capacity
tib-fib
  tibia and fibula
TIBV
  Tibrogargan virus

TIC
- ticarcillin
- Toxicology Information Center
- trypsin-inhibitory capability
- trypsin-inhibitory capacity
- tumor-inducing complex

tic
- (diver)tic(ulum)

TICA
- terminal internal carotid artery
- traumatic intracranial aneurysm

TICCC
- time interval between cessation of contraception and conception

TICH
- thrombolysis-related intracranial hemorrhage

TI-CMV
- tissue-invasive cytomegalovirus

TICS
- diverticulosis

TICU
- thoracic intensive care unit
- transplant intensive care unit
- trauma intensive care unit

TID
- three times a day [L. *ter in die*] (*See also* t.i.d.)
- time interval difference
- titrated initial dose
- transient ischemic dilation
- tubal inflammatory damage

t.i.d.
- three times a day [L. *ter in die*] (*See also* TID)

TIDA
- tuberoinfundibular dopaminergic neuron
- tuberoinfundibular dopamine (system)

TIDM
- three times daily with meals

TIE
- transient ischemic episode
- transient ischemic event

TIES
- The Instructional Environment Scale

TIF
- testicular interstitial fluid
- tracheal intubation fiberscope
- tropic immersion foot
- tumor-inducing factor
- tumor-inhibiting factor

TIF2
- transcriptional intermediary factor 2

TIF$_{50}$
- tidal inspiratory flow at 50% of tidal volume

TIFB
- thrombin-increasing fibrinopeptide B

TIg
- tetanus immune globulin
- tetanus immunoglobulin

TIGR
- trabecular meshwork-inducible glucocorticoid response

TIH
- time interval histogram
- tumor-inducing hypercalcemia

TII
- terminal ileum intubation

TIL, TILS
- tumor-infiltrating lymphocyte

TILV
- Tilligerry virus

TIM
- tissue-infiltrating macrophage
- transthoracic intracardiac monitoring
- triose isomerase

TIMC
- tumor-induced marrow cytotoxicity

TIME
- toddler and infant motor evaluation

TIMP
- Test of Infant Motor Performance
- tissue inhibitor of metalloproteinase

TIMP-1, TIMP-2, TIMP-3
- tissue inhibitor of metalloproteinase 1–3

TIMV
- Timbo virus

TIN
- three (times) in night [L. *ter in nocte*]
- Tone in Noise (test)
- tubulointerstitial nephritis
- tubulointerstitial nephropathy

tinc, tinct
- tincture

TIND
- Treatment Investigational New Drug (application)

NOTES

TINEM
there is no evidence of malignancy
TINU
tubulointerstitial nephritis and
uveitis (syndrome)
TINV
Tinaroo virus
TIP
terminal interphalangeal
thermal inactivation point
time to pregnancy
Toxicology Information Program
translation-inhibiting protein
tubularized incised plate
(urethroplasty)
tumor-inhibiting principle
TIPP
The Injury Prevention Program
TIPPB
transperineal interstitial permanent
prostate brachytherapy
TIPPS
tetraiodophenolphthalein sodium
TIPS, TIPSS
transjugular intrahepatic
portosystemic shunt
transjugular intrahepatic
portosystemic stent shunt
TIQ
tetrahydroisoquinoline
TIR
terminal innervation ratio
total immunoreactive
trophoblast in regression
TIRFM
total-internal reflection microscopy
TIS
tetracycline-induced stenosis
transdermal infusion system
trypsin-insoluble segment
tumor in situ
TISP
total immunoreactive serum
pepsinogen
TISS
Therapeutic Intervention Scoring
System
TIT
Treponema (pallidum)
immobilization test
triiodothyronine (*See also* T_3, TITh,
TRIT)
triple intrathecal therapy
TITh
triiodothyronine (*See also* T_3, TIT,
TRIT)
3,5,3′-triiodothyronine (*See also* T_3)

tI/tTOT
ratio of inspiration time and total
time of breathing cycle
TIU
trypsin-inhibiting unit
TIUP
term intrauterine pregnancy
TIUV
total intrauterine volume
TIVA
total intravenous anesthesia
TIVC
thoracic inferior vena cava
TIW, tiw, tiwk
three times a week
three times weekly
TJ
tendon jerk
tetrajoule
tight junction
triceps jerk
TJA
total joint arthroplasty
TJC
tender joint count
TJN
tongue jaw neck (dissection)
twin jet nebulizer
TJP
tracheojejunal puncture
TJR
total joint replacement
T-JTA
Taylor-Johnson Temperament
Analysis
TK
cytosolic thymidine kinase
through the knee
thymidine kinase
tourniquet (*See also* TQ)
toxicokinetics
transketolase
triose-kinase
TKA
total knee arthroplasty
total knee arthroscopy
transketolase activity
trochanter-knee-ankle
tyrosine kinase activity
TKD
thymidine kinase deficiency
tokodynamometer (*See also* TOCO)
TKE
terminal knee extension
TKG
tocodynagraph
TKIC
true knot in cord

TKLI
tachykinin-like immunoreactivity
TKM
thymidine kinase, mitochondrial
TKNO
to keep needle open
TKO
to keep open (vein for IV)
TKP
thermal keratoplasty
thermokeratoplasty
total knee prosthesis
TKR
total knee (a)rthroscopy
total knee replacement
TKRL
total knee replacement, left
TKRR
total knee replacement, right
TKS
thermokinetic selectivity
thymidine kinase, soluble
TKVO
to keep vein open (*See also* TKO)
TL
taper-lock
team leader
temporal lobe
terminal limen
theophylline
thermolabile
thermoluminescence
thoracolumbar
Thorndike-Lorge written frequency
threat to life
thymic lymphocyte antigen
thymus(-dependent) lymphocyte
thymus leukemia (antigen)
thymus lymphoma
time lapse
time limited
tolerance level
total laryngectomy
total lipids
transverse line
trial leave
tubal ligation
T/L
terminal latency (electromyography)
Tl
thallium

^{201}**Tl**
thallium-201
TLA
thigh-leg angle
tissue lactase activity
translaryngeal aspiration
translumbar aortogram
translumbar aortography
transluminal angioplasty
transperitoneal laparoscopic
adrenalectomy
trypsin-like amidase
TLAA
T-lymphocyte-associated antigen
TLAC
Test of Learning Accuracy in
Children
Test of Listening Accuracy in
Children
triple lumen Arrow catheter
TL BLT
tubal ligation, bilateral
TLC
Test of Language Competence
therapeutic lifestyle change
thin-layer chromatography
titanium linear cutter
T-lymphocyte choriocarcinoma
total L-chain concentration
total lung capacity
total lung compliance
total lymphocyte count
triple-lumen catheter
TLC-C
Test of Language Competence for
Children
^{201}**TlCl**
thallium chloride (radioisotope)
TLCO
carbon monoxide transfer factor
TLD
thermoluminescent dosimeter (rod)
thoracic lymphatic duct
transluminescent dosimeter
tumor lethal dose
T/LD$_{100}$
minimal dose causing 100% death
or malformation
minimum dose causing death or
malformation of 100% of fetuses
TLE
temporal lobe epilepsy

NOTES

807

TLE *(continued)*
    thin-layer electrophoresis
    total life expectancy
    total lipid extract
TLESR
    transient lower esophageal
      relaxation
TLI
    thymidine labeling index
    tonic labyrinthine inverted
    total lymphoid irradiation
    total lymphoid radiation
    Totman Loss Index
    translaryngeal intubation
    tritiated thymidine labeling index
    trypsin-like immunoactivity
TLK
    thermal laser keratoplasty
TLM
    torn lateral meniscus
TLN
    transperitoneal laparoscopic
      nephrectomy
TLNB
    term living newborn
TLND
    therapeutic lymph node dissection
TLNV
    Tlacotalpan virus
TLP
    time-limited psychotherapy
    total laryngopharyngectomy
    transitional living program
TLQ
    total living quotient
TLR
    target lesion reintervention
    target lesion revascularization
    tonic labyrinthine reflex
TLS
    thoracolumbosacral strain
    tight lens syndrome
    tumor lysis syndrome
^{201}Tl sestamibi
    thallium sestamibi
TLSO
    thoracolumbar spinal orthosis
    thoracolumbosacral orthosis
TLSO-FELR
    thoracolumbosacral orthosis—flexion,
      extension, lateral (bending), and
      (transverse) rotation
TLSSO
    thoracolumbosacral spinal orthosis
      (*See also* TLSO)
TLT
    tonsillectomy
    tryptophan load test

TLV
    threshold limit value
    tidal liquid ventilation
    total liquid ventilation
    total lung volume
TLW
    total lung water
TLX
    trophoblast-lymphocyte cross-reactive
    trophoblast-lymphocyte cross-
      reactivity
TM
    team member
    tectorial membrane
    telangiectatic matting
    temperature by mouth
    temporalis muscle
    temporomandibular (joint)
    teres major (muscle)
    term milk
    thalassemia major
    Thayer-Martin (medium)
    thrombomodulin
    thrombomodulin glycoprotein
    time and modifying
    time motion
    tirilazad mesylate
    tobramycin (*See also* TOB)
    trabecular meshwork
    trademark (unregistered)
    transitional mucosa
    transmediastinal
    transmetatarsal
    transport maximum
    transport mechanism
    transport medium
    transverse myelitis
    treadmill
    trimester (*See also* TRI)
    tropical medicine
    tubular myelin
    tumor
    tympanic membrane (*See also* MT)
    tympanometric
T&M
    type and crossmatch (*See also* TC,
      T&C)
TM$_{PAH}$
    maximal tubular (excretory capacity
      for) *para*-aminohippuric acid
T_m
    temperature midpoint (Kelvin)
    tubular maximal (excretory capacity
      of kidneys) (*See also* Tm)
    tubular transport maximum
Tm
    melting temperature
    temperature, muscle

thulium
transport maximum
tubular maximal
tubular maximal (excretory capacity of kidneys) (*See also* T_m)
tubular maximum
tumor-bearing mice

tM

time required to complete M phase of cell cycle

t_m, t_m

temperature midpoint (Celsius)

TMA

tetramethylammonium
thrombotic microangiopathy
thyroid microsomal antibody (*See also* TMAb)
transcription-mediated amplification
transmalleolar axis
transmetatarsal amputation
trimethoxyamphetamine
trimethoxyphenyl aminopropane
trimethylamine
trimethylxanthine amphetamine
true metatarsus adductus

T/MA

tracheostomy mask (anesthesia)

TMAb

thyroid microsomal antibody (*See also* TMA)

TMAF

temporary master apical file

TMAH

trimethylphenylammonium (anilinium) hydroxide

TMAI

trimethylphenylammonium (anilinium) iodide

TMAO

trimethylamine oxide

TMAS

Taylor Manifest Anxiety Scale

TMA-uria

trimethylaminuria

T-MAX, T-max

time of maximal (concentration) (*See also* T_{max})

T_{max}

maximum temperature
time of maximal concentration (*See also* T-MAX)

TMB

tetramethyl benzidine
tetramethylbenzidine
total monocular blindness
transient monocular blindness
trimethoxybenzoate
tris-maleate buffer

TMBA

trimethoxybenzaldehyde
trimethylbenzanthracene

TMC

transmural colitis
triamcinolone terramycin

TMCA

trimethylcolchicinic acid

TMCN

triamcinolone

TMD

temporomandibular disorder
temporomandibular dysfunction
transmural drainage
treating physician
trimethadione (*See also* TMO)

T-MDS, TMDS, t-MDS

therapy-related myelodysplasia
therapy-related myelodysplastic syndrome

TME

thermolysin-like metalloendopeptidase
total mesorectal excision
total metabolizable energy
transmissible mink encephalopathy
transmural enteritis
trapezium-metacarpal eburnation

TMEP

telangiectasia macularis eruptiva perstans

TMET

treadmill exercise test

TMEV

Tembe virus
Theiler murine encephalomyelitis virus

TMF

transformed mink fibroblast

TMG

toxic multinodular goiter

TmG, TM_G

maximal tubular reabsorption rate for glucose

NOTES

T

TMH

tetramethylammonium hydroxide
trainable mentally handicapped

TMI

threatened myocardial infarction
transmandibular implant
transmural infarction

TMIF

tumor-cell migration-inhibition factor
tumor-cell migratory inhibition
factor

TMIS

Technicon Medical Information
System

TMJ, TMJD

temporomandibular joint
(dysfunction) (*See also* TMD)

TMJ-OA

temporomandibular joint
osteoarthritis

TMJ-PDS

temporomandibular joint-pain
dysfunction syndrome

TMJS

temporomandibular joint syndrome

TMJ-SF

temporomandibular joint synovial
fluid

TML

terminal motor latency
tetramethyl lead
tongue midline
treadmill

TMLR

transmyocardial laser
revascularization (*See also* TMR)

TMM

torn medial meniscus
total muscle mass

Tmm

McKay-Marg tension

TMNG

toxic multinodular goiter

TMNST

tethered median nerve stress test

TMO

trimethadione (*See also* TMD)

TMP

ribothymidylic acid (*See also* rTMP)
thallium myocardial perfusion
thymidine monophosphate
thymolphthalein
transmembrane (hydrostatic) pressure
transmembrane potential
trimandibular plate
trimethoprim
trimethyl psoralen

TMPD

temporomandibular pain dysfunction
tetramethylparaphenylinediamine
transmucosal potential difference

TMPDS

temporomandibular pain (and)
dysfunction syndrome

TMP-SMX, TMP-SMZ

trimethoprim-sulfamethoxazole

TMR

laser transmyocardial
revascularization
temporomesial region
tetramethylrhodamine
tissue-maximum ratio
topical magnetic resonance
trainable mentally retarded
transmyocardial (laser)
revascularization (*See also* TMLR)
transmyocardial revascularization

TmrHisto

tumor histology

TMRI

tetramethylrhodamine isothiocyanate
tetramethylrhodamine isothionate

TMS

tetramethylsilane
thallium myocardial scintigraphy
thread mate system
transcranial magnetic stimulation
trimethylsilane
trimethylsilyl (*See also* TMSi)

TMS-1

Topographic Modeling System-1

TMSI

trimethylsilylimidazole

TMSi

trimethylsilyl (*See also* TMS)

TMST

treadmill stress test (*See also* TST)

TMT

tarsometatarsal
temporalis muscle temperature
teratoma with malignant
transformation
Trail-Making Test (psychiatry)
treadmill test
tympanic membrane thermometer

TMTC

too many to count

TMTD

tetramethylthiuram disulfide

TMTX

trimetrexate

TMU

tetramethylurea

TMUV

Tembusu virus

TMV
    tobacco mosaic virus
    tracheal mucous velocity

TMX
    trimazosin

TMZ
    temazepam
    transformation zone
    trimetazidine 1

TN
    (intraocular) tension, normal (*See also* Tn)
    talonavicular
    team nursing
    temperature normal
    tension
    tension, normal
    tiodazosin
    total negatives
    trigeminal neuralgia
    trigeminal nucleus
    trochlear nucleus
    true negative

T&N
    tension and nervousness

T/N
    tar and nicotine

T$_4$N
    normal serum thyroxine

Tn
    (intraocular) tension, normal (*See also* TN)
    ocular tension
    thoron
    transposon
    troponin

TNA
    total nutrient admixture

TNAB
    transthoracic needle biopsy

TNB
    term newborn
    transnasal butorphanol
    transrectal needle biopsy (of the prostate)
    transthoracic needle biopsy
    Tru-Cut needle biopsy

TNBP
    transurethral needle biopsy of the prostate

TNC
    turbid, no creamy (layer)

TNCB
    trinitrochlorobenzene

TND
    term normal delivery
    transient neonatal diabetes

TNDM
    transient neonatal diabetes mellitus

TNE
    transnasal esophagoscopy

TNEE
    titrated norepinephrine excretion

TNF
    tissue necrosis factor
    trinitrofluorenone
    true negative fraction
    tumor necrosis factor

TNF-α, TNFa, TNF-alpha
    tumor necrosis factor alpha

TNF-β, TNFb, TNF-beta
    tumor necrosis factor-beta

TNF-bp
    tumor necrosis factor-binding protein

TNFR
    tumor necrosis factor receptor

TNG
    toxic nodular goiter
    trinitroglycerol (nitroglycerin)

tng
    tongue
    training

TNH
    transient neonatal hyperammonemia

TNI
    total nodal irradiation

T/NK
    T/natural killer (cell)

TNKase
    tenecteplase

TNM
    (primary) tumor, (regional lymph) node, (remote) metastases (classification, staging)
    tumor, node, metastasis

TNMR
    tritium nuclear magnetic resonance

TNP
    total net positive
    trinitrophenyl

TNPM
    transient neonatal pustular melanosis

NOTES

TNR
>tonic neck reflex
>true negative rate

TNS
>tension night splint
>total nuclear score
>transcutaneous nerve stimulator
>transient neurologic symptoms
>tumor necrosis serum

TnSNPV
>*Trichoplusia ni* SNPV

TNT
>triamcinolone and nystatin
>trinitrotoluene

TnT
>troponin T

TNTC
>too numerous to count

TNU
>tobacco nonuser

TNV
>tobacco necrosis virus

TNVAD
>Test of Nonverbal Auditory Discrimination

TNY
>trichomonas and yeast

TO
>no evidence of primary tumor
>old tuberculin
>original tuberculin
>target organ
>telephone order
>temperature, oral (*See also* T(O))
>Theiler original (strain of mouse encephalomyelitis virus)
>thoracic orthosis
>time off
>time out
>tincture of opium (*See also* t.o.)
>total obstruction
>tracheoesophageal
>transfer out
>tuboovarian
>turned on
>turnover

T&O
>tandem and ovoids
>tubes and ovaries

T/O
>time out

T(O)
>oral temperature (*See also* TO)

TO₂
>oxygen transport rate

t.o.
>tincture of opium (*See also* TO)

TOA
>time of arrival
>tuboovarian abscess

TOAA
>to affected areas

TOAL
>Test of Adolescent Language

TOAPOT
>tuboovarian abscess after previous tubal occlusion

TOB
>tobacco
>tobramycin (*See also* TM)

TOBE
>tests of basic experience

TOBEC
>total body electrical conductivity

TOBI
>tobramycin solution for inhalation

TOBP
>tobramycin, peak

TobRV
>tobacco ringspot virus (*See also* TRSV)

TOC
>table of contents
>test of cure
>total organic carbon
>tuboovarian complex

TOCE
>transcatheter oily chemoembolization

TOCO
>tocodynamometer (*See also* TKD)

TOCP
>triorthocresyl phosphate

TOD
>tail-on detector (genetics)
>tension oculus dextra (tension of right eye)
>time of death
>time of departure
>Time-oriented Data (Bank)
>tubal occlusion device

TOE
>tracheoesophageal

TOES
>toxic oil epidemic syndrome

TOF
>tetralogy of Fallot (*See also* TET, TF)
>time of flight (radiology)
>time-of-flight
>total of four
>tracheoesophageal fistula
>train-of-four

TOFA
>time-of-flight and absorbance

TOFMS
>time-of-flight mass spectometry

TOGV
>transposition of great vessels

TOH
>throughout hospitalization
>Tower of Hanoi
>transient osteoporosis of hip

TOL
>Tower of London
>trial of labor

tol
>tolerance
>tolerated

TOLA
>temporary leave of absence

tolb
>tolbutamide

TOLD
>Test of Language Development

TOLD-I
>Test of Language Development-
>Intermediate

TOLD-I:2
>Test of Language Development -
>Intermediate, Second Edition

TOLD-P
>Test of Language Development-
>Primary

TOLD-P:2
>Test of Language Development -
>Primary, Second Edition

TOM
>therapeutic outcomes monitoring
>tomorrow
>transcutaneous oxygen monitor (*See
>also* TCOM)

tomo
>tomogram

TON
>tonight

TONAR
>oral-nasal acoustic ratio
>the oronasal acoustic ratio

TONE
>tilted optimized nonsaturating
>excitation

TONI
>Test of Nonverbal Intelligence

TOP
>temporal, occipital, parietal
>termination of pregnancy

>test orientation procedure
>tissue oncotic pressure
>Topografov (virus)
>total ossicular prosthesis

TOP-8
>Treatment Outcome PTSD (post-
>traumatic stress disorder) (scale)

top.
>topical (*See also* T)

TOPA
>topical oropharyngeal anesthesia

TOPL
>Test of Pragmatic Language

TOPO
>topographic simulated keratometric
>power

TOPO 1
>topoisermerase

TOPO I
>DNA topoisomerase I

TOPO II
>topoisomerase II

TOPO-II-alpha
>topoisomerase II-alpha

TOPOSS
>Tests of Perception of Scientists
>and Self

TOPS
>Take Off Pounds Sensibly

TopSS
>Topographic Scanning System

TopSS/ICG
>Topographic Scanning
>System/indocyanine green

TOPV
>trivalent oral poliovirus vaccine

TOR
>toremifene

TORC
>Test of Reading Comprehension

TORCH
>toxoplasmosis, other agents, rubella,
>cytomegalovirus, herpes simplex
>toxoplasmosis, other infections,
>rubella, cytomegalovirus, and
>herpes simplex

TOR inhibitor
>target of rapamycin inhibitor

TORP
>total ossicular (chain) replacement
>prosthesis

NOTES

TORP *(continued)*
  total ossicular reconstruction
    prosthesis
TOS
  tension oculus sinister (tension of
    left eye)
  thoracic outlet syndrome
  toxic oil syndrome
TOSV
  Toscana virus
TOT
  tincture of time
  tip-of-the-tongue
  total operating time
TOTAL-C
  total cholesterol
TOT BILI
  total bilirubin (*See also* TB, TBIL,
    T Bili)
TOTM
  trioctyltrimellitate
TOTP
  triorthotolyl phosphate
TOTPAR
  total pain relief
tot prot
  total protein (*See also* TP, T
    PROT)
TOV
  thrombosed oral varix
  trial of void
TOVA
  Test of Variables of Attention
TOWER
  testing, orientation, work,
    evaluation, rehabilitation
TOWL
  Test of Written Language
tox
  toxic
  toxicity (*See also* T)
  toxoid
TOXGR
  toxic granulation (differential)
TOXICON
  Toxicology Information
    Conversational On-Line Network
TOXLINE
  Toxicology Information On-Line
TOXO, toxo
  toxoplasmosis
TP
  tail pinch
  temperature and pressure
  temporal peak
  temporoparietal
  tender point
  terminal phalanx

  testosterone propionate
  tetanus-pertussis
  therapeutic pass
  thickly padded
  thought process
  threshold potential
  thrombocytopenic purpura
  thrombophlebitis
  thymic polypeptide
  thymidine phosphorylase
  thymus protein
  time to progression
  tissue pressure
  Todd paralysis
  toe pressure
  toilet paper
  total population
  total positives
  total protein (*See also* tot prot, T
    PROT)
  T piece
  trailing pole
  transforming principle
  transition point (*See also* T)
  transpyloric
  transverse polarization
  treating physician
  treatment period
  triamphenicol
  triazolophthalazine
  trigger point
  triphosphate
  true positive
  tryptophan (*See also* Tp, Trp, W)
  tryptophan pyrrolase
  tube precipitin
  tuberculin precipitate
  tuberculin precipitation
TP-1
  thymostimuline
TP5
  thymopoietin pentapeptide
T&P, T+P
  temperature and pulse
  turn and position
T:P
  trough-to-peak ratio
T$_p$P^T
  thrombus precursor protein
Tp
  tampon
tp
  physical half-life
TPA
  alteplase, recombinant (tissue
    plasminogen activator)
  12-O-tetradecanoylphorbol 13-acetate

tannic acid, polyphosphomolybdic acid, and amido acid (staining technique)

temporary portacaval anastomosis

temporopolar artery

third-party administrator

thrombotic pulmonary artery

tissue plasminogen activator (*See also* t-PA)

tissue polypeptide antigen

total parenteral alimentation

total phobic anxiety

Treponema pallidum agglutination

tumor polypeptide antigen

t-PA

tissue plasminogen activator (*See also* TPA)

TPAC

torso phased-array coil

TPAL

term (infants), premature (infants), abortions, living (children) (obstetric history)

TPB

transpalatal bar

tryptone phosphate broth

TPBA

thermal/perfusion balloon angioplasty

TPBF

total pulmonary blood flow

TPBS

three-phase bone scintigraphy

three-phase (radionuclide) bone scanning

TPC

target plasma concentration

telescoping plugged catheter

telopeptide-poor collagen

thenar palmar crease

thromboplastic plasma component

time to peak contrast

time-to-pulse-height converter

total patient care

total plasma catecholamines

total plasma cholesterol

treatment planning conference

Treponema pallidum complement

tympanocentesis

TPCC

Treponema pallidum cryolysis complement

TPCF

Treponema pallidum complement fixation

TPCV

total packed cell volume

TPD

temporary partial disability

thiamine propyldisulfide

title peritoneal dialysis

tropical pancreatic diabetes

tumor-producing dose

typhoid vaccine, not otherwise specified

TPDa

typhoid vaccine, attenuated live (oral Ty21a strain)

TPDAKD

typhoid vaccine, acetone-killed and dried (U.S. military)

TPDHP

typhoid vaccine, heat and phenol inactivated, dried

TPDVI

typhoid vaccine, Vi capsular polysaccharide

TPE

therapeutic plasma exchange

thermoplastic elastomer

tissue-protective, end-cutting

total placental estrogens

total protective environment

T-penia

thrombocytopenia

TPERM

time of peak emptying rate of mouth

TPERP

time of peak emptying rate of pharynx

TPEY

tellurite polymyxin egg yolk (agar)

TPF

temporoparietal fascial flap

thymus permeability factor

trained participating father (birth)

true positive fraction

TPFR

time to peak filling rate

TPFRE

time of peak filling rate of esophagus

NOTES

TPG
> therapeutic play group
> transmembrane potential gradient
> transplacental gradient
> transvalvular pressure gradient
> tryptophan peptone glucose (broth)

TPGYT
> trypticase-peptone-glucose-yeast
> extract-trypsin (medium)

TPH
> thromboembolic pulmonary
> hypertension
> trained participating husband (birth)
> transplacental hemorrhage
> transrectal prostatic hyperthermia
> treponemal hemagglutination
> *Treponema pallidum*
> hemagglutination
> tryptophan hydroxylase

TPHA
> *Treponema pallidum*
> hemagglutination (assay)
> *Treponema pallidum*
> hemagglutination (test)

TPHOS
> triple phosphate (crystal)

TPI
> Treatment Priority Index
> *Treponema pallidum* immobilization
> *Treponema pallidum* immobilization
> (test)
> trigger point injection
> triosephosphate isomerase
> triose phosphate isomerase

TPIA
> *Treponema pallidum* immobilization
> (immune) adherence

TPIT
> trigger point injection therapy

tpk
> time to peak

TPL
> triphosphate of lime
> tyrosine phenol-lyase

T plasty
> tympanoplasty

T-PLL
> T-cell prolymphocytic leukemia

TPLS
> The Primary Language Screen

TPLSM
> two-photon laser-scanning
> microscope

TPM
> temporary pacemaker
> thrombophlebitis migrans
> topiramate (Topamax)
> total particulate matter

> total passive motion
> triphenylmethane

TPMT
> thiopurine methyltransferase

TPMV
> Thottapalayam virus

TPN
> thalamic projection neuron
> total parenteral nutrition
> triphosphopyridine nucleotide

TPNH
> triphosphopyridine nucleotide,
> (reduced)

TPO
> temporoparietooccipital
> thrombopoietin
> thyroid peroxidase
> thyroperoxidase
> trial prescription order
> tryptophan peroxidase

TPO Ab
> thyroperoxidase antibody

TPP
> tetraphenylporphyrin
> thiamine pyrophosphate
> thiamin pyrophosphate
> thrust plate prosthesis
> transpulmonary pressure
> tubal perfusion pressure

TP&P
> time, place, and person

TpP, TpPT
> thrombus precursor protein

TPPase
> thiamine pyrophosphatase

TPPMMC
> trapezoidal paddle pectoralis major
> myocutaneous (flap)

TPPN
> total peripheral parenteral nutrition

TPPS
> Toddler-Preschooler Postoperative
> Pain Scale

TpPT (*var. of* TpP)

TPPV
> trans pars plana vitrectomy

TPR
> temperature
> temperature, pulse, respiration
> testosterone production rate
> Thompson-Parkridge-Richards (ankle
> orthosis)
> tissue-phantom ratio
> total peripheral resistance
> total pulmonary resistance
> transsphenoidal pituitary resection
> true positive rate

TPRI

    total peripheral resistance index

T-PRK

    tracker-assisted photorefractive
      keratectomy
    tracker-assisted PRK

T PROT

    total protein (*See also* tot prot, TP)

TPS

    titanium plasma sprayed
    trypsin
    tumor polysaccharide substance
    typhus (*Rickettsiae* sp.) vaccine

TPST

    true positive stress test

TPSV

    tumor peak systolic velocity

TPT

    Tactile Performance Test
    tetraphenyl tetrazolium
    time to peak tension
    total protein tuberculin
    transpyloric tube
    treadmill performance test
    trigger point therapy
    typhoid-paratyphoid (vaccine)

tPTEF

    time to peak expiratory flow

tPTEF/tE

    time to peak expiratory flow and
      total expiration time

TPTHS

    total parathyroid hormone secretion

tPTIF

    time to peak inspiratory flow

TPTX

    thyroid-parathyroidectomy
    thyroparathyroidectomy

TPTZ

    tripyridyltriazine

TPU

    tropical phagedenic ulcer

TPUR

    transperineal urethral resection

T-putty

    Theraputty

TPV

    tetanus-pertussis vaccine

TPVR

    total peripheral vascular resistance
    total pulmonary vascular resistance

TPWM

    temporoparietal white matter
    tympanoplasty with mastoidectomy

TPWOM

    tympanoplasty without
      mastoidectomy

TPZ

    tirapazamine

TQ

    time questionnaire
    tocopherolquinone
    tourniquet (*See also* TK)

TQM

    total quality management

TR

    recovery time
    rectal temperature (*See also* T(R))
    repetition time
    residual tuberculin
    to return
    terminal repeat
    tetrazolium reduction
    therapeutic radiology
    therapeutic reaction
    therapeutic recreation
    thioredoxin reductase
    thyroid hormone receptor
    timed release
    time to repeat
    tincture (*See also* T, Tr, tr)
    total repair
    total resistance
    total response (*See also* R)
    trace (*See also* T, Tr, tr)
    trachea
    transfusion reaction
    transplant recipient
    transverse relaxation
    treatment (*See also* Tr, tr, treat.,
      TX, Tx, treat., trt, trx)
    T_3 receptor
    tremor
    tricuspid regurgitation
    triradial
    tuberculin residue
    tuberculin R (new tuberculin)
    tuberculin Ruckland (new
      tuberculin)
    tubular reabsorption
    tumor registry
    turbidity reducing
    turnover rate

T

NOTES

T&R
    tenderness and rebound
T(R)
    rectal temperature (*See also* TR)
T(°R)
    absolute temperature on the
        Rankine scale
T$_r$
    radiologic half-life
    retention time
Tr
    tincture (*See also* T, TR, tr)
    trace (*See also* T, TR, tr)
    tragion
    treatment (*See also* TR, tr, treat.,
        trt, TX, trx)
    trypsin
tr
    tincture (*See also* T, TR, Tr)
    trace (*See also* T, TR, Tr, tr)
    traction
    treatment (*See also* TR, Tr, treat.,
        trt, TX, trx)
    tremor
TRA
    to run at
    therapeutic recreation associate
    total renin activity
    transaldolase
    trans-retinoic acid
    traumatic rupture of thoracic aorta
    tumor regression antigen
    tumor-resistant antigen
tra
    transfer
TRAb
    thyrotropin receptor autoantibody
    TSH receptor antibody
TRAC
    traction
trach
    trachea
    tracheal
    tracheostomy
    tracheotomy
TRAcP
    tartrate-resistant acid phosphatase
TRAF
    tumor (necrosis factor) receptor-
        associated factor
    tumor receptor-associated factor
TRAFO
    tone-reducing ankle-foot orthosis
TRAIDS
    transfusion-related AIDS
TRAIL
    TNF-related apoptosis inducing
        ligand

tumor necrosis factor-related
    apoptosis-inducing ligand
TRAJ
    timed repetitive ankle jerk
TRAK
    total reference air-kerma
TRALD
    transfusion-related acute lung injury
TRALI
    transfusion-associated lung injury
    transfusion-related acute lung injury
TRAM
    transverse rectus abdominis muscle
    transverse rectus abdominis
        musculocutaneous (flap)
    transverse rectus abdominis
        myocutaneous (breast
        reconstruction)
    Treatment Rating Assessment
        Matrix
    Treatment Response Assessment
        Method
TRAMP
    transverse rectus abdominis
        musculoperitoneal (flap)
TRAMPE
    tricho-rhino-auriculo-phalangeal
        multiple exostoses
    trichorhinophalangeal multiple
        exostoses
TRAN
    transfusion
TRANCE
    tumor necrosis factor-related
        activation-induced cytokine
trans
    transference
    transverse (*See also* T)
Trans D, trans D
    transverse diameter
transm
    transmission
    transmitted
transpl
    transplantation (*See also* TX)
    transplanted
TRANS Rx
    transfusion reaction
trans sect
    transverse section (*See also* TS, T
        sect)
transsex
    transsexual
TRAP
    tartrate-resistant acid phosphatase
    tartrate-resistant (leukocyte) acid
        phosphatase

telomere repeat amplification protocol

telomeric repeat amplification protocol

thrombin receptor-activating peptide

total peroxyl radical-trapping antioxidant potential

total radical-trapping antioxidant parameter

twin reverse arterial perfusion

twin reversed arterial perfusion

TRAP-6

thrombin receptor-activating peptide 6

TRAPS

tumor necrosis factor receptor-associated periodic syndrome

TRAS

transesophageal atrial stimulation

transplant renal artery stenosis

trau, traum

trauma

traumatic

TRB

return to baseline

terbutaline

TRb

trilateral retinoblastoma

TRBC

total red blood cells

TRBF

total renal blood flow

TRBV

Tribec virus

TRC

tanned red (blood) cell

total renin concentration

total respiratory conductance

total ridge count

TRCA

tanned red (blood) cell agglutination

TRCH

tanned red (blood) cell hemagglutination

TRCHI

tanned red (blood) cell hemagglutination inhibition

TRCV

total red cell volume

TRD

tinnitus relief device

tongue-retaining device

total-retinal detachment

tractional retinal detachment

traction retinal detachment

traumatic rupture of the diaphragm

treatment-related death

treatment-resistant depression

TRDN

transient respiratory distress of the newborn

TRDS

transient respiratory distress syndrome

TRE

negative T_3 response element

thyroid hormone-response element

thyroid response element

true radiation emission

T_3RE

T_3 responsive element

TREA

thoroughness, reliability, efficiency, analytic (ability)

triethanolamine

treat.

treatment (*See also* TR, Tr, tr, TX, trt, trx)

TREC

T-cell receptor-rearrangement excision circles

Tren, TREND

Trendelenburg (position) (*See also* TRND)

TRF

T-cell replacing factor

Teacher Rating Form

Teacher Report Form

thyrotropin release factor

thyrotropin-releasing factor

trf

transfer

TRFC

total rosette-forming cell

TRG

tumor regression grade

trg, trng

training

TRGI

Teacher's Reading Global Improvement (scale, test)

triglycerides incalculable

NOTES

TRH
protirelin (thyrotropin-releasing
hormone)
tension-reducing hypothesis
thyroid-releasing hormone
thyrotropin-releasing hormone
TRH-DE
TRH-degrading ectoenzyme
TRH-R
thyrotropin-releasing hormone
receptor
TRH-ST
thyrotropin-releasing hormone
stimulation test
TRI
intracytoplasmic tuboreticular
inclusion
tetrazolium reduction inhibition
total response index
transient radicular irritation
transient response imaging
trifocal
trimester (*See also* TM)
tubuloreticular inclusion
tri
tricentric
T₃RIA, T₃(RIA)
triiodothyronine radioimmunoassay
T₄RIA, T₄(RIA)
tetraiodothyronine (thyroxine)
radioimmunoassay
thyroxine radioisotope assay
TRIAC, triac
triiodothyroacetic acid
3,5,3′-triiodothyroacetic acid
TRIADS
time-resolved imaging by automatic
data segmentation
TRIC
trachoma (and) inclusion
conjunctivitis
TRICB
trichlorobiphenyl
TRICH, Trich
trichinosis
Trichomonas
TRICKS
time-resolved imaging contrast
kinetics
TRIG, trig
triglyceride (*See also* TG)
TRIMIS
Tri-Service Medical Information
System
TRIS, tris
tris (hydroxymethyl)aminomethane
(*See also* THAM)

TRISS
Trauma and Injury Severity Scores
TRIT
triiodothyronine (*See also* T₃, TIT)
Trit, trit
triturate
TRITC
tetramethylrhodamine isothiocyanate
tetrarhodamine isothiocyanate
TRK
total rotating knee
transketolase
TRL
triglyceride-rich lipoprotein
triglyceride-rich protein
TRLI
transfusion-related lung injury
TR-LSC
time-resolved liquid scintillation
counting
TRM
transplant-related mortality
treatment-related mortality
TRML, trml
terminal (*See also* ter, term.)
TRM-SMX
trimethoprim and sulfamethoxazole
tRNA
transfer ribonucleic acid
TRNBP
transrectal needle biopsy of the
prostate
TRND
Trendelenburg (position) (*See also*
Tren, TREND)
TRNG
tetracycline-resistant *Neisseria
gonorrhoeae*
TRO
to return to office
thyroid-related ophthalmopathy
tissue reflectance oximeter
TROCA
tangible reinforcement of operant
conditioned audiometry
TROCH, Troch
troche (lozenge)
troch
trochiscus
TROM
total range of motion
trop
tropical
TRP
Tactile Reproduction Pegboard
total refractory period
trichorhinophalangeal (syndrome)

tubular reabsorption of phosphate
tubular reabsorption phosphate
Trp
tryptophan (*See also* TP, Tp, W)
TRPA
tryptophan-rich prealbumin
TrPl
treatment plan
TRPM-2
testosterone repressed prostate
message-2
TRPS
trichorhinophalangeal syndrome
TrPs
trigger points
TRPT
theoretical renal phosphorus
threshold
TRR
total respiratory resistance
TRRP
Thackray Reading Readiness Profile
TR-RXR
thyroid hormone receptor-retinoid X
receptor
TRS
Therapeutic Recreation Specialist
total reducing sugars
tubuloreticular structure
TrS
traumatic surgery
TRSV
tobacco ringspot virus (*See also*
TobRV)
TRT
thermoradiotherapy
thoracic radiation therapy
total reading time
treatment-related toxicity
trt
treatment (*See also* TR, Tr, tr,
treat., TX, trx)
TRU
terminal respiratory unit
turbidity-reducing unit
T₃RU
T_3 resin uptake
triiodothyronine resin uptake
TRUS
transrectal ultrasonography
transrectal ultrasound-guided sextant
(biopsy)

transrectal ultrasound (scanning)
transurethral ultrasound
TRUSP
transrectal ultrasound of prostate
TRUST
toluidine red unheated serum test
TRUV
Trubanaman virus
TRV
Tanjong Rabok virus
tobacco rattle virus
TRW
teboroxime resting washout
TRX
thioredoxin
trx
treatment (prescription) (*See also*
TR, Tr, tr, treat., trt, TX)
TRZ
tartrozine
triazolam
TS
(2′-deoxy)thymidylate synthase
telomerase
temperature sensitive
temperature sensitivity
temporal stem
terminal sedation
terminal sensation
testosterone sulfate
test solution
thermostable
thiosporin
thoracic spine
thoracic surgery
throat swab
thymidylate synthase
tissue space
tocopherol supplemented
toe sign
total solids (in urine)
toxic substance
toxic syndrome
trabecular separation
tracheal sound
tracheal spiral
transitional sleep
transsexual
transverse section (*See also* trans
sect, T sect)
transverse sinus
Trauma Score

T

NOTES

TS (*continued*)
    treadmill score
    trichostasis spinulosa
    tricuspid stenosis
    trimethoprim-sulfamethoxazole
    triple strength
    tropical sprue
    Troyer syndrome
    trypticase soy (plate)
    T suppressor (cell)
    tuberous sclerosis
    tubular sound
    tumor specific
    Turner syndrome
    type specific

T-S
    type and screen

T/S
    thyroid to serum (iodide ratio)

Ts
    skin temperature
    tension by Schiotz (tonometer)
    T helper suppressor cell
    tosylate
    T suppressor

tS
    time required to complete S phase of cell cycle

ts, tsp
    teaspoon

TSA
    technical surgical assistance
    Test of Syntactic Ability
    tissue-specific antigens
    toluene sulfonic acid
    Total Severity Assessment
    total shoulder arthroplasty
    total solute absorption
    toxic shock antigen
    trypticase-soy agar
    tumor-specific antigen
    tumor-susceptible antigen
    type-specific antibody
    tyramide signal amplification

T$_4$SA
    thyroxine-specific activity

TSAb
    thyroid-stimulating antibody

TSAE
    transcatheter splenic arterial embolization

TSAH
    traumatic subarachnoid hemorrhage

TSAP
    toxic shock-associated protein

Tsaph
    temperature in saphenous (vein)

TSAS
    total severity assessment score

TSAT
    tube slide agglutination test

TSB
    total serum bilirubin
    trypticase soy broth
    tryptone soy broth

TSBA
    total serum bile acids

TSBAb
    thyroid stimulation-blocking antibody
    TSH stimulation blocking antibody

TSBB
    transtracheal selective bronchial brushing

TSBC
    Time-Sample Behavioral Checklist

TSBP
    testis-specific binding protein

TSC
    technetium sulfur colloid
    theophylline serum concentration
    thiosemicarbazide (stain)
    total static compliance
    total symptom complex
    transverse spinal sclerosis
    tuberous sclerosis complex

TSCA
    Toxic Substance Control Act

TSCC
    Trauma Symptom Checklist for Children

TSCS
    Tennessee Self-Concept Scale

TSD
    target-skin distance
    Tay-Sachs disease (*See also* TS)
    theory of signal detectability
    transfer summary dictated

TSDP
    tapered steroid dosing package

TSE
    targeted systemic exposure
    testicular self-examination
    total skin examination
    transmissible spongiform encephalopathy
    trisodium edetate
    turbo-spin echo

TSEB
    total skin electron beam

T sect
    transverse section (*See also* trans sect, TS)

TSEM
transmission scanning electron microscopy

TSF
thickness of skin fold
thrombopoiesis-stimulating factor
tissue-(coding) factor (*See also* TCF)
total systemic flow
triceps skinfold (thickness)
T-suppressor factor

TSFS
transseptal frontal sinusotomy

TSG
tumor-specific glycoprotein
tumor-suppressor gene

TSH
thyroid-stimulating hormone
thyrotropin-stimulating hormone

TSH-oma
TSH-secreting pituitary adenoma

TSH-R
thyroid-stimulating hormone receptor
thyrotropin receptor

TSHR
thyroid-stimulating hormone receptor
thyrotropin-receptor antibody

TSH-RAb
thyroid-stimulating hormone receptor antibody
thyroid-stimulating hormone receptor autoantibody
thyrotropin receptor-stimulating antibody

TSH-RF
thyroid-stimulating hormone-releasing factor

TSH-RH
thyroid-stimulating hormone-releasing hormone

TSI
Test of Social Inferences
thyroid-stimulating immunoglobulin
tobramycin solution for inhalation (TOBI)
triple sugar iron (agar) (*See also* TSIA)

TSIA
total small intestinal allotransplantation
triple sugar iron agar (*See also* TSI)

tSIDS
totally unexplained sudden infant death syndrome

T-SKULL
trauma skull

TSL
terminal sensory latency

TSLS
toxic shock-like syndrome

TSM
type-specific M protein

TSN
tryptophan peptone sulfide neomycin (agar)

TSNA
tobacco-specific nitrosamine

TSNP
two-step nested PCR

TSP
thrombospondin
tibial sesamoid position
topical skin protection
total serum protein
total suspended particulate
tribasic sodium phosphate
trisodium phosphate
tropical spastic paraparesis

TSP-1
thrombospondin-1

TSPA
thiophosphoramide (Thiotepa)

TSPAP
total serum prostatic acid phosphatase

TSP/HAM
tropical spastic paraparesis/HTLV-I associated myelopathy

T-spica
thumb spica (bandage)

T-spine, T/spine
thoracic spine

TSPP
technetium stannous pyrophosphate
tetrasodium pyrophosphate

TSR
testosterone-sterilized (female) rat
theophylline-sustained release
thyroid-serum ratio
total shoulder replacement
total systemic resistance
transfer
transient situational reaction

NOTES

TSRBC
trypsinized sheep red blood cell
TSRI
Teacher School Readiness Inventory
TS III ROP
threshold stage III of retinopathy of prematurity
TSRPC
totally stapled restorative proctocolectomy
TSRS
tissue-stone recognition system
TSS
total serum solids
toxic shock syndrome
transverse spinal sclerosis
tropical splenomegaly syndrome
tumor score system
TSSA
tumor-specific (cell) surface antigen
TSSE
toxic shock syndrome exoprotein
toxic shock syndrome exotoxin
TS-SPCL
transsclerally sutured posterior chamber lens
TS/SS
transverse/sigmoid sinus
TSST
toxic shock syndrome toxin
TSST-1
toxic shock syndrome toxin-1
TSSU
(operating) theatre sterile supply unit
TST
thromboplastin screening test
Titmus stereoacuity test
total sleep time
transition state theory
transscrotal testosterone
treadmill stress test (*See also* TMST)
tuberculin skin test
tumor skin test
Twenty Statements Test
TSTA
toxoplasmin skin test antigen
tumor-specific tissue antigen
tumor-specific transplantation antigen
TSTI
tumor-specific transplantation immunity
TSU
triple sugar urea (agar)
TSUV
Tsuruse virus

TSV
total stomach volume
total stroke volume
TSY
trypticase soy yeast
TT
tablet triturate
tactile tension
talar tilt
talking task
telephone device for the deaf
terminal transferase
Test Tape
tetanus toxin
tetanus toxoid (*See also* tet tox)
tetrathionate (broth)
tetrazol
text telephone
therapeutic touch
thrombin time
thrombolytic therapy
thromboplastin time
thymol turbidity
tibial tubercle
tibial tuberosity
tilt table
tine test
token test
tonometry
tooth treatment
total thyroidectomy
total thyroxine
total time
total transfer
trabecular thickness
transferred to
transfusion transmitted
transient tachypnea
transit time
transpupillary thermotherapy
transthoracic
transtracheal
triple therapy
tritiated thymidine (*See also* TTH)
tuberculin test
tube thoracostomy
tumor thrombus
turnover time
twitch tension
tympanic temperature
tyrosine transaminase
T-T
time-to-time
T&T
time and temperature
tobramycin and ticarcillin
touch and tone
tympanotomy and tube (insertion)

T/T
trace of/trace of (different substances on tests)

T$_i$/T$_{TOT}$, t$_i$/t$_{tot}$
duty cycle
ratio of inspiratory time to total cycle time

TT$_3$
total T$_3$

TT$_4$
total T$_4$
total thyroxine

TTA
tetanus toxoid antibody
timed therapeutic absence
tissue texture abnormality
total toe arthroplasty
transtracheal aspiration

T-TAC
transcervical tubal access catheter

TTAP
threaded titanium acetabular prosthesis

TTAT
toe touch as tolerated

TTBS
Tween-TRIS-buffered saline solution

TTBV
total trabecular bone volume

TTC
transtracheal catheter
triphenyltetrazolium chloride
triphenyl tetrazolium chloride
T-tube cholangiogram

TTCT
Torrance Tests of Creative thinking

TTD
tarsal tunnel decompression
temporary total disability
tetraethylthiuramdisulfide
tissue tolerance d
tissue tolerance dose
total temporary disability
total tumor dose
transient tic disorder
transverse thoracic diameter

TTD 2
trichothiodystrophy 2

TTDE
transthoracic color Doppler echocardiography

TTDF
time to distant failure

TTDM
thallium threadmill

TTDP
time-to-disease progression

TTE
total thoracic esophagectomy
transthoracic echocardiogram
transthoracic echocardiography
two-dimensional transthoracic echocardiography

TTF
thyroid transcription factor
time-to-treatment failure

TTF-1
thyroid transcription factor-1

TTF-2
thyroid transcription factor 2

TTFD
thiamine tetrahydrofurfuryl disulfide

TTG, TTGA
tellurite, taurocholate, gelatin agar
tellurite, taurocholate, gelatin (agar)

Ttg, tTG
tissue transglutaminase

TTGE
temporal temperature gradient gel electrophoresis
timed-temperature gradient electrophoresis

TTH
thyrotropic hormone (*See also* TH)
tritiated thymidine (*See also* TT)

TTI
Teflon tube insertion
tension-time index
time-tension index
tissue thromboplastin inhibition (test)
total time to intubation
transfer to intermediate
transtracheal insufflation

TTIB
tension-time index per beat

TTII
thyrotropin-binding inhibitory immunoglobulins

TTIT
tissue thromboplastin inhibition test

TTJV
transtracheal jet ventilation

NOTES

TTKG
>transtubular potassium concentration gradient

TTL
>total lymphocyte
>training and test lung

TTLC
>true total lung capacity

TTLF
>time to local failure

TTM
>total tumor mass
>transtelephonic (arrhythmia) monitoring
>transtelephonic (electrocardiographic) monitoring
>transtelephonic monitoring
>trichotillomania

TTMAD
>Testing-Teaching Module of Auditory Discrimination

TTN
>toxic thyroid nodule
>transient tachypnea of newborn (*See also* TTNB)

TTNA
>transthoracic needle aspiration

TTNAB
>transthoracic needle aspiration biopsy (*See also* TTNB)

TTNB
>transient tachypnea of newborn (*See also* TTN)
>transthoracic needle (aspiration) biopsy (*See also* TTNAB)

TTND
>time to nondetectable

TTO
>to take out
>tea tree oil
>time trade-off
>transfer to open
>transtracheal oxygen

TTOD
>tetanus toxoid outdated

TTOT
>transtracheal oxygen therapy

Ttot
>total respiratory time

T₃-toxicosis

T_3-toxicosis
>triiodothyronine toxicosis

TTP
>tender to palpation
>tender to pressure
>Testicular Tumor Panel
>thrombotic thrombocytopenic purpura
>thymidine triphosphate
>time to peak
>time to pregnancy
>time to tumor progression
>transtrabecular plane

TTPA
>triethylene thiophosphoramide

TTPD
>thoracic-pelvic-phalangeal dystrophy

TTP-HUS
>thrombotic thrombocytopenic purpura and hemolytic uremic syndrome

TTR
>tarsal tunnel release
>transthoracic resistance
>transthyretin
>Trauma Triage Rule
>triceps tendon reflex
>type-to-token ratio

T-trophic, T-tropic
>T-cell trophic
>T-cell-tropic

TTS
>tarsal tunnel syndrome
>temporary threshold shift
>testosterone transdermal system
>through the skin
>through-the-scope
>tight-to-shaft
>transdermal therapeutic system
>transfusion therapy service
>trigeminal trophic syndrome
>twin-to-twin transfusion syndrome (*See also* TTTS)

TTT
>thymol turbidity test
>tibial talar tilt/tibiotalar tilt
>tilt-table test
>tolbutamide tolerance test
>total tourniquet time
>total twitch time
>transpupillary thermal therapy
>turn-to-turn transfusion

TTTS
>twin-twin transfusion syndrome (*See also* TTS)

TTTT
>test tube turbidity test

T-TURP
>total transurethral resection of prostate

TTUTD
>tetanus toxoid up-to-date

TTV
>therapeutic trial visit
>tracheal transport velocity
>transfusion-transmitted virus
>TT virus

TTVP
temporary transvenous pacemaker
TTWB
touch-toe weightbearing
TTX
tetrodotoxin
TTx
thrombolytic therapy
TU
thiouracil
thiourea
thyroidal uptake
Todd unit
toxic unit
toxin unit
transmission unit
transrectal ultrasound
transurethral
tuberculin unit
turbidity unit
1-TU
1 tuberculin unit
5-TU
5 tuberculin unit
250-TU
250 tuberculin unit
T₃U
triiodothyronine uptake (*See also* T₃UP)
TUAV
Turuna virus
TUB
tuberculosis vaccine, not BCG
tubouterine (junction)
TUBA
transumbilical breast augmentation
TUBS
traumatic unidirectional Bankart lesion surgery
TUD
total urethral discharge
TUDC, TUDCA
tauroursodeoxycholate
tauroursodeoxycholic acid
TUDOR
transvaginal ultrasound-directed oocyte retrieval
TUE
transurethral extraction
TUEP, TUEVP
transurethral electrovaporization of prostate

transurethral evaporation of prostate (*See also* TUVP)
TUF
total ultrafiltration
TUG
timed up and go
total urinary gonadotropin
TUI
transurethral incision
TUIBN
transurethral incision of bladder neck
TUIP
transurethral incision of prostate
TUL
transurethral ureterolithotripsy
tularemia (*Francisella tularensis*) vaccine
TULIP
transurethral ultrasound-guided laser-induced prostatectomy
transurethral ultrasound-guided laser-induced prostatectomy (system)
TUMT
transurethral microwave thermotherapy
TUN
total urinary nitrogen
TUNA
transurethral needle ablation
TUNEL
TdT-mediated dUTP nick-end labeling
terminal deoxynucleotidyl transferase-mediated digoxigenin-dUTP nick-end labeling
terminal transferase-mediated dUTP-biotin nick-end labeling
TUP
transumbilical plane
T₃UP
triiodothyronine uptake (*See also* T₃U)
TUPR
transurethral prostatic resection
TUR
transurethral resection
T₃UR
triiodothyronine uptake ratio
TURB, TURBT
transurethral resection of bladder (tumor)

NOTES

turb
> turbid
> turbidity

TURBN
> transurethral resection of bladder neck

TUR-Cue photometer
> transurethral resection (*See also* TUR)

TURM
> transurethral microwave

TURP
> transurethral prostatectomy
> transurethral prostate procedure
> transurethral resection of prostate

TURS
> transurethral resection syndrome

TURV
> transurethral resection of valves
> Turlock virus

TURVN
> transurethral resection of vesical neck

TUSSI
> Temple University Short Syntax Inventory

TUU
> transureteroureterostomy

TUV
> transurethral valve

TUVP, TUVRP
> transurethral electrovaporization of prostate
> transurethral vaporization of prostate
> transurethral vaporization-resection of prostate

TV
> talipes varus
> target volume
> television
> Tellina virus
> temporary visit
> tetrazolium violet
> thoracic vertebra
> tick-borne virus
> tidal volume (*See also* TD, VT, V_T)
> total volume
> toxic vertigo
> transfer vesicle
> transvenous
> transverse
> trial visit
> *Trichomonas vaginalis*
> tricuspid valve
> trivalent
> true vertebra

> truncal vagotomy
> tuberculin volutin
> tubulovesicular

T/V
> touch/verbal

TV_I
> tidal inspiratory volume

TV_E
> tidal expiratory volume

TVA
> true visual acuity
> truncal vagotomy plus antrectomy

TVC
> third ventricle cyst
> timed ventilatory capacity
> timed vital capacity
> total viable cells
> total volume capacity
> transvaginal cone
> triple voiding cystogram
> true vocal cord

TVc
> tricuspid valve closure

TV-CDS
> transvaginal color Doppler sonography

TVD
> transmissible virus dementia
> triple vessel disease

TVDALV
> triple vessel disease with abnormal left ventricle

TVF
> tactile vocal fremitus
> Thiry-Vella fistula
> true vocal fold

TVG, TVGC
> time-varied gain
> time-varied gain control (*See also* TGC)

TVH
> total vaginal hysterectomy
> turkey virus hepatitis

TVHS
> transvaginal hysterosonography

TVI
> Temperament and Values Inventory
> time velocity integral
> total vascular isolation

T3/vind
> triiodothyronine to thyroxine index

TVL
> tenth value layer (radiation)

TVN
> tonic vibration response

TVO
> transtrochanteric valgus osteotomy

TVP
> tensor veli palatini
> textured vegetable protein
> transurethral electrovaporization of prostate
> transvenous pacemaker
> transvesical prostatectomy
> tricuspid valve prolapse
> truncal vagotomy (plus) pyloroplasty

TVR
> target vessel revascularization
> tonic vibration reflex
> total vascular resistance
> total vibration reflex
> tricuspid valve replacement

TVRSS
> total vasomotor rhinitis symptom score

TVS
> transvaginal sonography
> transvaginal suturing
> transvenous system
> trigeminovascular system

TVSC
> transvaginal (sector) scan

TVT
> tension-free vaginal tape
> transmissible vencreal tumor
> transvaginal tension-free
> tunica vaginalis testis

TVTV
> trivittatus virus

TVU
> total volume of urine
> transvaginal ultrasonography
> transvaginal ultrasound

TVUS, TV-UST
> transvaginal ultrasound

TW
> talked with
> tap water
> terminal web
> test weight
> thought withdrawal
> thymic weight
> total (body) water
> *Trophermyma whippleii*
> T-wave

TW2
> Tanner-Whitehouse mark 2 (bone-age assessment)

5TW
> five times a week

TWA
> time-weighted average
> total wrist arthroplasty
> T-wave alternans

TWAR
> Taiwan acute respiratory (agent)

T wave
> repolarization

Twb
> wet bulb temperature

TWBC
> total white blood cells

TWCS
> Test of Work Competency and Stability

TWD
> total white and differential (cell count)

TWE
> tap water enema
> tepid water enema

TWEAK
> TNF-weak homologue

TWETC
> tap water enema til clear

TWF
> Test of Word Finding

TWFD
> Test of Word Finding in Discourse

TWG
> total weight gain

TWHW
> toe walking and heel walking

TWI
> T-wave inversion

T1WI
> T1-weighted image

T2WI
> T2-weighted image

TwiST
> time without symptoms and toxicity

TWL
> transepidermal water loss (*See also* TEWL)

TWN
> twin

TWOC
> trial without catheter

NOTES

T

TWR
total wrist replacement
TWSTRS
Toronto Western Spasmodic
Torticollis Rating Scale
T1WT
T1 weighted image
TWWD
tap water wet dressing
TX
derivative of contagious tuberculin
thromboxane (*See also* TBX, Thx)
thyroidectomized
transplantation (*See also* transpl)
treatment (*See also* TR, Tr, tr,
treat., trt, trx)
T&X
type and crossmatch (*See also*
TXM)
Tx, T$_x$, tx
therapist
therapy
traction
transcription
transfuse
transplant
tympanostomy
TXA, TxA
thromboxane A
TXA2, TXA$_2$
thromboxane A2
TXB2, TXB$_2$
thromboxane B2
TxCAD
transplant coronary artery disease
TXE
Timoptic-XE
TXM
T-cell crossmatch
type and crossmatch (*See also*
T&X)
Txn
transplant
TXS
type and screen

Ty
thyroxine
type
typhoid
tyrosine (*See also* Tyr, Y)
TYCO
Tylenol with codeine
Tyk-2
tyrosine kinase-2
Tyl
Tylenol
tyloma
TYMP
tympanogram
tymp
tympanic
tympanicity (auscultation of chest)
tympanium
tympanostomy
typ
typical
TYR
tyramine
tyrode
Tyr
tyrosine (*See also* Ty, Y)
TyRIA
thyroid radioimmunoassay
TYUV
Tyuleniy virus
TZ
transition zone
triazolam
zymoplastic tuberculin [Ger.
Tuberculin zymoplastische]
TZD
thiazolidinedione
TZM
Kosher
T zone
transformation zone
TZT
triazinate

U

internal energy
kilurane (radioactivity unit)
Mann-Whitney rank sum statistic
potential difference (in volts)
ulna
ultralente (insulin)
uncertain
unerupted
unit
unknown (*See also* UK)
upper
uracil (*See also* URA, Ura)
uranium
urethra (*See also* UA, ureth)
uridine (*See also* Urd)
uridylic acid (*See also* UA)
urinary (*See also* ur)
urine (*See also* UR, ur)
urology (*See also* Urol)
uvula
wave on electrocardiogram

U/1

one fingerbreadth below umbilicus

U/3

upper third (of long bone)

24U

24 hour urine (collection)

U100

100 units per milliliter

1/U

one fingerbreadth above umbilicus

U/

at umbilicus

u

unified atomic mass unit

UA

Ulex agglutinin
ultra-audible (sound)
ultrasonic arteriogram
umbilical arterial
umbilical artery
unaggregated
unauthorized absence
uncertain about
unit of analysis
unrelated (children raised) apart
unstable angina
upper airway
upper arm
urethra (*See also* U, ureth)
uric acid (*See also* U/A, UR AC)
uridylic acid (*See also* U)
urinalysis
urinary aldosterone

urine aliquot
urocanic acid
uterine aspiration

U/A

uric acid (*See also* UA, UR AC)
uterine activity

UAC

umbilical artery catheter
underactive
upper airway congestion

UA/C

uric acid-creatinine (ratio)
urinary albumin to creatinine
(ratio)

UACL

ulcer-associated cell lineage

UACP

upper airway closing pressure

UAD

upper aerodigestive
upper airway disease
upper airway disorder

UADT

upper aerodigestive tract

UAE

unilateral absence of excretion
unsupported arm exercise
urinary albumin excretion
uterine artery embolization

UAG

uracil-adenine-guanine

UAI

uterine activity integral

UAL

ultrasonic-assisted lipoplasty
ultrasonic-assisted liposuction
ultrasound-assisted lipectomy
umbilical artery line
up (out of bed) as desired [up +
L. *ad libitum*] (*See also* UAT)

UALTE

unexplained apparent life-threatening
event

UA&M

urinalysis and microscopy

U-AMY

urinary amylase

UAN

uric acid nitrogen

UA/NQMI

unstable angina/non-Q-wave
myocardial infarction

UAO

upper airway obstruction
urine acid output

UAOP
　　upper airway opening pressure
UAP
　　unstable angina pectoris (*See also* USAP)
　　upper abdominal pain
UAPF
　　upon arrival patient found
UAPs
　　unlicensed assistive personnel
UAR
　　upper airway resistance
U-ARM
　　upper arm
UARS
　　upper airway resistance syndrome
　　upper airway respiratory syndrome
UAS
　　undifferentiated autoimmune syndrome
　　upper abdominal surgery
　　upstream activating sequence
UASA
　　upper airway sleep apnea
UAT
　　up (out of bed) as tolerated (*See also* UAL)
UAU
　　uterine activity unit
UAVC
　　univentricular atrioventricular connection
UB
　　ultimobranchial body
　　Unna boot
　　urinary bladder
ub
　　urinary bladder channel (acupuncture)
UBA
　　undenatured bacterial antigen
UBBC
　　unsaturated (vitamin) B_{12}-binding capacity
UBC
　　University of British Columbia (brace)
　　unsaturated binding capacity
UBD
　　universal blood donor
UBE
　　uniaxial balance evaluation
　　upper body ergometer
UbetaCF
　　urinary beta-core fragment
UBF
　　unknown black female
　　uterine blood flow

U-BFP
　　urinary basic fetoprotein
UBG
　　ultimobranchial gland
　　urobilinogen
UBI
　　ultraviolet blood irradiation
ubiq
　　ubiquitin
UBIS
　　ultrasound bone imaging sonometer
UBL
　　undifferentiated B-cell lymphoma
UBM
　　ultrasound backscatter microscopy
　　ultrasound biomicroscopy
　　unknown black male
　　urothelial basement membrane
UBO
　　unidentified bright object
UBP
　　Universal bone plate
　　ureteral back pressure
UBT
　　C-urea breath test
　　urea breath test
　　uterine balloon therapy
UBW
　　usual body weight
UC
　　ulcerative colitis
　　Uldall catheter
　　ultracentrifugal
　　umbilical cholesterol
　　umbilical cord
　　unchanged
　　unclassifiable
　　unconscious (*See also* UCS, ucs)
　　undifferentiated carcinoma
　　unfixed cryostat
　　unit clerk
　　unsatisfactory condition
　　untreated cell
　　urea clearance (*See also* UCL)
　　urethral catheterization
　　urinary catheter
　　urine concentrate
　　urine culture (*See also* U/C, UCX)
　　usual care
　　uterine contraction
U/C
　　umbilical artery to middle cerebral artery (pulsatility index ratio)
　　urine culture (*See also* UC, UCX)
U&C
　　urethral and cervical (cultures)
　　usual and customary

UCA
ultrasound contrast agent
unicystic ameloblastoma
UcA
urothelial carcinoma
UCAC
uterine cornual access catheter
UCAD
unstable coronary artery disease
U$_{Ca}$V
urinary calcium volume (excretion rate)
UCB
umbilical cord blood
unconjugated bilirubin (See also UCBR)
Unicorn Campbell Boy (orthotics)
unilateral calcaneal brace
UCBC
umbilical cord blood culture
UCBR
unconjugated bilirubin (See also UCB)
UCBT
unrelated cord-blood transplant
UCC
urgent care center
UCD
urine collection device
usual childhood diseases (See also UCHD, UDC)
UCE
upper completely edentulous
urea cycle enzymopathy
U-cell
undefined-cell
UCF
urinary free cortisol
UCG
ultrasonic cardiogram
ultrasonic cardiography
urinary chorionic gonadotropin
UCHD
usual childhood diseases (See also UCD, UDC, UCHI)
UCHI
usual childhood illnesses (See also UCI, UCHD)
UCHS
uncontrolled hemorrhagic shock
UCI
umbilical coiling index

urethral catheter in
urinary catheter in
usual childhood illnesses (See also UCHI)
UCL
ulnar collateral ligament
uncomfortable level
uncomfortable listening level (See also UCLL)
uncomfortable loudness level (See also ULL)
upper confidence limit
urea clearance (See also UC)
UCLL
uncomfortable listening level (See also UCL)
uncomfortable loudness level (See also UCL, ULL)
UCLP
unilateral cleft of lip and palate
UCN-01
7-hydroxystaurosporin
UCO
urethral catheter out
urinary catheter out
UCP
ultrasound catheter probe
umbilical cord prolapse
uncoupling protein
urethral closure pressure
urinary coproporphyrin
urinary C-peptide
UCP1
uncoupling protein 1
UCP2
uncoupling protein 2
UCP3
uncoupling protein 3
UCPP
urethral closure pressure profile
UCPs
urine collection pads
UCPT
urinary coproporphyrin test
UCR
unconditioned reflex (See also UR)
unconditioned response (See also UR)
usual, customary, and reasonable (fees)
UCRE
urine creatinine

NOTES

U

833

UCRP
Universal Control Reference Plasma
UCS
unconditioned stimulus (*See also* UDS, US)
unconscious (*See also* UC, ucs)
unicoronal synostosis
uterine compression syndrome
UC&S
urine culture and sensitivity
ucs
unconscious (*See also* UC, UCS)
UCT
ultrasound computed tomography
unchanged conventional treatment
UCTD
unclassifiable connective tissue disease
undifferentiated connective tissue disease
UCTS
undifferentiated connective tissue syndrome
UCU
urinary care unit
UCV
uncontrolled variable
UCVA
uncorrected visual acuity
UCX
urine culture (*See also* UC)
UD
ulcerative dermatosis
ulnar deviation
underdeveloped
undesirable discharge
unipolar depression
unit dose
urethral dilatation
urethral discharge
uridine diphosphate
urodynamics
uroporphyrinogen decarboxylase
uterine distention
uterus delivery
UDA
under direct vision
UDC
uninhibited detrusor (muscle) capacity
ursodeoxycholate
usual diseases of childhood (*See also* UCD, UCHD)
UDCA
ursodeoxycholic acid (*See also* URSO)
UDE
undetermined etiology

UDI
urinary diagnostic index
Urogenital Distress Inventory
UDMA
urethane dimethacrylate
UDN
updraft nebulizer
UDO
undetermined origin
UDP
unassisted diastolic pressure
uridine diphosphate
uridine 5′-diphosphate
urine drug panel
UDPG, UDPGlc
uridine diphosphoglucose
UDPGA, UDP-GlcUA
uridine diphosphoglucuronic acid
UDPGal
uridine diphosphogalactose
UDPGT
uridine diphosphate glucuronosyltransferase
uridine diphosphoglucuronyl transferase
UdR
uracil deoxyriboside (deoxyuridine)
UDRP
urine diribose phosphate
UDS
ultra–Doppler sonography
unconditioned stimulus (*See also* UCS, US)
unscheduled deoxynucleic acid synthesis
unscheduled deoxyribonucleic acid synthesis
urine drug screen
UDT
undescended testicle
UE
Ulex europaeus
uncertain etiology
under elbow
undetermined etiology
uninvolved epidermis
upper esophagus
upper extremity (*See also* U/E)
U/E
upper extremity (*See also* UE)
uE3
unconjugated estriol
UEA
upper extremity arterial
UEA-1
Ulex europaeus agglutinin I
UEC
uterine endometrial carcinoma

UEDs
unilateral epileptiform discharges
UEG
ultrasonic encephalography
unifocal eosinophilic granuloma
UEM
universal electron microscope
UEMC
unidentified endosteal marrow cell
UEP
urinary excretion of protein
UER
unaided equalization reference
UES
undifferentiated embryonal sarcoma
Unpleasant Events Schedule
upper esophageal sphincter
UESEP
upper extremity somatosensory
evoked potential
UESP
upper esophageal sphincter pressure
UESR
upper esophageal sphincter
relaxation
u/ext
upper extremity
UF
ulcerating form
ultrafiltrable
ultrafiltrate
ultrafiltration
ultrafine
ultrasonic frequency
unflexed
universal feeder
unknown factor
until finished
urea formaldehyde
UFA
unesterified fatty acid
unesterified free fatty acid (*See
also* FFA)
UFC
urinary free cortisol
urine free cortisol
UFCT
ultrafast computed tomography
UFD
ultrasonic flow detector
UFE
uniform food encoding

UFF
unusual facial features
UFFI
urea formaldehyde foam insulation
UFH
unfractionated heparin
UFISH
ultrasensitive fluorescence in situ
hybridization
UFN
until further notice
UFO
unflagged order
unidentified flying object
unidentified foreign object
Universal plantar fasciitis orthotic
UFOS
universal frame outer socket
UFOV
useful field of view
UFR
ultrafiltration rate
urine filtration rate
uFSH
urinary follicle-stimulating hormone
urinary FSH
UFV
ultrafiltration volume
unclassified fecal virus
UG
until gone
urinary glucose
urogastrone
urogenital
uteroglobulin
UGA
under general anesthesia
urogenital atrophy
UGCR
ultrasound-guided compression repair
UGD
urogenital diaphragm
UGF
unidentified growth factor
urinary gonadotropin fragment
UGH
uveitis, glaucoma, hyphema
(syndrome)
UGH+
uveitis, glaucoma, hyphema plus
(vitreous hemorrhage, syndrome)

U

NOTES

UGI
    upper gastrointestinal (tract) (*See also* UGIT)

UGIB
    upper gastrointestinal bleeding

UGIE
    upper gastrointestinal endoscopy

UGIH
    upper gastrointestinal (tract) hemorrhage

UGIS
    upper gastrointestinal series (*See also* UGI)

UGIT
    upper gastrointestinal tract (*See also* UGI)

UGI w/SBFT
    upper gastrointestinal (series) with small bowel follow through

UGK
    urine glucose ketone

UGNB
    ultrasonically guided needle biopsy

UGP
    urinary gonadotropin peptide

UGPP
    uridyl diphosphate glucose pyrophosphorylase

UGS
    urogenital sinus

UGSV
    Uganda S virus

UGVA
    ultrasound-guided vascular access

UH
    umbilical hernia
    unfavorable history
    upper half

UHBI
    upper hemibody irradiation

UHC
    ultrahigh carbon

UHD
    unstable hemoglobin disease

UHDDS
    Uniform Hospital Discharge Data Set

UHF
    ultrahigh frequency

u-hFSH
    urinary-derived human follicle-stimulating hormone

UHFV
    ultrahigh-frequency ventilation

UHL
    universal hypertrichosis lanuginosa

UHMM
    ultrahigh magnification mammography

UHMW
    ultrahigh molecular weight

UHMWPE
    ultrahigh molecular weight polyethylene

UHP
    University Health Plan

UHR
    underlying heart rhythm

UHT
    ultrahigh temperature

UHV
    ultrahigh vacuum
    ultrahigh voltage

UI
    Ulcer Index
    urinary incontinence
    uroporphyrin isomerase
    uteroplacental insufficiency

U/I
    unidentified

UIB
    Unemployment Insurance Benefits

UIBC
    unbound iron-binding capacity
    unsaturated iron-binding capacity

UID/S
    unilateral interfacetal dislocation or subluxation

UIEP
    urine immunoelectrophoresis

UIF
    undegraded insulin factor

UIFE
    urine immunofixation electrophoresis

UIP
    unusual interstitial pneumonitis
    usual interstitial pneumonia
    usual interstitial pneumonia (of Liebow)
    usual interstitial pneumonitis

UIQ
    upper inner quadrant

UIS
    Utilization Information Service

UJ
    uncovertebral
    universal joint (syndrome)

UJT
    unijunction transistor

UK
    unknown (*See also* U)
    urinary kallikrein (*See also* UKa)
    urine potassium
    urokinase

UKA
    unicompartmental knee arthroplasty
UKa
    urinary kallikrein (*See also* UK)
UK IC
    urokinase intracoronary
UKM
    urea kinetic modeling
UKO
    unknown origin
U_kV
    urinary potassium volume (excretion
        rate)
UL
    unauthorized leave
    undifferentiated lymphoma
    upper left
    upper lid
    upper limb
    upper limit
    upper lobe
    utterance length
U&L
    upper and lower (*See also* U/L)
U/L
    unit per liter
    upper body segment to lower body
        segment ratio
    upper and lower (*See also* U&L)
ULA
    undedicated logic array
ULBW
    ultralow birth weight
ULDR
    ultralow dose rate
ULE
    unilateral laterothoracic exanthem
uLH
    urinary luteinizing hormone
ULL
    uncomfortable loudness level (*See
        also* UCL)
ULLE
    upper lid left eye
ULM
    unprotected left main
ULMS
    uterine leiomyosarcoma
ULN
    upper limits of normal

uln
    ulna
    ulnar
ULO
    upper limb orthosis
ULP
    ultralow profile
    upper limb prosthesis
ULPA
    ultralow particulate air
ULPE
    upper lobe pulmonary edema
ULQ
    upper left quadrant
ULRE
    upper lid right eye
ULSB
    upper left sternal border
ULT
    ultralow temperature
ult
    ultimate
    ultimately
ULTT
    upper limb tension test
ULTT1
    upper limb tension test 1 (median
        nerve)
ULTT2a
    upper limb tension test 2a (medial
        nerve)
ULTT2b
    upper limb tension test 2b (radial
        nerve)
ULTT3
    upper limb tension test 3 (ulnar
        nerve)
ULV
    ultralow volume
ULYTES
    urine electrolytes
UM
    unmarried
    upper motor (neuron)
    uracil mustard
    Utilization Management
UMA
    urinary muramidase activity
UMAV
    Umatilla virus
Umax
    maximal urinary osmolality

U

NOTES

UMB, umb
umbilical
umbilicus

umb A line
umbilical artery line

UMBV
Umbre virus

umb ven
umbilical vein

umb V line
umbilical venous line

UMCD
uremic medullary cystic disease

UMCL
upper midclavicular line

$U_{Mg}V$
urinary magnesium volume (excretion rate)

UMI
uterine manipulator/injector

UMLS
Unified Medical Language System

UMN
upper motor neuron

UMNB
upper motor neurogenic bladder

UMNL
upper motor neuron lesion

UMP
undetermined malignant potential
uridine 5'-monophosphate
uridine monophosphate (uridylic acid)

UMPK
uridine monophosphate kinase

UMS
upper (fossa active), medial (knee pain), and short (leg on the side ipsilateral to the weak fossa)
urethral manipulation syndrome

UMT
unit of medical time

UN
ulnar nerve
undernourished
unilateral neglect
urea nitrogen
urinary nitrogen

UNA
urinary nitrogen appearance

U_{Na}, **UNa**
urinary concentration of sodium
urinary sodium

unacc
unaccompanied

UNAV
Una virus

UNaV
urinary sodium excretion

UNC
uncrossed
urine net charge

uncomp
uncompensated

uncond
unconditioned

uncor
uncorrected

UnCS, unCS
unconditioned stimulus (*See also* UnS)

UNCV
ulnar nerve conduction velocity

UNCVA
uncorrected visual acuity

UNDEL
undelivered

undet
undetermined

UNE
unopposed estrogen
urinary norepinephrine

UNG
uracil-N-glycosylase

U_{NH4^-}
urinary ammonium

UNHS, UNHSP
Universal Neonatal Hearing Screening
universal newborn hearing screening program

UNID
unidentified

unilat
unilateral

univ
universal

UNK, unk, unkn
unknown

UNL
upper normal limit

UN/P
unpatched eye

UN/P OD
unpatched right eye

UN/P OS
unpatched left eye

UNS, uns
unsatisfactory (*See also* unsat)
unsymmetrical (*See also* unsym)

UnS
unconditioned stimulus (*See also* UnCS, unCS)

unsat
> unsatisfactory (*See also* UNS, uns)
> unsaturated

unsym
> unsymmetrical (*See also* UNS)

UNTS
> unilateral nevoid telangiectasia syndrome

UNX
> uninephrectomy

UO
> under observation (*See also* U/O, u/o)
> undetermined origin
> ureteral orifice
> urinary output (*See also* UOP)

U/O, u/o
> under observation (*See also* UO)

UOAC
> uterine ostial access catheter

UOP
> urinary output (*See also* UO)

UOQ
> upper outer quadrant

UOS
> undifferentiated osteosarcoma

UOsm, Uosm
> urinary osmolality

UOV
> unit of variance

UOZ
> upper outer zone (quadrant)

UP
> ulcerative proctitis
> ultrahigh purity
> uniformly positive
> unipolar
> Unna-Pappenheim (stain)
> upright posture
> ureteropelvic
> uridine phosphorylase
> uroporphyrin
> uteroplacental

U/P
> up (out of bed) as desired [up + L. *ad libitum*] (*See also* UAL)
> urine-plasma ratio

uPA, u-PA
> urokinase plasminogen activator
> urokinase-type plasminogen activator

uPAR
> urokinase plasminogen activator receptor

UPC
> unknown primary carcinoma
> usual provider continuity

UPD
> uniparental disomy
> urinary production (rate)

UPDRS
> Unified Parkinson Disease Rating Scale

UPE
> upper partially edentulous

UPEP
> urine protein electrophoresis

UPF
> universal proximal femur (prosthesis)

UPG
> uroporphyrinogen

UPI
> uteroplacental insufficiency
> uteroplacental ischemia

UPIN
> unique physician (provided) identification number

UPJ
> ureteropelvic junction

UPL
> unusual position of limbs

UPLIF
> unilateral posterior lumbar interbody fusion

UPLIFT
> uterine positioning via ligament investment fixation truncation

UPN
> unique patient number

UPO
> metastatic carcinoma of unknown primary origin

UPOC
> Ultramatic Project-O-Chart projector

UPOR
> usual place of residence

UPOV
> Upolu virus

UPP
> urethral pressure profile
> urethral pressure profilometry
> uvulopalatoplasty

U

NOTES

UPPP
uvulopalatopharyngoplasty
UPPRA
upright peripheral plasma renin activity
UPRBC
unit of packed red blood cells
UPS
ultraviolet photoelectron spectroscopy
uninterruptible power supply
uroporphyrinogen synthase
uterine progesterone system
UPSC
uterine papillary serous carcinoma
Y
upsilon (20th letter of Greek alphabet), uppercase
υ, upsilon
kinematic viscosity (*See also* v)
upsilon (20th letter of Greek alphabet), lowercase
UPSIT
University of Pennsylvania Smell Identification Test
UPT
uptake
urine pregnancy test
UQ
ubiquinone
upper quadrant
UR
unconditioned reflex (*See also* UCR)
unconditioned response (*See also* UCR)
unrelated
upper respiratory
upper right
urinal
urinary retention
urine (*See also* U, ur)
urology
utilization review
ur
urinary (*See also* U)
urine (*See also* U, UR)
URA, Ura
unilateral renal agenesis
urethral resistance factor
UR AC, URC-A
uric acid
ur anal
urinalysis
urine analysis (*See also* UA)
URAS
unilateral renal artery stenosis

URC
upper rib cage
utilization review committee
URC SP
uric acid (urine) spot (test)
URD
undifferentiated respiratory disease
unrelated donor
upper respiratory disease
Urd
uridine (*See also* U)
UREA-S
urea nitrogen (urine) spot (test)
URED
unable to read (lab result)
URES
University Residence Environment Scale
ureth
urethra (*See also* U, UA)
URF
unidentified reading frame
uterine-relaxing factor
UR-FST
urine-fasting
urg
urgent
UR HR
urine (number of) hours (glucose tolerance)
URI
upper respiratory illness (*See also* URTI)
upper respiratory (tract) infection (*See also* URTI)
URIC A
uric acid
URIN
random urine
url
unrelated
UR&M
urinalysis, routine and microscopic
URO
upper respiratory obstruction
urology
uroporphyrin
uroporphyrinogen
UROB, UROBIL
urobilinogen
UROD
ultra-rapid opiate detoxification [under anesthesia]
uroporphyrinogen decarboxylase
URO-GEN
urogenital
URO-2H
urobilinogen—2 hours

Urol
> urologist
> urology (*See also* U)

UROS
> uroporphyrinogen synthetase

U-RPFA
> Ultegra rapid platelet function assay

URQ
> upper right quadrant (of abdomen)

URR
> upstream regulatory region
> urea reduction ratio

URS
> transurethral ureterorenoscopy
> ultrasonic renal scanning

URSB
> upper right sternal border

URSO
> ursodeoxycholic (acid) (*See also* UDCA)

URT
> upper respiratory tract
> uterine resting tone

URTI
> upper respiratory tract illness
> upper respiratory tract infection (*See also* URI)

UR-TIM
> urine-time

URUV
> Urucuri virus

URVD
> unilateral renovascular disease

UR VOL
> urine volume

US
> ultrasonic
> ultrasonography
> ultrasound (*See also* U/S)
> unconditional stimulus
> unconditioned stimulus (*See also* UCS, UDS)
> United States
> unit secretary
> upper segment
> Usher syndrome

U/S
> ultrasound (*See also* US)

USA
> unstable angina

USAP
> unstable angina pectoris (*See also* UAP)

USB
> upper sternal border

USC
> uterine serous carcinoma

US-CNB, USCNB
> ultrasonographically guided core needle biopsy
> ultrasound-guided core-needle biopsy

U-SCOPE
> ureteroscopy

USCVD
> unsterile controlled vaginal delivery

USE, USG
> ultrasonic echography (ultrasonography) (*See also* USG)
> ultrasonogram
> ultrasonography (*See also* USE)

US-FNAB
> ultrasound-guided fine-needle aspiration biopsy

USH
> usual state of health (*See also* USOH)

USI
> universal salt iodization
> urinary stress incontinence

USM
> ultrasonic mist

USN
> ultrasonic nebulizer
> unilateral spatial neglect

USO
> unilateral salpingo-oophorectomy

USOGH
> usual state of good health

USOH
> usual state of health (*See also* USH)

USP
> unassisted systolic pressure
> upper sternal border
> uterine-stimulating potency

USPDI
> United States Pharmacopeia Drug Information

USPIO
> ultrasmall-particle superparamagnetic iron oxide

NOTES

U

USR
    unheated serum reagin

USS
    ultrasound scanning
    Universal Spine System

UST
    upper single tooth

USUCVD
    unsterile uncontrolled vaginal
      delivery

USUV
    Usutu virus

USVMD
    urine specimen volume measuring
      device

USVMS
    urine specimen volume measuring
      system

USW
    ultrashort wave

UT
    unrelated (children raised) together
    untested
    untreated
    upper thoracic
    urea transporter
    urinary tract
    urticaria

uT
    unbound testosterone

ut
    uterus

UTA
    urinary tract anomaly

U_{TA}
    urinary titrable acidity

UTBG
    unbound thyroxine-binding globulin

UTD
    unable to determine
    up to date

UTF
    usual throat flora

UTI
    urinary tract infection
    urinary trypsin inhibitor

UTIV
    Utinga virus

UTJ
    uterotubal junction

UTL
    unable to locate

UTLD
    Utah Test of Language
      Development

UTM
    urinary tract malformation

UTO
    unable to obtain
    upper tibial osteotomy

UTP
    uridine triphosphate
    uridine 5'-triphosphate

UTPC
    usual type papillary carcinoma

UTR
    untranslated region
    5'-untranslated region

UTROSCT
    uterine tumor resembling an
      ovarian sex-cord tumor

UTS
    ulnar tunnel syndrome
    ultimate tensile strength
    ultrasound (*See also* UTZ)

UTTS
    ultrathin-walled two-stage

UTZ
    ultrasound (*See also* UTS)

UU
    urinary urea
    urine urobilinogen

UUD
    uncontrolled unsterile delivery

UUKV
    Uukuniemi virus

UUN
    urinary urea nitrogen excretion
    urine urea nitrogen

UUO
    unilateral ureteral obstruction
    unilateral ureteral occlusion

UUP
    urine uroporphyrin

U UREA
    urinary (concentration of) urea

UV
    ultraviolet
    ultraviolet (light)
    umbilical vein (*See also* uv)
    ureterovesical
    urinary volume

uv
    umbilical vein (*See also* UV)

UVA
    long-wavelength ultraviolet light
    ultraviolet A
    ultraviolet light, long wavelength
    ureterovesical angle

UVAC
    uterine vacuum aspirating curette

UVB
    ultraviolet B
    ultraviolet light, midrange-
      wavelength

UVC
  ultraviolet C
  umbilical vein catheter
  umbilical venous catheter
  urgent visit center
UVCP
  unilateral vocal cord paralysis
UVEB
  unifocal ventricular ectopic beat
UVER
  ultraviolet-enhanced reactivation
UVGI
  ultraviolet germicidal irradiation
UVH
  univentricular heart
UVI
  ultraviolet irradiation
UVJ
  ureterovesical junction
UVL
  ultraviolet light
  umbilical venous line
UV/MV
  umbilical vein to maternal vein

UVP
  ultraviolet photometry
UVR
  ultraviolet radiation
UW
  unilateral weakness
U/WB
  unit of whole blood
UWF
  unknown white female
UWL
  unstirred water layer
UWM
  unknown white male
  unwed mother
UW solution
  University of Wisconsin solution
UX
  uranium X (proactinium)
UYP
  upper yield point

NOTES

U

V

coefficient of variation
electrical potential (in volts)
gas volume
logical binary relation that is true if any argument is true and false otherwise
luminous efficiency
lung volume
minute volume (of air or blood)
potential energy (joules)
unipolar chest lead
vaccinated
vaccine
vagina (*See also* VAG, Vag, vag)
valine (*See also* VAL, Val)
valve
vanadium (element)
variable (*See also* var)
variation (*See also* var)
varnish
vector
vegetarian
vegetation
vein (*See also* v)
velocity (*See also* v)
venous
venous (blood)
ventilation
ventral
ventricle
ventricular (fibrillation)
ventricular (wave)
venule
verb
verbal (comprehension factor)
vertebral
vertex sharp transient (electroencephalography)
Viagra as in "vitamin V"
violet
viral (*See also* Vir)
viral (antigen)
virulence (*See also* VI, Vi)
virus (*See also* v, Vir)
vision
visual acuity (*See also* VA)
visual capacity
voice
volt
voltage
volume (of gas) (*See also* q, vol)
vomiting

V1

trigeminal (fifth cranial) nerve, ophthalmic division

V2

trigeminal (fifth cranial) nerve, maxillary division

V3

trigeminal (fifth cranial) nerve, mandibular division

V̇

gas volume per unit of time (gas flow)
ventilation

+V

positive vertical divergence (*See also* +VD)

V₁-V₆

precordial chest leads

v

rate of reaction catalyzed by an enzyme
specific volume
vein (*See also* V)
velocity (*See also* V)
venous (blood) (*See also* VB)
versus
very
virus (*See also* V, Vir)
vitamin

v̄

mixed venous (blood)

+v

positive vertical divergence

v-

vicinal isomer

VA

alveolar ventilation
alveolar volume
vacuum aspiration
valeric acid
valproic acid
vancomycin
variant angina
vasodilator agent
venoarterial
ventricular arrhythmia
ventriculoatrial
ventroanterior
vertebral artery
Veteran's Administration Hospital
viral antigen
visual activity
visual acuity (*See also* V)
visual aid
visual axis

V

845

VA *(continued)*
>volcanic ash
>volt-amp *(See also* va)
>volume, alveolar
>volume averaging

V&A
>vagotomy and antrectomy

V/A
>variety
>volt/ampere

V$_A$
>alveolar ventilation per minute

V̇$_A$
>alveolar ventilation *(See also* alv vent)

Va
>arterial gas volume
>visual acuity

va
>volt-ampere *(See also* VA)

VAA
>verbal-auditory agnosia

VABES
>vasoablative endothelial sarcoma

VABP
>venoarterial bypass pumping

VAC
>vacuum-assisted closure (dressings)
>ventriculoarterial connection
>ventriculoatrial condition
>ventriculoatrial conduction

vac
>vaccine
>vacuum

VACA
>valvuloplasty and angioplasty of congenital anomalies

VacA
>vacuolating toxin gene A

VACB
>vacuum-assisted core biopsy

VA cc, VA ccl
>distance visual acuity with correction *(See also* VA ccl)

vacc
>vaccination

VACE
>*Vitex agnus-castus* extract (Chaste tree berry extract)

VAC EXT
>vacuum extractor

VACig
>vaccinia immune globulin

VACTERL
>vertebral, anal, cardiac, tracheal, esophageal, renal, limb (abnormalities)

>vertebral, vascular, anal, cardiac, tracheoesophageal, renal, and limb (anomalies)

VACV
>vaccinia virus

VAD
>vascular access device
>vascular access dressing
>venous access device
>ventricular assist device
>vertebral artery dissection
>virus-adjusting diluent
>vitamin A deficiency

VaD
>vascular dementia

VADCS
>ventricular atrial distal coronary sinus

VADS
>Visual Aural Digit Span Test

VAE
>venous air embolism

V$_A$eff
>effective alveolar ventilation

VAER
>visual auditory evoked response

VAFD
>Vasceze Vascular Access Flush Device

VAG, Vag, vag
>vagina *(See also* V)
>vaginal *(See also* V)
>vascular access graft

VAG HYST
>vaginal hysterectomy *(See also* VH)

VAGM
>vein of Galen aneurysmal malformation

VAH
>vertebral ankylosing hyperostosis
>virilizing adrenal hyperplasia

VAHBE
>ventricular atrial His bundle electrocardiogram

VAHRA
>ventricular atrial height right atrium

VAHS
>virus-associated hemophagocytic syndrome

VAIN
>vaginal intraepithelial neoplasia
>vaginal intraepithelial neoplasm

VAKT
>visual, association, kinesthetic, tactile (reading)

VAL, Val
>valine *(See also* V)

val
> valve

VALE
> visual acuity, left eye

VALI
> ventilator-associated lung injury

VAM
> ventricular arrhythmia monitor

VAMP
> venous/arterial management
> protection

VAMS
> Visual Analogue Mood Scale

VAN
> vein, artery, nerve
> ventricular aneurysmectomy

VANCO/P
> vancomycin-peak

VANCO/T
> vancomycin-trough

VAOD
> visual acuity, right eye

VAOS
> visual acuity, left eye

VA OS LP with P
> visual acuity, left eye, left
> perception with projection

VAP
> average path velocity
> variant angina pectoris
> venous access port
> ventilator-associated pneumonia

vap
> vapor

VAPCS
> ventricular atrial proximal coronary
> sinus

VAPP
> vaccine-associated paralytic polio
> vaccine-associated paralytic
> poliomyelitis

VAPS
> visual analog pain score
> volume-assured pressure support

VAR
> variant angina pectoris
> varicella (chickenpox) (varicella
> zoster virus) vaccine
> visual auditory range

var
> variable (*See also* V)
> variant

variation (*See also* V)
variety

VARE
> visual acuity, right eye

VARPRO
> variable projection method

VAS
> vagus nerve stimulation
> vascular (*See also* vasc)
> vasculotropin
> vasectomy (*See also* vas)
> vesicle attachment site
> vestibular aqueduct syndrome
> vibratory acoustic stimulation
> vibroacoustic stimulation
> viral analog scale
> Visual Analogue Scale (pain)

vas
> vasectomy (*See also* VAS)

VASC
> Verbal Auditory Screen for
> Children
> Visual Auditory Screen for
> Children

VA sc, VA scl
> distance visual acuity without
> correction

vasc
> vascular (*See also* VAS)

vasodil
> vasodilation (*See also* VD)
> vasodilator (*See also* VD)

VASPI
> Visual Analogue Self Assessment
> Scales For Pain Intensity

VAS RAD
> vascular radiology

VAT
> variable antigen type
> vasoocclusive angiotherapy
> ventilatory anaerobic threshold
> ventricular activation time
> ventricular (pacing), atrial (sensing),
> triggered (mode, pacemaker)
> vertebral artery test
> vestibular autorotational testing
> vestibular autorotation test
> video-assisted thoracoscopy
> visceral abdominal fat
> visceral adipose tissue
> visual action time

NOTES

VAT *(continued)*
    visual apperception test
    Vocational Apperception Test
VATER
    vertebral (abnormality), anal
      (imperforation), tracheoesophageal
      (fistula), radial, ray, or renal
      (anomalies)
    vertebral, anus, tracheoesophageal,
      radial, and renal (abnormalities)
VATS
    video-assisted thoracic surgery
    video-assisted thoracoscopic surgery
    video-assisted thoracoscopy
    video-assisted transthoracic surgery
VATs
    variable antigen, surface
VAT:TAT ratio
    visceral abdominal fat to total
      abdominal fat ratio
VAX-D
    vertebral axial decompression
VB
    vagina bulbi
    valence bond
    Van Buren (catheter)
    venous blood (*See also* v)
    ventrobasal
    Veronal buffer
    viable birth
    virtual bronchoscopy
    voided bladder
VB$_1$
    first voided bladder specimen
VB$_2$
    second midstream bladder specimen
VB$_3$
    third midstream bladder specimen
VBAC
    vaginal birth after cesarean
      (section)
VBAC-TOL
    vaginal birth after cesarean—trial
      of labor
VBAI, VBAIN
    vertebrobasilar artery insufficiency
VBD
    Veronal-buffered diluent
VBEF
    VanB *Enterococcus faecium*
V-beta
    beta-chain variable region
VBG
    vagotomy and Billroth
      gastroenterostomy
    vascularized bone graft
    venous blood gas

    Veronal-buffered (serum with)
      gelatin
    vertical banded gastroplasty
VBI
    vertebrobasilar insufficiency
    vertebrobasilar ischemia
    vertebrobasilar territory ischemia
VBIO
    Video Binocular indirect
      ophthalmoscope
VBM
    vertebral bone mass
vBMD
    volumetric bone mineral density
VBMT
    vascularized bone marrow
      transplantation
VBOS
    Veronal-buffered oxalated saline
VBP
    venous blood pressure
    ventricular premature beat
VBR
    ventricle-to-brain ratio
    ventricular-brain ratio
VBS
    venous blood sample
    Veronal-buffered saline
    vertebrobasilar (artery) system
    videofluoroscopic barium swallow
      (evaluation)
VBS:FBS
    Veronal-buffered saline-fetal bovine
      serum
VBT
    vertebral body tenderness
VC
    colored vision
    color vision
    pulmonary capillary blood volume
    vascular change
    vasoconstriction
    vena cava
    venous capacitance
    venous capillary
    ventilatory capacity
    ventral column
    verbal comprehension
    verbal cues
    vertebral canal
    videocassette
    vinyl chloride
    vision, color
    visual capacity
    visual communication
    visual cortex
    vital capacity
    vocal cord

volume, capillary
volume control
voluntary closing
voluntary control
vomiting center
vowel-consonant

V/C

ventilation-to-circulation (ratio)

V&C

vertical and centric (bite)

V$_c$

pulmonary capillary blood volume

Vc

pulmonary capillary blood volume
pulmonary capillary gas volume
ventrocaudal nucleus

VCA

antiviral capsid antigen
vancomycin, colistin, and
   anisomycin
vasoconstrictor assay
viral capsid antigen

VCA-EB

viral capsid antigen, Epstein-Barr

VCAM

vascular cell adhesion molecule

VCAM-1

vascular cell adhesion molecule-1

VCB

ventricular capture beat

VCC

vasoconstrictor center
ventral cell column

Vcc

vision with correction

VCCA

velocity, common carotid artery

VCD

vacuum constriction device
vibrational circular dichroism
vocal cord dysfunction

VCDF

volume-cycled decelerating-flow
   ventilation

VCDQ

verbal comprehension deviation
   quotient

VCE

vagina, ectocervix, and endocervix
vaginal cervical endocervical
   (smear)

V$_{CE}$

velocity of contractile element

VCF

vaginal contraceptive film
velocity of circumferential fiber
   (shortening) (*See also* V$_{CF}$)
ventricular contractility function

V$_{CF}$

velocity of circumferential fiber
   (shortening) (*See also* VCF)

V$_{cf}$

fiber shortening velocity

VCFS

velocardiofacial syndrome

VCG

vectorcardiogram
vectorcardiography
voiding cystogram

VCI

volatile corrosion inhibitor

V-Cillin

penicillin V

VCIU

voluntary control (of) involuntary
   utterances

vCJD

variant Creutzfeldt-Jakob disease

VCL

curvilinear velocity
volar carpal ligament

VCM

vinyl chloride monomer

VCN

vancomycin (hydrochloride),
   colistimethate (sodium), nysatatin
   (medium)
vestibulocochlear nerve
Vibrio cholerae neuraminidase

VCO, V$_{CO}$
carbon monoxide (endogenous
   production)
ventilator CPAP oxyhood

VCO$_2$, V$_{CO2}$, V$_{CO2}$
carbon dioxide elimination (*See also*
   VECO$_2$)
carbon dioxide (output)
venous carbon dioxide (production)
volume, carbon dioxide
   (elimination)

VCP

vocal cord paralysis

NOTES

VCR
    vasoconstriction rate
    video cassette recorder
    volume clearance rate
VCS
    vasoconstrictor substance
    vesicocervical space
    Vocabulary Comprehension Scale
VCSA
    viral cell surface antigen
VCSF
    ventricular cerebrospinal fluid
VCSPS
    variable circumference suprapatellar
      socket
VCT
    venous clotting time
    voluntary counseling and testing
VCTS
    vitreal corneal touch syndrome
VCU, VCUG
    vesicoureterogram
    videocystourethrogram
    videocystourethrography
    voiding cystourethrogram
    voiding cystourethrograph
    voiding cystourethrography
VCV
    ventricular conduction velocity
    volume-controlled ventilation
    volume-control ventilation
    vowel-consonant-vowel
VD
    valvular disease
    vapor density
    vascular disease
    vasodilation (*See also* vasodil)
    vasodilator (*See also* vasodil)
    venereal disease
    ventricular dilator
    vertical deviation
    video densitometry
    video disk
    viral diarrhea
    voided
    volume of distribution
V&D
    vomiting and diarrhea
+VD
    positive vertical divergence
V_D
    ventilation per minute of dead
      space
    volume of dead space (*See also*
      VDS)
V_d
    apparent volume of distribution

Vd
    volume of distribution
vd
    double vibrations
VDA
    venous digital angiogram
    video dimensional analysis
    visual discriminatory acuity
V_DA
    ventilation of alveolar dead space
    volume of alveolar dead space
VDAC
    vaginal delivery after cesarean
    voltage-dependent anion channel
$V_D$an
    ventilation of anatomic dead space
    volume of anatomic dead space
VDBR
    volume of distribution of bilirubin
VDC
    vasodilator center
VDCC
    voltage-dependent calcium channel
VDD
    atrial synchronous ventricular
      inhibited pacing
VDDR
    pseudovitamin D deficiency rickets
    vitamin D-dependent rickets
VDDR-II
    vitamin D-dependent rickets type II
VDEM
    vasodepressor material
VDF
    ventricular diastolic fragmentation
VDG, VD-G
    venereal disease, gonorrhea
vdg
    voiding
VDH
    valvular disease of heart
    vascular disease of heart
VDI
    venous distensibility index
VDJ
    variable diversity joining
VDL
    vasodepressor lipid
    visual detection level
VDM
    vasodepressor material
VD or M
    venous distention or mass
V_{DM}
    volume of mechanical dead space
VDO
    varus derotational osteotomy

VDP
ventricular premature depolarization

VDPCA
variable-dose patient-controlled anesthesia

VDR
venous diameter ratio
vitamin D receptor
volumetric diffusive respirator

V$_D$rb
rebreathing ventilation

VDRE
vitamin D-response element

VDRF
ventilator-dependent respiratory failure

VDRL
Venereal Disease Research Laboratory (test)

VDRR
vitamin D-resistant rickets

VDRS
Verdun Depression Rating Scale

VDS, VD-S
vasodepressor syncope
vasodilator substance
venereal disease-syphilis
venous duplex scanning
ventral derotating spinal (implant)
ventral derotation spondylodesis
vindesine
volume of dead space (See also V$_D$)

VDT
video display terminal
visual display terminal
visual distortion test

VDTS
video display terminal simulator

VDU
video display unit
visual display unit

VDV
ventricular (end-)diastolic volume

VD/VT
dead-space gas volume to tidal gas volume (ratio)

VE
expired volume
vacuum extraction
vaginal examination
vasoepididymostomy
Venezuelan encephalitis (virus)
venous emptying
venous extension
ventilation
ventricular elasticity
ventricular escape
ventricular extrasystole
vertex
vesicular exanthema
Vietnam era
viral encephalitis
virtual endoscopy
visual efficiency
visual examination
vitamin E
vocational evaluation
volume ejection
volume of expired gas
voluntary effort

V&E
Vinethine and ether (anesthesia)

V/E
violence and eloper

V$_E$
environmental variance
minute ventilation
peak exercise ventilation
respiratory minute volume
(volume) airflow per unit of time
volume of expired gas

Ve
ventilation

VEA
ventricular ectopic activity
ventricular ectopic arrhythmia
viral envelope antigen
viscoelastic agent

VEB
ventricular ectopic beat
ventricular extra beat

VEC
vecuronium
velocity-encoded cine

VECG
vector electrocardiogram

VE-cMRI
velocity-encoded cine-magnetic resonance imaging

VECO$_2$
carbon dioxide elimination

V

NOTES

VECP
visual-evoked cortical potential
visually evoked cortical potential

vect
vector

VED
vacuum erection device
vacuum extraction delivery
ventricular ectopic depolarization
vital exhaustion and depression

VEDP
ventricular end-diastolic pressure

VEE
vagina, ectocervix, and endocervix
Venezuelan equine encephalitis
(virus)
Venezuelan equine encephalomyelitis
(virus)

VEEa
Venezuelan equine encephalitis
vaccine, attenuated live

V-EEG
vigilance-controlled
electroencephalogram

VEEI
Venezuelan equine encephalitis
vaccine, inactivated

VEF
ventricular ejection fraction
visually evoked field

VEFR
visually evoked flow response

VEG
vegetation (bacterial)

VEGF
vascular endothelial growth factor

VEGF2
vascular endothelial growth factor
2

VEGFR3
vascular endothelial growth factor
receptor 3

VEGF/VPF
vascular endothelial growth
factor/vascular permeability factor

VEGI
vascular endothelial cell growth
inhibitor

V_{EH}
extrahepatic distribution

vehic
vehicle

vel, veloc
velocity

VELS
Vane Evaluation of Language
Scale

VELV
Vellore virus

VEM
vasoexcitor material
vergence eye movements

$V_{E\ max}$
maximal flow per unit of time

VEN
venlafaxine

venostasis
visual evoked potential

vent
ventilation
ventilator
ventral
ventricular

vent fib
ventricular fibrillation (*See also* VF,
v fib)

ventilator
respirator

ventric
ventricle

VEOS
very early onset schizophrenia

VEP
visual evoked potential

VER
ventricular escape rhythm
veratridine
visual evoked response

VERP
ventricular effective refractory
period

VERT
velocity-enhanced resistance training

vert
vertebra
vertebral
vertical

VES
ventricular extrasystole
video-endoscopic surgery
vitamin E succinate

ves.
bladder [L. *vesica*]
vesicular
vessel

VESS
videoendoscopic swallowing study

VESV
vesicular exanthema of swine virus

VET
vestigial testis

vet
veteran
veterinarian
veterinary

VETS
    Veterans (Adjustment) Scale
VE/VCO$_2$
    ventilation/carbon dioxide production
VEWA
    Vocational Evaluation and Work
    Adjustment
VF
    left leg electrode for
        electrocardiogram
    ventricular fibrillation (*See also* vent
        fib, v fib)
    ventricular fluid
    ventricular flutter
    ventricular fusion
    vertical float (aquatic therapy)
    video frequency
    vigil, fatiguing
    visual field (*See also* F, Vf, VFD)
    vitreous fluorophotometry
    vocal fremitus
V$_f$
    variant frequency
Vf, vf
    visual field (*See also* F, VF, VFD)
VFA
    volatile fatty acid
Vfactor
    verbal (comprehension) factor
VFC
    Actis venous flow controller
    Vaccines for Children (program)
    venous flow controller
    ventricular function curve
VFCB
    vertical flow clean bench
VFD
    visual feedback display
    visual field
    vocal fold dysfunction
VFDF
    very fast death factor
VFDT
    Visual Form Discrimination Test
VFES
    videofluorographic evaluation of
        swallowing
VFFC
    visual fields full to confrontation
VFI
    visual field intact (*See also* VFIT)

Visual Functioning index
vocal fold injection
v fib
    ventricular fibrillation (*See also* vent
        fib, VF)
VFIT
    visual field intact (*See also* VFI)
VFL
    ventricular flutter
VFO
    variable flexion overhinge
VFP
    ventricular filling pressure
    ventricular fluid pressure
    vertical float progression (aquatic
        therapy)
    vitreous fluorophotometry
VFR
    voiding flow rate
VFS
    vascular fragility syndrome
VFSS
    videofluoroscopic swallowing study
VFT
    venous filling time
    ventricular fibrillation threshold
    Verbal Fluency Test
VFW
    velocity waveform
VG
    vein graft
    ventilated group
    ventricular gallop
    ventroglutcal
    very good
V&G
    vagotomy and gastroenterotomy
V$_G$
    genetic variance
VGA
    villoglandular adenocarcinoma
VGAD
    vein of Galen aneurysmal dilatation
VGAM
    vein of Galen aneurysmal
        malformation
VGB
    vigabatrin (Sabril)
VGCC
    voltage-gated calcium channel
VGE
    viral gastroenteritis

NOTES

853

VGH

very good health
veterinary general hospital

VGP

viral glycoprotein

VGPO

volume-guaranteed pressure option

VGTT

video graphic tool technology

VH

vaginal hysterectomy (*See also*
VAG HYST)
venous hematocrit
ventricular hypertrophy
vestibular hyperreactivity
viral hepatitis
visual hallucinations
vitreous hemorrhage
von Herrick (grading system)

V$_H$

hepatic distribution volume
variable domain of heavy chain
immunoglobulin

VH I

very narrow anterior chamber
angles

VH II

moderately narrow anterior chamber
angles

VH III

moderately wide open anterior
chamber angles

VH IV

wide open anterior chamber angles

VHC

valved holding chamber

VHD

valvular heart disease
vascular hemostatic device
ventricular heart disease
viral hematodepressive disease

VHDL

very high density lipoprotein

VHDPB

very high dose phenobarbital

VHF

very high frequency
viral hemorrhagic fever
visual half-field

VHI

voice handicap index

Vhigh

high regional wall motion velocity

vHL

von Hippel-Lindau (syndrome)

VHN

Vickers hardness number

VHP

vaporized hydrogen peroxide

VHSV

viral hemorrhagic septicemia virus

VI

inspired ventilation
untouched girl (virgin) [L. *virgo
intacta*]
vaginal irrigation
variable interval
vascular invasion
vastus intermedius
velocity index
ventilation index
virulence (*See also* V, Vi)
virulent (*See also* Vi, vir)
viscosity index
Visual Imagery
visual impairment
visual inspection
visually impaired
vitality index
volume index

V$_I$

volume of inspired gas (per
minute)

Vi

virulence (*See also* V, VI)
virulent (*See also* VI, vir)

VIA

virus-inactivating agent
virus infection-associated antigen

via

by way of

VIB

Vocational Interest Blank

vib

vibration

VIBS

vocabulary, information, block
(design), and similarities
(psychology)

VIC

Values Inventory for Children
vasoinhibitory center
vehicle for initial crawling
visual communication
visual communication (therapy)
voice intensity controller

VICA

velocity internal carotid artery

V-ICD

ventricular implantable cardioverter-
defibrillator

VID

vaginal intraepithelial dysplasia
videodensitometry

visible iris diameter
vitellointestinal duct
VIDA
vitiligo disease activity
VIESA
Vocational Interest, Experience, and
Skill Assessment
VIF
virus-induced interferon
VIG
vaccinia-immune globulin
vaccinia immunoglobulin
VIg
vaccinia immunoglobulin (*See also*
VIg)
vig
vigorous
VIH
Spanish and French abbreviation
for human immunodeficiency
virus
violence-induced handicap
VILI
ventilator-induced lung injury
VIM
ventralis intermedius
video-intensification microscopy
VIN
vaginal intraepithelial neoplasia
vinbarbital
vulvar intraepithelial neoplasia
VINV
Vinces virus
VIP
Validity Indicator Profile
vasoactive intestinal peptide
vasoactive intestinal polypeptide
vasoactive intracorporeal
pharmacotherapy
vasoinhibitory peptide
venous impedance plethysmography
very important patient
very important person
voluntary interruption of pregnancy
VIP-DAC
vaginal interruption of pregnancy
with dilatation and curettage
VIP-IR
vasoactive intestinal polypeptide
immunoreactivity

VIPoma
vasoactive intestinal peptide-
secreting tumor
vasoactive intestinal polypeptide
tumor
VIQ
Verbal Intelligence Quotient
Vocational Interest Questionnaire
VIR
virology
Vir
viral (*See also* V)
virus (*See also* V, v)
vir
green [L. *viridis*]
virulent (*See also* VI, Vi)
VIS
Vaccine Information Statement
vaginal irrigation smear
venous insufficiency syndrome
vertebral irritation syndrome
video imaging system
visceral manipulative treatment
visible
Visual Impairment Service
visual information storage
vocational interest schedule
vis
vision
visiting
visitor
visual
VISA
vancomycin-insensitive
Staphylococcus aureus
vancomycin-intermediate-resistant
Staphylococcus aureus
Vocational Interest and
Sophistication Assessment
VISC
vitreous infusion suction cutter
visc
viscera
visceral
viscosity
viscous
VISI
volar (flexed) intercalated segment
instability
Viso V
volume of Isoflow

V

NOTES

VIT
> venom immunotherapy
> vital (*See also* vit)
> vitamin (*See also* Vit)

Vit
> vitamin (*See also* VIT)

vit
> vital (*See also* VIT)
> vitrectomy
> vitreous

vital signs (*See also* VS, vs)

vit cap
> vital capacity
> vitamin capsule

vitel.
> yolk [L. *vitellus*]

vitr, vitr.
> glass [L. *vitrum*]
> vitreous

vits
> vitamins

VIU
> visual internal urethrotomy

viz
> visualized

viz.
> that is, namely [L. *videlicet*]

VJ
> ventriculojugular (shunt)
> Vogel-Johnson (agar)

VK
> vervet (African green monkey) kidney (cell)

VKC
> vernal keratoconjunctivitis

VKDB
> vitamin K deficiency bleeding

VKHS
> Vogt-Koyanagi-Harada syndrome

VL
> left arm electrode for electrocardiogram
> vastus lateralis
> ventralis lateralis
> ventrolateral
> vial
> viral load
> visceral leishmaniasis
> vision, left (eye)

V_L
> (actual) volume of lung
> variable domain of light chain immunoglobulin

VLA
> vanillacetic acid
> very late activation
> very-late antigen

> virus-like action
> virus-like agent

VLA-4
> very late antigen-4

VLAD
> variable life-adjusted display

VLAP
> vaporization laser ablation of the prostate
> visual laser ablation of prostate
> visual laser-assisted prostatectomy

VLBR
> very low birth rate

VLBW
> very low birth weight

VLBWPN
> very low birth weight preterm neonate

VLCAD
> very long chain acyl-CoA dehydrogenase
> very long chain acyl coenzyme A dehydrogenase

VLCD
> very low calorie diet

VLCFA
> very long chain fatty acid

VLD
> very low density

VLDL, VLDLP
> very low density lipoprotein

VLDL-C
> very low density lipoprotein C

VLDL-TG
> very low density lipoprotein-triglyceride

VLDS
> Verbal Language Development Scale

VLE
> vision left eye

VLF
> very low frequency

VLG
> ventral (nucleus of) lateral geniculate (body)

VLH
> ventrolateral (nucleus of) hypothalamus

VLIA
> virus-like infectious agent

VLM
> ventrolateral medulla
> virtual labor monitor
> visceral larva migrans

VLP
> ventricular late potential

ventriculolumbar perfusion
virus-like particle
VLPP
Valsalva leak point pressure
VLR
vastus lateralis release
VLS
vascular leak syndrome
VLSI
very large scale integration
VM
vasomotor
vastus medialis
vector magnitude
venous malformation
ventilated mask
Ventimask
ventricular mass
ventromedial
Venturi mask
vestibular membrane
viomycin
viral myocarditis
voltme
voltmeter
V/m
volt per meter
VMA
vanillylmandelic acid
vastus medialis advancement
V-mask
Venturi mask
VMAT
vesicular monoamine transporter
V$_{MAX}$
maximal velocity
V$_{max}$
maximal velocity
maximum velocity
peak flow velocity (Doppler)
VMC
vasomotor center
vinyl chloride monomer
void metal composite
von Meyenburg complex
VMCG
vector magnetocardiogram
VMD
vertical maxillary deficiency
VME
vertical maxillary excess

VMETH
volumetric multiple exposure
transmission holography
VMF
vasomotor flushing
VMGT
Visual-Motor Gestalt Test
VMH
ventromedial hypothalamic (neuron,
nuclei)
VMI
visual-motor integration
VMIT
visual-motor integration test
VMN
ventromedial nucleus
ventromedial nucleus of the
hypothalamus
VMO
vastus medialis oblique (muscle)
vastus medialis obliquus musculus
VMO:VL
vastus medialis obliquus:vastus
lateralis (ratio)
VMO:VL EMG
vastus medialis obliquus:vastus
lateralis (ratio) electromyographic
VMR
vasomotor response
vasomotor rhinitis
VMS
vanilla milkshake
Visual Memory Score
visual memory span
VMSC
Vineland Measurement of Social
Competence
VMST
Visual-Motor Sequencing Test
VMT
vasomotor tone
ventilatory muscle training
ventromedial tegmentum
VMU
vertebral motion unit
VN
vesical neck
vestibular neurectomy
vestibular nucleus
virus neutralization
virus-neutralizing
visceral nucleus

V

NOTES

VN *(continued)*
    visual naming
    vomeronasal

VNA
    virus-neutralizing antibody

VNC
    vesical neck contracture

VNDPT
    Visual Numerical Discrimination
      Pretest

VNE
    vascularization elsewhere in the
      retina
    verbal nonemotional stimuli
    video nasendoscopy

VNO
    vomeronasal organ

VNR
    ventral nerve root
    verbal, numerical, and reasoning
    vinorelbine

VNS
    vagus nerve stimulation
    villonodular synovitis

VNSSL
    video-assisted thoracic surgical non-
      rib-spreading lobectomy

VNTR
    variable numbers of tandem repeats

VO
    verbal order
    volume overload
    voluntary opening

VO$_2$
    aerobic capacity
    oxygen consumption (per minute)
    peak exercise oxygen consumption
    volume oxygen consumption
    volume of oxygen consumption per
      unit of time

V$_o$
    oral airflow in liters per second

Voa
    ventralis oralis anterior

VOC
    volatile organic compound

voc
    vocational

vocab
    vocabulary

VOCOR
    vasoocclusive crisis
    void on-call to operating room
      (*See also* VOCTOR)

VOCs
    volatile organic compounds

VOCTOR
    void on call to operating room
      (*See also* VOCOR)

VOD
    venoocclusive disease
    vision, right eye [L. *visio, oculus
      dexter*]

VOE
    vascular occlusive episode

VO$_2$ HR
    heart rate (pulse)

VOI
    Vocational Opinion Index

VO2I
    oxygen consumption index

vol
    volar
    volatile
    volume (*See also* q, V)
    volumetric
    voluntary
    volunteer

vol%
    volume percent

vol adm
    voluntary admission

vol/vol
    volume per volume (ratio)

VOM
    vinyl chloride monomer
    volt-ohm-millimeter

vom
    vomited

VO$_2$ max, VO$_2$max
    maximal oxygen consumption
    maximum oxygen consumption
    maximum oxygen uptake

VOO
    continuous ventricular asynchronous
      pacing

VOP
    venous occlusion plethysmography
    ventralis oralis posterior

VOR
    vestibuloocular reflex
    vestibuloocular response

VORP
    vibrating ossicular prosthesis

VOS
    vision, left eye [L. *visio oculus
      sinister*]
    voice outcome survey

VOSS
    visual observation shivering score

VOT
    Visual Organization Test
    voice onset time

VOU

vision, each eye [L. *visio oculus uterque*]

visio oculus uterque (vision of each eye)

voxel

volume element

VP

vapor pressure
variably positive
variegate porphyria
vascular permeability
vasopressin
velopharyngeal
venipuncture
venous pressure (*See also* Pv)
venous (volume) plethysmograph
ventricles to peritoneal cavity (shunt)
ventricular pacing
ventricular peritoneal
ventricular premature (beat)
ventriculoperitoneal (shunt)
ventroposterior
vertex potential
viral protein
virus protein
visual perception
Voges-Proskauer (medium, test)
voiding pressure
volume-pressure
vulnerable period

V&P

vagotomy and pyloroplasty
ventilation and perfusion

Vp

plasma volume
voltage peak
volumetric lung depth

vp

vapor pressure

VPA

valproic acid
ventricular premature activation
Vocal Profiles Analysis

v-PA

vascular plasminogen activator

V-Pad

sanitary napkin

VPAP

variable positive airway pressure

VPB

ventricular premature beat

VPC

vapor-phase chromatography
velopharyngeal competence
ventricular premature complex
ventricular premature contraction
volume of packed cells
volume-packed cells
volume percentage

VPCT

ventricular premature contraction threshold

VPD

velopharyngeal dysfunction
ventricular premature depolarization

VPd

venous dialysis pressure

VPDC

ventricular premature depolarization contraction

VPDF

vegetable protein diet (plus) fiber

V$_{pe}$

peak ejection velocity

VPF

vascular permeability factor

VPF/VEGF

vascular permeability factor/vascular endothelial cell growth factor

VPG

velopharyngeal gap
venting percutaneous gastrostomy

VPGSS

venous pressure gradient support stockings

VPI

vasopeptidase inhibitor
velopharyngeal incompetence
velopharyngeal insufficiency
ventral posterior inferior
ventroposteroinferior
Vocational Planning Inventory
Vocational Preference Inventory

VPL

ventral posterolateral (nucleus)
ventroposterolateral

VPM

Vantage Performance monitor
venous pressure module
ventilator pressure manometer

NOTES

V

VPM *(continued)*
    ventralis posteromedialis
    ventroposteromedial
vpm
    vibration per minute
7VPnC
    7-valent pneumococcal conjugate
VPO
    velopharyngeal opening
VPP
    viral porcine pneumonia
VPR
    virtual patient record
    volume-pressure response
vpr
    viral protein R
VPRC, VPRBC
    volume of packed red (blood) cells
VPS
    valvular pulmonic stenosis
    ventriculoperitoneal shunt
    visual pleural space
vps
    vibration per second
VPT
    vascularized patellar tendon
    vibration perception threshold
VPTEF/VT
    volume to peak expiratory flow
      and total expiratory volume
VQ
    voice quality
V̇/Q, V/Q, V̇/Q̇
    ventilation/perfusion
    ventilation/perfusion ratio
VQR
    ventilation/perfusion(-quotient) ratio
VR
    right arm electrode for
      electrocardiogram
    valve replacement
    valvular regurgitation
    variable rate
    variable ratio
    vascular resistance
    velocity ratio
    venous reflux
    venous resistance
    venous return
    ventilation rate
    ventilation ratio
    ventricular rate
    ventricular response
    ventricular rhythm
    verbal reprimand
    vesicular rosette
    vision, right (eye)
    visual reproduction

    vital record
    vitreoretinal
    vocal resonance
    vocational rehabilitation
V2R
    vasopressin receptor
Vr
    volume of relaxation
VRA
    visual reinforcement audiometry
    visual response audiometry
VRBC
    volume of red blood cells
VRC
    venous renin concentration
    vocational rehabilitation counselor
VRCP
    vitreoretinochoroidopathy
VRD
    ventricular radial dysplasia
VRE
    vancomycin-resistant *Enterococcus*
    vision right eye
VR&E
    vocational rehabilitation and
      education
VREF
    vancomycin-resistant *Enterococcus*
      faecium
VRG
    vertical ring gastroplasty
VRI
    viral respiratory infection
VRL
    ventral root, lumbar
VRNA
    viral ribonucleic acid
VRO
    varus rotational osteotomy
VROM
    voluntary range of motion
VRP
    very reliable product
    vocational rehabilitation program
VRR
    ventral root reflex
VRS
    viral rhinosinusitis
    volume reduction surgery
VRSA
    vancomycin-resistant *Staphylococcus*
      aureus
VRT
    variance of resident time
    venous refill time
    venous return time
    ventral root, thoracic
    vertical radiation topography

Visual Retention Test
vocational rehabilitation therapy

VRU

ventilator rehabilitation unit

VRV

ventricular rate variability
ventricular residual volume
Virgin River virus

VS

vaccination scar
vaccine serotype
vagal stimulation
Valsalva maneuver
valve system
variable softness
vasospasm
vegetative state
venesection
ventral subiculum
ventricular sense
ventricular septum
ventriculosubarachnoid
verbal scale
vertical shear
very sensitive
vesicular sound
vesicular stomatitis
vestibular schwannoma
veterinary surgeon
videostroboscopy
villonodular synovitis
visit
visited
visual storage
vital signs (*See also* vs)
volumetric solution
voluntary sterilization

V·s

volt-second

vs

single vibration
vibration-second
vital sign (*See also* VS)
voids

vs.

against [L. *versus*]

VSA

variant-specific surface antigen
vasospastic angina

VSADP

vocational skills assessment and
development program

VSAT

Visual Search and Attention Test

VSAV

vesicular stomatitis Alagoas virus

VSBE

very short below elbow (cast)

VSC

vertebral subluxation complex
volatile sulfur compound
voluntary surgical contraception

VSCC

voltage-sensitive calcium channel

VSCS

ventricular specialized conduction
system

VSD

Vaccine Safety Datalink
vascular septal defect
ventricular septal defect
ventriculoseptal defect
vesical external sphincter
dyssynergia
virtually safe dose

VSED

voluntarily stopping eating and
drinking

VSF

Vermont spinal fixator

VSFP

venous stop flow pressure

VSG

variant surface glycoprotein

VSHD

ventricular septal heart defect

VSI

visual motor integration

VSIV

vesicular stomatitis Indiana virus

VSL

straight line velocity

VSMC

vascular smooth muscle cell

VSMS

Vineland Social Maturity Scale

VSN

vital signs normal

vsn

vision

VSNJV

vesicular stomatitis New Jersey
virus

NOTES

VSO
vertical sagittal split osteotomy
vertical subcondylar oblique

VSOK
vital signs okay (normal)

VSP
variable screw placement
variable screw plate
variable spinal plating
vertical stabilization program

VSQOL
Vital Signs Quality of Life

VSR
venereal spirochetosis of rabbits
venous stasis retinopathy

VSS
apparent volume of distribution
videofluoroscopic swallowing study
vital signs stable

VSSAF
vital signs stable, afebrile

VST
visual search task

VSULA
vaccination scar upper left arm

VSV
vesicular stomatitis virus

VSW
ventricular stroke work

V SYNC
vertical synchronization pulse

Vsys
systolic wall motion velocity

VT
tetrazolium violet (stain)
tidal volume (*See also* TD, TV, V_T)
total ventilation
unsustained ventricular tachycardia
vacuum tube
vacuum tuberculin
validation therapy
vasotocin
venous thrombosis
ventricular tachyarrhythmia
ventricular tachycardia
verocytotoxin
verotoxin

V&T
volume and tension

V_T
tidal volume (*See also* TD, TV, VT)

V_t
pulmonary parenchymal tissue volume

VTA
ventral tegmental area
ventricular tachyarrhythmia

V_TA
alveolar tidal volume

V-TACH, V tach
ventricular tachycardia

VTBI
volume to be infused

VTCL
ventricular tachycardia cycle length

VTE
venous thromboembolism
ventricular tachycardia event

VTEC
verocytotoxin-producing *Escherichia coli*
verotoxin-producing *Escherichia coli*

VTED
venous thromboembolic disease

V-test
Voluter test (radiology)

VTG
volume thoracic gas

V_{TG}
thoracic gas volume

VTI
volume thickness index

VTL
viscerotropic leishmaniasis

VTM
mechanical tidal volume
variegated translocation mosaicism
virus transport medium

VT-NS
ventricular tachycardia nonsustained

VTO
visualized treatment objective

VTOP, VTP
voluntary termination of pregnancy

VTQS
Voc-Tech Quick Screener

VTS
vesicular transport system
volunteer transport service

VT-S
ventricular tachycardia sustained

VTSRS
Verdun Target Symptom Rating Scale

VTT
voice termination time

VT/VF
ventricular tachycardia/ventricular fibrillation

VTVM
vacuum tube voltmeter

VTX
vertex (presentation)
VU
varicose ulcer
very urgent
vesicoureteral (reflux)
volume unit (meter)
V/U
verbalize understanding
VUC
vacuum uterine cannula
voiding urine cytology
VUE
villitis of unknown etiology
VUJ
vesicoureteral junction
VUPM
voiding urethral pressure
measurement
VUPP
voiding urethral pressure
measurements
VUR
vesicoureteral reflux (grade I–V)
VURD
valves, unilateral reflux, dysplasia
VUSE
variable-angle uniform signal
excitation
VUV
vacuum ultraviolet
VV
vaccinia virus
varicose vein
venovenous
vesicovaginal (fistula) (*See also*
VVF)
V-V
ventriculovenous (shunt)
V/V
volume-to-volume (ratio)
V&V
vulva and vagina
V_{DS}/V_T
dead-space gas volume to tidal gas
volume ratio
vv
veins
venae
v/v
vice versa

VVA
venous-to-venous anastomosis
VVB
venovenous bypass
VVC
vulvovaginal candidiasis
VVD
vaginal vertex delivery
vascular volume of distribution
VVETP
Vietnam Veterans Evaluation and
Treatment Program
VVF
vesicovaginal fistula (*See also* VV)
VVFR
vesicovaginal fistula repair
VVG
Verhoeff-Van Gieson
VVI
ventricular demand pacing
vvi
vocal velocity index
VVL
varicose veins ligation
verruca vulgaris of the larynx
VVM
vertical vesicomyotomy
VVOR
visually enhanced vestibuloocular
reflex
visual vestibuloocular reflex
VVQ
verbalizer-visualization questionnaire
VVR
ventricular response rate
VvRI
venae rectales inferiores (*See also*
PRI)
VVS
vesicovaginal space
vulvar vestibulitis syndrome
VVT
ventricular synchronous pacing
VW
vascular wall
vessel wall
v/w
volume per weight
VWD
ventral wall defect
vWD, vWd
von Willebrand disease

V

NOTES

VWF

velocity waveform

vibration-induced white finger

VWFT

variable-width forms tractor

VWM

ventricular wall motion

VX-478

amprenavir

Vx

vertex

vitrectomy

V-XT

V-pattern exotropia

V-Y

shape of incisions in V-Y plasty

VZ, V-Z

varicella-zoster (virus) (*See also* VZV)

VZIg

varicella-zoster immune globulin

VZL

vinzolidine

VZV

chickenpox (varicella zoster virus)

varicella-zoster virus (*See also* VZ)

VZVV

varicella-zoster virus vaccine

W

dominant spotting (mouse)
energy (work)
section modulus
shape of surgical incisions (W-plasty)
tryptophan (*See also* TP, Tp, Trp)
tungsten
tungsten [Ger. *wolfram*]
wash
water
watt (*See also* w)
wearing glasses
Weber (test)
week (*See also* w, WK, wk)
wehnelt (aperture)
weight (*See also* w)
well
west
wetting
white (*See also* w, Wh, wh, wt)
white cell
whole (response) (*See also* WR)
widowed
width
wife
Wilcoxon rank sum statistic
Wistar (rat)
with (*See also* w, c̄, w/)
wolframium (tungsten)
word fluency
work

W-1

insignificant (allergies)

W-3

minimal (allergies)

W-5

moderate (allergies)

W-7

moderate-severe (allergies)

W-9

severe (allergies)

^{188}W

tungsten-188

W+

weakly positive

w

watt (*See also* W)
week (*See also* W, WK, wk)
weight (*See also* W)
white (*See also* W, Wh, wh, wt)
widowed
wife

WA

when awake
while awake
white American
wide awake (*See also* W/A)
with assistance

w/, w̄

with (*See also* W, c̄)

W/A

watt/ampere
wide awake (*See also* WA)

W or A

weakness or atrophy

WAB, WABT

Western Aphasia Battery
Western Aphasia Battery Test

WACH

wedge adjustable cushioned heel (shoe)

WADAO

weak and dizzy all over

WADIC

Wing Autistic Disorder Interview Checklist

WAF

weakness, atrophy, and fasciculation

WAGR

Wilms (tumor), aniridia, genitourinary (abnormalities), and (mental) retardation

WAI

Weinberger Adjustment Inventory
wheat amylase inhibitor

WAIHA

warm autoimmune hemolytic anemia

WAIS

Wechsler Adult Intelligence Scale

WAIS-III

Wechsler Adult Intelligence Scale-Third Edition

WAIS-R

Wechsler Adult Intelligence Scale, Revised

WAK

wearable artificial kidney

WALK

weight-activated locking knee (prosthesis)

WALV

Wallal virus

WAMBA

Wise areola mastopexy breast augmentation

WANV

Wanowrie virus

W

WAP
  wandering atrial pacemaker
  whole abdominopelvic irradiation
WAPT
  Weidel Auditory Processing Test
WAQ
  Work Attitudes Questionnaire
WARF
  warfarin
WARI
  wheezing associated respiratory
  infection
WARV
  Warrego virus
WAS
  Ward Atmosphere Scale
  (psychology)
  weekly activity summary
  whiplash-associated disorder
WASID
  Warfarin-Aspirin Symptomatic
  Intracranial Disease
WASO
  wake after sleep onset time
  wakefulness after sleep onset
WASP
  Weber Advanced Spatial Perception
  (test)
  white Anglo-Saxon Protestant
  Wiskott-Aldrich syndrome protein
Wass
  Wasserman (reaction, test)
WAT
  white adipose tissue
  Word Association Test
WB
  waist belt
  washable base
  washed bladder
  water bottle
  Wechsler-Bellevue (Scale)
  weightbearing
  well baby
  Western blot
  wet bulb
  whole blood (*See also* B, QB, W
  Bld)
  whole body
  Willowbrook
Wb
  weber (unit of magnetic flux)
WBA
  wax bean agglutinin
  whole-body activity
Wb/A
  weber per ampere
WBACT
  whole blood activated clotting time

WBAPTT
  whole-blood activated partial
  thromboplastin time
WBAT
  weightbearing as tolerated
WBC
  well-baby clinic
  white blood cell
  white blood corpuscle
WBC/hpf
  white blood cells per high-power
  field
WBCT
  whole-blood clotting time
WBD
  weeks by dates (for gestational
  age)
WBDS
  whole-body digital scanner
WBE
  weeks by examination (for
  gestational age)
  whole-body extract
WBF
  whole-blood folate
WBH
  weight-based heparin (dosing)
  whole-blood hematocrit
  whole-body hyperthermia
WBI
  whole body irradiation
  whole-bowel irrigation
  will be in
W Bld
  whole blood (*See also* B, QB,
  WB)
WBM
  whole boiled milk
Wb/m^2
  weber per square meter
WBN
  well-baby nursery
  well-born nursery
  wide band noise
WBNAA
  whole-brain N-acetylaspartate
WBOS
  wide base of support
WBP
  whole body protein
WBPTT
  whole-blood partial thromboplastin
  time
WBQC
  wide-base quad cane
WBR
  whole-body radiation
  whole-body retention

WBRS
    Ward Behavior Rating Scale
WBRT
    whole-blood recalcification time
    whole-brain radiation therapy
    whole-brain radiotherapy
WBS
    Wechsler-Bellevue Scale
    weeks by size (for gestational age)
    whole-body scan
    whole-body shower
    withdrawal body shakes
    wound-breaking strength
WBT
    wet bulb temperature
WBTT
    weightbearing to tolerance
WBUS
    weeks by ultrasound
WBV
    whole blood volume
WC
    ward confinement
    warm compress
    water closet
    wet compress
    wheelchair (*See also* W/C, wh ch,
      CH)
    when called
    white cell
    white (cell) cast
    white (cell) count
    whole complement
    whooping cough
    will call
    work capacity
    workers' compensation
    writer's cramp
W/C
    wheelchair (*See also* WC, wh ch,
      CH)
WCA
    work capacity assessment
WCB
    will call back
WCC
    well-child care
    white cell count
WCD
    wearable cardioverter-defibrillator

WCE
    white coat effect
    work capacity evaluation
WCH
    white coat hypertension
WCL
    whole-cell lysate
WC/LC
    warm compresses and lid scrubs
WCM
    whole cow's milk
WCOT
    wall coated open tubular
wcp
    whole chromosome paint
WCS
    Wisconsin Compression System
    work capacity specialist
WCST
    Wisconsin Card Sorting Test
WCT
    wide-complex tachycardia
WD
    wallerian degeneration
    ward
    warm and dry (*See also* W/D)
    well-developed (agar)
    well-differentiated
    wet dressing
    Whitney Damon (dextrose)
    with disease
    withdrawal dyskinesia
    without dyskinesia
    word (*See also* Wd)
    working distance
    wound (*See also* WND, wnd)
    wrist disarticulation
W4D
    Worth four-dot (test for fusion)
W/D
    warm (and) dry (*See also* WD)
    withdrawal
    withdrawn
W→D
    wet-to-dry (*See also* W-T-D)
Wd
    ward
    word (*See also* WD)
wd
    wound
    wounded

W

NOTES

WDCA
well-differentiated carcinoma

WDCC
well-developed collateral circulation

WDE
wound dressing emulsion

WDF
white divorced female

WDFA
well-differentiated fetal
adenocarcinoma

WDHA
watery diarrhea, hypokalemia, and
achlorhydria (syndrome)
watery diarrhea with hypokalemic
alkalosis

WDI
warfarin dose index

WDL
within defined limits
Wood-Downes-Lecks

WDRC
wide dynamic range compression

WDS
watery diarrhea syndrome
wet dog shakes (syndrome)
word discrimination score
wounds (*See also* wds)

wds
wounds (*See also* WDS)

WDWN, WD,WN
well-developed, well-nourished

WDXRF
wavelength-dispersive x-ray
fluorescence

WE
wage earner
wax ester
weekend (*See also* W/E)
Wernicke encephalopathy
whiskey equivalent

W/E
weekend (*See also* WE)

WEBINO
wall-eyed bilateral internuclear
ophthalmoplegia

WE-D
withdrawal-emergent dyskinesia

WEE
western equine encephalomyelitis
(virus)

WeeFIM
Functional Independence Measure
for Children

WEG
water-ethyleneglycol

WEMINO
wall-eyed monocular internuclear
ophthalmoplegia

WEP
weekend pass

WES
wall-echo shadow

WESR
Westergren erythrocyte
sedimentation rate
Wintrobe erythrocyte sedimentation
rate

WESSV
Wesselsbron virus

WEST
Weinstein enhanced sensory test
work evaluation systems technology

WEUP
willful exposure to unwanted
pregnancy

WF
well flexed
wet film
white female (*See also* W/F, wf)
wide field
Wistar-Furth (rat)
word fluency
Working Formulation for Clinical
Usage

W/F, wf
weakness and fatigue
white female (*See also* WF)

W FEEDS
with feedings

WFH
white-faced hornet

WFI
water for injection

WFL
within full limits
within functional limits

WFLC
white female living child

WF-O
will follow in office

WFR
wheal-and-flare reaction

WFRT
wide-field radiation therapy

WFSS
Wolpe Fear Survey Schedule

WG
water gauge
Wegener granulomatosis
Wright-Giemsa (stain)

WGA
wheat germ agglutinin

WGRV
Wongorr virus
WGTS
whole-gut transit scintigraphy
WH
walking heel (cast)
well-healed
well-hydrated
whole homogenate
wound healing
W/H
weight/height
Wh
white (*See also* W, w, wh, wt)
wh
whisper
whispered
white (*See also* W, w, Wh, wt)
wh
watt-hour
WHA
warmed, humidified air
WIIAV
Whataroa virus
wh ch
wheelchair (*See also* WC, W/C, CH)
white child
WHECS
wrist hand extension compression support
WHI
Women's Health Initiative
WHIS
War Head-Injury Score
WHMS
well-healed midline scar
WHNR
well-healed, no residuals
WHNS
well-healed, nonsymptomatic
well-healed, no sequelae
WHO
wrist-hand orthosis
WHOART
World Health Organization Adverse Reaction Terms (Terminology)
WHOQOL-100
World Health Organization Quality of Life 100-Item (instrument)
WHP, Whp, whp
whirlpool (*See also* WP, W/P)

WHPB
whirlpool bath (*See also* WPB)
WHR
(ratio of) waist to hip (circumference)
waist-to-hip ratio
whr
watt hour
WHS
Wolf-Hirschhorn syndrome
Women's Health Study
WHV
woodchuck hepatic virus
WHVP
wedge hepatic venous pressure
WHYMPI
Westhaven Yale Multidimensional Pain Inventory
WHZ
wheezes
WI
ventricular demand pacing
walk-in (patient)
wash-in
water ingestion
waviness index
weaning index
W/I
within
W&I
work and interest
WIA
wounded in action
WIC
Women, Infants, and Children (Program)
wid
widow
widowed
widower
WIED
walk-in emergency department
WIFC
widely invasive follicular carcinoma
win.
wound-induced
WIP
work in progress
WIPI
Word Intelligibility by Picture Identification

W

NOTES

WIQ
Waring Intimacy Questionnaire
WIS
Ward Incapacity Scale
Ward Initiation Scale
Wechsler Intelligence Scale
WISC
Wechsler Intelligence Scale for
Children
WISC-III
Wechsler Intelligence Scale for
Children III
WISC-R
Wechsler Intelligence Scale for
Children-Revised
WISH
Wistar Institute Susan Hayflick
(cell)
WIST
Whitaker Index of Schizophrenic
Thinking
WiST
time without symptoms of
progression or toxicity
WIT
water-induced thermotherapy
WITT
Wittenborn (Psychiatric Rating
Scale)
WITV
Witwatersrand virus
WJPB
Woodcock-Johnson
Psychoeducational Battery
WK
week (*See also* W, w, wk)
Wernicke-Korsakoff (syndrome)
work (*See also* wk)
wk
weak
week (*See also* W, w, WK)
work (*See also* WK)
WKD
Wilson-Kimmelstiel disease
WKF
well-known fact
W/kg
watt per kilogram
WKI
Wakefield Inventory
WKS
Wernicke-Korsakoff syndrome
WKY
Wistar-Kyoto (rat)
WL
waiting list
waterload (test)
wavelength (*See also* λ)

weight loss
workload
WLB
Western ligand blot
WLE
wide local excision
WLF
whole lymphocyte fraction
WLI
weight-length index
WLM
work-level month
WLR
within-list recognition
WLS
wet lung syndrome
WLT
waterload test
whole-lung tomography
WLU
workload unit
WM
Waldenström macroglobulinemia
wall motion
ward manager
warm, moist
wet mount
white male (*See also* W/M, wm)
white matter
whole milk (*See also* wm)
whole mount (microscopy) (*See also*
wm)
woman milk
W/M
white male (*See also* WM, wm)
w/m$_2$
watt per square meter
wm
white male (*See also* WM, W/M)
whole milk (*See also* WM)
whole mount (microscopy) (*See also*
WM)
WMA
wall motion abnormality
white matter signal abnormality
Wmax
peak work rate
WMC
weight-matched control
WMD
warm moist dressing (sterile)
weapons of mass destruction
white matter damage
WMFT
Wolf Motor Function Test
WMHI
white matter hyperintensity

WMI
wall motion index
weighted mean index

WML
white matter lesion (cerebral)

WMLC
white male living child

WMP
warm moist pack (unsterile)
weight management program

WMR
wedge matrix resection
work metabolic rate

WMS
wall-motion study
Wechsler Memory Scale
Wilson-Mikity syndrome

WMSI
wall motion score index

WMV
Wad Medani virus

WMX
whirlpool, massage, exercise

WN, W/N, w/n, wn
well-nourished

WND, wnd
wound (*See also* WD)

WNF
well-nourished female
West Nile fever

WNL
within normal limits

WNLS
weighted nonlinear least squares

WNL x 4
upper and lower extremities within
normal limits

WNM
well-nourished male
well-nourished man

WNR
within normal range

WNt50
Wagner-Nelson time 50 hours

WNV
West Nile encephalitis virus
West Nile virus

WO
wash-out
weeks old (*See also* wo)
wide open

without (*See also* ō, S, s̄, w/o,
wo)
written order

W/O
water (in) oil (emulsion)
water in oil

w/o
without (*See also* ō, S, s̄, WO,
wo)

wo
weeks old (*See also* WO)
without (*See also* ō, S, s̄, WO,
w/o)

WOB
work of breathing

WOMAC
Western Ontario and McMaster
Universities Osteoarthritis Index

WOMAC-PF
Western Ontario and McMaster
Universities Osteoarthritis Index
Physical Functioning subscale and
chair-performance

WONV
Wongal virus

WORC
Western Ontario Rotator Cuff

WORM
write once, read many

WOSI
Western Ontario Instability Index

WP
water packed
weakly positive
wet pack (*See also* WPk)
wettable powder
whirlpool (*See also* WHP, Whp,
whp, W/P)
white pulp
word processor
working point

W/P
water/powder (ratio)
whirlpool (*See also* WHP, Whp,
whp, WP)

WPB
whirlpool bath (*See also* WHPB)

WPCs
washed packed cells

WPCU
weighted patient care unit

NOTES

W

WPFM
Wright peak flowmeter
WPk
ward pack
wet pack (*See also* WP)
WPOA
wearing patch on arrival
WPPSI, WPP
Wechsler Preschool and Primary
Scale of Intelligence
WPPSI-R
Wechsler Preschool and Primary
Scale of Intelligence-Revised
WPRS
Wittenborn Psychiatric Rating Scale
WPSI
Wittenborn Psychiatric Symptoms
Inventory
WPT
marbled pure tone
WPV
within-person variability
WR
Waldeyer ring
washroom
Wassermann reaction (*See also* Wr)
water retention
weakly reactive (*See also* Wr)
whole response (*See also* W)
wide range
Wiedemann-Rautenstrauch
(syndrome)
wiping reaction
work rate
wrist
W/R
with respect (to)
Wr, wr
Wassermann reaction (*See also* WR)
weakly reactive (*See also* WR)
wrist
Wr^a
Wright antigen
WRA
with-the-rule astigmatism
WRAML
Wide Range Assessment of
Memory and Learning
WRAT
Wide Range Achievement Test
WRAT-R
Wide Range Achievement Test-
Revised
WRBC
washed red blood cell (*See also*
WRC)

WRC
washed red (blood) cell (*See also*
WRBC)
washed red cell
water-retention coefficient
WRE
whole ragweed extract
WRK
Woodward reagent K
WRMT
Woodcock Reading Mastery Test
WRST
Wilcoxon rank sum test
WRVP
wedged renal vein pressure
WS
walking speed
Wardenburg syndrome
Warthin-Starry (stain)
watermelon stomach
water soluble
water swallow
watt-second (*See also* W·s)
Werner syndrome
West syndrome
wet swallow
whole (response plus white) space
Wilder silver (stain)
Williams syndrome
work simplification
work simulation
work status
W&S
wound and skin
W·s
watt-second (*See also* WS)
WSA
water-soluble antibiotic
WSB
wheat soy blend
WSD
water seal drainage
weak syllable deletion
WSEP
Williams syndrome, early puberty
WSLP
Williams syndrome, late puberty
WSP
wearable speech processor
WSQ
wavelet scalar quantization
WSR
Westergren sedimentation rate
W/sr
watt per steradian
WSS
Weaver-Smith syndrome
wrinkly skin syndrome

WT
walking tank
walking training
wall thickness
water temperature
wild type (strain)
Wilms tumor
wisdom teeth
work therapy

0WT
zero work tolerance

wt
weight
white (*See also* W, w, Wh, wh)

WTD
wet tail disease

W-T-D
wet-to-dry (*See also* W→D)

WTE
whole time equivalent

WTF
weight transferral frequency

WTI
Wilms tumor 1

WTP
willingness to pay

WTS
whole tomography slice
Wilson-Turner syndrome

WTV
wound tumor virus

WTW
wet-to-wet (*See also* W-›W)

W/U, w/u
workup

WURS
Wender Utah Rating Scale

WV
walking ventilation
whispered voice

W/V, w/v
weight (of solute) per volume (of solution)

W$_v$
variable dominant spotting (mouse)

WV-MBC
walking ventilation to maximal breathing capacity (ratio)

WW
wet weight
wheeled walker

W/W, w/w
weight (of solute) per weight (of solvent)

W→W
wet-to-wet (*See also* WTW)

WWAC
walk with aid of cane

WW Brd
whole wheat bread

WWIF
warm water immersion foot

WWTP
wastewater treatment plant

WWW
World Wide Web

WX
wound of exit

WxB
wax bite

WxP
wax pattern

WY
women years

WY/NRT
Weidel Yes/No Reliability Test

WYOU
women years of usage

WYOV
Wyeomyia virus

WZa
wide zone alpha (hemolysis)

NOTES

W

χ, chi
chi (22nd letter of Greek alphabet), lowercase

X
androgenic (zone)
break
chi (22nd letter of Greek alphabet), uppercase
cross
cross-bite
crossed with
crossmatch (*See also* XM)
cross-section
decimal scale of potency or dilution
except
exophoria
exophoria distance (*See also* x)
exposure
extra
female sex chromosome
homeopathic symbol for decimal scale of potencies
ionization exposure rate
Kienböck unit (of x-ray exposure)
magnification
multiplication sign
reactance (electric current)
removal of
respirations (anesthesia chart)
start of anesthesia
ten
times
translocation between two X chromosomes
transverse
unknown quantity
xanthine
xanthosine (*See also* Xao)
xerophthalmia
X unit
Xylocaine

X2
chi-square

X3
(orientation as to) time, place and person

X′, x′
exophoria, near viewing

X+, X+#
xiphoid plus (number of fingerbreadths)

X
except
sample mean

x
axis of cylindric lens
except
exophoria distance (*See also* X)
horizontal axis of rectangular coordinate system
mole fraction
multiplied by
roentgen (rays)
sample mean

X-A
xylene-alcohol (mixture)

XA
xanthurenic acid

X:A
X chromosome to autosome (ratio)

Xa
chiasma

Xaa
unknown amino acid

Xan
xanthine

XANT
xanthochromic

Xanth
xanthomatosis

Xao
xanthosine (*See also* X)

XBT
xylose breath test

XC
excretory cystogram
excretory cystography

Xc
reactance (*See also* X)

XCCE
extracapsular cataract extraction (*See also* ECCE)

XCCL
exaggerated craniocaudal lateral (angle, view)

XCF
aortic cross clamp off

XCO
aortic cross clamp on

XCP
xanthogranulomatous pyelonephritis

Xc/R
reactance and resistance

XCT
x-ray computed tomography

XD
times daily
xanthoma disseminatum
X-linked dominant

X

X&D
    examination and diagnosis
X2d
    times two days
5xD
    five times a day
XDH
    xanthine dehydrogenase
XDP
    xanthine diphosphate
    xeroderma pigmentosum (*See also* XP)
XDR
    transducer
XDT
    defibrillation threshold (*See also* DFT)
    diversional therapy
Xe
    xenon
¹²⁷Xe
    xenon-127
¹³³Xe
    xenon-133
XeCl
    xenon chloride
XECT, XeCT, Xe-CT
    xenon-enhanced computed tomography
X-ed
    crossed
XEF
    excess ejection fraction
XEM
    Xonics electron mammography
xero
    xeromammography (*See also* XMM)
XES
    x-ray energy spectrometry
XF
    xerophthalmic fundus
XFER
    transfer
Xfmr
    transformer
XG
    xanthogranuloma
XGP
    xanthogranulomatous pyelonephritis (*See also* XPN)
XH
    extra high
ξ
    xi (14th letter of Greek alphabet), lowercase
Ξ
    xi (14th letter of Greek alphabet), uppercase

XIBV
    Xiburema virus
XIC
    X inactivation center
XIH
    idiopathic hypercalcuria
XIP
    x-ray in plaster
XIST, Xist
    X inactive, specific transcript
XKO
    not knocked out
XL
    excess lactate
    extended release (once a day oral solid dosage form)
    extra large
    inductive reactance
    xylose-lysine (agar base)
X-LA, XLA
    X-linked agammaglobulinemia
XLAS
    X-linked Alport syndrome
    X-linked aqueductal stenosis
XLCM
    X-linked cardiomyopathy
    X-linked (dilated) cardiomyopathy
XLD
    X-linked dominant
    xylose-lysine-deoxycholate (agar)
X-leg
    crossleg
XLFDP
    crosslinked fibrin degradation product
XLH
    X-linked hypophosphatemia
XLHN
    X-linked hypercalciuric nephrolithiasis
XLHR
    X-linked hypophosphatemic rickets
XLI
    X-linked ichthyosis
XLJR
    X-linked juvenile retinoschisis
XLMR
    X-linked mental retardation
XLMR/MCA
    X-linked mental retardation/multiple congenital anomaly
XLMTM
    X-linked myotubular myopathy
XLOS
    X-linked Opitz syndrome
XLP
    X-linked lymphoproliferative (disease) (*See also* XLS)

XLR
X-linked recessive
XLRP
X-linked retinitis pigmentosa
XLS
X-linked recessive lymphoproliferative syndrome (*See also* XLD)
XLT
X-linked thrombocytopenia
XM, X-mat., X-match
crossmatch (*See also* X)
X$_m$
magnetic susceptibility
XMG
x-ray mammogram
XML
extensible markup language
XMM
xeromammography (*See also* xero)
XMP
xanthine monophosphate
xanthosine 5'-monophosphate
XN
night blindness
Xn
Christian
XNA
xenoreactive natural antibody
XO
gonadal dysgenesis of Turner type
presence of only one sex chromosome
xanthine oxidase
XOAN
X-linked ocular albinism
XOM
extraocular movement
XOP
x-ray out of plaster
XOR
exclusive operating room
XP
xeroderma pigmentosum (*See also* XDP)
Xp
short arm of chromosome X
Xp-
deletion of short arm of chromosome X
XPA
xeroderma pigmentosum (group) A

XPC
xeroderma pigmentosum (group) C
XPN
xanthogranulomatous pyelonephritis (*See also* XGP)
XPS
x-ray photoemission spectroscopy
Xq
long arm of chromosome X
Xq-
deletion of long arm of chromosome X
XR
x-linked recessive
x-ray
XRA
x-ray arteriography
XRD
x-ray diffraction
XRE
xenobiotic-response element
XRF
x-ray fluorescence
XRITC
tetra-m cyclopropylrhodamine isothiocyanate
XRN
X-linked recessive nephrolithiasis
XRT
external radiation therapy
x-ray therapy (radiotherapy) (*See also* RT)
XS
corneal scar
cross-section
excess
excessive
xiphisternum
XSA
cross-sectional area
xenograph surface area
X-SCID, XSCID
X-linked severe combined immunodeficiency
XS-LIM
exceeds limits (of procedure)
XSLR
crossed straight leg raising (sign)
XSP
xanthoma striatum palmare
XT, xT
exotropia

NOTES

X

XT *(continued)*
> extract
> extracted

X(T), x(T)
> intermittent exotropia

X(T')
> intermittent exotropia at 33 cm

Xta
> chiasmata

Xtab
> crosstabulating

XTLE
> extratemporal-lobe epilepsy

XTM
> xanthoma tuberosum multiplex
> x-ray tomographic microscope

XTP
> xanthosine triphosphate

XU
> excretory urogram
> excretory urography
> X-unit (*See also* Xu)

Xu
> X-unit (*See also* XU)

XULN
> times upper limit of normal

XUV
> extreme ultraviolet

xvse
> transverse

XX
> double strength
> normal female sex chromosome
> type

XX/XY
> sex karyotypes

XY
> normal male sex chromosome type

Xy, Xyl
> xylose

XYL, XYLO
> Xylocaine

Xyzabcdef
> test terms barb

Y

    coordinate axis in plane
    male sex chromosome
    ordinate
    tyrosine (*See also* Ty, Tyr)
    vertical axis of rectangular coordinate system
    year (*See also* y)
    yellow
    young
    yttrium

^{50}Y

    yttrium-50

^{90}Y

    yttrium-90

y

    wave on phlebogram
    year (*See also* Y)
    yield

YA

    Yersinia arthritis

YAC

    yeast artificial chromosomes

YACP

    young adult chronic patient

YACV

    Yacaaba virus

YADH

    yeast alcohol dehydrogenase

YAG

    yttrium-aluminum-garnet (laser)
    yttrium, argon, garnet

YAPA

    young adult psychiatric assessment

YATAV

    Yata virus

Y/B

    yellow/blue

Yb

    ytterbium

YBOCS

    Yale-Brown Obsessive-Compulsive Scale

YBT

    Yerkes-Bridges Test (psychology)

YBV

    Yug Bogdanovac virus

YCB

    yeast carbon base

YCT

    Yvon coefficient test

yd

    yard

YDES

    yin deficiency-yang excess syndrome

YE

    yeast extract
    yellow enzyme

YEH$_2$

    reduced yellow enzyme

Yel, yel

    yellow

YET

    Youth Effectiveness Training

YF

    yellow fever

YFH

    yellow-faced hornet

YFI

    yellow fever immunization

YFV

    yellow fever virus

YF-VAX

    yellow fever vaccine

YGTSS

    Yale Global Tic Severity Scale

YHL

    years of healthy life

YHMD

    yellow hyaline membrane disease

YHT

    Young-Helmholtz theory

YHV

    Yaquina Head virus

YJV

    yellow jacket venom

Y2K

    year 2000

Yk

    York (antibody)

YLC

    youngest living child

YLD

    years of life with disability

YLF

    yttrium lithium fluoride

YLL

    years of life lost

YM

    yeast and mannitol

YMA

    yeast morphology agar

YMC

    young male Caucasian

YMRS

    Young Mania Rating Scale

Y

YMV
yam mosaic virus

Y/N
yes/no

YNB
yeast nitrogen base

YNS
yellow nail syndrome

YO, yo
years old

YOB
year of birth

YOD
year of death

YOGV
Yogue virus

YORA
younger-onset rheumatoid arthritis

YP
yeast phase
yield point
yield pressure

YPA
yeast, peptone, and adenine (sulfate)

YPC
YAG (yttrium aluminum garnet laser) posterior capsulotomy

YPLL
years of potential life lost (before age 65)

yr
year

YRBS
youth risk behavioral survey

YRD
Yangtze River disease

YRRM
Y chromosome RNA recognition motif

YS
yellow spot
yolk sac
Yoshida sarcoma

YSC
yolk sac carcinoma

YSR
youth self-report

YST
yeast (cells)
yolk sac tumor

YT
yttrium

YTD
year to date

YTDY
yesterday

YVS
yellow vernix syndrome

Z, zeta
atomic number (symbol)
contraction [Ger. *Zuckung*]
disk (band, line) that separates sacromeres [Ger. *Zwischenscheibe* intermediate disk]
glutamine
impedance
ionic charge number
no effect
point formed by line perpendicular to nasion-menton line through anterior nasal spine
proton number
section modulus
shape of surgical incision (Z-plasty)
standardized deviate
standard score
zero
zeta (sixth letter of Greek alphabet), uppercase
zone
zusammen

z
algebraic unknown or space coordinate
axis of three-dimensional rectangular coordinate system
catalytic amount
standardized device
standard normal deviate
zepto-

ZAAG
Zest Anchor Advanced Generation

ZAP
zoster-associated pain
zymosan-activated plasma (rabbit)

ZAPF
zinc adequate pair-fed

ZAS
zymosan-activated autologous serum

ZB
zebra body

ZC
zona compacta

ZCP
zinc chloride poisoning

ZD
zero defect
zero discharge
zinc deficient
zona drilling

ZDDP
zinc dialkyldithiophosphate

ZDO
zero differential overlap

ZDS
zinc depletion syndrome

ZDV
zidovudine

ZE, Z-E
Zollinger-Ellison (syndrome) (*See also* ZES)

ZEBRA
antibodies to the Epstein-Barr virus transactivator protein

ZEEP
zero end-expiratory pressure

ZEGV
Zegla virus

ZES
Zollinger-Ellison syndrome (*See also* ZE)

Z-ESR
zeta erythrocyte sedimentation rate

ζ
zeta (sixth letter of Greek alphabet), lowercase

ZF
zero frequency
zona fasciculata
zygomaticofrontal

ZFP
zero-flow pressure
zinc finger protein

ZG
zona glomerulosa

Z/G
zoster (serum) immunoglobulin (*See also* ZIG, ZIg)

ZGG
zinc gluconate glycine

ZGM
zinc glycinate marker

ZI
zona incerta

ZI^a
isotope with atomic number Z and atomic weight A

ZIG, ZIg
zoster immune globulin
zoster (serum) immunoglobulin (*See also* Z/G)

ZIKAV
Zika virus

ZIM
zimelidine

ZIP
zoster immune plasma

ZIRV
Zirqa virus

ZLN
zosteriform lentiginous nevus

Zm
zygomaxillare

ZMA
zinc meta-arsenite

ZMC
zygomatic malar complex
zygomatic maxillary complex
zygomaticomaxillary complex
zygomaxillary complex

ZN
Ziehl-Neelsen (method, stain)

Zn
zinc

^{65}Zn
zinc-65

Zn fl
zinc flocculation (test)

ZnO
zinc oxide

ZnOE, ZOE
zinc oxide-eugenol (white zinc)

ZnPc
zinc phthalocyanine

ZNPP
zinc protoporphyrin

ZNS
Ziehl-Neelsen stain
zonisamide

ZOG
zona glomerulosa protein

Zool
zoology

ZOOM
Guarana (herb)

ZOT, zot
zonula occludens toxin

ZP
zona pellucida

ZP1
zona pellucida 1

ZP2
zona pellucida 2

ZP3
zona pellucida 3

ZPA
zone of polarizing activity

ZPC
zero point of charge
zone of preparatory calcification
zopiclone

ZPG
zero population growth

Z-plasty
surgical relaxation of contracture

ZPLS
Zimmerman Preschool Language
Scale

ZPO
zinc peroxide

ZPP
zinc protoporphyrin

ZPP/H
zinc protoporphyrin/heme

ZPT
zinc pyrithione

ZR
zona reticularis

Zr
zirconium

ZrSiO$_4$
zirconium silicate

ZSB
zero stool (since) birth

ZSC
zone of slow conduction

ZSO
zinc suboptimal

ZSR
ζ sedimentation rate
zeta sedimentation rate

ZSRDS
Zung Self-Rating Depression Scale

ZT
Ziehen test

ZTGN
zheng ti guan nian

ZTN
zinc tannate (of) naloxone

ZTS
zymosan-treated serum

Z-TSP
zephiran-trisodium phosphate

ZTT
zinc turbidity test

ZTV
Zaliv Terpeniya virus

ZUMI
Zinnanti uterine manipulator-injector

ZVD
zidovudine

Zy
zygion

Zylo
Zyloprim

zz.
ginger [L. *zingiber*]

ZZR
zinc turbidity test

Z, Z′, Z″
increasing degrees of contraction
[Ger. *Zuckung*] (*See also* Z)

NOTES

Appendix 1
Angles, Triangles, and Circles

$\wedge$	above diastolic blood pressure (anesthesia records) elevated enlarged improved increased superior (position) upper	$<$	caused by derived from less severe than less than produced by proximal
		$\angle$	angle flexion flexor
$\vee$	below decreased deficiency deficit depressed deteriorated diminished down inferior (position) lower systolic blood pressure (anesthesia records)	∠̲ᴇ	angle of entry
		∠̲ˣ	angle of exit
		└	factorial product
		⌐	right lower quadrant
		¬	right upper quadrant
		⌐	left upper quadrant
		└	left lower quadrant
$>$	causes demonstrates distal followed by derived from greater than indicates leads to more severe than produces radiates to radiating to results in reveals shows to toward worse than yields	Δ	anion gap centrad prism change delta gap heat increment occipital triangle prism diopter temperature (anesthesia records)
		$\Delta +$	time interval
		ΔA	change in absorbance
		Δ dB	difference in decibels
		Δ H, H Δ	Hesselbach triangle
		Δ P	change in (intraocular) pressure
		Δ pH	change in pH
		Δ t	time interval

A1

Appendix 1

○	respiration (anesthesia records)	Ⓜ	murmur
♀	female female sex	ⓜ	by mouth mouth (temperature) murmur
♂	male male sex	√ⓜ	factitial murmur
Ⓐ , ⓐx	axilla (temperature)	Ⓞ	by mouth oral orally
Ⓗ , ⓗ	hypodermic hypodermically	Ⓡ	rectal rectally rectum (temperature) right
Ⓘm	intramuscular intramuscularly		
Ⓘv	intravenous intravenously	Ⓧ	end of anesthesia (anesthesia records) end of operation
Ⓛ	left		

Arrows

↑   above
elevated
elevation
enlarged
gas
greater than
improved
increase
increased
increases
more than
rising
superior (position)
up
upper

↑ g   increasing
rising

↑ V   increase due to in vivo
effect (lab)

↓   below
decrease
decreased
deficiency
deficit
depressed
depression
deteriorated
deteriorating
diminished
diminution
down
falling
inferior (position)
less than
low
normal plantar reflex
precipitate
precipitates
slower

↓ g   decreasing
diminishing
falling
lowering

↓ V   decrease due to in vivo effect (lab)

╱   deviated
displaced
increasing

╲   decreasing

→   approaches limit of
causes, demonstrates
direction of flow or reaction
distal
due to
followed by
indicates
leads to
produces
radiating to
results in
reveals
shows
to
to right
toward
yields

←   caused by
derived from
direction of flow or reaction
due to
produced by
proximal
resulting from
secondary to
to left

↑↑   extensor response (Babinski sign)
positive Babinski
testes undescended

Appendix 2

⇊	down bilaterally plantar response (Babinski sign) testes descended	⇕	reversible reaction up and down
		⇄ , ⇌	reversible (chemical) reaction

Genetic Symbols

□   male

○   female

◇   sex unspecified

□ ○   normal individuals

■ ● ◆   affected individual (with ≥ 2 conditions, the symbol is partitioned and shaded with a different fill defined in a key or legend)

5 ⑤ ◇5   multiple individuals, number known (number of siblings written inside symbol)

n ⓝ ◇n   multiple individuals, number unknown ("n" used in place of specific number)

□—○   mating

□═○   consanguinity

(+)   uncommon or uncertain mode of inheritance

I □—○
II □—○   parents and offspring, in generations

□ ○   dizygotic twins

□ ○   monozygotic twins

4 ③   number of children of sex indicated

(□)(○)   adopted individuals

□ ○   individual died without leaving offspring

□—○   no issue

■ ●   affected individuals

■ ●   proband or propositus (first affected family member coming to medical attention)

⬚⬚ examined professionally
    normal for trait

⬚ not examined
    dubiously reported to have trait

⬛⬚ not examined
    reliably reported to have trait

◨ ◐ heterozygotes for autosomal recessive

⊙ carrier of sex-linked recessive

⊠ ⊘ death

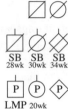
SB SB SB
28wk 30wk 34wk   stillbirth (SB)

⎍P⎍ ⓟ ⬠P
LMP 20wk
7/1/94

pregnancy (P); gestational age and karotype (if known) below
    symbol

⬚ ○
↗ ↗   consultand (individual seeking genetic counseling/testing)

male female ECT   spontaneous abortion (SAB); ECT below symbol indicates
    ectopic pregnancy

male female 16wk   affected SAB (gestational age, if known, below symbol, and
    key or legend used to define shading)

male female   termination of pregnancy (TOP)

▲ ▲ ▲
male female   affected TOP (key or legend used to define shading)

Source. Genetic symbols are public domain; we credit and gratefully acknowledge the *American Journal of Human Genetics* (56:746–747, 1995) as our source for these symbols.

Appendix 4
Numbers

0	completely absent (pulse) no response (reflexes)	3+	brisker than average (reflexes) moderate reaction (lab tests)
+1, 1+	markedly impaired (pulse)	+4, 4+	normal (pulse)
1+	low normal or somewhat diminished (reflexes) slight reaction or trace (lab tests)	4+	hyperactive (reflexes) large amount (lab tests) pronounced reaction (lab tests)
+2, 2+	moderately impaired (pulse)	$\overline{1}$	very brisk (reflexes) bowel movement (numeral indicates number of stools in a given period)
2+	average or normal (reflexcs) noticeable reaction or trace (lab tests)	1×	once one time
+3, 3+	slightly impaired (pulse)	2×, ×2	twice two times
		3×, ×3	three times, etc.

Arabic	Roman	Arabic	Roman
0		17	XVII
1	I, i	18	XVIII
2	II, ii	19	XIX
3	III, iii	20	XX
4	IV, iv	30	XXX
5	V, v	40	XL
6	VI, vi	50	L
7	VII, vii	60	LX
8	VIII, viii	70	LXX
9	IX, ix	80	LXXX
10	X, x	90	XC
11	XI, xi	100	C
12	XII, xii	1,000	M
13	XIII, xiii	5,000	$\overline{V}$
14	XIV, xiv	10,000	$\overline{X}$
15	XV	100,000	$\overline{C}$
16	XVI	1,000,000	$\overline{M}$

Appendix 5
Pluses, Minuses, and Equivalencies

+   acid (reaction)
added to
convex lens
decreased or diminished
(reflexes)
excess
less than 50%
inhibition of
hemolysis (Wassermann)
low normal (reflexes)
markedly impaired (pulse)
mild (severity)
plus
positive (lab tests)
present
slight reaction or trace
(lab tests)
sluggish (reflexes)
somewhat diminished
(reflexes)

(+)   significant

(+)ive   positive

+ to ++   slight pain

++   average (reflexes)
50% inhibition of
hemolysis
(Wassermann)
moderate (pain,
severity)
moderately impaired
(pulse)
normally active (reflexes)
noticeable reaction or
trace (lab tests)

+++   increased reflexes
75% inhibition of
hemolysis (Wassermann)
moderate amount

+++   moderate reaction (lab tests)
moderately hyperative
(reflexes)
moderately severe (pain,
severity)
brisker than average
(reflexes)
slightly impaired (pulse)

++++   complete inhibition of
hemolysis
(Wassermann)
large amount (lab tests)
markedly hyperactive
(reflexes)
markedly severe (pain,
severity)
normal (pulse)
pronounced reaction
(lab tests)
very brisk (reflexes)

−   absent
alkaline (reaction)
concave lens
deficiency
deficient
minus
negative (lab test)
none
subtract
without

(−)   insignificant

±   doubtful
either positive or negative
equivocal (reflexes,
qualitative tests)
flicker (reflexes)
indefinite
more or less
plus or minus

$\pm$	possibly significant questionable suggestive variable very slight (reaction, severity, trace) with or without	$\backsim$	combined with
		$\backsimeq$	equivalent
		$\not\backsimeq$	not equivalent to
		$\equiv$	identical identical with
$(\pm)$	possibly significant	$\not\equiv$	not identical not identical with
$\pm$ to $+$	minimal pain	$\doteqdot$	nearly equal to
$\mp$	minus or plus	$\doteq$	approximately equal

$\ddagger$	moderate (severity)
	normally active
	   (reflexes)
		$\cong$	approximately
			approximately
			   equal to
			congruent to

#	fracture gauge number pound(s) weight	$\doteq$	approaches
		$=$	equilateral
		$\triangleq$	equiangular
$\sim$	about approximate approximately proportionate to	$>$	greater than
		$\not>$	not greater than
		$<$	less than
$\approx$	approximately equal to	$\not<$	not less than
$=$	equal to	$\geq, \geqslant$	greater than or equal to
$\neq$	not equal to	$\leq, \leqslant$	less than or equal to

Primes, Checks, Dots, Roots, and Other Symbols

?	doubtful equivocal (reflexes) flicker (reflexes) not tested (severity) possible questionable question of suggested suggestive (severity) unknown	$\sqrt{c}$	check with
		$\sqrt{d}$	checked observed
		$\sqrt{g}, \sqrt{ing}$	checking
		$\sqrt{qs}$	voided sufficient quantity
!	factorial product	$\sqrt{}$	radical root
†	death deceased	$\sqrt[2]{}$	square root
/	divided by either meaning extension extensors fraction of per to	$\sqrt[3]{}$	cube root
		*	birth multiplication sign (genetics) not verified presumed supposed
'	foot hour univalent	°	degree measurement (1/360 of circle) severity (burns, wounds) temperature time (hour)
"	bivalent ditto inch minute second (1/60 degree)	:	is to ratio
		...	no data (in given category)
‴	line (1/12 inch) trivalent	∴	therefore
√	check observe for urine voided (urine)	∵	because since
∵√∴	urine and defecation voided and bowels moved	::	as equality between ratios proportion proportionate to

Statistical Symbols

α	probability of type I error significance level	p	probability of success in independent trials
β	probability of type II error	ρ	population correlation coefficient
$1-\beta$	power of statistical test	$P(A)$	probability that event A occurs
${}^nC_k; \left(\dfrac{n}{k}\right)$	binomial coefficient number of combination of n things taken k at a time	$P(A\backslash B)$	conditional probability that A occurs given that B has occurred
χ^2	chi-squared statistic	r	sample correlation coefficient, usually the Pearson product-moment correlation
E	expected frequency in cell of contingency table		
$E(X)$	expected value of random variable X	r^2	coefficient of determination
F	F statistic (variance ratio)	r_s	Spearman rank correlation coefficient
f	frequency	s	sample standard deviation
H_0	null hypothesis	s^2	sample variance
H_1	alternative hypothesis	SE	standard error of estimate
μ	population mean	σ	population standard deviation
N	population size		
n	sample size	σ^2	population variance
$n!$	n factorial	σdiff.	standard error of difference between scores
O	observed frequency in a contingency table	σest.	standard error of estimate
ϕ	ability continuum phi coefficient	σmeas.	standard error of measurement
P	probability		

t	Student t statistic Student test variable	$\neq$	not equal to
θ	latent trait	$\approx$	approximately equal to
U	Mann-Whitney rank sum statistic	$>$	greater than
		$\ngtr$	not greater than
W	Wilcoxon rank sum statistic	$<$	less than
$\overline{X}$	sample mean	$\nless$	not less than
$|x|$	absolute value of x	$\geq, \geqslant$	greater than or equal to
$\sqrt{x}$	square root of x	$\leq, \leqslant$	less than or equal to
z	standard score	∞	infinity

Appendix 8
Professional Titles and Degrees

AA
Anesthesiologist's Assistant

ADN
Associate Degree in Nursing

AHN
Army Head Nurse
Assistant Head Nurse

AHP
Assistant House Physician

AHS
Assistant House Surgeon

AMO
Assistant Medical Officer

ANP
Adult Nurse Practitioner
Advanced Nurse Practitioner

ARNP
Advanced Registered Nurse Practitioner

ART
Accredited Record Technician

ATh
Associate in Therapy

ATR
Activities Therapist, Registered

AuD
Doctorate of Audiology

BAMS
Bachelor of Ayurvedic Medicine and
 Surgery

BAO
Bachelor of the Art of Obstetrics

BChD
Bachelor of Dentistry

BCNP
Board-Certified Nuclear Pharmacist

BdentSci, BDSc
Bachelor of Dental Science

BDS
Bachelor of Dental Surgery

BHyg
Bachelor of Hygiene

BM, BMed
Bachelor of Medicine

BMedBiol
Bachelor of Medical Biology

BMedSci, BMS
Bachelor of Medical Science

BMET
Biomedical Equipment Technician

BMic
Bachelor of Microbiology

BMT
Bachelor of Medical Technology

BNEd
Bachelor of Nursing Education

BNSc
Bachelor of Nursing Science

BO
Bachelor of Osteopathy

BP, BPharm
Bachelor of Pharmacy

BPH
Bachelor of Public Health

BPHEng
Bachelor of Public Health Engineering

BPHN
Bachelor of Public Health Nursing

BS
Bachelor of Science
Bachelor of Surgery

BSc
Bachelor of Science

BSM
Bachelor of Science in Medicine

BSN
Bachelor of Science in Nursing

BSOT
Bachelor of Science in Occupational
   Therapy

BSPh
Bachelor of Science in Pharmacy

BSS
Bachelor of Sanitary Science

BVMS
Bachelor of Veterinary Medicine and
   Surgery

BVSc
Bachelor of Veterinary Science

CA
Certified Acupuncturist

CCRN
Critical Care Registered Nurse

CDA
Certified Dental Assistant

CDE
Certified Diabetes Educator

CDT
Certified Dental Technician

CEN
Certificate for Emergency Nursing

CEO
Chief Executive Officer

CFO
Chief Financial Officer

CFP
Clinical Fellowship Program

CGC
Certified Gastrointestinal Clinician

ChB
Bachelor of Surgery; Chirurgiae
   Baccalaureus

ChD, Chir. Doct.
Doctor of Surgery; Chirurgiae Doctor

ChM
Master of Surgery; Chirurgiae Magister

CHN
Certified Hemodialysis Nurse
Community Health Nurse

CHP
Coordinating Hospital Physician

CIC
Certified Infection Control

CIH
Certificate in Industrial Health

CLA
Certified Laboratory Assistant

CLA(ASCP)
Clinical Laboratory Assistant
(American Society of Clinical
Pathologists)

CLS(NCA)
Clinical Laboratory Scientist certified
by National Credentialing Agency

CLSP
Clinical Laboratory Specialist

CLT
Certified Laboratory Technician
Clinical Laboratory Technician
Clinical Laboratory Technologist

CLT(NCA)
Clinical Laboratory Technician certified
by National Credentialing Agency

CM
Master in Surgery; Chirurgiae Magister

CMA
Certified Medical Assistant

CMHN
Community Mental Health Nurse

CMO
Chief Medical Officer

CMT
Certified Medical Transcriptionist

CNM
Certified Nurse-Midwife

CNMT
Certified Nuclear Medicine Technologist

CNOR
Certified Nurse, Operating Room

CNP
Community Nurse Practitioner

CNRN
Certified Neuroscience Registered Nurse

CNS
Chief, Nursing Services
Clinical Nurse Specialist

CNSN
Certified Nutrition Support Nurse

CO
Certified Orthotist

COMA
Certified Ophthalmic Medical Assistant

CORD
Commissioned Officer Residency
Deferment

CORT
Certified Operating Room Technician

COS
Chief of Staff

COTA
Certified Occupational Therapy
Assistant

CP
Certified Prosthetist

CPAN
Certified Post-Anesthesia Nurse

CPed
Certified Pedorthist

CPH
Certificate in Public Health

CPNP/A
Certified Pediatric Nurse
Practitioner/Associate

CPO
Certified Prosthetist and Orthotist

CR
Chief Resident

CRL
Certified Record Librarian

CRNA
Certified Registered Nurse Anesthetist

CRNI
Certified Registered Nurse Intravenous

CRNP
Certified Registered Nurse Practitioner

CRT
Certified Respiratory Therapist

CRTT
Certified Respiratory Therapy
  Technician

CS
Chief of Staff

CST
Certified Surgical Technician

CSW
Certified Social Worker

CT
Cardiovascular Technologist
Cytotechnologist

CT(ASCP)
Cytotechnologist (American Society of
  Clinical Pathologists)

CVO
Chief Veterinary Officer

D, Dip
diplomate

DA
Dental Assistant
Diploma in Anesthetics

D&E
Diploma of Applied Parasitology and
  Entomology

DBIR
Director of Biotechnology Information
  Resources

DC
Doctor of Chiropractic

DCH
Diploma in Child Health

DCh
Doctor of Surgery; Doctor Chirurgiae

DchO
Doctor of Ophthalmic Surgery

DCM
Doctor of Comparative Medicine

DCO
Diploma of the College of Optics

DCP
Diploma in Clinical Pathology
Diploma in Clinical Psychology
District Community Physician

DD
Doctor of Divinity

DDH
Diploma in Dental Health

DDM
Diploma in Dermatological Medicine
Doctor of Dental Medicine

DDO
Diploma in Dental Orthopaedics

DDR
Diploma in Diagnostic Radiology

DDS
Director of Dental Services
Doctor of Dental Surgery

DDSc
Doctor of Dental Science

DGO
Diploma in Gynaecology and
  Obstetrics

DH
Dental Hygienist

DHg, Dhyg, DHy, DHyg, DrHyg
Doctor of Hygiene

DHMSA
Diploma of History of Medicine,
  Society of Apothecaries

Diet. Tech.
Dietetic Technician

Dip
diplomate

DipBact
Diploma in Bacteriology

DipChem
Diploma in Chemistry

DipClinPath
Diploma in Clinical Pathology

DipMicrobiol
Diploma in Microbiology

DipSocMed
Diploma in Social Medicine

DLO
Diploma in Laryngology and Otology

DM
Doctor of Medicine; Doctor
  Medicinae

DMA
Director of Medical Affairs

DMD
Doctor of Dental Medicine

DME
Director of Medical Education

DMJ
Diploma in Medical Jurisprudence

DMR
Diploma in Medical Radiology
Directorate of Medical Research

DMRE
Diploma in Medical Radiology and
  Electrology

DMS
Doctor of Medical Science

DMT
Doctor of Medical Technology

DMV
Doctor of Veterinary Medicine

DN
Diploma in Nursing
Diploma in Nutrition
District Nurse
Doctor of Nursing

DNB
Diplomate of the National Board (of
  Medical Examiners)

DNE
Director of Nursing Education
Doctor of Nursing Education

DNO
District Nursing Officer

DNS
Director of Nursing Services
Doctor of Nursing Services

DO
Diploma in Ophthalmology
Diploma in Osteopathy
Doctor of Ophthalmology
Doctor of Osteopathy

DOHyg
Diploma in Occupational
  Hygiene

DOM
Doctor of Oriental Medicine

DOMS
Diploma in Ophthalmic Medicine and
  Surgery
Doctor of Orthopedic Medicine and
  Surgery

DON
Director of Nursing

Doph
Doctor of Ophthalmology

DOPS
Director of Pharmacy Service(s)

Dorth
Diploma in Orthodontics
Diploma in Orthoptics

DOS
Doctor of Ocular Science
Doctor of Optical Science

DP
Doctor of Pharmacy
Doctor of Podiatry

DPD
Diploma in Public Dentistry

DPH
Diploma in Public Health
Doctor of Public Health/Hygiene

DPharm
Doctor of Pharmacy

DPhC
Doctor of Pharmaceutical Chemistry

DPhc
Doctor of Pharmacology

DPHN
Doctor of Public Health Nursing

Dphys
Diploma in Physiotherapy

DphysMed
Diploma in Physical Medicine

DPM
Diploma in Psychological Medicine
Doctor of Physical Medicine
Doctor of Podiatric Medicine
Doctor of Preventative Medicine
Doctor of Psychiatric Medicine

DPR
Department of Professional Regulation

DPsy
Doctor of Psychology

Dr, DR
doctor

DrHyg
Doctor of Hygiene

Dr Med
Doctor of Medicine

DrMT
Doctor of Mechanotherapy

DrPH
Doctor of Public Health
Doctor of Public Health/Hygiene

DS
Doctor of Science

DSC
Doctor of Surgical Chiropody

DSc
Doctor of Science

DSE
Doctor of Sanitary Engineering

DSIM
Doctor of Science in Industrial
    Medicine

DSM
Diploma in Social Medicine

DSSc
Diploma in Sanitary Science

DSur
Doctor of Surgery

DTCD
Diploma in Tuberculosis and Chest
    Diseases

D&D
Diploma in Venereology and
    Dermatology

DVM
Doctor of Veterinary Medicine

DVMS
Doctor of Veterinary Medicine and
    Surgery

DVR
Diploma in Vocational Rehabilitation
Doctor of Veterinary Radiology

DVS
Doctor of Veterinary Science
Doctor of Veterinary Surgery

DVSc
Doctor of Veterinary Science

EEG T
Electroencephalographic
    Technologist

EMT
Emergency Medical Technician

EMT-A
Emergency Medical Technician,
    Advanced
Emergency Medical Technician,
    Ambulance

EMT-B
Emergency Medical Technician,
    Basic

EMT-D
Emergency Medical Technician,
    Defibrillation

EMT-I
Emergency Medical Technician,
    Intermediate

EMT-M
Emergency Medical Technician,
    Military

EMT-P
Emergency Medical Technician,
    Paramedic

EN
Enrolled Nurse

FAAN
Fellow of the American Academy of
    Nursing

FAAP
Fellow of the American Academy of
Pediatrics

FACA
Fellow of the American College of
Anesthesiology

FACAG
Fellow of the American College of
Angiology

FACAI
Fellow of the American College of
Allergy and Immunology

FACAL
Fellow of the American College of
Allergy

FACAN
Fellow of the American College of
Anesthesiologists

FACAS
Fellow of the American College of
Abdominal Surgeons

FACC
Fellow of the American College of
Cardiologists

FACCP
Fellow of the American College of
Chest Physicians

FACCPC
Fellow of the American College of
Pharmacology and Chemotherapy

FACD
Fellow of the American College of
Dentists

FACEM
Fellow of the American College of
Emergency Medicine

FACEP
Fellow of the American College of
Emergency Physicians

FACFP
Fellow of the American College of
Family Physicians

FACFS
Fellow of the American College of Foot
Surgeons

FACG
Fellow of the American College of
Gastroenterology

FACHA
Fellow of the American College of
Hospital Administrators

FACLM
Fellow of the American College of
Legal Medicine

FACN
Fellow of the American College of
Nutrition

FACNM
Fellow of the American College of
Nuclear Medicine

FACNP
Fellow of the American College of
Neuropsychopharmacology
Fellow of the American College of
Nuclear Physicians

FACO
Fellow of the American College of
Otolaryngology

FACOG
Fellow of the American College of
Obstetricians and Gynecologists

FACOS
Fellow of the American College of
Orthopedic Surgeons

FACP
Fellow of the American College of
Physicians
Fellow of the American College of
Prosthodontists

FACPM
Fellow of the American College of
Preventative Medicine

FACR
Fellow of the American College of
Radiology

FACS
Fellow of the American College of
Surgeons

FACSM
Fellow of the American College of
Sports Medicine

FAMA
Fellow of the American Medical
Association

FANS
Fellow of the American Neurological
Society

FAPA
Fellow of the American Psychiatric
Association

FAPIIA
Fellow of the American Public Health
Association

FASHP
Fellow of the American Society of
Health-System Pharmacists

FCAP
Fellow of the College of American
Pathologists

FCGP
Fellow of the College of General
Practitioners

FChS
Fellow of the Society of Chiropodists

FCMS
Fellow of the College of Medicine and
Surgery

FCO
Fellow of the College of Osteopathy

FCPS
Fellow of the College of Physicians and
Surgeons

FCSP
Fellow of the Chartered Society of
Physiotherapy

FCST
Fellow of the College of Speech
Therapists

FDS
Fellow in Dental Surgery

FFA
Fellow of the Faculty of
Anaesthetists

FFCM
Fellow of the Faculty of Community
Medicine

FFD
Fellow in the Faculty of Dentistry

FFHom
Fellow of the Faculty of Homeopathy

FFOM
Fellow of the Faculty of Occupational
Medicine

FFR
Fellow of the Faculty of
Radiologists

FHA
Fellow of the Institute of Hospital
Administrators

FIAC
Fellow of the International Academy
of Cytology

FIB
Fellow of the Institute of Biology

FIC
Fellow of the Institute of Chemistry

FICD
Fellow of the International College of
Dentists

FICS
Fellow of the International College of
Surgeons

FIMLT
Fellow of the Institute of Medical
Laboratory Technology

FMCA
Forensic Medicine Consultant
Advisor

FMS
Fellow of the Medical Society

FNP
Family Nurse Practitioner

FPS
Fellow of the Pathological Society
Fellow of the Pharmaceutical Society

FRCP
Fellow of the Royal College of
Physicians (England)

FRCPC
Fellow of the Royal College of
Physicians of Canada

FRCPE
Fellow of the Royal College of
Physicians of Edinburgh

FRCP(I)
Fellow of the Royal College of
Physicians (Ireland)

FRSC
Fellow of the Royal Society, Canada

FSR
Fellow of the Society of Radiographers

GDMO
General Duties Medical Officer

GMO
General Medical Officer

GN
Graduate Nurse

GNP
Geriatric Nurse Practitioner
Gerontological Nurse Practitioner

GNS
Gerontological Nurse Specialist

GNT
Graduate Nurse Technician

GNTP
Graduate Nurse Transition Program

GPN
Graduate Practical Nurse

GRT
Graduate Respiratory Therapist

GRTT
Graduate Respiratory Therapist Technician

HAD
Hospital Administrator

HHA
Home Health Aid

HHD
Doctor of Holistic Health

HNC
Holistic Nurse Certified

HOC
Health Officer Certificate

HP
House Physician

HT
Histologic Technician

HT(ASCP)
Histologic Technician (American Society of Clinical Pathologists)

HTL(ASCP)
Histotechnologist (American Society of Clinical Pathologists)

ICN
Infection Control Nurse

ICP
Infection Control Practitioner

IEMT
Intermediate Emergency Medical Technician

IG
Inspector General

IME
Independent Medical Examiner

IMP
Individual Medicaid Practitioner

IMS
Indian Medical Service

JAR
Junior Assistant Resident

JHMO
Junior Hospital Medical Officer

JMS
Junior Medical Student

LAc
Licensed Acupuncturist

LCSW
Licensed Clinical Social Worker

LDS
Licentiate in Dental Surgery

LISW
Licensed Independent Social Worker

LM
Licentiate in Midwifery

LMFCC
Licensed Marriage, Family and Child Counselor

LMFT
Licensed Marriage and Family Therapist

LMT
Licensed Massage Therapist

LOT
Licensed Occupational Therapist

LPC
Licensed Professional Counselor

LPCC
Licensed Professional Certified
Counselor

LPN
Licensed Practical Nurse

LPT
Licensed Physical Therapist

LPTN
Licensed Psychiatric Technical Nurse

LRCP
Licentiate of the Royal College of
Physicians (England)

LRCP(E)
Licentiate of the Royal College of
Physicians (Edinburgh)

LRCP(I)
Licentiate of the Royal College of
Physicians (Ireland)

LRCS
Licentiate of the Royal College of
Surgeons

LSW
Licensed Social Worker

LT
Laboratory Technician

LVN
Licensed Visiting Nurse
Licensed Vocational Nurse

MA
Master of Arts
Medical Assistant

MACCC
Master Arts, Certified Clinical
Competence

MASc
Master of Ayurvedic Science

MBA
Master of Business Administration

MC
Master of Chirurgiae

MCE
Medicare Code Editor

MChD
Master of Dental Surgery

MChOrth
Master of Orthopaedic Surgery

MChOtol
Master of Otology

MClSci
Master of Clinical Science

MCommH
Master of Community Health

MD
Doctor of Medicine

MDD
Doctor of Dental Medicine

MDentSc
Master of Dental Science

MDS
Master of Dental Surgery

MDT
Mechanical Diagnostic Therapist

ME
Medical Examiner

MEDEX
extension of physician (physician assistant program using former medical corpsman; medicus)

MEDIHC
Military Experience Directed into Health Careers

MEDScD
Doctor of Medical Science

Med Tech
Medical Technician
Medical Technologist

MFCC
Marriage, Family, and Child Counselor

MFST
Medical Field Service Technician

MHT
Mental Health Technician

ML
Licentiate in Midwifery

MLDT
Manual Lymph Drainage Therapist

MLPN
Medical Licensed Practical Nurse

MLT
Medical Laboratory Technician (American Society of Clinical Pathologists)

MLT(AMT)
Medical Laboratory Technician (American Medical Technologists)

MLT(ASCP)
Medical Laboratory Technician certified by American Society of Clinical Pathologists

MMed
Master of Medicine

MMS, MMSc
Master of Medical Science

MMSA
Master of Midwifery, Society of Apothecaries

MMSc
Master of Medical Science

MNSc
Master of Nursing Science

MO
Master of Obstetrics
Master of Osteopathy

MOC
Medical Officer on Call

MOD
Medical Officer of the Day

MOH
Medical Officer of Health

MOOW
Medical Officer of the Watch

MPM
Master of Psychological Medicine

MPH
Master of Public Health

MPharm
Master in Pharmacy

MRad
Master of Radiology

MRC
Master of Rehabilitation Counseling

MRCP
Member of the Royal College of
 Physicians
Member of the Royal College of
 Physicians (of England)

MRCP(E)
Member of the Royal College of
 Physicians (Edinburgh)

MRCP(I)
Member of the Royal College of
 Physicians (Ireland)

MRCS
Member of the Royal College of
 Surgeons

MRL
Medical Records Librarian

MRT
Medical Records Technician

MS
Master of Science

MS I, II, III, IV
medical student: first, second, third, and
 fourth year

MSCCC
Master Sciences, Certified Clinical
 Competence

MScD
Doctor of Medical Science
Master of Dental Science

MScMed
Master of Science in Medicine

MScN
Master of Science in Nursing

MSD
Master of Science in Dentistry

MSHyg
Master of Science in Hygiene

MSM
Master of Medical Science

MSN
Master of Science in Nursing

MSPH
Master of Science in Public Health

MSPhar
Master of Science in Pharmacy

MS Rad
Master of Science in Radiology

MSSc
Master of Sanitary Science

MSSE
Master of Science in Sanitary
 Engineering

MSURG
Master of Surgery

MSW
Master of Social Welfare
Master of Social Work
Medical Social Worker

MT
Medical Technologist
Medical Transcriptionist
Monitor Technician

MTA
Medical Technical Assistant

MT(AMT)
Medical Technologist (American
 Medical Technologists)

MT(ASCP)
Medical Technologist (American
 Society of Clinical Pathologists)

MT(ASCP)SBB
Medical Technologist (American Society of Clinical Pathologists), Specialist Blood Bank

MTBC
Music Therapist-Board Certified

MTO
Medical Transport Officer

MTR
Music Therapist, Registered

MTRS
Licensed Master Therapeutic Recreation Specialist

MV
Veterinary Physician; Medicus Veterinarius

MVD
Doctor of Veterinary Medicine

NA
Network Administrator
Nurse Anesthetist

NCT
Nursing Care Technician

NCTMB
Nationally Certified Therapeutic Massage and Bodywork

ND
Doctor of Naturopathy
Naturopathic Doctor
Nursing Doctorate

NDP
Nurse Discharge Planner

NIRMP
National Intern and Resident Matching Program

NM(ASCP)
Technologist in Nuclear Medicine (American Society of Clinical Pathologists)

NMD
Doctor of Naturopathic Medicine

NMT(R)
Nuclear Medicine Technologist Registered

NOA
Nurse Obstetric Assistant

NOSTA
Naval Ophthalmic Support and Training Activity

NNP
Neonatal Nurse Practitioner

NP
Nurse Practitioner

NPOD
Neuropsychiatric Officer of the Day

OA
Orthopedic Assistant

OccTh
Occupational Therapist

OCN
Oncology Certified Nurse

OD
Doctor of Optometry
Officer-of-the-Day

OHN
Occupational Health Nurse

OHT
Occupational Health Technician

ON
Office Nurse
Orthopedic Nurse

ONC
Orthopedic Nursing Certificate

OphD
Doctor of Ophthalmology

ORN
Orthopedic Nurse

ORT
Operating Room Technician
Registered Occupational Therapist

Osteo
Osteopathologist

OTC
Orthopedic Technician, Certified

OTR
Occupational Therapist, Registered

OTRL
Occupational Therapist, Registered
   Licensed

PA
Physician Assistant

PA-C, PAC
Physician Assistant, Certified

PA-S
Physician Assistant, Student

PBM
Pharmacy Benefit Manager

PC
Psychiatric Counselor

PCLN
Psychiatric Consultation Liaison
   Nurse

PCMO
Principal Clinical Medical Officer

PD
Doctor of Pharmacy

Phar G
Graduate in Pharmacy

Pharm D
Doctor of Pharmacy; Pharmaciae
   Doctor

PhC
Pharmaceutical Chemist

PhD
Doctor of Pharmacy; Pharmaciae
   Doctor
Doctor of Philosophy; Philosophiae
   Doctor

PhG
Graduate in Pharmacy

PHN
Public Health Nurse

PHNC
Public Health Nurse Coordinator

PhTD
Doctor of Physical Therapy

PMO
Principal Medical Officer

PN
Practical Nurse

PNA
Pediatric Nurse Associate

PNC
Psychiatric Nurse Clinician

PNNP
Perinatal Nurse Practitioner

PNO
Principal Nursing Officer

PNP
Pediatric Nurse Practitioner

PNS
Practical Nursing Student

Pod D
Doctor of Podiatry

PSMT
Psychiatric Services Management Team

PST
Patient Service Technician

QMRP
Qualified Mental Retardation Professional

RACP
Royal Australasian College of Physicians

RCGP
Royal College of General Practitioners

RCP
Respiratory Care Practitioner

RCPT
Royal College of Physicians of Thailand

RCT
Registered Care Technologist

RD
Registered Dietician

RDA
Registered Dental Assistant

RDCS
Registered Diagnostic Cardiac Sonographer

RDH
Registered Dental Hygienist

RDMS
Registered Diagnostic Medical Sonographer

REEGT
Registered Electroencephalographic Technician

RGN
Registered General Nurse

RHIA
Registered Health Information Administrator

RHIT
Registered Health Information Technologist

RHU
Registered Health Underwriter

RKT
Registered Kinesiotherapist

RMA
Registered Medical Assistant

RMO
Resident Medical Officer
Responsible Medical Officer

RMT
Registered Music Therapist

RN
Registered Nurse

RNA
Registered Nurse Anesthetist

RNC
Registered Nurse, Certified

RNCD
Registered Nurse, Chemical Dependency

RNCNA
Registered Nurse, Certified in Nursing
Administration

RNCNAA
Registered Nurse, Certified in Nursing
Administration Advanced

RNCS
Registered Nurse, Certified Specialist

RNLP
Registered Nurse, license pending

RNMT
Registered Nuclear Medicine
Technologist

RNP
Registered Nurse Practitioner

RP
Registered Pharmacist

RPAC
Registered Physician's Assistant
Certified

RPFT
Registered Pulmonary Function
Therapist

RPh
Registered Pharmacist

RPT
Registered Physical Therapist

RPTA
Registered Physical Therapist Assistant

RRA
Registered Record Administrator

RRNA
Resident Registered Nurse Anesthetist

RRT
Registered Respiratory Therapist

RSCN
Registered Sick Children's Nurse

RSO
Resident Surgical Officer

RT
Radiologic Technologist
Registered Technologist
Respiratory Therapist

RT(ARRT)
Registered Technologist American
Registry of Radiologic Technologists

RT(N)
Registered Technologist in Nuclear
Medicine

RT(N)(AART)
Registered Technologist in Nuclear
Medicine American Registry of
Radiologic Technologists

RTR
Recreational Therapist, Registered

RT(R)(ARRT)
Registered Technologist in Radiography
American Registry of Radiologic
Technologists

RT(T)(AART)
Radiologic Technologist in Radiation
Therapy American Registry of
Radiologic Technologists

RVT
Registered Vascular Technologist

SA
Surgeon's Assistant
Surgical Assistant

SAC
Substance Abuse Counselor

SAMO
Senior Administrative Medical Officer

SAR
Senior Assistant Resident

ScD
Doctor of Science

SCM
State Certified Midwife

SCMO
Senior Clerical Medical Officer

SED
Surgeon, Emergency Department

SEN
State Enrolled Nurse

SEO
Surgical Emergency Officer

SG
Surgeon General

SGO
Society of Gynecologic Oncologists
Society of Gynecologic Oncology

SHMO
Senior Hospital Medical Officer

SHO
Senior House Officer

SM
Master of Science

SMI
Senior Medical Investigator

SMO
Senior Medical Officer

SMOH
Senior Medical Officer of Health

SN
Student Nurse

SNA
Student Nursing Assistant

SNM
Student Nurse Midwife

SNP
School Nurse Practitioner

SP
Speech Pathologist

SPA
Student Physician's Assistant

SPN
Student Practical Nurse

SR
Senior Resident

SRP
State Registered Physiotherapist

SRT
Stroke Rehabilitation Technician

TAS
Therapeutic Activities Specialist

TMA
Trained Medication Aide

UC
Unit Coordinator

UL
Unit Leader

USFMG
United States foreign medical graduates

USMG
United States medical graduate

Vet Med
Veterinary Medicine

Vet Sci
Veterinary Science

VMC
Village Malaria Communicator

VMD
Doctor of Veterinary Medicine;
    Veterinariae Medicinae Doctor

VN
Visiting Nurse
Vocational Nurse

VRTA
Vocational Rehabilitation Therapy
    Assistant

WC
Ward Clerk

WOC(ET)
Wound Ostomy Care, Enterostomal
    Therapy (nurse)

WS
Ward Secretary

XDFHom
Diploma of the Faculty of
    Homeopathy

XRT
X-Ray Technician

Professional Associations and Organizations

AABB
American Association of Blood Banks

AACAP
American Academy of Child and Adolescent Psychiatry

AACC
American Association for Clinical Chemistry

AACD
American Academy of Cosmetic Dentistry

AACN
American Association of Critical-Care Nurses

AACOM
American Association of Colleges of Osteopathic Medicine

AACR
American Association for Cancer Research

AACVPR
American Association of Cardiovascular and Pulmonary Rehabilitation

AAD
American Academy of Dermatology

AAE
American Association of Endodontists

AAFP
American Academy of Family Physicians

AAGP
American Association for Geriatric Psychiatry

AAHP
American Association of Homeopathic Pharmacists

AAHSA
American Association of Homes and Services for the Aging

AAI
American Association of Immunologists

AAM
American Academy of Microbiologists

AAMA
American Academy of Medical Acupuncture

AAMC
Association of American Medical Colleges

AAMD
American Association on Mental Deficiency

AAMFT
American Association for Marriage and Family Therapists

AAMI
American Association for Medical Instrumentation
Association for the Advancement of Medical Instrumentation

AAMR
American Association on Mental Retardation

AAMT
American Association for Medical Transcription

AAN
American Academy of Neurology
American Association of Neuropathologists

AANA
American Association of Nurse Anesthetists

AANP
American Association of Naturopathic Physicians

AAO
American Academy of Ophthalmology

AAOA
American Academy of Otolaryngic Allergy

AAO-HNS
American Academy of Otolaryngology-Head and Neck Surgery

AAOS
American Academy of Orthopaedic Surgeons

AAP
American Academy of Pediatrics
American Association of Pathologists

AAPA
American Association of Pathologist Assistants

AAPB
American Association of Pathologists and Bacteriologists
Association for Applied Psychophysiology and Biofeedback

AAPCC
American Association of Poison Control Centers

AAPMR
American Academy of Physical Medicine and Rehabilitation

AARP
American Association of Retired Persons

AASLD
American Association for the Study of Liver Diseases

AAST
American Association for the Surgery of Trauma

AAWC
American Academy of Wound Management

ABA
American Bar Association
American Board of Anesthesiology

ABC
American Botanical Council

ABIM
American Board of Internal Medicine

ABMTR
Autologous Bone Marrow Transplant Registry

ABPH
American Board of Psychological Hypnosis

ABPN
American Board of Psychiatry and Neurology

ABR
American Board of Radiology

ABS
American Board of Surgery

ABTA
American Brain Tumor Association

ACA
American Chiropractic Association
American Counseling Association

ACB
American Council of the Blind

ACC
American College of Cardiology

ACC/AHA
American College of Cardiology/American Heart Association

ACG
American College of Gastroenterology

ACGME
Accreditation Council for Graduate Medical Education
American College of Graduate Medical Education

ACIP
Advisory Committee on Immunization Practices

ACLA
American Clinical Laboratory Association

ACLPS
Academy of Clinical Laboratory Physicians and Scientists

ACNM
American College of Nurse-Midwives

ACNP
American College of Nurse Practitioners

ACOG
American College of Obstetricians and Gynecologists

ACP
American College of Pathologists

ACP-ASIM
American College of Physicians-American Society of Internal Medicine

ACR
American College of Radiology
American College of Rheumatology

ACS
American Cancer Society
American Chemical Society
American College of Surgeons
Association of Clinical Scientists

ACSM
American College of Sports Medicine

ACT
American College of Testing

ACTR
American Club of Therapeutic Radiologists

ADA
American Dental Association
American Diabetes Association
American Dietetic Association

ADAMHA
Alcohol, Drug Abuse, and Mental Health Administration

ADHF
American Digestive Health Foundation

AEC
American Endosonography Club
Atomic Energy Commission

AF
Arthritis Foundation

AFAR
American Federation of Aging Research

AFB
American Foundation for the Blind

AFIP
Armed Forces Institute of Pathology

AFRIMS
Armed Forces Research Institute of Medical Sciences

AFS
American Fertility Society

AGA
American Gastroenterological Association

AGD
Academy of General Dentistry

AGS
American Geriatrics Society

AHA
American Heart Association
American Hospital Association

AHAF
American Health Assistance Foundation

AHCA
American Health Care Association

AHCPR
Agency for Health Care Policy and Research

AHF
American Health Foundation

AHFS-DI
American Hospital Formulary Service-Drug Information

AHHA
American Holistic Health Association

AHRA
American Hospital Radiology Administrators

AHRQ
Agency for Healthcare Research and Quality

AHSC
Arizona Health Science Center

AHTA
American Horticultural Therapy Association

AIN
American Institute of Nutrition

AIP
American Institute of Physics

AIUM
American Institute of Ultrasound in Medicine

AJCC
American Joint Committee on Cancer

AJCCS
American Joint Committee on Cancer Staging

AJCC/UICC
American Joint Committee on Cancer/International Union Against Cancer

ALA
American Lung Association

ALF
American Liver Foundation

ALFA
Assisted Living Federation of America

AMA
American Medical Association

AMA-DE
American Medical Association Drug Evaluation

AMDA
American Medical Directors Association

AME
American Medical Electronics

AMF
American Menopause Foundation

AMPAC
Alternative Medicine Program Advisory Council

AMRA
American Medical Record Association

AMT
American Medical Technologists

AMTA
American Massage Therapy Association
American Music Therapy Association

AMVET
American Veterans of World War II

ANA
American Nurses Association

ANRC
American National Red Cross

ANSCII
American National Standard Code for Information Interchange

ANSI
American National Standards Institute

AO
Arbeitsgemeinschaft für Osteosynthesefragen

AoA
Administration on Aging

AOA
American Optometric Association
American Orthopaedic Association
American Osteopathic Association

AO-ASIF
Arbeitsgemeinschaft für Osteosynthesefragen-Association for the Study of Internal Fixation

AOFAS
American Orthopaedic Foot and Ankle Society

AONE
American Organization of Nurse Executives

AORN
Association of Perioperative Registered Nurses

AOTA
American Occupational Therapy Association, Inc.

APA
American Psychiatric Association
American Psychological Association

APDA
American Parkinson's Disease Association

APhA
Amcrican Pharmaceutical Association

APMA
American Podiatric Medical Association

APNA
American Psychiatric Nurses Association

APRL
Army Prosthetics Research Laboratory

APSA
American Pediatric Surgical Association

APTA
American Physical Therapy Association

ARA
American Rheumatism Association

ARC
American Red Cross
Association for Retarded Citizens

ARCBS
American Red Cross Blood Services

ARDMS
American Registry of Diagnostic Medical Sonographers

ARN
Association of Rehabilitation Nurses

ARSAC
Administration of Radioactive Substances Advisory Committee

ASA
American Society of Anesthesiologists
American Society on Aging
American Standards Association
American Stroke Association

ASAPS
American Society for Aesthetic Plastic Surgery

ASB
American Society of Bacteriologists

ASCCP
American Society for Colposcopy and Cervical Pathology

ASCI
American Society for Clinical Investigation

ASCIA
American Spinal Cord Injury Association

ASCLT
American Society of Clinical Laboratory Technicians

ASCP
American Society of Clinical Pathologists

ASCRS
American Society for Colon and Rectal Surgeons

ASDA
American Sleep Disorders Association

ASEP
American Society for Experimental Pathology

ASGE
American Society for Gastrointestinal Endoscopy

ASH
American Society of Hematology

ASHA
American Speech-Language-Hearing Association

ASIA
American Spinal Injury Association

ASIF
Association for the Study of Internal Fixation

ASIM
American Society of Internal Medicine

ASM
American Society for Microbiologists

ASP
American Society of Pathologists

ASPO
American Society of Preventive Oncology

ASPRS
American Society of Plastic and Reconstructive Surgeons

ASPS
American Society of Plastic Surgeons

ASRT
American Society of Radiologic Technologists
American Society of Registered Technologists

ASSH
American Society for Surgery of the Hand

ASTM
American Society for Testing and Materials

ASTRO
American Society for Therapeutic Radiology and Oncology

ASTS
American Society of Transplant Surgeons

ATA
American Tinnitus Association

ATPO
Association of Technical Personnel in Ophthalmology

ATS
American Thoracic Society

AUA
American Urological Association

AUR
Association of University Radiologists

AURT
Association of University Radiologic Technicians

BCA
Blue Cross Association

BCCG
British Cooperative Clinical Group

BCDSP
Boston Collaborative Drug Surveillance Program

BCHS
Bureau of Community Health Services

BCIA
Biofeedback Certification Institute of America

BCIC
Birth Control Investigation Committee

BCOA
Brookdale Center on Aging

BCTF
Breast Cancer Task Force

BDA
British Dental Association

BDAC
Bureau of Drug Abuse Control

BEAR
Biologic Effects of Atomic Radiation (Committee)

BHP
Bureau of Health Professions

BIPM
International Bureau of Weights and Measures; Bureau International des Poids et Mesures

BMD
Bureau of Medical Devices

BNA
Basle Nomina Anatomica

BNDD
Bureau of Narcotics and Dangerous Drugs

BNIST
National Bureau of Scientific Information; Bureau National d'Information Scientifique

BOD
Bureau of Drugs

BQA
Bureau of Quality Assurance

BSI
British Standards Institution

BTTP
British Testicular Tumour Panel

BVI
Better Vision Institute

BVM
Bureau of Veterinary Medicine

CAFMHS
Child, Adolescent, and Family Mental Health Service

CANE
Clearinghouse on Abuse and Neglect of the Elderly

CAP
College of American Pathologists

CARF
Commission on Accreditation of Rehabilitation Facilities

CAS
Center for Alcohol Studies
Child Assessment Schedule

CASCSP
Center for the Advancement of State Community Services Programs

CASH
Commission for Administrative Services in Hospitals

CBADAA
Certifying Board of the American Dental Assistants Association

CBBB
Council of Better Business Bureaus

CBER
Center for Biologics Evaluation & Research

CBIRF
Chemical Biological Incident Response Force (of the U.S. Marine Corps)

CBN
Commission on Biological Nomenclature

CBTC
Childhood Brain Tumor Consortium

CCAC
Continuing Care Accreditation Commission

CCC
Canadian Cardiovascular Coalition

CCDC
Canadian Communicable Disease Center

CCE
Council on Chiropractic Education

CCFA
Crohn's and Colitis Foundation of America

CCG
Children's Cancer Group

CCNSC
Cancer Chemotherapy National Service Center

CCS
Canadian Cardiovascular Society

CCUSA
Catholic Charities USA

CDC
Centers for Disease Control and Prevention
Communicable Disease Center

CDCP
Centers for Disease Control and Prevention

CDHNF
Children's Digestive Health and Nutrition Foundation

CDS
Christian Dental Society

CEM
Center for Molecular Epidemiology

CEQ
Council on Environmental Quality

CERAD
Consortium to Establish a Registry for Alzheimer's Disease

CF
Coalition for the Family

CFF
Cystic Fibrosis Foundation

CFH
Council on Family Health

CFS
Cystic Fibrosis Society

CFSTI
Clearinghouse for Federal Scientific and Technical Information

CGA
Catholic Golden Age

CHA
Catholic Hospital Association

CHAS
Center for Health Administration Studies

CHC
Community Health Council

CHEP
Cuban/Haitian Entrant Program

CHIP
Children's Health Insurance Program

CHSD
Children's Health Services Division

CHT
Center for Health Technology

CID
Central Institute for the Deaf

CIP
Carcinogen Information Program
Cardiac Injury Panel

CIS
Chemical Information Service

CLMA
Clinical Laboratory Management Association

CMB
Central Midwives' Board

CMHS
Center for Mental Health Services

CMS
Christian Medical Society
Council of Medical Staffs

CNME
Council on Naturopathic Medical Education

COCI
Consortium on Chemical Information

CODA
Codependents Anonymous

CODATA
Committee on Data for Science and Technology

COG
Central Oncology Group

COHSE
Confederation of Health Service Employees

COLA
Commission on Office Laboratory Accreditation

COTH
Council of Teaching Hospitals

COTRANS
Coordinated Transfer Application System

CPEHS
Consumer Protection and Environmental Health Service

CPHA
Commission on Professional and Hospital Activities

CPSC
Consumer Product Safety Commission

CREOG
Council on Resident Education in Obstetrics and Gynecology

CRHL
Collaborative Radiological Health Laboratory

CRRMP
Committee of Radiation from Radioactive Medicinal Products

CSCD
Center for Sickle Cell Disease

CSIN
Chemical Substances Information Network

CSM
Committee on Safety of Medicines

CSMB
Center for Study of Multiple Births

CSMMG
Chartered Society of Massage and Medical Gymnastics

CSTI
Clearinghouse for Scientific and Technical Information

CSU
Central Statistical Unit (of Venereal Disease Research Laboratory)

CTAA
Community Transportation Association of America

CTDTADA
The Council on Dental Therapeutics of the American Dental Association

CTVHCS
Central Texas Veterans Health Care System

CUOG
Canadian Urology Oncology Group

DAC
Division of Ambulatory Care

DAHEA
Department of Allied Health Education and Accreditation

DAHM
Division of Allied Health Manpower

DAIDS
Division of AIDS (of the National Institute of Allergy and Infectious Diseases, NIH)

DAV
Disabled American Veterans

DAWN
Drug Abuse Warning Network

DBS
Division of Biological Standards

DCC
Disaster Control Center

DCFS
Department of Children and Family Services

DCS
Department of Children's Services

DCYS
Department of Children and Youth Services

DDD
Division of Developmental Disabilities

DDNC
Digestive Disease National Coalition

DDPA
Delta Dental Plans Association

DEBRA
Dystrophic Epidermolysis Bullosa Research Association of America

DECAFS
Department of Children and Family Services

DEHS
Division of Emergency Health Services

DEM
Department of Emergency Medicine

DFCI
Dana-Farber Cancer Institute

DFS
Division of Family Services

DGMS
Division of General Medical Services

DHES
Division of Health Examination Statistics

DHEW
Department of Health, Education, and Welfare (now Department of Health and Human Services)

DHHS
Department of Health and Human Services

DHI
Dental Health International

DHS
Department of Human Services

DLC
Dental Laboratory Conference

DMH
Department of Mental Health
Department of Mental Hygiene

DMS
Department of Medicine and Surgery

DOD
Department of Defense

DOH
Department of Health

DOJ
Department of Justice

DOL
Department of Labor

DOSS
Department of Social Services

DOT
Department of Transportation

DPA
Department of Public Assistance

DPSS
Department of Public Social Services

DRME
Division of Research in Medical Education

DSHS
Department of Social and Health Services

DSMB
Data and Safety Monitoring Board

DSS
Department of Social Services

DTBE
Division of Tuberculosis Elimination

DTEG
Dermatology Teachers Exchange Group

DVA
Department of Veterans Affairs

DVCC
Disease Vector Control Center

DVH
Division for the Visually Handicapped

DVR
Division of Vocational Rehabilitation

EAB
Ethics Advisory Board

EBAA
Eye Bank Association of America

EC
Enzyme Commission (of International Union of Biochemistry)

ECaP
Exceptional Cancer Patients

ECFMG
Educational Commission on Foreign Medical Graduates

ECFMS
Educational Council for Foreign Medical Students

ECLAM
European Consensus Lupus Activity Measure

ECLM
European Confederation for Laboratory Medicine

EEOC
Equal Employment Opportunity Commission

EHA
Environmental Health Agency

EHPAC
Emergency Health Preparedness Advisory Committee

EIS
Epidemic Intelligence Service

ELS
European Laryngological Societies

ELSO
Extracorporeal Life Support Organization

EMCRO
Experimental Medical Care Review Organization

EMEA
European Medicines Evaluation Agency

ENAC
Emergency Notification and Assistance Convention System

ENTIS
European Network of Teratology Information Services

EORTC
European Organization for Research and Treatment of Cancer

EOS
European Orthodontic Society

EPA
Environmental Protection Agency

EPA/RCRA
Environmental Protection Agency Resource Conservation and Recovery Act

EPI
Expanded Program of Immunizations (World Health Organization)

ERDA
Energy Research and Development Administration

ESCOP
European Scientific Cooperative on Phytotherapy

ESPGHAN
European Society of Paediatric Gastroenterology, Hepatology, and Nutrition

EU
European Union

EULAR
European League Against Rheumatism

EURONET
European On-Line Network

EUROTOX
European Committee on Chronic Toxicity Hazards

FA
Families Anonymous

FACCT
Foundation for Accountability

FACMTA
Federal Advisory Council on Medical Training Aids

FACNHA
Foundation of American College of Nursing Home Administrators

FACOSH
Federal Advisory Committee on Occupational Safety and Health

FAH
Federation of American Hospitals

FAO
Food and Agriculture Organization

FBR
Foundation for Biomedical Research

FCER
Foundation for Chiropractic Education and Research

FCIC
Federal Consumer Information Center

FCMW
Foundation for Child Mental Welfare

FDA
Food and Drug Administration

FD&C
Food, Drug, and Cosmetic (Act)

FDCPA
Food, Drug, and Consumer Product Agency

FDD
Food and Drug Directorate

FEHBP
Federal Employee Health Benefits Program

FEMA
Federal Emergency Management Agency

FFS
Fight For Sight

FHC
Faith and Health Consortium

FIA
Family Independence Agency (formerly Department of Social Services)

FICA
Federal Insurance Contributions Act

FIGO
Federation International de Gynecologie et Obstetrique
International Federation of Gynecology and Obstetrics

FOA
Federation of Orthodontic Associations

FPO
Federation of Prosthodontic Organizations

FSA
Family Services Association

FSI
Food Sanitation Institute

FSOP
French Society of Pediatric Oncology

FWPCA
Federal Water Pollution Control Administration

GA
Gamblers Anonymous

GAO
General Accounting Office

GCWM
General Conference on Weights and Measures

GDB
Guide Dogs for the Blind

GDC
General Dental Council

GMENAC
Graduate Medical Education National Advisory Committee

GMS
General Medical Service

GNC
General Nursing Council

GOG
Gynecologic Oncology Group (of National Cancer Institute)

GPA
Global Program on AIDS

GRF
Glaucoma Research Foundation

GSA
Gerontological Society of America

GT
Generations Together

HAIC
Hearing Aid Industry Conference

HAP
Handicapped Aid Program

HASP
Hospital Admissions and Surveillance Program

HC
Hospital Corps

HCA
Hospital Corporation of America

HCFA
Health Care Financing Administration

HCIS
Health Care Information System

HCRE
Homeopathic Council for Research and Education

HCSD
Health Care Studies Division

HCTC
Health Care Technology Center

HDRF
Heart Disease Research Foundation

HDSA
Huntington's Disease Society of America

HEC
Health Education Council

HeCOG
Hellenic Cooperative Oncology Group

HER
HIV Epidemiology Research

HERS
Hysterectomy Educational Resources and Services Foundation

HEW
(Department of) Health, Education, and Welfare

HHCA
Home Health Care Agency

HHS
(Department of) Health and Human Services

HIAA
Health Insurance Association of America

HIBAC
Health Insurance Benefits Advisory Council

HIC
Heart Information Center

HICPAC
Hospital Infection Control Practices Advisory Committee

HII
Health Industries Institute
Health Insurance Institute

HISSG
Hospital Information Systems Sharing Group

HIVNET
Human Immunodeficiency Virus Project Network

HJD
Hospital for Joint Disease

HMAC
Health Manpower Advisory Council

HMSS
Hospital Management Systems Society

HNCCG
Head and Neck Cancer Cooperative Group

HRA
Human Resources Administration

HRRC
Human Research Review Committee

HRSA
Health Resources and Services Administration

HSA
Health Services Administration
Health Systems Agency

HSC
Hospital for Sick Children

HSMHA
Health Services and Mental Health Administration

HSQB
Health Standards and Quality Bureau

HSRC
Health Services Research Center
Human Subjects Review Committee

HSRI
Health Systems Research Institute

HTA
Herb Trade Association

IAB
Industrial Accident Board

IADR
International Association for Dental Research

IAEA
International Atomic Energy Agency

IAET
International Association for Enterostomal Therapy

IAG
International Academy of Gnathology

IAM
Institute of Aviation Medicine

IAO
International Association for Orthodontics

IAP
International Academy of Pathology

IAPAAS
International Association of Physical Activity, Aging, and Sports

IAPG
International Antimicrobial Project Group

IARC
International Agency for Research on Cancer

IASHS
Institute for Advanced Study in Human Sexuality

IASP
International Association for the Study of Pain

IAVI
International AIDS Vaccine Initiative

IBC
Institutional Biosafety Committee

IBCSG
International Breast Cancer Study Group

IBED
Inter-African Bureau for Epizootic Diseases

IBMTR
International Bone Marrow Transplant Registry

ICA
Institute of Clinical Analysis
International Chiropractic Association

ICAAC
Interscience Conference on Antimicrobial Agents and Chemotherapy

ICAO
International Civil Aviation Organization

ICCIDD
International Council for Control of Iodine Deficiency Disorder

ICCR
International Committee for Contraceptive Research

ICD
Institute for Crippled and Disabled

ICDRG
International Contact Dermatitis Research Group

ICH
International Council on Harmonization

ICHD
Inter-Society Commission for Heart Disease

ICHPPC
International Classification of Health Problems in Primary Care

ICIC
International Cancer Information Center

ICLH
Imperial College, London Hospital

ICOPER
International Cooperative Pulmonary Embolism Registry

ICR
Institute for Cancer Research

ICRC
International Committee of the Red Cross

ICRETT
International Cancer Research Technology Transfer

ICREW
International Cancer Research Workshop

ICRP
International Commission on Radiological Protection

ICRS
Index Chemicus Registry System

ICRU
International Commission on Radiological Units

ICS
International Continence Society

ICSH
International Committee for Standardization in Hematology

IDAMIS
Integrated Dose Abuse Management Informational Systems

IDARP
Integrated Drug Abuse Reporting Process

IDIC
Internal Dose Information Center

IDSA
Infectious Disease Society of America

IEC
Independent Ethics Committee

IFCC
International Federation of Clinical Chemistry

IFRP
International Fertility Research Program

IGCCCG
International Germ Cell Cancer Collaborative Group

IHCP
Institute of Hospital and Community Psychiatry

IHPP
Intergovernmental Health Project Policy

IHS
Indian Health Service
International Headache Society

IIME
Institute of International Medical Education

IIS
International Institute of Stress

IKDC
International Knee Documentation Committee

ILAE
International League Against Epilepsy

ILAR
International League of Associations for Rheumatology

ILO
International Labor Organization

ILSI
International Life Science Institute

IMA
Interchurch Medical Assistance

IMIC
International Medical Information Center

IMR
Institute for Medical Research
Institution for the Mentally Retarded

IMRG
Internal Microvascular Research Group

INCC
Institut National du Cancer du Canada

IOA
International Ostomy Association

IOM
Institute of Medicine

IP
L'Institut Pasteur

IPAR
Institute of Personality Assessment and Research

IRC
Institutional Review Committee (Board)
International Red Cross

IRH
Institute of Religion and Health
Institute for Research in Hypnosis

IRIS
International Research Information Service

IRRC
Institutional Research Review Committee

IRS
Information and Referral Society

IRSG
Intergroup Rhabdomyosarcoma Study Group

ISA
Incest Survivors Anonymous

ISCLT
International Society for Clinical Laboratory Technology

ISCP
International Society of Comparative Pathology

ISGyP
International Society of Gynecologic Pathologists

ISH
International Society of Hematology

ISHLT
International Society for Heart and Lung Transplantation

ISHT
International Society for Heart Transplantation

ISM
International Society of Microbiologists

ISMP
Institute for Safe Medication Practices

ISO
International Standards Organization

ISR
Institute for Sex Research
Institute of Surgical Research

ISSVD
International Society for the Study of Vulvar Diseases

ISUP
International Society for Urological Pathology

ITC
Interagency Testing Committee

ITF
International Tremor Foundation

ITI
International Team Implantologists

ITQB-IBET
Molecular Genetics Unit of the Institute of Biotechnology

IUPAC
International Union of Pure and Applied Chemistry

JACL
Japanese American Citizens League

JCAH
Joint Commission on Accreditation of Hospitals

JCAHO
Joint Commission on Accreditation of Healthcare Organizations

JCAHPO
Joint Commission on Allied Health Personnel in Ophthalmology

JCMHC
Joint Commission on Mental Health of Children

JCOG
Japanese Clinical Oncology Group

JDF
Juvenile Diabetes Foundation

JFS
Jewish Family Services

JOA
Japanese Orthopaedic Association

JRCOMP
Joint Review Committee for Ophthalmic Medical Personnel

JTF-CS
Joint Task Force for Civil Support (of the Defense Department)

KS-GEC
Kansas Geriatric Education Center

LAVA
Los Angeles Veterans Administration Hospital

LC
Library of Congress

LCB
Laboratory of Cancer Biology

LCDC
Laboratory Centre for Disease Control (Canada)

LCE
Legal Counsel for the Elderly

LCSSG
Laparoscopic Colorectal Surgery Group

LFA
Lupus Foundation of America

LHI
Labor Health Institute

LIA
Laser Institute of America

LLS
Leukemia and Lymphoma Society, Inc.

LNCVA
Lighthouse National Center for Vision and Aging

LRN
Laboratory Response Network

LSE
Legal Services for the Elderly

LSUMC
Louisiana State University Medical Center

MACDP
Metropolitan Atlanta Congenital Defects Program

MAO
Montana Academy of Ophthalmology

MAOP
Mid-Atlantic Oncology Program

MAP
Medical Assistance Program
Medical Audit Program

MASH
Mobile Army Surgical Hospital

MCA
Medicines Control Agency (United Kingdom)

MCB
Medicines Control Board

MCR
Medical Corps Reserve
Medicare Cost Report

MDA
Medical Devices Agency (United Kingdom)

MDACC
MD Anderson Cancer Center

MDBDF
March of Dimes Birth Defect Foundation

MDPH
Michigan Department of Public Health

MEB
Medical Evaluation Board

MEDICO
Medical International Cooperation

MERB
Medical Examination and Review Board

MFCU
Medicaid Fraud Control Unit

MFSS
Medical Field Service School

MGMA
Medical Group Management Association

MHA
Mental Health Association

MHCS
Mental Hygiene Consultation Service

MHHP
Minnesota Heart Health Program

MHI
Mental Health Institute

MHRI
Mental Health Research Institute

MIB
Medical Impairment Bureau

MIC
Medical Interfraternity Conference

MINE
Medical Information Network of Europe

MIR
Mallinckrodt Institute of Radiology

MLA
Medical Library Association

MMAP
Maine Medical Assessment Program

MMIS
Medicaid Management Information System

MMPNC
Medical Maternal Program for Nuclear Casualties

MMRS
Metropolitan Medical Response Systems

MOH
Ministry of Health

MORC
Medical Officers Reserve Corps

MOWAA
Meals on Wheels Association of America

MPA
Medical Procurement Agency
Medical Products Agency (Sweden)

MPU
Medical Practitioners Union

MRCL
Medical Research Council Laboratories

MRI
Medical Research Institute

MROD
Medical Research and Operations Directorate

MSA
Medical Services Administration

MSC
Medical Service Corps

MSKCC
Memorial Sloan-Kettering Cancer Center

MSS
Medicare Statistical System

MSSP
Maternal Support Services Program

MSTS
Musculoskeletal Tumor Society

MTF
Musculoskeletal Transplant Foundation

MTSO
Medical Transcription Service Organization

N4A
National Association of Area Agencies on Aging

NAACLS
National Accrediting Agency for Clinical Laboratory Sciences

NAAMM
North American Academy of Manipulative Medicine

NACDG
North American Contact Dermatitis Group

NACHC
National Association of Community Health Centers

NACI
National Advisory Committee on Immunization

NACSCAOM
National Accreditation Commission for Schools and Colleges of Acupuncture and
Oriental Medicine

NAD
National Association of the Deaf

NADL
National Association of Dental Laboratories

NAELA
National Academy of Elder Law Attorneys, Inc.

NAEPP
National Asthma Education and Prevention Program

NAFC
National Association for Continence

NAHC
National Association for Home Care

NAHD
National Association for Human Development

NAHF
National Association for Health & Fitness

NAHI
National Athletic Health Institute

NAHOF
National Association on HIV Over Fifty

NAMCS
National Ambulatory Medical Care Survey

NAMES
National Association of Medical Equipment Suppliers

NAMI
National Alliance for the Mentally Ill

NAMRU
Navy Medical Reserve Unit

NAMS
North American Menopause Society

NANASP
National Association of Nutrition and Aging Service Programs

NANDA
North American Nursing Diagnosis Association

NAPCA
National Asian Pacific Center on Aging

NAPGCM
National Association of Progressional Geriatric Care Managers

NAPNAP
National Association of Pediatric Nurse Associates and Practitioners

NAPNES
National Association for Practical Nurse Education and Services

NARIC
National Rehabilitation Information Center

NARMC
Naval Aerospace and Regional Medical Center

NASDAD
National Association of Seventh-Day Adventist Dentists

NAS-NRC
National Academy of Science-National Research Council

NASPGN
North American Society for Pediatric Gastroenterology and Nutrition

NASUA
National Association of State Units on Aging

NASW
National Association of Social Workers

NATR
National Association of Tumor Registrars

NBA
National Bar Association

NBCCG
National Bladder Cancer Collaborative Group

NBCE
National Board of Chiropractic Examiners

NBME
National Board of Medical Examiners

NBS
National Bureau of Standards

NBTF
National Biomedical Tracer Facility

NBTS
National Blood Transfusion Service

NC
Nurse Corps

NCADD
National Council on Alcoholism and Drug Dependence

NCAHE
National Council Against Health Fraud

NCAI
National Coalition for Adult Immunization

NCAMLP
National Certification Agency for Medical Laboratory Personnel

NCBA
National Caucus and Center on Black Aged, Inc.

NCCAM
National Center for Complementary and Alternative Medicine

NCCAN
National Center for Child Abuse and Neglect

NCCAOM
National Certification Committee for Acupuncture and Oriental Medicine

NCCDS
National Cooperative Collaborative Crohn's Disease Study

NCCLS
National Committee for Clinical Laboratory Standards

NCCN
National Comprehensive Cancer Network

NCCNHR
National Citizen's Coalition for Nursing Home Reform

NCCS
National Coalition for Cancer Survivorship

NCCTG
North Central Cancer Treatment Group

NCDB
National Cancer Data Base

NCEA
National Center on Elder Abuse

NCEP
National Cholesterol Education Program

NCHLS
National Council of Health Laboratory Services

NCHS
National Center for Health Statistics

NCI
National Cancer Institute

NCIC
National Cancer Institute of Canada

NCL
National Consumer's League

NCLEX-RN
National Council Licensure Examination for Registered Nurses

NCLR
National Council of La Raza

NCME
Network for Continuing Medical Education

NCMHD
National Center on Minority Health and Health Disparities (NIH)

NCMHI
National Clearinghouse for Mental Health Information

NCOA
National Council on Aging, Inc.

NCOG
North California Oncology Group

NCPIE
National Council on Patient Information and Education

NCPL
National Center on Poverty Law, Inc.

NCPSSM
National Committee to Preserve Social Security and Medicare

NCQA
National Commission for Quality Assurance

NCRA
National Cancer Registrars Association

NCRP
National Council on Radiation Protection and Measurements

NCRR
National Center for Research Resources (NIH)

NCTC
National Cancer Tissue Culture
National Collection of Type Cultures

NCYC
National Collection of Yeast Cultures

NDA
National Dental Association

NDC
National Data Communications
National Drug Code
Naval Dental Clinic

NDCD
National Drug Code Directory

NDDG
National Diabetes Data Group

NDDIC
National Digestive Diseases Information Clearinghouse

NDIC
National Diabetes Information Clearinghouse

NDS
Naval Dental School

NDSB
Narcotic Drugs Supervisory Board

NDTI
National Disease and Therapeutic Index

NECHI
Northeastern Consortium for Health Information

NEHCRC
Native Elder Health Care Resource Center

NEHEP
National Eye Health Education Program

NEI
National Eye Institute

NEISS
National Electronic Injury Surveillance System

NELS
National Educational Longitudinal Survey

NEOB
New England Organ Bank

NEOPO
Northeast Organ Procurement Organization

NERICP
New England Regional Infant Cardiac Program

NESO
Northeastern Society of Orthodontists

NFB
National Foundation for the Blind

NFCA
National Family Caregivers Association

NGNA
National Gerontological Nursing Association

NGTF
National Gay Task Force

NHCoA
National Hispanic Council on Aging

NHF
National Hospital Foundation

NHGRI
National Human Genome Research Institute (NIH)

NHIC
National Health Information Center

NHLBI
National Heart, Lung, and Blood Institute

NHPCO
National Hospice and Palliative Care Organization

NHPF
National Health Policy Forum

NHPPN
National Health Professions Placement Network

NHS
National Health Service (United Kingdom)

NHSR
National Hospital Service Reserve

NIA
National Institute on Aging (NIH)

NIA-RI
National Institute on Aging-Reagan Institute

NIAAA
National Institute on Alcohol Abuse and Alcoholism (NIH)

NIAID
National Institute of Acquired Immune Deficiency
National Institute of Allergy and Infectious Diseases (NIH)

NIAMD
National Institute of Arthritis and Metabolic Diseases (NIH)

NIAMS
National Institute of Arthritis and Musculoskeletal and Skin Diseases (NIH)

NIBIB
National Institute of Biomedical Imaging and Bioengineering

NICA
National Interfaith Coalition on Aging

NICE
National Institute for Clinical Excellence (United Kingdom)

NICHD
National Institute of Child Health and Human Development

NICOA
National Indian Council on Aging

NIDA
National Institute on Drug Abuse (NIH)

NIDCD
National Institute on Deafness and Other Communication Disorders

NIDCR
National Institute of Dental and Craniofacial Research

NIDDK
National Institute of Diabetes and Digestive and Kidney Disease

NIDR
National Institute of Dental Research

NIEHS
National Institute of Environmental Health Sciences (NIH)

NIGMS
National Institute of General Medical Sciences (NIH)

NIH
National Institutes of Health

NIH-ORBD-NRC
NIH Osteoporosis and Related Bone Diseases National Resource Center

NIHR
National Institute for Healthcare Research

NIIC
National Injury Information Clearinghouse

NIMH
National Institute of Mental Health (NIH)

NINDS
National Institute of Neurological Disorders and Stroke (NIH)

NINR
National Institute for Nursing Research (NIH)

NIOSH
National Institute of Occupational Safety and Health (NIH)

NIRSC
National Information and Referral Support Center

NIST
National Institute of Standards and Technology

NJCLD
National Joint Committee on Learning Disabilities

NKF
National Kidney Foundation

NKUDIC
National Kidney and Urological Diseases Information Clearinghouse

NLHEP
National Lung Health Education Program

NLM
National Library of Medicine (NIH)

NLSBPH
National Library Service for the Blind and Physically Handicapped

NMA
National Medical Association

NMAC
National Medical Audiovisual Center

NMC
National Medical Care

NMDP
National Marrow Donor Program

NMFI
National Master Facility Inventory

NMHA
National Mental Health Association

NML
National Medical Library

NMNRU
National Medical Neuropsychiatric Research Unit

NMRDC
Naval Medical Research and Development Command

NMRL
Naval Medical Research Laboratory

NMRT
National Medical Response Team

NMRU
Naval Medical Research Unit

NMS
Naval Medical School

NMSS
National Multiple Sclerosis Society

NMTCB
Nuclear Medicine Technology Certification Board

NNC
National Nutrition Consortium

NNDC
National Naval Dental Center

NNFA
National Nutritional Foods Association

NNIS
National Nosocomial Infections Surveillance

NOCSAE
National Operating Committee on Standards for Athletic Equipment

NOCTI
National Occupation Competency Testing Institute

NOF
National Osteoporosis Foundation

NORD
National Organization for Rare Disorders

NOVA
National Organization of Victim Assistance

NOVS
National Office of Vital Statistics

NPCTG
National Prostatic Cancer Treatment Group

NPF
National Psoriasis Foundation

NPI
Neuropsychiatric Institute

NPIN
National Prevention Information Network

NPRCWA
National Policy and Resource Center on Women and Aging

NPSF
National Patient Safety Foundation

NPTR
National Pediatric Trauma Registry

NRB
Noninstitutional Review Board

NRC
National Research Council
Nuclear Regulatory Commission

NRCC
National Registry in Clinical Chemistry

NRCDLTC
National Resource Center: Diversity and Long-Term Care

NRCNAA
National Resource Center on Native American Aging

NREMT-P
National Registry of Emergency Medical Technicians-Paramedic level

NRHA
National Rural Health Association

NRIC
National Resource and Information Center

NRM
National Registry of Microbiologists

NRMP
National Residency Matching Plan

NRPB
National Radiological Protection Board

NRSCC
National Reference System in Clinical Chemistry

NRSFPS
National Reporting System for Family Planning Services

NSA
National Stroke Association

NSCERC
National Senior Citizens' Education and Research Center

NSCIDRC
National Spinal Cord Injury Data Research Center

NSCLC
National Senior Citizens' Law Center

NSF
National Sleep Foundation

NSGA
National Senior Games Association

NSHC
National Self-Help Clearinghouse

NTIS
National Technical Information Service

NTL
National Training Laboratories

NTP
National Toxicology Program

NVAC
National Vaccine Advisory Committee

NWHIC
National Women's Health Information Center

NWHN
National Women's Health Network

OAA
Opticians Association of America

OAM
Office of Alternative Medicine

OASDHI
Old Age, Survivors, Disability, and Health Insurance

OCA
Organization of Chinese Americans

OCCAM
Office of Cancer Complementary and Alternative Medicine

OCD
Office of Child Development
Office of Civil Defense

OCHS
Office of Cooperative Health Statistics

OCIS
Oncology Center Information System

ODAC
Oncologic Drugs Advisory Committee (of the US Food and Drug Administration)

ODSS
Office of Disability Support Services

OGD
Office of Generic Drugs (of the Food and Drug Administration)

OHTA
Office of Health Technology Assessment

OIF
Osteogenesis Imperfecta Foundation

OIG
Office of the Inspector General

OME
Office of the Medical Examiner

ONS
Office for National Statistics (United Kingdom)
Oncology Nursing Society

OPD
Office of Orphan Products Development

OPO
Organ Procurement Organization

OPS
Ophthalmic Photographers Society

OPSR
Office of Professional Standards Review

OPST-BQA
Office of Professional Standards Review & Bureau of Quality Assurance

OPTN
Organ Procurement and Transplantation Network

ORLAU
Orthotic Research and Locomotor Assessment Unit

ORNL
Oak Ridge National Laboratory

OSEP
Office of Special Education Programs

OSH
Office on Smoking and Health

OSHA
Occupational Safety and Health Administration

OTIS
Organization of Teratology Information Services

OTOD
Organization of Teachers of Oral Diagnosis

OTSG
Office of the Surgeon General

OVR
Office of Vocational Rehabilitation

OWL
Older Women's League

PACE
Program of All-Inclusive Care for the Elderly

PACT
Philadelphia Association of Clinical Trials

PAHO
Pan American Health Organization

PAR
Program for Alcohol Recovery

PBA
Prevent Blindness America

PBTG
Philadelphia Bone Marrow Transplant Group

PCA
President's Council on Aging

PCAC
Physical Care Assessment Center

PCC
Poison Control Center

PCIC
Poison Control Information Center

PCPFS
President's Council on Physical Fitness and Sports

PDF
Parkinson's Disease Foundation

PFC
Partnership for Caring

PFF
Pulmonary Fibrosis Foundation

PFS
Patient and Family Services

PHD
Public Health Department

PHLS
Public Health Laboratory Service

PHO
Physician/Hospital Organization

PhRMA
Pharmaceutical Research and Manufacturers of America (formerly the Pharmaceutical Manufacturers Association)

PHS
Public Health Service

PHTS
Pediatric Home Treatment Service

PLSG
Pigmented Lesion Study Group

PMIS
PSRO (Professional Standards Review Organization) Management Information System

POCAAN
People of Color Against AIDS Network

PPFA
Planned Parenthood Federation of America

PPRC
Physician Payment Review Commission

PQRI
Product Quality Research Initiative

PRB
Prosthetics Research Board

PRC
Pension Rights Center

PRIME
Prematriculation Program in Medical Education

PRO
Peer Review Organization
Professional Review Organization

PROMIS
Problem-oriented Medical Information System

ProPAC
Prospective Payment Assessment Commission

PRSIS
Prospective Rate Setting Information System

PSEF
Plastic Surgery Educational Foundation

PSR
Physicians for Social Responsibility

PSRC
Plastic Surgery Research Council

PSRO
Professional Standards Review Organization

PWBA
Pension and Welfare Benefits Administration

PWP
Parents Without Partners

RABBI
Rapid Access Blood Bank Information

RC
Red Cross

RCAI
Restorative Care of America, Inc.

RCOG
Royal College of Obstetricians and Gynaecologists

RCP
Royal College of Physicians (of England)

RCPE
Royal College of Physicians of Edinburgh

RCPI
Royal College of Physicians of Ireland

RCS
Royal College of Surgeons of England

RCSED
Royal College of Surgeons of Edinburgh

RCSI
Royal College of Surgeons of Ireland

RDG
Research Discussion Group

REACH
Reassurance to Each (assistance to families of mentally ill)

ROPA
Regional Organ Procurement Agency

RTECS
Registry of Toxic Effects of Chemical Substances

SA
Sexaholics Anonymous

SADD
Students Against Drunk Driving

SAGES
Society of American Gastrointestinal Endoscopic Surgeons

SAMHSA
Substance Abuse and Mental Health Services Administration

SART
Society for Assisted Reproductive Technology

SASA
Sex Abuse Survivors Anonymous

SBH, SBOH
State Board of Health

SC
Sanitary Corps

SCHIP
State Children's Health Insurance Program

SCOI
Southern California Orthopedic Institute

SDA
Seventh Day Adventist

SERHOLD
(National Biomedical) Serials Holding Database

SESAP
Surgical Education and Self-Assessment Program

SHEA
Society for Healthcare Epidemiology of America

SHHH
Self-Help for Hard of Hearing People, Inc.

SHPDA
State Health Planning and Development Agency

SIECUS
Sex Information and Educational Council of the United States

SIOP
International Society of Pediatric Oncology

SJCRH
St. Jude Children's Research Hospital

SJM
St. Jude Medical

SK, SKI
Sloan-Kettering Institute

SLAA
Sex and Love Addicts Anonymous

SLICC
Systemic Lupus International Collaborating Clinics

SLT
Surgical Laser Technologies

SNDA
Student National Dental Association

SPP
Society for Pediatric Pathology

SPRY
Setting Priorities for Retirement Years (Foundation)

SRA
Science Research Associates

SSA
Social Security Administration

SSIE
Smithsonian Science Information Exchange

SSO
Society of Surgical Oncology

SSOP
Second Surgical Opinion Program

SWOG
Southwest Oncology Group

TAC
Toxicant Analysis Center

TCDB
Traumatic Coma Data Bank

TCSG
The Center for Social Gerontology

TDB
Toxicology Data Bank

TERIS
Teratogen Information System

TGA
Therapeutic Goods Administration (Australia)

TIRR
The Institute for Rehabilitation Research

TMIC
Toxic Materials Information Center

TRI
Thyroid Research Institute

TSRH
Texas Scottish Rite Hospital

UAPD
Union of American Physicians and Dentists

UCB
University of California, Berkeley

UCBL
University of California, Berkeley, Laboratory

UCI
University of California, Irvine

UCLA
University of California, Los Angeles

UH
University Hospital

UHSC
University Health Services Clinic

UICC
International Union Against Cancer

UKTSSA
United Kingdom Transplant Support Service Authority

UNAIDS
Joint United Nations Programme on HIV/AIDS

UNOS
United Network for Organ Sharing

UOA
United Ostomy Association

URAC
Utilization Review Accreditation Commission

USAFH
United States Air Force Hospital

USAFRHL
United States Air Force Radiological Health Laboratory

USAFSAM
United States Air Force School of Aerospace Medicine

USAH
United States Army Hospital

USAHC
United States Army Health Clinic

USAIDR
United States Army Institute of Dental Research

USAMEDS
United States Army Medical Service

USAMRIID
United States Army Medical Research Institute of Infectious Disease

USAMRMC
United States Army Medical Research and Material Command

USAN
United States Adopted Names (Council)

USASI
United States of America Standards Institute

USBS
United States Bureau of Standards

USD
United States Dispensary

USDA
United States Department of Agriculture

USDHHS
United States Department of Health and Human Services

USFDA
United States Food and Drug Administration

USH
United Services for Handicapped

USHC
United Seniors Health Council

USHL
United States Hygienic Laboratory

USMH
United States Marine Hospital

USNH
United States Naval Hospital

USPHS
United States Public Health Service

USRDS
United States Renal Data System

USVH
United States Veterans Hospital

VA
Department of Veterans Affairs
Veterans Administration

VAAESS
Vaccine-Associated Adverse Events Surveillance System (Canada)

VACO
Veterans Administration Central Office

VAD
Veterans Administration Domiciliary

VAERS
Vaccine Adverse Events Reporting System

VAH
Veterans Administration Hospital

VAMC
Veterans Administration Medical Center

VAPC
Veterans Administration Prosthetic Center

VC
Veterinary Corps

VDEL
Venereal Disease Experimental Laboratory

VDRL
Venercal Disease Research Laboratories

VEDA
Vestibular Disorders Association

VH
Veteran's Hospital

VHA
Veterans Health Administration

VIBS
Victims Information Bureau Service

VICP
Vaccine Injury Compensation Program

VNA
Visiting Nurse Association

VNAA
Visiting Nurse Association of America

VNS
Visiting Nursing Service

VRS
Vocational Rehabilitation Services

WARDS
Working for Animals Used in Research Drugs and Surgery

WASP
World Association of Societies of Pathology

WEH/CHOP
Wills Eye Hospital/Children's Hospital of Philadelphia

WFC
World Federation of Chiropractic

WHO
World Health Organization

WHO/ILAR
World Health Organization/International League of Associations for Rheumatology

WMR
World Medical Relief

WOCN
Wound, Ostomy, and Continence Nurses (Society)

WRAIR
Walter Reed Army Institute of Research

WRAMC
Walter Reed Army Medical Center

WRARU
Walter Reed Army Research Unit

WW
Weight Watchers

YMCA
Young Men's Christian Association

YWCA
Young Women's Christian Association

Chemotherapy and Other Drug Regimens

ABCM
Adriamycin, bleomycin, cyclophosphamide, mitomycin C

ABCVEP-I
Adriamycin, bleomycin, cyclophosphamide, vincristine, etoposide, prednisolone I

ABCVEP-II
Adriamycin, bleomycin, cyclophosphamide, vincristine, etoposide, prednisolone II

ABCX
Adriamycin, bleomycin, cisplatin, radiation therapy

ABDV
Adriamycin, bleomycin, vinblastine, dacarbazine

ABP
Adriamycin, bleomycin, prednisone

ABV
actinomycin D, bleomycin, vincristine
Adriamycin, bleomycin, vinblastine

ABVD
Adriamycin, bleomycin, vinblastine, dacarbazine

ABVD-MP
Adriamycin, bleomycin, vinblastine, dacarbazine, methylprednisolone

ABVE
Adriamycin, bleomycin, vincristine, etoposide

5-AC
5-azacytidine

AC
Adriamycin, cyclophosphamide

aC
arabinosylcytosine

ACC$_\beta$
acetyl-CoA carboxylase

ACD
actinomycin D (dactinomycin)

ACE
Adriamycin, cyclophosphamide, etoposide

ACFUCY
actinomycin D, fluorouracil, cyclophosphamide

ACM
aclarubicin, cyclophosphamide, methotrexate

ACNU
nimustine

ACOAP
Adriamycin, cyclophosphamide, Oncovin, cytosine, arabinoside, prednisone

ACOP
Adriamycin, cyclophosphamide, Oncovin, prednisone

ACOPP
Adriamycin, cyclophosphamide, Oncovin, prednisone, procarbazine

ACTC, Act-C
actinomycin C

ACTD, Act-D
actinomycin D
dactinomycin

act-FU-Cy
actinomycin D, fluorouracil, cyclophosphamide

ACV
amifostine, cisplatin, vinblastine

ACVBP
Adriamycin, cyclophosphamide, vindesine, bleomycin, prednisone

ADCONFU
Adriamycin, cyclophosphamide, Oncovin, fluorouracil

ADE
Ara-C, daunorubicin, etoposide

ADIC
Adriamycin, DTIC

ADM, ADR, ADRIA, Adria
Adriamycin

AdOAP
Adriamycin, Oncovin, arabinosylcytosine, prednisone

AFM
Adriamycin, fluorouracil, methotrexate

AFP
Adriamycin, fluorouracil, cisplatin

ALOMAD
Adriamycin, Leukeran, Oncovin, methotrexate, actinomycin D, dacarbazine

AMD
actinomycin D

AOPA
Ara-C, Oncovin, prednisone, asparaginase

AOPE
Adriamycin, Oncovin, prednisone, etoposide

APC
amsacrine, prednisone, chlorambucil

APE
Ara-C, Platinol, etoposide

APO
Adriamycin, prednisone, Oncovin

Ara
arabinose

Ara-A, araA
arabinosyladenine

Ara-AMP
adenine arabinoside monophosphate

Ara-C, araC, aC
arabinosylcytosine
cytarabine cytosine arabinoside

araC-Hu
arabinosylcytosine, hydroxyurea

ara-U
arabinosyluracil

ASAP
Adriamycin, Solu-Medrol, Ara-C, Platinol

A-SHAP
Adriamycin, Solu-Medrol, high-dose Ara-C, Platinol

ASP
asparaginase

AU
azauridine

AV
Adriamycin, vincristine

AVCF
Adriamycin, vincristine, cyclophosphamide, fluorouracil

AVDP
asparaginase, vincristine, daunorubicin, prednisone

AVLP
anhydrovinblastine

AVM
Adriamycin, vinblastine, methotrexate

AVP
Adriamycin, vincristine, procarbazine

5-AZA
5-azacytidine

AzC
azacytosine

AZG
azaguanine

AZQ
aziridinylbenzoquinone

AZU
azauridine

AZUR, AzUr
azauridine

BAC
BCNU, ara-C, cyclophosphamide

BACO
bleomycin, Adriamycin, CCNU, Oncovin

BACON
bleomycin, Adriamycin, CCNU, Oncovin, nitrogen mustard

BACOP
bleomycin, Adriamycin, cyclophosphamide, Oncovin, prednisone
bleomycin, Adriamycin, Cytoxan, Oncovin, prednisone

BACT
BCNU, ara-C, cyclophosphamide, 6-thioguanine
BCNU, ara-C, Cytoxan, 6-thioguanine
bleomycin, Adriamycin, Cytoxan, tamoxifen citrate

BAP
bleomycin, Adriamycin, prednisone

BAVIP
bleomycin, Adriamycin, vinblastine, imidazole carboxamide, prednisone

BBVP-M
BCNU, bleomycin, VePesid, prednisone, methotrexate

BCAP
BCNU, cyclophosphamide, Adriamycin, prednisone

B-CAVe
bleomycin, CCNU, Adriamycin, Velban

BCD
bleomycin, cyclophosphamide, dactinomycin

BCNU
bischloroethylnitrosourea

BCP
BCNU, cyclophosphamide, prednisone

BCVPP
BCNU, cyclophosphamide, vinblastine, procarbazine, prednisone
bleomycin, cyclophosphamide, vincristine, procarbazine, prednisone

B-DOPA
bleomycin, dacarbazine, Oncovin, prednisone, Adriamycin

BEAC
BCNU, etoposide, ara-C, cyclophosphamide

BEAM
BCNU, etoposide, ara-C, melphalan

BELD
bleomycin, Eldisine, lomustine, dacarbazine

BEMP
bleomycin, Eldisine, mitomycin, Platinol

BEP
bleomycin, etoposide, Platinol

BHD
BCNU, hydroxyurea, dacarbazine

BHD-V
BCNU, hydroxyurea, dacarbazine, vincristine

BiCNU
carmustine

BIP
bleomycin, ifosfamide, Platinol

BLEO, BLM
bleomycin

BLEO-MOP
bleomycin, mechlorethamine, Oncovin, prednisone

BMP
BCNU, methotrexate, procarbazine

BOLD
bleomycin, Oncovin, lomustine, dacarbazine

BOP
bleomycin, Oncovin, Platinol
bleomycin, Oncovin, prednisone

BOPAM
bleomycin, Oncovin, prednisone, Adriamycin, methotrexate

BOSE
bleomycin, Oncovin, streptozotocin, etoposide

BU-CY, BU/CY
busulfan and Cytoxan
busulfan-cyclophosphamide

BVAP
BCNU, vincristine, Adriamycin, prednisone

BVD
BCNU, vincristine, dacarbazine

C
carboplatin
chloramphenicol

CABOP, CA-BOP
cyclophosphamide, Adriamycin, bleomycin, Oncovin, prednisone

CAC
cisplatin, ara-C, caffeine

CA/CAF
cyclophosphamide, doxorubicin with or without fluorouracil

CACP
cisplatin

CAD
cyclophosphamide, Adriamycin, dacarbazine
cytosine arabinoside daunorubicin

CADIC
cyclophosphamide, Adriamycin, dacarbazine

CAE
cyclophosphamide, Adriamycin, etoposide

CAF
cyclophosphamide, Adriamycin, fluorouracil
Cytoxan, Adriamycin, fluorouracil

CAFP
cyclophosphamide, Adriamycin, fluorouracil, prednisone

CAFTH
Cytoxan, Adriamycin, fluorouracil, tamoxifen, Halotestin

CAFVP
cyclophosphamide, Adriamycin, fluorouracil, vincristine, prednisone

CALF
Cytoxan, Adriamycin, leucovorin calcium, fluorouracil

CALF-E
Cytoxan, Adriamycin, leucovorin calcium, fluorouracil, ethinyl estradiol

CALLF
Cytoxan, Adriamycin, leucovorin calcium, fluorouracil

CAM
Cytoxan, Adriamycin, methotrexate

CAMB
Cytoxan, Adriamycin, methotrexate, bleomycin

CAMBO-VIP
Cytoxan, Adriamycin, methotrexate, bleomycin, Oncovin, vinblastine, ifosfamide,
  Platinol

CAMEO
cyclophosphamide, Adriamycin, methotrexate, etoposide, Oncovin

CAMF
cyclophosphamide, Adriamycin, methotrexate, fluorouracil

CAMP
cyclophosphamide, Adriamycin, methotrexate, procarbazine

CAP-BOP
cyclophosphamide, Adriamycin, procarbazine, bleomycin, Oncovin, prednisone

CAPPR
Cytoxan, Adriamycin, Platinol, prednisone

CAT
chloramphenicol acetyltransferase
cytosine arabinoside, Adriamycin, thioguanine

CAV
cyclophosphamide, Adriamycin, vincristine

CAVe
CCNU, Adriamycin, vinblastine

CAVP
cyclophosphamide, Adriamycin, vincristine, prednisone

CAVP16
Cytoxan, Adriamycin, VP-16

CAV-P-VP
cyclophosphamide, Adriamycin, vincristine, Platinol, VP-16

Cb
carboplatin

CBP
cyclophosphamide, bleomycin, cisplatin

CBPPA
cyclophosphamide, bleomycin, procarbazine, prednisone, Adriamycin

CBV
cyclophosphamide, BCNU, VP-16
Cytoxan, BCNU, VP-16

CCFE
cyclophosphamide, cisplatin, fluorouracil, estramustine

CCM
cyclophosphamide, CCNU, methotrexate

CCNU
chloroethylcyclohexylnitrosourea

CCOF
CCNU, Oncovin, prednisone

CCV
CCNU, cyclophosphamide, vincristine

CCVB
CCNU, cyclophosphamide, vincristine, bleomycin

CCVPP
CCNU, cyclophosphamide, vinblastine, procarbazine, prednisone

CD
cytarabine, daunorubicin

CDDP
cis-diamminedichloroplatinum
cisplatin

CE
carboplatin, etoposide

CEB
carboplatin, etoposide, bleomycin

CECA
cisplatin, etoposide, Cytoxan, Adriamycin

CEF
Cytoxan, epirubicin, fluorouracil

CEOP
cyclophosphamide, epirubicin, Oncovin, prednisone
cyclophosphamide, epirubicin, Oncovin, prednisolone

CEOP-B
cyclophosphamide, epirubicin, Oncovin, prednisone, bleomycin

CEP
cyclophosphamide, etoposide, Platinol

CEV
cyclophosphamide, etoposide, vincristine

CFL
cisplatin, fluorouracil, leucovorin calcium

CFM
cyclophosphamide, fluorouracil, mitoxantrone

CFPT
cyclophosphamide, fluorouracil, prednisone, tamoxifen

CFR
citrovorum-factor rescue

CHAD
cyclophosphamide, hexamethylmelamine, Adriamycin, DDP

CHAM-OCA
cyclophosphamide, hydroxyurea, actinomycin D, methotrexate, Oncovin, citrovorum factor, Adriamycin

CHAP
cyclophosphamide, hexamethylmelamine, Adriamycin, Platinol

CHF
cyclophosphamide, hexamethylmelamine, fluorouracil

CHL
chlorambucil
chloramphenicol

ChlVPP
chlorambucil, vinblastine, procarbazine, prednisone

CHO
cyclophosphamide, hydroxydaunorubicin, Oncovin

CHOD
Cytoxan, hydroxydaunomycin, Oncovin, dexamethasone

CHOP
cyclophosphamide, hydroxydaunomycin, Oncovin, prednisone

CHOP-BLEO
cyclophosphamide, hydroxydaunorubicin, Oncovin, prednisone, bleomycin

CHOPE
Cytoxan, Halotestin, Oncovin, prednisone, etoposide

CHOR
cyclophosphamide, hydroxydaunorubicin, Oncovin, radiation

CISCA
cisplatin, cyclophosphamide, Adriamycin

cis-DDP
cis-diamminedichloroplatinum
cisplatin

CL286558
zeniplatin

CL287110
enloplatin

CLB
chlorambucil

CLINPROT
Clinical Cancer Protocols

CLS
cisplatinum, Lipiodol, Spongel

ClVPP
chlorambucil, vinblastine, procarbazine, prednisone

CMC
chloramphenicol
cyclophosphamide, methotrexate, CCNU

CMED
cyclophosphamide, methotrexate, etoposide, dexamethasone

CMF
cyclophosphamide, methotrexate, fluorouracil
Cytoxan, methotrexate, fluorouracil

CMFH
cyclophosphamide, methotrexate, fluorouracil, hydroxyurea

CMFP
cyclophosphamide, methotrexate, fluorouracil, prednisone
Cytoxan, methotrexate, fluorouracil, prednisone

CMFPT
Cytoxan, methotrexate, fluorouracil, prednisone, tamoxifen

CMFPTH
cyclophosphamide, methotrexate, fluorouracil, prednisone, tamoxifen, Halotestin

CMF-TAM
cyclophosphamide, methotrexate, fluorouracil, tamoxifen

CMFV
cyclophosphamide, methotrexate, fluorouracil, vincristine

CMFVP
cyclophosphamide, methotrexate, fluorouracil, vincristine, prednisone
Cytoxan, methotrexate, fluorouracil, vincristine, prednisone

CMH
Cytoxan, m-AMSA, hydroxyurea

C-MOPP
cyclophosphamide, mechlorethamine, Oncovin, procarbazine, prednisone

CMV
cisplatin, methotrexate, Velban
cisplatin, methotrexate, vinblastine

CNF
cyclophosphamide, Novantrone, fluorouracil

CNOP
Cytoxan, Novantrone, Oncovin, prednisone

CNV
colistimethate, nystatin, vancomycin

COAP
cyclophosphamide, Oncovin, arabinosylcytosine, prednisone
Cytoxan, Oncovin, ara-C, prednisone

COB
cisplatin, Oncovin, bleomycin

CODE
cisplatin, vincristine, doxorubicin, etoposide

COF/COM
Cytoxan, Oncovin, fluorouracil plus Cytoxan, Oncovin, methotrexate

COM
cyclophosphamide, Oncovin, methotrexate
cyclophosphamide, Oncovin, methyl-CCNU

COMB
cyclophosphamide, Oncovin, methyl-CCNU, bleomycin

COMLA
cyclophosphamide, Oncovin, methotrexate, leucovorin, arabinosylcytosine

COMP
cyclophosphamide, Oncovin, methotrexate, prednisone

CONPADRI I
cyclophosphamide, Oncovin, L-phenylalanine mustard, Adriamycin

CONPADRI II
CONPADRI I plus high dose methotrexate

CONPADRI III
CONPADRI II plus intensified doxorubicin

COP
cyclophosphamide, Oncovin, prednisone

COPA
cyclophosphamide, Oncovin, prednisone, Adriamycin

COP-BLAM
cyclophosphamide, Oncovin, prednisone, bleomycin, Adriamycin, Matulane

COP-BLEO
cyclophosphamide, Oncovin, prednisone, bleomycin

COPE
Cytoxan, Oncovin, Platinol, etoposide

COPP
cyclophosphamide, Oncovin, procarbazine, prednisone

COPPA
cyclophosphamide, Oncovin, procarbazine, prednisone, Adriamycin

COPP/ABVD
cyclophosphamide, Oncovin, procarbazine, prednisone, Adriamycin, bleomycin, vinblastine, dacarbazine

CPA
cyclophosphamide

CPB
cyclophosphamide, Platinol, BCNU

CPC
Cytoxan, Platinol, carboplatin

CPDD
cis-platinum diamminedichloride

CPM
CCNU, procarbazine, methotrexate

CPT
cisplatin

CPV
cyclophosphamide, Platinol, VP-16

CROP
cyclophosphamide, rubidazone, Oncovin, prednisone

CSA, CsA
cyclosporin A

CTCb
cyclophosphamide, thiotepa, carboplatin
Cytoxan, thiotepa, carboplatin

14C-TOPO
14C-Topotecan

CTX, ctx
Cytoxan

CV
cisplatin, VePesid

CVA
cyclophosphamide, vincristine, Adriamycin

CVA-BMP
cyclophosphamide, vincristine, Adriamycin, BCNU, methotrexate, procarbazine

CVAD
Cytoxan, vincristine, Adriamycin, dexamethasone

CVB
CCNU, vinblastine, bleomycin

CVD
cisplatin, vinblastine, dacarbazine

CVEB
cisplatin, vinblastine, etoposide, bleomycin

CVM
cyclophosphamide, vincristine, methotrexate

CVP
cyclophosphamide, vincristine, prednisone

CVPP
cyclophosphamide, vincristine, prednisone, procarbazine
Cytoxan, vinblastine, procarbazine, prednisone

CY, Cy
cyclophosphamide
cytarabine

CyA
cyclosporin A

CyADIC
cyclophosphamide, Adriamycin, DIC

CYC
cyclophosphamide

CYCLO, CyClo
cyclophosphamide
cyclopropane

CyHOP
cyclophosphamide, Halotestin, Oncovin, prednisone

CYP
cyclophosphamide

CY/TBI
Cytoxan/total body irradiation

CY-VA-DIC
cyclophosphamide, vincristine, Adriamycin, DTIC

D-3+7
cytarabine, daunorubicin

DAC
deoxyazacytidine

DACE
dexamethasone, ara-C, carboplatin, etoposide

DACT
dactinomycin
actinomycin D

DAIP
dexamethasone, ifosfamide, cisplatin, cytarabine

DAP
dianhydrogalactitol, Adriamycin, Platinol

DAT
daunorubicin, ara-C, thioguanine

DATVP
daunomycin, ara-C, thioguanine, vincristine, prednisone

DAUNO
daunorubicin

DAVA
desacetyl vinblastine amide

DAVH
dibromodulcitol, Adriamycin, vincristine, Halotestin

DAVTH
dibromodulcitol, Adriamycin, vincristine, tamoxifen, Halotestin

DBD
dibromodulcitol

DBH
dacarbazine, carmustine, hydroxyurea

DBPT
dacarbazine, carmustine, cisplatin, tamoxifen
DTIC, BCNU, Platinol, tamoxifen

DCCMP
daunorubicin, cyclocytidine, 6-metacaptopurine, prednisone

DCDA
deuterium with cesium dihydrogen arsenate

DCHN
dicyclohexylamine nitrite

DCMP
daunorubicin, cytarabine, 6-mercaptopurine, prednisone

DCNU
chlorozotocin

DCPM
daunorubicin, cytarabine, prednisolone, mercaptopurine

DCT
daunorubicin, cytarabine, thioguanine

DCV
dacarbazine, CCNU, vincristine

DDP
cis-diamminedichloroplatinum

DFV
DDP, fluorouracil, VePesid

DHAP
dexamethasone, high-dose cytarabine, cisplatin

DIC
dimethyltriazenoimidazole carboxamide

DICE
dexamethasone, ifosfamide, cisplatin, etoposide

DICEP
dose-interactive cyclophosphamide, etoposide, Platinol

DMC
dactinomycin, methotrexate, cyclophosphamide

DNM
daunomycin

DNR
daunorubicin

DOAP
daunorubicin, Oncovin, ara-C, prednisone

DRB
daunorubicin

DSF
doxorubicin, streptozocin, fluorouracil

DTC-101
cytarabine

DTIC
dacarbazine
dimethyltriazcnoimidazole carboxamide

DTIC-Dome
dimethyl triazeno imidazole carboxamide-Dome

DVB
cis-diamminedichloroplatinum, vindesine, bleomycin

DVLP
daunomycin, vincristine, L-asparaginase, prednisone

DVPA
daunorubicin, vincristine, prednisone, L-asparaginase

DVPL-ASP
daunorubicin, vincristine, prednisone, L-asparaginase

DXR
doxorubicin

DZAPO
daunorubicin, azacytidine, ara-C, prednisone, Oncovin

EAP
etoposide, Adriamycin, Platinol

EBV
epirubicin, bleomycin, vinblastine

ECF
epirubicin, cisplatin, fluorouracil

ECHO
etoposide, cyclophosphamide, hydroxydaunomycin, Oncovin

ECMV
etoposide, Cytoxan, methotrexate, vincristine

EDAP
etoposide, dexamethasone, ara-C, Platinol

EFP
etoposide, fluorouracil, Platinol

ELF
etoposide, leucovorin, fluorouracil

EMA-CO
etoposide, methotrexate, actinomycin D, citrovorum factor
etoposide, methotrexate-leucovorin, actinomycin D, cyclophosphamide, Oncovin

EMP
estramustine phosphate

E-MVAC
escalated methotrexate, vinblastine, Adriamycin, cisplatin
escalated methotrexate, vinblastine, Adriamycin, cisplatin or cyclophosphamide
escalated methotrexate, vinblastine, Adriamycin, Cytoxan

EP, EPEG
etoposide

EPIC
early postoperative intraperitoneal chemotherapy
etoposide, prednisolone, ifosfamide, cisplatin

epiDX
epidoxorubicin

EPISODE
etoposide, cisplatin

EPOCH
etoposide, prednisone, Oncovin, Cytoxan, Halotestin

ESAP
etoposide, Solu-Medrol, Ara-C, Platinol

ESHAP
etoposide, Solu-Medrol, high-dose ara-C, Platinol

ETO, ETP
etoposide

EV
etoposide and vincristine

EVA
etoposide, vinblastine, Adriamycin

FABQ
5-fluorouracil, Adriamycin, cyclophosphamide

FAC
fluorouracil, Adriamycin, cyclophosphamide

FAC-LEV
fluorouracil, Adriamycin, cyclophosphamide, levamisole

FAC-M
fluorouracil, Adriamycin, Cytoxan, methotrexate

FAM
fluorouracil, Adriamycin, mitomycin C

FAM-CF
fluorouracil, Adriamycin, mitomycin, citrovorum factor

FAMe
fluorouracil, Adriamycin, methyl-CCNU

FAMM
fluorouracil, Adriamycin, mitomycin C, methyl-CCNU

FAMP
fludarabine monophosphate

FAM-S
fluorouracil, Adriamycin, mitomycin C, streptozotocin

FAMTX
fluorouracil, Adriamycin, methotrexate

FAP
fluorouracil, Adriamycin, Platinol

F-ara-A
fludarabine phosphate

5-FC
5-flucytosine, 5-fluorocytosine

FCE
fluorouracil, cisplatin, etoposide

F-CL
fluorouracil, calcium leucovorin

FCP
fluorouracil, cyclophosphamide, prednisone

FEC
fluorouracil, epirubicin, cyclophosphamide
fluorouracil, epirubicin, Cytoxan
fluorouracil, etoposide, cisplatin

FED
fluorouracil, etoposide, cisplatin

FEPP-B
vindesine, etoposide, procarbazine, prednisone, bleomycin

F-FU
F-labeled fluorouracil

FHX
fluorouracil, hydroxyurea, radiotherapy

FIME
fluorouracil, ICRF-159, methyl-CCNU

FIVB
fluorouracil, imidazole, vincristine, BCNU

FLAC
fluorouracil, leucovorin calcium, Adriamycin, Cytoxan

FLAG-ida
fludarabine, ara-C, G-CSF, idarubicin

FLAP
fluorouracil, leucovorin, doxorubicin, cisplatin

FLe
fluorouracil, levamisole

FLEP
fluorouracil, leucovorin, Platinol

FMD
fludarabine, mitoxantronc, dexamethasone

FMV
fluorouracil, methyl-CCNU, vincristine

FND
fludarabine, mitoxantrone, dexamethasone

FNM
fluorouracil, Novantrone, methotrexate

FOMI
fluorouracil, Oncovin, mitomycin C

FRACON
framycetin, colistin, nystatin

Ft
ftorafur

FU, 5-FU
fluorouracil
5-fluorouracil

FUdR
floxuridine

FUFA
fluorouracil and leucovorin (folinic acid)

FUFOL
fluorouracil and leucovorin calcium (folinic acid)

5FU/LV
fluorouracil and leucovorin

FUM
fluorouracil methotrexate

FUMIR
fluorouracil, mitomycin C, radiation

FUR
fluorouracil, riboside

FURAM
ftorafur, Adriamycin, mitomycin C

FUVAC
5-fluorouracil, vinblastine, Adriamycin, Cytoxan

FY
framycetin

GEM
gemcitabine

Gepardo
German preoperative Adriamycin, docetaxel

HAC
hexamethylmelamine, Adriamycin, cyclophosphamide

HA-IA
nebacumab

HAM
hexamethylmelamine, Adriamycin, melphalan

H-CAP
hexamethylmelamine, cyclophosphamide, Adriamycin, Platinol

HDAC, HDARAC
high-dose ara-C

HDC-ABMT
high-dose chemotherapy with autologous bone marrow transplantation

HDC/ASCR
high-dose chemotherapy with autologous bone marrow or stem cell rescue

HDC-ASCS
high-dose chemotherapy with autologous stem cell support

HDCC
high-dose combination chemotherapy

HD-CNVp
high-dose cyclophosphamide, mitoxantrone, VP-16

HD-CPA
high-dose cyclophosphamide

HDCPT
high-dose cyclophosphamide therapy

HDC-SCR
high-dose chemotherapy with stem-cell rescue

HDMTX
high-dose methotrexate

HDMTX-CF
high-dose methotrexate, citrovorum factor

HDMTX-LV
high-dose methotrexate, leucovorin

HDPEB
high-dose Platinol, etoposide, bleomycin

HD-VAC
high-dose methotrexate, vinblastine, Adriamycin, cisplatin

Hex, HM, HMM
hexamethylmelamine

Hexa-CAF
hexamethylmelamine, cyclophosphamide, amphotericin B, fluorouracil
hexamethylmelamine, cyclophosphamide, Adriamycin, fluorouracil

HI-DAC
high-dose cytosine arabinoside

HN2
mechlorethamine
nitrogen mustard

HOAP-BLEO
hydroxydaunomycin, Oncovin, ara-C, prednisone, bleomycin

HOM
hexamethylmelamine, Oncovin, methotrexate

HOP
hydroxydaunomycin, Oncovin, prednisone

HXM
hexamethylmelamine

ICE
ifosfamide, carboplatin, etoposide

ID
ifosfamide, mesna uroprotection, doxorubicin

IDA, IDR
idarubicin

IE
ifosfamide, and etoposide with mesna

IF, IFO, IFOS, IFX
ifosfamide

IMAC
ifosfamide, mesna uroprotection, Adriamycin, cisplatin

IMF
ifosfamide, mesna uroprotection, methotrexate, fluorouracil

IMV
ifosfamide, methotrexate, vincristine

IMVP-16
ifosfamide, mesna uroprotection, methotrexate, etoposide

IPA
ifosfamide, Platinol, Adriamycin

ITM, ITMTX
intrathecal methotrexate

ITN
irinotecan

ITP
Ifex, Taxol, Platinol

IU
iodouracil

IUDR
idoxuridine

JM-9
iproplatin

LAM
L-asparaginase, methotrexate

LAPOCA
L-asparaginase, prednisone, Oncovin, cytarabine, Adriamycin

L-ASP
L-asparaginase

L-CF
leucovorin-citrovorum factor

LCR
leurocristine

LE
liposomal encapsulated doxorubicin

LEU, LCV, LV, LVR
leucovorin

Leu-Dox
N-1-leucyldoxorubicin

LMF
Leukeran, methotrexate, fluorouracil

LOHP
oxaliplatin

LOMAC
leucovorin, Oncovin, methotrexate, Adriamycin, cyclophosphamide

LPAM
L-phenylalanine mustard

L-Spar
asparaginase (Elspar)

L-VAM
leuprolide acetate, vinblastine, Adriamycin, mitomycin

LVFU
leucovorin and fluorouracil

M
methotrexate

M2, M&2
vincristine, carmustine, cyclophosphamide, melphalan, prednisone

3M
mitomycin, mitoxantrone, methotrexate

M-3+7
mitoxantrone, cytarabine

MABOP
Mustargen, Adriamycin, bleomycin, Oncovin, prednisone

MAC
methotrexate, actinomycin D, chlorambucil
methotrexate, actinomycin D, cyclophosphamide

MACC
methotrexate, Adriamycin, cyclophosphamide, CCNU
methotrexate, ara-C, cyclophosphamide, CCNU

MACHO
methotrexate, asparaginase, Cytoxan, hydroxydaunomycin, Oncovin

MACOB
methotrexate, Adriamycin, cyclophosphamide, Oncovin, bleomycin

MACOP-B
methotrexate, Adriamycin, cyclophosphamide, Oncovin, prednisone, bleomycin
methotrexate-leucovorin, Adriamycin, cyclophosphamide, Oncovin, prednisone,
 bleomycin

MADDOC
mechlorethamine, Adriamycin, dacarbazine, DDP, Oncovin, cyclophosphamide

MAID
mesna, Adriamycin, ifosfamide, dacarbazine
mesna, Adriamycin, interleukin-3, dacarbazine

MAZE
mAMSA, azacitidine, etoposide

M-BACOD
methotrexate, bleomycin, Adriamycin, cyclophosphamide, Oncovin,
 dexamethasone
moderate-dose methotrexate, bleomycin, Adriamycin, cyclophosphamide, Oncovin,
 dexamethasone

M-BACOS
methotrexate, bleomycin, Adriamycin, cyclophosphamide, Oncovin, Solu-Medrol

MBC
methotrexate, bleomycin, cisplatin

MBD
methotrexate, bleomycin, DDP

MCBP
melphalan, cyclophosphamide, BCNU, prednisone

MCCNU, MeCCNU
methyl-CCNU
methyl chloroethyl cyclohexylnitrosourea

M-CH
mitomycin (adsorbed onto activated) charcoal

MCP
melphalan, cyclophosphamide, prednisone

MCV
methotrexate, cisplatin, vinblastine

MDLO
metoclopramide, dexamethasone, lorazepam, ondansetron

MeCP
methyl-CCNU, cyclophosphamide, prednisone

MECY
methotrexate, cyclophosphamide

MEFA
methyl-CCNU, fluorouracil, Adriamycin

MEP
mitomycin C, etoposide, Platinol

MF
mitomycin, fluorouracil

MFL
mitoxantrone, fluorouracil, leucovorin

MICE
mesna, ifosfamide, carboplatin, etoposide

MIFA
mitomycin-C, fluorouracil, Adriamycin

MIME
mesna, ifosfamide, mitoxantrone, etoposide
mitoguazone, ifosfamide, methotrexate, etoposide with mesna
mini-VAB

MIT, Mi
mitomycin

MITO-C, MIT-C, MMC
mitomycin C

MMM
mitoxantrone, methotrexate, mitomycin

MMOPP
methotrexate, mechlorethamine, Oncovin, procarbazine, prednisone

MOAD
methotrexate, Oncovin, L-asparaginase, dexamethasone

MOB
mechlorethamine, Oncovin, bleomycin

MOB-PT
mitomycin C, Oncovin, bleomycin, cisplatin

MOCA
methotrexate, Oncovin, Cytoxan, Adriamycin

MOF
MeCCNU, Oncovin, fluorouracil
methotrexate, Oncovin, fluorouracil

MOP
methotrexate, Oncovin, prednisone
methylprednisolone, Oncovin, procarbazine

MOP-BAP
Mustargen, Oncovin, prednisone, bleomycin, Adriamycin, procarbazine

MOPP
Mustargen, Oncovin, procarbazine, prednisone

MOPP/ABV
mechlorethamine, Oncovin, procarbazine, prednisone, Adriamycin, bleomycin, vinblastine

MP
melphalan, prednisolone

6-MP
6-mercaptopurine

MPC
meperidine, promethazine, chlorpromazine

m-PFL
methotrexate, cisplatin (Platinol), fluorouracil, and leucovorin

MPL
melphalan

MPR
mercaptopurine riboside

MTC
metoclopramide
mitomycin C

MTX, MTRX
methotrexate

MV
mitoxantrone, VePesid

MVAC
methotrexate, vinblastine, Adriamycin, cisplatin

MVB
methotrexate and vinblastine

MVC
mitoxantrone, vinblastine, cyclophosphamide

M-VEC
methotrexate, vinblastine, epirubicin, cisplatin

MVH
methotrexate, VP-16, hexamethylmelamine

MVP
mitomycin, vinblastine, Platinol

MVPP
mechlorethamine, vinblastine, procarbazine, prednisone
mustine, vinblastine, procarbazine, prednisone

MVVPP
mechlorethamine, vincristine, vinblastine, procarbazine, prednisone
Mustargen, vincristine, vinblastine, procarbazine, prednisone

NAC
nitrogen mustard, Adriamycin, CCNU

9-NC
rubitecan
9-nitrocamptothecin

NCAS, NCS
neocarzinostatin
zinostatin

NH2
topical nitrogen mustard

NOVP
mitoxantrone, Oncovin, vinblastine, prednisone

NVB
Navelbine

OAP
Oncovin, ara-C, prednisone

ODAP
Oncovin, dianhydrogalactitol, Adriamycin, Platinol

OEPA
Oncovin, etoposide, prednisone, Adriamycin

OM, OSM
oncostatin M

OMAD
Oncovin, methotrexate, Adriamycin, dactinomycin

7-OMEN
menogaril

OPAL
Oncovin, prednisone, L-asparaginase

OPEN
Oncovin, prednisone, etoposide, Novantrone

OPP
Oncovin, procarbazine, prednisone

OPPA
Oncovin, procarbazine, prednisone, Adriamycin

OPPA/COPP
Oncovin, procarbazine, prednisone, Adriamycin, cyclophosphamide, Oncovin,
  procarbazine, prednisone

OxPt
oxaliplatin

PAB-Esc-C
Platinol, Adriamycin, bleomycin, escalating doses of Cytoxan

PAC-1, PAC-V
Platinol, Adriamycin, cyclophosphamide

PATCO
prednisone, ara-C, thioguanine, cyclophosphamide, Oncovin

PAVe
L-phenylalanine mustard, vinblastine
procarbazine, Alkeran, Velban

PBV
Platinol, bleomycin, vinblastine

PCB
procarbazine

PCE
Platinol, Cytoxan, etoposide

PCV
procarbazine, CeeNU, vincristine

PCZ
procarbazine

PDD
platinum, diamminedichloride

PDOX
pegylated doxorubicin

PE
Platinol, etoposide

PEB
Platinol, etoposide, bleomycin

PEF
Platinol AQ, epirubicin, fluorouracil

PEI
Platinol, etoposide, ifosfamide

PELF
cisplatin, epirubicin, folinic acid, fluorouracil

PFE
Platinol, fluorouracil, etoposide

PFL
Platinol, fluorouracil, leucovorin

PFL-IFN, PFL + IFN
Platinol, fluorouracil, leucovorin, interferon alfa-2b

PFT
prednisone, fluorouracil, tamoxifen

PHRT
procarbazine, hydroxyurea, radiotherapy

PIzA
Platinol, ifosfamide, Adriamycin

PM
prednimustine

P-MVAC
Platinol, methotrexate, vinblastine, Adriamycin, carboplatin

POACH
prednisone, Oncovin, ara-C, cyclophosphamide, hydroxydaunomycin

POC
procarbazine, Oncovin, CCNU

POCC
procarbazine, Oncovin, CCNU, Cytoxan

POMP
prednisone, Oncovin, methotrexate, Purinethol

PR
epirubicin
procarbazine

ProMACE
prednisone, Cytoxan, methotrexate, leucovorin, Adriamycin, cyclophosphamide,
etoposide

ProMACE-CytaBOM
prednisone, Cytoxan, Adriamycin, cyclophosphamide, etoposide + cytarabine,
bleomycin, Oncovin

ProMACE-MOPP
prednisone, Cytoxan, Adriamycin, cyclophosphamide, etoposide + mustargen,
Oncovin, procarbazine, prednisone

PSC 833/VAD
PSC 833/vincristine, doxorubicin, dexamethasone

PTU
propylthiouracil

PTX
paclitaxel

PVA
prednisone, vincristine, asparaginase

PVB
Platinol, vinblastine, bleomycin

PVC
paclitaxel, vinblastine, cisplatin

PVDA
prednisone, vincristine, daunorubicin, asparaginase

PVP
Platinol, VP-16

P-VP-B
cisplatin, etoposide, bleomycin

PXL
paclitaxel

RIDD
recombinant interleukin-2, dacarbazine, diamminedichloroplatinum

SDI
Sandimmune (cyclosporine)

SIM
Sandimmune

SMF
streptozotocin, mitomycin, fluorouracil

Stanford V
mechlorethamine, doxorubicin, vinblastine, vincristine, bleomycin, etoposide, prednisone

STEAM
streptonigrin, thioguanine, cyclophosphamide, actinomycin, mitomycin

T-2
dactinomycin, doxorubicin, vincristine, cyclophosphamide

T-10
cyclophosphamide, dactinomycin

TAM
tamoxifen

TC
thioguanine and cytarabine

TCA
thioguanine, cytarabine

TEC
thiotepa, etoposide, carboplatin

TEM
Temodal

TEMP
tamoxifen, etoposide, mitoxantrone, Platinol

TFL
trimetrexate, fluorouracil, leucovorin

6TG
6-thioguanine

TG, 6-TG
thioguanine

THPCOP
THP-doxorubicin, cyclophosphamide, Oncovin, prednisone

TIC
Taxol, ifosfamide, cisplatin

6-T-MOP
6-thioguanine, methotrexate, Oncovin, prednisone

TMX
tamoxifen

TMZ
temozolomide

TNT
thiotepa, mitoxantrone, paclitaxel

TOAP
thioguanine, Oncovin, ara-C, prednisone

TPCH
6-thioguanine, procarbazine, CCNU, hydroxyurea

TPDCV
6-thioguanine, procarbazine, dibromodulcitol, CCNU, vincristine

TPT
topotecan

TRAMPCOL
6-thioguanine, rubidomycin, ara-C, methotrexate, prednisolone, cyclophosphamide, Oncovin

TRAP
thioguanine, rubidomycin, ara-C, prednisone

TT
thiotepa

TXL
paclitaxel

TXT
docetaxel

TZ
temozolomide

TZM
temozolomide

UFT
uracil, fluorouracil, tegafur

URA
uracil

VAB
Velban, actinomycin-D, bleomycin
vincristine, actinomycin D, bleomycin

VAB-6
vinblastine, actinomycin D, bleomycin, cisplatin, cyclophosphamide

VAB-II
Velban, actinomycin D, bleomycin, platinum

VAB-VI
cyclophosphamide, Velban, actinomycin D, bleomycin, platinum

VAC
vincristine, actinomycin D, cyclophosphamide
vincristine, Adriamycin, cisplatin
vincristine, Adriamycin, cyclophosphamide

VACA
vincristine, actinomycin A, cyclophosphamide, Adriamycin

VACAD
vinblastine, Adriamycin, Cytoxan, actinomycin D, dacarbazine

VACP
VePesid, Adriamycin, Cytoxan, Platinol

VADA
vincristine, Adriamycin, dexamethasone, actinomycin D

VAdCA + I/E
vincristine, doxorubicin, cyclophosphamide, dactinomycin + ifosfamide with mesna

VADRIAC
vincristine, doxorubicin, cyclophosphamide

VAD/V
vinblastine, Adriamycin, dexamethasone, verapamil

VAFAC
vincristine, Adriamycin, fluorouracil, amethopterin, cyclophosphamide

VAI
vinblastine, actinomycin D, ifosfamide

VALOP-B
etoposide, doxorubicin, cyclophosphamide, vincristine, prednisone, bleomycin

VAM
vinblastine, Adriamycin, mitomycin C
VP-16, Adriamycin, methotrexate

VAMP
vincristine, actinomycin, methotrexate, prednisone
vincristine, Adriamycin, methylprednisolone

VAP
vincristine, Adriamycin, prednisone, procarbazine
vincristine, Adriamycin, procarbazine

VAPA
vincristine, Adriamycin, prednisone, ara-C

VAT
vinblastine, Adriamycin, thiotepa

VATH
vinblastine, Adriamycin, thiotepa, Halotestin, fluoxymesterone

VAV
VP-16, Adriamycin, vincristine

VB
vinblastine, bleomycin

VBAP
vincristine, BCNU, Adriamycin, prednisone

VBC
vincristine, bleomycin, cisplatin

VBL
vinblastine

VBM
vinblastine, bleomycin, methotrexate

VBMCP
vincristine, BCNU, melphalan, cyclophosphamide, prednisone

VBMF
vinblastine, bleomycin, methotrexate, fluorouracil

VBMPC
vinblastine, BCNU, melphalan, prednisone, Cytoxan

VBP
vinblastine, bleomycin, Platinol

VCAP
vincristine, cyclophosphamide, Adriamycin, prednisone

VCMP
vincristine, cyclophosphamide, melphalan, prednisone

VCP
vincristine, cyclophosphamide, prednisone

VCPC
vindesine, Cytoxan, cisplatin, CCNU

VCR
vincristine

VDBCC
vincristine, dactinomycin, bleomycin, cisplatin, cyclophosphamide

VDC
vincristine, doxorubicin, cyclophosphamide

VDD
vincristine, doxorubicin, dexamethasone

VDP
vinblastine, dacarbazine, Platinol
vincristine, daunorubicin, prednisone

VEEP
vincristine, epirubicin, etoposide, prednisolone

VeIP
vinblastine, ifosfamide, Platinol

VEMP
vincristine, Endoxan, mercaptopurine, prednisone

VEPA
vinblastine, etoposide, prednisone, Adriamycin

VEPA-B
VEPA, bleomycin

VEPA-M
vincristine, etoposide, prednisone, Adriamycin, methotrexate

VFAM
vincristine, fluorouracil, Adriamycin, mitomycin C

VFL
vinflunine

VICE
vincristine, ifosfamide, carboplatin, etoposide

VIE
vinblastine, ifosfamide, etoposide

VIG
vinblastine, ifosfamide, gallium (nitrate)

VIMB
VP-16, ifosfamide, mitoxantrone, bleomycin

VIP
VePesid, ifosfamide (with mesna rescue), Platinol

VIP-B
VP-16, ifosfamide, Platinol, bleomycin

VLB
vincaleukoblastine

VLP
vincristine, L-asparaginase, prednisone

VM-26
teniposide

VMCP
vincristine, melphalan, cyclophosphamide, prednisone

VMP
VePesid, mitoxantrone, prednimustine

VNB
vinorelbine

VP
vincristine, prednisone

VP-16
etoposide

VPCA
vincristine, prednisone, cyclophosphamide, ara-C

VPCMF
vincristine, prednisone, cyclophosphamide, methotrexate, fluorouracil

VPP
VP-16, Platinol

VRB
vinorelbine (Navelbine)

VRL
vinorelbine

Chemotherapy abbreviations and acronyms are built on a basic group of drugs, using generic, brand, and/or chemical names to create an acronym or easily remembered word. The table below lists the generic name of the chemotherapy drug and some of the many other names that are commonly used.

GENERIC NAME	BRAND, TRADE, MISCELLANEOUS NAMES
aclarubicin	Aclacin, aclacinomycin A
aldesleukin	Proleukin, IL-2, Interleukin-2
altretamine	Hexalen
amifostine	Ethyol, Ethiofos, Gammaphos

GENERIC NAME

BRAND, TRADE, MISCELLANEOUS NAMES

amsacrine	mAMSA
ara-A	arabinosyladenine, Vidarabine Anhydrous, Vira-A
ara-C	*See* cytarabine
asparaginase	Elspar, Oncaspar, Pegaspargase
azacytidine	5 AZC , 5-Azacytidine, 5-AC, 5-ACZR
bleomycin	Blenoxane
capecitabine	Xeloda
carboplatin	Paraplatin, CBDCA
carmustine	BCNU, BiCNU, Gliadel
chlorambucil	Leukeran
chlormethine	Mustine
chloroethylcyclohexylnitrosourea	*See* lomustine, CCNU
cladribine	Leustatin
citrovorum factor	*See* leucovorin
cisplatin	Platinol, diammine dichloroplatinum, CDDP
cyclophosphamide	Cytoxan, CytoxanIV, Neosar, CTX
cytarabine	Cytosar-U, ara-C, Cytosine arabinoside, DepoCyt, arabinosylcytosine
dacarbazine	DTIC, DTIC-Dome, dimethyltriazenoimidazolecarboxamide
dactinomycin	Cosmegen, actinomycin-D
desacetylvinblastine amide	DAVA, DVA, VDS
diaziquone	AZQ, CI-904, Diaziquone, NSC-182986
docetaxel	Taxotere
doxorubicin	Adriamycin, Rubex, hydroxydaunorubicin HCl, 14-hydroxydaunomycin
epirubicin	Ellence
etoposide	Toposar, VP-16, VePesid, EPE, Epipodophyllotoxin, VP 16–213
fludarabine	Fludara
fluorouracil	Adrucil, Efudex, Fluoroplex, Fluorouracil IV, 5-FU
gemcitabine	Gemzar
granisetron	Kytril
hydroxyurea	Hydrea
idarubicin	Idamycin
ifosfamide	Ifex, isophosphamide
interferon alfa	Alferon N, Intron A, Roferon-A, Wellferon
irinotecan	Camptosar, Cpt-11, HCL

GENERIC NAME	BRAND, TRADE, MISCELLANEOUS NAMES
levamisole	Ergamisol
leucovorin calcium	Folinic acid
leucovorin	Wellcovorin, Wellcovorin IM/IV, Leucovorin, Leucovorin IM/IV
liposomal doxorubicin	Doxil, Evacet
lomustine	CeeNU, CCNU
mechlorethamine	*See* nitrogen mustard
megestrol	Megace, Pallace, megestrol acetate
melphalan	Alkeran
mercaptopurine	Purinethol, 6-MP
mesna	Mesnex
methotrexate	Abitrexate, amethopterin
methotrexate Injection	MTX Injection
metoclopramide	Reglan
mitomycin	Mutamycin, Mitomycin-C
mitotane	Lysodren
mitoxantrone	Novantrone
neocarzinostatin	zinostatin
nitrogen mustard	Mustargen, mechlorethamine
oxaliplatin	Eloxatin
paclitaxel	Paxene, Taxol
pirarubicin	THP-doxorubicin
razoxane	ICRF-159
rituximab	Rituxan
streptonigrin	SN, rufochromomycin, bruneomycin
streptozoticin	STZ, Zanosar, 2-deoxy-2-methylnitrosoaminocarbonylamino-d-glucopyranos
tamoxifen	Nolvadex
thioguanine	Tabloid, 6-TG, TG
topotecan hydrochloride	Hycamtin
trastuzumab	Herceptin
vinblastine	Velban, Vinblastine, vincaleukoblastine
vincristine	Oncovin, Vincasar
vindesine	Eldisine
vinorelbine tartrate	Navelbine

Clinical Trials

AAASPS
African American Antiplatelet Stroke Prevention Study

AASK
African American Study of Kidney Disease and Hypertension

ABACAS
Adjunctive Balloon Angioplasty Following Coronary Atherectomy Study

ACAPS
Asymptomatic Carotid Artery Plaque Study

ACAS
Asymptomatic Carotid Atherosclerosis Study

ACCESS
Acute Candesartan Clinical Evaluation of Stroke Survivors

ACIT
Asymptomatic Cardiac Ischemia Trial

ACME
Angioplasty Compared to Medicine

ACOVE
Assessing Care of Vulnerable Elders

ACTG
AIDS Clinical Trials Group

ACTG 214
AIDS Clinical Treatment Group 214

ACTG 325
AIDS Clinical Treatment Group 325

ACTG 334
AIDS Clinical Treatment Group 334

ACTG 349
AIDS Clinical Treatment Group 349

ACUTE
Assessment of Cardioversion Utilizing Transesophageal Echocardiography

ADMIT
Arterial Disease Multiple Intervention Trial

AFCAPS/TexCAPS
Air Force/Texas Coronary Atherosclerosis Prevention Study

AFFIRM
Atrial Fibrillation Followup Investigation of Rhythm Management

AIDSTRIALS
Clinical Trials of Acquired Immunodeficiency Syndrome Drugs

AIPRI
Angiotensin-Converting Enzyme Inhibition in Progressive Renal Insufficiency

AIRE
Acute Infarction Ramipril Efficacy
Acute Infarction Reperfusion Efficacy

ALIVE
AIDS Link to Intravenous Experiences

ALLHAT
Antihypertensive and Lipid-Lowering Treatment to Prevent Heart Attack Trial

AMIABLE
Acute Myocardial Infarction Angioplasty Bolus Lysis Evaluation

AMIS
Aspirin in Myocardial Infarction Study

AMISTAD
Acute Myocardial Infarction Study of Adenosine

APASS
Antiphospholipid Antibodies in Stroke Study

APLAUSE
Antiplatelet Treatment after Intravascular Ultrasound-Guided Optimal Stent
   Expansion

APRICOT
Antithrombotics in the Prevention of Reocclusion in Coronary Thrombolysis
Aspirin versus Coumadin Trial

APT
Atherosclerosis Prevention and Treatment

ARK
Analysis of Radial Keratotomy

ASIST
Atenolol Silent Ischemia Trial

ASPECT
Anticoagulants in Secondary Prevention of Events in Coronary Thrombosis

ASPIRE
Action on Secondary Prevention by Intervention to Reduce Events

ASS
Acute Stroke Study

ASSIST
American Stop Smoking Intervention Study (for Cancer Prevenion)

ATLAS
Aspirin and Ticlid versus Anticoagulation for Stents
Assessment of Treatment with Lisinopril and Survival

AVEG
AIDS Vaccine Evaluation Group

AVEU
AIDS Vaccine Evaluation Unit

AVID
Amiodarone Versus Implantable Defibrillators
Angiography versus Intravascular Ultrasound-Directed Coronary Stent Placement
Antiarrhythmics versus Implantable Defibrillators

BARACCO
Balloon Angioplasty versus Rotational Angioplasty in Chronic Coronary Occlusion

BARI
Bypass Angioplasty Revascularization Investigation

BAROCCO
Balloon Angioplasty versus Rotacs for Total Chronic Coronary Occlusion

BASIS
Basal Antiarrhythmic Study of Infarct Survival

BCDDP
Breast Cancer Detection Demonstration Project

BCPT
Breast Cancer Prevention Trial

BECAIT
Bezafibrate Coronary Atherosclerosis Intervention Trial

BEHAVE-AD
Behavioral Pathology in Alzheimer Disease

BEST
beStent clinical trial
Beta-Blocker Evaluation of Survival Trial
Beta-Blocker Stroke Trial
Bolus Dose-Escalation Study of Tissue-Type Plasminogen Activator
Bucindolol Evaluation of Survival Trial

BEST+ICD
Beta-Blocker Strategy Plus Implantable Cardioverter-Defibrillator

beta-WRIST
Beta-Washington Radiation for In-Stent Restenosis Trial

BHAT
Beta-Blocker Heart Attack Trial

BHFS
Benazepril Heart Failure Study

BHS
Bogalusa Heart Study

BOAT
Balloon versus Optimal Atherectomy Trial

BOING
Body Oscillation Integrates Neuromuscular Gain

BRILLIANT
Blood Pressure, Renal Effects, Insulin Control, Lipids, Lisinopril, and Nifedipine Trial

BTSG
Brain Tumor Study Group

CABG Patch
Coronary Artery Bypass Graft Surgery With/Without Simultaneous Epicardial
  Patch for Automatic Implant

CABRI
Coronary Angioplasty versus Bypass Revascularization Investigation
Coronary Artery Bypass Revascularization Investigation

CACHET
Comparison of Abciximab Complications with Hirulog (and Back-Up Abciximab)
  Events Trial

CADILLAC
Controlled Abciximab and Device Investigation to Lower Late Angioplasty Complications

CADS
Captopril and Digoxin Study

CAFS
Canadian Atrial Fibrillation Study

CAMI
Canadian Assessment of Myocardial Infarction

CAMIAT
Canadian Amiodarone Myocardial Infarction Arrhythmia Trial
Canadian Myocardial Infarction Amiodarone Trial

CAPIT
Core Assessment Program for Intracerebral Transplantation

CAPPP
Captopril Prevention Project

CAPRIE
Clopidogrel versus Aspirin in Patients at Risk of Ischemic Events

CAPS
Cardiac Arrhythmia Pilot Study

CAPTURE
Chimeric 7E3 Antiplatelet in Unstable Angina Refractory to Standard Treatment

CAR
Cardiac Ablation Registry

CARAFE
Cocktail Attenuation of Rotational Ablation Flow Effects

CARAT
Coronary Angioplasty and Rotablator Atherectomy Trial

CARAT II
Coronary Angioplasty and Rotablator Atherectomy Trial II

CARDIA
Coronary Artery Risk Development in Young Adults

CARE
Calcium Antagonist in Reperfusion

CARES
Cancer Rehabilitation Evaluation System

CARET
Carotene and Retinol Efficacy Trial

CASANOVA
Carotid Artery Stenosis with Asymptomatic Narrowing: Operation versus Aspirin
    Study

CASCADE
Cardiac Arrest in Seattle: Conventional versus Amiodarone Drug Evaluation
Conventional Antiarrhythmic versus Amiodarone in Survivors of Cardiac Arrest
    Drug Evaluation

CASES
Canadian Activase for Stroke Effectiveness Study

CASS
Coronary Artery Surgery Study

CAST
Cardiac Arrhythmia Suppression Trial
Chinese Acute Stroke Trial

CAST II
Cardiac Arrhythmia Suppression Trial II

CATCH
Child and Adolescent Trial of Cardiovascular Health
Community Actions to Control High Blood Pressure

CATS
Canadian American Ticlopidine Study
Captopril and Thrombolysis Study

CAVATAS
Carotid and Vertebral Artery Transluminal Angioplasty Study

CAVEAT
Coronary Angioplasty versus Excisional Atherectomy Trial

CCABOT
Cornell Coronary Artery Bypass Outcomes Trial

CCAIT
Canadian Coronary Atherosclerosis Intervention Trial

CCAT
Canadian Coronary Atherectomy Trial

CCP
Cooperative Cardiovascular Project

CCSG
Children's Cancer Study Group

CCSS
Childhood Cancer Survivor Study

CCTAT
Cooperative Clinical Trials in Adult Transplantation

CCTPT
Cooperative Clinical Trials in Pediatric Transplantation

CDP
Coronary Drug Project

CHAPS
Carvedilol Heart Attack Pilot Study

CHF-STAT
Congestive Heart Failure-Survival Trial of Antiarrhythmic Therapy

CHIC
Cardiovascular Health in Children

CIBIS
Cardiac Insufficiency Bisoprolol Study

CIDS
Canadian Implantable Defibrillator Study

CIGTS
Collaborative Initial Glaucoma Treatment Study

CLAS
Cholesterol Lowering Atherosclerosis Study

CLASP
Carolinas Laparoscopic Advanced Surgery Program

CLASS
Celecoxib Long-Term Arthritis Safety Study
Clomethiazole Acute Stroke Study

CLASSIC
Clopidogrel Aspirin Stent International Cooperative

CLEK
Collaborative Longitudinal Evaluation of Keratoconus

CLOUT
Clinical Outcomes with Ultrasound Trial
Core Laboratory Ultrasound Analysis

COBALT
Continuous Infusion versus Bolus Alteplase Trial
Continuous Infusion versus Double-Bolus Administration of Alteplase

COMS
Collaborative Ocular Melanoma Study

CONSENSUS
Cooperative North Scandinavian Enalapril Survival Study

CONVINCE
Controlled Onset Verapamil Investigation for Cardiovascular Endpoints

COPERNICUS
Carvedilol Prospective Randomized Cumulative Survival

CORAMI
Cohort of Rescue Angioplasty in Myocardial Infarction

CPPT
Coronary Primary Prevention Trial

CPS
Collaborative Perinatal Study

CRC
Cancer Research Campaign

CREST
Carotid Revascularization Endarterectomy versus Stenting Trial

CRISP
Cholesterol Reduction in Seniors Program

CRISP-US
Cholesterol Reduction in Seniors Program, United States

CRTP
Consciousness Research and Training Project

CRUISE
Can Routine Ultrasound Influence Stent Expansion

CRUSADE
Coronary Revascularization Ultrasound Angioplasty Device

CSSCD
Cooperative Study of Sickle Cell Disease

CSSRD
Cooperative Systematic Studies of the Rheumatic Disease

CTAC
Cancer Treatment Advisory Committee

CURE
Clopidogrel in Unstable Angina to Prevent Recurrent Ischemic Events

CURN
Conduct and Utilization of Research in Nursing

DAIS
Diabetes Atherosclerosis Intervention Study

DART
Dilation versus Ablation Revascularization Trial

DASH
Delay in Accessing Stroke Healthcare
Dietary Approaches to Stop Hypertension

DAVID
Dual-Chamber and VVI Implantable Defibrillator (trial)

DCCT
Diabetes Control and Complications Trial

DENIS
Deutsch Nicotinamide Diabetes Intervention Study

DESAD
(National Collaborative) Diethylstilbestrol Adenosis (Project, Study)

DESTINI-CFR
Doppler Endpoints Stenting International Investigation: Coronary Flow Reserve

DIAD
Detection of Ischemia in Asymptomatic Diabetics

DIG
Digitalis Investigation Group

DIGAMI
Diabetes Mellitus Insulin Glucose Infusion in Acute Myocardial Infarction

DIG-CAPTOPRIL
Canadian Digoxin Captopril

DIMT
Dutch Ibopamine Multicenter Trial

DOQI
Dialysis Outcomes Quality Initiative

DORC
Dutch Ophthalmic Research Center

DOUBLE
Double Bolus Lytic Efficacy

DPT-1
Diabetes Prevention Trial Type 1 Diabetes

DRS
Diabetes Retinopathy Study

DUCCS
Duke University Clinical Cardiology Study

DUET
Dispatch Urokinase Efficacy Trial

EARTS
European Anti-ICAM Renal Transplant Study

EAST
Emory Angioplasty versus Surgery Trial

EBMT
European Group for Bone Marrow Transplantation

ECAT
European Concerted Action on Thrombosis

ECOG
Eastern Cooperative Oncology Group

ECST
European Carotid Surgery Trial

ELITE
Evaluation of Losartan in the Elderly

ELLDOPA
Early versus Later L-DOPA

EMCRO
Experimental Medical Care Review Organization

EMIAT
European Myocardial Infarct Amiodarone Trial

EMIP
European Myocardial Infarction Project

ENDIT
European Nicotinamide Diabetes Intervention Trial

ENTICES
Enoxaparin and Ticlopidine after Elective Stenting

ENTIRE
Enoxaparin and TNK-t-PA with/without GP IIb/IIIa Inhibitor as Reperfusion
    Strategy in ST-Elevation Myocardial Infarction

EORTC QLQ
European Organization for Research and Treatment of Cancer Quality of Life
    Questionnaire

EPILOG
Evaluation of PTCA to Improve Long-Term Outcome by c7E3 GPIIb/IIIa Receptor
    Blockade

EPISTENT
Evaluation of Platelet IIb-IIIa Inhibitors for Stenting

EQOL
Economics and Quality of Life Substudy of GUSTO

ERA
Enoxaparin Restenosis after Angioplasty

ERASE
Emergency Room Assessment of Sestamibi for Evaluation of Chest Pain

EROTIC
European Organization for Research and Treatment of Cancer

ESCOBAR
Emergency Stenting Compared to Conventional Balloon Angioplasty

ESPRIT
European/Australian Stroke Prevention in Reversible Ischaemia Trial

ESSENCE
Efficacy and Safety of Subcutaneous Enoxaparin in Non-Q-Wave Coronary Events

ESVEM
Electrophysiology Study versus Electrocardiographic Monitoring

ETDRS
Early Treatment Diabetic Retinopathy Study

EUP
Experimental Use Permit

EXACTO
Excimer Laser Angioplasty in Coronary Total Occlusion

EXCEL
Expanded Clinical Evaluation of Lovastatin

FACET
Flosequinan ACE Inhibitor Trial
Fosinopril versus Amlodipine Cardiovascular Events Randomized Trial

FASTER
Fibrinolytic and Aggrastat ST Elevation Resolution

FATS
Familial Atherosclerosis Treatment Study

FCVDS
Framingham Cardiovascular Disease Survey

FHRS
Familial Hypercholesterolemia Regression Study

FHS
Framingham Heart Study

FICSIT
Frailty and Injuries: Cooperative Studies of Interventional Techniques

FIR.S.T.
First Seizure Trial Group

FLUENT
Fluvastatin Long-Term Extension Trial

FOOD
Feed or Ordinary Diet

FREIR
Federal Research on Biological and Health Effects of Ionizing Radiation

FRISC
Fast Revascularization During Instability in Coronary Artery Disease
Fragmin During Instability in Coronary Artery Disease

GABI
German Angioplasty Bypass Surgery Investigation

GISSI
Gruppo Italiano Per lo Studio Della Streptokinase Nell'Infarto Miocardio

GITSG
Gastrointestinal Tumor Study Group

GIVIO
Gruppo Interdisciplinare Valutazione Interventi in Oncologia

GRACE
Gianturco-Roubin Stent Acute Closure Evaluation

GRAMI
Gianturco-Roubin in Acute Myocardial Infarction

GREAT
Grampian Region Early Anistreplase Trial

GTSG
Gastrointestinal Tumor Study Group

GUIDE
Guidance by Ultrasound Imaging for Decision Endpoints

GUIDE II
Guidance by Ultrasound Imaging for Decision Endpoints II

GUSTO
Global Utilization of Streptokinase and t-PA for Occluded Coronary Arteries

GUSTO-1
Global Utilization of Streptokinase and Tissue Plasminogen Activator for Occluded
Coronary Arteries

HALT
Heroin Antagonist and Learning Therapy

HARP
Harvard Atherosclerosis Reversibility Project

HART
Heparin Aspirin Reperfusion Trial
Hypertension Audit of Risk Factor Therapy

HEAP
Heparin in Early Patency

HEART
Healing and Early Afterload Reducing Therapy
Health Evaluation and Risk Tabulation

HERO
Hirulog Early Reperfusion/Occlusion

HIPS
Heparin Infusion Prior to Stenting

HIT
Hirudin for the Improvement of Thrombolysis

HOPE
Heart Outcomes Prevention Evaluation
Hospital Outcomes Reversibility for the Elderly

HOT
Hypertensive Optimal Treatment Trial

HVTN
HIV Vaccine Trials Network

HWRS
Habits of Work and Recreation Survey

ICARUS
Islet Cell Antibody Registry of Users Study

ICSS
International Carotid Stenting Study

IMAGE
International Multicenter Angina Exercise

IMPACT
Integrilin to Minimize Platelet Aggregation and Coronary Thrombosis

IMPACT-Stent
Integrilin to Minimize Platelet Aggregation and Coronary Thrombosis in Stenting

INRC
International Neuroblastoma Response Criteria

INTEGRITI
Integrilin and Tenecteplase in Acute Myocardial Infarction

INTIME
Intravenous t-PA for Treatment of Infarcting Myocardium Early

IONDT
Ischemic Optic Neuropathy Decompression Trial

IPSS
International Pilot Study of Schizophrenia

IPTR
International Pancreas Transplant Registry

IRAS
Insulin Resistance Atherosclerosis Study

ISAM
Intravenous Streptokinase in Acute Myocardial Infarction

ISAR
Intracoronary Stenting and Antithrombotic Regimen

ISIS
International Study of Infarct Survival

ISIS-2
Second International Study of Infarct Survival

IST
International Stroke Trial

KIGS
Kabi International Growth Study

KIHD
Kuopio Ischemia Heart Disease Risk Factor Study

LAARS
LDL Apheresis Atherosclerosis Regression Study

LACI
Laser Angioplasty for Critical Ischemia

LAPIS
Late Potential Italian Study

LARS
Laser Angioplasty for Restenosed Stents

LASAR
Local Alcohol and Stent Against Restenosis

LATE
Late Assessment of Thrombolytic Efficacy

LESG
Late Effects Study Group

LIFE
Longitudinal Interval Followup Evaluation

LIMIT
Leicester Intravenous Magnesium Intervention Trial

LIMITS
Liquaemin in Myocardial Infarction during Thrombolysis with Saruplase

LIPID
Long-Term Intervention with Pravastatin in Ischemic Disease

LONG WRIST
Washington Radiation for In-Stent Restenosis Trial for Long Lesions

MAAS
Multicenter Antiatheroma Study
Multicenter Antiatherosclerotic Study

MACE
Mayo Asymptomatic Carotid Endarterectomy

MACS
Multicenter AIDS Cohort Study

MAPS
Multivessel Angioplasty Prognosis Study

MARCATOR
Multicenter American Research Trial with Cilazapril after Angioplasty to Prevent
   Transluminal Coronary Obstruction and Restenosis

MARISA
Monotherapy Assessment of Ranolazine in Stable Angina

MARS
Mevacor Atherosclerosis Regression Study
Monitored Atherosclerosis Regression Study

MASS
Medicine, Angioplasty, or Surgery Study

MAST
Multicenter Acute Stroke Trial

MATE
Medicine versus Angioplasty for Thrombolytic Exclusions

MDC
Metoprolol in Dilated Cardiomyopathy

MDPIT
Multicenter Diltiazem Post-Infarction Trial

MDRD
Modification of Diet in Renal Disease

MEET
Multistage Exercise Electrocardiographics Test

MERCATOR
Multicenter European Research Trial with Cilazapril after Angioplasty to Prevent Transluminal Coronary Obstruction and Restenosis

MERFS
Multicenter European Radiofrequency Survey

MERIT-HF
Metoprolol CR/XL Controlled Release Randomized Intervention Trial in Heart Failure

MEXIS
Metoprolol and Xamoterol Infarction Study

MFS
Minnesota Followup Study

M-HEART
Multi-Hospital Eastern Atlantic Restenosis Trial

MIDAS
Multicenter Isradipine/Diuretic Atherosclerosis Study
Myocardial Infarction Data Acquisition System

MILIS
Multicenter Investigation for the Limitation of Infarct Size

MILTS
Multicentre International Liver Tumor Study

MIRAGE
Multi-Institutional Research in Alzheimer Genetic Epidemiology

MITRA
Maximal Individual Therapy in Acute Myocardial Infarction

MOCHA
Multicenter Oral Carvedilol in Heart Failure Assessment

MOS
Medical Outcomes Study

MOS-HIV
Medical Outcomes Study-Human Immunodeficiency Virus

MOS sf-20
Medical Outcomes Study, short form, 20 items

MOS sf-36
Medical Outcomes Study, short form, 36 items

MOST
Mode Selection Trial in Sinus Node Dysfunction

MPRG
Multicenter Postinfarction Research Group

MPS
Macular Photocoagulation Study

MRFIT
Multiple Risk Factor Intervention Trial

MUSIC
Multicenter Ultrasound Stent in Coronary Artery Disease

MUST
Multicenter Stent Study
Multicenter Stents Ticlopidine
Medication Use Studies

MUSTT
Multicenter Unsustained Tachycardia Trial

NABTT
New Approaches to Brain Tumor Therapy

NACI DCA
New Approaches to Coronary Intervention Registry Directional Coronary Atherectomy

NACI Gianturco-Roubin
New Applications for Coronary Interventions, Gianturco-Roubin

NACPTAR
North American Cerebral Transluminal Angioplasty Registration

NADE
New Animal Drug Evaluation

NAMIS
Nifedipine Angina Myocardial Infarction Study

NAPRTCS
North American Pediatric Renal Transplant Cooperative Study

NASCET
North American Symptomatic Carotid Endarterectomy Trial

NASTRA
North American Study of Treatment for Refractory Ascites

NCGS
National Cooperative Growth Study

NCIC-CTG
National Cancer Institute of Canada Clinical Trials Group

NCI-CTC
National Cancer Institute Common Toxicity Criteria

NEET
Nordic Enalapril Exercise Trial

NETT
National Emphysema Treatment Trial

NFS
National Fertility Study

NHANES
National Health and Nutrition Examination Survey

NHANES II
Second National Health and Nutrition Examination Survey

NHBPEP
National High Blood Pressure Education Program

NHDS
National Hospital Discharge Survey

NHIS
National Health Interview Survey

NHLBI/NAEPP
National Heart, Lung, Blood Institute/National Asthma Education Prevention
    Program

NINDS-TPAST
National Institutes of Neurological Disorders and Stroke-Tissue Plasminogen
    Activator Stroke Trial

NIP
National Immunization Program
National Inpatient Profile

NIS-2
Second National Incidence Study

NIT
National Intelligence Test

NKF-DOQI
National Kidney Foundation-Data Outcomes Quality Initiative

NLTCORC
National Long-Term Care Ombudsman Research Center

NLTCRC
National Long-Term Care Research Center

NMCUES
National Medical Care Utilization and Expenditure Survey

NNHS
National Nursing Home Survey

NRMI
National Registry of Myocardial Infarction

NSABP
National Surgical Adjuvant Breast and Bowel Project

OARS
Optimal Atherectomy Restenosis Study

OASIS
Organization to Assess Strategies for Ischemic Syndromes

OCBAS
Optimal Coronary Balloon Angioplasty versus Stent

OMERACT
Outcome Measures in Rheumatology Clinical Trial

ONTT
Optic Neuritis Treatment Trial

OPERA
Omapatrilat in Persons with Enhanced Risk of Atherosclerotic Events

OPTIMA
Oxford Project to Investigate Memory and Aging

OPTIMAAL
Optimal Therapy in Myocardial Infarction with the Angiotensin II Antagonist Losartan
Optimal Trial in Myocardial Infarction with the Angiotensin II Antagonist Losartan

OPTIME-CHF
Outcomes of a Prospective Trial of Intravenous Milrinone for Exacerbations of Chronic Heart Failure

OPUS
Orbofiban in Patients with Unstable Coronary Syndromes

ORBIT
Oral Glycoprotein IIb/IIIa Receptor Blockade to Inhibit Thrombosis

ORCHID
Optimal Regimen Cures *Helicobacter*-Induced Dyspepsia

PACTG
Pediatric AIDS Clinical Trial Group Protocol

PAMI
Primary Angioplasty in Myocardial Infarction

PARAGON
Platelet IIb/IIIa Antagonist for the Reduction of Acute Coronary Syndrome Events
in a Global Organization Network

PARIS
Peripheral Artery Radiation Investigational Study
Persantine and Aspirin Reinfarction Study
Port Access Recovery Improvement Study

PART
Prevention of Atherosclerosis with Ramipril Therapy

PAS
Physician's Activity Study
Professional Activities Study

PASE
Physical Activity Scale for the Elderly Evaluation

PAS/MAP
Professional Activities Study Medical Audit Program (medical records)

PASS
Piracetam in Acute Stroke Study
Postural Assessment Scale for Stroke Patient
Practical Applicability of Saruplase Study

PATENT
Prourokinase and t-PA Enhancement of Thrombolysis

PATH
Partnership Approach to Health

PCIVOT
Prostate Cancer Intervention versus Observation Trial

PEA
Pulseless Electrical Study

PEACE
Prevention of Events with ACE Inhibition

PEPI
Postmenopausal Estrogen/Progestin Intervention

PERI
Psychiatric Epidemiology Research Interview

PICS
Pacing in Cardiomyopathy Study

PICSS
Patent Foramen Ovale in Cryptogenic Stroke Study

PICTURE
Post Intracoronary Treatment Ultrasound Result Evaluation

PILOT
Preliminary Investigation of Local Therapy Using Porous PTCA Balloons and
  Low-Molecular-Weight Heparin

PIOPED
Prospective Investigation of Pulmonary Embolism Diagnosis

PIVOT
Prostate Cancer Intervention versus Observation Trial

PLAC
Pravastatin Limitation of Atherosclerosis in Coronary Arteries
Pravastatin, Lipids, and Atherosclerosis in the Carotid Arteries

PLAC-2
Pravastatin, Lipids, and Atherosclerosis in the Carotid Arteries

POEM
Patency, Outcomes and Economics of MIDCAB
Patient-Oriented Evidence That Matters

PORTS
Patient Outcomes Research Team Study

POSCH
Program on the Surgical Control of Hyperlipidemias

POST
Posterior Stroke Trial
Potassium-Channel Opening Stroke Trial

PRAISE
Prospective Randomized Amlodipine Survival Evaluation

PRCCT
Prospective Randomized Controlled Clinical Trials

PRECISE
Prospective Randomized Evaluation of Carvedilol in Symptoms and Exercise

PREDICT
Prospective Randomized Evaluation of Diltiazem CD Trial

PREVENT
Prevention of Recurrent Venous Thromboembolism
Program in Ex Vivo Vein Graft Engineering via Transfection
Proliferation Reduction with Vascular Energy Trial
Prospective Randomized Evaluation of the Vascular Effects of Norvasc Trial

PRISM
Platelet Receptor Inhibition for Ischemic Syndrome Management
Prospective Record of the Impact and Severity of Menstrual Symptoms

PRISM-PLUS
Platelet Receptor Inhibition for Ischemic Syndrome Management in Patients
    Limited to Very Unstable Signs and Symptoms

PROGRESS
Perindopril (Aceon) Protection against Recurrent Stroke Study

PROOF
Prevent Recurrence of Osteoporotic Fractures

PURSUIT
Platelet Glycoprotein IIb/IIIa in Unstable Angina; Receptor Suppression Using
    Integrilin Therapy
Platelet IIb/IIIa Underpinning the Receptor for Suppression of Unstable Ischemia
    Trial

PVSG
Polycythemia Vera Study Group

QOLHS
Quality of Life Hypertension Study

QoLITY
Quality of Life Trial Hypertension

QUIET
Quinapril Ischemic Event Trial

R3
ReoPro Readministration Registry

RACE
Ramipril Angiotensin Converting Enzyme Inhibition

RADAR
Rapid Assessment of Disease Activity in Rheumatology

RADIANCE
Randomized Assessment of Digoxin on Inhibitors of Angiotensin-Converting Enzyme

RALES
Randomized Aldactone Evaluation Study

RAPPORT
ReoPro in Acute Myocardial Infarction and Primary PTCA Organization and Randomized Trial

RAVES
Reduced Anticoagulation in Vein Graft Stent

REGRESS
Regression Growth Evaluation Statin Study

REIN
Ramipril Efficacy in Nephropathy

RESCUE
Randomized Evaluation of Salvage Angioplasty with Combined Utilization of Endpoints

REST
Restenosis Stent Trial

RESTORE
Randomized Efficacy Study of Tirofiban for Outcomes and Restenosis

RIGHT
Cerivastatin Gemfibrozil Hyperlipidemia Treatment

RISC
Research on Instability in Coronary Artery Disease

RITA
Randomized Intervention in the Treatment of Angina

ROCKET
Regionally Organized Cardiac Key European Trial

ROSTER
Rotational Atherectomy versus Balloon Angioplasty for Diffuse In-Stent Restenosis

4S
Scandinavian Simvastatin Survival Study

SAVE
Survival and Ventricular Enlargement

SCAT
Simvastatin/Enalapril Coronary Atherosclerosis Regression Trial

SCD-HeFT
Sudden Cardiac Death in Heart Failure Trial

SCRIP
Stanford Coronary Risk Intervention Project

SCRIPPS
Scripps Coronary Radiation to Inhibit Proliferation Post Stenting

SECURE
Study to Evaluate Carotid Ultrasound Changes with Ramipril and Vitamin E

SENIC
Study on Efficacy of Nosocomial Infection Control

SEPS
Submaximal Exercise Performance Substudy

SEQOL
Study of Economics and Quality of Life

SHEP
Systolic Hypertension in the Elderly Program

SHS
Strong Heart Study

SICCO
Stenting in Chronic Coronary Occlusion

SMART
Second Manifestations of Arterial Disease
Serum Markers Acute Myocardial Infarction and Rapid Treatment
Study of Medicine versus Angioplasty Reperfusion Trial
Study of Microstent's Ability to Limit Restenosis Trial
Study of Monoclonal Antibody Radioimmunotherapy

SMILE
So Much Improvement with a Little Exercise
Survival of Myocardial Infarction: Long-Term Evaluation

SNAP
Study of Nitroglycerin and Chest Pain

SOLVD
Studies of Left Ventricular Dysfunction

SPAF
Stroke Prevention in Atrial Fibrillation

SPAF TEE
Stroke Prevention in Atrial Fibrillation III Transesophageal Echocardiogram

SPINAF
Stroke Prevention in Nonrheumatic Atrial Fibrillation

SPORT
Stent Implantation Post Rotational Atherectomy Trial

SPRINT
Secondary Prevention Reinfarction Israeli Nifedipine Trial

SSSS
Scandinavian Simvastatin Survival Study

STAMI
Stenting for Acute Myocardial Infarction

STAMP
Solid Tumor Autologous Marrow Transplant Program

STAR
Study of Tamoxifen and Raloxifene

STARS
Stent Antithrombotic Regimen Study
St. Thomas' Atherosclerosis Regression Study

START
Saruplase and Taprostene Acute Reocclusion Trial
Selection of Thymidine Analog Regimen Therapy
Stents and Radiation Therapy
Stent versus Angioplasty Restenosis Trial
Stent versus Directional Coronary Atherectomy Randomized Trial
St. Thomas Atherosclerosis Regression Trial
Study of Thrombolytic Therapy with Additional Response Following Taprostene

STaRT
Screening Test for the Assignment of Remedial Treatment

STENTIM
Stenting in Acute Myocardial Infarction

STENTIM-2
Stenting with Elective Wiktor Stent in Acute Myocardial Infarction

STENT PAMI
Stent Primary Angioplasty for Myocardial Infarction

STICH
Surgical Treatment for Intracerebral Hemorrhage

STOP
Stenting of Total Occlusion versus PTCA

STOP-AF
Systemic Trial of Pacing to Prevent Atrial Fibrillation

STOP-ROP
Supplemental Therapeutic Oxygen for Prethreshold Retinopathy of Prematurity

STRATAS
Study to Determine Rotablator and Transluminal Angioplasty Strategy

STRESS
Stent Restenosis Study

SUMIT
Streptokinase-Urokinase Myocardial Infarction Trial

SURE
Serial Ultrasound Analysis of Restenosis

SVCP
Special Virus Cancer Program

SWIFT
Should We Intervene Following Thrombolysis

SWORD
Survival with Oral d-sotalol

SYMPHONY
Sibrafiban versus Aspirin to Yield Maximum Protection from Ischemic Heart Events Post-Acute Coronary Syndromes

TACS
Thrombolysis and Angioplasty in Cardiogenic Shock

TACT
Ticlopidine Angioplasty Coronary Trial

TACTICS
Thrombolysis and Counterpulsation to Improve Cardiogenic Shock Survival
Treat Angina with Aggrastat and Determine Costs of Therapy with Invasive or
    Conservative Strategies

TAIM
Trial of Antihypertensive Interventions and Management

TAM
Total Atherosclerosis Management

TAMI
Thrombolysis and Angioplasty in Myocardial Infarction

TASC
Trial of Angioplasty and Stents in Canada

TASS
Ticlopidine Aspirin Stroke Study

TASTE
Ticlopidine Aspirin Stent Evaluation

TAUSA
Thrombolysis and Angioplasty in Unstable Angina

TEAM
Thrombolytic Trial of Eminase in Acute Myocardial Infarction
Training in Expanded Auxiliary Management

TECBEST
Transluminal Extraction Catheter Before Stent

TIBBS
Total Ischemic Burden Bisoprolol Study

TIBET
Total Ischaemic Burden European Trial

TIMI
Thrombin Inhibition in Myocardial Infarction
Thrombolysis in Myocardial Infarction

TIMI-7
Thrombin Inhibition in Myocardial Ischemia

TOAST
Treatment of Acute Stroke Trial

TOHP
Trials of Hypertension Prevention

TOPIT
Transluminal Extraction Catheter or PTCA in Thrombus

TRACE
Trandolapril Cardiac Evaluation

TREAT
Tranilast Restenosis Following Angioplasty Trial

TREND
Trial Reversing Endothelial Dysfunction

TRIM
Thrombin Inhibition in Myocardial Ischemia

TUMMY
Trial Using Medicinal Microbiotic Yogurt

UGDP
University Group Diabetes Program

UKPDS
United Kingdom Prospective Diabetes Study

USPET
Urokinase-Streptokinase Pulmonary Embolism Trial

VA-HIT
Veterans Administration High-Density Lipoprotein Intervention Trial

Val-HeFT
Valsartan Heart Failure Trial

VALIANT
Valsartan in Acute Myocardial Infarction Trial

VALUE
Valsartan Antihypertensive Long-Term Use Evaluation

VANQWISH
Veterans Affairs Non-Q-Wave Infarction Strategies in Hospital

VAS
Verapamil Angioplasty Study

VASIS
Vasovagal Syncope International Study

VEGAS
Vein Graft AngioJet Study

VEGAS I
Vein Graft AngioJet Study-Phase I

VEGAS II
Vein Graft AngioJet Study-Phase II

VeHF
Veterans Heart Failure

VEST
Vesnarinone Survival Trial

V-HeFT
Veterans Administration Heart Failure Trial

V-HeFT II
Vasodilator Heart Failure Trial II
Veterans Administration Heart Failure Trial II

VHS
Veterans Health Study

VIGOR
Vioxx Gastrointestinal Outcomes Research

VISP
Vitamin Intervention for Stroke Prevention

VITATOPS
Vitamins to Prevent Stroke

VOTE
Value of Transesophageal Echocardiography

VPS
Vaccine Preparedness Study

WALK
Walking with Angina-Learning is Key

WESDR
Wisconsin Epidemiologic Study of Diabetic Retinopathy

WEST
Women's Estrogen for Stroke Trial

WIHS
Women's Interagency HIV Study

WINS
Women's Intervention Nutrition Study

WITS
Women and Infants Transmission Study

WRIST
Washington Radiation for In-Stent Restenosis Trial